# Epidemiology

T0272044

# Textbook of Bladder Cancer

# Textbook of Bladder Cancer

Edited by

## Seth P Lerner MD, FACS

Associate Professor of Urology, Beth and Dave Swalm Chair in Urologic Oncology,
Scott Department of Urology, Baylor College of Medicine, Houston, TX, USA

## Mark P Schoenberg MD

Professor of Urology and Oncology, Director of Urologic Oncology, James Buchanan Brady
Urological Institute, The Johns Hopkins Medical Institutions, Baltimore, MD, USA

## Cora N Sternberg MD, FACP

Chairman, Division of Medical Oncology, San Camillo Forlanini Hospital, Rome, Italy

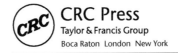

## CRC Press
Taylor & Francis Group
Boca Raton  London  New York

CRC Press is an imprint of the
Taylor & Francis Group, an **informa** business

CRC Press
Taylor & Francis Group
6000 Broken Sound Parkway NW, Suite 300
Boca Raton, FL 33487-2742

First issued in paperback 2019

© 2006 by Taylor & Francis Group, LLC
CRC Press is an imprint of Taylor & Francis Group, an Informa business

No claim to original U.S. Government works

ISBN-13: 978-1-84184-382-7 (hbk)
ISBN-13: 978-0-367-39122-5 (pbk)

A CIP record for this book is available from the British Library

Library of Congress Cataloging-in-Publication Data
Data available on application

Composition by Phoenix Photosetting, Chatham, Kent, UK

**Visit the Taylor & Francis Web site at**
**http://www.taylorandfrancis.com**

**and the CRC Press Web site at**
**http://www.crcpress.com**

# Contents

## SECTION 1: Epidemiology

## SECTION 2: Pathology

## SECTION 5:    Treatment

SECTION 6:   **T2-4**

SECTION 7:   **Primary bladder sparing therapy**

## SECTION 8: Urinary tract reconstruction

## SECTION 9: Treatment of regionally advanced and metastatic bladder cancer

# Contributors

Hassan Abol-Enein, MD, PhD
Professor of Urology, Director of Urology and
Nephrology Center, Mansoura University, Mansoura,
Egypt

Alex F Althausen, MD
Clinical Professor of Urology, Harvard Medical School,
Department of Urology, Massachusetts General
Hospital, Boston, MA, USA

Gilad E Amiel, MD
Monical Fellow in Oncology and Minimally Invasive
Surgery, Scott Department of Urology, Baylor College of
Medicine, Houston, TX, USA

Aristotelis G Anastasiadis, MD
Associate Professor of Urology, Department of Urology,
University Hospital, University of Tuebingen,
Tuebingen, Germany

Marco A Arap, MD, PhD
Assistant Professor of Urology, School of Medicine,
University of Sao Paulo, Sao Paulo, Brazil

Sami Arap, MD
Professor of Urology, School of Medicine, University of
Sao Paulo, Sao Paulo, Brazil

Anthony Atala, MD
W Boyce Professor and Chair, Department of Urology;
Director, Institute for Regenerative Medicine, Wake
Forest University Medical Center, Winston-Salem, NC,
USA

Jessie L-S Au, PharmD, PhD
Distinguished University Professor, College of
Pharmacy, The Ohio State University, Columbus, OH,
USA

Jelle Barentsz, MD
Professor of Radiology, Chair for Research, Department
of Radiology, University Medical Center St Radboud,
Nijmegen, The Netherlands

Joaqim Bellmunt, MD, PhD
Vall d'Hebron University Hospital, Barcelona, Spain

William Benedict, MD
Professor of Cancer Medicine, Department of
Genitourinary Medical Oncology, UT MD Anderston
Cancer Center, Houston, TX, USA

Gail Bentley, MD
Professor and Chairman, Department of Pathology,
Karmanos Cancer Institute and Wayne State University
Detroit, MI, USA

Bernard H Bochner, MD
Associate Attending Physician, Department of Urology,
Memorial Sloan-Kettering Cancer Center, New York, NY,
USA

Andreas Böhle, MD
Professor of Urology, Helios Agnes Karll Hospital, Bad
Schwartau, Germany

David G Bostwick, MD, MBA
Medical Director, Bostwick Laboratories, Glen Allen, VA,
USA

Michelle Boyar, MD
Clinical Fellow in Medical Oncology and Hematology,
Columbia University Medical Center, New York, NY,
USA

Sven Brandau, MD
Head, Division of Immunotherapy, Research Center
Borstel, Borstel, Germany

Robert Bristow, MD, PhD, FRCP(C)
Associate Professor, Departments of Radiation Oncology and Medical Biophysics, University of Toronto; Clinician-Scientist, Radiation Oncology and Applied Molecular Oncology, Princess Margaret Hospital/University Health Network, Toronto, ON, Canada

Theresa Chan, MD
Staff Pathologist, Quest Diagnostics, Baltimore, MD, USA

Lian Cheng, MD
Associate Professor of Pathology and Urology, Indiana University School of Medicine, Indianapolis, IN, USA

Marc S Chuang, MD
Chief Resident in Urology, The University of Chicago, Chicago, IL, USA

Noel Clarke MBBS, ChM, FRCS(Urol)
Consultant Urologist, Christie Hospital Manchester and Hope Hospital, Salford, UK

John J Coen, MD
Assistant Professor of Radiation Oncology, Harvard Medical School; Genitourinary Oncology Unit, Department of Radiation Oncology, Massachusetts General Hospital, Boston, MA, USA

Richard J Cote, MD, FRCPath
Professor, Department of Pathology and Urology, USA/Norris Comprehensive Cancer Center, Los Angeles, CA, USA

Roland Dahlem
General Hospital Hamburg, Hamburg, Germany

Guido Dalbagni, MD, FACS
Associate Attending Surgeon, Department of Urology, Memoral Sloan-Kettering Cancer Center, New York, NY, USA

Atreya Dash, MD
Fellow, Department of Urology, Memorial Sloan-Kettering Cancer Center, New York, NY, USA

Ram H Datar, PhD
Assistant Professor of Clinical Pathology, USC Keck School of Medicine, Los Angeles, CA, USA

George L Delclos, MD, MPH
Professor and Director, Division of Environmental and Occupational Health Sciences, University of Texas School of Public Health, Houston, TX, USA

Arline D Deitch, PhD
Emeritus Professor, Department of Urology, University of California, Davis, CA, USA

Colin P Dinney, MD
Professor, Chair of Urology, The University of Texas, MD Anderson Cancer Center, Houston, TX, USA

S Machele Donat, MD, FACS
Associate Attending Urology, Memorial Sloan-Kettering Cancer Center, Cornell-Weill Medical College, New York, NY, USA

Michael J Droller, MD
Katherine and Clifford Goldsmith Professor of Urology and Professor of Oncology, The Mount Sinai Medical Center, New York, NY, USA

Paolo Emiliozzi
San Giovanni Hospital, Rome, Italy

Jonathan I Epstein, MD
Professor of Pathology, Urology and Oncology, The Reinhard Professor of Urological Pathology, Director of Surgical Pathology, The Johns Hopkins Hospital, Baltimore, MD, USA

Andrew J Evans, MD, PhD, FRCP(C)
Assistant Professor of Pathology, Department of Pathobiology and Laboratory Medicine, Princess Margaret Hospital and the University of Toronto, Toronto, ON, Canada

Sarah A Felknor, DrPH, MS
Assistant Professor of Occupational Health, Division of Environmental and Occupational Health Sciences, University of Texas School of Public Health, Houston, TX, USA

Fernando A Ferrer, MD
Director Pediatric Urologic Surgery, Assistant Professor Surgery, Pediatrics and Oncology, Connecticut Children's Medical Center, University of Connecticut School of Medicine, Farmington, CT, USA

Susan Feyerabend, MD
Department of Urology, University Hospital, University of Tuebingen, Tuebingen, Germany

Margit Fisch, MD
Professor of Urology, Director of the Center of Urology and Pediatric Urology, General Hospital Harburg, Hamburg, Germany

Ben George, MD
Resident, Gundersen Lutheran Medical Center, Department of Internal Medicine, LaCrosse, WI, USA

Robert H Getzenberg, PhD
Professor of Urology and Oncology, Director of Urology Research, James Buchanan Brady Urological Institute, Johns Hopkins Medicine, Baltimore, MD, USA

Mohamed A Ghoneim, MD, MD(Hon)
Professor of Urology, Mansoura University, Mansoura, Egypt

Inderbir S Gill, MD, MCh
Professor of Surgery, Head, Section of Laparoscopic and Robotic Urology, Glickman Urological Institute, Cleveland, OH, USA

Mary K Gospodarowicz, MD, FRCP(C)
Professor and Chair, Department of Radiation
Oncology, University of Toronto; Medical Director,
Oncology Programs, and Chief, Radiation Medicine
Program, Princess Margaret Hospital, Toronto, ON,
Canada

Donald P Griffith, MD
Chief of the Urology Service, Michael E DeBakey
Veterans Affairs Medical Center, Houston, TX, USA

David Grignon, MD
Professor and Chairman, Department of Pathology,
Karmanos Cancer Institute and Wayne State University,
Detroit, MI, USA

Jian Gu, PhD
Instructor, Department of Epidemiology, The University
of Texas MD Anderson Cancer Center, Houston, TX,
USA

Mary Ellen Haisfield-Wolfe, RN, MSN, OCN
Research Nurse Coordinator, Department of Surgery,
Johns Hopkins Medical Institutions, Baltimore, MD,
USA

Richard E Hautmann, MD, MDHon
Professor of Urology, Chairman Department of Urology,
University of Ulm, Ulm, Germany

Aditi Hazra, PhD, MPH
Research Fellow, Department of Epidemiology, Harvard
School of Public Health, Boston, MA, USA

George P Hemstreet III, MD, PhD
Chief, Section of Urologic Surgery, Malashock Chair of
Urology, Nebraska Medical Center, Omaha, NE, USA

Niall M Heney, MD
Clinical Professor of Urology, Harvard Medical School,
Departmentof Urology, Massachusetts General Hospital,
Boston, MA, USA

Harry W Herr, MD
Attending Surgeon, Department of Urology, Memorial
Sloan-Kettering Cancer Center; Professor of Urology,
Cornell University of Medical College, New York, NY,
USA

Tzong-Tyng Hung, BSc(Hons)
PhD Student, Oncology Research Centre, Prince of
Wales Hospital, Randwick, NSW, Australia

Maha Hussain, MD, FACP
Professor of Medicine and Urology, University of
Michigan Comprehensive Cancer Center, Ann Arbor, MI,
USA

Thomas Jarrett, MD
Associate Professor of Urology, Co-Director,
Endourology Fellowship; Chief, Division of
Endourology and Laparoscopy, Johns Hopkins Hospital,
Baltimore, MD, USA

Michael AS Jewett, MD, FRCS(C)
Professor of Surgery, Division of Urology and
Department of Surgical Oncology, Princess Margaret
Hospital and the University of Toronto, Toronto, ON,
Canada

James O Jin, MD, PhD
Fellow, Section of Hematology/Oncology, Department
of Medicine, University of Chicago, Chicago, IL, USA

Jeffrey A Jones, MD, MS, FACS
Flight Surgeon, Space Medicine & Healthcare Systems,
NASA, Johnson Space Center; Adjunct Associate
Professor, Baylor College of Medicine, Surgery/Urology
Staff, Michael E DeBakey Veterans Administration
Medical Center, Houston, TX, USA

A Karim Kader, MD, PhD, FRCS(C)
Fellow in Urologic Oncology, MD Anderson Cancer
Center, Houston, TX, USA

Wassim Kassouf, MD
Assistant Professor, Division of Urology, McGill
University Health Center, Montreal, PQ, Canada

Donald S Kaufman, MD
Clinical Professor of Medicine, Harvard Medical School;
Director, Genitourinary Oncology Clinic, Massachusetts
General Hospital, Boston, MA, USA

Melissa R Kaufman, MD
Resident in Urology, Vanderbilt University Medical
Center, Nashville, TN, USA

Lambertus A Kiemeney, PhD, MSc
Professor, Departments of Epidemiology & Urology,
Radboud University Nijmegen Medical Centre,
Nijmegen, The Netherlands

Laurence Klotz, MD FRCS(C)
Professor, Department of Surgery, University of Toronto;
Chief, Division of Urology, Sunnybrook and Women's
College Health Sciences Centre, Toronto, ON, Canada

Deborah W Knapp, DVM, MS, Dipl ACVIM
Professor of Comparative Oncology, Department of
Veterinary Clinical Sciences, Purdue University, West
Lafayette, IN, USA

Margaret Knowles, BSc, PhD
Professor of Experimental Cancer Research, University of
Leeds; Associate Director, Cancer Research UK Clinical
Centre in Leeds, St James's University Hospital, Leeds,
UK

Martin Kriegmair, Prof Dr Med
Director and Professor, Urological Clinic München-
Planegg, Planegg, Germany

Markus A Kuczyk, MD
Professor of Urology and Vice Chairman, Department of
Urology, University Hospital, University of Tuebingen,
Tuebingen, Germany

Donald L Lamm, MD, FACS
President, Bladder Cancer Genitourinary Oncology, Phoenix, AZ, USA

Seth P Lerner, MD, FACS
Associate Professor of Urology, Beth and Dave Swalm Chair in Urologic Oncology, Scott Department of Urology, Baylor College of Medicine, Houston, TX, USA

Frederik Liedberg, MD
Senior Registrar, Department of Urology, University Hospital, Lund, Sweden

Guillermo Lima, MD
Fellow, Department of Urology, Johns Hopkins Hospital, Baltimore, MD, USA

Scott M Lippman, MD
Professor, Chairman, Clinical Cancer Prevention Department, The University of Texas MD Anderson Cancer Center, Houston, TX, USA

Vinata B Lokeshwar, PhD
Associate Professor, Departments of Urology and Cell Biology and Anatomy, University of Miami School of Medicine, Miami, FL, USA

Antonio Lopez-Beltran, MD
Professor of Pathology, Unit of Anatomic Pathology, Cordoba University School of Medicine, Cordoba, Spain

Yair Lotan, MD
Assistant Professor of Urology, Department of Urology, University of Texas Southwestern Medical Center, Dallas, TX, USA

Gary R MacVicar, MD
Instructor, Department of Medicine, Division of Hematology/Oncology, Feinberg School of Medicine and the Robert H Lurie Comprehensive Cancer Center Northwestern University, Chicago, IL, USA

David J McConkey, PhD
Professor, Department of Cancer Biology, University of Texas MD Anderson Center, Houston, TX, USA

Laurence B McCullough, PhD
Professor of Medicine and Medical Ethics, Associate Director of Education, Center for Medical Ethics and Health Policy, Baylor College of Medicine, Houston, TX, USA

S Bruce Malkowicz, MD
Professor of Urology, University of Pennsylvania, School of Medicine, Philadelphia, PA, USA

Per-Uno Malmström, MD, PhD
Professor, Department of Urology, University Hospital, Uppsala, Sweden

Åsa Månsson, RN, PhD
Senior Lecturer, Department of Health Sciences, Medical Faculty, Lund University, Sweden

Wiking Månsson, MD, PhD
Associate Professor, Senior Consultant, Department of Urology, University Hospital, Lund, Sweden

Michael J Manyak, MD, FACS
Professor of Urology, Engineering, Microbiology and Tropical Medicine, The George Washington University, Washington, District of Columbia; Vice President of Medical Affairs, Cytogen Corporation, Princeton, NJ, USA

Edward M Messing, MD, FACS
WW Scott Professor, Chairman of Urology, Professor of Oncology and Pathology, Deputy Director, James P Wilmot Cancer Center, University of Rochester School of Medicine and Dentistry, Rochester, MN, USA

Robert D Mills, FRCS(Urol)
Consultant Urologist, The Norfolk and Norwich University Hospital, Norwich, Norfolk, UK

Michael F Milosevic, MD FRCP(C)
Associate Professor, Department of Radiation Oncology, University of Toronto; Clinician-Scientist, Radiation Medicine Program, Princess Margaret Hospital/University Health Network, Toronto, ON, Canada

Rodolfo Montironi, MD
Professor of Pathology, Institute of Pathological Anatomy and Histophathology, University of Ancona School of Medicine, Ancona, Italy

Paula MJ Moonen, MD, DRS
Department of Urology, Radboud University Nijmegen Medical Center, Nijmegen, The Netherlands

Yoshifumi Narumi, MD, PhD
Department of Radiology, Osaka University Hospital, Osaka, Japan

Alan M Nieder, MD
Assistant Professor, Department of Urology, University of Miami Miller School of Medicine, Miami, FL, USA

Unyime O Nseyo, MD, FACS
Professor, Urology Division, Virginia Commonwealth University Medical Center, Richmond, VA, USA

Willem Oosterlinck, PhD, MD
Professor of Urology, Head of the Department of Urology, Ghent University Hospital, Ghent, Belgium

Torben F Orntoft, MD, DMSci
Professor; Chief Physician, Head, Department of Clinical Biochemistry, Aarhus University Hospital at Skejby, Aarhus, Denmark

Juan Palou, MD, PhD
Chief of Urologic Oncology, Associate Professor of Urology, Fundació Puigvert, Autonomus University of Barcelona, Barcelona, Spain

Vito Pansadoro, MD
President, Vincenzo Pansadoro Foundation, Rome, Italy

Angela Papageorgiou, PhD
Fellow, Department of Cancer Biology, University of Texas MD Anderson Cancer Center, Houston, TX, USA

Daniel P Petrylak, MD
Associate Professor of Medicine, Director, Genitourinary Oncology Program, College of Physicians and Surgeons, Columbia Presbyterian Medical Center, New York, NY, USA

Lori A Pinke MD
Urologist, Urology Associates Ltd., Phoenix, AZ, USA

George R Prout Jr, MD
Professor Emeritus of Surgery, Harvard Medical School; Consultant in Urology, 1800 River Watch Lane, Annapolis, Maryland; Consultant, Division of Cancer Control and Population Sciences, National Cancer Institute, Bethesda, MD, USA

Junqi Qian, MD
Director of Molecular Diagnostics, Bostwick Laboratories, Glen Allen, VA, USA

Michael Ritchey, MD, FACS
Professor of Urology, Mayo Clinic College of Medicine, Scottsdale, AZ, USA

Ronald Rodriguez, MD, PhD
Assistant Professor of Urology, Medical Oncology, Cellular and Molecular Medicine, Viral Oncology; Director, Urology Residency Program, Johns Hopkins University School of Medicine, Baltimore, MD, USA

Randall C Rowland, MD, PhD
Professor and Chief, Division of Urology, University of Kentucky, Lexington, KY, USA

Pamela J Russell, BSc, MSc, PhD, DipEd
Conjoint Professor of Medicine, University of New South Wales; Director, Oncology Research Centre, Prince of Wales Hospital, Randwick, NSW, Australia

Anita L Sabichi, MD
Associate Professor, Department of Clinical Cancer Prevention, The University of Texas, MD Anderson Cancer Center, Houston, TX, USA

Arthur I Sagalowsky, MD
Professor and Chief of Urologic Oncology, Dr. Paul Peters Chair in Urology in Memory of Rumsey and Louis Strickland, Department of Urology, University of Texas Southwestern Medical Center, Dallas, TX, USA

Guido Sauter, Prof Dr Med
Director, Department of Pathology, University Medical Center Hamburg-Eppendorf, Hamburg, Germany

Mark P Schoenberg, MD
Professor of Urology and Oncology, Director of Urologic Oncology, James Buchanan Brady Urological Institute, The Johns Hopkins Medical Institutions, Baltimore, MD, USA

Barthold PH Schrier, MD
Urologist, Fellow of the European Board of Urology, Department of Urology, Jeroen Bosch Hospital, 's Hertogenbosch, The Netherlands

José Segarra, MD
Fundació Puigvert, Autonomus University of Barcelona, Barcelona, Spain

Avishay Sella, MD
Professor, Head, Department of Oncology, Asaf Harofeh Medical Center, Zerifin, Tel-Aviv University, Israel

Sharon Sharir, MD, MPH, FRCS(C)
Assistant Professor of Surgery, Divisions of Urology and Surgical Oncology, Sunnybrook and Women's College Health Sciences Center and the University of Toronto, Toronto, ON, Canada

Amir Sherif, MD, PhD
Senior Consultant, Department of Urology, Karolinska University Hospital, Solna, Karolinska Institute, Stockholm, Sweden

William U Shipley, MD
Andres Soriano Professor of Radiation Oncology, Harvard Medical School; Head, Genitourinary Oncology Unit, Department of Radiation Oncology, Massachusetts General Hospital, Boston, MA, USA

Marissa Shrader, PhD
Fellow, Department of Cancer Biology, University of Texas MD Anderson Center, Houston, TX, USA

Donald G Skinner, MD
Professor and Chairman of Urology, Department of Urology, University of Southern California Keck School of Medicine, Norris Comprehensive Cancer Center, Los Angeles, CA, USA

Eila C Skinner, MD
Associate Professor of Urology, Department of Urology, University of Southern California Keck School of Medicine, Norris Comprehensive Cancer Center, Los Angeles, CA, USA

Joseph A Smith Jr, MD
Professor and Chairman, Department of Urologic Surgery, Vanderbilt University Medical Center, Nashville, TN, USA

Mark S Soloway, MD
Professor and Chairman, Department of Urology, University of Miami Miller School of Medicine, Miami, FL, USA

Eduardo Solsona, MD
Chief of Urology, Valencia Oncology Institute, Valencia, Spain

Walter M Stadler, MD
Associate Professor, Director of Genitourinary Oncology, University of Chicago, Departments of Medicine and Surgery, Sections of Hematology/Oncology and Urology, Maryland, Chicago, IL, USA

John P Stein, MD, FACS
Associate Professor of Urology, Department of Urology, University of Southern California Keck School of Medicine, Norris Comprehensive Cancer Center, Los Angeles, CA, USA

Gary D Steinberg, MD, FACS
Associate Professor of Surgery/Urology, Director of Urologic Oncology, The University of Chicago, Chicago, IL, USA

Arnulf Stenzl, MD
Professor and Chairman, Department of Urology, University Hospital, University of Tuebingen, Tuebingen, Germany

Cora N Sternberg, MD, FACP
Chairman, Division of Medical Oncology, San Camillo Forlanini Hospital, Rome, Italy

Urs E Studer, MD
Professor and Chair Department of Urology, University of Bern, Bern, Switzerland

Tung-Tien Sun, PhD
Rudolf L. Baer Professor of Dermatology, Professor of Pharmacology and Urology, New York University Medical School, New York, NY, USA

David A Swanson, MD
Clinical Professor of Urology, The University of Texas MD Anderson Cancer Center, Houston, TX, USA

Richard J Sylvester, ScD
Assistant Director, Biostatistics, European Organisation for Research and Treatment of Cancer Data Center, Brussels, Belgium

Dan Theodorescu, MD, PhD
Paul Mellon Professor of Urology and Molecular Physiology; Director, Paul Mellon Prostate Institute, University of Virginia, VA, USA

Joachim W Thüroff, MD
Professor and Chairman, Department of Urology and Paediatric Urology, Johannes Gutenberg-University Medical School, Mainz, Germany

Ingolf Tuerk, MD, PhD
Clinical Professor for Urology, Director for Minimal Invasive Laparoscopic Urology, Institute of Urology, Lahey Clinic Medical Center, Burlington, MA, USA

Hendrik van Poppel, MD, PhD, FEBU
Professor and Chairman of Urology, Department of Urology, University Hospital of the Catholic University of Leuven, Leuven, Belgium

Adrian PM van der Meijden, MD, PhD
Consultant, Department of Urology, Jeroen Bosch Hospital, 's Hertogenbosch, The Netherlands.

Robert W Veltri, PhD
Associate Professor, Department of Urology, Brady Urological Institute, Marburg, Baltimore, MD, USA

Frederick M Waldman, MD, PhD
Professor, Departments of Laboratory Medicine, Urology and Cancer Center, University of California San Francisco, San Francisco, CA, USA

Joanne Walker RN, MS, CWOCN
Wound, Ostomy and Continence Nurse, The Johns Hopkins Hospital, Baltimore, MD, USA

Zhiping Wang, PhD, MD
Professor of Urology and Cell Biology; Chairman, Institute of Urology, 2nd Hospital of Lanzhou University, Lanzhou, PR China

Ralph W DeVere White, MD
Professor and Chair, Department of Urology; Director, UC Davis Cancer Center, University of California, Davis, CA, USA

M Guillaume Wientjes, PhD
Professor, College of Pharmacy, James Cancer Hospital and Solove Research Institute, The Ohio State University, Columbus, OH, USA

Christoph Wiesner, MD
Department of Urology and Pediatric Urology, Johannes Gutenberg-University Medical School, Mainz, Germany

J Alfred Witjes, MD, PhD
Professor, Department of Urology, Radboud University Nijmegen Medical Center, Nijmegen, The Netherlands

David P Wood Jr, MD
Chief of Urologic Oncology, Professor, Department of Urology, University of Michigan, Ann Arbor, MI, USA

Xifeng Wu, MD, PhD
Professor of Epidemiology, Department of Epidemiology, The University of Texas MD Anderson Cancer Center, Houston, TX, USA

Xue-Ru Wu, MD
Associate Professor, Departments of Urology and Microbiology, New York University School of Medicine, New York, NY, USA

Takuhiro Yamaguchi, PhD
Assistant Professor, Department of
Biostatistics/Epidemiology and Preventive Health
Sciences, School of Health Sciences and Nursing,
University of Tokyo, Tokyo, Japan

Anthony L Zietman, MD
Professor of Radiation Oncology, Harvard Medical
Schoool, Genitourinary Oncology Unit, Department of
Radiation Oncology, Massachusetts General Hospital,
Boston, MA, USA

# Preface

Urothelial cancer comprises many neoplastic diseases affecting the urethra, bladder and upper urinary tract. Discoveries in the basic sciences are advancing our understanding of these complex diseases. Technological advances in endoscopy, imaging, intravesical therapy, surgery and urinary tract reconstruction have dramatically improved patient care and clinical outcomes. Despite effective chemotherapy, long-term cure can be elusive for patients with metastatic disease offering opportunities for new drug development and application of targeted therapeutics.

This textbook was conceived to bring a state-of-the-art comprehensive analysis of urothelial cancer to students, physicians, scientists and health professionals at all stages of medical education. Leading authorities were brought together for each subject in order to provide multiple and often contrasting viewpoints.

Urothelial cancer is a substantial world health problem. We hope this textbook proves informative, thought provoking and a valuable resource for research and patient care for health care professionals across many disciplines.

Seth P Lerner
Mark P Schoenberg
Cora N Sternberg

# Acknowledgments

The editors wish to thank the over 150 authors who have contributed the outstanding manuscripts with over 70 chapters to create a truly comprehensive textbook. We congratulate the team at Taylor & Francis and especially wish to acknowledge Alan Burgess and Rupal Malde, and, at Naughton Project Management, Sarah Abel, for their patience and guidance.

We could not have completed this project without the editorial contributions of Carolyn Schum and project coordination leadership of Valerie R Price from the Scott Department of Urology at Baylor College of Medicine.

# Epidemiology of bladder cancer

1

*Michael J Droller*

## INTRODUCTION

### CLINICAL OVERVIEW

Of the various types of cancer that occur in the urinary bladder, most retain the histologic appearance of their transitional cell origin.[1] Less than 5% develop as squamous cell carcinoma, and even fewer as adenocarcinoma.[2] Exceptions to this occur in areas in which schistosomiasis is endemic and in which squamous cell cancers occur in substantially higher numbers.[3]

Bladder cancer ranks fourth in incidence among cancers in men in North America and eighth in women,[4] with an overall annual incidence of over 64,000 cases and a male:female ratio of 2–3:1. Although the number of deaths attributable to bladder cancer is estimated at >12,000 per year, the case:fatality ratio of approximately 4.4:1 indicates that most cases are not life threatening[5]; rather, the more problematic issue with most cases of bladder cancer is their recurrence and far fewer are likely to progress (see Chapter 24).

In a 1999 survey of cancer diagnoses through 1990, urothelial bladder cancer was found to account for approximately 3% to 3.5% of the 8 million new cases of cancer diagnosed worldwide each year, making it the ninth most frequent cancer.[6] This represented an incidence of approximately 260,000 new cases involving men and women in a 3.5:1 ratio.[7] In this survey, approximately 115,000 patients (in an approximately 3:1 ratio of men:women) died of the disease annually,[8] suggesting that it may be diagnosed in a more aggressive form or at a later stage in women. This also suggested

that the prevalence would approximate the accumulation of all those that had not died of the disease, estimated to approach 800,000 over 5 years. Figures recently published by WHO[9] indicated an increase in new diagnoses in 2002 (nearly 356,500 cases—approximately 273,800 in men and 82,700 in women) and a parallel increase in annual deaths (approximately 145,000 with 108,300 in men and 36,700 in women) (Table 1.1). The male:female ratios with these figures (3.1:1 in new diagnoses and 2.95:1 in cancer deaths) were virtually identical to previously published figures. Whether the apparent increase in new cases and mortality represents increased industrialization and exposure to carcinogens (taking into account such changes having occurred many years previously with a lag phase in the development of urothelial cancer), increased awareness by the public of this problem with improved access to healthcare and diagnostic activities, inclusion of those patients with aggressive forms of the disease and limited hope of cure in this segment of the bladder cancer population, and other uncharacterized factors is unknown.

The variable frequency in different areas of the world suggests that environmental and lifestyle factors are important in determining the incidence of the disease.

**Table 1.1** Bladder cancer: worldwide incidence/prevalence (WHO 2002)

|  | Cases | Deaths | 1-year prevalence | 5-year prevalence |
|---|---|---|---|---|
| Male | 273,858 | 108,310 | 224,742 | 860,299 |
| Female | 82,699 | 36,699 | 64,673 | 249,966 |
| Total | 356,557 | 145,009 | 289,415 | 1,110,265 |

Data from Ferlay et al.[9] Online. Available: www-dep.iarc.fr

The highest age-adjusted incidence rates in men occur in North America (23.3/100,000), Northern Africa (23.3/100,000), and Southern Europe (22.0/100,000), with corresponding rates of 5.4, 4.8, and 3.2/100,000 in women. The lowest rates occur in Melanesia and Middle Africa (2.7 and 2.8/100,000 in men; 0.6 and 0.5/100,000 in women, respectively).[6] Although the complexity of factors contributing to the diagnosis of bladder cancer and the quality of such information must qualify the reliability of these numbers and the strength of their interpretation, the critical factors of industrialization, cigarette smoking, and schistosomiasis (in Northern Africa) stand out as dominant risk factors for the development of bladder cancer. Indeed, the global incidence of bladder cancer appears to have increased in the Third World in parallel with increased industrialization and use of tobacco. Nonetheless, substantial variation still exists, probably reflecting absolute and differential access to healthcare, longevity (bladder cancer occurs with increasing frequency with age), the prolonged time between exposure to carcinogens and the clinical expression of urothelial cancer, and various host factors that may predispose or protect in the ultimate development of disease.[4,5]

Over time, the cancer will recur in 50% to 70% of all bladder cancer patients.[10] Further, rapidity and multiplicity of recurrence will likely be increased if the first recurrence takes place early in life, if the initial tumor is large, or if there are multiple tumors present.[11-13] Since prevalence reflects the total number of individuals with a particular condition at a specific point in time, the problem of recurrence places bladder cancer as the second most prevalent cancer among men, led only by prostate cancer.[5]

Of the 64,000 new cases of urothelial cancer diagnosed in North America each year, 70% to 75% (37,800–40,800) present as 'superficial', i.e. not invasive of the muscularis propria.[14,15] These often recur but the majority are not likely to become life threatening (see Chapter 24). The remaining 25% to 30% (14,500–16,000) are deeply invasive, extending into the bladder wall muscle or through it to the perivesical tissues. These do represent a potentially life-threatening situation since at least 50% have occult metastases which often become apparent within 2–3 years of initial diagnosis.[16,17]

Of the superficial cancers, 70% (26,000–28,500) are confined to the bladder mucosa.[10,14,15] Although three-fourths of these will recur (an event more likely in the setting of large or multiple tumors), less than 5% (1300–1400) will progress to invasive cancer.[14,15,18,19] Those that do are predominantly high grade.

The remaining 30% of 'superficial' tumors (11,000–12,000) are invasive of the lamina propria.[10,15] If we exclude the 10% to 20% of these (1000–2000) that are actually found to be invasive of the muscularis propria on repeat resection,[20,21] it is predominantly those that are high grade and deeply invasive of the lamina pro-

pria (approximately 50%, or 5000–6000 cases) that have a high risk of progression to muscle invasion.[22-24] Taken together, a life-threatening situation is encountered in approximately 22,000–25,500 cases overall (14,500–16,000 with muscle invasion at initial diagnosis and an additional 7000–9500 of high-grade lesions with extensive lamina propria invasion). The remaining 20,500–32,000 newly diagnosed patients have a 70% risk of recurrence but are unlikely to progress.

The bladder is a reservoir for urine and its waste product contents. It can be inferred from this that bladder cancer is associated with cumulative exposure to a variety of potentially etiologic carcinogens.[25,26] This has been supported by reports of high rates of bladder cancer in industrialized regions of the world, presumably as a result of exposure to carcinogenic substances used in manufacturing or occurring as the by-products of various manufacturing processes.[27-29] A parallel association has been suggested by the high rates of bladder cancer reported in cigarette smokers. This association has been based upon the high concentrations of known urothelial carcinogens contained in cigarette smoke and their inhalation, either directly or as second-hand smoke.[30-32] The increased general incidence of bladder cancer worldwide can be ascribed to both of these factors.[33]

The incidence of bladder cancer increases with age, presumably reflecting cumulative exposures to carcinogens with time.[34] Most cases occur in patients over the age of 50 years. In fact, bladder cancer is unusual in individuals younger than 40 years, and those that occur in the much younger age group tend to be of lower grade and mucosally confined, i.e. less aggressive biologically.[35,36] Once excised, such lesions rarely recur. On the other hand, cancers that occur in individuals above the age of 40 behave in a fashion similar to those that develop in older patients.[37]

Over the past 15 years, a nearly 40% increase has been observed in the incidence of bladder cancer in the US.[34] Since screening programs have not been sufficiently implemented to account for this, and since tumors detected only at autopsy, and therefore considered incidental, are not common,[38] epidemiologists have postulated that increased carcinogen exposure may account for this escalation.[39,40] Unfortunately, although many associations have been described, their documentation often has not been validated.[41] For example, over the past 30–40 years, tobacco exposure among women has increased dramatically as has the entry of women into the workforce.[42] While a corresponding increase in their incidence of lung cancer has occurred, increased rates of bladder cancer that might have been predicted in association with an increased exposure to carcinogens has not materialized.[43] This has prompted suggestions that cumulative exposures to environmental substances (shown to be carcinogenic in laboratory investigations) were the likely underlying reasons for the increases that were seen.[39,40]

On the other hand, causation postulated solely on the basis of carcinogen exposure has not appeared sufficient to account for the incidence of bladder cancer. An additional factor might be particular host characteristics that could conceivably affect mechanisms by which carcinogens induce neoplastic transformation (see discussion below).[44,45] This could explain some of the discrepancies seen in the incidence of bladder cancer and quantification of exposures to putative carcinogens. This could also account for some of the racial differences that characterize the incidence of urothelial bladder cancer. Thus, Caucasian men and women are 2.8 and 1.5 times more likely to be diagnosed with bladder cancer than African–American men and women, respectively.[34,46] Correspondingly, Caucasian men overall have a 3.9% chance of developing bladder cancer compared with a 0.8% chance in African–American women.[46] Further observations have suggested that urothelial cancers among African–Americans are more likely to be aggressive.[47] How this relates to issues of carcinogen exposure, 'protective' characteristics of the urothelium in various populations, genetic and/or enzymatic vulnerability to certain risk factors, access to healthcare by specific ethnic groups, and socioeconomic issues is unknown.

## CRITERIA IN ESTABLISHING EPIDEMIOLOGIC ASSOCIATIONS

The fundamental issue in epidemiology is causation.[5] The risk of contracting a condition or disease may vary in different areas and in different populations. This suggests an influence of environmental exposure, and this is likely in the context of particular genetic or molecular susceptibility. Historically, the issue of exposure to carcinogens and the bladder's role as a reservoir for the accumulation of waste products in the urine made environmental carcinogens the critical suspects as likely causes of urothelial (and squamous cell) carcinoma.[48] This was based on the original report by Rehn in 1895 of an increased incidence of bladder cancer in factory workers exposed to aniline dyes,[49] subsequent reports of industrial exposures to aromatic amines and bladder cancer development,[50,51] and laboratory studies of carcinogen induction of urothelial cancer in animal models.[52,53] However, many of the earlier reports have been criticized on the basis of questions regarding the application of epidemiologic investigational methods, the use of data that were unreliable or incomplete, concerns about the application of statistical analysis, and arguably misleading interpretations and conclusions.[5]

In addressing these issues, criteria that might be used to demonstrate causal relationships between urothelial cancer and exposure to a particular carcinogen have been proposed by Hill,[54] as recently reviewed by Fleshner and Kondylis,[5] to include the following:

1. The *strength* of association between exposure to carcinogens (cumulative doses) and the development of disease.
2. The *consistency* of association between exposure to carcinogens and disease development (notwithstanding studies in which varying methodologies and populations are examined).
3. The need for exposure to a causal agent to *precede* development of the cancer.
4. The *specificity* of exposure to a particular carcinogen to be seen in association with development of a particular cancer.
5. The *dose* of exposure, implying a greater risk of disease development with increasing or cumulative exposure to an agent considered causal (though possibly influenced by thresholds and critical periods of exposure during particular intervals of enhanced susceptibility).
6. The need for a putative causal association to be *biologically plausible*.
7. The requirement that a valid association have *coherence*, i.e. that it should not conflict with issues involving the natural history of the cancer.
8. The understanding that an association can be strengthened through *analogy*, i.e. similar mechanisms underlying causation in other conditions.
9. An appreciation that experimental studies that provide evidence confirming an association (though ethically and practically impossible to do) should be replaceable by a *preventive approach* to address the causal association, through which protection from or removal of a carcinogen leads to decreased rates of cancer development.

Although these criteria have been used to assess the validity of epidemiologic studies, such studies have often been limited by the absence of experimental controls associated with diverse genetic, geographic, and quantitative or qualitative exposure issues. Pitfalls in fundamental study design, acquisition of data, analysis of information, and unforeseen or unknown biases in the populations being studied have influenced our ability to interpret data meaningfully and have led to the generation of associations and conclusions that often have been found to be spurious or inconsistent with interpretations in other studies.[5,55] Recent epidemiologic investigations suggesting associations between exposure to putative carcinogens and development of urothelial cancer have therefore been subjected to a more cautious interpretation through consideration of various confounding variables that might have influenced documentation of exposures and characterization of a cancer in a particular individual or in variably defined population groups.

## TYPES OF EPIDEMIOLOGIC INVESTIGATION

The types of study that have been designed to explore and characterize associations between exposures in particular populations and the development of a specific disease include etiologic, case-control, and cohort studies.[5,56] The advantages and disadvantages in establishing the causal nature in a risk-disease association have recently been reviewed extensively by Fleshner and Kondylis[5] and include the following.

- 'Etiologic' studies examine groups of individuals and attempt to correlate incidence or mortality rates of a particular disease and levels of carcinogen exposure. These studies may be considered 'international' in being targeted towards populations in different countries, 'regional' in being focused on a particular region, or 'time-trend' if exploring a change of disease incidence and changing levels of exposure within the same population.[5] Such studies may be weakened by a paucity of information on individual exposure, the substitution of proxy measures of actual exposure, and the possible occurrence of exposures to other substances that themselves may induce carcinogenesis through cumulative exposures and confound the postulated association of a particular agent with the development of disease.
- 'Case-control' studies incorporate controls in exploring causal associations between specific exposures and development of disease.[5] These studies compare the exposure of individuals with a particular disease to the agent in question with exposures in individuals that do not have the disease. Results represent a comparison between the odds of exposure in individuals *with* disease and the odds of exposure in control individuals *without* disease, and are generally expressed as an 'odds ratio'.
- 'Cohort' studies compare rates of disease in individuals exposed to particular agents with rates of disease in individuals that have not been exposed.[5] Results are expressed as 'relative risks'. In these studies, individuals in each group are identified on the basis of their exposure and then studied *prospectively* for the development of disease. Such studies are considered the most representative of a controlled trial. Their major advantage is that exposure is determined *prior* to disease development. Therefore, the potential bias created by the need to recall exposure once the disease has developed in other types of study should not influence results in cohort studies. However, these studies are costly and often require a long time for the development of disease. As a consequence, individuals accessioned for study may be lost to follow-up.

## CARCINOGENS AND UROTHELIAL CANCER

Information on the epidemiology of urothelial and squamous cell cancer of the urinary bladder has been obtained through analysis of results of epidemiologic studies and from studies of the development of bladder cancer in animals exposed to specific carcinogens. Dating from the earliest observations suggesting an association between carcinogen exposure and development of bladder cancer by Rehn,[49] additional associations have been reported in other studies linking exposure to carcinogens in certain industries with development of bladder cancer.[50,51] Observations documenting carcinogen ingestion with urothelial cancer development in animal models confirmed these early associations.[52,53] Eventually, they prompted the implementation of legislative measures to decrease the intensity and cumulative nature of these exposures in attempts to decrease the risk of developing urothelial cancer.

That the incidence of bladder cancer has continued to increase[34] may reflect a continued cumulative exposure to carcinogens, an increased awareness of bladder cancer, and the significance of hematuria and of irritative urinary symptoms by the public and healthcare workers (presumably prompting patients to seek evaluation), and an increased access to healthcare by individuals that may have been exposed to carcinogens and taken advantage of screening programs. Most likely, this increase reflects progressive worldwide industrialization, the increase in cigarette smoking seen worldwide, and introduction of increased levels of carcinogens in the air, water, and general food supply.[57-59] Indeed, despite an increased awareness of risk factors, regulatory and other preventive measures, and programs designed for earlier diagnosis, the continued high rate of cigarette smoking worldwide and the consequent increased interaction with high concentrations of carcinogens through direct and second-hand exposures over many more years as deaths from noncancer causes may actually have decreased and lifespans increased is probably primarily responsible for this.[30-32,60] Moreover, because epidemiologic studies have often been insufficiently powered to document causality with a single agent, cumulative exposure to many carcinogenic substances may be the principal contributing factor to the increased incidence of bladder cancer around the world.[39-41,55]

### CIGARETTE SMOKING

The association between cigarette smoking and urothelial cancer appears to have become the major issue responsible for the genesis of bladder cancer throughout the world,[60] often confounding the efficacy ascribed to protective and preventive measures that have been legislated for industry to reduce exposures occasioned by carcinogens in the workplace.[30,55,61,62] Some have suggested that at least 50% of bladder cancers in men might not have occurred if these individuals had not smoked cigarettes.[63] An at least two- to four-fold increased risk for bladder cancer among cigarette smokers has been suggested.[64,65] Dose–response relationships and time trends in addressing the Hill criteria have documented that the number of cigarettes smoked, the degree of inhalation, the use of cigarette filters, and the cessation of cigarette smoking have each had effects in defining and characterizing the causal relationships associated with the development of urothelial cancer.[31,32,60] Other studies have shown that the type of tobacco used (blond versus black), representing the manner by which tobacco is cured and responsible for the concentrations of carcinogens that remain, correlate with bladder cancer risk.[66–69] Thus, adducts between DNA and 4-aminobiphenyl have been reported to be higher among smokers of air-cured tobacco (black) than among smokers of flue-cured tobacco (blond).[68,70] The combustion products of black versus blond tobaccos have been found to have correspondingly higher levels of carcinogens, respectively.[68,69]

Several reports have suggested that former smokers may be at lower risk for the development of bladder cancer than those that continue to smoke.[32,71] The precise role of cessation of smoking on incidence, recurrence, and progression of urothelial cancer in these studies, however, is unclear.[5] Further confounding interpretation of these studies has been the delayed development of urothelial cancer from the time that an individual may have smoked or been exposed to second-hand smoke, their exposure to additional environmental carcinogens through air, water, and food pollution, and possible individual susceptibilities contingent upon host genetic and enzymatic characteristics.[5]

Molecular studies have identified polycyclic aromatic hydrocarbons, aromatic and arylamines (e.g. 4-aminobiphenyl), unsaturated aldehydes (e.g. acrolein), and oxygen-free radicals in cigarette smoke as carcinogens associated with urothelial cancer.[55,68,72] Amongst these, 4-aminobiphenyl has been suggested to be the most important of these carcinogens.[68]

## AROMATIC AMINES

Historically, the identification of aromatic amines as carcinogens was based on associations between exposure through production or use of particular substances in various industries or through certain occupations associated with a statistically increased development of urothelial cancer. Most prominent among these were the chemical dye, rubber, and plastic manufacturing industries, all of which involved the use and production of aromatic amines in their manufacturing processes.[39,41,50,51,73–75] Some reports described an over 100-fold increased risk associated with exposure to the compounds used in these industries, with risk determined both by intensity and duration of exposure.[76] These associations prompted numerous laboratory studies using animal models and in vitro cellular protocols that corroborated the carcinogenic activities of these substances.[52,53] This in turn led to various governmental guidelines and regulations regarding ventilation, protective clothing, and monitoring/avoidance measures to reduce exposures to workers in these industries and decrease their risk for developing urothelial malignancies.

Nonetheless, the potential for exposure and the consequent cancer risk remain in many areas. Thus, workers in the textile, dry cleaning, hairdressing (use of hair dyes), and coal gasification/tar distillation/carbon black industries appear to have an increased risk for development of urothelial cancer because of the carcinogens generated in manufacturing or used in processing.[77–81] For example, perchloroethylene (an organic solvent used in dry cleaning), chemical dyes and aromatic amines (used in the textile industry),[77,78] and hair dyes that contain chemical carcinogens[78] have an apparent association with genesis of urothelial cancer as documented through clinical/epidemiologic studies and corroborated in laboratory investigations. Further, polycyclic aromatic hydrocarbons are found in high levels in processes involved in coal gasification and tar distillation, apparently producing a higher risk for the development of urothelial cancer among workers in these industries.[79–81]

Unfortunately, reports suggesting these increased risks have remained inconclusive in a definitive sense as they often have not documented duration and amount of exposure.[81] Furthermore, they have often been confounded by the high rate of cigarette smoking seen in many of the workers that have developed urothelial cancer.[55,61,62] The latter could conceivably outweigh the risk from carcinogens specifically involved in these industries. Although the cumulative exposure to carcinogens may be an important factor in this setting, the specific association with any one of the carcinogens may be difficult to define and verify.

## ENVIRONMENTAL AND 'LIFESTYLE' CARCINOGEN EXPOSURE

Outside of the workplace, and as the result of certain exposures through everyday life in various parts of the world, other substances have been reported to have an association with the development of bladder cancer. These include arsenic levels in the water supply in Taiwan,[82] use of the Chinese herb *Aristolochia fangchi*,[83] and ingestion of ochratoxin A in bracken fern in the Balkans.[84]

- The association of high levels of arsenic in the ground water in Southwestern Taiwan with a 15-fold increased risk for development of bladder cancer was confirmed in experimental studies of rats fed high levels of arsenic.[85]
- Ingestion of *A. fangchi* in China was associated with development of bladder cancer when nearly 50% of individuals that had used this herb as part of a weight loss program developed end-stage renal disease and either urothelial dysplasia or bladder cancer.[83]
- In the Balkan States, ingestion of ochratoxin A through intake of milk products from animals that had ingested bracken fern (a plant endemic in this region) was associated with the development of urothelial cancer of the upper tracts and of the bladder.[86]

Other epidemiologic studies have suggested potential risks with tryptophan intake,[87] coffee drinking,[88,89] and the use of artificial sweeteners.[87] Analyses of this work and subsequent investigations, however, have failed to validate these specific associations,[5] suggesting that confounding variables such as cigarette smoking may have been responsible for the increased risks hypothesized.

## MEDICAL EXPOSURE AND UROTHELIAL CANCER

Other reports have described associations between various medications or medical treatments and the development of bladder cancer. These have included the use of phenacetin and acetaminophen,[90,91] cyclophosphamide,[92,93] and pelvic radiation therapy.[94] These associations have appeared to depend largely upon cumulative exposures.

- The association between phenacetin and urothelial cancer of the upper tracts and the bladder was suggested by the development of renal pelvic cancers (transitional cell and squamous cell) in workers that had ingested large quantities of phenacetin to treat their migraine headaches.[90,95] Although this drug is currently no longer available, acetaminophen (paracetamol)—a metabolite of phenacetin—is available in 'over-the-counter' preparations. However, no epidemiologic studies have documented a potential risk of this substance as carcinogenic.
- An association between high cumulative doses of cyclophosphamide (Cytoxan) to treat various pediatric and adult malignancies (lymphoma, leukemia) and development of urothelial cancer (often high grade) has been reported and confirmed in several studies.[93,96] Attempts to reduce the intensity of the bladder's exposure to the metabolic

products of cyclophosphamide and presumably the later development of cancer have consisted of the use of reducing agents, hydration, and catheter drainage of the bladder during and immediately after treatment. Systematic studies of the preventive benefit of these measures, however, have not been done.

- Radiation to the cervix and to the prostate, commonly used treatments for cancers of these organs, has been associated with an approximately 10% increased risk for the development of urothelial cancer.[94,97,98] Efforts to reduce this risk other than by attempting to improve the focus of radiation on the target organ and reduce exposure of the bladder have not been reported.

An association between infection by *Schistosoma haematobium* and the development of urothelial cancer (largely squamous cell cancer but also transitional cell cancer) has been documented in many reports.[99,100] Some have suggested that the inflammatory response to the deposition of ova in the periureteral areas of the bladder is responsible for inducing bladder cancer. Others have suggested that concomitant infection with bacteria that may convert nitrates to nitrites and nitrosamines may be responsible for the development of urothelial cancer in these instances.[101] In addition, these patients may also have had a high exposure to carcinogen-containing fertilizers.[101] However, many had also smoked large quantities of cigarettes,[100] which also probably contributed to their increased risk for bladder cancer.

## CARCINOGENESIS

### HOST FACTORS

Although intensity, duration, and cumulativeness of exposure to carcinogenic substances may be critical in the development of bladder cancer, these factors need to be placed in the context of host molecular and enzymatic factors that may also play a role in this process by creating a greater susceptibility to the development of a urothelial malignancy. Thus, the metabolism of carcinogenic substances may be affected by individual and race-specific cellular enzymatic capabilities, either increasing or reducing their carcinogenic activity.[102,103]

In bladder cancer, acetylation of aromatic amines as a potential mechanism for carcinogen inactivation has drawn the most attention in this regard. The ability of the urothelium to detoxify carcinogens by their acetylation is determined by genes known as NAT1 and NAT2, which are responsible for the generation of the enzyme N-acetyl transferase. These determine whether an individual is a 'slow acetylator' or a 'fast acetylator'.[103] NAT2 expression has been suggested to be the predominant gene involved in this function. Individuals homozygous for the expression of NAT2 (designated slow acetylators) have a two- to four-fold increased risk for developing urothelial cancer,[104] presumably because they do not inactivate carcinogens rapidly enough to prevent their interactions with urothelial DNA in inducing mutations and carcinogenesis. Correspondingly, heterozygosity of this gene, which characterizes fast acetylators, has been associated with a lesser risk for the development of bladder cancer.[104,105] Fast acetylators are less likely to be affected by exposure to aromatic amines than slow acetylators.[105] The variable potential predisposition to bladder cancer development in different racial and ethnic groups has been suggested to reflect not only socioeconomic-based differences in carcinogen exposure patterns but also possible variability in expression of these enzymes.[106-108]

The p450 cytochrome oxidase system may also be important in the metabolism and detoxification of urothelial carcinogens.[107,108] This system may be vested in hepatocytes, determining the ability of the liver to detoxify potential carcinogens before they are passed into the urine. Individuals deficient in this system appear to have an increased risk of developing urothelial cancer.[109] Within the p450 enzyme group is the CYP1A2 isoenzyme, which may be particularly important in the metabolism of aromatic amines.[108] This isoenzyme activates 4-aminobiphenyl by hydroxylation of its N-radical. Individuals with greater or lesser expression of enzymes within this family are at greater or lesser risk, respectively, for development of urothelial cancer.[110]

Recent studies have also suggested a possible role of glutathione S transferase M1 (GSTM1) in the metabolism and detoxification of polycyclic aromatic hydrocarbons.[111] For example, smokers or workers exposed to aromatic amines deficient in this enzyme may have a 30% to 50% increased risk for developing urothelial cancer.[112,113] Ethnic and racial variation in this enzyme may also predispose certain groups to bladder cancer development on exposure to various carcinogens.[107,114,115]

## CARCINOGENESIS IN UROTHELIAL CANCER

Carcinogenesis is the process whereby malignant transformation occurs by introduction of a genetic defect into a cell, proliferation of that cell with perpetuation of the defect in the progeny of that transformed cell, and genesis of a tumor or 'growth' that either remains confined to the urothelium or invades and metastasizes.[116] Mechanisms for programmed cell death can come into play to eliminate that abnormal cell.[117] However, cancers may also contain genetic defects in areas that govern the cell cycle and programmed cell death (apoptosis).[118] These processes then no longer

serve as controls to eliminate abnormal cells, i.e. cells susceptible to normal controls that govern proliferation and growth and direct the organization of a particular cell type in the overall structure of organs within the host's body. This results in these abnormal cells surviving, proliferating, and producing a tumor that ultimately becomes clinically evident. If the genetic and biochemical capabilities are present, cells from this tumor mass may invade the structure of the origin and disseminate to other sites, proliferating at those sites and ultimately subsuming the metabolism and vital processes of the host.[119] Biologically, the tumor requires a compatible environment so that further proliferation can take place and the resulting tumors or growths can survive at the site of origin and at those distant sites.

Introduction of a specific genetic defect, or increased multiplicity of a variety of genetic defects, may be associated with a more aggressive biologic capability.[120] In this, the cells not only proliferate to generate a localized mass, but also penetrate the connective tissue scaffold that supports their epithelial origin, i.e. the urothelial lining of the bladder. Cells that are poorly differentiated may escape the constraints ordinarily imposed on a tumor mass (cohesion between adjacent cells and adhesion to the connective tissue framework).[121] These cells, while penetrating into and through the connective tissue scaffold, may then disseminate through channels created by formation of new blood vessels and new lymphatics (angiogenesis).[122] Although such cells may encounter a hostile environment in the circulation, the survival of some and the subsequent colonization of distant structures (metastasis) is the process whereby death of the host may ultimately result. Despite investigations designed to explore the processes involved in carcinogenesis, malignant transformation, the development of proliferative and metastatic tumors, and the factors that induce or inhibit these processes, little is known of the details of these events or of the means by which tumor growth and progression can be prevented.[123,124]

The field of epidemiology explores associations between exposure of normal cells to substances that can induce malignant transformation and the actual development of a malignancy.[5] Although epidemiologic studies attempt to correlate exposure to specific substances with the generation of malignancies, little is known of the actual processes involved, of the genetic changes that occur in response to specific exposures, and of how these lead to the clinical expression of tumors with distinct biologic behavior. Translation of genetic and biochemical correlates of carcinogenesis to the pathogenesis of different forms of cancer may provide an understanding of the intrinsic biologic potential of the various forms of disease. Unique host characteristics may also be important in determining what type of malignancy is likely to develop in response to exposure to a particular carcinogen. Each of these may ultimately become relevant in exploiting epidemiologic principles and developing preventive efforts to address the occurrence of different types of urothelial cancer following exposure to specific carcinogens.

## CONCLUSION

Associations between exposures to various substances that act as carcinogens and the development of urothelial cancer make this form of cancer one that may be preventable by strict adherence to public health measures and avoidance of exposure to specific substances. While reduced exposure to potential carcinogens in the workplace may decrease the cumulative risk presented by carcinogens in certain industries, individuals also need to be cognizant of their own responsibility to avoid exposure to substances (e.g. cigarette smoking) that fall outside the realm of strict legislative preventive measures.

Additionally, studies will be needed to define epidemiologic risks in the context of individual host factors and specific exposures as these may relate to the development of different forms of bladder cancer. An understanding of these factors may ultimately help prevent the development of the more devastating forms of this disease.

## REFERENCES

1. Murphy WM, Farrow GM, Beckwith B. Renal and Bladder Tumors. AFIP Fascicle Series. Washington DC: American Registry of Pathology, 1994.
2. Kantor AF, Hartge P, Hoover RN, et al. Epidemiologic characteristics of squamous cell carcinoma and adenocarcinoma of the bladder. Cancer Res 1988;48:3853–3855.
3. El Sabai I. Cancer of the bladder in Egypt. Proc Int Symp Bilharziasis (Cairo) 1996;1:709–723.
4. Jemal A, Tiwari RC, Murray T, et al. Cancer statistics, 2004. CA Cancer J Clin 2004;54:8–29.
5. Fleshner N, Kondylis F. Demographics and epidemiology of urothelial cancer of the urinary bladder. In Droller MJ (ed): Urothelial Tumors. Hamilton, Ontario: Decker, 2004, pp 1–16.
6. Parkin DM, Pisani P, Ferlay J. Estimates of the worldwide incidence of 25 major cancers in 1990. Int J Cancer 1999;80:827–841.
7. Pisani P, Parkin DM, Bray F, Ferlay J. Estimates of the worldwide mortality from 25 cancers in 1990. Int J Cancer 1999;83:18–29.
8. Landis SH, Murray T, Bolden S, Wingo PA. Cancer statistics. CA Cancer J Clin 1998;48:6–29.
9. Ferlay F, Bray F, Pisani P, et al. GLOBOCAN 2002: Cancer Incidence, Mortality and Prevalence Worldwide. IARC CancerBase No. 5. Version 2.0. Lyon: IARC Press, 2004.
10. Heney NM, Ahmed S, Flanigan MJ, et al. Superficial bladder cancer: progression and recurrence. J Urol 1983;130:1083–1086.
11. Fitzpatrick JM, West AB, Butler MR, et al. Superficial bladder tumor (stage pTa grades 1 & 2): the importance of recurrence pattern following initial resection. J Urol 1986;135:920–924.
12. Holmang S, Hedelin H, Anderstrom C, et al. The relationship among multiple recurrences, progression and prognosis of patients with stages Ta and T1 transitional cell carcinoma of the bladder followed for at least 20 years. J Urol 1995;153:18–24.
13. Parmar MKB, Friedman LS, Hargreave TB, et al. Prognostic factors for recurrence follow-up policies in the treatment of superficial bladder cancer: report from the British Medical Research Council Subgroup on Superficial Bladder Cancer. J Urol 1989;142:284–288.
14. Fitzpatrick JM. Superficial bladder cancer: natural history, evaluation, and management AUA Update Series 1989;8:82–90.
15. Heney NM, Nocks BN, Daly JJ, et al. Ta and T1 bladder cancer: location, recurrence, and prognosis. Brit J Urol 1982;54:152–157.
16. Prout GR Jr, Griffin PP, Shipley WU. Bladder carcinoma as a systemic disease. Cancer 1979;43:2532–2539.
17. Kaye KW, Lange PH. Mode of presentation of invasive bladder cancer: reassessment of the problem. J Urol 1982;128:31–33.
18. Abel PD. Follow-up of patients with 'superficial' transitional cell carcinoma of the bladder: the case for a change in policy. Brit J Urol 1993;72:135–142.
19. Pagano F, Garbeglio A, Milani C, et al. Prognosis of bladder cancer. I: Risk factors in superficial transitional cell carcinoma. Eur Urol 1987;13:145–148.
20. Klain R, Loy V, Huland H. Residual tumor discovered in routine second transurethral resection in patients with stage T1 transitional cell carcinoma of the bladder. J Urol 1991;146:316–318.
21. Langenstroer P, See W. The role of a second transurethral resection for high-grade bladder cancer. Curr Urol Rep 2000;1:204–207.
22. Smits G, Schaafsma E, Kiemeney L, et al. Microstaging of pT1 transitional cell carcinoma of the bladder: identification of subgroups with distinct risks of progression. Urology 1998;52:1009–1013.
23. Younes M, Sussman J, True LD. The usefulness of the level of muscularis mucosa in the staging of invasive transitional cell carcinoma of the urinary bladder. Cancer 1990;66:543–548.
24. Hassui Y, Osada Y, Kitada S, et al. Significance of invasion to the muscularis mucosa on the progression of superficial bladder cancer. Urology 1994;43:782–786.
25. Steineck G. Demographic and epidemiologic aspects of bladder cancer. In Droller MJ (ed): Bladder Cancer: Current Diagnosis and Treatment. Totowa, NJ: Humana Press, 2001, pp 1–24.
26. Cohen SM, Shirai T, Steineck G. Epidemiology and etiology of premalignant and malignant urothelial changes. Scand J Urol Nephrol Suppl 2000;205:105–115.
27. Steineck G, Plato N, Norell SE, et al. Urothelial cancer and some industry-related chemicals: an evaluation of the epidemiologic evidence. Am J Ind Med 1990;17:371–391.
28. Silverman DT, Hoover RN, Mason TJ, et al. Motor exhausts-related occupations and bladder cancer. Cancer Res 1986;46:2113–2116.
29. Schulte PA, Ringen K, Hemstreet GP, et al. Occupational cancer of the urinary tract. Occup Med 1987;2:85–107.
30. Mannetje A, Kogevinas M, Chang-Claude J, et al. Smoking as a confounder in case-control studies of occupational bladder cancer in women. Am J Ind Med 1999;36:75–82.
31. Lopez-Abente G, Gonzalez CA, Errezola M. Tobacco smoke inhalation pattern, tobacco type, and bladder cancer in Spain. Am J Epidemiol 1999;134:830–842.
32. Hartge P, Silverman D, Hoover R, et al. Changing cigarette habits and bladder cancer risk: a case-control study. J Natl Cancer Inst 1987;78:1119–1125.
33. Parker DM, Pisani P, Ferlay J. Estimates of the worldwide incidence of 25 major cancers in 1990. Int J Cancer 1999;80:827–841.
34. Ries LAG, Eisner MP, Kosary CL, et al. SEER Cancer Statistics Review, 1975–2000. Bethesda, MD: National Cancer Institute, 2003.
35. Fitzpatrick JM, Reda M. Bladder carcinoma in patients 40 years old or less. J Urol 1986;135:53–54.
36. Iori F, DeDomineis C, Liberti M, et al. Superficial bladder tumors in patients under 40 years of age: clinical, prognostic, and cytogenetic aspects. Urol Int 2001;67:224–227.
37. Cutler SJ, Heney NM, Freidell GH. Longitudinal study of patients with bladder cancer: factors associated with disease recurrence and progression. In Bonney WW, Prout GR (eds): Bladder Cancer. Baltimore: Williams & Wilkins, 1982, p 35.
38. Shirai T, Fukushima S, Hirose M, et al. Epithelial lesions of the urinary bladder in 313 autopsy cases. Jpn J Cancer Res (Gann) 1987;98:1073–1080.
39. Silverman DT, Rothman N, Devesa SS. Epidemiology of bladder cancer. In Syrigos KN, Skinner DG (eds): Bladder Cancer: Biology, Diagnosis and Management. New York: Oxford University Press, 1999, pp 11–55.

40. Cohen SM. Urinary bladder carcinogenesis. Toxicol Pathol 1998;26:121–127.

41. Johansson SL, Cohen SM. Epidemiology and etiology of bladder cancer. Semin Surg Oncol 1997;13:291–298.

42. Mannitje A, Kogevinas M, Chang-Claude J, et al. Smoking as a confounder in case-control studies of occupational bladder cancer in women. Am J Ind Med 1999;36:75–82.

43. Mannitje A, Kogevinas M, Chang-Claude J, et al. Occupation and bladder cancer in European women. Cancer Causes Control 1999;10:209–217.

44. Talalay P. Mechanisms of induction of enzymes that protect against chemical carcinogenesis. Adv Enzyme Regul 1989;28:237–250.

45. Wourmboudt LW, Commandeur JN, Vermeulen NP. Genetic polymorphisms of human N-acetyltransferases, cytochrome P450, glutathione-S-transferase and epoxide hydrolase enzymes: relevance to xenobiotic metabolism and toxicity. Crit Rev Toxicol 1999;29:59–134.

46. Miller BA, Kolonel LN, Bernstein L, et al. Racial/ethnic patterns of cancer in the United States, 1988–92 (NIH Publication). Bethesda, MD: National Cancer Institute, 1996, pp 96–104.

47. Prout GR, Wesley M, Greenberg RS, et al. Bladder cancer: race differences in extent of disease at diagnosis. Cancer 2000;15:1349–1358.

48. Kabat GC, Dieck GS, Wynder EL. Bladder cancer in non-smokers. Cancer 1986;57:362–367.

49. Rehn L. Blasengeschwulste bei Fuchsin–Arbeitern. Arch Klin Chir 1895;50:588–600.

50. Case RAM, Hosker ME, McDonald DB, et al. Tumors of the urinary bladder in workmen engaged in the British chemical industry. Role of arylbenzidine, alpha-naphthylamine, and beta-naphthylamine. Br J Intern Med 1954;11:75–92.

51. Steineck G, Plato N, Gerhardsson M, et al. Urothelial cancer and some industry-related chemicals: an evaluation of the epidemiologic evidence. Am J Ind Med 1990;17:379–391.

52. Hueper WC, Wiley FH, Wolfe HD. Experimental production of bladder tumors in dogs by administration of beta-naphthylamine. J Ind Hyg Toxicol 1936;20:46–48.

53. Hicks RM, Wright R, Wakefield JSJ. The induction of rat bladder cancer by 2-naphthylamine. Br J Cancer 1982;46:646–661.

54. Hill AB. The environment and disease: association or causation? Proc Roy Soc Med 1965;58:295–300.

55. Wynder EL, Goldsmith R. The epidemiology of bladder cancer: a second look. Cancer 1977;40:1246–1253.

56. Rothman KJ. Modern Epidemiology. Boston: Little Brown, 1986.

57. Kunze E, Chang-Claude J, Frentzel-Beyme R. Life style and occupational risk factors for bladder cancer in Germany. Cancer 1992;69:176–190.

58. Cantor KP, Hoover R, Mason TJ, et al. Bladder cancer, drinking water source, and tap water consumption: a case-control study. J Natl Cancer Inst 1987;79:1269–1279.

59. Silverman DT, Hoover RN, Mason TJ, et al. Motor exhaust-related occupations and bladder cancer. Cancer Res 1986;46:2113–2116.

60. Morrison AS, Buring JE, Verhoeck WG, et al. An international study of smoking and bladder cancer. J Urol 1984;131:650–654.

61. D'Avanzo B, Negri E, LaVecchia C, et al. Cigarette smoking and bladder cancer. Eur J Cancer 1990;26:714–718.

62. Cole P, Manson RR, Haring H, et al. Smoking and cancer of the lower urinary tract. N Engl J Med 1971;284:129–134.

63. Silverman DT, Hartge P, Morrison AS, et al. Epidemiology of bladder cancer. Hematol Oncol Clin North Am 1992;6:1–30.

64. Chyou PA, Nomura AMY, Stemmemann GN. A prospective study of diet, smoking, and lower urinary tract cancer. Ann Epidemiol 1993;3:211–216.

65. Fleshner N, Garland J, Moadel A, et al. Influence of smoking status on the disease-related outcomes of patients with tobacco-associated superficial transitional cell cancer of the bladder. Cancer 1999;86:1337–1345.

66. Vineis P, Esteve J, Hartge P, et al. Effects of timing and type of tobacco in cigarette-induced bladder cancer. Cancer Res 1998;48:3849–3852.

67. Clavel J, Cordier S, Boccon-Gibod L, et al. Tobacco and bladder cancer in males: increased risk for inhalers and smokers of black tobacco. Int J Cancer 1989;44:605–610.

68. Bartsch H, Malaveile C, Friesen M, et al. Black (air-cured) and blond (flue-cured) tobacco cancer risk. IV. Molecular dosimetry studies implicate aromatic amines as bladder carcinogens. Eur J Cancer 1993;29:1199–1208.

69. Burch JD, Rohan TE, Howe GR, et al. Risk of bladder cancer by source and type of tobacco exposure: a case control study. Int J Cancer 1989;44:622–628.

70. Bartsch H, Caporaso N, Coda M, et al. Carcinogen hemoglobin adducts, urinary mutagenicity, and metabolic phenotype in active and passive cigarette smokers. J Natl Cancer Inst 1990;82:1826–1831.

71. Thompson IM, Peck M, Rodriguez FR. The impact of cigarette smoking on stage, grade, and number of recurrences of transitional cell carcinoma of the bladder. J Urol 1987;137:401–403.

72. Bernardini S, Adessi GL, Chezy E, et al. Influence of cigarette smoking on p53 gene mutations in bladder carcinomas. Anticancer Res 2001;21:3001–3004.

73. La Vecchia C, Airoldi L. Human bladder cancer: epidemiological, pathological, and mechanistic aspect. IARC Sci Publ 1999;147:139–157.

74. Silverman DT, Levin LI, Hoover RN, et al. Occupational risks of bladder cancer in the United States: I. White men. J Natl Cancer Inst 1989;81:1472–1480.

75. Vineis P, Magnani C. Occupation and bladder cancer in males: a case-control study. Int J Cancer 1985;35:599–606.

76. Bulbulyan MA, Figgs LW, Zahn SH, et al. Cancer incidence and mortality among beta-naphthylamine and benzidine dye workers in Moscow. Int J Epidemiol 1995;24:266–275.

77. Weiss NS. Cancer in relation to occupational exposure to perchloroethylene. Cancer Causes Control 1995;6:257–266.

78. Gago-Dominguez M, Castelao JE, Yuan JM, et al. Use of permanent hair dyes and bladder cancer risk. Int J Cancer 2001;91:575–579.

79. Wong O, Raabe GK. A critical review of cancer epidemiology in the petroleum industry, with a meta-analysis of a combined database of more than 350,000 workers. Regul Toxicol Pharmacol 2000;32:78–98.

80. Boffetta P, Jourenkova N, Gustavsson P. Cancer risk from occupational and environmental exposure to polycyclic aromatic hydrocarbons. Cancer Causes Control 1997;8:444–472.

81. Steineck G, Plato N, Norell SE, et al. Urothelial cancer and some industry-related chemicals: an evaluation of the epidemiologic literature. Am J Ind Med 1990;17:371–391.

82. Brown KG, Beck BD. Arsenic and bladder cancer mortality. Epidemiology 1996;7:667–669.

83. Nortier JL, Martinez MC, Schmeiser HH, et al. Urothelial carcinoma associated with the use of a Chinese herb (Aristolochia fangchi). N Engl J Med 2000;342:1686–1692.

84. Pfohl-Leszkowicz J, Petkova-Bocharova T, Chernozemsky IN, et al. Balkan endemic nephropathy and associated urinary tract tumors: a review on aetiological causes and the potential role of mycotoxins. Food Addit Contam 2002;18:282–302.

85. Chiou HY, Chiou ST, Hsu Y, et al. Incidence of transitional cell carcinoma and arsenic in drinking water: a follow-up study of 8,102 residents in an arseniasis-endemic area in northeastern Taiwan. Am J Epidemiol 2001;153:411–418.

86. Cukuranovic R, Ignjatovic M, Stefanovic V. Urinary tract tumors and Balkan nephropathy in the South Monrovia River basin. Kidney Int Suppl 1991;34:580–584.

87. Bryan GT. The role of urinary tryptophan metabolites in the etiology of bladder cancer. Am J Clin Nutr 1971;24:841–852.

88. Donato F, Boffetta P, Fazioli R, et al. Bladder cancer, tobacco smoking, coffee and alcohol drinking in Brescia, Northern Italy. W Eur J Epidemiol 1997;13:795–800.

89. Woolcott CG, King WD, Marrett LD. Coffee and tea consumption and cancers of the bladder, colon and rectum. Eur J Cancer 2002;11:137–145.

90. Piper JM, Tonascia J, Matanowski GM. Heavy phenacetin use and bladder cancer in women aged 20 to 49 years. N Engl J Med 1985;313:292–295.

91. McCredie M, Stewart JH. Does paracetamol cause urothelial cancer or renal papillary necrosis? Nephron 1988;49:196–200.

92. Valaovic P, Jewett MA. Cyclophosphamide-induced bladder cancer. Can J Urol 1999;6:745–748.

93. Agarwala S, Hemal AK, Seth A, et al. Transitional cell carcinoma of the urinary bladder following exposure to cyclophosphamide in childhood. Eur J Pediatr Surg 2001;11:207–210.

94. Quilty PM, Kerr GR. Bladder cancer following low or high dose pelvic radiation. Clin Radiol 1987;38:583–586.

95. Johansson S, Wahlquist L. Tumors of the urinary bladder and ureter associated with abuse of phenacetin-containing analgesics. Acta Pathol Microbiol Scand 1977;85:768–774.

96. Pederson-Bjergaard J, Ersboll J, Hansen V, et al. Carcinoma of the urinary bladder after treatment with cyclophosphamide for non-Hodgkin's lymphoma. N Engl J Med 1988;318:1028–1032.

97. Duncan RE, Bennett DW, Evans AT, et al. Radiation induced bladder tumors. J Urol 1977;188:43–45.

98. Neugut AI, Ahsan H, Robinson E, et al. Bladder carcinoma and other second malignancies after radiotherapy for prostate carcinoma. Cancer 1997;79:1600–1604.

99. Tawfik HN. Carcinoma of the urinary bladder associated with schistosomiasis in Egypt: the possible casual relationship. Princess Tahamatsu Symp 1987;18:197–209.

100. Mostafa MH, Sheweita SA, O'Conner PJ. Relationship between schistosomiasis and bladder cancer. Clin Microbiol Rev 1999;12:97–111.

101. Tricker AR, Mostafa MH, Spiegelhalder B, et al. Urinary excretion of nitrate, nitrite and v-nitroso compounds in schistosomiasis and bilharzia bladder cancer patients. Carcinogenesis 1989;10:547–552.

102. Cartwright RA, Glashan RW, Rogers HJ, et al. The role of N-acetyl transferase in bladder carcinogenesis: a pharmacogenetic epidemiological approach to bladder cancer. Lancet 1982;2:842–845.

103. Mommsen S, Barfod NM, Aagaard J. N-acetyl transferase phenotypes in the urinary bladder carcinogenesis of a low-risk population. Carcinogenesis 1985;6:199–201.

104. Risch A, Wallace DM, Bathers S, et al. Slow N-acetylation genotype is a susceptibility factor in occupational and smoking related bladder cancer. Hum Mol Genet 1995;4:231–236.

105. Hayes RB, Rothman N. N-acetylation phenotype and genotype and risk of bladder cancer in benzidine-exposed workers. Carcinogenesis 1993;14:675–678.

106. Bell DA, Taylor JA, Butler MA, et al. Genotype/phenotype discordance for human arylamine N-acetyl transferase (NAT2) reveals a new slow actylator allele common in African–Americans. Carcinogenesis 1993;14:1689–1692.

107. Theodorescu D. Molecular carcinogenesis and pathogenesis of proliferative and progressive (invasive) urothelial cancer. In Droller MJ (ed): Urothelial Tumors. Hamilton, Ontario: Decker, 2004, pp 28–43.

108. Butler MA, Iwasaki M. Guengerich FP, et al. Human cytochrome P-450 PA (P450IA2), the phenacetin O-deethylase, is primarily responsible for the hepatic 3-demethylation of caffeine and N-oxidation of carcinogenic arylamines. Proc Acad Sci USA 1989;86:7696–7700.

109. Bryant MS, Vineis P, Skipper PL, et al. Hemoglobin adducts of aromatic amines: associations with smoking status and type of tobacco. Proc Natl Acad Sci USA 1988;85:9788–9791.

110. Kalow W, Tang BK. Caffeine as a metabolic probe: exploration of the enzyme-inducing effect of cigarette-smoking. Clin Pharmacol Ther 1991;49:44–48.

111. Yu ME, Ross RK, Chan KK, et al. Glutathione S-transferase M1 genotype affects amino-biphenyl-hemoglobin adduct levels in white, black, and Asian smokers and non-smokers. Cancer Epidemiol Biomarkers Prev 1995;4:861–864.

112. Jong Jeong H, Jin Kim H, Young Seo I, et al. Association between glutathione S-transferase M1, and T1 polymorphisms and increased risk for bladder cancer in Korean smokers. Cancer Lett 2003;202:193–199.

113. Shen M, Hung RJ, Brennan P, et al. Polymorphisms of the DNA repair and bladder cancer risk in a case-control study in Northern Italy. Cancer Epidemiol Biomarkers Prev 2003;12:1234–1240.

114. Board P, Coggan M, Johnston P, et al. Genetic heterogeneity of the human glutathione transferases: a complex of gene families. Pharmacol Ther 1990;48:357–369.

115. Bell DA, Taylor JA, Paulson DF, et al. Genetic risk and carcinogen exposure: a common inherited defect of the carcinogen-metabolism gene glutathione S-transferase M1 (GSTM1) that increases susceptibility to bladder cancer. J Natl Cancer Inst 1993;85:1159–1164.

116. Reeder JE, Messing EM. Cell-cycle aberrations in human bladder cancer. In Droller MJ (ed): Urothelial Tumors. Hamilton, Ontario: Decker, 2004, pp 17–27.

117. Reed JC. Apoptosis and cancer. In Kufe DW, Pollack RE, Weichselbaum RR, et al (eds): Cancer Medicine. Hamilton, Ontario: Decker, 2003, pp 41–52.

118. Kastan M. On the trail from p53 to apoptosis? Nat Genet 1997;17:130–131.

119. Behrens J. Cadherins and catenins: role in signal transduction and tumor progression. Cancer Metastasis Rev 1999;18:15–30.

120. Cohen SM, Ellwein LB. Genetic error, cell proliferation, and carcinogenesis. Cancer Res 1991;51:6493–6500.

121. Mareel M, Boterberg T, Noe V, et al. E-cadherin/catenin/cytoskeleton complex: a regulator of cancer invasion. J Cell Physiol 1997;173:271–274.

122. Brown LF, Berse B, Jackman RW, et al. Increased expression of vascular permeability factor (vascular endothelial growth factor) and receptors in kidney and bladder carcinoma. Am J Pathol 1993;143:1255–1262.

123. Cordon-Cardo C. Mutation of cell cycle regulators—biological and clinical implications for human neoplasia. Am J Pathol 1995;147:545–560.

124. Habuchi T, Ogawa O, Kakehi Y, et al. Accumulated allelic losses in the development of invasive urothelial cancer. Int J Cancer 1993;53:579–584.

# Occupational risk factors

2

*Sarah A Felknor, George L Delclos*

## INTRODUCTION

The first knowledge that selected occupations could pose a risk for the development of bladder cancer was published in 1895, when the German surgeon Rehn described a cluster of cases among Frankfurt workers involved in the manufacture of coal tar-derived magenta and auramine dyes.[1,2] Since then, occupation-related bladder cancer has largely followed the development of the industrialized world. In the United States, the first bladder cancer cases associated with occupation were identified in the 1930s. In 1938, Hueper et al provided animal evidence of the carcinogenicity of β-naphthylamine (also known as 2-naphthylamine) in dogs.[3] In 1954, Case and colleagues published the first formal epidemiologic study of bladder cancer, showing increases in mortality in a cohort of British chemical workers that ranged from 8 to 87 times that of nonexposed persons, depending on the specific chemical.[4,5]

Bladder cancer was recognized as a compensable occupational disease in the United Kingdom in the early 1950s and, in the mid-1960s, the British government banned the production and use of β-naphthylamine. In the US, the advent of Occupational Safety and Health Administration (OSHA) in 1970 led to the regulation of β-naphthylamine as a carcinogen, resulting in the nearly complete elimination of its manufacture for purposes other than research.[6] Similar strict regulations have been in place for benzidine and 4-aminobiphenyl in many developed countries over the past 40 years, primarily affecting the rubber and textile dye manufacturing industries, and have presumably resulted in a decreased burden of occupational exposure to these compounds.[7]

In most cases, the substitution of less toxic materials has allowed these industries to remain productive while controlling exposure to these well-established human carcinogens. As more manufacturing processes are transferred from developed to developing countries, however, it is less certain whether the benefits of these control technologies are being transferred to the same degree. This, combined with less stringent enforcement of worker protections, weaker surveillance systems, and the small body of occupational health research conducted in developing nations, raises important new questions regarding the burden of occupational bladder cancer in these countries.[8-10]

## OCCUPATIONAL EXPOSURES

To date, over 40 different occupations and more than 200 chemicals have been identified as risk factors for bladder cancer, although the strength of the evidence varies from one compound to another.[11] Across the various industries, the chemicals most frequently linked to occupational bladder cancer are the aromatic amines, most notably β-naphthylamine, 4-aminobiphenyl, and benzidine. Aromatic amines have many industrial uses, primarily as intermediary compounds in the production of textile dyes and as antioxidants in the manufacture of rubber. They can also be present as contaminants in several industrial environments, including aluminum production, chemical manufacturing, and the automobile industry.[8,12]

The International Agency for Research on Cancer (IARC) has classified seven specific aromatic amines as either Group 1 (definite) or Group 2A (probable) human carcinogens. Group 1 carcinogens are 4-aminobiphenyl, benzidine, β-naphthylamine, and N,N-bis(2-chloroethyl)-2-naphthylamine (chlornaphazine).

The Group 2A carcinogens are ortho-toluidine, 4-chloro-ortho-toluidine and 4,4´-methylene bis(2-chloroaniline) (MOCA). In addition, the IARC lists the rubber industry and both magenta and auramine manufacturing as Group 1 exposure circumstances. Benzidine-based dyes, as a general class of industrial compounds, and occupational exposure to them by barbers or hairdressers, are listed as Group 2A carcinogenic exposure circumstances.[13,14] In the course of their work, barbers and hairdressers potentially are exposed to various permanent hair dyes, which can contain various aromatic amines. Interestingly, personal hair dye use has not been found to be a risk factor.[7,15]

Several excellent recent reviews of the fairly large body of epidemiologic evidence that forms the scientific basis linking selected chemicals, occupations, and industries to bladder cancer are available.[7,8,15,16] Historically, the most consistently identified at-risk industries are aromatic amine manufacture, dyestuff manufacture, the rubber industry, painting, leather tanneries, different segments of the automobile industry, and aluminum production.

Even though increased risks have been documented repeatedly in these industries, identification of the specific chemical link to the risk has not always been straightforward, except possibly in the chemical manufacturing and rubber industries. In most cases, the presumed carcinogens have been aromatic amines, benzidine-based azo dyes and/or nitrosamines present as intermediary compounds, additives or workplace contaminants, as is the case with the painting and leather industries.[17-21] In the case of the automobile industry—including motor vehicle parts and supplies, mechanics, machinists, and transportation—identification of the offending chemicals is more speculative, and includes diesel exhaust and polycyclic aromatic hydrocarbons present in degreasing solvents and various machining fluids.[12,22] In the aluminum industry, for some time, exposures to coal tar pitch volatiles and other polycyclic aromatic hydrocarbons have been identified as the most likely carcinogens.[23] However, in a recent study of aluminum (cryolite) workers with elevated bladder cancer risk conducted in Denmark, in which exposure to polycyclic aromatic hydrocarbons was deemed to be insignificant, the role of other causal agents such as fluoride has been raised.[24] Notwithstanding the uncertainty, however, the aluminum industry has largely acknowledged the excess cancer risk, and is implementing various controls and screening programs for its workers.[25]

In addition, there are several other potential at-risk industries for which the data are either incomplete or which may represent new areas of concern. Exposure to diesel exhaust has been examined as a cause of bladder cancer, but data are still inconclusive. In a large record-linkage study conducted with data from Sweden, Boffetta and colleagues did not find an increased risk of bladder cancer in either men or women exposed to diesel emissions.[26] Boffetta and Silverman also conducted a meta-analysis of 35 studies of diesel exhaust exposure, mainly focusing on truck drivers and bus drivers.[27] Based on 15 studies, the summary relative risk for truck drivers was 1.17 (95% CI: 1.06–1.29); for bus drivers, based on 10 studies, the summary relative risk was 1.33 (95% CI: 1.22–1.45). The authors concluded that, although an association between diesel exhaust exposure and bladder cancer was possible, the magnitude of the effect was such that the effects of bias or confounding could not be completely discounted.

A few studies have examined bladder cancer risk within the petroleum industry, with conflicting results. Gun and colleagues, in a prospective study of the Australian petroleum industry, detected an increased standardized incidence rate of 1.37 (95% CI: 1.00–1.83).[28] In contrast, Lewis and colleagues failed to find a similar excess among Canadian petroleum workers.[29] In a general study of cancer mortality among acrylonitrile-exposed workers in a nitrogen products manufacturing plant within the petrochemical industry, Marsh and colleagues found an unexpected excess of bladder cancer cases among the non-acrylonitrile-exposed control group, although the actual agent so far has not been conclusively identified.[30]

In a meta-analysis of 40 studies of foundry workers, Gaertner and Theriault identified small increases in the summary risk estimates, in the range of 1.11–1.16, depending on the quality of the studies.[31] The authors believed that this small increase in risk was susceptible to confounding and bias, and recommended additional studies, focused on the evaluation of dose–response patterns.

Marine engineers are potentially exposed to various oil and petroleum products over the course of a working lifetime. Rafnsson and Sulem performed a cancer cohort study of 6603 marine engineers from Iceland followed from 1955 to 1998, and, after allowing for a latency of 40 years and consideration of smoking, found an increased standardized incidence ratio of 1.3 (95% CI: 1.0–1.8).[32]

Although the manufacture and use of β-naphthylamine have been strictly regulated in the US for several decades, potential exposure to this compound has been detected in new settings, including Superfund sites and as a contaminating by-product in the polyethylene pipe manufacturing industry.[33,34] Similarly, although benzidine production is controlled in developed countries, high rates of occupational bladder cancer continue to be detected in countries such as China, which still employs a large number of workers in this industry.[9] In each of these high-risk populations, screening programs were implemented, some of which include state-of-the-art biomarkers, hopefully to allow the earlier detection of this curable disease.[9,33,34] (For a more detailed discussion of the role of screening for bladder cancer, see Chapter 23.)

## MAGNITUDE OF THE RISK

As is the case with bladder cancer in general, occupationally acquired bladder cases are more common in men than in women, largely because of the historically higher prevalences of smoking and employment in at-risk industries among men. However, increased risks have also been documented in women, including those employed in the rubber industry.[35] In addition, Pelucchi et al, in a case-control study of northern Italian women, found a greater than three-fold odds of a history of occupational exposure to chemical, dye/paints, and the pharmaceutical industry among women with bladder cancer.[36] In a population-based case-control study conducted in Iowa, female secondary school teachers, record clerks, domestic service employees, and workers in the laundering and dry cleaning business had elevated risks of bladder cancer.[12]

Overall, bladder cancer is highest in non-Hispanic whites.[7] Minorities have been less well studied, particularly with respect to occupational bladder cancer. Based on data from the National Bladder Cancer Study, a population-based case-control study conducted in 10 states, Silverman and colleagues estimated that bladder cancers of between 21% and 25% in white men, and 27% in nonwhite men, were occupationally related, although this difference was not statistically significant.[37,38] In a recent proportional mortality study of US national data from 21 states, Schulz and Loomis found elevated proportional mortality ratios for African–American men and women and Latino males in various occupations, most notably within the metal industry, for Asian males in sales, and for Asian women employed in the personal services industry, when compared with workers of the same gender and ethnic–racial group.[39]

Estimates of the at-risk worker population in the US have been based on two surveys conducted by the National Institute for Occupational Safety and Health (NIOSH) in 1972–1974 (National Occupational Hazard Survey) and in 1981–1983 (National Occupational Exposure Survey) and may, therefore, be somewhat outdated. By crosslinking these data sets, which provide information on potential hazards by industry and occupation, against lists of known and suspected bladder carcinogens from the Registry of Toxic Effects of Chemical Substances (RTECS) and from the IARC, Ruder and colleagues estimated that 1.8 million workers in the 1970s and approximately 3.5 million in the 1980s experienced some level of exposure to occupational bladder carcinogens.[11]

With respect to histology, virtually all occupational bladder cancers are transitional cell carcinomas, as is the case with non-occupational bladder cancer.[40] Two studies have provided some evidence that occupationally acquired bladder cancer is more frequently an invasive, high-grade tumor that may develop on average 15 years ahead of non-occupational bladder cancer.[41,42] However, in general, epidemiologic studies have rarely distinguished between preneoplastic and invasive tumors, or examined tumor grade, so it cannot be stated with certainty whether a specific cell type predominates in occupationally induced bladder cancer as compared to non-occupational cancer.

Cigarette smoking is clearly the most important modifiable risk factor causally linked to bladder cancer, accounting for 50% to 60% of the attributable risk in developed nations.[7] Estimates of the fraction attributable to occupational exposures, with the exception of a few studies suggesting figures in the range of 0% to 3%, have ranged from 16% to 25% in many more studies, almost all of which have been conducted in developed countries.[8,43] The attributable risk in developing nations is less well characterized, but may well be higher than in developed countries because of a greater proportion of workers employed in the secondary sector of the economy (which includes manufacturing) and lower enforcement of regulatory standards.

## INDIVIDUAL RISK

As is the case with most occupational disease, individual risk is dependent on the intensity of the occupational exposure and on factors that indicate an individual susceptibility—genetic or acquired—to the development of bladder cancer. Exposure intensity, in turn, is determined by the level of daily exposure to a given chemical carcinogen and the overall duration of exposure. Epidemiologic studies of occupational bladder cancer have generally not included quantitative measures of personal exposure to chemicals which, although unfortunate, is not unusual in these types of study. Instead, surrogates of personal exposure, such as job title within an industry, are frequently used.[15]

Duration of exposure is generally characterized both by the time spent (in months or years) in an at-risk occupation or industry, and by latency, i.e. the length of time (generally in years) that has elapsed between the onset of exposure to an occupational carcinogen and the measurement of the health outcome. Although the length of time spent in an at-risk job or industry, for most cases of occupational bladder cancer, was many months to years, there have been isolated case reports suggesting that the duration of exposure to a bladder carcinogen could be as brief as 3 months.[42] However, in this same large study of over 1000 dye workers in Wakayama City, Japan, the mean duration of exposure to carcinogenic chemicals was around 5 years. With respect to latency, most studies have found that risk is rarely increased before at least 20 years have elapsed from the onset of exposure.[42,44] In some occupational groups, the increased risk has not been detected before 30 or even 40 years have elapsed, such as in Tokyo dyestuff workers or

Icelandic marine engineers.[32,45] In addition, the age at which the exposure began is likely to be important. For example, among Italian dyestuff manufacturing workers with exposure to various aromatic amines, higher risks were detected among workers exposed at younger ages, even after controlling for duration of exposure, suggesting latency is critical.[15,42]

After the skin and respiratory surfaces, the bladder is the main internal body surface affected by occupational carcinogens. The initial routes of exposure for bladder carcinogens can be via inhalation, ingestion, or absorption through the skin. Aromatic amines, the main class of bladder chemical carcinogens, must be metabolically activated in order to bind to DNA. This activation is mediated by selected enzymes whose expression varies in human populations, making some individuals potentially more predisposed to the development of cancer than others. The reactive species are excreted in urine, enabling them to come in contact with the urothelium.[2,15,16] Several enzyme systems have been studied in bladder cancer, most notably N-acetyltransferase (NAT). In the 1950s, in studies of the metabolism of the antituberculosis agent isoniazid, it was found that approximately 50% of whites metabolized this drug more slowly than the rest of the population, and were referred to as 'slow acetylators'.[46] This was later linked to a low activity rate of the NAT enzyme. N-acetylation transforms aromatic amine compounds into less reactive metabolites and, hence, may protect against carcinogenesis. Several studies have suggested that slow acetylators may also be at an increased risk of bladder cancer in the presence of aromatic amine exposure, and have been reviewed recently by IARC.[47,48]

NAT enzyme activity is determined by two genes, NAT1 and NAT2, each of which has various polymorphisms, some of which may be protective.[49] Vineis and colleagues conducted a pooled analysis of case-control studies and case series in Europe, with a total of 1530 cases and 731 controls, to evaluate the association between NAT2 genotypes and bladder cancer.[46] Overall, the authors found evidence for a significant association between NAT2 and bladder cancer (odds ratio 1.42, 95% CI: 1.14–1.77), and confirmed that the highest risks occurred among smokers, persons with occupational exposure to bladder carcinogens and, especially, slow acetylators. Their findings suggested an interactive effect between the NAT2 genotype, smoking, and occupation, where the genotype might be modulating the effects of the environmental carcinogens.

Glutathione S-transferase M1 (GSTM1) is another enzyme involved in detoxification pathways for carcinogens, and its deficiency has been linked to an increased risk of bladder cancer, although the magnitude of this effect is unclear.[15] Shinka and colleagues studied 137 dyestuff workers in Japan and found that the prevalence of GSTM1 deficiency did not differ significantly between those with and without urothelial cancer, although a trend test was positive.[50] The effects of occupational factors, namely a history of working in small factories and greater duration of exposure, however, were greater than the contribution of the enzyme deficiency.

For a more in-depth discussion of genetic susceptibility and bladder cancer, the reader is referred to Chapter 4.

## CONCLUSION

The association between exposure to selected chemical carcinogens, occupations or industries and bladder cancer is well established, and it is estimated that 20% to 27% of bladder cancers are attributable to occupational exposures. The risk of occupational bladder cancer is dependent not only on the intensity and characteristics of the workplace exposures, but also on individual susceptibility to these cancers. In developed countries, strict regulatory controls are likely to have resulted in a decreased burden of exposure to bladder carcinogens in the workplace. However, the situation is less clear in developing countries where some of these risky technologies may have been transferred, and where enforcement of regulations and worker protections are likely to be less stringent.

## REFERENCES

1. Rehn L. Blasengeschwuelste bei Fuchsinarbeitern. Arch Klin Chur 1895;50:588–600.

2. Weisburger JH. Comments on the history and importance of aromatic and heterocyclic amines in public health. Mutat Res 2002;506–507:9–20.

3. Hueper WC, Wiley F, Wolfe HD. Experimental production of bladder tumors in dogs by administration of β-naphthylamine. J Indust Hyg Toxicol 1938;20:46–84.

4. Case RAM, Hosler ME. Tumours of the urinary bladder in workmen engaged in the manufacture and use of certain dyestuff intermediates in the British chemical industry. Part I. The role of aniline, benzidine, 1-naphthylamine and 2-naphthylamine. Br J Ind Med 1954;11:75–104.

5. Case RAM, Pearson JT. Tumours of the urinary bladder in workmen engaged in the manufacture and use of certain dyestuff intermediates in the British chemical industry. Part II. Further considerations of the role of aniline and of the manufacture of auramine and magenta (fuchsin) as possible causative agents. Br J Industr Med 1954;11:213–216.

6. Verma DK, Purdham JT, Roels HA. Translating evidence about occupational conditions into strategies for prevention. Occup Environ Med 2002;59:205–214.

7. Yu MC, Skipper PL, Tannenbaum SR, Chan KK, Ross RK. Arylamine exposures and bladder cancer risk. Mutat Res 2002;506–507:21–28.

8. Vineis P, Piratsu R. Aromatic amines and cancer. Cancer Causes Control 1997;8:346–355.

9. Hemstreet GP, Yin S, Ma Z, et al. Biomarker risk assessment and bladder cancer detection in a cohort exposed to benzidine. J Natl Cancer Inst 2001;93:427–436.

10. Delclós J, Betancourt O, Marqués F, Tovalín H. Globalización y salud laboral. Arch Prev Riesgos Labor 2003;6:4–9.

11. Ruder AM, Fine LJ, Smith DS. National estimates of occupational exposure to animal bladder tumorigens. J Occup Med 1990;32:797–805.

12. Zheng T, Cantor KP, Zhang Y, Lynch CF. Occupation and bladder cancer: a population-based, case-control study in Iowa. J Occup Environ Med 2002;44:685–691.

13. International Agency for Research on Cancer. Overall evaluations of carcinogenicity to humans. Group 1: carcinogenic to humans. Online. Available: www.cie.iarc.fr/monoeval/crthall.html.

14. International Agency for Research on Cancer. Overall evaluations of carcinogenicity to humans. Group 2A: probably carcinogenic to humans. Online. Available: www-cie.iarc.fr/monoeval/crthall.html.

15. Negri E, La Vecchia C. Epidemiology and prevention of bladder cancer. Eur J Cancer Prev 2001;10:7–14.

16. Monson R, Christiani D. Summary of the evidence: occupation and environment and cancer. Cancer Causes Control 1997;8:529–531.

17. Teschke K, Morgan MS, Checkoway H, Franklin G, Spinelli JJ, van Belle G, Weiss NS. Surveillance of nasal and bladder cancer to locate sources of exposure to occupational carcinogens. Occup Environ Med 1997;54:443–451.

18. Chen R, Seaton A. A meta-analysis of painting exposure and cancer mortality. Cancer Detection Prev 1998;22:533–539.

19. Steenland K, Palu S. Cohort mortality study of 57 000 painters and other union members: a 15 year update. Occup Environ Med 1999;56:315–321.

20. Morris Brown L, Moradi T, Gridley G, Plato N, Dosemeci M, Fraumeni JF. Exposures in the painting trades and paint manufacturing industry and risk of cancer among men and women in Sweden. J Occup Environ Med 2002;44:258–264.

21. Montanaro F, Ceppi M, Demers P, Puntoni R, Bonassi S. Mortality in a cohort of tannery workers. Occup Environ Med 1997;54:588–591.

22. Park RM, Mirer FE. A survey of mortality at two automotive engine manufacturing plants. Am J Ind Med 1996;30:664–673.

23. Farant JP, Ogilvie D. Investigation of the presence of amino and nitro polycyclic aromatic hydrocarbons in a Soderberg primary aluminum smelter. AIHA J 2002;63:721–725.

24. Grandjean P, Olsen J. Extended follow-up of cancer incidence in fluoride-exposed workers. J Natl Cancer Inst 2004;96:802–803.

25. Molloy T. ALCOA warns of cancer risk. The Associated Press. Online. Available: http://www.fluorideaction.org/pollution/1375.html.

26. Boffetta P, Dosemeci M, Gridley G, Bath H, Moradi T, Silverman D. Occupational exposure to diesel engine emissions and risk of cancer in Swedish men and women. Cancer Causes Control 2001;12:365–374.

27. Boffetta P, Silverman DT. A meta-analysis of bladder cancer and diesel exhaust exposure. Epidemiol 2001;12:125–130.

28. Gun RT, Pratt NL, Griffith EC, Adams GG, Bisby JA, Robinson KL. Update of a prospective study of mortality and cancer incidence in the Australian petroleum industry. Occup Environ Med 2004;61:150–156.

29. Lewis RJ, Schnatter AR, Drummond, et al. Mortality and cancer morbidity in a cohort of Canadian petroleum workers. Occup Environ Med 2003;60:918–928.

30. Marsh GM, Gula MH, Youk AO, Cassidy LD. Bladder cancer among chemical workers exposed to nitrogen products and other substances. Am J Ind Med 2002;42:286–295.

31. Gaertner RR, Theriault GP. Risk of bladder cancer in foundry workers: a meta-analysis. Occup Environ Med 2002;59:655–663.

32. Rafnsson V, Sulem P. Cancer incidence among marine engineers, a population-based study (Iceland). Cancer Causes Control 2003;14:29–35.

33. Marsh GM, Callahan C, Pavlock D, Leviton LC, Talbott EO, Hemstreet G. A protocol for bladder cancer screening and medical surveillance among high-risk groups: the Drake Health Registry experience. J Occup Med 1990;32:881–886.

34. Felknor SA, Delclos GL, Lerner SP, Burau KD, Wood SM, Lusk CM, Jalayer AD. Bladder cancer screening program for a petrochemical cohort with potential exposure to β-naphthylamine. J Occup Environ Med 2003;45:289–294.

35. Carpenter L, Roman E. Cancer and occupation in women: identifying associations using routinely collected national data. Environ Health Perspect 1999;107(Suppl):299–303.

36. Pelucchi C, La Vecchia C, Negri E, Dal Maso L, Franceschi S. Smoking and other risk factors for bladder cancer in women. Prev Med 2002;35:114–120.

37. Silverman DT, Levin LI, Hoover RN, Hartage P. Occupational risks of bladder cancer in the United States. I. White men. J Natl Cancer Inst 1989;81:1472–1480.

38. Silverman DT, Levin LI, Hoover RN. Occupational risks of bladder cancer in the United States. II. Nonwhite men. J Natl Cancer Inst 1989;81:1480–1483.

39. Schulz MR, Loomis D. Occupational bladder cancer mortality among racial and ethnic minorities in 21 states. Am J Ind Med 2000;38:90–98.

40. Cohen SM, Shirai T, Steineck G. Epidemiology and etiology of premalignant and malignant urothelial changes. Scan J Urol Nephrol 2000;205(Suppl):105–115.

41. Cartwright RA, Gadian T, Garland JB, Bernard SM. The influence of malignant cell cytology on the survival of industrial bladder cancer cases. J Epidemiol Community Health 1981;35:35–38.

42. Shinka T, Sawada Y, Morimoto S, Fujinaga T, Nakamura J, Ohkawa T. Clinical study on urothelial tumors of dye workers in Wakayama City. J Urol 1991;146:1504–1507.

43. Vineis P, Simonato L. Proportion of lung and bladder cancers in males resulting from occupation: a systematic approach. Arch Environ Health 1991;46:6–15.

44. Sorahan T, Hamilton L, Jackson JR. A further cohort study of workers employed at a factory manufacturing chemicals for the rubber industry, with special reference to the chemicals 2-mercaptobenzothiazole (MBT), aniline, phenyl-β-naphthylamine and o-toluidine. Occup Environ Med 2000;57:106–115.

45. Miyakawa M, Tachibana M, Miyakawa A. Re-evaluation of the latent period of bladder cancer in dyestuff-plant workers in Japan. Int J Urol 2001;8:423–430.

46. Vineis P, Marinelli D, Autrup H, et al. Current smoking, occupation, N-acetyltransferase-2 and bladder cancer: a pooled analysis of genotype-based studies. Cancer Epidemiol Biomarkers Prev 2001;10:1249–1252.

47. Vineis P, Landi MT, Caporaso N. Metabolic polymorphisms and the cancer risk: the evaluation of epidemiological studies. Medicina del Lavoro 1992;83:557–575.

48. Vineis P, Caporaso N, Cuzick J, Lang M, Malats N, Boffetta P. Genetic susceptibility to cancer: metabolic polymorphisms. IARC Scientific Publ No. 148. Lyon, France: IARC Press, 1999.

49. Cascorbi I, Roots I, Brockmuller J. Association of NAT1 and NAT2 polymorphisms to urinary bladder cancer: significantly reduced risk in subjects with NAT1*10. Cancer Res 2001;61:5051–5056.

50. Shinka T, Ogura H, Morita T, Nishikawa T, Fujimaga T, Ohkawa T. Relationship between glutathione S-transferase M1 deficiency and urothelial cancer in dye workers exposed to aromatic amines. J Urol 1998;159:380–383.

# Familial bladder cancer

3

*Lambertus A Kiemeney*

## INTRODUCTION

In Western countries, bladder cancer is one of the most common cancers among men. Bladder cancer is less frequent among women and, for as yet undetermined reasons, blacks experience only half the risk of whites. As early as 1895, certain occupational exposures were associated with an increased risk of bladder cancer. The most carcinogenic of these chemicals are now banned from the workplace. In addition to occupational exposures, cigarette smoking is by far the most important risk factor, leading to a two- to four-fold increase in risk. Cigarette smoking accounts for approximately 30% to 50% of all cases of bladder cancer. Other risk factors for which evidence is accumulating are urinary tract infections, radiation therapy, cyclophosphamide use, and quality of drinking water (chlorination by-products and arsenic).

In addition to these environmental risk factors, genetic susceptibility may be responsible for a considerable part of all bladder cancers. Polymorphisms in genes coding for carcinogen metabolizing enzymes (e.g. GSTM1 and NAT2) have consistently been shown to increase the risk of bladder cancer. In theory, these polymorphisms should modify the effect of smoking, i.e. smokers with slower acting variants of such detoxifying genes are expected to run a higher risk than smokers with faster acting variants. Unfortunately, until now, there have been few empirical data to illustrate such gene–environment interactions. Worldwide, many research groups are now studying the role of genetic variants in bladder cancer. The emphasis is not only on carcinogen-metabolizing enzymes but also on genes involved in cell cycle control, DNA repair, and immune response. Almost without exception, these genetic

variants have a low penetrance. Although they may increase the risk of bladder cancer, their effect is too modest to cause clustering of bladder cancer in families, which is the focus of this chapter. For the last two decades, much attention has been paid to hereditary subtypes of common cancers, and many high-penetrance tumor suppressor genes and DNA repair genes have been discovered. Familial bladder cancer has received less attention, and the role of familial transmission has yet to be completely explored.

## CASE REPORTS OF FAMILIAL BLADDER CANCER

The first indication for the existence of an inherited subtype of bladder cancer comes from case reports. Thelen and Schaeuble were the first to report familial clustering of transitional cell carcinoma (TCC), when in 1957 they described identical male twins, both smokers, with 'benign transitional cell papillomas' of the bladder.[1] Fraumeni and Thomas reported four cases of bladder cancer in a family of Russian–Jewish origin.[2] The father was diagnosed with invasive bladder cancer at the age of 54 years; three sons had bladder cancer at the ages of 57, 59, and 64 years (two had well-differentiated noninvasive papillary tumors; one had metastatic squamous cell carcinoma). All affected individuals in this kindred were heavy smokers but none was employed in a high-risk occupation. Benton and Henderson presented the occupational histories of nine individuals with TCC of the bladder diagnosed before the age of 25 years. One patient was a 19-year-old repairman with exposure to glues and solvents. The father, a welder, was diagnosed with TCC of the bladder 1 year before the diagnosis in the son.[3] Although chance occurrence is a possible explanation in this family, the early age at onset of disease strongly favors an inherited etiology.

Familial bladder TCC was also reported by McCullough et al in six members of a two-generation family. Four affected patients were diagnosed before the age of 50 years and two before the age of 40. Two of these patients later had upper urinary tract TCC and five had other tumors (basal cell, stomach, prostate, cervix uteri, and unknown primary). Other tumors were also diagnosed among the nonaffected siblings in this kindred, including one with leukemia at the age of 20 and one with breast cancer at the age of 40. Interestingly, an identical twin of a patient in this kindred with TCC died of melanoma at the age of 63 years.[4] Although four individuals with TCC were smokers and two had high-risk occupations (painter and printer), a germline mutation in one of the unaffected parents of three affected brothers seems likely in this extraordinary pedigree.

Three interesting case reports appeared in the late 1970s and early 1980s: Lynch et al reported on three siblings diagnosed with bladder cancer before the age of 50 years[5]; Mahboubi et al also reported on three cases of TCC in a nuclear family[6]; and Purtilo et al described 13 cases of bladder TCC in six unrelated families from Massachusetts.[7] This last study is interesting because five of the six families were identified from a registration of 162 incident cases of bladder cancer, yielding a 3% prevalence estimate of familial bladder cancer. Furthermore, all three affected individuals in one of the families were diagnosed with disease at very early ages (19, 28, and 33 years).

In a study from the Netherlands, 96 families with more than one bladder cancer patient were identified and, of these, 30 families had a pedigree suggestive of a genetic origin.[8]

All of these case reports clearly suggest but cannot prove the existence of an inherited subtype of bladder cancer. More formal evidence for familial aggregation and segregation patterns must come from epidemiologic studies while linkage studies and/or modern molecular biology methods are needed for the mapping and identification of susceptibility genes.

## FAMILIAL UPPER URINARY TRACT TCC

There are several case reports of familial TCC of the upper urinary tract, the rarity of which favors a genetic origin.[9] Some of these reports were published before it became known that the risk of this tumor is increased in families with hereditary nonpolyposis colon cancer (HNPCC).[10] For that reason, it is difficult to determine whether familial TCC of the ureter and renal pelvis may occur in a site-specific manner. In most cases of familial upper urinary tract TCC, however, there is also a co-occurrence of colorectal cancers. Most of these families fulfill the Amsterdam or Bethesda criteria of HNPCC. The International Collaborative Group on HNPCC advises screening for upper urinary tract tumors if such tumors have been diagnosed in a HNPCC family. The screening should consist of ultrasonography and urine analysis annually or biannually, starting at the age of 30.

Although TCC of the upper and lower urinary tract resemble each other morphologically, the risk of bladder cancer is not increased in HNPCC families.[10] HNPCC is caused by one or more mutations in DNA mismatch repair genes leading to microsatellite instability (MSI). MSI typical of HNPCC is defined with mono- and dinucleotide repeat microsatellites. A second variety of instability can be seen at selective tetranucleotide repeats, i.e. elevated microsatellite alterations at select tetranucleotides (EMAST). Recently, it was shown that, as for colorectal cancer, the pattern of MSI varies with location in the urinary tract. In bladder cancer, the mono- and dinucleotide MSI was rare, whereas EMAST was common. In upper urinary tract tumors, MSI occurred frequently, whereas EMAST was seen less frequently than in bladder cancer.[11]

Strong familial clustering of TCC of the upper and lower urinary tract has also been found in some rural areas of the Balkan states of eastern Europe.[12] It is likely that the familial clustering of such tumors in these areas is related to Balkan endemic nephropathy, caused by exposure to ochratoxin A, a toxin produced by some species of Penicillium and Aspergillus in cereal grains. The high risk of TCC among consanguineous married persons, and the low risk among relatives that moved to nonendemic villages, strongly argue against a genetic origin.

## BLADDER CANCER AND RETINOBLASTOMA

Bladder cancer within a familial context is sometimes seen in association with carcinomas of nongenitourinary origin. The association with retinoblastoma is especially noteworthy. Chan and Pratt described the family of an 11-year-old white girl with bilateral retinoblastoma and multiple nonradiation-induced osteosarcomas.[13] The mother had unilateral retinoblastoma. The maternal grandfather and one of his brothers were diagnosed with bladder TCC at the ages of 60 and 47 years, respectively. Aherne described a family with retinoblastoma and osteosarcoma in which the mother of two affected children had bladder cancer at the age of 40 years.[14] He also summarized five other British cases of retinoblastoma. The father of one patient died of bladder cancer at the age of 50.

Three relatively small cohort studies in the 1980s confirmed the increased risk of bladder cancer among relatives of retinoblastoma patients.[15-17] This increased risk appeared to be confined to known carriers of the mutated retinoblastoma gene. Because the protein encoded by the retinoblastoma 1 gene (p105 Rb) functions in cell proliferation, DNA replication, DNA repair, and cell-cycle checkpoint control, and because RB1 mutations are frequently found in bladder tumors, it is possible that hereditary retinoblastoma survivors run an increased risk of bladder cancer.

The first studies of the risk of second primary tumors among retinoblastoma survivors did not find such an increased risk of bladder cancer. Most of these studies, however, included relatively young patient groups.[18] Recently, in a long-term follow-up study from the UK, five bladder cancer cases were found among 144 hereditary retinoblastoma cases, an observed-to-expected ratio of 26.3 (95% CI: 8.5–61.4).[19] This study shows that bladder cancer should be put on the list of tumors for which hereditary retinoblastoma patients should be checked during lifetime follow-up. Recent case reports also suggest the occurrence of leiomyosarcomas of the bladder among retinoblastoma survivors.[20-22]

# EPIDEMIOLOGIC STUDIES ON FAMILIAL BLADDER CANCER

## CASE CONTROL STUDIES

Although many studies have examined familial clustering of bladder cancer, most only did so as one of many research hypotheses, making familial bladder cancer not the prime subject of interest.[9] In a number of these studies, an ill-defined definition of family history was used, leading to an inability to distinguish between several types of genitourinary cancer among relatives. Additionally, in most of these studies, the occurrence of bladder cancer among relatives was not verified. In this review, only a few of those studies will be highlighted.

The largest study is a population-based examination of 2982 patients and 5782 controls conducted in 1978 (the United States National Bladder Cancer Study or US-NBCS).[23] Six percent of the cases versus 4% of the controls identified at least one member in the immediate family (parents and siblings) that had genitourinary cancer. The odds ratio (OR) adjusted for race, sex, smoking, and age was 1.5 (95% CI: 1.2–1.8), which can be interpreted as a 50% increased risk of bladder cancer if there is a first degree relative with cancer of the genitourinary tract. This risk appeared to be somewhat higher in persons younger than 45 years (OR = 2.7, 95% CI: 0.8–2.9) and in female patients (OR = 1.8, 95% CI: 1.1–2.7). Unfortunately, as stated before, examination of

family history was not a major objective of this study. Therefore, the authors were unable to distinguish bladder cancer from kidney cancer, and were unable to verify reports of familial cancer.

Piper et al performed a case-control study in Baltimore among young women, the group with a greater than average odds ratio for family history in the aforementioned US-NBCS.[24] A total of 162 women with bladder cancer, 20–49 years of age, were matched to population controls and asked about a history of bladder or kidney cancer (renal cell and TCC) in first degree relatives. Four patients (2.5%) and one control (0.6%) reported a positive family history, yielding an insignificant odds ratio of 4.0. Only one individual reported bladder cancer in a parent, and one reported that a sister had papillary cancer of the kidney and ureter. The remaining two patients and one control reported kidney cancer in the father. Thus, there is a striking difference between the prevalence of a positive history in this study and that in the US-NBCS. Of course, young women usually have young relatives with a low risk of bladder cancer. However, in the US-NBCS the prevalence was also much higher among female controls only (3.3%) and among controls younger than the age of 45 years (2.0%). The reason for this difference remains unknown.

In a German study conducted by Kunze et al, 675 patients with histologically confirmed benign or malignant epithelial tumors of the bladder, ureter, renal pelvis, and urethra were compared to matched controls with non-neoplastic diseases of the lower urinary tract (predominantly prostatic hyperplasia in men and urinary tract infection in women).[25] An interviewer-administered questionnaire noted bladder cancer in first degree relatives. In a multivariable analysis, controlling for smoking status, occupational exposures, and phenacetin use, a positive family history showed an odds ratio of 2.5 (95% CI: 1.1–5.8) in men and a statistically insignificant odds ratio of 1.5 in women. This higher risk in men is in contrast with the findings from the US-NBCS.[23]

## COHORT STUDIES

A disadvantage of the aforementioned case-control studies is that the exposure (bladder cancer in the family) was examined by simple questions asked of the patients and controls. No adjustment could be made for total number of relatives, age, sex, smoking status, and age of the relatives. However, a few studies specifically addressed the issue of familial bladder cancer. Kramer et al collected demographic data and cigarette smoking status on all first degree relatives of 319 men with bladder cancer diagnosed in New York State and 319 neighborhood controls.[26] The two cohorts of relatives were then linked to the New York State Tumor Registry in order to obtain valid data on cancer occurrence: 14 cases of bladder cancer were found among 1619 relatives of patients, while 7 were found among 1773 relatives of controls. In a multivariable proportional hazards regression model with age, sex, and smoking status, the hazard ratio of case-control status was 1.9 (90% CI: 0.9–4.1). According to the authors, there were no instances in which more than one first degree relative within a family was affected. Thus, the prevalence of a positive family history among the controls can be estimated at 2.2%. In a small hospital-based study by Lynch et al, the cumulative risk of bladder cancer among first and second degree relatives of 49 consecutively ascertained bladder cancer cases was compared to the expected risk based on the United States Third National Cancer Survey.[27] The cumulative risk among relatives of the patients was 1.6 times higher than expected. In an additional analysis, the authors found significant heterogeneity of risk across families; only 3 of the 49 families studied (6%) were at high risk.

Kiemeney et al identified the first to third degree relatives of 190 patients with bladder, ureter or renal pelvis TCC diagnosed between 1983 and 1992 in Iceland through the Icelandic Cancer Family Resource. The records of these 12,328 relatives were subsequently linked to the 1965–1994 cancer registry. In 41 of the 190 pedigrees, at least one relative had TCC of the urinary tract; 38 of the probands had only one, and three had two affected relatives. The prevalence of family history of TCC was 3% in first degree and 10% in first or second degree relatives. The risk of TCC among all relatives was slightly elevated (observed-to-expected ratio 1.2, 95% CI: 0.9–1.7). Surprisingly, the observed-to-expected ratio was higher among second and third degree relatives than among first degree relatives. This argues against the existence of a hereditary subtype of bladder TCC, at least in the founder population of Iceland.[28]

The largest study, specifically designed to study familial bladder cancer, was also conducted by the group of Kiemeney in the Netherlands. With use of a family case-control design, 1193 patients, newly diagnosed with TCC of the bladder, ureter, renal pelvis or urethra, were contacted. Information on the patients' first degree relatives was collected by postal questionnaire and subsequent telephone calls. The patients' partners filled out a similar questionnaire on their relatives. All reported occurrences of TCC among the 8014 first degree case-relatives and 5673 control-relatives were verified using medical records. Disease occurrence among case-relatives and control-relatives was compared in order to obtain the familial risk. Random effect proportional hazards regression analyses were used to calculate this familial risk while adjusting for age, sex, and smoking behavior. Among the case-relatives, 101 individuals were diagnosed with cancer of the bladder (n=97), ureter (n=3), and renal pelvis (n=1), compared to 38 individuals among the control-relatives (bladder n=36, ureter n=1, and urethra n=1). In six case-families and two control-families, two

affected first degree relatives were found. Overall, 8% of the patients had a positive family history of TCC compared to 4% of the controls. The mean age at diagnosis of patients with a positive family history was similar to that of patients with a negative family history (62 years). The mean age at diagnosis of TCC among affected case-relatives was only slightly lower than that of affected control-relatives (64 versus 66 years). The cumulative risk of TCC among case-relatives was 3.8% compared to 2.1% among control-relatives. The age, sex, and smoking adjusted hazard ratio (HR) of TCC for case-relatives compared to control-relatives was 1.8 (95% CI: 1.3–2.7). This risk appeared to be higher among women (HR=3.2) and among nonsmokers (HR=3.9). When only parents were included in the analyses, the hazard ratio increased (HR=2.2), whereas it decreased when only siblings were included (HR=1.5). After stratification by tumor site in the probands (upper versus lower urinary tract), the adjusted HR was 1.8 among relatives of probands with upper urinary tract TCC and 1.9 among relatives of probands with bladder TCC. When all the relatives of probands with a pTa tumor were excluded from the analyses, the HRs increased only slightly to 2.0. The same was found when the relatives of probands older than 60 years were excluded from the analyses (HR=2.4). A striking clustering of tumors at other sites among the case-relatives was not found, although an increased risk was observed for tumors of the hematolymphopoietic system (HR=1.9, 95% CI: 1.2–3.0). Familial clustering with other tumors was also evaluated among the relatives of probands with a positive family history of TCC. There was some (nonsignificant) suggestion of a clustering of tumors of the female genital organs, non-TCC urinary tract tumors, and cancer of the hematolymphopoietic system.[29]

The latter observation was also made in a study by Goldgar and associates.[30] They estimated familial relative risks from the Utah Population Database by identifying all cases of cancer in first degree relatives of patients. These observed values were compared with those expected on the basis of cohort-specific internal rates calculated from 399,786 relatives of all individuals in the Utah Population Database known to have died in Utah. The first degree relatives of bladder cancer probands were found to have an increased risk of bladder cancer of 1.5 (95% CI: 1.0–2.2) (not adjusted for smoking). When only relatives of young probands (age <60 years) were considered, the familial risk was 5.1 (95% CI: 1.0–12.5). Among these relatives of young probands, a 3.7-fold increase (95% CI: 1.1–7.4) in the risk of lymphocytic leukemia was found.

## THE CAUSE OF FAMILIAL CLUSTERING

From the epidemiologic studies it can be concluded that the risk of bladder cancer is increased approximately two-fold with a positive family history of bladder cancer. The next question, of course, is whether this is caused by genetic susceptibility or shared environment. In a study of Danish twins, published in 1963, no differences were found between the concordance rate of urinary system cancers in 1528 monozygotic (MZ) twin pairs and in 2609 same sexed, dizygotic (DZ) twin pairs.[31] In fact, in neither group was a pair found with both twins affected. This result has been used as an argument against an inherited subtype of bladder cancer. However, the concordance rates of breast cancer and intestinal tumors (for which hereditary forms are known to exist) were also not greater in MZ twins. By contrast, in a more recent twin study from Scandinavia (Denmark, Sweden, and Finland) Lichtenstein et al reported five concordant and 146 discordant pairs of bladder cancers among 7231 MZ male twin pairs. Among 13,769 DZ male twin pairs, two concordant pairs and 253 discordant pairs were found. The relative risk of bladder cancer among MZ twins was 6.6 (95% CI: 2.6–16.9; the relative risk among DZ twins was 1.7 (95% CI: 0.4–6.9). The concordance rate was three times higher among MZ twins (6%) than among DZ twins (2%). Assuming that the correlation in environmental risk factors is similar among MZ and DZ twins, this finding suggests the existence of a genetic etiology of bladder cancer.[32]

Dong and Hemminki used the Swedish Family-Cancer Database to quantify the risk of cancer in more than 5.5 million offspring from more than 2 million nuclear families if one of the parents had cancer or if one or more of the siblings had cancer.[33] The risk of bladder cancer for offspring was increased by a factor 1.5 (95% CI: 1.1–2.0) if one of the parents had bladder cancer. If one of the siblings had bladder cancer, the risk was increased by a factor 3.3 (95% CI: 1.7–5.8). The higher (relative) risk in the case of an affected sibling was considered to be an indication for a recessive or X-linked transmission model. Because only 1 of the 12 offspring with bladder cancer with an affected sibling was female, the authors suggested that an X-linked model was most likely.[33] On the other hand, ascertainment bias due to cohort effects in, for example, diagnostic procedures and data quality, may also result in higher risks for siblings. The same holds for a higher correlation in environmental exposures between siblings compared to parents and offspring. With respect to the latter possibility, in a later study on the Swedish Family-Cancer Database by the same group, it was estimated that 7% of the occurrence of bladder cancer is due to genetic effects, 12% to shared environmental effects, 4% to childhood environmental effects, and 77% to nonshared environmental effects.[34]

The family case-control study from the Netherlands performed complex segregation analysis in order to evaluate the segregation pattern of bladder cancer within the 1193 families of probands with TCC. Strong evidence for a Mendelian inheritance pattern of TCC through a single major gene was not found. The 'no major gene' (or sporadic) model seemed to be the most parsimonious one to describe the occurrence of TCC in these families. However, none of the Mendelian models could be clearly rejected, which means that an inherited subtype of TCC cannot be excluded. A major gene may segregate in some families but this effect may have been masked in a background of high sporadic incidence. Also, the families consisted of first degree relatives only, which makes the power of segregation analyses fairly limited, despite the large number of families.[35]

The same group also evaluated whether mutagen sensitivity plays a role in developing TCC, and whether this sensitivity is different in familial and nonfamilial cases. Intrinsic susceptibility was quantified by a mutagen sensitivity assay (mean number of chromatid breaks per cell (PBLs) after damage induction with bleomycin in the late S–G2 phase of the cell cycle). In this study, 25 sporadic patients, 23 familial patients (2 patients in one nuclear family), and 13 hereditary patients (2 patients <60 years or 3 patients in one nuclear family) were selected and compared with control subjects without a history of cancer. TCC patients showed a higher mutagen sensitivity score compared to control subjects (mean number of chromatid breaks per cell: 0.91, 95% CI: 0.84–0.97, and 0.74, 95% CI: 0.69–0.79, respectively; p=0.001). Sporadic and familial patients exhibited the highest susceptibility (0.94, 95% CI: 0.82–1.06, and 0.93, 95% CI: 0.83–1.03, respectively). Hereditary patients (0.79, 95% CI: 0.72–0.86) showed susceptibility similar to controls.[36] From this study, it can be concluded that mutagen sensitivity (i.e. genetic susceptibility) increases the risk of nonhereditary TCC. The relatively low mutagen sensitivity score among hereditary patients may point to a different carcinogenic pathway.

## THE FIRST HIGH-PENETRANCE BLADDER CANCER SUSCEPTIBILITY GENE

Recently, a new bladder cancer gene was discovered by the collaborative group of Drs Schoenberg and Sidransky in Baltimore.[37] In 1996, the Baltimore group identified a family in which a male was diagnosed with grade 2 superficial TCC of the bladder at the age of 29 years. He subsequently developed renal pelvis TCC. His mother died of metastatic TCC of the bladder at the age of 65. Because both the proband's wife and his mother had a history of miscarriages, a karyogram was made which showed a balanced germline translocation t(5;20)(p15;q11).[38] Dr Sidransky's laboratory zoomed in at the breakpoints of this translocation, which finally resulted in the discovery of a new bladder cancer gene at 20q11.[37] This gene, CDC91L1, encoding the CDC91L1 protein–also called phosphatidylinositol glycan class U

(PIG-U)—has a role in the glycosylphosphatidylinositol (GPI) anchoring pathway. Further research suggested that the gene is amplified and overexpressed in as many as one-third of bladder cancers and primary tumors. CDC91L1 should therefore be regarded as an oncogene. The translocation led to overexpression of the gene and, probably, to both bladder cancers in this pedigree. Carriers of the translocation in this family were therefore genetically susceptible for bladder cancer. Because the exact translocation site should be regarded as an extremely rare phenomenon, this gene should not be considered as a candidate for the genetic cause of hereditary bladder cancer in many patients. For that, tumor suppressor or DNA mismatch repair genes have yet to be discovered.

## SCREENING IN FAMILIES WITH BLADDER CANCER

The cumulative risk of developing non-pTa bladder cancer before the age of 75 is approximately 1.8% and 0.4% for white males and females, respectively. In case of one first degree relative with bladder cancer, these risks are doubled.[29] The absolute risk of bladder cancer for a person with a positive family history is, therefore, still very small, and probably not a reason for screening. There are too few data to deduce the absolute risk of bladder cancer for persons with two first degree relatives with bladder cancer (or one first and one second degree relative in either the paternal or maternal lineage). There are also no data supporting the efficacy of screening unaffected relatives of (at least) two patients. Nevertheless, it seems logical to offer a routine check-up for such relatives. The protocol for such a screening may be:

- starting at the age of 40, or 5 years younger than the age of the youngest patient in the family
- ultrasonography of the bladder and upper urinary tract at the first screening only
- sediment and cytology once annually (possibly including a marker such as NMP22).

## CONCLUSION

There is clear evidence that TCC of the ureter and renal pelvis is related to HNPCC. A large number of case reports suggest that TCC of the bladder clusters in families. Epidemiologic studies have shown that the risk of bladder cancer is increased approximately two-fold when there is a positive family history. The cause of this familial clustering is still subject to speculation but several lines of evidence suggest a contributing genetic factor. This genetic factor is rare but its penetrance may

be quite high, although not as high as in hereditary breast, prostate, or colorectal cancer. The effect of the genetic factor is probably site-specific: there is no strong clustering of other types of cancer in bladder cancer families.

The study of hereditary forms of common cancers has yielded important clues about the etiology and pathogenesis of both inherited and sporadic forms of these tumors. It has also led to possibilities for genetic testing, early detection, and even primary prevention of cancer, as in the case of colorectal cancer and breast cancer. A worldwide collaborative effort to identify and study families at high risk of bladder cancer seems necessary in order to move forward in the field of hereditary bladder cancer.

## REFERENCES

1. Thelen A, Schaeuble J. Gleichzeitiges Vorkommen von Blasenpapillomen bei eineiigen Zwillingen. Z Urol 1957;50:188–195.
2. Fraumeni JF Jr, Thomas LB. Malignant bladder tumors in a man and his three sons. JAMA 1967;201:507–509.
3. Benton B, Henderson BE. Environmental exposure and bladder cancer in young males. J Natl Cancer Inst 1973;51:269–270.
4. McCullough DL, Lamm DL, McLaughlin AP III, Gittes RF. Familial transitional cell carcinoma of the bladder. J Urol 1975;113:629–635.
5. Lynch HT, Walzak MP, Fried R, Domina AH, Lynch JF. Familial factors in bladder carcinoma. J Urol 1979;122:458–461.
6. Mahboubi AO, Ahlvin RC, Mahboubi EO. Familial aggregation of urothelial carcinoma. J Urol 1981;126:691–692.
7. Purtilo DT, McCarthy B, Yang JP, Friedell GH. Familial urinary bladder cancer. Semin Oncol 1979;6:254–256.
8. Aben KK, Macville MV, Smeets DF, Schoenberg MP, Witjes JA, Kiemeney LA. Absence of karyotype abnormalities in patients with familial urothelial cell carcinoma. Urology 2001;57(2):266–269.
9. Kiemeney LALM, Schoenberg M. Familial transitional cell carcinoma. J Urol 1996;156:867–872.
10. Watson P, Lynch HT. Extracolonic cancer in hereditary nonpolyposis colorectal cancer. Cancer 1993;71:677–685.
11. Catto JW, Azzouzi AR, Amira N, et al. Distinct patterns of microsatellite instability are seen in tumours of the urinary tract. Oncogene 2003;22(54):8699–8706.
12. Chernozemsky IN, Petkova-Bocharova T, Nikolov IG, Stoyanov IS. Familial aggregation of urinary system tumors in a region with endemic nephropathy. Cancer Res 1978;38:965–968.
13. Chan H, Pratt CB. A new familial cancer syndrome? A spectrum of malignant and benign tumors including retinoblastoma, carcinoma of the bladder, and other genitourinary tumors, thyroid adenoma, and a probable case of multifocal osteosarcoma. J Natl Cancer Inst 1977;58:205–207.
14. Aherne G. Retinoblastoma associated with other primary malignant tumours. Trans Ophthalmol Soc UK 1974;94:938–944.
15. Tarkkanen A, Karjalainen K. Excess of cancer deaths in close relatives of patients with bilateral retinoblastoma. Ophthalmologica 1984;189:143–146.
16. DerKinderen DJ, Koten JW, Nagelkerke NJ, Tan KE, Beemer FA, Den Otter W. Non-ocular cancer in patients with hereditary retinoblastoma and their relatives. Int J Cancer 1988;41:499–504.
17. Sanders BM, Jay M, Draper GJ, Roberts EM. Non-ocular cancer in relatives of retinoblastoma patients. Br J Cancer 1989;60(3):358–365.
18. Moll AC, Imhof SM, Bouter LM, et al. Second primary tumors in patients with hereditary retinoblastoma: a register-based follow-up study, 1945–1994. Int J Cancer 1996;67(4):515–519.
19. Fletcher O, Easton D, Anderson K, Gilham C, Jay M, Peto J. Lifetime risks of common cancers among retinoblastoma survivors. J Natl Cancer Inst 2004;96(5):357–363.

20. Liang SX, Lakshmanan Y, Woda BA, Jiang Z. A high-grade primary leiomyosarcoma of the bladder in a survivor of retinoblastoma. Arch Pathol Lab Med 2001;125(9):1231–1234.

21. Bleoo SL, Godbout R, Rayner D, Tamimi Y, Moore RB. Leiomyosarcoma of the bladder in a retinoblastoma patient. Urol Int 2003;71(1):118–121.

22. Venkatraman L, Goepel JR, Steele K, Dobbs SP, Lyness RW, McCluggage WG. Soft tissue, pelvic, and urinary bladder leiomyosarcoma as second neoplasm following hereditary retinoblastoma. J Clin Pathol 2003;56(3):233–236.

23. Kantor AF, Hartge P, Hoover RN, Fraumeni JF Jr. Familial and environmental interactions in bladder cancer risk. Int J Cancer 1985;35:703–706.

24. Piper JM, Matanoski GM, Tonascia J. Bladder cancer in young women. Am J Epidemiol 1986;123:1033–1042.

25. Kunze E, Chang-Claude J, Frentzel-Beyme R. Life-style and occupational risk factors for bladder cancer in Germany. A case-control study. Cancer 1992;69:1776–1790.

26. Kramer AA, Graham S, Burnett WS, Nasca P. Familial aggregation of bladder cancer stratified by smoking status. Epidemiology 1991;2:145–148.

27. Lynch HT, Kimberling WJ, Lynch JF, Brennan K. Familial bladder cancer in an oncology clinic. Cancer Genet Cytogenet 1987;27:161–165.

28. Kiemeney LA, Moret NC, Witjes JA, Schoenberg MP, Tulinius H. Familial transitional cell carcinoma among the population of Iceland. J Urol 1997;157(5):1649–1651.

29. Aben KK, Witjes JA, Schoenberg MP, Hulsbergen-van de Kaa C, Verbeek AL, Kiemeney LA. Familial aggregation of urothelial cell carcinoma. Int J Cancer 2002;98(2):274–278.

30. Goldgar DE, Easton DF, Cannon-Albright LA, Skolnick MH. Systematic population-based assessment of cancer risk in first-degree relatives of cancer probands. J Natl Cancer Inst 1994;86(21):1600–1608.

31. Harvald B, Hauge M. Heredity of cancer elucidated by a study of unselected twins. JAMA 1963;186:749–753.

32. Lichtenstein P, Holm NV, Verkasalo PK, et al. Environmental and heritable factors in the causation of cancer—analyses of cohorts of twins from Sweden, Denmark, and Finland. N Engl J Med 2000;343(2):78–85.

33. Dong C, Hemminki K. Modification of cancer risks in offspring by sibling and parental cancers from 2,112,616 nuclear families. Int J Cancer 2001;92(1):144–150.

34. Czene K, Lichtenstein P, Hemminki K. Environmental and heritable causes of cancer among 9.6 million individuals in the Swedish Family-Cancer Database. Int J Cancer 2002;99(2):260–266.

35. Aben KKH, Baglietto L, Baffoe-Bonnie A, et al. Segregation analysis of urothelial cell carcinoma. Eur J Cancer (in press).

36. Aben KK, Cloos J, Koper NP, Braakhuis BJ, Witjes JA, Kiemeney LA. Mutagen sensitivity in patients with familial and non-familial urothelial cell carcinoma. Int J Cancer 2000;88(3):493–496.

37. Guo Z, Linn JF, Wu G, et al. CDC91L1 (PIG-U) is a newly discovered oncogene in human bladder cancer. Nat Med 2004;10(4):374–381.

38. Schoenberg M, Kiemeney L, Walsh PC, Griffin CA, Sidransky D. Germline translocation t(5;20)(p15;q11) and familial transitional cell carcinoma. J Urol 1996;155:1035–1036.

# Pathology

# Genetic susceptibility to bladder cancer

# 4

*Aditi Hazra, Jian Gu, Xifeng Wu*

## INTRODUCTION

Bladder cancer (BC), like lung cancer, is an archetype of an environmentally induced disease. Cigarette smoking is the predominant risk factor for BC and is estimated to cause up to half the cases in men and a third in women. Many of the tobacco carcinogens, most notably aromatic amines, are also found in the chemical industrial work environment, making occupational exposure the second major risk factor for BC.[1] Vineis and Simonato[2] estimated that the proportion of BC attributable to occupational exposure ranged between 0% and 3% in some studies and 16% and 24% in others. Arsenic in drinking water, prolonged exposure to chlorinated surface water, and the use of hair dyes are other risk factors for BC. Because most substances and their metabolites, including carcinogens, are excreted via the urinary tract, diet may also play a role in the carcinogenesis of BC.

Despite the overwhelming evidence that most BC occurrences are attributable to carcinogenic exposures in tobacco smoke and occupational environments, only a small percentage of individuals exposed to carcinogens develop BC. The underlying hypothesis is that genetic factors may render certain individuals more susceptible to BC upon carcinogen exposure. Inherited predisposition to cancer is recognized clinically, principally by family history. Results from case reports and large epidemiologic studies—including the clustering of transitional cell carcinoma in families, an extremely early age at disease onset, and a two-fold increase in risk for first degree relatives—provide evidence for the role of genetic predisposition factors in BC etiology.[3]

It is apparent that gene–environment interactions play central roles in BC occurrence. The study of human cancer risk through molecular epidemiology bridges the most recent advances in molecular biology and cancer genetics with epidemiology. Unlike classic epidemiologic methodology, whose 'black-box' approach to studying the association between exposures and cancer often limits the evaluation of host susceptibility factors to age, sex, and ethnicity, molecular epidemiology strives to identify potential gene–environment interactions in cancer causation.

Carcinogenesis is a multistep process. From carcinogen exposure to cancer initiation, multiple genetically controlled cellular functions are involved, including the metabolism (activation and detoxification) of carcinogens, maintenance of genomic stability (DNA repair, cell cycle checkpoints, apoptosis, and telomere integrity), and control of microenvironmental factors, such as inflammation. Epigenetic events also contribute to carcinogenesis. Most of the genes that control these molecular processes have been identified and are polymorphic in the human population. Some polymorphic forms have been shown to alter gene function. Therefore, individuals with adverse genotypes and/or phenotypes in one or more of these cellular functions may be at a higher risk than the general population of developing BC from carcinogenic exposures. This chapter will summarize recent advances in the identification of genetic susceptibility factors that contribute to risk assessment and clinical outcome prediction in BC.

# GENETIC VARIATIONS IN CANCER RISK

## CARCINOGEN METABOLISM

Most environmental carcinogens are chemically inert and require metabolic activation. The balance between carcinogen activation and detoxification is believed to affect cancer development, since accumulation of active carcinogen metabolites and increased DNA adduct formation contribute to a higher BC risk. Therefore, susceptibility to BC depends, at least partly, on genetic differences in the ability to metabolize carcinogens.

Of specific interest are the genetic variations in phase I activation enzymes, which are involved in the conversion of carcinogenic substrates to genotoxic electrophilic intermediates, and phase II enzymes, which mostly detoxify by conjugating phase I enzyme-produced genotoxic intermediates to water-soluble derivatives. The remainder of this section will discuss associations between BC risk and polymorphisms of genes that code for various phase I and phase II enzymes.

### CYP

The cytochrome P450 family, encoded by the CYP family of genes, are classic phase I activation enzymes. Specifically, they are involved in the initial oxygenation of carcinogenic substrates. Of the 17 human CYP families identified so far, members of the CYP 1, 2, and 3 families play major roles in the metabolic activation of various environmental carcinogens. Polymorphisms of several CYP family genes, including CYP1A1, CYP1B1, CYP2D6, and CYP2E1, have been investigated in relation to various cancers. Although several different studies found associations between polymorphisms and modified risk for certain cancers, the overall results were inconsistent. For instance, two single nucleotide polymorphisms (SNPs), T3801C and A2455G in CYP1A1 gene, were significantly associated with increased risk for lung cancer but not BC.[4–6] One study found that the variant allele of a SNP of CYP2E1 (C1019T in the 5' flanking region) was associated with increased BC risk.[7] Other published studies failed to find significant associations between polymorphisms of other CYP family genes, such as CYP1B1, CYP2D6, and CYP2E1, and BC risk.[5,8,9]

### GST

The glutathione-S-transferases (GSTs) are a class of phase II enzymes that protect against DNA damage and adduct formation by conjugating glutathiones to electrophilic intermediates, thereby yielding a hydrophilic, less reactive metabolite that can be excreted. Different GST families exist—$\alpha$, $\mu$, $\pi$, and $\theta$.[10] Large variations in enzymatic activity have been reported for several GSTs. Across different populations, it is relatively common for deletions of either GSTM1 or GSTT1 to lead to enzyme activity loss. The results of numerous studies investigating GSTM1's role in cancer risk have been fairly consistent for the different cancers studied. The null genotype of GSTM1 repeatedly correlates with increased risk for BC: in a recent meta-analysis that included 17 studies, 2149 patients, and 3646 controls, GSTM1 null alleles were associated with increased BC risk with an odds ratio (OR) of 1.44 (95% CI: 1.23–1.68).[11] GSTT1 metabolizes the monohalomethanes and ethylene oxide found in tobacco smoke. The null homozygote of GSTT1 is associated with BC risk in two recent reports (OR=1.74, 95% CI: 1.02–2.95; OR=2.54, 95% CI: 1.32–4.98, respectively).[9,12] Individuals with both GSTM1 and GSTT1 null genotypes experienced an even greater risk (OR=2.58, 95% CI: 1.27–5.23).[9]

### NAT

Carcinogenic aromatic amines are metabolized by N-acetyltransferases (NATs). Two distinct NATs, NAT1 and NAT2, have been identified in the activation and detoxification of aromatic amines. Several widely studied polymorphisms of the NAT2 gene result in slow or fast acetylation. Slow acetylators are hypothesized to increase BC risk because a decreased rate of inactivation leads to carcinogen accumulation. Studies have consistently supported this hypothesis: in a meta-analysis of data from 21 published case-control studies, the pooled OR of BC association with slow-acetylator status was 1.31 (95% CI: 1.11–1.55).[13] There is also evidence for a multiplicative interaction between smoking and the NAT2 genotype.[14] A recent study[9] reported a borderline BC risk (OR=1.50, 95% CI: 0.99–2.27) for the NAT2 slow genotype but found a three-fold increase in risk for the joint effect with occupational exposure to aromatic amines (OR=3.26, 95% CI: 1.06–9.95).

### NQO1

NAD(P)H:quinone oxidoreductase (NQO1) is a cytosolic phase II enzyme involved in the two-electron reduction of quinine substrates. This enzyme facilitates metabolic activation and detoxification of carcinogenic compounds from tobacco, most notably benzo(a)pyrene. Immunohistochemical analysis has revealed a broad spectrum of NQO1 expression in BC patients.[15,16] A C609T transition (Pro187Ser) is associated with reduced NQO1.[17,18] Three studies have examined the relationship between this NQO1 polymorphism and BC risk, and the results were contradictory. In the first study, the variant genotypes (C/T + T/T) appeared to be a risk factor,[19] in the second, a protective factor,[7] and, in the third, a borderline risk factor.[20] Larger studies are needed to clarify the relationship between this polymorphism and BC risk.

### SULT

Sulfotransferase 1A1 (SULT1A1) belongs to a gene superfamily that metabolizes carcinogens via sulfonation. O-sulfation is a common step in phase II detoxification. SULT1A1 is involved in the metabolism of polycyclic aromatic hydrocarbons (PAHs) and aromatic amines. A G-to-A transition in SULT1A1 results in an Arg-to-His substitution (Arg213His) and decreased activity and thermal stability of the SULT1A1 enzyme. The His allele frequency was higher in BC cases compared to healthy controls.[21] The combined variant alleles (Arg/His + His/His) conferred a statistically significant reduced risk of BC (OR=0.72, 95% CI: 0.54–0.97) compared to individuals with the Arg/Arg allele. A recent study reported a marginal protective effect for this polymorphism.[9]

## Others

Other phase I and phase II enzymes have also been studied. Hung et al[20] assessed the relationship of BC risk with polymorphisms in genes that modulate oxidative stress, including myeloperoxidase (MPO), catechol-O-methyltransferase (COMT), and manganese superoxide dismutase (MnSOD). The homozygous variant of the G-463A SNP of MPO was associated with a reduced BC risk (OR=0.31, 95% CI: 0.12–0.80). The Val/Val genotype of the Ala16Val SNP of MnSOD increased the BC risk with OR of 1.91 (95% CI: 1.20–3.04); the COMT Val108Met SNP was not associated with BC.

## DNA DAMAGE AND REPAIR

The integrity of genomic DNA is relentlessly under assault from a plethora of other endogenous and exogenous sources, such as reactive oxygen species of cellular metabolism, errors in replication or recombination, ionizing radiation, and therapeutic drugs. The majority of activated environmental carcinogens form DNA adducts by covalently binding to DNA strand. Cells can respond to DNA lesions by activating cell cycle checkpoint and repair mechanisms or triggering apoptosis. DNA repair mechanisms must be continuously vigilant against the constant barrage of genotoxic assaults. A compromised DNA repair system—characterized by the accumulations of mutations in the genome—is associated with increased cancer risk. Wood et al[22] compiled a comprehensive list of DNA repair genes based on the draft of the human genomic sequence and identified approximately 130 human DNA repair genes. The products of these genes are mainly involved in four major human DNA repair pathways: mismatch repair (MMR), nucleotide excision repair (NER), base excision repair (BER), and double-strand break (DSB) repair. Each of these pathways initializes specialized protein complexes to detect and repair DNA damage[23]:

- NER removes mainly bulky DNA adducts, which are typically generated after exposure to environmental genotoxic agents, e.g. ultraviolet light and benzo(a)pyrene
- the BER pathway excises oxidized DNA bases, which may arise spontaneously, during inflammatory responses, or from interactions with exogenous agents

- the DSB repair pathway fixes double-strand breaks caused by a plethora of pathologic stimuli, including ionizing radiation, chemotherapeutic drugs, free radicals, and telomere dysfunction.

DNA repair capacity (DRC) varies substantially within the human population. Defects in DRC may lead to genetic instability and carcinogenesis. An increasing number of publications are suggesting that common polymorphisms in DNA repair genes alter protein function, contribute to the interindividual differences in DRC, and thus modulate cancer risks.

## POLYMORPHISMS IN DNA REPAIR GENES

### NER

The key NER genes include XPA, XPC, XPD, XPG, and XPF. All of these genes contain a considerable number of polymorphisms, some of which have potential functional significance and have been investigated in a variety of cancer types, including BC. XPA recognizes damage and plays a crucial role in assembling the remainder of the repair machinery. Wu et al[24] studied an XPA polymorphism (A→G transition) in the 5' noncoding region and found that the presence of one or two copies of the G allele was associated with a reduced lung cancer risk. The relationship between XPA polymorphisms and BC has not yet been studied.

The XPC protein was identified as a DNA damage sensor and NER recruitment factor. A polymorphism in XPC exon 15, an A→C transition resulting in a lysin-to-glutamine amino acid change at codon 939 (Lys939Gln), was associated with a significant increase in BC risk (OR=1.49, 95% CI: 1.16–1.92).[12]

The XPD protein opens the DNA double helix to allow for excision of the damaged DNA fragment. The XPD codon 751 SNP (Lys751Gln) is of special interest, and its relationship with several cancers has been investigated. Positive associations were reported for some cancer types, but BC studies have consistently failed to find a significant association of this polymorphism with BC risk.[12,25-27]

XPG and XPF/ERCC1 are two endonucleases that cut damaged DNA at the opened site. The XPG Asp1104His exon 15 homozygous variant was initially associated with a decreased risk of BC; however, the association did not retain statistical significance after the Bonferroni correction for multiple comparisons.[12] The genotype distribution of XPF Arg415Gln differed significantly between cases and controls in a breast cancer study.[28] No study has yet assessed the relationship between XPF polymorphisms and BC.

### BER

The major genes involved in BER include XRCC1, OGG1, and APEX. The product of XRCC1 stimulates endonuclease activity and acts as a scaffold in the subsequent sealing steps of the apurinic/apyrimidinic (AP) sites. Several studies reported no association between an XRCC1 polymorphism in exon 10 (Arg399Gln) and BC risk.[12,25,27,29,30] Stern et al[29] also studied two more XRCC1 polymorphisms, Arg194Trp and Arg280His. No significant association was observed for the Arg280His polymorphism, but a slight protective effect was observed for individuals carrying at least one variant allele for the Arg194Trp polymorphism.

OGG1 codes for a protein that catalyzes the excision of the 8-oxoguanine adduct. Attenuated OGG1 enzyme activity reduces ability to excise 8-oxoguanine and thereby leads to accumulation of oxidation-induced mutations. Association of a common polymorphism in OGG1 (Ser326Cys) with cancer was assessed in a number of studies, and the variant Cys/Cys genotype has consistently been shown to be associated with significantly increased risks for several cancers.[31] However, OGG1 polymorphisms have not yet been studied in relation to BC.

In the initial step of BER, APEX—a DNA glycosylase—recognizes and removes damaged bases by hydrolyzing the N-glycosidic bond. Two polymorphisms in APEX (Glu148Asp and Gln50His) have been identified,[32] but no studies have been performed to assess their associations with any types of cancer.

## DSB repair

Homologous recombination (HR) and nonhomologous end-joining (NHEJ) are the two complementary pathways of DSB repair. Many genes are involved in these two pathways,[33] but only a few polymorphisms have been examined in relation to cancer risk. Studies assessing the relationship of BC risk to polymorphisms of XRCC3, which is involved in the HR pathway, have yielded inconsistent findings. During HR, the XRCC3 protein enables the Rad51 protein complex to assemble at the site of damage. A common C→T polymorphism in XRCC3 codon 241 (Thr241Met) has been studied in relation to BC, but the results were inconsistent. Matullo et al[25] reported a positive association between the Met allele and BC risk, especially among former smokers and nonsmokers compared to current smokers. Shen et al[27] observed that the variant Met allele protected against BC (OR=0.63, 95% CI: 0.42–0.93). Two other studies[12,30] did not find any significant association between the Met allele and BC. Larger epidemiologic studies are needed to clarify the relationship between XRCC3 polymorphisms and BC risk.

## PHENOTYPIC ASSAYS USED TO MEASURE DNA REPAIR

Phenotypic assays, which measure the efficiency of multiple DNA repair steps, usually are time- and labor-intensive and require highly trained technicians to perform. Various phenotypic assays have been applied to assess genetic instability and DNA repair capacity in population-based studies, including those that detect DNA adducts, metaphase chromosomal aberrations, micronuclei, sister chromatid exchanges, DNA damage, and host-cell reactivation.[34]

## DNA adduct detection

The C8-deoxyguanosine derivative of 4-aminobiphenyl (4-ABP) is a major product of carcinogen–DNA adducts in the bladder.[35] Performing immunohistochemical analyses of human bladder biopsy samples with an antibody specific to the 4-ABP–DNA adduct, Curigliano et al[36] found an association between staining levels and smoking history. Adduct levels were significantly higher in current smokers than in nonsmokers (p<0.0001), and there was a linear relationship between mean levels of relative staining and number of cigarettes smoked per day. For PAHs and other carcinogens with strong fluorescent properties, fluorescence detection of adducts in either DNA or products of DNA hydrolysis can be used. Mass spectrometry can detect specific chemicals in certain DNA adducts. Airoldi et al[37] applied gas chromatography–mass spectrometry to detect the DNA adducts of 4-ABP in 75 bladder cancer biopsies, and their results showed that detectable 4-ABP–DNA adducts were clearly associated with current smoking in higher tumor grades.

Finally, electrochemical detection can be used for recognizing minor DNA damage, such as the presence of 8-oxoguanine, which is formed in DNA by oxidative processes. A meta-analysis of 691 cancer patients and 632 controls from five lung cancer studies, one oral cancer study, and one BC study, illustrates the importance of phenotypic assays in molecular epidemiology. In this meta-analysis, bulky DNA adducts were measured by [32]P-postlabeling and ELISA. Patients that were current smokers had 83% higher adduct level compared to controls that currently smoked (95% CI: 0.44–1.22).[38] These findings suggest that current smokers with high levels of DNA adducts are at an increased risk for lung and bladder cancers.

## Mutagen sensitivity assay

Inherited susceptibility increases vulnerability to damage by environmental carcinogens and thereby elevates cancer risk. Hsu et al developed mutagen sensitivity, an in vitro short-term lymphocyte culture assay that indirectly assesses the DRC of different pathways by counting the number of induced chromatid breaks after exposure to an array of mutagens.[39,40] For example, exposure of the host genome to γ-radiation, which induces single- and double-stranded breaks, allows for evaluation of the BER and DSB pathways. In contrast, benzo(a)pyrene diolepoxide (BPDE), which forms covalent adducts when it interacts with DNA, triggers the NER repair pathway. Therefore, exposing the host genome to BPDE will test the effectiveness of the NER repair pathway. A series of epidemiologic studies[41-45] have clearly established mutagen sensitivity as an indicator of predisposition to various cancers including BC.

## Comet assay

The comet assay is a quick, accurate method for detecting both single- and double-stranded breaks, as well as for measuring the DRC of individual cells.[46,47] The comet assay has several advantages: it requires a relatively small number of cells, has the potential to be high throughput, and uses image analysis, which reduces the potential for observer bias and permits both densitometric and geometric measurements. A mutagen-challenged comet assay was used to measure baseline, BPDE-induced, and γ-radiation-induced DNA damage in individual peripheral blood lymphocytes of BC patients and controls.[48] Levels of all three types of DNA damage were statistically or borderline significantly associated with BC risk: at baseline (OR=1.84, 95% CI: 1.07–3.15), after γ-radiation (OR=1.81, 95% CI: 1.04–3.14), and after BPDE treatment (OR=1.69, 95% CI: 0.98–2.93).

## Host-cell reactivation assay

In this phenotypic assay, which measures DNA damage and repair, lymphocytes are transfected with damaged, nonreplicating recombinant plasmid DNA that contains a reporter gene. The host-cell reactivation assay has been successfully applied to a number of epidemiologic studies, mostly examining lung cancer.[34] We recently developed the use of the luciferase reporter gene in the host-cell reactivation assay to measure DRC after 4-ABP-induced damage. Utilizing this new technique, we found that BC patients exhibited poor DRC compared to healthy controls (13.0% versus 14.4%, p=0.006); furthermore, individuals with poor DRC had a 3.42-fold increased risk for BC (95% CI: 1.07–10.91) (unpublished data).

## CELL CYCLE CHECKPOINT

Cells can temporarily arrest at cell cycle checkpoints to repair damage, discharge an exogenous cellular stress signal, or acquire essential growth factors, hormones, or nutrients.[49] Checkpoint signaling may also trigger activation of apoptotic pathways if cellular damage cannot be properly repaired. Defects in cell cycle checkpoints can result in gene mutations, chromosome damage, and aneuploidy, all of which may contribute to tumorigenesis. Many genes are involved in cell cycle control, and many of them contain polymorphisms. Only a few have been studied in association with BC: CCND1, p53, and p21.

## CCND1

CCND1 is an important positive regulator of the G1/S checkpoint. One common CCND1 polymorphism, an A→G transition at nucleotide 870, which is found in the conserved splice donor region of exon 4, causes two different mRNA transcripts (a and b). Two studies have assessed the association between this CCND1 genotype and BC risk, but the results are inconsistent.[50,51] In a hospital-based case-control study of native Japanese (222 cases and 317 controls), Wang et al[50] found a significant 1.76-fold increased BC risk among individuals with the A/A genotype (95% CI: 1.09–2.84). In a larger study of non-Hispanic whites (515 cases and 612 controls), Cortessis et al[51] did not find a significantly increased BC risk for the A/A genotype (AA versus GG: OR=0.90, 95% CI: 0.60–1.33). The discrepancy between these two studies could have resulted from differences in populations studied, study design, and sample sizes. Further studies are needed to assess the relationship between this polymorphism and BC risk.

## p53

The association between p53 polymorphisms and cancer risk was highlighted in several lung cancer studies.[52,53] Studies of the association between BC and the Arg72Pro polymorphism have produced inconsistent results. From their Greek study of 50 cases and 99 controls, Soulitzis et al[54] concluded that the Arg/Arg genotype was associated with an increased BC risk (OR=4.69, 95% CI: 2.13–10.41). Kuroda et al,[55] on the other hand, found an association between the Pro/Pro genotype and increased BC risk (OR=1.86, 95% CI: 0.98–3.54); this Japanese study had a sample size of 112 cases and 175 controls. Two additional studies, performed independently in Tunisia and Turkey, used similar small sample sizes but found no association between the Arg72Pro polymorphism and BC risk.[56,57] Larger studies are needed to clarify the association of this polymorphism and BC risk.

## p21

p21/WAF1 is a cyclin-dependent kinase inhibitor. The link between a common p21 polymorphism (Ser31Arg) and cancer risk was examined in a Taiwanese BC study carried out by Chen et al[58] who reported that the variant allele (Arg) was associated with increased BC risk. However, the small sample size of this study, 53 cases and 119 controls, limits the validity of its findings.

## APOPTOSIS

Apoptosis is an integral physiologic mechanism designed to purge damaged cells. Deficient apoptotic potential not only encourages tumorigenesis but also renders cancer cells resistant to therapeutic treatment. Two distinct pathways—the extrinsic (death receptor) and the intrinsic (mitochondrial)—initiate apoptosis in mammalian cells. The apoptotic pathways depend on the interaction of many proteins. The capacity to induce apoptosis may be modulated by genetic polymorphisms in critical genes of these pathways. The National Center for Biotechnology Information SNP database and the National Cancer Institute SNP500Cancer database suggest that most genes from both apoptotic pathways contain a considerable number of SNPs. However, only a few studies have investigated the association of SNPs in apoptotic pathway genes with cancer risk.[59-61] So far, only one published case-control study has reported a significant correlation between SNPs in apoptotic pathway genes and BC. Hazra et al reported that a C→G SNP (C626G) at amino acid 209 (T209R), in exon 4 of the death receptor 4 (DR4) gene, conferred a 42% decreased BC risk among Caucasians.[61] This reduction in risk was more evident in women, younger individuals, and light smokers. Given that apoptosis signaling is critical, not only in eliminating damaged cells but also in mediating the therapeutic actions of many anticancer drugs, we expect a dramatic increase in molecular epidemiologic studies of SNPs in the apoptotic pathway.

## TELOMERES

In eukaryotic cells, telomeres form the protective DNA–protein complexes that cap chromosome ends.[62,63] Telomeres preclude nucleolytic degradation, end-to-end fusion, irregular recombination, and other fatal cellular events. Telomere dysfunction increases mutation rate and genomic instability.[64] In addition, telomeres may also be involved in chromosomal repair, as shown by the recruitment or de novo synthesis of telomere repeats at double-stranded breaks and by the ability of yeast telomeres to serve as repositories of essential components of the DNA repair machinery, particularly those involved in NHEJ.[65,66]

Because telomere dysfunction leads to genetic instability, individuals with such dysfunction may be at a higher risk for developing cancer. Wu et al developed an improved quantitative laser scanning cytometer-based approach, Q-FISH[LSC], for evaluating telomere length distribution in individual cells and investigated whether telomere dysfunction, as assessed by telomere length, was associated with risk of BC and other cancers.[67] Telomeres were statistically significantly shorter in patients with BC than in controls. An increasing risk for BC correlated with decreasing telomere length. Stratified analysis also suggested a greater-than-additive interaction between smoking status and telomere length. In addition, in a joint analysis using available DNA damage data, as measured by comet assay from 32 BC patients and 72 controls, telomere length was significantly inversely associated with baseline and mutagen-induced genetic instability.[67] These data provided the first epidemiologic evidence for the association between shortened telomeres and increased cancer risk.

## INFLAMMATION GENES

Acute inflammation is usually self-limiting because anti-inflammatory cytokines are produced soon after the release of proinflammatory cytokines. In contrast, chronic inflammation deregulates cellular homeostasis and can drive carcinogenesis. Inflammation due to chronic infection may be responsible for as much as 25% of cancer cases worldwide.

Genetic polymorphisms in inflammation genes, including IL6, IL8, PPARG, and TNFα, have been studied in relationship with cancer risk. A G→C transversion at −174 of IL6 affects the transcription of the gene and alters the amount of released IL6.[68] PPARG has a polymorphism in the coding region (C34G) that results in an amino acid change (Pro12Ala), which might affect its ability to encode a nuclear transcription factor. In a case-control study, Wang et al observed that the variant IL6 genotype is associated with increased risk of BC (OR=1.52, 95% CI: 1.02–2.28).[69] Furthermore, individuals with variant genotypes for both IL6 (C/C) and PPARG (C/G + G/G) had an even higher BC risk (OR=2.76, 95% CI: 1.42–5.35).

## GENETIC VARIATIONS AND CLINICAL OUTCOMES

Recently, there has been an emerging awareness of the role of genetics in predicting the patient's natural history of cancer and therapeutic response. Genetic susceptibility modulates tumor etiology and pathogenesis, including factors such as tumor histopathology, cancer stage, rate of disease progression, and propensity for metastasis. Genetic variations also influence individual response to chemoprevention, chemotherapy, and radiotherapy. Differences in therapeutic response come from interindividual variation in drug metabolism, DNA damage repair, cell cycle checkpoints, expression of drug receptors, and bioavailability of the chemotherapeutic agent.

## GENETIC VARIATIONS AND THE NATURAL HISTORY OF BC

Studying BC patients, Inatomi et al showed that the NAT2 slow genotype was associated with a greater likelihood of developing a high-grade (G3) or an advanced stage (pT2–pT4) tumor.[70] Two small Taiwanese studies compared the genotype frequencies of the p53 Arg72Pro and p21 Ser31Arg polymorphisms in two patient groups: those with invasive tumors and those with noninvasive tumors.[58,71] Performing Fisher's exact test, they reported that p53 Pro/Pro homozygotes were more frequently found in invasive tumors than in noninvasive tumors (25% and 2.9%, respectively, p<0.001); they also found that the p21 Ser/Arg heterozygote was more prominent in invasive tumors. In a study of 172 BC patients, Sakano et al examined two 3′ UTR polymorphisms in the CDKN2A (p16) gene, C500G and C540T, and found that the tumor-specific survival was significantly shorter in patients with either the 500 C→G or the 540 C→T polymorphism, as compared to those with wild-type (C/C) alleles (p=0.02).[72] Marsh et al studied two polymorphisms in the tumor necrosis factor (TNF) gene, G488A and C859T, in 196 BC patients.[73] A significant association between TNF 488A and TNF 859T and BC risk was detected. Furthermore, these polymorphisms were associated with grade of tumor at presentation, although there was no significant effect on subsequent tumor behavior.[73]

## PHARMACOGENETICS

Even though interindividual variations in drug response can result from differences in age, sex, and disease stage, genetic factors influence both the efficacy of a drug and the extent of an adverse reaction. Specifically, genetic variations in drug metabolism enzyme and DNA repair genes significantly affect therapeutic response. The cytochrome P450 family enzymes are responsible for the metabolism of a broad range of chemotherapeutic agents. For example, a polymorphism in the CYP3A affects the metabolism of several agents used to treat BC, including ifosfamide, vinblastine, paclitaxel, and docetaxel.[74] The GST family enzymes conjugate platinum, alkylating agents, and other anticancer drugs to glutathione.[75] Genetic variations that cause attenuated or enhanced metabolic activity will affect the bioavailability of therapeutic agents and thereby modulate individual therapeutic response.

Cytotoxic effects from treatment result from the DNA damage induced by radiotherapy and several chemotherapeutic agents, including cisplatin and cyclophosphamide. It is believed that individuals with defective DRCs are more sensitive to DNA-damaging drugs than those with normal DRC. Bosken et al found that defective host DRC was associated with poorer survival when patients with non-small cell lung cancer were treated with platinum-based chemotherapy.[76] Research on the effects of DRC in BC treatment is expected to explode in the next decade.

Immunotherapeutic response may be altered by genetic variants in inflammation genes. Bacillus Calmette–Guérin (BCG) is the prevailing choice of immunotherapy for superficial BC. BCG stimulates the immune system, in particular interferon-γ production. We studied a number of polymorphisms in inflammation genes and found that the variant allele of a common IL6 promoter polymorphism, G174C, was associated with an increased risk of recurrence among individuals receiving maintenance BCG (unpublished data).

## EPIGENETIC EVENTS AND CANCER

Recently there has been a surge of research validating the hypothesis that both genetic and epigenetic alterations are critical events in tumorigenesis.[77] Epigenetic changes in DNA methylation, such as global hypomethylation and region-specific hypermethylation, have been described in various cancer types, including bladder cancer, where each tumor type possesses its own distinct pattern of methylation. Although much remains to be learned about the precise mechanisms underlying alterations of methylation patterns, it is known that the key players in CpG island methylation and resulting transcription silencing are DNA methyltransferases (DNMTs)—which are responsible for the de novo synthesis and maintenance of methylation—and methyl-binding proteins (MBD)—which bind to methylated DNA and recruit repression complexes containing histone deacetylases. Given that aberrant promoter methylation plays an important role in tumorigenesis, polymorphisms in methylation-related genes may modify cancer risk by interfering with the normal methylation process. Shen et al identified a C→T transition at a novel promoter region of the DNMT3B gene; this polymorphism significantly increased promoter activity.[78] Hazra et al studied this SNP in BC and found that the variant allele (TT), compared to the CC and CT variants, had a marginal protective effect for women (OR=0.51, 95% CI: 0.24–1.09) which was more evident in women who were never smokers (OR=0.41, 95% CI: 0.21–0.79).[79] Further studies are needed to clarify the relationship of this SNP with BC risk. Although there have been no reports on MBD polymorphisms and cancer risk, a recent study by Zhu et al showed that high levels of MBD2 expression were associated with a significantly reduced BC risk (OR=0.43, 95% CI: 0.21–0.90).[80]

Like proteins that are directly involved in DNA methylation and transcription silencing, methyl group metabolism genes also affect the rate of DNA methylation. S-adenosylmethionine (SAM) is the primary methyl group donor for DNA methylation. The major proteins involved in the recycling of SAM include methylene-tetrahydrofolate reductase (MTHFR) and methionine synthase (MS), both of which are also major folate metabolism proteins. Two functional SNPs in MTHFR genes, C667T (Ala222Val) and A1298C (Glu429Ala), have been studied in many cancer sites, but the results were inconsistent.[81-83] Two studies comparing BC patients and controls failed to find significant differences for genotype distributions and allele frequencies in the C667T SNP.[12,84] Kimura et al also did not find a significant association of a functional SNP in MS, A2756G (Asp919Gly), with BC risk.[84] However, Lin et al recently investigated the joint effects of MTHFR and MS polymorphisms, dietary folate intake, and cigarette smoking on BC risk.[85] Genotype data were analyzed in a subset of 410 Caucasian cases and 410 controls. Compared with individuals with the MTHFR C677T wild type (CC) and a high folate intake, those with the variant genotype (CT or TT) and a low folate intake were at a 3.51-fold increased risk of BC (95% CI: 1.59–6.52). When genotype was analyzed alongside smoking status, it was found that current smokers with the variant genotype had a 6.56-fold increased risk (95% CI: 3.28–13.12) compared to never smokers with the MTHFR 677 wild type. Analyses of the MTHFR A1298C and MS A2756G SNPs revealed similar results, suggesting that polymorphisms of the MTHFR and MS genes act together with low folate intake and smoking to increase BC risk.[85]

## CONCLUSIONS AND FUTURE DIRECTIONS

Over the past decade, molecular cancer epidemiology has uncovered the potential gene–gene and gene–environment interactions in cancer causation, thereby rising to prominence in the field of cancer research. As this chapter has illustrated, considerable progress has been made in our understanding of genetic susceptibility factors for BC. Extensive comparisons of genetic polymorphisms between BC patients and controls have identified a number of low-penetrance risk factors for BC which will facilitate attempts to identify high-risk populations. In addition, a fascinating new research field, pharmacogenetics, has emerged from current research on genetic predisposition and is rapidly advancing.

Despite molecular cancer epidemiology's many successes, numerous challenges must be met before recently identified genetic susceptibility factors can be established as having a causal association with specific environmental carcinogens:

1. Large, well-designed studies of common polymorphisms are needed to avoid false-positive and false-negative results.
2. Given that carcinogenesis is a multifactorial and multistep process, it may be necessary to use pathway-based concurrent genotyping of a comprehensive list of polymorphisms to evaluate the relative importance of each gene and the potential gene–gene interactions. This strategy is advantageous because it is difficult to detect subtle differences in a phenotype based on a single polymorphism.
3. Since the entire human genome contains millions of polymorphisms, computational algorithms are needed to select the polymorphisms that are most likely to cause phenotypic changes and contribute to carcinogenesis. SIFT (sorting intolerant from tolerant) and POLYPHEN (polymorphism phenotyping) are two programs that can prioritize polymorphisms for research.[86]

4. Since haplotype may provide more information than individual genotypes, more effort should be put into haplotyping to complement genotyping.
5. High-throughput, cost-effective phenotypic assays are needed to measure the collective effects of multigenic and multistep pathways in large-scale epidemiologic studies.
6. Biomarker validation will need to keep pace with the rapid identification of genetic susceptibility markers.

Although molecular epidemiology has grown rapidly in the past decade, few markers have been validated for application to risk assessment or clinical outcome prediction. As molecular cancer epidemiologists, we have much work to do before we can reach our ultimate goal: a practical risk assessment model to predict both cancer occurrence in high-risk populations and clinical outcomes of cancer patients. Such a model will have enormous preventive and clinical implications. In the next decade, we will undoubtedly move closer to this goal.

## REFERENCES

1. Anton-Culver H, Lee-Feldstein A, Taylor TH. Occupation and bladder cancer risk. Am J Epidemiol 1992;136:89–4.
2. Vineis P, Simonato L. Proportion of lung and bladder cancers in males resulting from occupation: a systematic approach. Arch Environ Health 1991;46:6–15.
3. Kiemeney LA, Schoenberg M. Familial transitional cell carcinoma. J Urol 1996;156:867–872.
4. Katoh T, Inatomi H, Nagaoka A, Sugita A. Cytochrome P4501A1 gene polymorphism and homozygous deletion of the glutathione S-transferase M1 gene in urothelial cancer patients. Carcinogenesis 1995;16:655–657.
5. Brockmöller J, Cascorbi I, Kerb R, Roots I. Combined analysis of inherited polymorphisms in arylamine N-acetyltransferase 2, glutathione S-transferases M1 and T1, microsomal epoxide hydrolase, and cytochrome P450 enzymes as modulators of bladder. Cancer Res 1996;56:3915–3925.
6. Vineis P, Veglia F, Benhamou S, et al. CYP1A1 T3801 C polymorphism and lung cancer: a pooled analysis of 2451 cases and 3358 controls. Int J Cancer 2003;104:650–657.
7. Choi JY, Lee KM, Cho SH, et al. CYP2E1 and NQO1 genotypes, smoking and bladder cancer. Pharmacogenetics 2003;13:349–355.
8. Anwar WA, Abdel-Rahman SZ, El Zein RA, Mostafa HM, Au WW. Genetic polymorphism of GSTM1, CYP2E1 and CYP2D6 in Egyptian bladder cancer patients. Carcinogenesis 1996;17:1923–1929.
9. Hung RJ, Boffetta P, Brennan P, et al. GST, NAT, SULT1A1, CYP1B1 genetic polymorphisms, interactions with environmental exposures and bladder cancer risk in a high-risk population. Int J Cancer 2004;110:598–604.
10. Hayes JD, Pulford DJ. The glutathione-S-transferase supergene family: regulation of GST and the contribution of the isoenzymes to cancer chemoprevention and drug resistance. Crit Rev Biochem Mol Biol 1995;30:445–600.
11. Engel LS, Taioli E, Pfeiffer R, et al. Pooled analysis and meta-analysis of glutathione S-transferase M1 and bladder cancer: a HuGE review. Am J Epidemiol 2002;156:95–109.
12. Sanyal S, Festa F, Sakano S, et al. Polymorphisms in DNA repair and metabolic genes in bladder cancer. Carcinogenesis 2004;25:729–734.
13. Marcus PM, Vineis P, Rothman N. NAT2 slow acetylation and bladder cancer risk: a meta-analysis of 22 case-control studies conducted in the general population. Pharmacogenetics 2000;10:115–122.

14. Marcus PM, Hayes RB, Vineis P, et al. Cigarette smoking, N-acetyltransferase 2 acetylation status, and bladder cancer risk: a case-series meta-analysis of a gene–environment interaction. Cancer Epidemiol Biomarkers Prev 2000;9:461–467.

15. Basu S, Brown JE, Flannigan GM, et al. Immunohistochemical analysis of NAD(P)H:quinone oxidoreductase and NADPH cytochrome P450 reductase in human superficial bladder tumours: relationship between tumour enzymology and clinical outcome following intravesical mitomycin C therapy. Int J Cancer 2004;109:703–709.

16. Choudry GA, Stewart PA, Double JA, et al. A novel strategy for NQO1 (NAD(P)H:quinone oxidoreductase, EC 1.6.99.2) mediated therapy of bladder cancer based on the pharmacological properties of EO9. Br J Cancer 2001;85:1137–1146.

17. Ross D, Traver RD, Siegel D, Kuehl BL, Misra V, Rauth AM. A polymorphism in NAD(P)H:quinone oxidoreductase (NQO1): relationship of a homozygous mutation at position 609 of the NQO1 cDNA to NQO1 activity. Br J Cancer 1996;74:995–996.

18. Siegel D, McGuinness SM, Winski SL, Ross D. Genotype–phenotype relationships in studies of a polymorphism in NAD(P)H:quinone oxidoreductase 1. Pharmacogenetics 1999;9:113–121.

19. Park SJ, Zhao H, Spitz MR, Grossman HB, Wu X. An association between NQO1 genetic polymorphism and risk of bladder cancer. Mutat Res 2003;536:131–137.

20. Hung RJ, Boffetta P, Brennan P, et al. Genetic polymorphisms of MPO, COMT, MnSOD, NQO1, interactions with environmental exposures and bladder cancer risk. Carcinogenesis 2004;25:973–978.

21. Zheng L, Wang Y, Schabath MB, Grossman HB, Wu X. Sulfotransferase 1A1 (SULT1A1) polymorphism and bladder cancer risk: a case-control study. Cancer Lett 2003;202:61–69.

22. Wood RD, Mitchell M, Sgouros J, Lindahl T. Human DNA repair genes. Science 2001;291:1284–1289.

23. Christmann M, Tomicic MT, Roos WP, Kaina B. Mechanisms of human DNA repair: an update. Toxicology 2003;193:3–34.

24. Wu X, Zhao H, Wei Q, et al. XPA polymorphism associated with reduced lung cancer risk and a modulating effect on nucleotide excision repair capacity. Carcinogenesis 2003;24:505–509.

25. Matullo G, Palli D, Peluso M, et al. XRCC1, XRCC3, XPD gene polymorphisms, smoking, and 32P-DNA adducts in a sample of healthy subjects. Carcinogenesis 2001;22:1437–1445.

26. Stern MC, Johnson LR, Bell DA, Taylor JA. XPD codon 751 polymorphism, metabolism genes, smoking, and bladder cancer risk. Cancer Epidemiol Biomarkers Prev 2002;11:1004–1011.

27. Shen M, Hung RJ, Brennan P, et al. Polymorphisms of the DNA repair genes XRCC1, XRCC3, XPD, interaction with environmental exposures, and bladder cancer risk in a case-control study in northern Italy. Cancer Epidemiol Biomarkers Prev 2003;12:1234–1240.

28. Smith TR, Levine EA, Perrier ND, et al. DNA-repair genetic polymorphisms and breast cancer risk. Cancer Epidemiol Biomarkers Prev 2003;12:1200–1204.

29. Stern MC, Umbach DM, van Gils CH, Lunn RM, Taylor JA. DNA repair gene XRCC1 polymorphisms, smoking, and bladder cancer risk. Cancer Epidemiol Biomarkers Prev 2001;10:125–131.

30. Stern MC, Umbach DM, Lunn RM, Taylor JA. DNA repair gene XRCC3 codon 241 polymorphism, its interaction with smoking and XRCC1 polymorphisms, and bladder cancer risk. Cancer Epidemiol Biomarkers Prev 2002;11:939–943.

31. Goode EL, Ulrich CM, Potter JD. Polymorphisms in DNA repair genes and associations with cancer risk. Cancer Epidemiol Biomarkers Prev 2002;12:1513–1530.

32. Pieretti M, Khattar NH, Smith SA. Common polymorphisms and somatic mutations in human base excision repair genes in ovarian and endometrial cancers. Mutat Res 2001;432:53–59.

33. Khanna KK, Jackson SP. DNA double-strand breaks: signaling, repair and the cancer connection. Nat Genet 2001;27:247–254.

34. Spitz MR, Wei Q, Dong Q, Amos CI, Wu X. Genetic susceptibility to lung cancer: the role of DNA damage and repair. Cancer Epidemiol Biomarkers Prev 2003;12:689–698.

35. Talaska G, al-Juburi AZ, Kadlubar FF. Smoking related carcinogen-DNA adducts in biopsy samples of human urinary bladder: identification of N-(deoxyguanosin-8-yl)-4-aminobiphenyl as a major adduct. Proc Natl Acad Sci USA 1991;88:5350–5354.

36. Curigliano G, Zhang YJ, Wang LY, et al. Immunohistochemical quantitation of 4-aminobiphenyl-DNA adducts and p53 nuclear overexpression in T1 bladder cancer of smokers and nonsmokers. Carcinogenesis 1996;17:911–916.

37. Airoldi L, Orsi F, Magagnotti C, et al. Determinants of 4-aminobiphenyl-DNA adducts in bladder cancer biopsies. Carcinogenesis 2002;25:861–866.

38. Veglia F, Matullo G, Vineis P. Bulky DNA adducts and risk of cancer: a meta-analysis. Cancer Epidemiol Biomarkers Prev 2003;12:157–160.

39. Hsu TC. Genetic predisposition to cancer with special reference to mutagen sensitivity. In Vitro Cell Dev Biol 1987;23:591–603.

40. Hsu TC, Johnston DA, Cherry LM, et al. Sensitivity to genotoxic effects of bleomycin in humans: possible relationship to environmental carcinogenesis. Int J Cancer 1989;43:403–409.

41. Spitz MR, Hsu TC, Wu X, Fueger JJ, Amos CI, Roth JA. Mutagen sensitivity as a biological marker of lung cancer risk in African Americans. Cancer Epidemiol Biomarkers Prev 1995;4:99–103.

42. Wu X, Gu J, Patt Y, Hassan M, Spitz MR, Beasley RP, Hwang LY. Mutagen sensitivity as a susceptibility marker for human hepatocellular carcinoma. Cancer Epidemiol Biomarkers Prev 1998;7:567–570.

43. Wu X, Gu J, Amos CI, Jiang H, Hong WK, Spitz MR. A parallel study of in vitro sensitivity to benzo[a]pyrene diol epoxide and bleomycin in lung carcinoma cases and controls. Cancer 1998;83:1118–1127.

44. Wu X, Gu J, Hong WK, et al. Benzo[a]pyrene diol epoxide and bleomycin sensitivity and susceptibility to cancer of upper aerodigestive tract. J Natl Cancer Inst 1998;90:1393–1399.

45. Wu X, Lippman SM, Lee JJ, et al. Chromosome instability in lymphocytes: a potential indicator of predisposition to oral premalignant lesions. Cancer Res 2002;62:2813–2818.

46. Rojas E, Lopez MC, Valverde M. Single cell gel electrophoresis assay: methodology and applications. J Chromatogr B Biomed Sci Appl 1999;722:225–254.

47. Tice RR, Agurell E, Anderson D, et al. Single cell gel/comet assay: guidelines for in vitro and in vivo genetic toxicology testing. Environ Mol Mutagen 2000;35:206–221.

48. Schabath MB, Spitz MR, Grossman HB, Zhang K, Dinney CP, Zheng PJ, Wu X. Genetic instability in bladder cancer assessed by the comet assay. J Natl Cancer Inst 2003;95:540–547.

49. Laiho M, Latonen L. Cell cycle control, DNA damage checkpoints and cancer. Ann Med 2003;35:391–397.

50. Wang L, Habuchi T, Takahashi T, et al. Cyclin D1 gene polymorphism is associated with an increased risk of urinary bladder cancer. Carcinogenesis 2002;23:257–264.

51. Cortessis VK, Siegmund K, Xue S, Ross RK, Yu MC. A case-control study of cyclin D1 CCND1 870A—>G polymorphism and bladder cancer. Carcinogenesis 2003;24:1645–1650.

52. Wu X, Zhao H, Amos CI, et al. P53 genotypes and haplotypes associated with lung cancer susceptibility and ethnicity. J Natl Cancer Inst 2002;94:681–690.

53. Matakidou A, Eisen T, Houlston RS. TP53 polymorphisms and lung cancer risk: a systematic review and meta-analysis. Mutagenesis 2003;180:377–385.

54. Soulitzis N, Sourvinos G, Dokianakis DN, Spandidos DA. P53 codon 72 polymorphism and its association with bladder cancer. Cancer Lett 2002;179:175–183.

55. Kuroda Y, Tsukino H, Nakao H, Imai H, Katoh T. P53 codon 72 polymorphism and urothelial cancer risk. Cancer Lett. 2003;189:77–83.

56. Mabrouk I, Baccouche S, El-Abed R, et al. No evidence of correlation between p53 codon 72 polymorphism and risk of bladder or breast carcinoma in Tunisian patients. Ann N Y Acad Sci 2003;1010:764–770.

57. Toruner GA, Ucar A, Tez M, Cetinkaya M, Ozen H, Ozcelik T. P53 codon 72 polymorphism in bladder cancer—no evidence of association with increased risk or invasiveness. Urol Res 2001;29:393–395.

58. Chen WC, Wu HC, Hsu CD, Chen HY, Tsai FJ. P21 gene codon 31 polymorphism is associated with bladder cancer. Urol Oncol 2002;7:63–66.

59. Fisher MJ, Virmani AK, Wu L, et al. Nucleotide substitution in the ectodomain of trail receptor DR4 is associated with lung cancer and head and neck cancer. Clin Cancer Res 2001;7:1688–1697.

60. Wang LE, Cheng L, Spitz MR, Wei Q. Fas A670G polymorphism, apoptotic capacity in lymphocyte cultures, and risk of lung cancer. Lung Cancer 2003;42:1–8.

61. Hazra A, Chamberlain RM, Grossman HB, Zhu Y, Spitz MR, Wu X. Death receptor 4 and bladder cancer risk. Cancer Res 2003;63:1157–1159.

62. McEachern MJ, Krauskopf A, Blackburn EH. Telomeres and their control. Annu Rev Genet 2000;34:331–358.

63. Blackburn EH. Switching and signaling at the telomere. Cell 2001;106:661–673.

64. Hackett JA, Feldser DM, Greider CW. Telomere dysfunction increases mutation rate and genomic instability. Cell 2001;106:275–286.

65. Haber JE. Sir-Ku-itous routes to make ends meet. Cell 1999;97:829–832.

66. Martin SG, Laroche T, Suka N, Grunstein M, Gasser SM. Relocalization of telomeric Ku and SIR proteins in response to DNA strand breaks in yeast. Cell 1999;97:621–633.

67. Wu X, Amos CI, Zhu Y, et al. Telomere dysfunction: a potential cancer predisposition factor. J Natl Cancer Inst 2003;95:1211–1218.

68. Fishman D, Faulds G, Jeffery R, et al. The effect of novel polymorphisms in the interleukin-6 (IL-6) gene on IL-6 transcription and plasma IL-6 levels, and an association with systemic-onset juvenile chronic arthritis. J Clin Invest 1998;102:1369–1376.

69. Wang Y, Lerner S, Leibovici D, Dinney CP, Grossman HB, Wu X. Polymorphisms in the inflammatory genes IL-6, IL-8, TNF-α, NFKB1, and PPARG and bladder cancer risk. Proc Am Assoc Cancer Res 2004;Abstract 3979.

70. Inatomi H, Katoh T, Kawamoto T, Matsumoto T. NAT2 gene polymorphism as a possible marker for susceptibility to bladder cancer in Japanese. Int J Urol 1999;6:446–454.

71. Chen WC, Tsai FJ, Wu JY, Wu HC, Lu HF, Li CW. Distributions of p53 codon 72 polymorphism in bladder cancer—proline form is prominent in invasive tumor. Urol Res 2000;28:293–296.

72. Sakano S, Berggren P, Kumar R, et al. Clinical course of bladder neoplasms and single nucleotide polymorphisms in the CDKN2A gene. Int J Cancer 2003;104:98–103.

73. Marsh HP, Haldar NA, Bunce M, et al. Polymorphisms in tumour necrosis factor (TNF) are associated with risk of bladder cancer and grade of tumour at presentation. Br J Cancer 2003;89:1096–1101.

74. Royer I, Monsarrat B, Sonnier M, Wright M, Cresteil T. Metabolism of docetaxel by human cytochromes P450: interactions with paclitaxel and other antineoplastic drugs. Cancer Res 1996;56:58–65.

75. Waxman DJ. Glutathione S-transferases: role in alkylating agent resistance and possible target for modulation chemotherapy—a review. Cancer Res 1990;50:6449–6454.

76. Bosken CH, Wei Q, Amos CI, Spitz MR. An analysis of DNA repair as a determinant of survival in patients with non-small-cell lung cancer. J Natl Cancer Inst 2002;94:1091–1099.

77. Jones PA, Baylin SB. The fundamental role of epigenetic events in cancer. Nat Rev Genet 2002;3:415–428.

78. Shen H, Wang L, Spitz MR, Hong WK, Mao L, Wei Q. A novel polymorphism in human cytosine DNA-methyltransferase-3B promoter is associated with an increased risk of lung cancer. Cancer Res 2002;62:4992–4995.

79. Hazra A, Gu J, Zhu Y, Grossman HB, Spitz MR, Wu X. DNMT3b and bladder cancer risk: from genotype to phenotype. Proc Am Assoc Cancer Res 2004;Abstract 1604.

80. Zhu Y, Spitz MR, Zhang H, Grossman HB, Frazier ML, Wu X. Methyl-CpG-binding domain 2: a protective role in bladder carcinoma. Cancer 2004;100:1853–1858.

81. Jeng YL, Wu MH, Huang HB, et al. The methylenetetrahydrofolate reductase 677C—>T polymorphism and lung cancer risk in a Chinese population. Anticancer Res 2003;23:5149–5152.

82. Shen H, Spitz MR, Wang LE, Hong WK, Wei Q. Polymorphisms of methylene-tetrahydrofolate reductase and risk of lung cancer: a case-control study. Cancer Epidemiol Biomarkers Prev 2001;10:397–401.

83. Stolzenberg-Solomon RZ, Qiao YL, Abnet CC, et al. Esophageal and gastric cardia cancer risk and folate- and vitamin B(12)-related polymorphisms in Linxian, China. Cancer Epidemiol Biomarkers Prev 2003;12:1222–1226.

84. Kimura F, Florl AR, Steinhoff C, et al. Polymorphic methyl group metabolism genes in patients with transitional cell carcinoma of the urinary bladder. Mutat Res 2001;458:49–54.

85. Lin J, Spitz MR, Wang Y, et al. Polymorphisms of folate metabolic genes and susceptibility to bladder cancer: a case-control study. Carcinogenesis 2004;25(9):1639–1647.

86. Zhu Y, Spitz MR, Amos CI, Lin J, Schabath MB, Wu X. An evolutionary perspective on single-nucleotide polymorphism screening in molecular cancer epidemiology. Cancer Res 2004;64:2251–2257.

# Urothelial carcinoma and its variants

5

*Antonio Lopez-Beltran, Liang Cheng*

## INTRODUCTION

Urothelial carcinoma of the bladder traditionally has been classified into two groups: superficial tumors and muscle-invasive tumors. Approximately 80% of patients with primary urothelial carcinoma will display a relatively indolent, low-grade tumor confined to the superficial mucosa. Despite the relatively indolent nature of superficial urothelial tumors, the recurrence rate can be as high as 70%, thus necessitating long-term follow-up. In addition, more than one-third of recurrent superficial tumors may eventually progress to a higher grade and/or stage.[1-5] The most important predictors of clinical course are the depth of invasion at presentation, multiplicity, early recurrent tumors, tumor size, histologic grade, and pathologic stage.[1,6-11] From a pathologist's point of view, tumor configuration (papillary versus nonpapillary), vascular invasion and, even more importantly, the level of lamina propria invasion, or thickness of tumor invasion as measured by an ocular micrometer, are important predictors for invasive urothelial carcinomas.[4,8,12,13]

Three basic diagnostic categories are identified in the urinary bladder on the basis of the pattern of growth of the urothelial tumors (flat, papillary non-invasive, or infiltrative). Their clinical behaviors are also related to the degree of architectural, cytologic, and molecular alterations of the urothelium.[9,14] Several classifications have been reported in the literature, and current genetic data suggest two major pathways that correspond to morphologically defined entities.[15-19] The genetically stable category includes non-invasive, low-grade papillary tumors (pTa, G1, and G2). The genetically unstable category contains non-invasive, high-grade (including pTa, G3, and CIS) and infiltrating carcinomas (stage pT1-4). Non-invasive low-grade bladder neoplasms have fewer genomic alterations and are therefore viewed as genetically stable.[18] Invasive tumors appear to be genetically unstable and have more chromosomal aberrations. The potential value for this classification also depends on accurate diagnosis and consistent separation of pTa from pT1 tumors.

Recognition of early invasion (stage pT1) in urothelial neoplasia is one of the most challenging areas in bladder pathology, and reproducibility between pathologists is a major issue.[8] This fact, together with the proposal by some urologists to treat early invasive tumors more aggressively, makes the accurate diagnosis of pT1 tumors even more relevant in clinical practice. The emerging role of flat intraepithelial lesions as precursors of bladder cancer at both morphologic and molecular levels—in particular flat urothelial hyperplasia, urothelial dysplasia, and carcinoma in situ—will be considered in this chapter, together with the role of infiltrating urothelial carcinoma and non-invasive papillary urothelial neoplasia. Grading of papillary urothelial neoplasia, including 1973 and 2004 World Health Organization (WHO) classification and staging, will be discussed in Chapter 6.

## FLAT INTRAEPITHELIAL LESIONS

### NORMAL UROTHELIUM

The urothelium is composed of basal, intermediate, and superficial cells without cytologic atypia (Figure 5.1). The number of cell layers may vary (usually less than seven) due to tangential sectioning. Malignancy-associated cellular change (MACC) is a recently

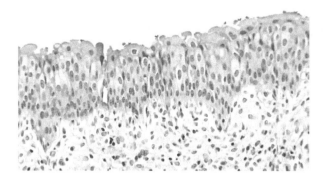

**Fig. 5.1**
Normal urothelium.

introduced concept, encompassing urothelial abnormalities of bladders harboring neoplastic lesions that are not detectable by routine light microscopy.[14,20] However, MACC is detectable when chromatin analysis or genetic studies are performed. Most reports show chromosome 9 alterations in MACC, similar to those in the coexistent carcinoma.[14] The clinical relevance of MACC remains to be established.

## UROTHELIAL HYPERPLASIA

Urothelial hyperplasia is characterized by markedly thickened mucosa without cytologic atypia (Figure 5.2). It may be seen adjacent to low-grade urothelial papillary tumors. Within the spectrum of hyperplasia, a papillary architecture may be present; most of these patients have concomitant papillary tumors.[21,22] When seen by itself, there is no evidence suggesting that it has a premalignant potential.[20] However, molecular analyses have shown that the lesion, at least in bladder cancer patients, may be clonally related to the papillary tumors.[22] Molecular alterations can also be seen in histologically 'normal appearing' urothelium and stroma in bladders from cancer patients.[23,24]

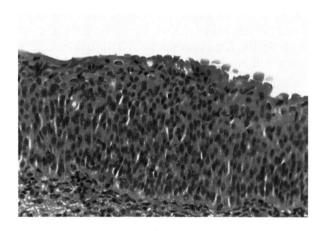

**Fig. 5.2**
Urothelial hyperplasia.

## UROTHELIAL DYSPLASIA

Dysplasia is an intraurothelial lesion with appreciable cytologic and architectural changes that are believed to be preneoplastic but which fall short of carcinoma in situ (CIS). The urothelium of dysplasia typically shows cohesive cells characterized by nuclear/nucleolar changes that include irregular nuclear crowding and nuclear hyperchromasia (Figure 5.3A). Nucleoli may be prominent, and mitotic figures, when present, are generally basally located. The umbrella cells are usually present. Most cellular abnormalities in dysplasia are restricted to the basal and intermediate cell layers. There may be an increased number of cell layers. Nuclear and architectural features are considered most useful in distinguishing between reactive urothelial atypia and dysplasia.[20] Cytokeratin 20 may be of value in its recognition (Figure 5.3B).[25] Alterations of p53 and allelic losses, particularly in chromosome 9, have been demonstrated to occur in dysplasia.[25,26]

Dysplasia is most relevant in non-invasive papillary neoplasms, where its presence indicates urothelial instability and is a marker for recurrence or progression.[27,28] De novo dysplasia progresses to bladder neoplasia in about 15% to 19% of cases.[29,30] The use of the term atypia as synonymous with

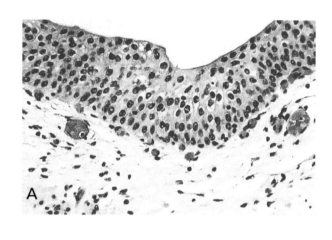

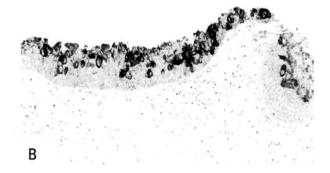

**Fig. 5.3**
**A** Urothelial dysplasia. **B** Abnormal cytokeratin 20 expression in urothelial dysplasia.

urothelial dysplasia is discouraged. Due to inherent inter- and intraobserver variability, grading of urothelial dysplasia is not recommended.

## UROTHELIAL CARCINOMA IN SITU

CIS is a non-papillary flat lesion in which the surface epithelium contains cells that are cytologically malignant (Figure 5.4).[20,31] The morphologic diagnosis of CIS requires the presence of severe cytologic atypia.[3,29] Full thickness change is not essential, although it is usually present. Prominent disorganization of cells is characteristic, with loss of cellular polarity and cohesiveness (Figure 5.5A). The tumor cells tend to be large and pleomorphic, with moderate to abundant cytoplasm, although they are sometimes small with a high nuclear to cytoplasmic ratio. The chromatin tends to be coarse and clumped.[20,31,32] Nucleoli are usually large and prominent in at least some of the cells, and may be multiple. Mitotic figures are also seen in the uppermost layers of the urothelium, and may be atypical.[9,33] Superficial (umbrella) cells may be present.

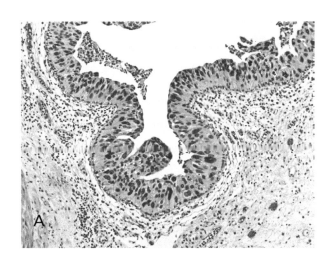

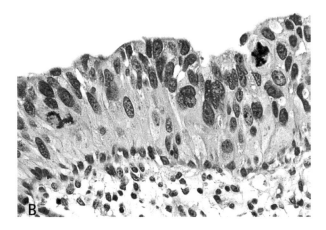

**Fig. 5.4**
**A, B** Urothelial carcinoma in situ.

Several patterns and/or variants have been described. Individual neoplastic cells may be seen scattered amidst normal urothelium (pagetoid pattern) (Figure 5.5B).[20,31] Loss of intercellular cohesion of CIS may result in the so-called 'denuding cystitis' or in residual neoplastic cells attached to the surface ('clinging' pattern) (Figure 5.5C). Small and large cell variants have been described. CIS cells may involve von Brunn's nests and cystitis cystica.

Cytokeratin 20 is abnormally expressed in CIS. Abnormal expression of p53 (Figure 5.5D) and RB protein may correlate with progression of CIS or response to bacillus Calmette–Guérin (BCG) therapy.[17,25] The nuclear matrix protein NMP22 is present in CIS. Cytogenetically, CIS shows close similarities to invasive tumors.[15,34]

Primary (de novo) CIS accounts for 1% to 3% of urothelial neoplasms and is most commonly seen in the bladder.[3] Approximately 15% of patients with CIS of the bladder will have prostatic urethral involvement; a recurrent tumor may occasionally be found in the urethral stump after cystectomy. The distal ureters are involved in 6% to 60%, the prostatic urethra in 20% to 67%, and the prostate ducts and acini in up to 40%.[20] Primary CIS is less likely to progress to invasive disease than secondary CIS.[20] Approximately 45% to 65% of patients with CIS and concomitant invasive tumors will die of the disease, as compared to 7% to 15% of patients with primary CIS with or without concomitant non-invasive papillary tumors. CIS with aneuploid karyotypes appears to be at high risk of progression.

## NON-INVASIVE PAPILLARY UROTHELIAL NEOPLASIA

The topic of the best contemporary classification and grading system of the non-invasive papillary neoplasia has been debated and should still be considered unsettled. From the practical point of view, the use of both the 1973[35] (Box 5.1) and 2004 WHO classifications (former WHO/ISUP 1998)[36] (Box 5.2) have been recommended until the latter is sufficiently validated[37,38] (Figure 5.6).

Bladder cancer may develop via a variety of pathways.[6,23,30,39–41] Most tumors have a papillary

| **Box 5.1** Grading of non-invasive papillary urothelial neoplasia according to the WHO 1973 grading system |
| --- |
| Urothelial papilloma |
| Grade 1 papillary urothelial carcinoma |
| Grade 2 papillary urothelial carcinoma |
| Grade 3 papillary urothelial carcinoma |

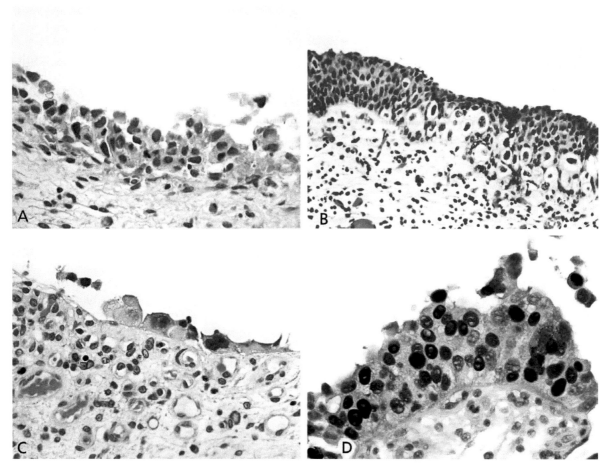

**Fig. 5.5**
**A** Loss of cellular polarity and cohesiveness in urothelial carcinoma in situ (CIS). **B** Pagetoid spread of urothelial CIS. **C** Urothelial CIS, clinging type. **D** P53 overexpression in urothelial CIS.

---

**Box 5.2** Grading of non-invasive papillary urothelial neoplasia according to the WHO 2004 grading system

Urothelial papilloma

Papillary urothelial neoplasm of low malignant potential

Low-grade papillary urothelial carcinoma

High-grade papillary urothelial carcinoma

---

configuration at diagnosis.[21] Such low-grade, mucosal-confined tumors may recur, but have a low progression rate.[37] Additional genetic changes may induce the development of higher grade papillary lesions. The WHO 2004 classification recommends stratifying patients according to stage, i.e. non-invasive papillary (stage Ta) and invasive (stage T1–4).[7,8] Approximately 80% of patients with primary non-invasive urothelial carcinoma will display a relatively indolent low-grade tumor with a recurrence rate as high as 70%, thus necessitating frequent, costly, long-term follow-up.[42,43] In addition, up to one-third of recurrent superficial tumors may eventually progress to a higher grade and/or stage.[37]

Clearly, urothelial carcinoma represents a heterogeneous entity with significant malignant potential.[2] The most important predictors of clinical course in non-invasive urothelial tumors are pathologic grade, multiplicity, early recurrence, and tumor size, but the presence of dysplasia and CIS in the adjacent urothelium can also be relevant.[3,20,30,31] Several classifications have been reported in the literature, and current genetic data suggest two major pathways that correspond to morphologically-defined entities. The genetically stable category includes low-grade (grade 1 and some grade 2, WHO 1973 scheme) non-invasive papillary tumors[7,21]; the genetically unstable category contains high-grade (some grade 2 and all grade 3, WHO 1973 scheme) non-invasive and CIS, and invasively growing carcinomas (stage T1–4). Non-invasive low-grade bladder neoplasms have only few genomic alterations and are therefore viewed as genetically stable.

Some classifications and grading schemes of the urothelial neoplasms have been reported in the literature.[2,44] The recent WHO 2004 (former WHO/ISUP 1998) classification reflects work in progress.[21] The WHO

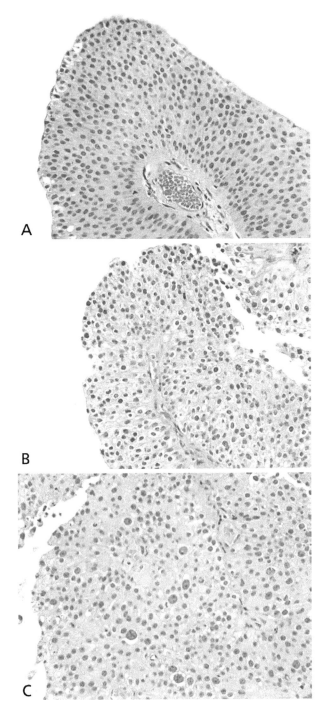

**Fig. 5.6**
Grading of non-invasive papillary urothelial neoplasia. **A** Papillary urothelial neoplasm of low malignant potential (formerly designated as WHO 1973 grade 1 urothelial carcinoma). **B** Low-grade urothelial carcinoma (formerly designated as WHO 1973 grade 2 urothelial carcinoma). **C** High-grade urothelial carcinoma (formerly designated as WHO 1973 grade 3 urothelial carcinoma).

1973 classification is preferred by some authors as it allowed valid comparison of results between different clinical centers. The standard WHO 1973 classification and grading of bladder tumors is a robust, clinically

proven, widely-used, time-tested, and reasonably reproducible method for pathologic reporting, and therefore is still recommended.[9,45] Some controversies followed the introduction of the WHO/ISUP 1998 classification of bladder tumors, mainly because of lack of validation, reproducibility, and translation studies. In particular, there is a poor interobserver agreement for papillary urothelial neoplasms of low malignant potential (PUNLMP) and low-grade urothelial carcinoma ($\kappa=0.12-0.50$).[46] After structured training for the new WHO/ISUP 1998 grading system, Murphy et al concluded that neither refinements of morphologic criteria nor additional education would significantly decrease interpretive discrepancy in the grading of urothelial carcinoma.[46] In a recent study, Bol et al found that agreement among three experienced pathologists on the diagnosis of PUNLMP was 0%.[47] Using the WHO 1999 classification system, the distribution of papilloma, PUNLMP, and grade 1, 2, and 3 urothelial carcinoma was 0.8%, 0%, 50.8%, 25.4%, and 23% respectively, after second review among three pathologists.[47] Oyasu believed that the new term 'PUNLMP' should not be used in bladder classification, considering that bladder cancer is a disease of field change and that progression to a high-grade cancer is a common event among patients who are constantly exposed to carcinogens.[48]

The natural history shows that bladder cancer is actually two diseases. The first is non-invasive, low-grade papillary urothelial tumors (PUNLMP and low grade), previously classified as grade 1 and characterized by genetic stability with common chromosome 9 alterations and frequent FGFR3 mutations.[49] These tumors have a high propensity to recur but rarely invade or metastasize. The second type of bladder cancer is the high-grade lesion that originates as urothelial dysplasia and begins as CIS or non-invasive high-grade papillary carcinoma (grade 3 and some grade 2, WHO 1973 scheme). They have common alterations at the TP53 and RB tumor suppressor genes. Both types of neoplasm can develop in the same patient, either simultaneously or sequentially.

According to the WHO 2004 classification, non-invasive papillary urothelial lesions distinguish urothelial papilloma and inverted papilloma, PUNLMP, and non-invasive low- and high-grade urothelial carcinoma.[21,50] The main clinicopathologic features of these categories follow.

## UROTHELIAL PAPILLOMA, INVERTED PAPILLOMA AND DIFFUSE PAPILLOMATOSIS

Urothelial papilloma is a benign exophytic neoplasia composed of a delicate fibrovascular core covered by normal-looking urothelium[51,52] (Figure 5.7). The superficial cells are often prominent. Mitoses are absent to rare and, if present, are located in the basal cell layer.

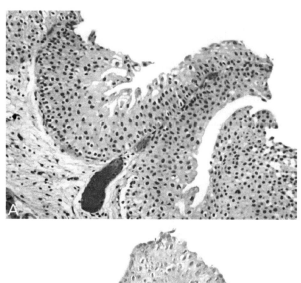

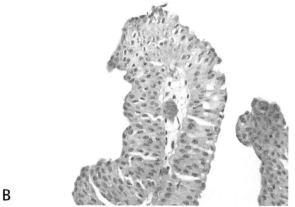

**Fig. 5.7**
A, B Urothelial papilloma.

The stroma may show edema and/or inflammatory cells. Diffuse papillomatosis applies when the mucosa is extensively involved by small delicate papillary processes creating a velvety cystoscopic appearance. Papillomas are diploid with low proliferation, uncommon p53 expression, and frequent (75%) FGFR3 mutation.[49] Cytokeratin 20 expression is limited to the superficial (umbrella) cells as is usual in normal urothelium.[25] The incidence is below 1% of all bladder tumors and the male:female ratio is 1.9:1. Hematuria is common. Most papillomas are single and occur in younger patients (mean age 46 years), close to the ureteric orifices in most cases. Urothelial papilloma may recur; however, it does not progress.

Inverted papilloma applies to a benign urothelial tumor that has an inverted growth pattern with normal to minimal cytologic atypia of the cells.[51,53] Most cases are solitary polypoid lesions, <3 cm, and arise in the bladder trigone; however, they can also be found along the urinary tract. At histology, inverted papilloma has a smooth surface covered by normal urothelium, and endophytic cords of urothelial cells invaginating extensively from the surface urothelium into the subjacent lamina propria but not into the muscular bladder wall. Trabecular and glandular have been described. Foci of nonkeratinizing squamous metaplasia

and neuroendocrine differentiation have been reported. Focal minor cytologic atypia may be present but mitotic figures are not seen or are very rare. Inverted papilloma may coexist with carcinoma. The male:female ratio is 4–5:1. The age of patients ranges from 10 to 94 years. Hematuria or obstructive symptoms are common and less than 1% of cases recur.[53]

## PAPILLARY UROTHELIAL NEOPLASM OF LOW MALIGNANT POTENTIAL

Papillary urothelial neoplasm of low malignant potential (PUNLMP) is a controversial lesion defined as non-invasive papillary urothelial tumor which resembles exophytic urothelial papilloma but shows increased cellularity exceeding the thickness of normal urothelium. At cystoscopy, most cases are solitary, 1–2 cm in diameter and located in the lateral or posterior wall, close to the ureteric orifices.[54] The papillae are slender without fusion and lined by multilayered urothelium with minimal to absent cytologic atypia. The cell polarity is preserved with minimal variation in the architecture. The nuclei are slightly enlarged. The superficial cell layer is often preserved. Mitoses are rare and have a basal location.

These tumors are considered non-invasive grade 1 papillary urothelial carcinoma in the WHO 1973 scheme. Most are diploid with a low proliferation rate, but show frequent FGFR3 mutation and allelic loss in 80% and 81% of cases, respectively.[16,49] Gross or microscopic hematuria is frequent.[54] The male:female ratio is 5:1 and the mean age at diagnosis is 65 years (range 29–94 years). Mean reported tumor recurrence, stage progression, and tumor-related mortality occur in approximately 35%, 4%, and 2% of patients, respectively.[37] In some series, stage progression can be as high as 8%.[37,55]

## NON-INVASIVE PAPILLARY UROTHELIAL CARCINOMA, LOW AND HIGH GRADE

### LOW-GRADE TUMOR

A low-grade neoplasm of urothelium lining papillary fronds shows recognizable variations in architecture and cytology. The tumor shows slender papillae with frequent branching, minimal fusion, and variations in nuclear polarity, size, shape, and chromatin pattern and with presence of nucleoli. Mitoses may occur at any level in those cases of low grade.[21,37,50] These cases are considered as grade 1 or grade 2 in the WHO 1973 classification scheme. Altered expression of cytokeratin 20, CD44, p53, and p63 is frequent, some tumors being diploid. FGFR3 mutations are seen in about the same frequency as that for PUNLMP.[49] The male:female ratio is 2.9:1 and the mean age at diagnosis is 70 years (range 28–90 years). Most patients present with hematuria and have a single tumor in the posterior or lateral wall; however, 22% of them have two or more tumors. Tumor recurrence, stage progression, and tumor-related mortality are approximately 50%, 10%, and 5%, respectively, but stage progression can be as high as 13% in some series.

## HIGH-GRADE TUMOR

In high-grade tumors (all grade 3 and some grade 2, WHO 1973 scheme) the urothelium lining papillary fronds show a predominant disorder with moderate-to-marked architectural and cytologic atypia with the papillae frequently fused and variations in architectural and cytologic features that are easily recognizable even at scanning power.[37,50] The nuclei are often pleomorphic with prominent nucleoli and altered polarity. Mitoses are frequent. The thickness of the urothelium varies considerably. Carcinoma in situ is frequent in the adjacent mucosa. Changes in cytokeratin 20, p53, and p63 expression and aneuploidy are more frequent than in previous categories. Molecular alterations in these tumors show a frequency of p53, HER2 or EGFR overexpression, and p21Waf1 or p27Kip1 loss comparable to that seen in invasive cancers.[56,57] Genetically, high-grade non-invasive lesions (pTa G3) resemble invasively-growing tumors. A comparative genomic hybridization-based study showed deletions at 2q, 5q, 10q, and 18q as well as gains at 5p and 20q.[21] Hematuria is common and the endoscopic appearance varies from papillary to nodular/solid single or multiple tumors. Progression in terms of stage and death due to disease can be observed in as many as 65% of patients.[37]

## INFILTRATING UROTHELIAL CARCINOMA

Infiltrating urothelial carcinoma is defined as a urothelial tumor that invades beyond the basement membrane. Infiltrative carcinomas grossly span a range of morphology including papillary, polypoid, nodular, solid, ulcerative or transmural diffuse. They may be solitary or multifocal.

The histology of infiltrating urothelial carcinomas is variable and includes pT1–4 tumors. Most pT1 carcinomas are papillary, low or high grade, whereas most pT2–4 carcinomas are infiltrating and high grade, and therefore will be discussed separately. According to the new WHO 2004 classification,[36] infiltrating urothelial carcinomas are graded as low or high, depending upon the degree of nuclear anaplasia and architectural abnormalities. The WHO 1973 grading system (grade 1, 2, and 3)[35] has also been widely used by pathologists and will be discussed in Chapter 6.

## BLADDER CARCINOMA WITH EARLY STROMAL INVASION (STAGE T1)

Stage is the single most important prognostic indicator in urothelial carcinoma.[1,6,58] Infiltrating urothelial carcinoma is defined by the World Health Organization as a urothelial tumor that invades beyond the basement membrane. The 2002 TNM (tumor, lymph nodes, and metastasis) staging system defines pT1 tumors of the bladder as those invading the lamina propria but not the muscularis propria.[7,59] Although pT1 tumors have a less favorable prognosis than pTa (non-invasive) tumors, clinically they are both usually lumped together under the term 'superficial' bladder tumors,[14,60,61] a practice no longer recommended.[9,50] Muscularis mucosae is often present in the lamina propria and consists of thin and wavy fascicles of smooth muscle, which are frequently associated with large caliber blood vessels (Figure 5.8A). Muscularis mucosae invasion (pT1) (Figure 5.8B) should not be mistaken for muscularis propria invasion (pT2). It is unacceptable to simply state 'smooth muscle invasion' in the pathology

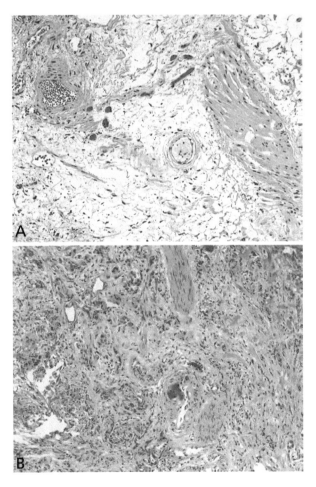

**Fig. 5.8**
**A** Muscularis mucosae in the urinary bladder. **B** pT1 tumor with muscularis mucosae invasion.

report. The presence or absence of muscularis propria should also be mentioned in the pathology report for the adequacy of resection.

The nature of submitted specimens is important in assessing pT1 tumors.[8] Most bladder tumors are frequently excised by cold-cup biopsies and transurethral resection of bladder tumor (TURBT). The resulting hematoxylin and eosin (H&E) sections in cold-cup biopsies usually contain urothelial neoplasm (usually <1 cm in diameter), the lamina propria, and sometimes the superficial muscularis propria with maintained orientation, thus facilitating assessment of early invasion. Larger tumors (>1 cm) usually require TURBT, in which the urologist should include a generous sampling of the underlying muscularis propria in order to enable adequate pathologic staging. The specimens resulting from this procedure are often fragmented, heavily cauterized, and tangentially sectioned with frequent disruption of the tumor architecture, and thus may be difficult to orient. While examining and reporting on both types of specimen, it is important to note the presence or absence of muscularis propria in the pathology report in order to assess involvement by the neoplastic process, and to provide feedback to the urologist regarding adequacy of resection.

An additional feature of importance in the evaluation of bladder tumor specimens is the presence of vascular invasion, which can involve blood vessels or lymphatic channels[62] (Figure 5.9A). The identification of vascular/lymphatic invasion can be difficult because, on conventional evaluation, it can be confused with artifactual clefting around nests of invasive carcinoma.[8] Because vascular invasion is frequently overdiagnosed in H&E stained slides, the reported prognostic significance of that factor remains uncertain.[63,64] In suspicious cases, blood vessels should be highlighted by immuno-peroxidase staining for factor VIII related antigen or, more appropriately, by using monoclonal antibodies against CD31 or CD34 (Figure 5.9B). Staining will not resolve the problem of differentiating lymphatic versus artifactual space entrapment by tumor cells in selected cases, and this type of involvement should be reported as indeterminate for vascular invasion.[8] The incidence of vascular/lymphatic invasion is variable and has been reported to range from 5% to 10% of stage pT1 cases in immunohistochemical studies.[63,65] In one study, 5-year survival was 81% for pT1 patients without vascular invasion and 44% for those with vascular invasion, suggesting that vascular invasion is an independent predictor of poor outcome regardless of tumor grade.[63] Vascular invasion is more frequent in larger, high-grade tumors without papillary configuration.

The clinical significance of vascular invasion in advanced infiltrating disease is controversial, with some authors reporting differences in biologic behavior. Leissner et al[66] and Bassi et al[67] found blood vessel

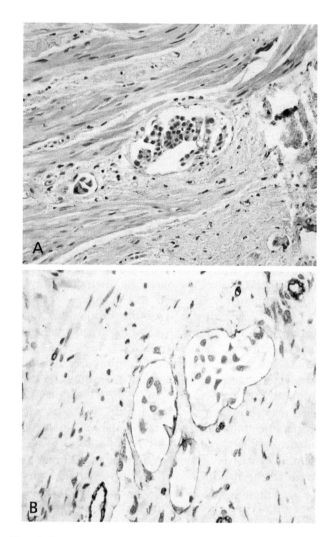

**Fig. 5.9**
A Vascular invasion. B CD34 immunostaining highlights endothelial cells.

invasion, as well as nodal status and tumor stage, to be an independent predictor in patients treated with radical cystectomy. Also, vascular/lymphatic invasion might be an independent prognostic factor in organ-confined invasive bladder cancer (Lerner SP, personal communication). Therefore, the presence of vascular/lymphatic invasion should be included in the pathology report.[38]

It is of paramount importance to distinguish T1 from Ta tumors. The main morphologic diagnostic criteria for invasion into the lamina propria are discussed briefly in the following section.

## DIAGNOSIS OF LAMINA PROPRIA INVASION: GENERAL FEATURES

The recognition of lamina propria invasion by urothelial carcinoma is one of the most challenging fields in surgical pathology, and the pathologist should follow strict criteria in its assessment.[8] While evaluating tumor invasion, it is important to focus on the following features (Box 5.3).

---

**Box 5.3**  Diagnosis of lamina propria invasion (T1)

1. General features
   - Histologic grade
   - Stroma–epithelial interface (morphologic appearance of the basement membrane)
   - Invading epithelium
   - Stromal response

2. Lamina propria invasion in specific bladder tumors
   - Carcinoma in situ with microinvasion (CISmic)
   - Papillary urothelial carcinoma with microinvasion
   - Papillary urothelial carcinoma with invasion into the 'stalk'
   - Well-established invasion into underlying lamina propria
   - Urothelial carcinoma with endophytic or broad front growth pattern

3. Pitfalls in the diagnosis of stage pT1 bladder carcinoma
   - Tangential sectioning and poor orientation
   - Obscuring inflammation
   - Thermal injury
   - CIS involving von Brunn's nests
   - Muscle invasion indeterminate for type of muscle
   - Variants of urothelial carcinoma with deceptively bland cytology
   - Pseudoinvasive nests of benign proliferative urothelial lesions

---

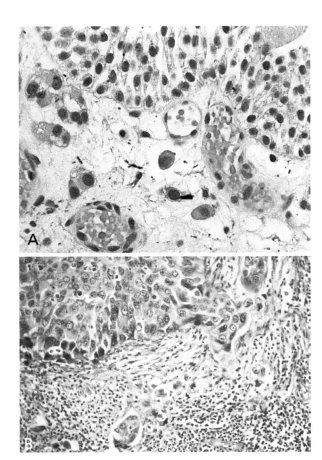

**Fig. 5.10**
**A** Early invasion of urothelial carcinoma (pT1). **B** Individual tumor cells percolating through the stroma in microinvasive urothelial carcinoma (pT1).

## HISTOLOGIC GRADE

Lamina propria invasion should be carefully evaluated in all high-grade papillary carcinomas.[68] While invasion is not necessarily an unexpected finding in low grade tumors, it is much more commonly encountered in high-grade lesions, reaching 70% to 96% in some series.[9,61,68]

## STROMA–EPITHELIAL INTERFACE (MORPHOLOGIC APPEARANCE OF THE BASEMENT MEMBRANE)

Tangentially sectioned, densely packed, non-invasive papillary tumors exhibit a stroma–epithelial interface that is smooth and regular.[69] In instances of true invasion, variably sized and irregularly-shaped nests or individual tumor cells percolating through the stroma are likely to be seen (Figure 5.10). When the specimen includes tangential sections through non-invasive tumor, or when urothelial carcinoma involves von Brunn's nests, the basement membrane preserves a regular contour, whereas it is frequently absent or disrupted in cases of true invasion. This feature may be assessed on H&E stains; however, in many cases, additional clues are needed, including the detection of a parallel array of thin-walled vessels that evenly line the

basement membrane of non-invasive nests, these being absent in patients with invasive tumors.

## HISTOLOGIC CHARACTERISTICS OF THE INVADING EPITHELIUM

The invasive front of the neoplasm may show one of several features: single cells or irregularly shaped nests of tumor within the stroma, and sometimes tentacular or finger-like extensions can be seen arising from the base of the papillary tumor. Frequently, the invading nests appear morphologically different from cells at the base of the non-invasive component of the tumor, with more abundant cytoplasm and often with a higher degree of nuclear pleomorphism.[8] In some cases, particularly in microinvasive disease, the invasive tumor cells may acquire abundant eosinophilic cytoplasm. At low to medium power magnification, these microinvasive cells seem to be more differentiated than the overlying non-invasive disease, a feature known as paradoxical differentiation (Figure 5.11).[69]

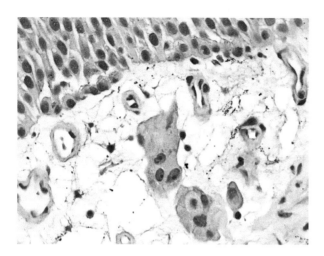

**Fig. 5.11**
Paradoxical differentiation in microinvasive urothelial carcinoma.

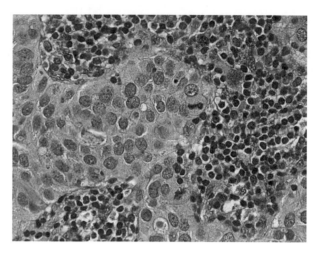

**Fig. 5.13**
Tumor cells may elicit heavy inflammatory response in the stroma.

## STROMAL RESPONSE

The stromal reaction in the lamina propria associated with invasive tumor may be inflammatory, myxoid, or fibrous, and assessment of this provides an important diagnostic clue. Although the majority of bladder tumors with unquestionable lamina propria invasion exhibit some sort of stromal reaction, microinvasive disease usually does not, making its identification even more difficult.

In some cases, a retraction artifact around superficially invasive individual tumor cells may mimic angiolymphatic invasion (Figure 5.12). Often, this finding is focal, and may itself be one of the early signs of invasion into the lamina propria. Lamina propria invasion may elicit a brisk inflammatory response (Figure 5.13). Numerous inflammatory cells in the

lamina propria may obscure the interface between epithelium and stroma. This makes small nests or single-cell invasion difficult to recognize.

In other cases, a cellular stroma with spindled fibroblasts, variable collagenization, inflammation, and/or a hypocellular stroma with myxoid background may be seen in invasive urothelial carcinomas. Rarely, the tumor induces an exuberant proliferation of fibroblasts, which may display alarming cellular atypia (similar to giant cell cystitis). This feature, although a helpful clue to invasion, should not be mistaken for the spindle cell component of a sarcomatoid urothelial carcinoma.

## INVASIVE UROTHELIAL CARCINOMA, CONVENTIONAL TYPE (STAGE T2–4)

Invasive urothelial carcinoma may present as polypoid, sessile, ulcerated or infiltrative tumor (Figure 5.14A) in which the neoplastic cells invade the bladder wall as nests, cords, trabeculae, small clusters or single cells that are often separated by a desmoplastic stroma. The tumor sometimes grows in a more diffuse, sheet-like pattern, but, even in these cases, focal nests and clusters are generally present. The cells show moderate to abundant amphophilic or eosinophilic cytoplasm and large hyperchromatic nuclei (Figure 5.14B,C). In larger nests, palisading of nuclei may be seen at the edges of the nests. The nucleus is typically pleomorphic and often has irregular contours with angular profiles. Nuclear grooves may be identified in some cells. Nucleoli are highly variable in number and appearance, with some cells containing single or multiple small nucleoli and others having large eosinophilic nucleoli. Foci of marked pleomorphism may be seen, with bizarre and

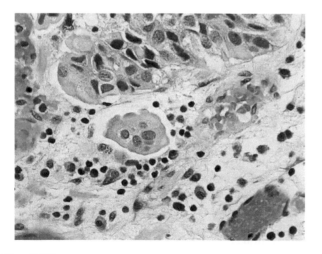

**Fig. 5.12**
Artifactual retraction of tumor cells may mimic vascular invasion.

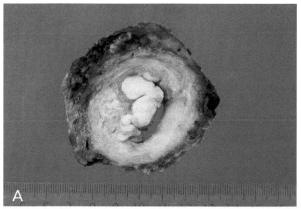

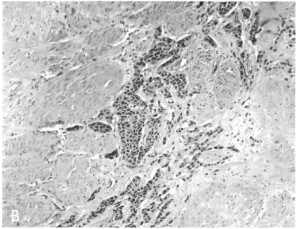

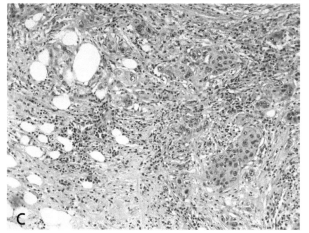

**Fig. 5.14**
Invasive urothelial carcinoma. **A** Gross appearance of papillary invasive urothelial carcinoma. **B** Urothelial carcinoma invading into muscularis propria wall. **C** Extravesical adipose tissue involvement by urothelial carcinoma.

multinuclear tumor cells. Mitotic figures are common, with numerous abnormal forms.

Invasive tumors are invariably high grade, although there is a spectrum of some cases exhibiting marked anaplasia with focal giant cell formation. A subset of invasive urothelial carcinomas may exhibit vascular invasion. The most important morphology-based prognostic factors in patients with advanced bladder

cancer are tumor stage and lymph node status. In an attempt to identify new parameters for assessing prognosis in bladder cancer patients more accurately, Jimenez et al have recently introduced a new morphologic classification of invasive bladder tumors, distinguishing three patterns of growth: nodular, trabecular, and infiltrative.[68] Tumors with an infiltrative growth pattern are associated with a worse prognosis than tumor displaying a non-infiltrative (nodular or trabecular) growth pattern.

## HISTOLOGIC VARIANTS OF UROTHELIAL CARCINOMA

Urothelial carcinoma has a propensity for divergent differentiation, with the most common being squamous, followed by glandular. Virtually the whole spectrum of bladder cancer variants may be seen in variable proportions accompanying otherwise typical urothelial carcinoma. The clinical outcome of some of these variants differs from typical urothelial carcinoma; therefore, recognition of these variants is important (Box 5.4).

## UROTHELIAL CARCINOMA WITH MIXED DIFFERENTIATION

About 20% of urothelial carcinomas contain areas of squamous or glandular differentiation.[70]

---

**Box 5.4**  Variants of urothelial carcinoma

1. Mixed differentiation
   - With squamous differentiation
   - With glandular differentiation
   - Other (specify type and %)
2. Small cell carcinoma
3. Nested variant
4. Micropapillary carcinoma
5. Microcystic carcinoma
6. Lymphoepithelioma-like carcinoma
7. Plasmacytoid/lymphoma-like carcinoma
8. Inverted papilloma-like carcinoma
9. Urothelial carcinoma with syncytiotrophoblastic giant cells
10. Giant cell carcinoma
11. Clear cell (glycogen-rich) urothelial carcinoma
12. Sarcomatoid carcinoma (carcinosarcoma)
13. Lipoid-cell variant
14. Undifferentiated carcinoma
15. Urothelial carcinoma with unusual stromal reactions
    - Pseudosarcomatous stroma
    - Stromal osseous or cartilaginous metaplasia
    - Osteoclast-type giant cells
    - Prominent lymphoid infiltrate

## SQUAMOUS DIFFERENTIATION

Defined by the presence of intercellular bridges or keratinization, squamous differentiation occurs in 21% of urothelial carcinomas of the bladder. Its frequency increases with grade and stage. Detailed histologic maps of urothelial carcinoma with squamous differentiation have shown that the proportion of the squamous component may vary considerably, with some cases having urothelial CIS as the only urothelial component. These cases may have a less favorable response to therapy than pure urothelial carcinoma.[71–74] Of 91 patients with metastatic carcinoma, 83% with mixed adenocarcinoma and 46% with mixed squamous cell carcinoma experienced disease progression despite intensive chemotherapy, whereas it progressed in <30% of patients with pure urothelial carcinoma.[74] Low-grade urothelial carcinoma with focal squamous differentiation has a higher recurrence rate.[73] Tumors with any identifiable urothelial element are classified as urothelial carcinoma with squamous differentiation, and an estimate of the percentage of squamous component should be provided (Figure 5.15A).[8] Cytokeratin 14, L1 antigen and caveolin-1 have been reported as immunohistochemical markers of squamous differentiation.[8,75]

## GLANDULAR DIFFERENTIATION

Glandular differentiation (Figure 5.15B) is less common than squamous differentiation and may be present in about 6% of urothelial carcinomas of the bladder.[73] Glandular differentiation is defined as the presence of true glandular spaces within the tumor. These may be tubular or enteric glands with mucin secretion. A colloid–mucinous pattern characterized by nests of cells 'floating' in extracellular mucin, occasionally with signet ring cells, may be present.[73] Cytoplasmic mucin-containing cells are present in 14% to 63% of typical urothelial carcinoma and are not considered to represent glandular differentiation.[76,77] The diagnosis of adenocarcinoma is reserved for pure tumors. A tumor with mixed glandular and urothelial differentiation is classified as urothelial carcinoma with glandular differentiation, and an estimate of the percentage of glandular component should be provided.[8] The expression of MUC5AC-apomucin may be useful as an immunohistochemical marker of glandular differentiation in urothelial tumors.[76,77] When small cell carcinoma is present in association with urothelial carcinoma, even focally, it portends a poor prognosis. Small cell carcinoma is an important finding and usually dictates more aggressive therapy (see following section).[78]

## SMALL CELL CARCINOMA

Small cell carcinoma is a malignant neuroendocrine neoplasm derived from the urothelium that histologically mimics its pulmonary counterpart. Patients with small cell carcinoma of the urinary bladder have a dismal prognosis. In a recent series of 64 cases of small cell carcinoma of the urinary bladder,[78] the mean age at diagnosis was 66 years and the male:female ratio was 3.3:1; 88% presented with hematuria. All the patients except one had muscle-invasive disease at presentation. Thirty-eight patients (59%) underwent cystectomy and 66% of patients had lymph node metastasis at the time of cystectomy, with regional lymph nodes, bone, liver, and lung being the most common locations. Twenty cases (32%) were pure small cell carcinoma; 44 cases (68%) consisted of small cell carcinoma with other histologic types (urothelial carcinoma, 35 cases; adenocarcinoma, 4 cases; sarcomatoid urothelial carcinoma, 2 cases; and 3 cases with both adenocarcinoma and urothelial carcinoma). None of the clinicopathologic parameters (age, sex, presenting symptoms, smoking history, the presence of a non-small cell carcinoma component, chemotherapy or radiation therapy) was associated with survival. No significant survival difference was found

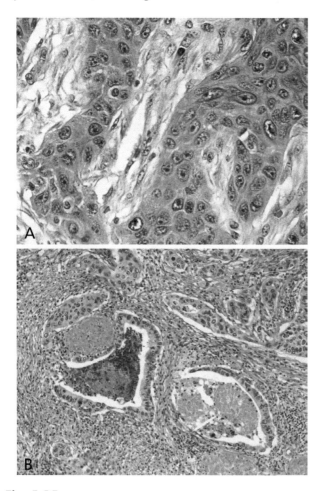

**Fig. 5.15**
Urothelial carcinoma with mixed differentiation. **A** Squamous differentiation. **B** Glandular differentiation.

between patients who underwent cystectomy and those who did not receive cystectomy (p=0.65).[78] Patients with organ-confined cancers had marginally better survival than those with non-organ-confined cancer (p=0.06). Overall, 12-month, 18-month, 3-year, and 5-year cancer-specific survivals were 56%, 41%, 23%, and 16%, respectively. The prognosis of small cell carcinoma of the urinary bladder remains poor irrespective of therapy. Electrolyte abnormalities such as hypercalcemia or hypophosphatemia, and ectopic secretion of ACTH have also been reported as part of the paraneoplastic syndrome associated with primary small cell carcinoma of the bladder.

At gross examination, most tumors appear as large, solid, isolated, polypoid, nodular masses with or without ulceration, and may extensively infiltrate the bladder wall. The vesical lateral walls and the dome are the most frequent topographies but rare cases may arise in a diverticulum.[7] At histology, tumors consist of small, rather uniform cells, with nuclear molding, scant cytoplasm, and nuclei containing finely stippled chromatin and inconspicuous nucleoli (Figure 5.16).

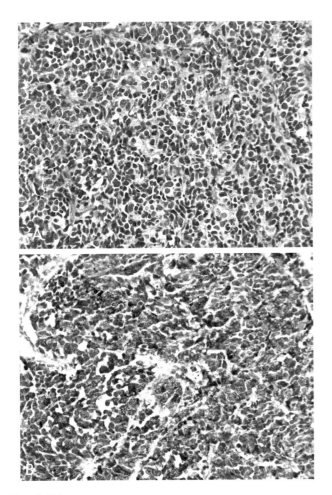

**Fig. 5.16**
A Small cell carcinoma of the urinary bladder. B Neuro-endocrine marker (chromogranin A) was positive in this tumor.

Mitoses are present and may be frequent. Necrosis is common, and there may be DNA encrustation of blood vessel walls (Azzopardi phenomenon). Most patients have areas of urothelial carcinoma, sometimes in the form of flat urothelial CIS, and, exceptionally, squamous cell carcinoma, adenocarcinoma or sarcomatoid carcinoma. This is important, because the presence of these differentiated areas does not contradict the diagnosis of small cell carcinoma.[79] Neuroendocrine granules are found with electron microscopy, but the immunohistochemical profile reveals neuronal-specific enolase in 87% of cases, and chromogranin A in only a third of cases. Some cases are also reactive against synaptophysin, PGP 9.5, thyroid transcription factor-1 (TTF1), p53 (DO7), and Ki67 (MIB1).[80–82]

The diagnosis of small cell carcinoma can be made on morphologic grounds alone, even if neuro-endocrine differentiation cannot be demonstrated. Frequently, small cell carcinoma expresses cytokeratin which supports the hypothesis of urothelial origin. The recent finding of c-kit and c-erbB2 expression by immunohistochemistry opens new possibilities for therapy in small cell carcinoma of the bladder.[82,83] Data obtained by comparative genomic hybridization suggest that urinary bladder small cell carcinoma is a genetically unstable tumor, typically exhibiting a high number of cytogenetic abnormalities. The differential diagnosis is metastasis of a small cell carcinoma from another site, lymphoma, lympho-epithelioma-like carcinoma, plasmacytoid carcinoma, and a poorly differentiated urothelial carcinoma.[84]

## NESTED VARIANT

The nested variant of urothelial carcinoma is an aggressive neoplasm with fewer than 50 reported cases. There is a marked male predominance, and 70% of patients died 4–40 months after diagnosis, in spite of therapy.[85] This rare pattern of urothelial carcinoma was first described as a tumor with a 'deceptively benign' appearance that closely resembles Brunn's nests infiltrating the lamina propria (Figure 5.17A).[86,87] Some nests have small tubular lumens that eventually can predominate. Nuclei generally show little or no atypia, but invariably the tumor contains foci or unequivocal cancer with cells exhibiting enlarged nucleoli and coarse nuclear chromatin. This feature is most apparent in the deeper aspects of the cancer.[87–92] The differential diagnosis of the nested variant of urothelial carcinoma includes prominent Brunn's nests, cystitis cystica and glandularis, inverted papilloma, nephrogenic metaplasia, carcinoid tumor, paraganglionic tissue, and paraganglioma.[93–95]

## MICROPAPILLARY CARCINOMA

Micropapillary carcinoma (Figure 5.17B) is a distinct variant of urothelial carcinoma that resembles papillary serous carcinoma of the ovary; approximately 60 cases have been reported in the literature. There is a male predominance and the patients' ages range from the fifth to the ninth decade with a mean age of 66 years. The most common presenting symptom is hematuria. The first description of micropapillary carcinoma consisted of 18 patients whose ages ranged from 47 to 81 years (mean 67 years) with a male:female ratio of 5:1.[90,96,97] Seven patients died of carcinoma. The micropapillary component is found in association with non-invasive papillary or invasive urothelial carcinoma in 80% of reported cases, consisting of slender delicate filiform processes or small papillary clusters of tumor cells; when

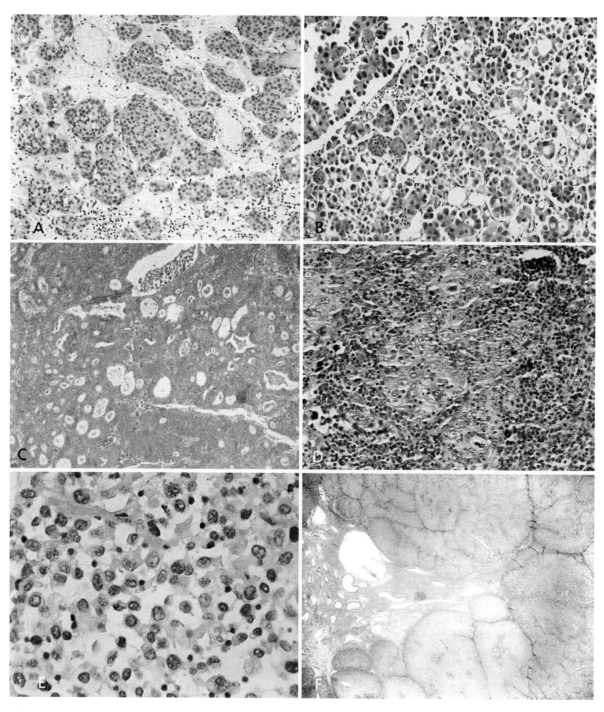

**Fig. 5.17**
Variants of urothelial carcinoma. **A** Nested variant. **B** Micropapillary variant. **C** Microcystic variant.
**D** Lymphoepithelioma-like carcinoma. **E** Plasmacytoma-like carcinoma. **F** Inverted papilloma-like carcinoma.

present in invasive carcinoma, it is composed of infiltrating tight clusters of micropapillary aggregates that are often within lacunae that are negative for endothelial markers.[98] Twenty-five percent of cases show glandular differentiation, and some authors consider it as a variant of adenocarcinoma.[99] Psammoma bodies are infrequent. Vascular and lymphatic invasion are common, and most cases show invasion of the muscularis propria or deeper, often with metastases. Immunohistochemical studies in one large series disclosed immunoreactivity of the micropapillary carcinoma in 20 of 20 cases for epithelial membrane antigen (EMA), cytokeratin 7 and 20, and Leu-M1. The presence of a surface micropapillary component in bladder biopsy specimens with cancer is an unfavorable prognostic feature, and deeper biopsies may be useful to determine the level of muscle invasion. The main differential consideration is serous micropapillary ovarian carcinoma in women or mesothelioma in both genders.[96]

## MICROCYSTIC CARCINOMA

The microcystic variant of invasive urothelial carcinoma is characterized by the formation of microcysts, macrocysts, or tubular structures with cysts ranging from microscopic up to 1–2 cm in diameter (Figure 5.17C).[97] The cysts and tubules may be empty or contain necrotic debris or mucin that stains with periodic acid–Schiff stain with diastase predigestion. This variant of cancer may be confused with benign proliferations such as florid polypoid cystitis cystica and glandularis and nephrogenic metaplasia. This pattern should be separated from the nested variant of urothelial carcinoma with tubular differentiation.[91]

## LYMPHOEPITHELIOMA-LIKE CARCINOMA

Carcinoma that histologically resembles lympho-epithelioma of the nasopharynx has recently been described in the urinary bladder, with fewer than 40 cases reported.[84,90,100,101] Disease in the urinary bladder is more common in men than in women (3:1 ratio) and occurs in late adulthood (range 52–81 years; mean 69 years).[101,102] Most patients present with hematuria. The tumor is solitary and usually involves the dome, posterior wall, or trigone, often with a sessile growth pattern. Histologically, it may be pure or mixed with typical urothelial carcinoma, the latter being focal and inconspicuous in some instances. Glandular and squamous differentiation may be seen. The tumor is composed of nests, sheets, and cords of undifferentiated cells with large pleomorphic nuclei and prominent nucleoli (Figure 5.17D). The cytoplasmic borders are poorly defined, imparting a syncytial appearance. The

background consists of a prominent lymphoid stroma that includes T and B lymphocytes, plasma cells, histiocytes, and occasional neutrophils or eosinophils. Epstein–Barr virus infection has not been identified in lymphoepithelioma-like carcinoma of the bladder.[84,103] Thus far, this tumor has been found to be responsive to chemotherapy when it is encountered in its pure form.[84] The epithelial cells stain with several cytokeratin markers—AE1/AE3, CK8, CK7—and are rarely positive for CK20. The major differential diagnostic considerations are poorly differentiated urothelial carcinoma with lymphoid stroma, poorly differentiated squamous cell carcinoma, and lymphoma. Immuno-histochemistry reveals cytokeratin immunoreactivity in the malignant cells, confirming their epithelial nature. Most reported cases of the urinary bladder had a relatively favorable prognosis when pure or predominant, but when lymphoepithelioma-like carcinoma is focally present in an otherwise typical urothelial carcinoma, the disease behaves as it does in patients with conventional urothelial carcinoma of the same grade and stage.

## LYMPHOMA-LIKE OR PLASMACYTOMA-LIKE CARCINOMA

Zukerberg et al[104] described two patients with bladder carcinoma that diffusely permeated the bladder wall and was composed of cells with a monotonous appearance, mimicking lymphoma. The tumor cells were medium sized, with eosinophilic cytoplasm and eccentric nuclei producing a plasmacytoid appearance (Figure 5.17E). The epithelial nature of the malignancy was confirmed by immunohistochemistry. Differential diagnostic considerations include lymphoma (plasmacytoid type) and multiple myeloma. Identification of an epithelial component confirms the diagnosis. In a series report of six cases, the male:female ratio was 2:1, and the age range was 54–73 years. All cases stained positively for cytokeratin cocktail, cytokeratin 20 and 7, and all were negative for leukocyte common antigen. Five of six patients died of disease (mean survival, 23 months).[105]

## INVERTED PAPILLOMA-LIKE CARCINOMA

The potential for misinterpretation of urothelial carcinoma with endophytic growth as inverted papilloma is high.[87,106,107] By definition, this variant of urothelial carcinoma has significant nuclear pleomorphism, mitotic figures, and architectural abnormalities consistent with low- or high-grade urothelial carcinoma (Figure 5.17F). In most cases, the overlying epithelium has similar abnormalities and often contains typical urothelial carcinoma. Inverted papilloma-type carcinomas with minimal cytologic and architectural abnormalities have high mitotic activity. An exophytic papillary or invasive component is often associated with the inverted element. However, in cases of inverted papilloma fragmented during transurethral resection, a pseudoexophytic pattern may result. In some instances, both inverted papilloma and inverted papilloma-type carcinoma are intimately mixed.[108] Large papillary tumors with prominent endophytic growth 'invade' the lamina propria with a pushing border. Unless this pattern is accompanied by true destructive stromal invasion, the likelihood of metastasis is minimal because the basement membrane is not truly breached.[106]

## UROTHELIAL CARCINOMA WITH SYNCYTIOTROPHOBLASTIC GIANT CELLS

Syncytiotrophoblastic giant cells are present in up to 12% of cases of urothelial carcinoma, producing substantial amounts of immunoreactive beta-human chorionic gonadotropin (HCG) indicative of syncytiotrophoblastic differentiation (Figure 5.18).[109–114] The number of HCG-immunoreactive cells is inversely associated with cancer grade.[115,116] Secretion of HCG into the serum may be associated with a poor response to radiation therapy.[117] The most important differential diagnostic consideration is choriocarcinoma; most but not all cases previously reported as primary choriocarcinoma of the bladder represent urothelial carcinoma with syncytiotrophoblasts.[118]

## GIANT CELL CARCINOMA

High-grade urothelial carcinoma may contain epithelial tumor giant cells or the tumor may appear undifferentiated, resembling giant cell carcinoma of the lung (Figure 5.19). This variant is very infrequent.[119] Malignant giant cells in urothelial carcinoma, when present in great numbers, portend a poor prognosis, similar to that associated with giant cell carcinoma in the lung. The giant cells display cytokeratin and vimentin immunoreactivity. The differential diagnosis includes giant cells associated with trophoblastic differentiation, osteoclast-type giant cells in invasive high-grade urothelial carcinoma, sarcomatoid carcinoma with giant cells, and metastatic giant cell carcinoma to the bladder.[120–122]

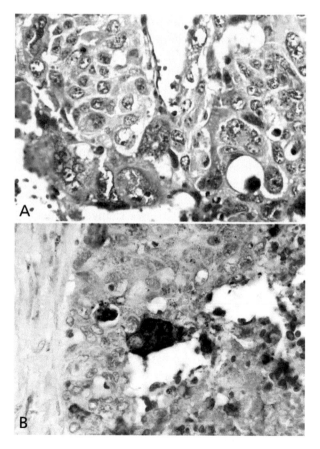

**Fig. 5.18**
**A** Urothelial carcinoma with syncytiotrophoblastic giant cells.
**B** HCG immunostaining highlights the giant cells.

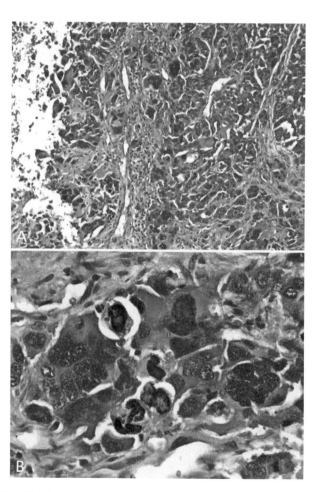

**Fig. 5.19**
**A, B** Giant cell carcinoma.

## CLEAR CELL (GLYCOGEN-RICH) CARCINOMA

Up to two-thirds of cases of urothelial carcinoma have foci of clear cell change resulting from abundant glycogen (Figure 5.20). The glycogen-rich clear cell 'variant' of urothelial carcinoma, recently described, appears to represent the extreme end of the morphologic spectrum, consisting predominantly or exclusively of cells with abundant clear cytoplasm that stains for cytokeratin 7.[90,123–125] Recognition of this pattern avoids confusion with clear cell adenocarcinoma of the bladder and metastatic clear cell carcinoma of the kidney and prostate.[122]

## SARCOMATOID CARCINOMA WITH/WITHOUT HETEROLOGOUS ELEMENTS (CARCINOSARCOMA, METAPLASTIC CARCINOMA)

The term sarcomatoid variant of urothelial carcinoma should be used for all biphasic malignant neoplasms exhibiting morphologic and/or immunohistochemical evidence of epithelial and mesenchymal differentiation (with the presence or absence of heterologous elements acknowledged in the report).[7] There is considerable confusion and disagreement in the literature regarding nomenclature and histogenesis of these tumors. As with other organs, various terms have been used for these neoplasms, including carcinosarcoma, sarcomatoid carcinoma, pseudosarcomatous transitional cell carcinoma, malignant mesodermal mixed tumor, spindle cell carcinoma, giant cell carcinoma, and malignant teratoma.[126,127] In some series, both carcinosarcoma and sarcomatoid carcinoma are included as 'sarcomatoid carcinoma'; in others they are regarded as separate entities. A previous history of

carcinoma treated by radiation or the exposition to cyclophosphamide therapy is common.[128]

The gross appearance is characteristically 'sarcoma-like'—dull gray with infiltrative margins (Figure 5.21A). The tumors are often polyploid with large intraluminal masses. Microscopically, sarcomatoid carcinoma is composed of urothelial, glandular or small cell components showing variable degrees of differ-

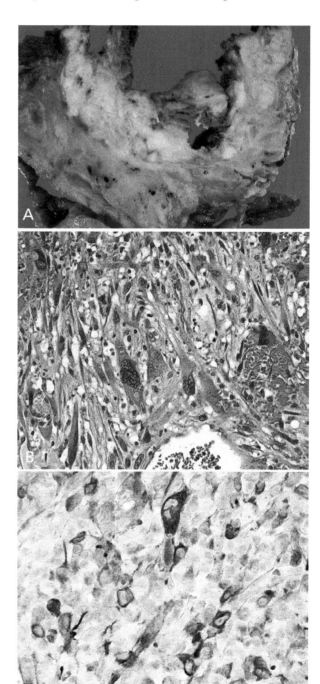

**Fig. 5.21**
Sarcomatoid carcinoma. **A,** Gross and **B,** microscopic appearance of sarcomatoid urothelial carcinoma. **C** Epithelial nature of tumor cells was confirmed by cytokeratin staining.

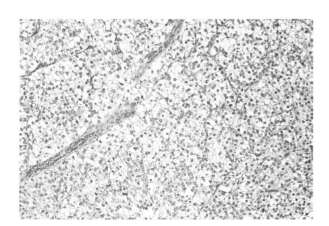

**Fig. 5.20**
Clear cell (glycogen-rich) carcinoma.

entiation.[128] Carcinoma in situ is present in 30% of cases and occasionally is the only apparent epithelial component.[128–130] A small subset of sarcomatoid carcinoma may have a prominent myxoid stroma.[126,131] The mesenchymal component most frequently observed is a undifferentiated high-grade spindle cell neoplasm (Figure 5.21B). The most common heterologous element is osteosarcoma followed by chondrosarcoma, rhabdomyosarcoma, leiomyosarcoma, liposarcoma, and angiosarcoma; alternatively, multiple types of heterologous differentiation may be present.[128,130] By immunohistochemistry, epithelial elements react with cytokeratins (Figure 5.21C), whereas stromal elements react with vimentin or specific markers corresponding to the mesenchymal differentiation. The sarcomatoid phenotype retains the epithelial nature of the cells by immunohistochemistry or electronmicroscopy.[126,128,131]

Recent molecular studies strongly argue for a monoclonal origin of both components in sarcomatoid carcinoma and carcinosarcoma.[127,132–135] These two categories have similar clinical characteristics, including patient age, sex, presentation, and outcome. The most frequent presenting signs and symptoms are hematuria, dysuria, nocturia, acute urinary retention, and lower abdominal pain. The mean age is 66 years (range 50–77 years).[128,129,136,137] Pathologic stage is the best predictor of survival in sarcomatoid carcinoma.

The major differential diagnostic consideration is urothelial carcinoma with pseudosarcomatous stroma,[138] a rare entity with reactive stroma.[137–140] In cases with exclusively spindle cells, the main differential diagnostic consideration is sarcoma, particularly leiomyosarcoma. The rarity of primary bladder sarcoma warrants that any malignant spindle cell tumor in the urinary bladder in an adult be considered sarcomatoid carcinoma until proven otherwise. Immunostaining with cytokeratin is helpful in this setting. Sarcomatoid carcinoma with prominent myxoid and sclerosing stroma may be mistaken for inflammatory pseudo-tumor.[131,140]

## LIPOID-CELL VARIANT

Lipoid-cell variant is a rare neoplasm defined by the WHO (1999, 2004) as a urothelial carcinoma which exhibits transition to a cell type resembling signet-ring lipoblasts (Figure 5.22). It is currently considered to be an ill-defined tumor variant, and whether it should be classified as carcinosarcoma remains to be established. Clinicopathologic features and the immunohisto-chemical findings in seven reported cases showed gross hematuria as the initial symptom. All patients were elderly men (mean age 74 years; range 63–94 years). On microscopic examination, the extension of the lipid cell pattern varied from 10% to 30% of the tumor specimen, with associated micropapillary (n=1), plasmacytoid

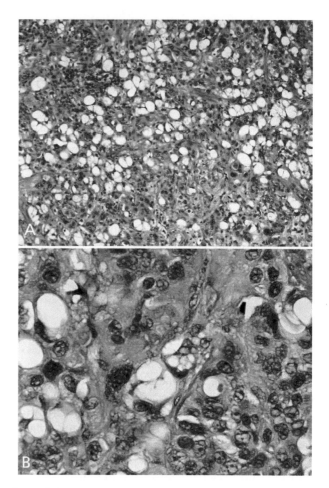

**Fig. 5.22**
**A, B** Urothelial carcinoma, lipoid cell variant.

(n=2), and grade 3/3 conventional urothelial carcinomas (n=4). The immunohistochemical results showed an epithelial phenotype of the lipoid cell component characterized by diffuse staining with cytokeratins AE1/AE3. The reported cases were pathologic stage T2 (n=2), T3a (n=1), T3b (n=3), and T4 (n=1). Patient follow-up showed one dead and two alive with disease at 58, 14, and 55 months, respectively; two patients showed no evidence of disease at 11 and 29 months; and two patients died of other causes at 10 and 15 months.

## UNDIFFERENTIATED CARCINOMA

This category contains tumors that cannot be otherwise classified. To our knowledge, they are extremely rare. Earlier literature has reported small cell carcinoma, giant cell carcinoma, and lymphoepithelioma-like carcinoma in this category, but these tumors are now recognized as specific tumor variants (see respective sections). Large cell undifferentiated carcinomas as in the lung are rare in the urinary tract, and those with neuroendocrine features should be recognized as a specific tumor variant.[7]

## UROTHELIAL CARCINOMA WITH UNUSUAL STROMAL REACTION

Infiltrating urothelial carcinoma may be associated with a variety of stromal reactions, which are occasionally pronounced.

- Urothelial carcinoma may have a *pseudosarcomatous stroma*, which rarely displays sufficient cellularity, cytologic atypia, spindle cell proliferation or myxoid appearance to raise serious concern about sarcomatoid carcinoma.[138,141] The stromal cells reveal immunohistochemical evidence of fibroblastic or myofibroblastic differentiation and invariably are cytokeratin negative or focally positive.
- Tumor-associated *osseous and/or chondroid metaplasia* is present in some cases of urothelial carcinoma and its metastases,[142–144] and this should be differentiated from osteosarcoma and chondro-sarcoma. The metaplastic bone or cartilage is histologically benign.[145]
- Zukerberg et al[146] described the presence of *osteoclast-type giant cells* in two cases of invasive high-grade urothelial carcinoma. The giant cells had abundant eosinophilic cytoplasm and numerous small, round, regular nuclei and displayed immunoreactivity for vimentin and CD68 but not for epithelial markers. It seems not to be related to prognosis.
- An inflammatory cell response in the stroma adjacent to invasive tumor is relatively common. This response usually takes the form of a *lymphocytic infiltrate* with a variable admixture of plasma cells. Generally, this cellular reaction is mild to moderate, but occasionally it may be dense. Sometimes, a neutrophilic response is observed, with or without extensive eosinophilic infiltrate,[147–151] suggesting that, in the absence of a cellular response, the carcinoma is likely to be more aggressive.[151] In a recent study, intense inflammation in bladder carcinoma was found to be associated with tumor angiogenesis and indicative of a good prognosis.[152] Exclusion of lymphoepithelioma-like carcinoma of the urinary bladder is mandatory when there is extensive inflammation in the stroma.[84]

## CONCLUSION

Accurate diagnosis and classification of urothelial tumors are critical for patient management. Detailed pathologic evaluation of urothelial carcinoma of the bladder remains of paramount importance since it provides useful information to guide urologists in daily clinical practice.

Appropriate evaluation of important predictors of clinical course such as tumor multiplicity, vascular invasion, tumor size, depth of invasion, histologic grade, and, most importantly, pathologic staging will continue to be included as main issues in the final report. The inclusion of novel approaches in clinical practice that provide better results in pathologic substaging of T1 tumors—for example, the use of a micrometer for measurement of the depth of tumor invasion, or the identification of novel biomarkers—should continue to expand in the near future, thus providing an accurate diagnosis and consistent separation and stratification of pT1 tumors.

Agreement on the best contemporary tumor grading system is desirable. Also, morphologic clinically relevant variants of bladder cancer should be recognized and reported by the practicing pathologist. The emerging role of flat intraepithelial lesions as precursors of bladder cancer at both the morphologic and the molecular levels—in particular flat urothelial hyperplasia, urothelial dysplasia, and CIS—will be the target of important research in the near future. Finally, the clinical significance of genetic anomalies found in normal-looking urothelium needs to be addressed in coming years.

## REFERENCES

1. Cheng L, Weaver AL, Leibovich BC, et al. Predicting the survival of bladder carcinoma patients treated with radical cystectomy. Cancer 2000;88:2326–2332.
2. Cheng L, Neumann RM, Nehra A, et al. Cancer heterogeneity and its biologic implications in the grading of urothelial carcinoma. Cancer 2000;88:1663–1670.
3. Cheng L, Cheville JC, Leibovich BC, et al. Survival of patients with carcinoma in situ of the urinary bladder. Cancer 1999;85:2469–2474
4. Cheng L, Neumann RM, Weaver AL, Spotts B, Bostwick DG. Predicting cancer progression in patients with stage T1 bladder carcinoma. J Clin Oncol 1999;17:3182–3187.
5. Jordan AM, Weingarten J, Murphy WM. Transitional cell neoplasms of the urinary bladder. Can biologic potential be predicted from histologic grading? Cancer 1987;60:2766–2774.
6. Droller MJ. Bladder cancer: state-of-the-art care. CA Cancer J Clin 1998;48:269–284.
7. Lopez-Beltran A, Sauter G, Gasser T, et al. Urothelial tumors: infiltrating urothelial carcinoma. In Eble JN, Sauter G, Epstein JI, Sesterhenn IA (eds): World Health Organization Classification of Tumors. Pathology and Gentics of Tumors of the Urinary System and Male Genital Organs. Lyon: IARC Press, 2004.
8. Lopez-Beltran A, Cheng L. Stage pT1 bladder carcinoma: diagnostic criteria, pitfalls and prognostic significance. Pathology 2003;35:484–491.
9. Bostwick DG, Ramnani D, Cheng L. Diagnosis and grading of bladder cancer and associated lesions. Urol Clin North Am 1999;26:493–507.
10. Cheng L, Neumann RM, Scherer BG, et al. Tumor size predicts the survival of patients with pathologic stage T2 bladder carcinoma: a critical evaluation of the depth of muscle invasion. Cancer 1999;85:2638–2647.
11. Cheng L Neumann RM, Weaver AL, et al. Grading and staging of bladder carcinoma in transurethral resection specimens. Correlation with 105 matched cystectomy specimens. Am J Clin Pathol 2000;113:275–279.
12. Cheng L, Weaver AL, Neumann RM, et al. Substaging of T1 bladder carcinoma based on the depth of invasion as measured by micrometer. A new proposal. Cancer 1999;86:1035–1043.

13. Cheng L Weaver AL, Bostwick DG. Predicting extravesical extension of bladder carcinoma: a novel method based on micrometer measurement of the depth of invasion in transurethral resection specimens. Urology 2000;55:668–672.

14. Montironi R, Lopez-Beltran A, Mazzuchelli R, Bostwick DG. Classification and grading of the non-invasive neoplasms: recent advances and controversies. J Clin Pathol 2003;56:91–95.

15. Simon R, Jones PA, Sidransky D, et al. Genetics and predictive factors of non-invasive urothelial neoplasias. In Eble JN, Sauter G, Epstein JI, Sesterhenn IA (eds). World Health Organization Classification of Tumors. Pathology and Gentics of Tumors of the Urinary System and Male Genital Organs. Lyon: IARC Press, 2004.

16. Cheng L, MacLennan GT, Zhang S, et al. Laser capture microdissection analysis reveals frequent allelic losses in papillary urothelial neoplasm of low malignant potential of the urinary bladder. Cancer 2004;101:183–188.

17. Cordon-Cardo C, Cote RJ, Sauter G. Genetic and molecular markers of urothelial premalignancy and malignancy. Scand J Urol Nephrol 2000;205:82–93.

18. Richter J, Jiang F, Gorog JP, et al. Marked genetic differences between stage pTa and stage pT1 papillary bladder cancer detected by comparative genomic hybridization. Cancer Res 1997;57:2860–2864.

19. Richter J, Wagner U, Schraml P, et al. Chromosomal imbalances are associated with a high risk of progression in early invasive (pT1) urinary bladder cancer. Cancer Res 1999;59:5687–5691.

20. Lopez-Beltran A, Cheng L, Andersson L, et al. Preneoplastic non-papillary lesions and conditions of the urinary bladder: an update based on the Ancona International Consultation. Virchows Arch 2002;440:3–11.

21. Sauter G, Algaba F, Amin MB, et al. Non-invasive urothelial neoplasias. In Eble JN, Sauter G, Epstein JI, Sesterhenn IA (eds): World Health Organization Classification of Tumors. Pathology and Gentics of Tumors of the Urinary System and Male Genital Organs. Lyon: IARC Press, 2004.

22. Hartmann A, Moser K, Kriegmair M, et al. Frequent genetic alterations in simple urothelial hyperplasias of the bladder in patients with papillary urothelial carcinoma. Am J Pathol 1999;154:721–727.

23. Paterson RF, Ulbright TM, MacLennan GT, et al. Molecular genetic alterations in the laser-capture microdissected stroma adjacent to bladder carcinoma. Cancer 2003;98:1830–1836.

24. Muto S, Horie S, Takahashi S, et al. Genetic and epigenetic alterations in normal bladder epithelium in patients with metachronous bladder cancer. Cancer Res 2000;60:4021–4025.

25. Harnden P, Eardley I, Joyce AD, et al. Cytokeratin 20 as an objective marker of urothelial dysplasia. Br J Urol 1996;78:870–875.

26. Hartmann A, Schlake G, Zaak D, et al. Occurrence of chromosome 9 and p53 alterations in multifocal dysplasia and carcinoma in situ of human urinary bladder. Cancer Res 2002;62:809–818.

27. Wolf H, Hojgaard K. Urothelial dysplasia concomitant with bladder tumours as a determinant factor for future new occurances. Lancet 1983;2:134–136.

28. Kiemeney L, Witjes J, Heibroek R, et al. Dysplasia in normal-looking urothelium increases the risk of tumour progression in primary superficial bladder cancer. Eur J Cancer 1994;30A:1621–1625.

29. Cheng L, Cheville JC, Neumann RM, et al. Flat intraepithelial lesions of the urinary bladder. Cancer 2000;88:625–631.

30. Cheng L, Cheville JC, Neumann RM, et al. Natural history of urothelial dysplasia of the bladder. Am J Surg Pathol 1999;23:443–447.

31. Lopez-Beltran A, Luque RJ, Moreno A, et al. The pagetoid variant of bladder urothelial carcinoma in situ: a clinicopathological study of 11 cases. Virchows Arch 2002;441:148–153.

32. McKenney JK Gomez JA, Desai S, Lee MW, Amin MB. Morphologic expressions of urothelial carcinoma in situ. Am J Surg Pathol 2001;25:356–362.

33. Helpap B, Kollermann J. Assessment of basal cell status and proliferative patterns in flat and papillary urothelial lesions: a contribution to the new WHO classification of the urothelial tumors of the urinary bladder. Hum Pathol 2000;31:745–750.

34. Stampfer DS, Carpinito GA, Rodriguez-Villanueva J, et al. Evaluation of NMP22 in the detection of transitional cell carcinoma of the bladder. J Urol 1998;159:394–398.

35. Mostofi FK, Sobin LH, Torloni H. Histological typing of urinary bladder tumours. Geneva: World Health Organization, 1973.

36. Eble JN, Sauter G, Epstein JI, Sesterhenn IA (eds) World Health Organization Classification of Tumours: Pathology and Genetics of Tumours of the Urinary System and Male Genital Organs. Lyon: IARC Press, 2004.

37. Lopez-Beltran A, Montironi R. Non-invasive urothelial neoplasms: according to the most recent WHO classification. Eur Urol 2004;46:170–176.

38. Lopez-Beltran A, Bassi P, Pavone-Macaluso M, et al. Handling and pathology reporting of specimens with carcinoma of the urinary bladder, ureter, and renal pelvis. Eur Urol 2004;45:257–266.

39. Cheng L, MacLennan GT, Pan CX, et al. Allelic loss of the active X chromosome during bladder carcinogenesis. Arch Pathol Lab Med 2004;128:187–190.

40. Cheng L, Gu J, Ulbright TM, et al. Precise microdissection of human bladder carcinomas reveals divergent tumor subclones in the same tumor. Cancer 2002;94:104–110.

41. Cheng L, Bostwick DG, Li G, et al. Conserved genetic findings in metastatic bladder cancer: a possible utility of allelic loss of chromosome 9p21 and 17p13 in diagnosis. Arch Pathol Lab Med 2001;125:1197–1199.

42. Holmang S, Andius P, Hedelin H, et al. Stage progression in Ta papillary urothelial tumors: relationship to grade, immunohistochemical expression of tumor markers, mitotic frequency and DNA ploidy. J Urol 2001;165:1124–1128; discussion 1128–1130.

43. Holmang S, Johansson SL. Stage Ta-T1 bladder cancer: the relationship between findings at first followup cystoscopy and subsequent recurrence and progression. J Urol 2002;167:1634–1637.

44. Cheng L, Bostwick DG. World Health Organization and International Society of Urological Pathology classification and two-number grading system of bladder tumors: reply. Cancer 2000;88:1513–1516.

45. Bostwick DG, Mikuz G. Urothelial papillary (exophytic) neoplasms. Virchows Arch 2002;441:109–116.

46. Murphy WM, Takezawa K, Maruniak NA. Interobserver discrepancy using the 1998 World Health Organization/International Society of Urologic Pathology classification of urothelial neoplasms: practical choices for patient care. J Urol 2003;168:968–972.

47. Bol M, Baak J, Buhr-Wildhagen S, et al. Reproducibility and prognostic variability of grade and lamina propria invasion in stages Ta, T1 urothelial carcinoma of the bladder. J Urol 2003;169:1291–1294.

48. Oyasu R. World Health Organization and International Society of Urological Pathology Classification and two-number grading system of bladder tumors. Cancer 2000;88:1509–1512.

49. van Rhijn BW, Montironi R, Zwarthoff EC, et al. Frequent FGFR3 mutations in urothelial papilloma. J Pathol 2002;198:245–251.

50. Epstein JI, Amin MB, Reuter VR, et al. The World Health Organization/International Society of Urological Pathology consensus classification of urothelial (transitional cell) neoplasms of the urinary bladder. Bladder Consensus Conference Committee. Am J Surg Pathol 1998;22:1435–1448.

51. Cheville JC, Wu K, Sebo TJ, et al. Inverted urothelial papilloma: is ploidy, MIB-1 proliferative activity, or p53 protein accumulation predictive of urothelial carcinoma? Cancer 2000;88:632–636.

52. Cheng L, Darson M, Cheville JC, et al. Urothelial papilloma of the bladder. Clinical and biologic implications. Cancer 1999;86:2098–2101.

53. Sauter G. Inverted papilloma. In Eble JN, Sauter G, Epstein JI, Sesterhenn IA (eds): World Health Organization Classification of Tumors. Pathology and Gentics of Tumors of the Urinary System and Male Genital Organs. Lyon: IARC Press, 2004.

54. Cheng L, Neumann RM, Bostwick DG. Papillary urothelial neoplasms of low malignant potential. Clinical and biologic implications. Cancer 1999;86:2102–2108.

55. Samaratunga H, Makarov DV, Epstein JI. Comparison of WHO/ISUP and WHO classification of noninvasive papillary urothelial neoplasms for risk of progression. Urology 2002;60:315–319.

56. Lopez-Beltran A, Luque RJ, Alvarez-Kindelan J, et al. Prognostic factors in stage T1 grade 3 bladder cancer survival: the role of G1-S

modulators (p53, p21Waf1, p27kip1, Cyclin D1, and Cyclin D3) and proliferation index (ki67-MIB1). Eur Urol 2004;45:606–612.

57. Lopez-Beltran A, Luque RJ, Alvarez-Kindelan J, et al. Prognostic factors in survival of patients with stage Ta and T1 bladder urothelial tumors: the role of G1-S modulators (p53, p21Waf1, p27Kip1, cyclin D1, and cyclin D3), proliferation index, and clinicopathologic parameters. Am J Clin Pathol 2004;122:444–452.

58. Herr HW. Staging invasive bladder tumors. J Surg Oncol 1992;51:217–220.

59. Greene FL, Page DL, Fleming ID, et al. AJCC Cancer Staging Manual, 6th ed. New York: Springer-Verlag, 2002.

60. Abel PD, Henderson D, Bennett MK, et al. Differing interpretations by pathologists of the pT category and grade of transitional cell cancer of the bladder. Br J Urol 1988;62:339–342.

61. Malmstrom PU, Busch C, Norlen BJ. Recurrence, progression, and survival in bladder cancer. A retrospective analysis of 232 patients with greater than or equal to 5-year follow-up. Scand J Urol Nephrol 1987;21:185–195.

62. Lapham RL, Grignon D, Ro JY. Pathologic prognostic parameters in bladder urothelial biopsy, transurethral resection, and cystectomy specimens. Semin Diagn Pathol 1997;14:109–122.

63. Lopez JI, Angulo JC. The prognostic significance of vascular invasion in stage T1 bladder cancer. Histopathology 1995;27:27–33.

64. Song TY, Razvi H, McLean CA, et al. Prognostic value of angiogenesis and vascular invasion in muscle-invasive bladder cancer. Can J Urol 1996;3:229–234.

65. Ramani P, Birch BR, Harland SJ, et al. Evaluation of endothelial markers in detecting blood and lymphatic channel invasion in pT1 transitional carcinoma of bladder. Histopathology 1991;19:551–554.

66. Leissner J, Koeppen C, Wolf HK. Prognostic significance of vascular and perineural invasion in urothelial bladder cancer treated with radical cystectomy. J Urol 2003;169:955–960.

67. Bassi P, Ferrante GD, Piazza N, et al. Prognostic factors of outcome after radical cystectomy for bladder cancer: a retrospective study of a homogeneous patient cohort. J Urol 1999;161:1494–1497.

68. Jimenez RE, Keany TE, Hardy HT, et al. pT1 Urothelial carcinoma of the bladder: criteria for diagnosis, pitfalls, and clinical implications. Adv Anat Pathol 2000;7:13–25.

69. Reuter V. Bladder: risk and prognostic factors. A pathologist's perspective. Urol Clin North Am 1999;26:481–492.

70. Sakamoto N, Tsuneyoshi M, Enjoji M. Urinary bladder carcinoma with a neoplastic squamous component: a mapping study of 31 cases. Histopathology 1992;21:135–141.

71. Akdas A, Turkeri L. The impact of squamous metaplasia in transitional cell carcinoma of the bladder. Int Urol Nephrol 1991;23:333–336.

72. Ayala A, Ro J. Premalignant lesions of the urothelium and transitional cell tumors. In Young R (ed): Pathology of the Urinary Bladder. Philadelphia: Churchill Livingstone, 1989.

73. Lopez-Beltran A, Martin J, Garcia J, et al. Squamous and glandular differentiation in urothelial bladder carcinomas. Histopathology, histochemistry and immunohistochemical expression of carcinoembryonic antigen. Histol Histopathol 1988;3:63–68.

74. Ro JY, Staerkel GA, Ayala AG. Cytologic and histologic features of superficial bladder cancer. Urol Clin North Am 1992;19:435–453.

75. Fong A, Garcia E, Gwynn L, et al. Expression of caveolin-1 and caveolin-2 in urothelial carcinoma of the urinary bladder correlates with tumor grade and squamous differentiation. Am J Clin Pathol 2003;120:93–100.

76. Kunze E, Francksen B, Schulz H. Expression of MUC5AC apomucin in transitional cell carcinomas of the urinary bladder and its possible role in the development of mucus-secreting adenocarcinomas. Virchows Arch 2001;439:609–615.

77. Kunze E, Francksen B. Histogenesis of nonurothelial carcinomas of the urinary bladder from pre-existent transitional cell carcinomas. A histopathological and immunohistochemical study. Urol Res 2002;30:66–78.

78. Cheng L, Pan CX, Yang XJ, et al. Small cell carcinoma of the urinary bladder: a clinicopathologic analysis of 64 patients. Cancer 2004;101:957–962.

79. Cheng L, Jones TD, McCarthy RP, et al. Molecular genetic evidence for a common clonal origin of urinary bladder small cell carcinoma and co-existing urothelial carcinoma. Am J Pathol 2005;166(5):1533–1539.

80. Wang X, Jones TD, MacLennan GT, et al. P53 expression in small cell carcinoma of the urinary bladder: biological and prognostic implications. (submitted)

81. Jones TD, Kernek KM, Yang XJ, et al. Thyroid transcription factor-1 expression in small cell carcinoma of the urinary bladder: an immunohistochemical profile of 44 cases. Am J Clin Pathol 2005 (in press).

82. Soriano P, Navarro S, Gil M, et al. Small-cell carcinoma of the urinary bladder. A clinico-pathological study of ten cases. Virchows Arch 2004;445:292–297.

83. Pan CX, Yang XJ, Lopez-Beltran A, et al. c-kit Expression in small cell carcinoma of the urinary bladder: prognostic and therapeutic implications. Mod Pathol 2005;18(3):320–323.

84. Lopez-Beltran A, Luque RJ, Vicioso L, et al. Lymphoepithelioma-like carcinoma of the urinary bladder: a clinicopathologic study of 13 cases. Virchows Arch 2001;438:552–557.

85. Holmang S, Johansson SL. The nested variant of transitional cell carcinoma—a rare neoplasm with poor prognosis. Scand J Urol Nephrol 2001;35:102–105.

86. Murphy WM, Deana DG. The nested variant of transitional cell carcinoma: a neoplasm resembling proliferation of Brunn's nests. Mod Pathol 1992;5:240–243.

87. Talbert ML, Young RH. Carcinomas of the urinary bladder with deceptively benign-appearing foci. A report of three cases. Am J Surg Pathol 1989;13:374–381.

88. Drew PA, Furman J, Civantos F, et al. The nested variant of transitional cell carcinoma: an aggressive neoplasm with innocuous histology. Mod Pathol 1996;9:989–994.

89. Paik SS, Park MH. The nested variant of transitional cell carcinoma of the urinary bladder. Br J Urol 1996;78:793–794.

90. Young RH, Eble JN. Unusual forms of carcinoma of the urinary bladder. Hum Pathol 1991;22:948–965.

91. Young RH, Oliva E. Transitional cell carcinomas of the urinary bladder that may be underdiagnosed. A report of four invasive cases exemplifying the homology between neoplastic and non-neoplastic transitional cell lesions. Am J Surg Pathol 1996;20:1448–1454.

92. Tatsura H, Ogawa K, Sakata T, et al. A nested variant of transitional cell carcinoma of the urinary bladder: a case report. Jpn J Clin Oncol 2001;31:287–289.

93. Cheng L, Cheville JC, Sebo TJ, et al. Atypical nephrogenic metaplasia of the urinary tract: a precursor lesion? Cancer 2000;88:853–861.

94. Cheng L, Leibovich BC, Cheville JC, et al. Paraganglioma of the urinary bladder: can biologic potential be predicted? Cancer 2000;88:844–852.

95. Lopez-Beltran A, Luque RJ, Quintero A, et al. Hepatoid adenocarcinoma of the urinary bladder. Virchows Arch 2003;442:381–387.

96. Amin MB, Ro JY, el-Sharkawy T, et al. Micropapillary variant of transitional cell carcinoma of the urinary bladder. Histologic pattern resembling ovarian papillary serous carcinoma. Am J Surg Pathol 1994;18:1224–1232.

97. Young RH, Zukerberg LR. Microcystic transitional cell carcinomas of the urinary bladder. A report of four cases. Am J Clin Pathol 1991;96:635–639.

98. Maranchie JK, Bouyounes BT, Zhang PL, et al. Clinical and pathological characteristics of micropapillary transitional cell carcinoma: a highly aggressive variant. J Urol 2000;163:748–751.

99. Johansson SL, Borghede G, Holmang S. Micropapillary bladder carcinoma: a clinicopathological study of 20 cases. J Urol 1999;161:1798–1802.

100. Amin MB, Ro JY, Lee KM, et al. Lymphoepithelioma-like carcinoma of the urinary bladder. Am J Surg Pathol 1994;18:466–473.

101. Holmang S, Borghede G, Johansson SL. Bladder carcinoma with lymphoepithelioma-like differentiation: a report of 9 cases. J Urol 1998;159:779–782.

102. Dinney CP, Ro JY, Babaian RJ, et al. Lymphoepithelioma of the bladder: a clinicopathological study of 3 cases. J Urol 1993;149:840–841.

103. Gulley ML, Amin MB, Nicholls JM, et al. Epstein–Barr virus is detected in undifferentiated nasopharyngeal carcinoma but not in lymphoepithelioma-like carcinoma of the urinary bladder. Hum Pathol 1995;26:1207–1214.

104. Zukerberg LR, Harris NL, Young RH. Carcinomas of the urinary bladder simulating malignant lymphoma. A report of five cases. Am J Surg Pathol 1991;15:569–576.

105. Tamboli P, Amin MB, Mohsin SK, et al. Plasmocytoid variant of non-papillary urothelial carcinoma [abstract]. Mod Pathol 2000;13:107A.

106. Amin MB, Gomez JA, Young RH. Urothelial transitional cell carcinoma with endophytic growth patterns: a discussion of patterns of invasion and problems associated with assessment of invasion in 18 cases. Am J Surg Pathol 1997;21:1057–1068.

107. Cameron KM, Lupton CH. Inverted papilloma of the lower urinary tract. Br J Urol 1976;48:567–577.

108. Goertchen R, Seidenschnur A, Stosiek P. Clinical pathology of inverted papillomas of the urinary bladder. A complex morphologic and catamnestic study. Pathologe 1994;15:279–285.

109. Campo E, Algaba F, Palacin A, et al. Placental proteins in high-grade urothelial neoplasms. An immunohistochemical study of human chorionic gonadotropin, human placental lactogen, and pregnancy-specific beta-1-glycoprotein. Cancer 1989;63:2497–2504.

110. Fowler AL, Hall E, Rees G. Choriocarcinoma arising in transitional cell carcinoma of the bladder. Br J Urol 1992;70:333–334.

111. Grammatico D, Grignon DJ, Eberwein P, et al. Transitional cell carcinoma of the renal pelvis with choriocarcinomatous differentiation. Immunohistochemical and immunoelectron microscopic assessment of human chorionic gonadotropin production by transitional cell carcinoma of the urinary bladder. Cancer 1993;71:1835–1841.

112. Seidal T, Breborowicz J, Malmstrom P. Immunoreactivity to human chorionic gonadotropin in urothelial carcinoma: correlation with tumor grade, stage, and progression. J Urol Pathol 1993;1:397–410.

113. Shah VM, Newman J, Crocker J, et al. Ectopic beta-human chorionic gonadotropin production by bladder urothelial neoplasia. Arch Pathol Lab Med 1986;110:107–111.

114. Bastacky S, Dhir R, Nangia AK, et al. Choriocarcinomatous differentiation in a high-grade urothelial carcinoma of the urinary bladder: case report and litterature review. J Urol Pathol 1997;6:223–234.

115. Yamase HT, Wurzel RS, Nieh PT, et al. Immunohistochemical demonstration of human chorionic gonadotropin in tumors of the urinary bladder. Ann Clin Lab Sci 1985;15:414–417.

116. Oyasu R, Nan L, Smith DP, et al. Human chorionic gonadotropin beta-subunit synthesis by undifferentiated urothelial carcinoma with syncytiotrophoblastic differentiation. Arch Pathol Lab Med 1994;118:715–717.

117. Martin JE, Jenkins BJ, Zuk RJ, et al. Human chorionic gonadotrophin expression and histological findings as predictors of response to radiotherapy in carcinoma of the bladder. Virchows Arch A Pathol Anat Histopathol 1989;414:273–277.

118. Cho JH, Yu E, Kim KH, et al. Primary choriocarcinoma of the urinary bladder—a case report. J Korean Med Sci 1992;7:369–372.

119. O'Connor RC, Hollowell CM, Laven BA, et al. Recurrent giant cell carcinoma of the bladder. J Urol 2002;167:1784.

120. Serio G, Zampatti C, Ceppi M. Spindle and giant cell carcinoma of the urinary bladder: a clinicopathological light microscopic and immunohistochemical study. Br J Urol 1995;75:167–172.

121. Amir G, Rosenmann E. Osteoclast-like giant cell tumour of the urinary bladder. Histopathology 1990;17:413–418.

122. Bates AW, Baithun SI. The significance of secondary neoplasms of the urinary and male genital tract. Virchows Arch 2002;440:640–647.

123. Braslis KG, Jones A, Murphy D. Clear-cell transitional cell carcinoma. Aust N Z J Surg 1997;67:906–908.

124. Kotliar SN, Wood CG, Schaeffer AJ, et al. Transitional cell carcinoma exhibiting clear cell features. A differential diagnosis for clear cell adenocarcinoma of the urinary tract. Arch Pathol Lab Med 1995;119:79–81.

125. Oliva E, Amin MB, Jimenez R, et al. Clear cell carcinoma of the urinary bladder: a report and comparison of four tumors of mullerian origin and nine of probable urothelial origin with discussion of histogenesis and diagnostic problems. Am J Surg Pathol 2002;26:190–197.

126. Jones E, Young R. Nonneoplastic and neoplastic spindle cell proliferations and mixed tumors of the urinary bladder. J Urol Pathol 1994;2:105–134.

127. Torenbeek R, Blomjous CE, de Bruin PC, et al. Sarcomatoid carcinoma of the urinary bladder. Clinicopathologic analysis of 18 cases with immunohistochemical and electron microscopic findings. Am J Surg Pathol 1994;18:241–249.

128. Lopez-Beltran A, Pacelli A, Rothenberg HJ, et al. Carcinosarcoma and sarcomatoid carcinoma of the bladder: clinicopathological study of 41 cases. J Urol 1998;159:1497–1503.

129. Lopez-Beltran A, Escudero AL, Cavazzana AO, et al. Sarcomatoid transitional cell carcinoma of the renal pelvis. A report of five cases with clinical, pathological, immunohistochemical and DNA ploidy analysis. Pathol Res Pract 1996;192:1218–1224.

130. Young RH, Wick MR, Mills SE. Sarcomatoid carcinoma of the urinary bladder. A clinicopathologic analysis of 12 cases and review of the literature. Am J Clin Pathol 1988;90:653–661.

131. Jones EC, Young RH. Myxoid and sclerosing sarcomatoid transitional cell carcinoma of the urinary bladder: a clinicopathologic and immunohistochemical study of 25 cases. Mod Pathol 1997;10:908–916.

132. Fossa S. Rare and unusual tumors of the genitourinary tract. Curr Opin Oncol 1992;4:463–468.

133. Lahoti C, Schinella R, Rangwala AF, et al. Carcinosarcoma of urinary bladder: report of 5 cases with immunohistologic study. Urology 1994;43:389–393.

134. Perret L, Chaubert P, Hessler D, et al. Primary heterologous carcinosarcoma (metaplastic carcinoma) of the urinary bladder: a clinicopathologic, immunohistochemical, and ultrastructural analysis of eight cases and a review of the literature. Cancer 1998;82:1535–1549.

135. Torenbeek R, Hermsen MA, Meijer GA, et al. Analysis by comparative genomic hybridization of epithelial and spindle cell components in sarcomatoid carcinoma and carcinosarcoma: histogenetic aspects. J Pathol 1999;189:338–343.

136. Sen SE, Malek RS, Farrow GM, et al. Sarcoma and carcinosarcoma of the bladder in adults. J Urol 1985;133:29–30.

137. Ikegami H, Iwasaki H, Ohjimi Y, et al. Sarcomatoid carcinoma of the urinary bladder: a clinicopathologic and immunohistochemical analysis of 14 patients. Hum Pathol 2000;31:332–340.

138. Bannach G, Grignon D, Shum D. Sarcomatoid transitional cell carcinoma vs pseudosarcomatous stromal reaction in bladder carcinoma: an immunohistochemical study. J Urol Pathol 1993;1:105–113.

139. Lopez-Beltran A, Lopez-Ruiz J, Vicioso L. Inflammatory pseudotumor of the urinary bladder. A clinicopathological analysis of two cases. Urol Int 1995;55:173–176.

140. Iczkowski KA, Shanks JH, Gadaleanu V, et al. Inflammatory pseudotumor and sarcoma of urinary bladder: differential diagnosis and outcome in thirty-eight spindle cell neoplasms. Mod Pathol 2001;14:1043–1051.

141. Mahadevia PS, Alexander JE, Rojas-Corona R, et al. Pseudosarcomatous stromal reaction in primary and metastatic urothelial carcinoma. A source of diagnostic difficulty. Am J Surg Pathol 1989;13:782–790.

142. Eble JN, Young RH. Stromal osseous metaplasia in carcinoma of the bladder. J Urol 1991;145:823–825.

143. Kinouchi T, Hanafusa T, Kuroda M, et al. Ossified cystic metastasis of bladder tumor to abdominal wound after partial cystectomy. J Urol 1995;153:1049–1050.

144. Lopez-Beltran A, Nogales F, Donne CH, et al. Adenocarcinoma of the urachus showing extensive calcification and stromal osseous metaplasia. Urol Int 1994;53:110–113.

145. Lamm K. Chondroid and osseous metaplasia in carcinoma of the bladder. J Urol Pathol 1995;3:255–262.

146. Zukerberg LR, Armin AR, Pisharodi L, et al. Transitional cell carcinoma of the urinary bladder with osteoclast-type giant cells: a report of two cases and review of the literature. Histopathology 1990;17:407–411.

147. Feeney D, Quesada ET, Sirbasku DM, et al. Transitional cell carcinoma in a tuberculous kidney: case report and review of the literature. J Urol 1994;151:989–991.

148. Flamm J. Tumor-associated tissue inflammatory reaction and eosinophilia in primary superficial bladder cancer. Urology 1992;40:180–185.

149. Lipponen PK, Eskelinen MJ, Jauhiainen K, et al. Tumour infiltrating lymphocytes as an independent prognostic factor in transitional cell bladder cancer. Eur J Cancer 1992;29A:69–75.

150. Sarma KP. The role of lymphoid reaction in bladder cancer. J Urol 1970;104:843–849.

151. Lopez-Beltran A, Morales C, Reymundo C, et al. T-zone histiocytes and recurrence of papillary urothelial bladder carcinoma. Urol Int 1989;44:205–209.

152. Offersen BV, Knap MM, Marcussen N, et al. Intense inflammation in bladder carcinoma is associated with angiogenesis and indicates good prognosis. Br J Cancer 2002;87:1422–1430.

# WHO/ISUP grading system

# 6

*Theresa Chan, Jonathan I Epstein*

## INTRODUCTION

In December 1998, members of the World Health Organization (WHO) and the International Society of Urologic Pathologists (ISUP) published the WHO/ISUP consensus classification of urothelial (transitional cell) neoplasms of the urinary bladder.[1] This new classification system arose out of the need to develop a universally acceptable classification system for bladder neoplasia that could be used effectively by pathologists, urologists, and oncologists. Before this classification system was developed, numerous diverse grading schemes for bladder cancer existed, and the same lesion seen by different pathologists might result in very different diagnoses solely because of differences in definitions. A strength of the consensus classification system is that it provides detailed histologic criteria for papillary urothelial lesions. In contrast, earlier grading systems for bladder tumors were vague and subjective. This classification system covered not only neoplastic conditions but also preneoplastic lesions (Box 6.1).

## NORMAL AND HYPERPLASTIC UROTHELIUM

Many pathologists overuse the diagnosis of 'mild dysplasia' to describe flat lesions with a minimally disordered growth pattern or cellular hyperchromasia due to variation in tissue fixation, staining, or specimen orientation. The consensus classification states that the term 'mild dysplasia' should not be used and that flat lesions with minimal cytologic atypia and architectural disorder should be diagnosed as 'normal'.

**Box 6.1** The WHO/ISUP consensus classification of urothelial (transitional) cell lesions

1. Normal
   - Normal*
2. Hyperplasia
   - Flat hyperplasia
   - Papillary hyperplasia
3. Flat lesions with atypia
   - Reactive (inflammatory) atypia
   - Dysplasia
   - Carcinoma in situ†
4. Papillary neoplasms
   - Papilloma
   - Papillary neoplasm of low malignant potential (PUNLMP)
   - Non-invasive papillary carcinoma, low grade
   - Non-invasive papillary carcinoma, high grade

\* May include cases formerly diagnosed as 'mild dysplasia'.
† May include cases formerly diagnosed as 'severe dysplasia'.

Flat urothelial hyperplasia consists of a markedly thickened mucosa without cytologic atypia, and may be seen adjacent to low-grade papillary urothelial neoplasms, but there are no data regarding its premalignant potential when seen by itself.

Papillary urothelial hyperplasia is characterized by urothelium of variable thickness with undulating growth. In contrast to papillary urothelial tumors, these lesions lack distinct fibrovascular cores. Papillary urothelial hyperplasia without cytologic atypia, because of its frequent association with either a prior or concurrent history of a low-grade papillary bladder neoplasm, is thought to be a precursor lesion of these neoplasms.[2] Papillary urothelial hyperplasia may also be lined by cytologically atypical urothelium, ranging from dysplasia to flat carcinoma in situ (CIS), which is often associated with and thought to be a precursor of high-grade papillary urothelial carcinomas.[3]

## FLAT LESIONS WITH ATYPIA

Prior to the consensus classification, pathologists used the terms 'atypia' and 'dysplasia' interchangeably to denote either inflammatory atypia or a preneoplastic condition. The WHO/ISUP system described the histologic findings associated with inflammatory atypia and designated these lesions as 'reactive atypia' which should not be considered neoplastic.

Dysplasia (intraurothelial neoplasia) was defined as a lesion with appreciable cytologic and architectural abnormalities believed to be neoplastic, yet falling short of the diagnostic threshold for CIS. There is evidence along several lines of investigation that dysplasia may be a precursor of invasive carcinoma.[4–9]

Carcinoma in situ is a flat lesion of the urothelium, and a documented precursor of invasive cancer in many cases (Figure 6.1). Before use of the consensus classification, CIS was frequently underdiagnosed and described as moderate dysplasia or atypia. The WHO/ISUP system described the key histologic features of CIS, including its more subtle variations that had often been under-recognized. Under the WHO/ISUP system, all CIS are, by definition, high-grade lesions.

## PAPILLARY UROTHELIAL NEOPLASMS: CLASSIFICATION

The classification of papillary urothelial neoplasms has been a long-standing source of controversy.[10] One area of controversy is the grading of papillary urothelial carcinomas. There are numerous grading systems, all of

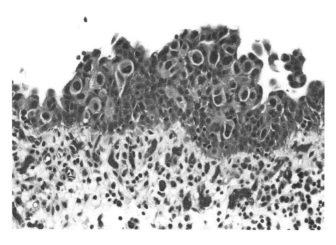

**Fig. 6.1**
Flat urothelial carcinoma in situ.

which have poor interobserver reproducibility, with most cases falling into the intermediate category.[11–18] The WHO/ISUP system is a modified version of the scheme proposed by Malmström et al.[16] A major limitation of the WHO 1973 grading system is the vague definition and lack of specific histologic criteria of the various grades. The following statement is the sole description of the difference between WHO grades 1, 2, and 3, as written in the original WHO 1973 book[13]:

> Grade 1 tumors have the least degree of anaplasia compatible with the diagnosis of malignancy. Grade 3 applies to tumors with the most severe degrees of cellular anaplasia, and Grade 2 lies in between.

Detailed histologic description of the various grades, employing specific cytologic and architectural criteria, is one of the major contributions of the WHO/ISUP system. These criteria are based on the architectural features of the papillae and the overall organization of the cells. Cytologic features encompassed in the WHO/ISUP system include nuclear size, nuclear shape, chromatin content, nucleoli, mitoses, and umbrella cells. The terminology used in the WHO/ISUP system parallels that used in urine cytology. Having a classification used in both cytology and histopathology is also advantageous. A website (www.pathology.jhu.edu/bladder) illustrating examples of the various grades was developed to further improve accuracy in using the WHO/ISUP system.

## RELATION OF WHO 1973 TO WHO/ISUP

A major misconception is that there is a one-to-one translation between the WHO/ISUP and the WHO 1973 classification systems. Only at the extremes of grades in the WHO 1973 classification does this correlation hold true. Lesions called papilloma in the WHO classification system would also be called papilloma in the WHO/ISUP system. At the other end of the grading spectrum, lesions called WHO grade 3 are by definition high-grade carcinoma in the WHO/ISUP system. However, for WHO grades 1 and 2, there is no direct translation to the WHO/ISUP system. Some lesions classified as WHO grade 1 in the 1973 system, upon review show no cytologic atypia, some nuclear enlargement, and merely thickened urothelium, so are classified as papillary urothelial neoplasms of low malignant potential (PUNLMP) in the WHO/ISUP system. However, other WHO grade 1 lesions showing slight cytologic atypia and mitoses are diagnosed in the WHO/ISUP system as low-grade papillary urothelial carcinomas.

WHO grade 2 is a very broad category. It includes lesions that are relatively bland, which in some places are diagnosed as WHO grade 1–2; these lesions in the

WHO/ISUP system would be called low-grade papillary urothelial carcinoma. In other cases, WHO grade 2 lesions border on higher grade lesions, which in many institutions are called WHO grade 2–3; these lesions in the WHO/ISUP classification system would be called high-grade papillary urothelial carcinoma.

## PAPILLOMA

Using the WHO 1973 system, some experts applied very restrictive criteria for the diagnosis of urothelial papilloma, in part based on the number of cell layers, and regarded all other papillary neoplasms as carcinomas. Others applied a broader definition of 'urothelial papilloma' so as not to label all patients with papillary lesions with minimal cytologic and architectural atypia as having carcinoma. The WHO/ISUP system has very restrictive histologic criteria for the diagnosis of papilloma when normal-appearing urothelium lines papillary fronds. Defined in this way, papilloma is a rare benign condition, typically occurring as a small, isolated growth seen primarily in younger patients. The majority of these lesions, once excised, will not recur.[19]

## PAPILLARY UROTHELIAL NEOPLASM OF LOW MALIGNANT POTENTIAL (PUNLMP)

The category of PUNLMP was derived to describe lesions that do not have cytologic features of malignancy, yet have thickened urothelium thicker than that with papilloma (Figure 6.2). Having a category of PUNLMP avoids labeling patients as having cancer with its psychosocial and financial (i.e. insurance) implications, though they are not diagnosed as having a benign lesion (i.e. papilloma) that might lead to their being followed

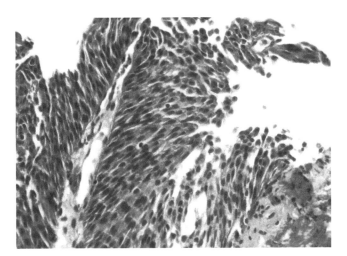

**Fig. 6.2**
Papillary neoplasm of low malignant potential (PUNLMP).

less closely. The prognosis of patients with these lesions and other papillary tumors in the WHO/ISUP system will be discussed later in this work. The current classification system allows for designation of a lesion (papillary urothelial neoplasm of low malignant potential) which biologically has a very low risk of progression, yet is not entirely benign. In the past, these lesions were a source of controversy, as some experts would label such lesions as malignant, while others, not wanting to label a patient with such a low-grade papillary lesion as having carcinoma, would diagnose these lesions as papilloma. This intermediate category allows both schools of thought to diagnose a lesion as not fully malignant, while still documenting the need for additional follow-up.

## LOW- AND HIGH-GRADE PAPILLARY CARCINOMA

In an attempt to simplify the WHO 1973 system and avoid an intermediate cancer grade group (WHO grade 2), which is often the default diagnosis for many pathologists, the WHO/ISUP system classifies papillary urothelial carcinoma into only two grades:

- Low-grade papillary urothelial carcinomas exhibit an orderly appearance overall but have minimal variability in architecture and/or cytologic features that are easily recognizable at scanning magnification (Figure 6.3).
- High-grade papillary urothelial carcinomas are characterized by a disorderly appearance resulting from marked architectural and cytologic abnormalities, recognizable at low magnification (Figure 6.4).

It is important to remember that a single papillary urothelial neoplasm may contain a spectrum of cytologic and architectural abnormalities. In tumors with variable histology, the tumor should be graded according to the highest grade, although current practice is to ignore minuscule areas of higher grade tumor. Studies are needed to determine how significant a minor component must be in order to have an impact on prognosis.

## PAPILLARY UROTHELIAL NEOPLASMS: PROGNOSIS

One of the earliest papers reported to have used the WHO/ISUP system has led to misconceptions regarding the classification system. A manuscript was submitted for publication in October 1998 and eventually published in *Cancer* entitled 'Papillary urothelial neoplasms of low malignant potential'.[20] This article was

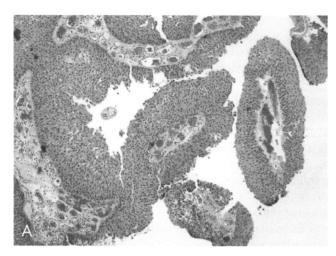

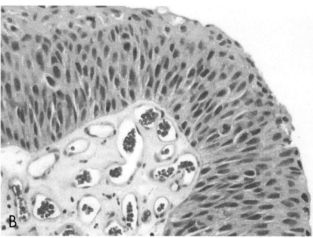

**Fig. 6.3**
A, B Non-invasive papillary carcinoma, low grade.

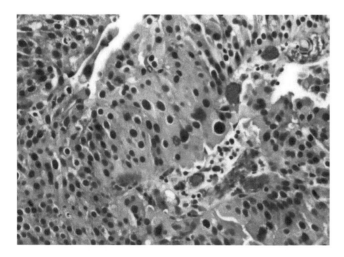

**Fig. 6.4**
Non-invasive papillary carcinoma, high grade.

submitted before the WHO/ISUP classification system was even published and before there were detailed illustrations or descriptions of how to use the new system. The authors took lesions that were formerly called WHO grade 1 and designated them as PUNLMP. As described above, there is not a one-to-one translation between the WHO/ISUP and WHO 1973 classification systems. If these lesions were analyzed correctly using the WHO/ISUP classification system, many would not be classified as PUNLMP, but would be diagnosed as low-grade urothelial carcinomas. It is no surprise that the cases they classified as PUNLMP had an increased risk of recurrence, progression, and death from bladder cancer. This article has been cited as an argument against the use of the WHO/ISUP system. However, given that WHO grade 1 cancers were simply renamed as PUNLMP in that study, it should not even be considered as having used the WHO/ISUP system.

Before discussing the prognosis for patients based on the WHO/ISUP system, it is worthwhile to briefly highlight differences amongst studies in terms of their inclusion criteria and definition of progression. Some reports restrict their study only to cases without invasion (Ta). Although stage T1 disease is still considered to be 'superficial bladder cancer', once lamina propria invasion is identified, these patients are at an increased risk of subsequently developing detrusor muscle (muscularis propria) invasion (stage T2). Consequently, including Ta (non-invasive) and T1 (superficially invasive) tumors leads to a heterogeneous group of patients.

Another difference in inclusion criteria is that some studies include patients with CIS, while others do not. CIS is one of the more aggressive lesions in the bladder despite its flat morphology. Including patients with CIS in a study of patients with non-invasive or minimally invasive papillary carcinomas adds an additional variable, which must be taken into account when analyzing prognosis. The definition of progression also varies amongst studies. Some include progression from Ta to T1, while others require evolution to T2. In some but not other studies a change in grade or the development of CIS is considered progression.

The first article to use the WHO/ISUP system, as it was meant to be used and to correlate its lesions with prognosis, was published by Desai et al in 2000.[21] The authors examined 120 Ta and T1 tumors. However, it was not clear if patients with a history of CIS were excluded. Desai et al[21] showed significant differences in prognosis amongst the various categories. While papillomas did not recur or progress, and LMP tumors recurred but did not progress, patients with low-grade and, to a greater extent, high-grade carcinomas experienced progression (Table 6.1).[21]

In 2001, Alsheikh et al examined 49 patients with Ta tumors that did not receive any additional treatment after an initial transurethral resection.[22] The authors

**Table 6.1** Relation of WHO/ISUP grades to progression

| | Papilloma (%) (n=8) | PUNLMP (%) (n=8) | Low grade (%) (n=42) | High grade (%) (n=62) |
|---|---|---|---|---|
| Recurrence | 0 | 33.3 | 64.1 | 56.4 |
| Any stage progression | 0 | 0 | 10.5 | 27.1 |
| Lamina propria invasion | 0 | 0 | 2.6 | 8.3 |
| Detrusor muscle invasion | 0 | 0 | 5.3 | 6.3 |
| Metastases/death | 0 | 0 | 10.6 | 25.0 |

Based on data from Desai et al.[21]

focused on the differences between the 20 PUNLMPs and 29 low-grade carcinomas: 25% of the PUNLMPs recurred, in contrast to 48% of the low-grade carcinomas. Of the two patients whose disease progressed to high-grade muscle-invasive carcinoma, both initially had low-grade carcinomas. One other patient whose disease progressed to CIS also had low-grade carcinoma initially.

The largest study to date using the WHO/ISUP classification system is that by Holmang et al.[23] Three hundred and sixty-three Ta tumors were evaluated and 83% of the patients were treated only with transurethral resection of the bladder tumor. Progression was considered to have occurred when tumors developed invasion beyond the muscularis mucosae (deep lamina propria, formerly stage T1B) or metastatic disease. Most patients with PUNLMP had no evidence of recurrence, and only a small percentage of patients had tumor at last follow-up, with no one dying of disease. In contrast, patients with low grade carcinoma had an increased risk of recurrence, and a small percentage of patients died of the disease. Patients with high-grade carcinoma had a greater risk (16%) of dying of disease (Table 6.2).[23] Low- and high-grade carcinomas had a similar risk of recurrence, which contrasted with a lower risk with PUNLMPs. In terms of progression, PUNLMPs and low-grade carcinomas had similar risks compared with an increased risk with high-grade carcinomas. The difference between the risk of progression in WHO

grade 2 and grade 3 lesions was greater than the difference between low- and high-grade carcinomas as classified in the WHO/ISUP system. Since most WHO grade 3 cases are aggressive tumors and already have coexisting invasive cancer, very few patients with WHO grade 3 tumors initially satisfied the criteria of having non-invasive papillary carcinoma (Ta); of the 363 with non-invasive papillary carcinomas, only 3.6% were classified as WHO grade 3. Furthermore, some of patients with WHO grade 3 non-invasive papillary cancers had coexistent CIS. With the WHO/ISUP system, Holmang et al classified 28% of the patients as having high-grade carcinoma, with an increased risk of progression.

Pich et al also focused their investigations on differences between PUNLMPs and low-grade carcinomas.[24] In addition to recurrence and progression, p53 expression and proliferation markers were analyzed. In their study, p53 and MIB1 (a proliferation marker) immunostaining were considered positive in all the reactive nuclei, regardless of the staining intensity, and the fraction of positive cells was recorded. A case was considered positive if >10% of the cells stained. Sixty-two Ta tumors were studied. No patients received adjuvant therapy until recurrence. Progression was defined as any invasion or metastasis, which occurred in five patients. Differences in recurrence were noted between PUNLMPs and low-grade cancers, with recurrence rates of 47.4% and 76.7%, respectively. While none of the PUNLMPs progressed, 11.6% of the low-grade carcinomas progressed. There was also a difference in the recurrence-free interval between PUNLMPs and low-grade carcinomas, with 76 and 15 months' recurrence-free intervals, respectively. Statistically significant differences were also noted between the two WHO/ISUP grades in their p53 expression, mitoses, and MIB1 activity. The relationship of the markers to recurrence was not directly analyzed.

We have also analyzed tumors using the WHO/ISUP classification system for p53 expression and proliferation as measured by Ki67.[25] In this study, 200 cells from the most immunoreactive regions of each lesion were visually counted and the percentage of cells

**Table 6.2** Relation of WHO/ISUP grades to progression

| | PUNLMP (%) (n=95) | Low grade (%) (n=160) | High grade (%) (n=108) |
|---|---|---|---|
| No evidence of disease | 94 | 76 | 67 |
| Alive with disease | 3 | 10 | 9 |
| Dead with disease | 1 | 6 | 7 |
| Dead of disease | 0 | 4 | 16 |
| No follow-up | 2 | 4 | 1 |

Based on data from Holmang et al.[23]

positive for p53 and Ki67—labeling index (LI)—was tabulated without knowledge of the WHO/ISUP diagnosis. Immunohistochemical positivity was defined as strong, homogenous nuclear staining; nonspecific staining of umbrella cells was excluded. An increase in p53 expression of 0.4%, 2.9%, and 25.7% was documented in cases of LMP, low-grade carcinoma, and high-grade carcinoma, respectively. Proliferation (Ki67 labeling index) also increased amongst the three grades: 2.5%, 7.3%, and 15.7%, respectively.

In a separate study, 134 patients with Ta tumors without prior or concurrent CIS or invasion were analyzed.[26] Progression was defined as tumor recurrence with any invasion (T1 or T2), or CIS. The 90-month actuarial risks of progression for WHO papilloma, and carcinomas grade 1, 2, and 3 were 0%, 11%, 24%, and 60%, respectively. The corresponding progression rates for WHO/ISUP papilloma, PUNLMP, and low-grade and high-grade carcinomas were 0%, 8%, 13%, and 51%, respectively. WHO grade (p=0.003) and tumor size (p=0.03) and WHO/ISUP (p=0.002) and tumor size (p=0.04) independently predicted progression. Although WHO grade 3 cancers had a more rapid progression rate and a slightly worse long-term progression rate compared to WHO/ISUP high-grade cancer, only 4.5% of tumors were WHO grade 3 whereas 21.6% were classified as WHO/ISUP high grade. Our findings are similar to those in Holmang et al's study, where only 3.6% of tumors were classified as WHO (1973) grade 3, as compared with 28% classified as WHO/ISUP high-grade carcinoma.[23] As patients with non-invasive high-grade papillary carcinoma are not treated with definitive therapy (i.e. cystectomy), the goal should not be to restrict this high-risk group to a very small population, but to expand it to include all patients at significant risk of progression to be monitored closely.

## INVASIVE UROTHELIAL CARCINOMA

Confusion in terminology is not limited to the diagnostic entities in the various classification schemes, as it also exists for the descriptive terminology applied to invasive urothelial lesions. Various terms include 'superficial muscle invasion', 'deep muscle invasion', 'muscle invasion (not otherwise specified)', and 'superficial bladder cancer'. The last term is particularly confusing as it could be applied to CIS, non-invasive papillary neoplasms, or truly invasive urothelial carcinoma (T1). Because of variations in treatment and prognostic significance related to the depth of invasion of bladder tumors, the consensus group developed several recommendations to provide clinicians with this essential information in an unambiguous manner.

Invasion of the lamina propria is characterized by nests, clusters, or single urothelial cells which have breached the epithelial basement membrane. A useful feature in identifying invasion is the presence of marked retraction artifacts around the infiltrating cellular clusters, which may closely mimic lymphovascular invasion. Since vascular invasion is uncommon in urothelial carcinomas limited to the lamina propria, care should be taken not to overinterpret this artifact. As invasion extends into the mid-level of the lamina propria, carcinoma will eventually infiltrate into wispy smooth muscle bundles, the muscularis mucosae. Although several studies have shown that the depth of lamina propria invasion with respect to the muscularis mucosae has prognostic significance, the consensus committee chose to make substaging of lamina propria invasion optional. Pathologists are encouraged, however, to assess the extent of invasion (i.e. focal versus extensive) to help guide urologists to an appropriate treatment plan.

The distinction between invasion of the muscularis mucosae and muscularis propria (detrusor muscle) is critical but may be difficult. The presence of numerous blood vessels admixed with small bundles of smooth muscles favors muscularis mucosae whereas large dense bundles of smooth muscle characterize the muscularis propria. The depth of invasion cannot be accurately determined in all instances. When biopsies are equivocal, pathologists should convey their uncertainty to the urologist, who is likely to initiate a restaging procedure.

Three final comments on depth of invasion are warranted:

1. The pathologist has accomplished the task if able to discriminate between invasion of the muscularis mucosae and muscularis propria on a bladder biopsy specimen. Attempts at substaging the depth of invasion of the muscularis propria on a biopsy specimen are neither required nor expected. Definitive assessment of the depth of invasion should be reserved for the final resection specimen.
2. The presence of adipose tissue admixed with tumor on a biopsy specimen is not necessarily indicative of extravesical spread of tumor. In fact, fat may be present at any level of the bladder, including both the lamina propria and muscularis propria.
3. The consensus committee recommends mentioning the presence or absence of muscularis propria in all bladder biopsy specimens as this provides useful feedback to the urologist regarding biopsy technique and adequacy.

## CONCLUSION

The potential advantages of the WHO/ISUP system are:

- acceptance across a broad spectrum of urologic pathologists, allowing for uniform terminology and common definitions

- detailed definitions of various preneoplastic conditions and various grades of tumor, hopefully leading to greater interobserver reproducibility
- use of terminology that is more or less consistent with what is used in urine cytology, creating a consensus classification between cytology and histopathology
- creation of a category (PUNLMP) for tumors with a negligible risk of progression, and thus avoiding a diagnosis of cancer with its psychosocial and financial (i.e. insurance) implications; these patients also are not diagnosed as having a benign lesion (i.e. papilloma) that might not be followed as closely
- identification of a larger group of patients at high risk for progression for urologists to follow more closely
- recommendations for reporting extent of invasive carcinoma in an unambiguous manner, essential for proper treatment and management.

In 2004, the WHO made its recommendations on the classification of non-invasive urothelial lesions.[27] The recommendations are essentially the same as the WHO/ISUP 1998 system, and thus there is now only one unified nomenclature system.

## REFERENCES

1. Epstein JI, Amin MB, Reuter VE, Mostofi FK. The World Health Organization/International Society of Urological Pathology consensus classification of urothelial (transitional cell) neoplasms of the urinary bladder. Bladder Consensus Conference Committee. Am J Surg Pathol 1998;12:1435–1448.
2. Taylor DC, Bhagavan BS, Larsen MP, Cox JA, Epstein JI. Papillary urothelial hyperplasia. A precursor to papillary neoplasms. Am J Surg Pathol 1996;20:1481–1488.
3. Swierczynski SL, Epstein JI. Prognostic significance of atypical papillary urothelial hyperplasia. Hum Pathol 2002;33(5):512–517.
4. Althausen AF, Prout GRJ, Dal JJ. Noninvasive papillary carcinoma of the bladder associated with carcinoma in-situ. J Urol 1976;116:575–580.
5. Farrow GM, Utz DC, Rife CC. Morphological and clinical observations of patients with early bladder cancer treated with total cystectomy. Cancer Res 1976;36:2495–2501.
6. Koss LG. Mapping of the urinary bladder: its impact on the concepts of bladder cancer. Hum Pathol 1979;10:533–548.
7. Smith G, Elton RA, Beynon LL, Newsam JE, Chisolm GD, Hargreave TB. Prognostic significance of biopsy results of normal-looking mucosa in cases of superficial bladder cancer. Br J Urol 1983;55:665–669.
8. Heney NM, Ahmed S, Flanagan MJ, et al. Superficial bladder cancer: progression and recurrence. J Urol 1983;130:1083–1086.
9. Hofstäder F, Delgado R, Jakse G, Judmaier W. Urothelial dysplasia and carcinoma in situ of the bladder. Cancer 1986;57:356–361.
10. Eble JN, Young RH. Benign and low-grade papillary lesions of the urinary bladder: a review of the papilloma–papillary carcinoma controversy and a report of 5 typical papillomas. Semin Diagn Pathol 1989;6:351–371.
11. Broders AC. Epithelium of the genito-urinary organs. Ann Surg 1922;75:574–604.
12. Bergkvist A, Ljungqvist A, Moberger G. Classification of bladder tumours based on the cellular pattern. Acta Chir Scand 1965;130:371–378.
13. Mostofi FK, Sobin LH, Torloni H. Histological typing of urinary bladder tumours. International classification of tumors 19. Geneva: World Health Organization, 1973.
14. Ooms ECM, Anderson WAAD, Alons CL, Boon ME, Veldhuizen RW. Analysis of the performance of pathologists in the grading of bladder tumors. Hum Pathol 1983;14:140–143.
15. Jordan AM, Weingarten J, Murphy WM. Transitional cell neoplasms of the urinary bladder. Can biologic potential be predicted from histologic grading? Cancer 1987;60:2766–2774.
16. Malmström P-U, Busch C, Norlén BJ. Recurrence, progression and survival in bladder cancer: a retrospective analysis of 232 patients with 5-year follow-up. Scand J Urol Nephrol 1987;21:185–195.
17. Abel PD, Henderson D, Bennett, Hall RR. Differing interpretations by pathologists of the pT category and grade of transitional cell cancer of the bladder. Br J Urol 1988;62:339–342.
18. Carbin B-E, Ekman P, Gustafson H, Christensen NJ, Silfversward C, Sandstedt B. Grading of human urothelial carcinoma based on nuclear atypia and mitotic frequency. II: Prognostic importance. J Urol 1991;145:972–976.
19. McKenney JK, Amin MB, Young RH. Urothelial (transitional cell) papilloma of the urinary bladder: a clinicopathologic study of 25 cases. Mod Pathol 2002;15:174A.
20. Cheng L, Newman RM, Bostwick DG. Papillary urothelial neoplasms of low malignant potential. Cancer 1999;86:2102–2108.
21. Desai S, Lim SD, Jiminez RE, et al. Relationship of cytokeratin 20 and CD44 protein expression with WHO/ISUP grade in pTa and pT1 papillary urothelial neoplasia. Mod Pathol 2000;13:1315–1323.
22. Alsheikh A, Mohamedali Z, Jones E, et al. Comparison of the WHO/ISUP classification and cytokeratin 20 expression in predicting the behavior of low-grade papillary urothelial tumors. Mod Pathol 2001;14:267–272.
23. Holmang S, Andius P, Hedelin H, et al. Stage progression in TA papillary urothelial tumors: relationship to grade, immunohistochemical expression of tumor markers, mitotic frequency and DNA ploidy. J Urol 2001;165:1124–1130.
24. Pich A, Chiusa L, Formiconi A, Galliano D, Bortolini P, Navone R. Biologic differences between noninvasive papillary urothelial neoplasms of low malignant potential and low grade (grade 1) papillary carcinomas of the bladder. Am J Surg Pathol 2001;25:1528–1533.
25. Cina SJ, Lancaster-Weiss KJ, Lecksell K, et al. Correlation of ki-67 and p53 with the new World Health Organization/International Society of Urological Pathology classification system for urothelial neoplasia. Arch Pathol Lab Med 2001;125:646–651.
26. Samaratunga H, Makarov, DV, Epstein JI. Comparison of WHO/ISUP and WHO classification of non-invasive papillary urothelial neoplasms for risk of progression. Urology 2002;60(2):315–319.
27. Eble JN, Sauter G, Epstein JI, Sesterhenn IA (eds). World Health Organization Classification of Tumours. Pathology and Genetics of Tumours of the Urinary System and Male Genital Organs. Lyon: IARC Press, 2004.

# Urothelial bladder tumor pathology

## Contemporary consensus classification and diagnosis based on the World Health Organization (WHO) 1973 classification

7

*David G Bostwick, Rodolfo Montironi, Junqi Qian, Antonio Lopez-Beltran, Liang Cheng*

## INTRODUCTION

The WHO 1973 classification of bladder cancer is the most widely used system in the world today. The main criticism of this classification has been its imprecise histopathologic diagnostic criteria. The Ancona 2001 refinement is a contemporary consensus description ('telescopic ramification') of the WHO 1973 classification with expanded diagnostic criteria that are fully compatible with all related publications for the past 3 years.

Urothelial tumors are divided into two main groups based on growth pattern: flat and papillary. Flat tumors form a morphologic continuum whose classification includes reactive changes, dysplasia, and carcinoma in situ (CIS); subgrading of CIS is not recommended. Papillary tumors include papilloma, and carcinoma grade 1, 2 and 3. The diagnostic criteria for each of these categories were refined and optimized in the Ancona 2001 consensus refinement. New classification and grading schemes were found to be fraught with conflicting definitions and varying translations with the WHO 1973 standard, rendering them ineffective and confusing. Terms recently introduced for these grading schemes, including 'low malignant potential' and 'atypia of uncertain clinical significance', are discouraged.

We conclude that the WHO 1973 standard for classification and grading of bladder tumors is a robust, clinically proven, widely used, time-tested, and reasonably reproducible method for pathologic reporting, and is recommended with only minor modifications.

## CLASSIFICATION AND GRADING SYSTEMS

The World Health Organization (WHO) 1973 classification and grading system for bladder tumors has been repeatedly validated and is near-universally used.[1-3] Nonetheless, multiple new classification and grading schemes for bladder cancer were formally introduced and promoted by their respective architect pathologists in the past few years without validation and with little or no input from urologists, oncologists, radiation therapists, or any nonpathologists (Table 7.1, Figure 7.1).[4-7] Marked variation in interpretation and definitions of all of these new schemes has resulted in confusion and frustration among pathologists and clinicians; for example, careful examination revealed multiple different published definitions of the WHO/ISUP 1998 scheme and two definitions of the new WHO 1999 scheme (Table 7.1), none of which has been validated. These new grading systems often depart considerably from the popular standard of the 1973 World Health Organization, introducing new terms, as described above, amid controversy. These terms have encountered great resistance among clinician users, and both were formally abandoned by consensus at the Ancona conference, similar to the recommendation of Oyasu.[2]

New grading efforts for bladder tumors were intended to create universal standards of terminology and criteria to allow comparison of results from different centers and promote cooperation. However, the laudable goals of the recent efforts for change have not been attained, and these new schemes appear to have little hope of

**Table 7.1** Classification of papillary urothelial neoplasms: comparison with and translation from the WHO 1973 classification

| WHO 1973 Standard | WHO/ISUP 1998-A* | WHO/ISUP 1998-B† | WHO/ISUP 1998-C‡ | WHO 1999-A§ | WHO 1999-B+ | WHO 1973, Ancona 2001# |
|---|---|---|---|---|---|---|
| Papilloma | Papilloma | Papilloma | Papilloma | Papilloma and LMP | Papilloma | Papilloma |
| Grade 1 carcinoma | LMP | LMP | LMP and low-grade carcinoma | LMP and new grade 1 carcinoma | LMP and new grade 1 carcinoma | Grade 1 carcinoma |
| Grade 2 carcinoma | Low-grade carcinoma | Low- and high-grade carcinoma | Low- and high-grade carcinoma | Grade 2 carcinoma (unchanged) | New grade 1 carcinoma and new grade 2 carcinoma | Grade 2 carcinoma |
| Grade 3 carcinoma | High-grade carcinoma | High-grade carcinoma | High-grade carcinoma | Grade 3 carcinoma (unchanged) | New grade 3 carcinoma | Grade 3 carcinoma |

ISUP, International Society of Urologic Pathologists; LMP, urothelial tumor of low malignant potential; WHO, World Health Organization.
* WHO/ISUP 1998-A: Refers to definitions and translations from International Society of Urologic Pathologists meeting minutes, March 1998 consensus conference, published in Bostwick & Lopez-Beltran[77]; Cheng et al.[78]
† WHO/ISUP 1998-B: Refers to translation in Reuter & Melamed.[46]
‡ WHO/ISUP 1998-C: Refers to translation in Holmang et al[6]; also to translation in Yin & Leong.[79]
§ WHO 1999-A: Refers to definitions and translations in Mostofi et al.[5]
+ WHO 1999-B: Refers to translation in Holmang et al.[6]
# The Ancona 2001 refinement of WHO 1973 uses the same terminology for papillary neoplasms as WHO 1973; the definitions are also identical, but have been merely expanded to allow greater precision in separation of each of the diagnostic categories.[1]

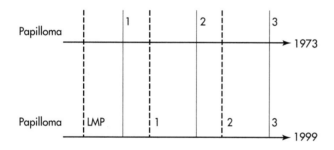

**Fig. 7.1**
Comparison of World Health Organization (WHO) grading schemes for papillary urothelial tumors. The spectrum of tumors is a continuum that ranges from benign papilloma (left side) to grade 3 carcinoma (right side); the continuum is represented by the horizontal lines. Note that the cut points for grade 1 and grade 2 cancer in 1973 (solid vertical lines) are shifted to the right in the 1999 scheme (dotted vertical lines), with the additional category of papillary tumor of low malignant potential (LMP) between papilloma and grade 1 carcinoma.

widespread acceptance. A recent study of reproducibility revealed that WHO 1973 was identical to WHO/ISUP 1998.[8] A smaller report noted 'moderate' reproducibility between two pathologists with the WHO/ISUP 1998 classification.[9] Further, we believe that the WHO 1973 standard, the most widely used system in the world, was not 'broken' to begin with, and thus did not require substantial repairs or alterations; we believe that minor modifications and refinements are sufficient based on our current knowledge.

The main criticism of the WHO 1973 classification has been the imprecise histopathologic diagnostic criteria.[6,10] However, at least one group of authors erroneously reported that the description was only '6 lines' of text, failing to observe additional text elsewhere in the original WHO publication.[6]

In an effort to improve the precision and utility of the WHO 1973 classification, we present herein an expanded and refined description of the scheme. This effort was inspired by discussions during the consensus meeting, and is thus considered the Ancona (Italy) refinement, following the suggestions of the TNM staging committee for 'telescopic ramification' of existing systems rather than complete abandonment of previous systems (Box 7.1).[11]

Remarkably, the collected authors, assembled from multiple countries from around the world and multiple disciplines, easily reached agreement on these criteria.

Grading of bladder tumors, particularly papillary tumors, may be difficult owing to intratumoral heterogeneity, and two caveats are recognized:

1. Grading is based on the highest level of abnormality noted. No formal recommendation has been previously made regarding the amount or extent of a higher grade needed for upgrading, but we require at least one high-power field (40× magnification with additional 20× eyepieces); further study of this suggestion is indicated.

2. Tangential cutting of urothelium at the base results in the appearance of fused papillae and sheets of cells with large nuclei and increased number of mitotic figures that may lead to overdiagnosis or overgrading.[12]

# FLAT LESIONS

## REACTIVE CHANGES

### Diagnostic criteria

Reactive changes are almost always associated with acute or chronic inflammation in the lamina propria. This results from a variety of inciting agents, including bacteria, calculi, trauma, chemicals and toxins, or no apparent cause (idiopathic). In early acute cystitis resulting from bacterial infection, there is vascular dilation and congestion, erythematous and hemorrhagic mucosa, and moderate to severe edema. With time, polypoid or bullous cystitis may develop, sometimes with ulceration. The urothelium may be hyperplastic or metaplastic, and, when ulcerated, is often covered by a fibrinous membrane with neutrophils and bacterial colonies. Stromal edema and chronic inflammation gradually become more pronounced, particularly in the lamina propria. If the acute inflammation persists, chronic cystitis usually develops, sometimes with prominent mural fibrosis. In chronic cystitis, the mucosa may be thin, hyperplastic, or ulcerated, often with reactive changes (Figure 7.2). Follicular cystitis is an uncommon but distinctive variant of chronic cystitis. Granulation tissue is often conspicuous in the early stages, and may be replaced by dense scarring, particularly in the late healing stages. This process may be transmural and involve perivesicular tissue.

### Clinical significance

Patients with reactive changes are not at increased risk for the development of dysplasia, CIS, or urothelial

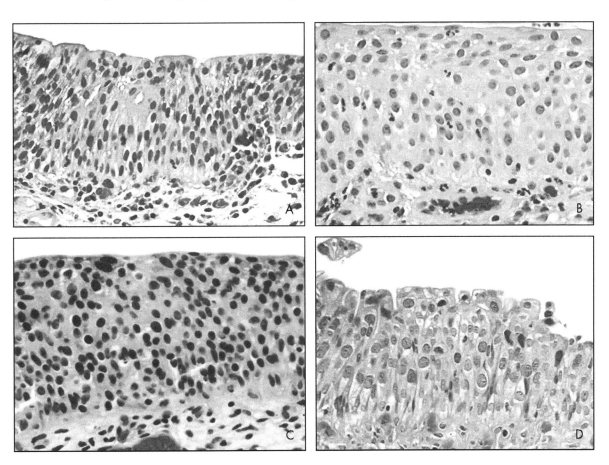

**Fig. 7.2**
**A** Reactive urothelial changes. **B** Reactive urothelial changes. **C** Urothelial dysplasia. **D** Urothelial dysplasia bordering on CIS.

carcinoma.[13,14] This category of reactive changes now incorporates the WHO/ISUP 1998 category of 'atypia of unknown clinical significance'. Cheng et al studied 35 patients with 'atypia of unknown clinical significance' followed for a mean of 3.7 years and found no increased risk for recurrence or progression; they recommended abandoning the term and compressing the category into reactive changes, and we concur.[13]

## DYSPLASIA

### Diagnostic criteria

The cytologic abnormalities in dysplasia are less severe than in CIS, and are usually restricted to the basal and intermediate layers (see Figure 7.2). The abnormalities include cell crowding and disorganization with nuclear enlargement, coarsely clumped chromatin, variation in nuclear shape, and scattered notching of chromatinic rims. Nucleoli are usually small and inconspicuous or rarely enlarged. Mitotic figures are usually absent. The superficial cell layer is intact. Nuclear and architectural features are most useful in distinguishing reactive changes and dysplasia.[15]

### Clinical significance

Urothelial dysplasia is a marker for cancer risk. Cheng et al studied 36 patients with isolated dysplasia of the bladder and found that 19% developed biopsy-proven cancer progression (11% with CIS and 8% invasive cancer) with a mean follow-up of 8.2 years; three patients developed muscle-invasive cancer.[16] Zuk et al studied 15 patients with dysplasia that were followed for a mean of 4.8 years, finding that 15% of patients developed CIS.[17] Similarly, Baithun and colleagues found that 14% of patients with dysplasia developed CIS.[18] These results emphasize the need for careful monitoring of patients with dysplasia by endoscopy and cytology; treatments such as intravesical chemotherapy or bacillus Calmette–Guérin (BCG) are not currently recommended because the side effects of these agents may outweigh the potential and unknown benefits.

## CARCINOMA IN SITU

### Diagnostic criteria

Urothelial CIS is characterized by flat disordered proliferation of urothelial cells with marked cytologic abnormalities (Figure 7.3). In most cases, CIS is multifocal, appearing cystoscopically as erythematous velvety or granular patches, although it may be visually undetectable.[19] The cells of CIS may form a layer that is only one cell layer thick, of normal thickness (up to seven cells), or the thickness of hyperplasia (more than seven cells). The diagnosis of CIS requires the presence of severe cytologic atypia (nuclear anaplasia); full thickness change is not essential, although it is usually present. Interobserver agreement with CIS is good to very good.

Prominent architectural disorganization of the urothelium is characteristic, with loss of cell polarity and cohesiveness. Superficial (umbrella) cells may be present except in areas of full thickness abnormality. The tumor cells tend to be large and pleomorphic, with moderate to abundant cytoplasm, although they are sometimes small with a high nucleus to cytoplasmic ratio. The chromatin tends to be coarse and clumped. Morphometrically, the cells display increased nuclear area, nuclear perimeter, and maximum nuclear diameter. Nucleoli are usually large and prominent in at least some of the cells, and may be multiple. Mitotic figures are often seen in the uppermost urothelium, and may be atypical. The adjacent mucosa often contains lesser degrees of cytologic abnormality.

The small cell pattern of CIS is usually associated with an increased number of cell layers. In such cases, the cytoplasm is scant and nuclei are enlarged and hyperchromatic, with coarse, unevenly distributed chromatin; scattered prominent nucleoli are distorted and angulated. Mitotic figures are frequently present, often with abnormal forms. The cells are randomly oriented and disorganized, often with striking cellular discohesion, that, in some cases, results in few or no recognizable epithelial cells on the surface, a condition referred to as denuding cystitis.[14] Careful search of all residual mucosa is important in biopsies that have little or no mucosa in order to exclude the denuding cystitis of CIS.

CIS is often associated with focal discontinuity of the basement membrane. There may be intense chronic inflammation in the superficial lamina propria in some cases, and vascular ectasia and proliferation of small capillaries are frequent. In denuded areas, residual CIS may involve von Brunn's nests. Rarely, CIS exhibits pagetoid growth, characterized by large single cells or small clusters of cells within otherwise normal urothelium, in squamous metaplasia, or within prostatic ducts.[20-23] Individual cells showing pagetoid spread have enlarged nuclei with coarse chromatin, single or multiple nucleoli, and abundant pale to eosinophilic cytoplasm that is mucin negative. Careful search should be made for subepithelial invasion (microinvasion), often appearing as single cells or small nests of cells with retraction artifact. Microinvasion may be masked by chronic inflammation, denuded mucosa, or stromal fibrosis.

### Clinical significance

Urothelial CIS has a high likelihood of progressing to invasive carcinoma if untreated, occurring in up to 83% of cases.[24] Cystectomy reveals foci of microinvasion in 34% of bladders with CIS, and muscle-invasive cancer in up to 9%.[20-22] Patients with CIS treated by radical

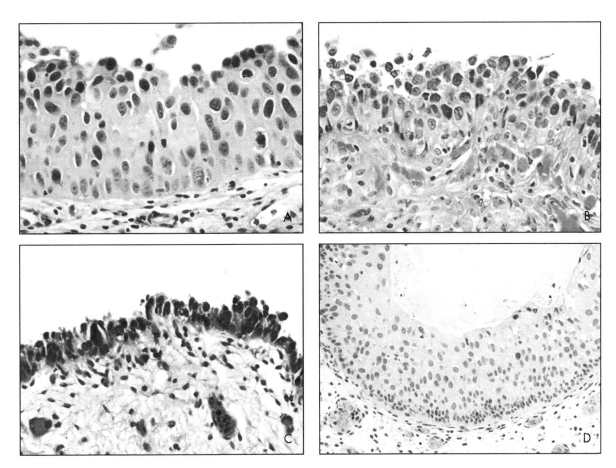

**Fig. 7.3**
**A** CIS displays disorderly proliferation of malignant urothelial cells with high nuclear cytoplasmic ratio, nuclear pleomorphism, irregular nuclear contours, coarsely granular chromatin, and prominent nucleoli. **B** CIS with early cellular discohesion. **C** CIS with partially denuded urothelium. **D** CIS involving Brunn's nests.

cystectomy have up to 100% 5-year survival.[25] Intravesical therapy is also commonly employed, including thiotepa, mitomycin C, and BCG.[26]

Primary CIS has a lower risk of progression (28% versus 59%) and death (7% versus 45%) than secondary CIS.[23] Factors predictive of high risk of progression include multifocality, coexistent bladder neoplasm, prostatic urethral involvement, and recurrence after treatment. Concomitant ureteral CIS is uncommon, present in 8% of patients undergoing radical cystectomy.[27] In a recent study, frozen sections failed to detect CIS of the ureteral margin in 17% of cases, but was only rarely associated with local morbidity; the authors questioned the value of frozen section examination of ureteral margins, and recommended reliance on urine cytology.[27]

The clinical course of patients with urothelial CIS is variable; up to 83% of patients will develop invasive cancer, and up to 38% of patients will die of bladder cancer.[13,19-23,25,27-44] Melamed et al first described the natural history of urothelial CIS and found that 9 of 25 patients (36%) developed invasive carcinoma within 5 years after the initial diagnosis; others (16 patients)

received cystectomy.[35] Stanisic et al treated 26 patients with intravesical therapy for CIS.[40] At 5 years, 50% of their patients progressed to deeply invasive (muscle or beyond) or metastatic cancer, and 27% died. In a study of 62 patients with CIS, Utz and Farrow showed that 60% of patients developed invasive cancer, and 38% died of cancer within a period of 5 years.[43] In detailed mapping studies of 21 cystectomy specimens removed from patients with CIS, invasive cancer was identified in 20% of cases and extensive mucosal involvement was seen in every case.[43] These results, in conjunction with the findings of Cheng et al,[13,28] indicate that urothelial CIS is a significant risk factor for the development of invasive cancer and subsequent death due to cancer.

Isolated urothelial CIS in the absence of papillary urothelial carcinoma is less common. Orozco et al studied 102 patients with urothelial CIS and found that 73 patients (72%) had coexistent urothelial carcinoma, including 27 patients with coexistent non-invasive papillary urothelial carcinoma.[23] With less than 5 years of follow-up, 2 of 29 patients with isolated urothelial CIS died of bladder cancer; 33 of 73 patients (45%) with secondary CIS died of bladder cancer. Among 27 patients with coexistent non-invasive papillary urothelial carcinoma, 12 patients (44%) died of bladder cancer. Cheng et al found that there was no outcome difference between patients with isolated CIS (80 patients) and those with coexistent non-invasive papillary urothelial carcinoma (58 patients).[28] Fifteen year cancer-specific survival was 72% for those with isolated CIS compared to 78% for those with coexistent non-invasive papillary urothelial carcinoma.

## PAPILLARY LESIONS

### PAPILLOMA

#### Diagnostic criteria

In 1973 the World Health Organization recommended restrictive criteria for papilloma,[1] and these diagnostic features are now internationally accepted; standardized criteria should eliminate much of the confusion regarding the incidence and diagnosis of this lesion (Table 7.2). The WHO criteria for papilloma include the following five main features: 1) small (<2 cm in greatest dimension; 2) usually solitary papillary lesion with one or more delicate fibrovascular cores; 3) lined by cytologically and architecturally normal urothelium with orderly maturation; 4) an intact superficial (umbrella) cell layer and no mitotic figures; and 5) occurring in patient usually less than 50 years of age (Figure 7.4).[1] The urothelium is usually of normal thickness, although factitious appearance of thickening may be observed owing to tangential cutting at the base of the papilloma. There is little or no variation in nuclear size, shape, or spacing when compared with normal urothelium, and the chromatin texture is finely granular without nucleolar enlargement. Slight deviation from one of these criteria may be acceptable with an otherwise typical papilloma; for example, the presence of mild to moderate cytologic atypia of the superficial cells does not exclude the diagnosis of papilloma, particularly when accompanied by an explanatory inflammatory infiltrate. Papilloma should not be confused with grade 1 urothelial carcinoma despite the suggestion of a small number of authors to the contrary.[45,46]

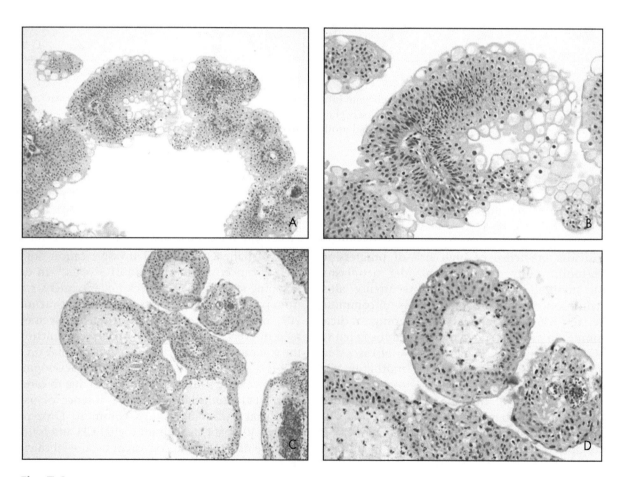

**Fig. 7.4**
**A–D** Papilloma: urothelial papilloma is characterized by a papillary lesion with delicate fibrovascular cores lined by cytologically and architecturally normal urothelium. The papillae are lined by urothelial cells that are less than seven cell layers in thickness.

**Table 7.2** Diagnostic features of urothelial papilloma and grade 1 carcinoma

|  | Papilloma | Grade 1 carcinoma |
|---|---|---|
| Age (years) | Younger (usually <50) | Older (usually >50) |
| Sex (male:female) | 2:1 | 3:1 |
| Size | Small, usually <2 cm | Larger |
| *Microscopic findings* |  |  |
| Well-formed papillae | Present | Present |
| Thickness of urothelium | ≤7 layers | Usually >7 layers |
| Superficial umbrella cells | Present | Usually present |
| Cytology: | Minimal or absent | Mild |
|   nuclear enlargement | Rare or none | Slight to moderate |
|   nuclear hyperchromasia | Rare or none | Slight |
|   chromatin | Fine granular | Slightly coarse or granular |
|   nucleolar enlargement | Absent | May be present |
| Mitotic figures | None | Rare |
| Stromal invasion | Absent | Uncommon |

Inverted urothelial papilloma shares many features with exophytic papilloma, but is well defined elsewhere and was not the focus of the Ancona refinement. Rare cases have combined features of typical exophytic papilloma and inverted papilloma, and, when encountered, these varied findings should be included in the pathologist's report.

## Clinical significance

Papilloma is uncommon, representing less than 3% of papillary urothelial tumors.[47] Such lesions usually occur in patients less than 50 years of age, but rare cases with otherwise typical features can be seen in patients in their upper fifties. An otherwise typical papilloma occurring in an older patient (well beyond 50 years) is best considered to be grade 1 urothelial carcinoma.

With the restrictive definition of the WHO 1973 classification, urothelial papilloma has a low recurrence rate and very infrequent association with the development of invasive urothelial carcinoma and cancer death; it does not have the capacity to invade or metastasize.[48,49] However, it is neoplastic, with a small but significant potential for recurrence.[50,51] Eble and Young reviewed 80 years of published studies of benign and low-grade urothelial neoplasms of the urinary bladder and concluded that urothelial papillomas '...are rare tumors somehow fundamentally different from noninvasive low-grade carcinomas'.[47] These authors believed that 'true papillomas of the bladder that are distinct from grade 1 papillary carcinoma do occur rarely'. Miller et al found that none of 26 patients with papilloma developed recurrence or urothelial carcinoma.[52] Bergkvist et al reported no cancer deaths in 12 patients with urothelial papilloma (referred to as

grade 0 carcinoma); recurrence rate and the rate of developing urothelial carcinoma were not reported.[53] Buerger believed in 1915 that 'many of the other loosely accepted notions regarding the malignancy of papilloma *per se* were found to be fallacious'.[54]

Cheng et al studied 52 patients with papilloma that were followed for a mean of 9.8 years; 20 patients (38%) had more than 8 years of follow-up.[55] The tumor was solitary in 49 (94%) patients and multiple in 3 (6%) patients. Four (8%) patients developed recurrent papilloma (mean interval from the diagnosis to recurrence, 3.2 years); one developed grade 1 carcinoma 6 years after the initial diagnosis of papilloma. None of the other patients developed dysplasia, CIS, or urothelial carcinoma, and none died of bladder cancer.

## GRADE 1 UROTHELIAL CARCINOMA

### Diagnostic criteria

Grade 1 papillary carcinoma consists of an orderly arrangement of normal urothelial cells lining delicate papillae with minimal architectural abnormalities and minimal nuclear atypia (Figure 7.5). There may be some complexity and fusion of the papillae, but this is usually not prominent. The urothelium is often thickened, with more than seven cell layers, but may be normal; formal counting of the number of cells in thickness in routine practice is discouraged, recognizing that there is no absolute cut point for normal and abnormal. Regardless of thickness, the urothelium displays normal maturation and cohesiveness, with an intact superficial cell layer. Nuclei tend to be uniform in shape and spacing, although there may be some enlargement and elongation. The chromatin texture is finely granular, similar to papilloma, without significant nucleolar enlargement. Mitotic figures are rare or absent.

### Clinical significance

Grade 1 carcinoma appears to have a predilection for the ureteric orifice,[56] referred to as the 'typical primary site' by Page et al.[57] Sixty-nine percent of grade 1 urothelial carcinomas were centered around the ureteric orifice and tumor was found in the anterior wall in two patients (1%).[56] The dome appears to be an uncommon location for grade 1 cancer (3%).

Patients with grade 1 carcinoma are at risk of local recurrence, progression, and dying of bladder cancer.[48] Cheng et al reported the Mayo Clinic experience with 122 untreated patients with grade 1 urothelial carcinoma that were followed for a mean of 12.8 years.[58] Thirty-three (29%) patients had recurrence or progression, with mean interval from diagnosis to recurrence or progression of 4.1 years. Twelve patients had biopsy-proven non-invasive urothelial carcinoma (Ta); 17 patients had cystoscopically detected recurrences (all were treated by fulguration without

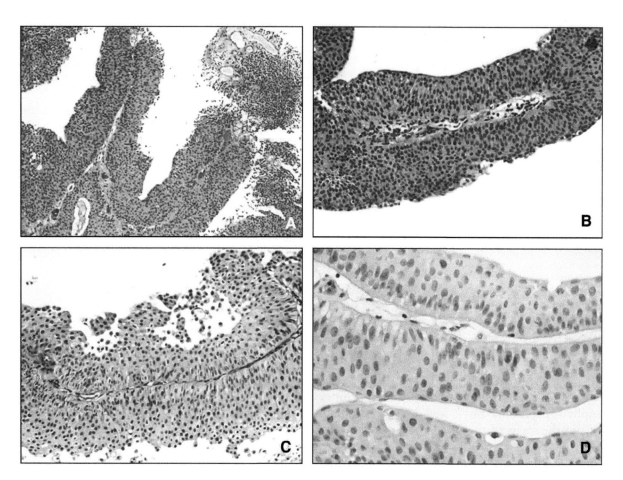

**Fig. 7.5**
**A–C** Grade 1 carcinoma characterized by an orderly proliferation of urothelial cells without significant cytologic atypia. The papillae are well formed and are lined by urothelial cells that are usually more than seven cell layers in thickness. **D** High-power view of grade 1 carcinoma.

biopsy); and 4 patients developed invasive urothelial carcinoma, including 2 with muscle-invasive carcinoma. Twelve (75%) of 16 patients with biopsy-proven recurrence or progression had cancer dedifferentiation and resulting higher grade cancer than initial biopsies. Mean interval from initial diagnosis to development of invasive carcinoma was 13.3 years (range 10–14 years). Three patients (3%) died of bladder cancer.

With 20 years of follow-up, Holmang et al found that 14% of patients with non-invasive grade 1 urothelial carcinoma (pTa G1) died of bladder cancer.[59] In Greene et al's study of 100 patients with grade 1 cancer, 10 (10%) patients died of bladder cancer after more than 15 years; of 73 patients that had recurrences, 22% of recurrent cancer was higher grade than the original.[60] The mean interval from initial diagnosis to the development of invasive cancer (10 patients) was 8 years. Malmström et al reported that 5 of 45 (11%) patients with stage pTa grade 1 urothelial carcinoma developed invasive urothelial carcinoma during a mean follow-up of 6.5 years.[61] Prout et al reviewed a series of 178 patients with pTa grade 1 bladder cancer for the National Bladder Cancer Study Group and followed for

a median of 4.8 years; they found that 61% subsequently developed other papillary tumors, 16% progressed to higher grade, 4% developed invasive cancer, including three with muscle-invasive cancer, and one patient (0.5%) died of bladder cancer.[62] They concluded that '...there are little data to support the use of the term papilloma to describe stage Ta grade 1 tumors without reservation' and '...grade 1 tumors might best be referred to as Ta, grade 1 transitional cell tumors' rather than classified as papilloma. In England et al's study of 135 patients with grade 1 urothelial carcinoma (mean follow-up 9 years), 70% of patients had recurrence, including seven with cancer progression, and four died of bladder cancer; the mean interval from the time of diagnosis to cancer progression was 6 years.[63] Five-year recurrence-free survival was only 25% in Pocock et al's report of 34 patients with Ta grade 1 urothelial carcinoma.[64] Nine (5%) patients died of bladder cancer among 155 patients with grade 1 urothelial carcinoma.[65] Mufti et al reviewed 198 patients with grade 1 urothelial carcinoma, and found that only 53% of patients remained cancer-free at 5 years; the actuarial cancer mortality rate was 4%.[56] Jordan et al studied 91 patients with grade 1 papillary urothelial (transitional cell) tumors and found 40% of patients had recurrence.[49] Twenty percent of patients with recurrences developed high-grade (grade 3) cancer, and four patients died of bladder cancer. Long-term follow-up is recommended for patient management. In a recent review of 152 patients with Ta grade 1 urothelial carcinoma, Leblanc et al found that 83 patients (55%) had tumor recurrence after initial diagnosis, including 37% with cancer progression.[66] Patients that remained tumor-free for 1 year still had a 43% chance of late recurrence. In light of high risk for late recurrence and the potential to progress into muscle-invasive cancer, the authors concluded that Ta grade 1 tumor should be considered carcinoma, and that lifelong periodic examination is warranted.[66]

Papillary tumor of low malignant potential was found to have a high level of genetic changes that commonly occur in advanced bladder carcinoma, including loss of heterozygosity in 81% of patients (41% with D9S177, 32% with IFNA, 29% with TP53, 26% with D12S1051, and 44% with D3S3050).[67]

## GRADE 2 UROTHELIAL CARCINOMA

### Diagnostic criteria

Grade 2 carcinoma retains some of the orderly architectural appearance and maturation of grade 1 carcinoma, but displays at least focal moderate variation in orderliness, nuclear appearance, and chromatin texture that should be apparent at low magnification (Figure 7.6). Cytologic abnormalities are invariably present in grade 2 carcinoma, with moderate nuclear crowding, moderate variation in cell polarity, moderate nuclear hyperchromasia, moderate anisonucleosis, and mild nucleolar enlargement. Mitotic figures are usually limited to the lower half of the urothelium, but this is inconstant. Superficial cells are usually present, and the mucosa is predominantly cohesive, although variation may be present. Some tumors may be extremely orderly, reminiscent of grade 1 carcinoma, with only a small focus of obvious disorder or irregularity in cell spacing; these are considered grade 2 cancer, recognizing that grade is based on the highest level of abnormality

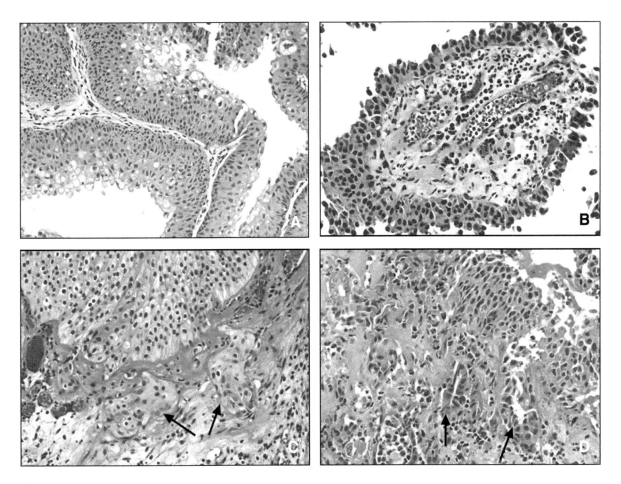

**Fig. 7.6**
**A, B** Grade 2 papillary urothelial carcinoma. **C, D** Early lamina propria invasion (arrows) with papillary grade 2 carcinoma (different cases).

present. Grade 2 carcinomas represent a wide spectrum of tumors that span the morphologic continuum from grade 1 to grade 3.

## Clinical significance

Most cases of urothelial carcinoma are WHO grade 2, and the outcome is significantly worse than those with lower grade papillary cancer. Recurrence risk for patients with non-invasive grade 2 cancer is 45% to 67%, with invasion occurring in up to 20% and cancer-specific death in 13% to 20% following surgical treatment.[48,51] Patients with grade 2 cancer and lamina propria invasion are at even greater risk, with recurrence in 67% to 80% of cases, development of muscle-invasive cancer, in 21% to 49%, and cancer-specific death in 17% to 51% of those treated surgically.[48]

In order to improve stratification of the large WHO grade 2 group, some investigators subdivided these cases into two subgroups based on the degree of nuclear deviation and polarity of cells. In one study, grade 2A consisted of urothelial cancer with slight cellular deviation, some variation in nuclear size, and normal polarity of cells, whereas grade 2B cancer had obvious variability in nuclear size and shape, with some loss of normal polarity.[68] Using this modification, the authors identified tumor progression in 4% and 33% of grade 2A and 2B cancer, respectively (all pTa and pT1).[68] This subdivision of grade 2 was also of prognostic significance for muscle-invasive cancer.[68,69]

Other investigators considered both nuclear pleomorphism and mitotic count as criteria for subdividing grade 2 urothelial cancer, and were successful in identifying groups of cancers with different outcomes.[70] Grade 2A bladder cancer had a 5-year survival rate of 92%, similar to grade 1 cancer, whereas grade 2B cancer was comparable to grade 3 cancer, with a 5-year survival rate of 43%.[71-73] This subdivision of grading was reproducible, with interobserver agreement of more than 90%.[70] Others found that mitotic index was the single most useful criterion for bladder cancer grading.[74,75]

A recent study of 151 cancers treated by radical cystectomy revealed that the separation of low- and high-grade cancer by the WHO/ISUP 1998 classification was unable to predict cancer stage or cancer-specific survival.[76]

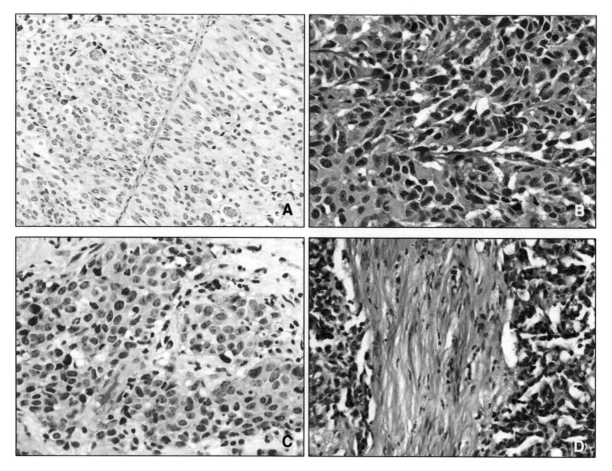

**Fig. 7.7**
**A–C** Grade 3 carcinoma. **D** Grade 3 carcinoma with muscularis propria invasion.

## GRADE 3 UROTHELIAL CARCINOMA

### Diagnostic criteria

Grade 3 carcinoma displays the most extreme nuclear abnormalities among papillary urothelial cancers, similar to those seen in CIS (Figure 7.7). The obvious urothelial disorder and loss of polarity is present at scanning magnification, and often includes loss of normal architecture and cell polarity, loss of cell cohesion, and frequent mitotic figures. Cellular anaplasia, characteristic of grade 3 carcinoma, is defined as increased cellularity, nuclear crowding, disturbance of cellular polarity, absence of differentiation from the base to the mucosal surface, nuclear pleomorphism, irregularity in the size of the cells, variation in nuclear shape and chromatin pattern, increased number of mitotic figures throughout the mucosa, and the occasional presence of neoplastic giant cells.[1] The superficial cell layer is usually partially or completely absent with grade 3 carcinoma, often accompanied by prominent cellular discohesion.

### Clinical significance

Recurrence risk for patients with non-invasive grade 3 cancer is 65% to 85%, with invasion occurring in 20% to 52% and cancer-specific death in up to 35% following surgical treatment.[48,77] Patients with grade 3 cancer and lamina propria invasion recur in 46% to 71% of cases, develop muscle-invasive cancer in 24% to 48%, and cancer-specific death in 25% to 71% of those treated surgically.[48]

## CONCLUSION

The robust WHO 1973 standard for classification and grading of bladder tumors is recommended with minor modifications (as noted above) for international use to allow valid comparison of results between different clinical centers. As with all existing classification and grading methods, the Ancona 2001 refinement of the WHO classification should be regularly reviewed and updated as appropriate when new and confirmed data emerge.

### REFERENCES

1. Mostofi FK, Sobin LH. Histologic typing of urinary bladder tumors. Geneva: World Health Organization; 1973.
2. Oyasu R. World Health Organization and International Society of Urological Pathology classification and two-number grading system of bladder tumors. Cancer 2000;88:1509–1512.
3. Sobin LH. The WHO histological classification of urinary bladder tumours. Urol Res 1978;6:193–195.
4. Reuter VE, Epstein JI, Amin MB, Mostofi FK. The 'WHO/ISUP Consensus Classification of Urothelial (Transitional Cell) Neoplasms': continued discussion. Hum Pathol 1999;30:879–880.
5. Mostofi FK, Davis CJ, Sesterhenn IA. Histologic typing of urinary bladder tumors. World Health Organization. Berlin: Springer-Verlag, 1999, pp 7–11.
6. Holmang S, Andius P, Hedelin H, Wester K, Busch C, Johansson SL. Stage progression in Ta papillary urothelial tumors: relationship to grade, immunohistochemical expression of tumor markers, mitotic frequency and DNA ploidy. J Urol 2001;165:1124–1128; discussion 1128–1130.
7. Epstein JI, Amin MB, Reuter VR, Mostofi FK. The World Health Organization/International Society of Urological Pathology consensus classification of urothelial (transitional cell) neoplasms of the urinary bladder. Bladder Consensus Conference Committee. Am J Surg Pathol 1998;22:1435–1448.
8. Yorukoglu K, Tuna B, Dikicioglu E, et al. Reproducibility of the 1998 World Health Organization/International Society of Urologic Pathology classification of papillary urothelial neoplasms of the urinary bladder. Virchows Arch 2003;443:734–740.
9. Campbell PA, Conrad RJ, Campbell CM, Nicol DL, MacTaggart P. Papillary urothelial neoplasm of low malignant potential: reliability of diagnosis and outcome. BJU Int 2004;93:1228–1231.
10. Epstein JI. The new World Health Organization/International Society of Urological Pathology (WHO/ISUP) classification for TA, T1 bladder tumors: is it an improvement? Crit Rev Oncol Hematol 2003;47:83–89.
11. Schroder FH, Hermanek P, Denis L, Fair WR, Gospodarowicz MK, Pavone-Macaluso M. The TNM classification of prostate cancer. Prostate 1992;4(Suppl):129–138.
12. Lopez-Beltran A, Cheng L. Stage pT1 bladder carcinoma: diagnostic criteria, pitfalls and prognostic significance. Pathology 2003;35:484–491.
13. Cheng L, Cheville JC, Neumann RM, Bostwick DG. Flat intraepithelial lesions of the urinary bladder. Cancer 2000;88:625–631.
14. Elliott GB, Moloney PJ, Anderson GH. 'Denuding cystitis' and in situ urothelial carcinoma. Arch Pathol 1973;96:91–94.
15. Murphy WM, Soloway MS. Urothelial dysplasia. J Urol 1982;127:849–854.
16. Cheng L, Cheville JC, Neumann RM, Bostwick DG. Natural history of urothelial dysplasia of the bladder. Am J Surg Pathol 1999;23:443–447.
17. Zuk RJ, Rogers HS, Martin JE, Baithun SI. Clinicopathological importance of primary dysplasia of bladder. J Clin Pathol 1988;41:1277–1280.
18. Baithun SI, Rogers HS, Martin JE, Zuk RJ, Blandy JP. Primary dysplasia of bladder. Lancet 1988;1:483.
19. Zincke H, Utz DC, Farrow GM. Review of Mayo Clinic experience with carcinoma in situ. Urology 1985;26:39–46.
20. Farrow GM. Pathology of carcinoma in situ of the urinary bladder and related lesions. J Cell Biochem 1992;161(Suppl):39–43.
21. Farrow GM, Utz DC, Rife CC, Greene LF. Clinical observations on sixty-nine cases of in situ carcinoma of the urinary bladder. Cancer Res 1977;37:2794–2798.
22. Farrow GM, Barlebo H, Enjoji M, et al. Transitional cell carcinoma in situ. Prog Clin Biol Res 1986;221:85–96.
23. Orozco RE, Martin AA, Murphy WM. Carcinoma in situ of the urinary bladder. Clues to host involvement in human carcinogenesis. Cancer 1994;74:115–122.
24. Hudson MA, Herr HW. Carcinoma in situ of the bladder. J Urol 1995;153:564–572.
25. Amling CL, Thrasher JB, Frazier HA, Dodge RK, Robertson JE, Paulson DF. Radical cystectomy for stages Ta, Tis and T1 transitional cell carcinoma of the bladder. J Urol 1994;151:31–35; discussion 35–36.
26. Witjes JA. Bladder carcinoma in situ in 2003: state of the art. Eur Urol 2004;45:142–146.
27. Silver DA, Stroumbakis N, Russo P, Fair WR, Herr HW. Ureteral carcinoma in situ at radical cystectomy: does the margin matter? J Urol 1997;158:768–771.
28. Cheng L, Cheville JC, Neumann RM, et al. Survival of patients with carcinoma in situ of the urinary bladder. Cancer 1999;85:2469–2674.
29. Koss LG. Carcinoma of the bladder in situ. JAMA 1969;207:1919.

30. Koss LG, Tiamson EM, Robbins MA. Mapping cancerous and precancerous bladder changes. A study of the urothelium in ten surgically removed bladders. JAMA 1974;227:281–286.

31. Koss LG, Nakanishi I, Freed SZ. Nonpapillary carcinoma in situ and atypical hyperplasia in cancerous bladders: further studies of surgically removed bladders by mapping. Urology 1977;9:442–455.

32. Koss LG. Evaluation of patients with carcinoma in situ of the bladder. Pathol Annu 1982;17:353–359.

33. Koss LG. Minimal neoplasia as a challenge for early cancer detection. Recent Results Cancer Res 1988;106:1–8.

34. Lamm DL. Carcinoma in situ. Urol Clin North Am 1992;19:499–508.

35. Melamed MR, Grabstald H, Whitmore WF Jr. Carcinoma in situ of bladder: clinico-pathologic study of case with a suggested approach to detection. J Urol 1966;96:466–471.

36. Melamed MR, Voutsa NG, Grabstald H. Natural history and clinical behavior of in situ carcinoma of the human urinary bladder. 1964 CA Cancer J Clin 1993;43:348–370.

37. Nagy GK, Frable WJ, Murphy WM. Classification of premalignant urothelial abnormalities. A Delphi study of the National Bladder Cancer Collaborative Group A. Pathol Annu 1982;17(Pt 1):219–233.

38. Murphy WM, Busch C, Algaba F. Intraepithelial lesions of urinary bladder: morphologic considerations. Scand J Urol Nephrol 2000;205(Suppl):67–81.

39. Riddle PR, Chisholm GD, Trott PA, Pugh RC. Flat carcinoma in situ of bladder. Br J Urol 1975;47:829–833.

40. Stanisic TH, Donovan JM, Lebouton J, Graham AR. 5-year experience with intravesical therapy of carcinoma in situ: an inquiry into the risks of 'conservative' management. J Urol 1987;138:1158–1161.

41. Utz DC, Hanash KA, Farrow GM. The plight of the patient with carcinoma in situ of the bladder. J Urol 1970;103:160–164.

42. Utz DC, Zincke H. The masquerade of bladder cancer in situ as interstitial cystitis. J Urol 1974;111:160–161.

43. Utz DC, Farrow GM. Management of carcinoma in situ of the bladder: the case for surgical management. Urol Clin North Am 1980;7:533–541.

44. Utz DC, Farrow GM. Carcinoma in situ of the urinary tract. Urol Clin North Am 1984;11:735–740.

45. Murphy WM, Farrow GM, Beckwith B. Renal and Bladder Tumors. Washington, DC: American Registry of Pathology, 1994.

46. Reuter VE, Melamed MR. The urothelial tract: renal pelvis, ureter, urinary bladder, and urethra. In Sternberg SS (ed): Diagnostic Surgical Pathology, 3rd ed. Philadelphia: Lippincott Williams & Wilkins, 1999, pp 1853–1972.

47. Eble JN, Young RH. Benign and low-grade papillary lesions of the urinary bladder: a review of the papilloma–papillary carcinoma controversy, and a report of five typical papillomas. Semin Diagn Pathol 1989;6:351–371.

48. Bostwick DG. Natural history of early bladder cancer. J Cell Biochem 1992;161(Suppl):31–38.

49. Jordan AM, Weingarten J, Murphy WM. Transitional cell neoplasms of the urinary bladder. Can biologic potential be predicted from histologic grading? Cancer 1987;60:2766–2774.

50. McKenney JK, Amin MB, Young RH. Urothelial (transitional cell) papilloma of the urinary bladder: a clinicopathologic study of 26 cases. Mod Pathol 2003;16:623–629.

51. Sebe P, Lebret T, Molinie V, et al. [Superficial grade G2 tumors of the bladder: recurrence, progression, prognosis]. Prog Urol 2003;13:608–612.

52. Miller A, Mitchell JP, Brown NJ. The Bristol Bladder Tumour Registry. Br J Urol 1969;41(Suppl):1–64.

53. Bergkvist A, Ljungqvist A, Moberger G. Classification of bladder tumours based on the cellular pattern. Preliminary report of a clinical–pathological study of 300 cases with a minimum follow-up of eight years. Acta Chir Scand 1965;130:371–378.

54. Buerger L. The pathological diagnosis of tumors of the bladder with particular reference to papilloma and carcinoma. Surg Gynecol Oncol 1915;21:179–198.

55. Cheng L, Darson M, Cheville JC, et al. Urothelial papilloma of the bladder. Clinical and biologic implications. Cancer 1999;86:2098–2101.

56. Mufti GR, Virdi JS, Singh M. 'Solitary' Ta–T1 G1 bladder tumour—history and long-term prognosis. Eur Urol 1990;18:101–106.

57. Page BH, Levison VB, Curwen MP. The site of recurrence of non-infiltrating bladder tumours. Br J Urol 1978;50:237–242.

58. Cheng L, Neumann RM, Bostwick DG. Papillary urothelial neoplasms of low malignant potential. Clinical and biologic implications. Cancer 1999;86:2102–2108.

59. Holmang S, Hedelin H, Anderstrom C, Johansson SL. The relationship among multiple recurrences, progression and prognosis of patients with stages Ta and T1 transitional cell cancer of the bladder followed for at least 20 years. J Urol 1995;153:1823–1826; discussion 1826–1827.

60. Greene LF, Hanash KA, Farrow GM. Benign papilloma or papillary carcinoma of the bladder? J Urol 1973;110:205–207.

61. Malmström P-U, Busch C, Norlen BJ. Recurrence, progression and survival in bladder cancer. A retrospective analysis of 232 patients with greater than or equal to 5-year follow-up. Scand J Urol Nephrol 1987;21:185–195.

62. Prout GR Jr, Barton BA, Griffin PP, Friedell GH. Treated history of noninvasive grade 1 transitional cell carcinoma. The National Bladder Cancer Group. J Urol 1992;148:1413–1419.

63. England HR, Paris AM, Blandy JP. The correlation of T1 bladder tumour history with prognosis and follow-up requirements. Br J Urol 1981;53:593–597.

64. Pocock RD, Ponder BA, O'Sullivan JP, Ibrahim SK, Easton DF, Shearer RJ. Prognostic factors in non-infiltrating carcinoma of the bladder: a preliminary report. Br J Urol 1982;54:711–715.

65. Gilbert HA, Logan JL, Kagan AR, et al. The natural history of papillary transitional cell carcinoma of the bladder and its treatment in an unselected population on the basis of histologic grading. J Urol 1978;119:488–492.

66. Leblanc B, Duclos AJ, Benard F, et al. Long-term followup of initial Ta grade 1 transitional cell carcinoma of the bladder. J Urol 1999;162:1946–1950.

67. Cheng L, MacLennan GT, Zhang S, Wang M, Pan CX, Koch MO. Laser capture microdissection analysis reveals frequent allelic losses in papillary urothelial neoplasm of low malignant potential of the urinary bladder. Cancer 2004;101:183–188.

68. Pauwels RP, Schapers RF, Smeets AW, Debruyne FM, Geraedts JP. Grading in superficial bladder cancer (1). Morphological criteria. Br J Urol 1988;61:129–134.

69. Schapers RF, Pauwels RP, Wijnen JT, et al. A simplified grading method of transitional cell carcinoma of the urinary bladder: reproducibility, clinical significance and comparison with other prognostic parameters. Br J Urol 1994;73:625–631.

70. Carbin BE, Ekman P, Gustafson H, Christensen NJ, Sandstedt B, Silfversward C. Grading of human urothelial carcinoma based on nuclear atypia and mitotic frequency. I. Histological description. J Urol 1991;145:968–971.

71. Jakse G, Loidl W, Seeber G, Hofstadter F. Stage T1, grade 3 transitional cell carcinoma of the bladder: an unfavorable tumor? J Urol 1987;137:39–43.

72. Kakizoe T, Friedell GH, Soloway MS, Suemasu K, Shimosato Y, Mukai K. Report of the 1991 International Meeting on Fundamental and Clinical Research in Urogenital Cancer. Jpn J Clin Oncol 1992;22:60–65.

73. Takashi M, Sakata T, Murase T, Hamajima N, Miyake K. Grade 3 bladder cancer with lamina propria invasion (pT1): characteristics of tumor and clinical course. Nagoya J Med Sci 1991;53:1–8.

74. Lipponen PK, Eskelinen MJ, Kiviranta J, Pesonen E. Prognosis of transitional cell bladder cancer: a multivariate prognostic score for improved prediction. J Urol 1991;146:1535–1540.

75. Lipponen PK, Eskelinen MJ, Nordling S. Progression and survival in transitional cell bladder cancer: a comparison of established prognostic factors, S-phase fraction and DNA ploidy. Eur J Cancer 1991;27:877–881.

76. Kruger S, Thorns C, Bohle A, Feller AC. Prognostic significance of a grading system considering tumor heterogeneity in muscle-invasive urothelial carcinoma of the urinary bladder. Int Urol Nephrol 2003;35:169–173.

77. Bostwick DG, Lopez-Beltran A. Bladder Biopsy Interpretation. Glen Allen: United Pathologists Press, 1999.

78. Cheng L, Neumann RM, Nehra A, Spotts BE, Weaver AL, Bostwick DG. Cancer heterogeneity and its biologic implications in the grading of urothelial carcinoma. Cancer 2000;88:1663–1670.

79. Yin H, Leong AS. Histologic grading of noninvasive papillary urothelial tumors: validation of the 1998 WHO/ISUP system by immunophenotyping and follow-up. Am J Clin Pathol 2004;121:679–687.

# Molecular biology

SECTION 3

# Non-urothelial tumors

8

*David Grignon, Gail Bentley*

## INTRODUCTION

Urothelial tumors account for more than 90% of primary neoplasms in the adult patient population. A minority of primary epithelial tumors are non-urothelial in type. Clinical features and treatment of this group of neoplasms are dealt with elsewhere in the text (Chapters 69 and 70). This chapter focuses exclusively on the pathology of these lesions.

## PRIMARY ADENOCARCINOMA

Adenocarcinoma may arise primarily from the urinary bladder; however, secondary involvement from tumors developing in adjacent organs is more common. Primary adenocarcinoma accounts for 0.5% to 2% of all malignant bladder tumors.[1-4] The largest published series, with 72 and 185 cases respectively, were reported by Grignon et al[5] and El-Mekresh et al.[6] Adenocarcinomas of the bladder usually fall into one of two major categories defined on the basis of presumed site of origin: those arising in the bladder proper and those arising from the urachal remnants. For clinical and pathologic reasons, urachal and non-urachal adenocarcinoma will be addressed in separate sections. Specific variants of clinical significance (signet ring cell carcinoma and clear cell adenocarcinoma) are dealt with individually.

## URACHAL ADENOCARCINOMA

### Introduction

Approximately one-third of primary bladder adenocarcinomas arise in the urachus. The histologic

distinction in separating urachal from non-urachal adenocarcinoma may be difficult and requires correlation of clinical and pathologic findings. The clinicopathologic criteria for urachal origin have been well described. The criteria of Johnson et al[7] are perhaps most practical:

- the tumor should be located anteriorly or in the dome
- there should be a sharp demarcation between tumor and normal epithelium
- a primary tumor elsewhere must be excluded.

There are no specific pathologic features that distinguish urachal from non-urachal tumors, and immunohistochemistry has not been helpful in making this distinction.

### Pathologic features

The vast majority of urachal adenocarcinomas form discrete masses within the dome of the bladder. The epicenter is located in the wall of the bladder rather than being mucosally based, as is typical for non-urachal tumors. The bladder mucosa may be intact or ulcerated with the cut surface having a glistening mucoid appearance due to the abundant mucin secretion; less commonly the tumor appears solid. The tumor may extend along the urachal tract and be found within the abdominal wall.

Urachal adenocarcinoma appears in a variety of histologic forms. The most common is mucinous (colloid) carcinoma, in which there are single cells, and nests of malignant cells floating within extracellular mucin (Figure 8.1). The cells can have a columnar or signet ring morphology. The next most frequently observed is enteric adenocarcinoma, with features typical of colorectal adenocarcinoma. An uncommon

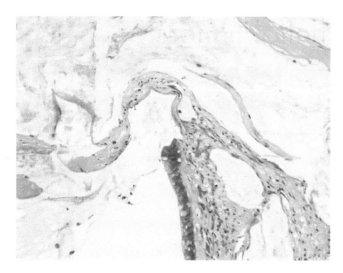

**Fig. 8.1**
Urachal adenocarcinoma composed of abundant extravasated mucin with a strip of neoplastic enteric-type epithelium in keeping with the mucinous (colloid) pattern of adenocarcinoma most typical of these tumors.

pattern is that of linitis plastica-like signet ring cell carcinoma (discussed below).[8] Histochemical stains reveal neutral and acid (sulfated and nonsulfated) mucin in these tumors.[5] Urachal adenocarcinoma expresses cytokeratin (including CK20), carcino-embryonic antigen (CEA), Leu-M1, and epithelial membrane antigen (EMA).[3,5] There is consistent nonreactivity for vimentin, OC125, and HER-2/neu.[3] The tumors are prostate specific antigen (PSA) and prostate specific acid phosphatase (PSAP) negative.[3,9]

## Differential diagnosis

The major differential diagnostic considerations are non-urachal bladder adenocarcinoma and metastatic adenocarcinoma. As noted earlier, these distinctions require clinicopathologic correlation. Primary colonic neoplasms account for 20% of all secondary tumors involving the urinary bladder. Urachal adenocarcinoma should be distinguished from urachal villous adenoma,[10] a lesion that is histologically identical to those found in the gastrointestinal tract.

## NON-URACHAL ADENOCARCINOMA

## Pathologic features

Primary non-urachal adenocarcinoma can appear as an exophytic, papillary, solid, sessile, ulcerating, or infiltrative mass. The signet ring variant frequently shows diffuse thickening of the bladder wall, producing a linitis plastica-like appearance, and urothelial mucosal biopsies may be negative.

Definitions of adenocarcinoma vary. Most reports in the literature have excluded any case containing a

recognizable urothelial carcinoma component, preferring to classify these as urothelial carcinoma with glandular differentiation.[4,5] Although others have included these cases as adenocarcinoma if this pattern predominated,[11] the former approach is recommended and is endorsed in the 2004 World Health Organization classification.[12] Grignon et al[5] recognized six histologic variants of adenocarcinoma of the urinary bladder:

1. adenocarcinoma of no specific type, when the tumor did not resemble another recognized pattern
2. enteric, when the cancer was composed of pseudostratified columnar cells forming glands, often with central necrosis typical of colonic adenocarcinoma (Figure 8.2)
3. mucinous (colloid), when the tumor cells were single or in nests floating in extracellular mucin
4. signet ring, when the tumor consisted of signet ring cells diffusely infiltrating the bladder wall
5. clear cell, when the tumor was composed of papillary and tubular structures with cytologic features identical to mesonephric adenocarcinoma
6. mixed, when two or more of the described patterns were found.

For non-urachal tumors, the nonspecific and enteric types were most common.

A uniform grading system has not been applied to adenocarcinoma of the bladder.[2,13] Anderstrom et al[13] found grade to be a significant prognostic indicator, whereas Thomas et al[2] did not find a correlation between grade and outcome. In the former system, grade was based on the degree of gland formation, with two specific histologic subtypes (pure colloid and signet ring) considered to be poorly differentiated. The histologic pattern did not correlate with outcome in The

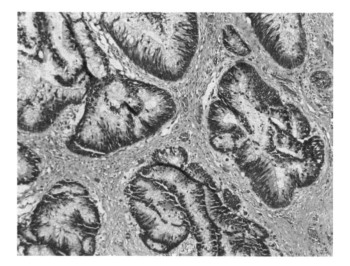

**Fig. 8.2**
Non-urachal adenocarcinoma composed of invasive nests of tumor cells with a wreath-like arrangement and areas of necrosis identical to the appearance characteristic of adenocarcinomas of gastrointestinal (enteric) origin.

University of Texas M.D. Anderson Cancer Center series, although the poor prognosis of the signet ring variant was noted.[5]

## Differential diagnosis

The differential diagnosis of adenocarcinoma is extensive. First, benign mimics of adenocarcinoma need to be excluded. In some cases, cystitis cystica and cystitis glandularis may be florid, producing pseudopapillary or polypoid lesions, which may mimic a tumor. In unusual cases, extracellular mucin is present, and careful evaluation for malignant cells is necessary. Villous adenoma rarely occurs in the urinary bladder,[14] and shows the cytologic and architectural abnormalities of adenomatous epithelium without stromal invasion. Nephrogenic adenoma must be distinguished from adenocarcinoma, particularly the clear cell variant. Endometriosis often involves the bladder and should be considered in females of childbearing age. Other müllerian types of glandular tissue have been described in the urinary bladder under the terms müllerianosis and endocervicosis.[15,16] As for urachal adenocarcinoma, secondary involvement of the bladder must be excluded. Cervical and endometrial adenocarcinomas can extend to the urinary bladder, but this is rare. Prostatic adenocarcinoma is more common. Clinicopathologic correlation should always be obtained.

## SIGNET RING CELL ADENOCARCINOMA

### Introduction

Primary signet ring cell carcinoma of the urinary bladder is a rare tumor, with fewer than 100 cases reported to date.[8,17] To warrant this diagnosis, at least a focal component of diffuse, linitis plastica-like signet ring cell adenocarcinoma should be present,and there should be no element of urothelial carcinoma.

### Pathologic features

In almost half of all cases, cystoscopy does not show a mucosal or mass lesion, with the mucosa most often being described as 'edematous' or 'bullous'. Histologically, two variants have been identified: one type is composed of signet ring cells floating in a pool of mucin and separated by cores of fibrous stroma; the second type features diffuse permeation by single signet ring cells, some with single cytoplasmic vacuoles and others with a bubbly cytoplasm, associated with a scirrhous stroma identical to linitis plastica of the stomach (Figure 8.3).[17] In some cases, the cytoplasm is pale and eosinophilic with the nucleus pushed to one end, a pattern referred to as monocytoid.[8,18] Mixtures of the two patterns have been reported.[17] Results of immunohistochemical staining for the signet ring cells show positive reactivity with pancytokeratin, Cam 5.2, CK20, EMA, CEA, 115D8, and OVTL 12/30.[19]

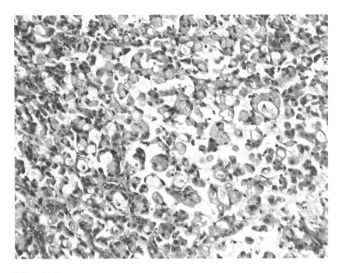

**Fig. 8.3**
Signet ring cell carcinoma composed of dispersed cells and clusters of cells in the bladder submucosa, the majority of which contain a single cytoplasmic mucin vacuole or have bubbly, finely vacuolated cytoplasm.

### Differential diagnosis

The presence of a predominant signet ring cell component in a urinary bladder tumor should prompt a thorough search to exclude a primary tumor in another area. Patients with bladder involvement by metastasis usually have extravesical symptoms, whereas patients with primary adenocarcinoma of the bladder commonly experience symptoms related to the bladder.[19] Prostatic adenocarcinoma may contain signet ring cells, and it is important to eliminate the prostate as a primary source in male patients.

## CLEAR CELL ADENOCARCINOMA

### Introduction

Primary clear cell adenocarcinoma of the urinary bladder is rare, with fewer than 25 well-documented cases in the English language literature.[20-24] In contrast to the bladder, the urethra is a relatively common site for clear cell adenocarcinoma, particularly in females.[25]

### Pathologic features

Grossly, the tumors are solid or papillary, and are most often located in the trigone or posterior wall. Histologically, the tumor cells proliferate in papillary, solid, or tubular patterns (Figure 8.4). There are two distinct populations of cells: the papillary component consists of cells having a distinct 'hobnail' appearance; the second component consists of clear cells in an alveolar or tubular pattern. The tubules may be cystically dilated. The cells have significant nuclear pleomorphism with frequent mitotic figures. Special stains demonstrate

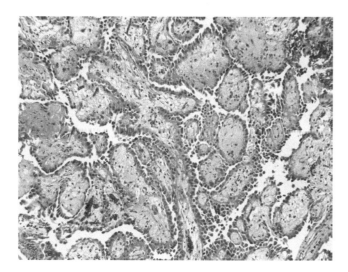

**Fig. 8.4**
Clear cell adenocarcinoma with papillary structures lined with neoplastic cells, some of which have the typical hobnail morphology.

abundant cytoplasmic glycogen, and, in most, focal cytoplasmic and luminal mucin.

## Differential diagnosis

The major differential diagnostic considerations are nephrogenic adenoma and metastatic clear cell carcinoma. Nephrogenic adenoma is typically small and has both papillary and tubular components that are lined by a single layer of flattened, cuboidal, low columnar or hobnail cells, with scant amphophilic cytoplasm.[26] Metastatic clear cell (mesonephric) carcinoma should be excluded in all female patients and requires clinical correlation. Renal cell carcinoma can metastasize to the bladder.[27] Recognition of the typical sinusoidal vascular pattern, lack of tubular differentiation, and the absence of mucin, as well as relevant clinical features, should resolve this differential.

## SQUAMOUS CELL CARCINOMA

Squamous cell carcinoma of the urinary bladder is relatively rare in Western countries, representing only 3% to 5% of all bladder tumors.[4,12,28] However, the prevalence of squamous cell carcinoma in areas of Africa and the Middle East, where schistosomiasis is endemic, is much higher, with squamous cell carcinoma accounting for up to 80% of bladder cancers.[29]

## Pathologic features

Grossly, most squamous cell carcinomas are bulky, polypoid, solid, necrotic masses, often filling the bladder lumen; however, some are predominantly flat and irregularly bordered, or ulcerated and infiltrating.[30,31] The presence of necrotic material and keratin debris on the surface is relatively constant.

The diagnosis of squamous cell carcinoma has been restricted by most authors to pure tumors,[15,30,32,33] an approach recently endorsed by the WHO (2004).[12] The tumors may be well-differentiated lesions, in which histologically well-defined islands of squamous cells with keratinization, prominent intercellular bridges, and minimal nuclear pleomorphism or atypia are found. Poorly differentiated tumors exhibit marked nuclear pleomorphism with only focal evidence of squamous differentiation (Figure 8.5). Squamous metaplasia is identifiable in the adjacent epithelium in 17% to 60% of cases from Europe and North America.[33] Squamous cell carcinoma of the bladder is graded according to the amount of keratinization present, as well as the degree of nuclear pleomorphism.[32,34] Histologic grade may correlate with stage and outcome,[32,35] although this relationship has not been uniform.[34]

## Differential diagnosis

The major consideration in the differential diagnosis of squamous cell carcinoma is urothelial carcinoma with squamous differentiation, which occurs in up to 20% of high-grade urothelial carcinomas.[36,37] In North America, Europe, and other regions where primary squamous cell carcinoma is uncommon, such tumors should be carefully studied for a urothelial component. If an identifiable urothelial element, including urothelial carcinoma in situ (CIS), is found, the tumor should be classified as urothelial carcinoma with squamous differentiation.[37] The presence of keratinizing squamous metaplasia, especially if associated with dysplasia, favors a diagnosis of squamous cell carcinoma. Secondary invasion of the bladder by adjacent primary disease, such as squamous cell carcinoma of the cervix or vagina, should always be considered and excluded clinically.

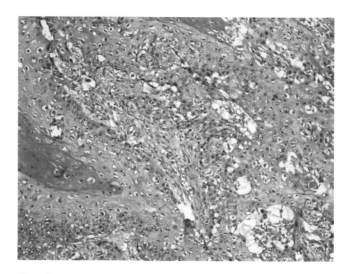

**Fig. 8.5**
Moderately well-differentiated squamous cell carcinoma with abundant keratinization.

## VERRUCOUS CARCINOMA

Rare cases of verrucous carcinoma of the urinary bladder have been described.[38-41] Most are in association with bilharzial cystitis, accounting for 3% of bladder cancers in one such series.[29] Only eight cases have been reported in the literature not associated with bilharzial infection. Limited data indicate that human papilloma virus is not important pathogenetically. Grossly, verrucous carcinoma is a wart-like, fungating, exophytic mass. Microscopically, there is well-differentiated hyper-keratotic squamous epithelium, extending down toward the submucosa in large, broad, bulbous projections that push the tissue rather than invade. There is minimal nuclear and architectural atypia. The criteria established by Ackerman[42] for the oral cavity include: 1) it must be exophytic with multiple warty surface projections composed of well-differentiated squamous epithelium; 2) it must lack features of anaplasia; and 3) the advancing margin must push, not infiltrate. We would apply the same criteria in the urinary bladder.

## BASALOID SQUAMOUS CELL CARCINOMA

Basaloid squamous cell carcinoma is a recently described variant of squamous cell carcinoma. It arises predominantly in the upper aerodigestive tract. Vakar-Lopez et al[43] have described a basaloid squamous cell carcinoma arising in the urinary bladder. Grossly, the mass was tan-brown, sessile, and multilobulated, involving the posterior wall. Microscopically, the tumor was composed of nests of small basaloid cells with peripheral palisading, central necrosis, and a pseudoglandular pattern. Cytologically, the cells have little cytoplasm, a high nuclear:cytoplasmic ratio with dense hyperchromatic nuclei, and numerous mitotic and apoptotic figures. Squamous differentiation and microscopic focus of transitional cell carcinoma were present. The remaining bladder had extensive squamous metaplasia with foci of dysplasia and squamous CIS. Basaloid squamous carcinomas in other organs have had a more aggressive course, and a worse prognosis, than the usual squamous cell carcinoma. Given the rarity of this histology in the bladder, there is no information regarding behavior or optimal treatment.

## SMALL CELL CARCINOMA

### Introduction

Small cell carcinoma of the urinary bladder is described as histologically identical to that occurring in the lung. To date there are well over 150 reported cases.[44-47] The tumor has been estimated to represent 0.5% to 1% of bladder malignancies.[48,49]

### Pathologic features

There are no specific gross features separating small cell carcinomas from other carcinomas of the bladder. They are usually polypoid or solid lesions, frequently ulcerating, and range in size from 2 to 10 cm. They can develop at any location, including in the dome and within diverticula. They usually show diffuse infiltration into the bladder wall, and occasionally extend into the perivesical adipose tissue.

Microscopically, the tumor has two major patterns. The oat cell type consists of a relatively uniform population of cells with scant cytoplasm, hyperchromatic nuclei with dispersed chromatin, and no or inconspicuous nucleoli. The intermediate cell type has more abundant cytoplasm and larger nuclei with less hyperchromasia, but dispersed chromatin and no or inconspicuous nucleoli (Figure 8.6). In some instances, the intermediate type of small cell carcinoma contains elongated or spindled cells. Both types have extensive necrosis, prominent nuclear molding, and frequent mitotic figures. In 23% to 67% of cases, the cells are mixed with cells having other histologic patterns.[44,45,50] A urothelial carcinoma component (papillary or nonpapillary) is most common, but glandular and squamous differentiation have been observed. In some cases, the adjacent urothelium has severe dysplasia or urothelial CIS. In contrast to urothelial carcinoma with squamous or glandular distinction, pure and mixed tumors are reported as small cell carcinoma with other histologic patterns, when present.[12]

In most reported cases studied by electron microscopy, dense core neurosecretory granules have been found.[46] In the majority of cases, evidence of

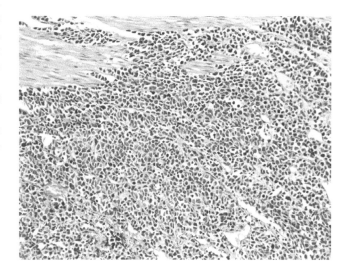

**Fig. 8.6**
Small cell carcinoma with sheets of poorly cohesive cells having uniform small nuclei, fine chromatin, and inconspicuous nucleoli with scanty cytoplasm.

neuroendocrine differentiation can be found immunohistochemically, with neuron-specific enolase immunoreactivity being the most frequently expressed, followed by synaptophysin and chromogranin.[46,48,51] Although cytokeratin is present in most tumors, some are nonreactive; a 'dot-like' pattern for cytokeratin has been noted in some cases.[46,51]

### Differential diagnosis

The major considerations for differential diagnosis are small cell carcinoma from another site and malignant lymphoma. Small cell carcinoma may arise in the prostate gland, and in about 50% of cases there is a coexistent adenocarcinoma component; positive staining of this element for PSA and PSAP would indicate prostatic origin. The small cell component usually is negative for these markers; in pure cases, therefore, clinical correlation may be essential to separate primary prostate tumors from primary bladder tumors. Metastases from other sites also need to be considered. Interestingly, symptomatic bladder metastasis from bronchogenic small cell carcinoma is a rare occurrence,[52] but clinical evaluation is necessary to exclude this possibility. The identification of a urothelial component, including urothelial CIS, would strongly support the theory of primary bladder origin.[46] Malignant lymphoma should be distinguishable in most cases on the basis of pathology.

# MESENCHYMAL TUMORS

Virtually all types of benign and malignant mesenchymal tumors have been reported as arising primarily in the urinary bladder.[53] There is nothing unique about the pathology of these tumors, and morphologically they resemble their counterparts at other locations. Overall, mesenchymal tumors account for less than 1% of primary urinary bladder neoplasms.

## BENIGN MESENCHYMAL TUMORS

The most common benign mesenchymal tumors arising in the urinary bladder are leiomyomas and hemangiomas:

- Leiomyomas occur predominantly in adults, with women being affected more often than men.[54,55] They frequently occur with obstructive symptoms because of a ball valve effect of the pedunculated tumor.[56] Most are submucosal with a polypoid or pedunculated appearance. Histologically, they are composed of fascicles of cells with eosinophilic cytoplasm and fusiform, blunt-ended nuclei. The presence of frequent mitoses, any abnormal mitoses, or necrosis indicates malignant potential.[55]

- Hemangiomas often occur in the pediatric population but may appear in adults.[57,58] Most patients have hematuria, but irritation, pain, and obstruction may also occur. In up to 30% there are associated cutaneous hemangiomas, and these are reported in association with Klippel–Trenaunay and Sturge–Weber syndromes.[59] Grossly, hemangiomas may be single or multiple, small or large, and they can be superficial or involve the full thickness of the bladder wall. Cystoscopically, they often appear to be lobulated and are a deep purple–red in color. Histologically, they consist of vascular spaces containing blood and thrombi. Depending on the pattern, hemangiomas are classified as cavernous, capillary, venous, or racemose, with cavernous being most common.

## MALIGNANT MESENCHYMAL TUMORS

The most common malignant mesenchymal tumors are rhabdomyosarcoma in children and leiomyosarcoma in adults:

- Rhabdomyosarcomas occur almost exclusively in children, with boys being affected more often than girls.[60] They most often are associated with hematuria or obstructive symptoms and cystoscopically appear as a polypoid mass filling the bladder lumen. Histologically, most are embryonal rhabdomyosarcoma, with diffuse infiltration of small blue round cells with scant cytoplasm. In the sarcoma botryoides type, the cells are scattered in a loose myxoid stroma, with condensation of rhabdomyoblasts beneath the surface epithelium in a cambium layer. Although rare rhabdoid or strap cells containing cross-striations may be found, this is not necessary for the diagnosis.

- Leiomyosarcomas are the most common sarcomas of the bladder in adults.[55,61] They occur in slightly more men than women and in patients in a wide age range, with most patients being between 40 and 60 years of age. Leiomyosarcomas may be polypoid and lobulated, or ulcerated and infiltrative. Histologically, the majority have the typical appearance of leiomyosarcoma, composed of interweaving fascicles of spindle-shaped cells with long blunt-ended nuclei and eosinophilic cytoplasm (Figure 8.7). Nuclear pleomorphism is variable as is the mitotic rate. Necrosis may be present. In a few cases, the tumor has had a myxoid or epithelioid morphology.

# MALIGNANT LYMPHOMA

Involvement of the bladder by malignant lymphoma is usually secondary to systemic lymphoma. Much less

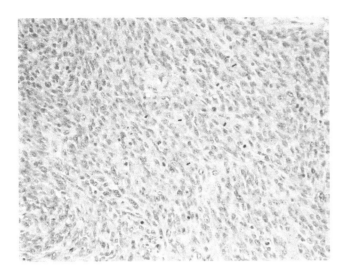

**Fig. 8.7**
Leiomyosarcoma with fascicles of malignant spindle cells.

frequent is the development of primary malignant lymphomas in the bladder in the absence of systemic lymphomas.[62,63] Such cases account for only 0.2% of all cases of extranodal malignant lymphoma. The majority of patients with primary lymphoma of the bladder are women (male:female ratio, 1:6.5), usually in the seventh and eighth decades (median age, 64 years). Most patients have gross hematuria, but may complain of dysuria or irritative symptoms.

Cystoscopically, the tumor may be single or multiple, and sessile or polypoid. Occasionally, diffuse involvement without formation of a discrete mass may be observed. The presence of intact mucosa overlying the mass is a useful clue to the diagnosis. Histologically, the tumor consists of a diffuse, infiltrative proliferation of lymphoid cells surrounding and permeating normal structures rather than replacing them.

The most common types are diffuse, large-cell and small lymphocytic lymphoma; less frequently, follicular, plasmacytoid, mantle zone, and monocytoid are found. More recently, the occurrence of mucosa-associated lymphoid tissue (MALT) type has been described.[64]

## SECONDARY TUMORS

Secondary involvement of the urinary bladder is most often by direct extension of tumors from adjacent organs such as the prostate gland, colorectum, and uterine cervix.[27,53] Less often metastases from distant sites may involve the bladder. While metastasis from almost all organs has been reported, among the most common are malignant melanoma and carcinomas of the lung, breast, and kidney.[27,65–66] The tumors in these cases resemble those of the primary origin. In many cases differentiation from urothelial carcinoma can be difficult and requires clinical correlation.

REFERENCES

1. Jacobo E, Loening S, Schmidt JD, Culp DA. Primary adenocarcinoma of the bladder: a retrospective study of 20 patients. J Urol 1977;117:54–56.
2. Thomas DG, Ward AM, Williams JL. A study of 52 cases of adenocarcinoma of the bladder. Br J Urol 1971;43:4–15.
3. Torenbeek R, Ladendijk JH, Van Diest PJ, Bril H, van de Molengraft FJ, Meijer CJ. Value of a panel of antibodies to identify the primary origin of adenocarcinomas presenting as bladder carcinoma. Histopathology 1998;32:20–27.
4. Grignon DJ. Neoplasms of the urinary bladder. In Bostwick DG, Eble JN (eds): Urologic Surgical Pathology. Philadelphia: Mosby-Year Book, 1996.
5. Grignon DJ, Ro JY, Ayala AG, Johnson DE, Ordonez NG. Primary adenocarcinoma of the urinary bladder: a clinicopathologic analysis of 72 cases. Cancer 1991;67:2165–2172.
6. El-Mekresh MM, el-Baz MA, Abol-Enein H, Ghoneim MA. Primary adenocarcinoma of the urinary bladder: a report of 185 cases. Br J Urol 1998;82:206–212.
7. Johnson DE, Hogan JM, Ayala AG. Primary adenocarcinoma of the urinary bladder. South Med J 1972;65:527–530.
8. Grignon DJ, Ro JY, Ayala AG, Johnson DE. Primary signet-ring cell carcinoma of the urinary bladder. Am J Clin Pathol 1991;95:13–20.
9. Abenoza P, Manivel C, Fraley EE. Primary adenocarcinoma of urinary bladder: clinicopathologic study of 16 cases. Urology 1987;29:9–14.
10. Eble JN, Hull MT, Rowland RG, Hotstetter M. Villous adenoma of the urachus with mucusuria: a light and electron microscopic study. J Urol 1986;135:1240–1244.
11. Mostofi FK, Thomson RV, Dean AL Jr. Mucous adenocarcinoma of the urinary bladder. Cancer 1955;8:741–758.
12. Eble JN, Sauter G, Epstein JI, Sesterhenn IA (eds). World Health Organization Classification of Tumours: Pathology and Genetics of Tumours of the Urinary System and Male Genital Organs. Lyons: IARC Press, 2004.
13. Anderstrom C, Johansson SL, von Schultz. Primary adenocarcinoma of the urinary bladder: a clinicopathologic and prognostic study. Cancer 1983;52:1273–1280.
14. Saleh HA, Papas P, Khatib G. Villous adenoma of the urinary bladder presenting as gross hematuria: a morphologic, histochemical and immunohistochemical study. J Urol Pathol 1996;4:299–306.
15. Nazeer T, Ro JY, Tornos C, Ordonez NG, Ayala AG. Endocervical type glands in urinary bladder: a clinicopathologic study of six cases. Hum Pathol 1996;27:816–820.
16. Young RH, Clement PB. Mullerianosis of the urinary bladder. Mod Pathol 1996;9:731–737.
17. Holmang S, Borghede G, Johansson SL. Primary signet ring cell carcinoma of the bladder: a report on 10 cases. Scand J Urol Nephrol 1997; 31:145–148.
18. Saphir O. Signet-ring cell carcinoma of the urinary bladder. Am J Pathol 1955;31:223–231.
19. Torenbeek R, Koot RA, Blomjous CE, De Bruin PC, Newling DW, Meijer CJ. Primary signet-ring cell carcinoma of the urinary bladder. Histopathology 1996; 28:33–40.
20. Chor PJ, Gaum LD, Young RH. Clear cell adenocarcinoma of the urinary bladder: report of a case of probable Müllerian origin. Mod Pathol 1993;6:225–228.
21. Young RH, Scully RE. Clear cell adenocarcinoma of the bladder and urethra: a report of three cases and review of the literature. Am J Surg Pathol 1985;9:816–826.
22. Drew PA, Murphy WM, Civantos F, Speights VO. The histogenesis of clear cell adenocarcinoma of the lower urinary tract: case series and review of the literature. Hum Pathol 1996;27:248–252.
23. Honda N, Yamada Y, Nanaura H. Mesonephric adenocarcinoma of the urinary bladder: a case report. Acta Urol Japn 2000;45:27–31.
24. Oliva E, Amin MB, Jiminez R, Young RH. Clear cell carcinoma of the urinary bladder: a report and comparison of four tumors of Müllerian origin and nine of probable urothelial origin with discussion of histogenesis and diagnostic problems. Am J Surg Pathol 2002;26:190–197.
25. Oliva E, Young RH. Clear cell adenocarcinoma of the urethra: a clinicopathologic analysis of 19 cases. Mod Pathol 1996;9:513–520.

26. Gilcrease MZ, Delgado R, Vuitch F, Albores-Saavedra J. Clear cell adenocarcinoma and nephrogenic adenoma of the urethra and urinary bladder: a histopathologic and immunohistochemical comparison. Hum Pathol 1998;29:1451–1456.

27. Goldstein AG. Metastatic carcinoma to the bladder. J Urol 1967;98:209–215.

28. Serretta V, Pomara G, Piazza F, Gange E. Pure squamous cell carcinoma of the bladder in western countries: report on 19 consecutive cases. Eur Urol 2000;37:85–89.

29. El-Bolkainy MN, Mokhtar NM, Ghoneim MA, Hussein MH. The impact of schistosomiasis on the pathology of bladder carcinoma. Cancer 1981;48:2643–2648.

30. Sarma KP. Squamous cell carcinoma of the bladder. Int Surg 1970;53:313–318.

31. Johnson DE, Schoenwald MB, Ayala AG, Miller LS. Squamous cell carcinoma of the bladder. J Urol 1976;115:542–544.

32. Faysal MH. Squamous cell carcinoma of the bladder. J Urol 1981;126:598–599.

33. Bessette PL, Abell MR, Herwig KR. A clinicopathologic study of squamous cell carcinoma of the bladder. J Urol 1974;112:66–67.

34. Newman DM, Brown JR, Jay AC, Pontius EE. Squamous cell carcinoma of the bladder. J Urol 1968;100:470–473.

35. Richie JP, Waisman J, Skinner DG, Dretler SP. Squamous carcinoma of the bladder: treatment by radical cystectomy. J Urol 1976;115:670–672.

36. Martin JE, Jenkins BJ, Zuk RJ, Blandy JP, Baithun SI. Clinical importance of squamous metaplasia in invasive transitional cell carcinoma of the bladder. J Clin Pathol 1989;42:250–253.

37. Sakamoto N, Tsuneyoshi M, Enjoji M. Urinary bladder carcinoma with neoplastic squamous component: a mapping study of 31 cases. Histopathology 1992;21:135–141.

38. Wyatt JK, Craig I. Verrucous carcinoma of urinary bladder. Urology 1980;16:97–99.

39. Ellsworth PI, Schned AR, Heaney JA, Snyder PM. Surgical treatment of verrucous carcinoma of the bladder unassociated with bilharzial cystitis: case report and literature review. J Urol 1995;153:411–414.

40. Wiedemann A, Diekmann WP, Holtmann G, Kracht H. Report of a case with giant condyloma (Buschke–Lowenstein tumor) localized in the bladder. J Urol 1995;153:1222–1224.

41. Oida Y, Yasuda M, Kajiwara H, Onda H, Kawamura N, Osamura RY. Double squamous cell carcinomas, verrucous type and poorly differentiated type, of the urinary bladder unassociated with bilharzial infection. Pathol Int 1997;47:651–654.

42. Ackerman LV. Verrucous carcinoma of the oral cavity. Surg 1948;23:670–678.

43. Vakar-Lopez F, Abrams J. Basaloid squamous cell carcinoma occurring in the urinary bladder. Arch Pathol Lab Med 2000;124:455–459.

44. Angulo JC, Lopez JI, Sanchez-Chapado M, et al. Small cell carcinoma of the urinary bladder: a report of two cases with complete remission and a comprehensive literature review with emphasis on therapeutic decisions. J Urol Pathol 1996;5:1–19.

45. Trias I, Algaba F, Condom E, et al. Small cell carcinoma of the urinary bladder: presentation of 23 cases and review of 134 published cases. Eur Urol 2001;39:85–90.

46. Grignon DJ, Ro JY, Ayala AG, et al. Small cell carcinoma of the urinary bladder: a clinicopathologic analysis of 22 cases. Cancer 1992;69:527–536.

47. Holmang S, Borghede G, Johansson SL. Primary small cell carcinoma of the bladder: a report of 25 cases. J Urol 1995;153;60:1820–1822.

48. Blomjous CEM, Vos W, De Voogt HJ, Van der Valk P, Meijer CJ. Small cell carcinoma of the urinary bladder: a clinicopathologic, morphometric, immunohistochemical, and ultrastructural study of 18 cases. Cancer 1989;64:1347–1357.

49. Lohrisch C, Murray N, Pickles T, Sullivan L. Small cell carcinoma of the bladder: long term outcome with integrated chemoradiation. Cancer 1999;86:2346–2352.

50. Mills SE, Wolfe JT 3rd, Weiss MA, et al. Small cell undifferentiated carcinoma of the urinary bladder: a light-microscopic, immunocytochemical, and ultrastructural study of 12 cases. Am J Surg Pathol 1987;11:606–617.

51. Atkin NB, Baker MC, Wilson D. Chromosome abnormalities and p53 expression in a small cell carcinoma of the bladder. Eur Urol 1999;35:323–326.

52. Coltart RS, Stewart S, Brown CH. Small cell carcinoma of the bronchus: a rare cause of haematuria from a metastasis in the urinary bladder. J Roy Soc Med 1985;78:1053–1054.

53. Murphy WM, Grignon DJ, Perlman EJ. Tumors of the Kidney, Bladder, and Related Urinary Structures. AFIP Atlas of Tumor Pathology, Series 4. Washington, DC: American Registry of Pathology, 2004.

54. Knoll LD, Segura JW, Scheithauer BW. Leiomyoma of the bladder. J Urol 1986;136:906–908.

55. Martin SA, Sears DL, Sebo TJ, Lohse CM, Cheville JC. Smooth muscle neoplasms of the urinary bladder: a clinicopathologic comparison of leiomyoma and leiomyosarcoma. Am J Surg Pathol 2002;26:292–300.

56. Kabalin JN, Freiha FS, Neibel JD. Leiomyoma of bladder. Urology 1990;35:210–212.

57. Jahn H, Nissen HM. Haemangioma of the urinary tract: review of the literature. Br J Urol 1991;68:113–117.

58. Cheng L, Leibovich BC, Cheville JC, et al. Hemangioma of the urinary bladder. Cancer 1999;86:498–504.

59. Hall BD. Bladder hemangiomas in Klippel–Trenaunay–Weber syndrome. N Engl J Med 1971;285:1032–1033.

60. Dehner LP. Pathology of the urinary bladder in children. In: Young RH (ed): Pathology of the Urinary Bladder. New York: Churchill Livingstone, 1989, pp 179–211.

61. Mills SE, Bova SG, Wick MR, Young RH. Leiomyosarcoma of the urinary bladder. Am J Surg Pathol 1989;13:480–489.

62. Abraham NZ Jr, Maher TJ, Hutchison RE. Extra-nodal monocytoid B-cell lymphoma of the urinary bladder. Mod Pathol 1993;6:145–149.

63. Ohsawa M, Aozasa K, Horiuchi K, Kanamarua A. Malignant lymphoma of bladder: report of three cases and review of the literature. Cancer 1993;72:1969–1974.

64. Al-Maghrabi J, Kamel-Reid S, Jewett M, Gospodarowicz M, Wells W, Banerjee D. Primary low-grade B-cell lymphoma of mucosa-associated lymphoid tissue type arising in the urinary bladder: report of 4 cases with molecular genetic analysis. Arch Pathol Lab Med 2001;125:332–336.

65. Berger Y, Nissenblatt M, Salwitz J, Lega B. Bladder involvement in metastatic breast carcinoma. J Urol 1992;147:137–139.

66. Sim SJ, Ro JY, Ordonez NG, Park YW, Kee KH, Ayala AG. Metastatic renal cell carcinoma to the bladder: a clinicopathologic and immunohistochemical study. Mod Pathol 1999;12:351–355.

# Gene discovery (overview)   9

*Margaret Knowles*

## INTRODUCTION

Our understanding of the molecular changes underlying the development of bladder cancer has progressed rapidly during the past 15 years. Not only do we now have a long list of genetic and gene expression changes found in tumors, but we also have a proposed model for the pathogenesis of urothelial cell carcinoma (UCC) based on molecular information. This chapter will consider the importance of molecular characterization and will summarize the information currently available, with particular emphasis on aspects that will not be covered in subsequent chapters.

Why study the molecular biology of cancer? Beyond the basic quest for information fueled by curiosity, there are compelling reasons to understand the molecular changes that occur in cancer cells. It is clear that the genotype to a very great extent determines what phenotype will be displayed, and, in turn, the phenotype of the cancer cell dictates the clinical course of disease. The diversity of clinical phenotype in bladder cancer has been outlined in earlier chapters and will become even more apparent in later chapters dealing with treatments and responses.

The various genetic and epigenetic changes that represent the primary heritable changes present in a cancer and the resulting wide range of secondary changes in gene expression represent a series of molecular markers that can be used to advantage in a number of ways in the clinical setting. These include classification of tumors at diagnosis, monitoring the course of the disease, and, by known associations, predicting prognosis and/or response to therapy. These changes also provide the key to development of individualized therapies based on the molecular profile of the tumor; for example, the development of drugs that inhibit specific targets, the development of reagents that potentiate the immune response to specific antigens, or gene therapy strategies that replace the function of damaged genes or utilize specific molecular features of a tumor to elicit cytotoxic effect.

Gene discovery has been a key objective of molecular studies of bladder cancer over the past two decades. Some of the genes identified are already being exploited for clinical benefit and others are being validated as useful markers or therapeutic targets. However, as will be indicated below, there remain some critical gaps in our knowledge of the molecular basis for bladder cancer development and this requires continued efforts to identify the genes concerned.

## APPROACHES TO CANCER GENE DISCOVERY

Several approaches have been used to discover genes involved in UCC development. Initial information came from classic cytogenetic analyses which indicated the likely location of key genes. Information available during the 1980s and 1990s revealed several common alterations: −9 or 9q−, +7, 1p−, 1q−, 5q−, i(5p), 11p−, 6p−, 6q−, 17p−, 2q−, 3p−, +8, +11, 21q− and −Y. Notably, monosomy 9 was identified as a frequent event, sometimes the only change seen in low grade/stage near diploid tumors (reviewed in Sandberg & Berger,[1] and discussed in more detail in Chapter 11).

Subsequent molecular studies that have focused on these genomic regions have involved a range of approaches. Some have looked directly at known oncogenes or tumor suppressor genes within the regions; for example, mutation analysis of *TP53* rapidly implicated p53 as the protein affected in tumors with deletions of 17p. Others have systematically screened regions of interest for either DNA copy number changes or for loss of heterozygosity (LOH). Increased DNA copy number, particularly high-level amplification, indicates the likely location of a relevant oncogene, whereas deletions imply the loss of copies of a tumor suppressor gene. Comparative genomic hybridization (CGH) provides a genome-wide method to map copy number changes, and, with the advent of array-based CGH, this can be achieved at very high resolution, leading to rapid mapping of both amplifications and deletions. Inactivation of tumor suppressor genes commonly requires biallelic loss of function in the tumor. This can be achieved by physical deletion of one copy and a small mutation of the second allele. Deletion of one allele can be detected as LOH in the tumor and this has been used to map regions of the genome that may contain relevant tumor suppressor genes. Some cases of LOH are not accompanied by physical deletion; as when reduplication of the chromosome has taken place or when LOH has occurred following mitotic recombination. CGH and LOH analyses provide complementary approaches for the localization of tumor suppressor genes.

The recent application of genome-wide screening of tumors at both the DNA level using CGH and single nucleotide polymorphism (SNP) arrays and at the RNA and protein expression levels using expression arrays and proteomic approaches is providing a wealth of information (see Chapters 11 and 12) that is likely to transform our understanding. Already some genetic events such as copy number gains and losses where the target gene(s) are not yet identified can be linked to particular tumor phenotypes and show potential for application as markers in the clinic.

## GENES IMPLICATED IN UCC DEVELOPMENT

There is now a long list of genes known to be genetically or epigenetically altered at significant frequency in UCC. Known tumor suppressor genes and oncogenes altered in bladder tumors are shown in Table 9.1.[2-33] These

**Table 9.1** Genetic alterations of known genes in transitional cell carcinoma

| Gene (cytogenetic location) | Alteration | Frequency/clinical association (reference) |
|---|---|---|
| **Oncogenes** | | |
| HRAS (11p15) | Activating mutation | 10–15% overall (2–4) |
| FGFR3 (4p16) | Activating mutation | 30–80% low grade/stage (5,6) |
| ERBB2 (17q23) | Amplification/overexpression | Amplified 10–14% high grade/stage (7–9) |
| CCND1 (11q13) | Amplification/overexpression | 10–20% all grades/stages (10,11) |
| MDM2 (12q13) | Amplification/overexpression | 4% amplification, high grade ~30% overexpression, low grade (12,13) |
| **Tumor suppressor genes** | | |
| INK4A-ARF (9p21) | Homozygous deletion/methylation/mutation | 20–30% high grade/stage (14–16) LOH 60% all grades/stages immortalization in vitro (17) |
| RB1 (13q14) | Deletion/mutation | 10–15% overall (18–20) 37% muscle invasive |
| TP53 (17p13) | Deletion/mutation | 70% muscle invasive (21–23) High grade and stage |
| PTEN (10q23) | Homozygous deletion/mutation | 10q LOH in 35% muscle invasive (24,25) 6.6% superficial |
| PTCH (9q22) | Deletion/mutation | LOH 60% all grades/stages (26,27) Mutation frequency low |
| TSC1 (9q34) | Deletion/mutation | LOH 60% all grades/stages (28–30) Mutation frequency low |
| DBC1 (9q32–33) *DCC/SMAD (18q) | Deletion/methylation Deletion | LOH 60% all grades/stages (31,32) LOH 30% high grade/stage (33) No mutation analysis to date |

LOH, loss of heterozygosity.
* Candidate gene; no tumor-specific mutations detected to date.

include genes encoding key G1 checkpoint proteins that are mutated in many tumor types (*TP53, RB, CDKN2A/ARF, CCND1*). The majority of these genes are altered only in invasive bladder tumors. Many other nonrandom genetic alterations have been identified in UCC, including deletions identified by LOH and CGH analyses and DNA amplification, identified by CGH analysis. Some specific examples of these will be described below (see also Chapter 10).

## ONCOGENES

Oncogenes are defined as genes that act in a dominant way to contribute to the cancer cell phenotype. Cellular proto-oncogenes represent the normal counterparts of these genes. Activation of proto-oncogenes can occur via overexpression of the normal gene, as achieved following gene amplification, or via translocations that place the gene under control of strong promoter elements, as is common in hematologic malignancies. Activation can also occur via mutations that alter the structure and function of the gene.

Proto-oncogenes of the ras family (*HRAS, NRAS,* and *KRAS2*) are activated in human tumors by mutations affecting a small number of codons that give rise to proteins with altered function. These small, highly related proteins are GDP/GTP binding proteins that cycle between the GDP- and GTP-bound state. In the GTP-bound state ras proteins activate downstream signaling pathways, particularly the MAP kinase pathway that can have profound effects on the cell, including increased proliferation and resistance to apoptosis.[34]

### HRAS

*HRAS* is mutated in some UCCs (see Table 9.1),[2-33] but there are conflicting estimates of the frequency of mutation that may be related to the techniques used for mutation detection. Tissue culture experiments on human tumor cells have shown that HRAS can upregulate EGFR expression (commonly found in invasive UCC) and induce an invasive phenotype.[35,36] However, transgenic mice engineered to express mutant HRAS in the urothelium develop papillary tumors rather than muscle-invasive tumors.[37] Further studies in animal models may help to clarify whether HRAS can participate in the development of both major forms of UCC. No clear association of *HRAS* mutation with tumor phenotype has been described. *NRAS* and *KRAS2* have not been adequately studied, but a few mutations of each have been reported. A comprehensive examination of a single tumor series for mutations in all three ras genes is merited.

### ERBB2

*ERBB2* (17q23) encodes a receptor tyrosine kinase of the EGFR/ERBB gene family. It is amplified in 10% to 20% and overexpressed in 10% to 50% of invasive UCC.[7,8,38,39]

Thus, in contrast to the situation in breast carcinoma, many cases of UCC show increased protein expression in the absence of gene amplification. The underlying mechanism has not yet been elucidated. A similar situation exists in the case of the EGF receptor, where 30% to 50% of invasive bladder tumors overexpress EGFR and this is associated with poor prognosis[40]; however, only a small percentage show gene amplification.

### MDM2

*MDM2* (12q14) is amplified in a few cases of UCC (4–6%).[12] MDM2 acts in an autoregulatory loop with p53, and its overexpression represents an alternative mechanism by which p53 function may be inactivated in some UCCs (see Chapter 10). Immunohistochemical studies have shown upregulation of expression of MDM2 in up to 44% of UCC samples but there is no consensus on the relation of this to tumor grade, stage, or prognosis.[41-43]

### CCND1

Amplification at 11q13 has been identified in UCC by various approaches.[10,11,44] The cyclin D1 gene (*CCND1*), which is involved in the regulation of progression from G1 to S phase of the cell cycle via the Rb pathway, is believed to be the target gene. Protein expression studies indicate that overexpression of cyclin D1 is more frequent than gene amplification. Initial studies showed no obvious correlation of 11q13 amplification with clinicopathologic data, but immunohistochemical studies indicate that there may be an inverse correlation of expression with tumor grade,[45,46] and a positive association with a papillary growth pattern.[45,47] Thus, CCND1 is implicated early in the development of superficial papillary UCC. The absence of high levels of expression in more advanced tumors may indicate that early involvement of this protein determines subsequent tumor pathogenesis.

Interestingly, cyclin D1 is a possible target of the Wnt/β-catenin pathway and recently it was reported that some high-grade bladder tumors (3/59 studied) had mutations in β-catenin.[48] This represents an alternative mechanism for cyclin D1 activation in these tumors that is accompanied by myc overexpression and appears to be associated with a more aggressive phenotype than the overexpression associated with gene amplification, found in low-grade tumors with papillary architecture.[47]

To date, the role of cyclin D1 has not been extensively explored in UCC. This association is similar to that observed for FGFR3 mutation (see below). Its participation in a pivotal cell cycle control mechanism and this association with papillary UCC provide a strong impetus for further study.

### MYC

Copy number gains of 8q have been identified in many studies, resulting in gain of *MYC*. High-level amplification has been reported in only a small number of cases.[49] However, myc protein levels showed no relationship to gains of 8q, suggesting that this does not represent a genetic mechanism for increasing *MYC* expression. This is borne out by a detailed amplicon mapping study that excluded *MYC* from the region of amplification.[50] Nevertheless, overexpression of the myc protein, unrelated to gene amplification, is found in a large proportion of UCC samples including non-recurrent papillary superficial tumors.[51,52]

## FGFR3

Fibroblast growth factor (FGF) receptor 3 (*FGFR3*) has recently been identified as an oncogene that is activated by mutation in UCC.[5,53–55] *FGFR3* maps to 4p16.3 within a common region of LOH in UCC,[56] but mutations do not appear to be related to LOH status.[6] Instead, FGFR3 appears to act as an oncogene in UCC. The frequency of *FGFR3* mutations detected varies (see Table 9.1).[2–33] Mutation is strongly associated with low tumor grade and stage, with up to 80% of low-grade pTa tumors showing mutation.[53] Mutation appears to indicate lower risk of tumor recurrence in these non-invasive UCCs.[55] Mutations have also been found in urothelial papilloma, indicating that this may be a very early event in urothelial cell transformation.[57] Recently two studies that assessed both *FGFR3* and *TP53* mutation in the same samples showed that these events are virtually mutually exclusive.[58,59] The possibility must be considered that *FGFR3* mutation in some way protects superficial UCC from progression. Functional analyses and studies of *FGFR3* signaling in urothelial cells, now in progress, may help to clarify this.

The *FGFR3* mutations found in UCC are the same as germline mutations found in inherited dwarfism syndromes (reviewed in Passos-Bueno et al[60]). The most common mutation found in UCC is S249C, which, when present in the germline, causes thanatophoric dysplasia type I, a lethal form of achondroplasia. All of the mutations found are confined to a few hot spots in exons 7, 10, and 15 of the gene and the predicted effect of mutation is constitutive activation of the kinase activity of the receptor[61] (Figure 9.1).

Interestingly, despite quite extensive studies of other major adult tumor types, *FGFR3* mutation is found at significant frequency only in bladder cancer. A small number of mutations have been described in multiple myeloma where they occur in association with the translocation t(4;14) and also in cervical carcinoma,[5] but none in a wide range of the common adult solid tumors.[54,62] This dramatic bladder tumor specificity may represent a significant opportunity for the development of tumor-specific therapy. The predominance of mutation in superficial bladder tumors lends itself well to the development of novel forms of intravesical therapy.

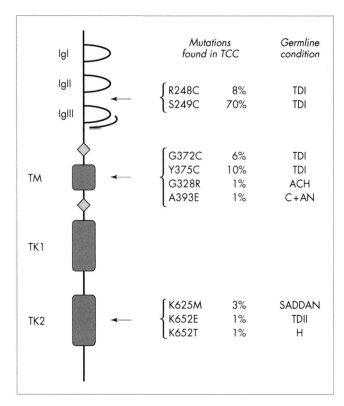

### Fig. 9.1

Structure of the FGFR3 protein showing positions and frequency of mutations identified in transitional cell carcinoma (TCC) and the corresponding germline conditions. ACH, achondroplasia; C+AN, Crouzon syndrome with acanthoma nigracans; H, hypochondroplasia with milder radiological features than N540K; IgI, II, III, immunoglobulin domains; SADDAN, severe achondroplasia with developmental delay and acanthosis nigracans; TDI, thanatophoric dysplasia type I; TDII, thanatophoric dysplasia type II; TK1, TK2, tyrosine kinase domains; TM, transmembrane domain.

*FGFR3* mutation may be a useful prognostic marker, as the recurrence rate for tumors with mutation appears lower than for tumors without mutation.[55] In a recent study, a combination of *FGFR3* mutation status and immunohistochemistry for MIB1 was found to be superior to pathologic grading for prediction of outcome (recurrence, progression, and disease-free survival).[63] *FGFR3* mutation screening has also been applied to urine sediments. Mutations were detected in 67% of patients undergoing transurethral resection UCC and in 28% of patients that subsequently underwent cystectomy.[64] *FGFR3* mutation screening outperformed cytology in both groups but in the low-grade superficial tumors was markedly better than cytology (68% versus 32%). In another prospective study, paired tumor and urine samples were analysed for *FGFR3* mutation and for microsatellite alterations. Identical alterations were detected in tumor and urine from the same patients and combined sensitivity was 89% for all types of tumor.[65]

## TUMOR SUPPRESSOR GENES

Tumor suppressor genes are genes whose functional inactivation contributes to tumor development. They have a wide range of negative regulatory functions, ranging from control of cell cycle progression to effects on cellular adhesion. Several of the tumor suppressor genes implicated in invasive UCC, including *TP53*, *RB*, *CDKN2A/ARF* (also altered in many superficial tumors), and *PTEN*, are major players in other human cancers.

### Chromosome 9 genes

The cytogenetic finding of monosomy 9 in many bladder cancers led to examination of this chromosome for LOH in UCC. Initial studies showed that more than 50% of tumors have LOH for markers on chromosome 9,[66,67] and commonly all markers studied showed LOH, in accord with cytogenetic observations. The finding in many studies of LOH for markers on both arms of chromosome 9[68-70] led to the hypothesis that there are relevant bladder tumor suppressor genes on both arms of this chromosome. The high frequency of LOH in tumors of all grades and stages,[68] and also in normal and hyperplastic urothelium,[71] suggests that at least one of these genes may be involved at a very early stage in tumor development.

Much effort has been expended to identify these genes. Many large tumor series have been studied for LOH to define the location of the target genes. This has proved difficult due to the large number of tumors with loss of an entire parental homologue. However, some tumors with smaller defined regions of LOH have allowed critical regions to be mapped. Currently, one region of loss is mapped on 9p (9p21) and at least three regions on 9q (at 9q22, 9q32–q33, and 9q34).[26,72-75] Candidate genes within these regions are *CDKN2A/ARF* (p16/p14ARF) and *CDKN2B* (p15) at 9p21,[14,15,76-78] *PTCH* (Gorlin syndrome gene) at 9q22,[26,27] *DBC1* (a novel gene) at 9q32–q33,[72,79,80] and *TSC1* (tuberous sclerosis syndrome gene 1) at 9q34.[28-30]

The CDKN2A/ARF locus (9p21) encodes two proteins—p16 and p14ARF—both of which are key cell cycle regulators (Figure 9.2A). These genes share a coding region in exon 2 but have distinct exons 1. The protein products are translated in different reading frames to generate two entirely different proteins: one, p16, plays a key role in the Rb pathway and the other, p14[ARF], is important in the p53 pathway (Figure 9.2B). Both genes are commonly inactivated in UCC via homozygous co-deletion. In the same region of 9p21 is the related gene *CDKN2B* encoding the cell cycle regulator p15, and, in many cases, though not all, this gene is also homozygously deleted. Point mutations of p16 are infrequent but hypermethylation of the promoter is found as a mechanism of inactivation of the second allele.[81,82] It is still unclear whether 9p21 deletion is related to UCC grade and stage. LOH of 9p21

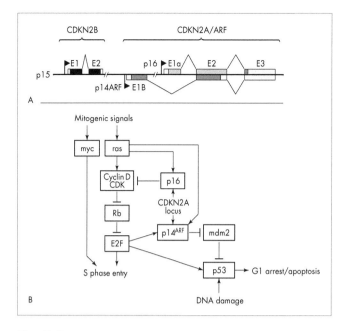

**Fig. 9.2**

**A** Organization of the *CDKN2A/ARF* and *CDKN2B* loci on 9p21. The transcript for p16 is derived from *CDKN2A* exons 1α, 2, and 3 and for p14[ARF] from exons 1β, 2, and 3. The protein products show no homology. **B** Relationship of the p53 and Rb pathways in controlling cell cycle progression and response to stress (DNA damage). The *CDKN2A* locus encodes both p16 and p14[ARF] and links the two pathways. All the genes shown are commonly altered either genetically or at the expression level in transitional cell carcinoma.

is as common in low-grade pTa as in invasive (≥pT2) UCC, although homozygous deletion is reported to be associated with larger tumor size and reduced recurrence-free interval.[83] This may indicate that, as suggested by knockout mouse studies (reviewed in Serrano[84]) and *in vitro* experiments on mouse cells,[85] haploinsufficiency of p16 and/or p14[ARF] is significant.

Three 9q genes are implicated as tumor suppressor genes:

- *PTCH*, the Gorlin syndrome gene, maps within a small region of deletion at 9q22. Although mutations are infrequent in UCC,[27] reduction in mRNA expression is common, and it has been suggested that *PTCH* may be haploinsufficient in the urothelium.[26]
- The novel gene *DBC1* is the only gene within the common region of deletion at 9q33. Homozygous deletion has been found in a few tumors,[79,80] and although mutational inactivation has not been described, transcriptional silencing by hypermethylation of the promoter is common.[31,72] The function of DBC1 is not yet clear, but ectopic expression induces a nonapoptotic form of cell death,[86] and, in cells that survive and express the protein, there is a delay in the G1 phase of the cell cycle.[87]

• The third gene, at 9q34, is TSC1. Germline mutation of TSC1 is associated with the familial hamartoma syndrome tuberous sclerosis complex (TSC). In bladder tumors, TSC1 mutations are found in approximately 13% of cases,[28,29] some in tumors without 9q34 LOH, again indicating the possible role of haploinsufficiency.[28] The TSC1 protein hamartin acts in a complex with the TSC2 protein tuberin in the PI3-kinase pathway to negatively regulate mTOR, a central molecule in the control of protein synthesis and cell growth[88] (Figure 9.3).

## PTEN

*PTEN* (**p**hosphatase and **ten**sin homologue deleted on chromosome **ten**) maps to 10q23, a region of common LOH in UCC of high grade and stage.[24,89,90] PTEN has a phosphatase domain that acts on both lipid and protein substrates. The major substrate appears to be the signaling lipid PtIns(3,4,5)P$_3$, a major product of PI3-kinase that is activated by various tyrosine kinase receptors. Thus PTEN is a negative regulator of this major signaling pathway, which affects cell phenotype in various ways including effects on proliferation, apoptosis. and cell migration.[91] Heterozygous knockout mice (PTEN +/−) show widespread proliferative changes, suggesting that loss of one allele in tumors may provide an advantage at the cellular level. Mutation screening in UCC has revealed some mutations of the second allele

in tumors with LOH and in bladder cell lines.[25,92,93] Some homozygous deletions have also been found. Gene replacement studies have been carried out in two bladder tumor cell lines that lack functional PTEN. In both cases this suppressed proliferation and induced G1 arrest.[94]

It should be noted that PTEN and TSC1 inactivation could represent alternative ways to inactivate the PI3-kinase pathway (see Figure 9.3), though it is not yet clear whether these are mutually exclusive events in UCC. However, it is anticipated that inactivation of PTEN is likely to have more profound effects as it acts upstream of AKT, which signals via several pathways in addition to that controlling cell growth via mTOR.

## TP53 and RB

The interconnecting pathways controlled by p53 and Rb regulate cell cycle progression and responses to stress, processes that are almost universally deregulated in malignant cells. As these are discussed in detail in Chapter 10, only a brief comment is given here. p53 plays a key role in determining cellular response to various stress signals. In the absence of stress stimuli, p53 protein levels are low; however, when activated, protein levels rise and transcription of a wide range of genes is activated. p53 activation induces apoptosis in some circumstances and cell cycle arrest in others, depending on the cell type and the nature of the

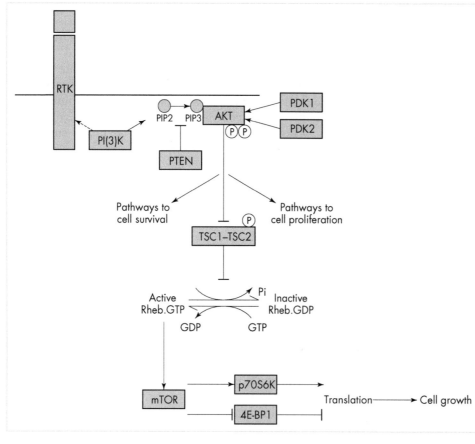

**Fig. 9.3**
The role of PTEN and TSC1 in control of cell growth via the PI3-kinase pathway. The TSC1 product hamartin in complex with the TSC2 product tuberin is a negative regulator of Rheb, which in turn is an activator of mTOR, linking nutrient sensing to control of protein translation and cell growth. PTEN is a lipid phosphatase that acts as a negative regulator of PtIns(3,4,5)P$_3$ (PIP3) production at the top of the pathway. RTK, receptor tyrosine kinase; PI(3)K, phosphoinositide 3-kinase; PDK1 and PDK2, 3-phosphoinositide-dependent kinases 1 and 2; mTOR, mammalian target of rapamycin.

stimulus. Mutation of *TP53* is found in many muscle-invasive bladder cancers.[21-23,95,96] As many mutations increase the half-life of the protein, detection of high levels of protein by immunohistochemistry provides a useful surrogate marker for mutation,[97] and this approach has been used extensively to measure p53 alteration. p53 accumulation has been associated with adverse prognosis in all types of UCC.[98-101] There are clear indications for the use of p53 both as a marker and as a therapeutic target in UCC (see Chapter 10).

Rb acts in a pathway that regulates progression from the G1 to S phase of the cell cycle (see Figure 9.2). It binds to members of the E2F transcription factor family, and this complex recruits histone deacetylases (HDACs) to E2F responsive promoters. Cdk-mediated phosphorylation of Rb prevents association with E2F and enables E2F-mediated gene expression and progression into S phase. The *RBI* gene is large and has not been screened for small mutations, but some homozygous deletions, LOH of 13q14, and loss of Rb protein expression have been detected in UCC. The frequency of loss of Rb, as for inactivation of p53, is higher in tumors of high grade and stage.[18-20,102]

The finding of frequent involvement of p53 and Rb, together with the finding that p16 and p14[ARF] are commonly deleted in UCC of all grades and stages, has generated much excitement. All of these proteins impact on cell cycle control and this validates the concept that the same cellular phenotype may be generated by different combinations of genetic events. p16 and p14[ARF] interact with and link the Rb and p53 pathways; inactivation of both of these together is likely to provide freedom from the G1 checkpoint more extensive than that conferred by either p53 or Rb inactivation alone. There are, therefore, several ways in which tumors may evade the checkpoint and it would be predicted that those with p53 and Rb or p16 loss would be more aggressive than those with either p53 or Rb loss alone. Rb and p53 have been assessed together in several studies and this prediction is borne out with double mutant tumors showing worse prognosis.[103-106] To date, an assessment of all genes known to be involved in this G1 checkpoint has not been carried out on a single patient series, but such an analysis may achieve much greater predictive power than single- or two-marker analyses.

## DNA REPAIR GENES

Defects in DNA repair processes may generate a mutator phenotype. In recent years mechanisms of mammalian DNA repair have been studied in great detail and there is now much information on the processes and genes involved. More than 125 gene products are involved in DNA repair.[107] Genes involved in several DNA repair pathways have been implicated in human cancer. A detailed discussion is beyond the scope of this chapter but several recent findings point to a role for defects in these pathways in the development of bladder cancer (see also Chapter 4). It is predicted that examination of these processes will reveal a major role in UCC development.

A hallmark of defects in DNA repair is genetic instability. In human cancers this can be manifested as microsatellite instability (MSI), resulting from defects in mismatch repair (MMR), and the role of defects in mismatch repair efficiency has been well documented in hereditary non-polyposis colorectal cancer (HNPCC). Alternatively, there may be widespread chromosomal instability (CIN) in which, at the cytogenetic level, there are multiple translocations, deletions, and rearrangements. Commonly, these two forms of instability appear to be mutually exclusive, implying that either is sufficient for carcinogenesis.[108]

Although widespread MSI is not common in UCC of the bladder,[109] recent studies have indicated that it is common in tumors of the upper tract,[110] particularly those with an inverted growth pattern,[111] and indeed upper urinary tract cancer is found at higher frequency in HNPCC kindreds.[112] Recently, the finding of a high level of instability at tetranucleotide repeats (30%), rather than mono- or dinucleotide repeats, suggests that there are distinct forms of microsatellite instability and that this second form, termed EMAST (elevated microsatellite alterations at selected tetranucleotide loci), may be an important mechanism in the bladder. Currently, the cause is unknown, although an association with *TP53* mutation has been reported in lung cancer, suggesting that this may be related to loss of a p53-mediated repair function.[113]

Cytogenetic, CGH, and LOH studies all report frequent aneuploidy, chromosomal deletions and rearrangements in advanced UCC. Currently, the molecular mechanisms that generate this phenotype are not well elucidated. The large number of breakpoints involved indicates that some form of aberrant double strand break repair or increased frequency of recombination may be involved. Amongst the many genes involved in the two mechanisms of double strand break repair (nonhomologous end joining and homologous recombination) are genes known to be mutated or whose expression is altered in cancer-prone syndromes and/or sporadic cancers (e.g. *BRCA1*, *BRCA2*, *ATM*, *BLM*, and *MRE11*). To date, these genes have not been examined systematically for alterations in bladder cancer. However, it is notable that the map locations of some of these genes coincide with regions known to show copy number changes in UCC. There is also some evidence that germline polymorphisms in DNA repair genes increase the risk of bladder cancer.[114] A detailed assessment of the impact of defective DNA repair mechanisms on the complement of genomic alterations in UCC represents a major area for future investigation.

# MOLECULAR PATHWAYS TO TUMOR DEVELOPMENT

Most UCCs (70–80%) are superficial papillary tumors at presentation and, despite the frequent development of recurrences (~70%), few of these progress to muscle invasion. Prognosis for patients with such superficial disease is good, though disease monitoring is costly and the associated morbidity and anxiety for patients is high. In contrast, for the 20% of tumors that are invasive at diagnosis, prognosis is much less favorable (50% survival at 5 years). The more common precursor lesion for these tumors is believed to be carcinoma *in situ* (CIS). The distinct clinical behaviour of these two groups of tumors has been predicted to indicate distinct underlying molecular differences. During the past decade this has been shown to be the case and genetic information has suggested a reappraisal of the previous practice of categorization of bladder cancer into 'superficial' and 'invasive' depending on the degree of invasion of the submucosa and the muscle wall of the bladder. Current genetic data indicate that low-grade superficial papillary tumors (pTa G1/2) should be considered as distinct from those tumors that have penetrated the basement membrane and invaded the submucosa (pT1), and from the high-grade lesion CIS, all of which have been grouped together in the past.

These are high-risk lesions that commonly progress to invade muscle.[115] High-grade Ta tumors (pTa G3) are also at increased risk of progression to invasion, and this is reflected in a spectrum of molecular changes and genetic instability similar to that seen in T2 tumors. A grouping into genetically stable (low-grade pTa) and genetically unstable superficial tumors is therefore appropriate.

Based on molecular and histopathologic observations, a model for molecular pathogenesis of UCC has developed (Figure 9.4). Although this ultimately may be found to be too simple, it does provide a useful anchor for genetic studies. A key observation is that most of the genetic changes described to date are found in high-grade/stage tumors. Low-grade (G1–2) pTa tumors show few molecular alterations. Despite efforts of many laboratories that have examined hundreds of such tumors, only two common alterations are found: deletions involving chromosome 9 and mutations of *FGFR3*. Mutation of *FGFR3* appears to define the large group of superficial tumors, and two recent studies confirm that *FGFR3* and *TP53* mutation are virtually mutually exclusive, each confined to one of the two major groups of UCC.[58,59] Chromosome 9 alterations are found in all types of UCC, suggesting that this is a pivotal alteration required for tumor development. The finding of chromosome 9 deletions in apparently normal urothelium in

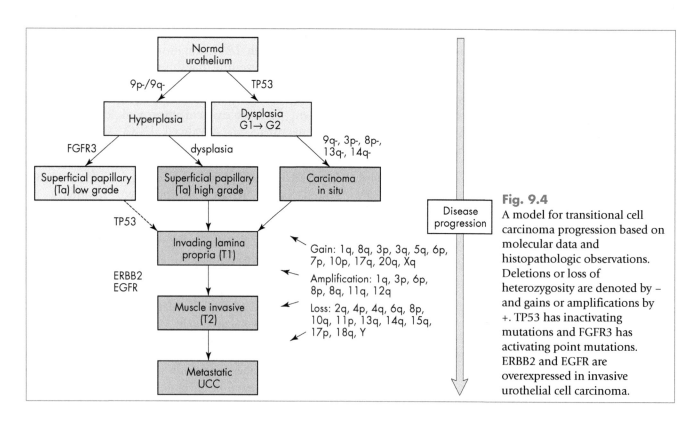

**Fig. 9.4**
A model for transitional cell carcinoma progression based on molecular data and histopathologic observations. Deletions or loss of heterozygosity are denoted by – and gains or amplifications by +. TP53 has inactivating mutations and FGFR3 has activating point mutations. ERBB2 and EGFR are overexpressed in invasive urothelial cell carcinoma.

individuals with bladder cancer and in hyperplastic urothelium, which is a likely precursor lesion for superficial papillary UCC, suggests that this may be a very early event. *FGFR3* mutation also occurs early, but to date there have been no reports of mutation in normal or hyperplastic urothelium. Low-grade pTa tumors are genetically very stable. There have been several studies of synchronous or metachronous tumors from the same patient, and in general these show a striking identity in the genetic alterations found.[116,117] Chromosome 9 LOH is the least divergent event, and other genetic events differ in different tumors from the same patient. This indicates that LOH of chromosome 9 is likely to be an early change whereas other events occur during independent evolution of different tumor clones.[117]

CIS is a fragile lesion that is difficult to sample as unfixed tissue. By definition, CIS has normal urothelial thickness, and commonly the cells, which are highly anaplastic, are only weakly adherent and tend to fragment during cystoscopy. Thus most specimens are only recognized retrospectively in paraffin-embedded samples. For this reason, only a few studies have attempted to assess genetic changes in such lesions. In general, the findings are similar to those for invasive tumors,[118] and this is considered an aggressive and high-risk lesion.

## GAPS IN KNOWLEDGE

Much work on UCC to date has been based on studies of panels of tumors at one point in their development. This has given information about frequent genetic alterations in UCC, but provides only one snapshot in the genetic evolution of each tumor. What is lacking at present is a clear view of the sequence and time course of the accumulation of molecular changes that culminate in tumor development.

The simple model for UCC pathogenesis shown in Figure 9.4 reveals other gaps in our current understanding. As bladder cancer is a disease of the middle to late decades of life, it is predicted that multiple heritable changes are required for tumor development. Thus it is surprising that so few changes have been identified in low-grade pTa tumors, which represent the major group at diagnosis. Efforts are in progress using expression and genomic microarray technology to identify other genetic or epigenetic events that may contribute to the development of these tumors, but as yet no other common changes have been described.

Another outstanding question concerns the significance of pT1 tumors. Are these merely muscle-invasive tumors caught in their journey towards the muscle, or do they represent a distinct group? Genetic

findings tend to support the former conclusion, but perhaps differences remain to be identified using novel approaches that will define these as a clear entity. No significant differences have yet been found between CIS, muscle-invasive UCC, and the metastases that develop from them. Possibly this reflects the early migration of cells to distant sites without the requirement for additional changes, or there may be determinants of progression and metastasis yet to be identified.

## FUTURE PROSPECTS: FEATURES OF CANCER CELLS

If our aim is to use tumor molecular biology as a means to improve clinical management, it is desirable that we identify those molecular changes that have most impact on tumor cell phenotype. This requires an understanding of the key features of tumor cells that are likely to influence their behaviour. Six key traits have been identified and discussed in detail in an excellent review by Hanahan and Weinberg.[119] These characteristics are self-sufficiency in growth signals, insensitivity to antigrowth (inhibitory) signals, evasion of apoptosis, acquisition of limitless replicative potential, sustained angiogenesis, and ability to invade and metastasize. Advanced bladder cancers commonly show all of these features. Examples of molecular alterations associated with some of these phenotypic traits will be discussed in subsequent chapters. Armed with extensive lists of genes and genetic alterations commonly found in such tumors, we are now in a position to begin to identify the links between genotype and phenotype and to exploit this understanding in the clinic.

## REFERENCES

1. Sandberg AA, Berger CS. Review of chromosome studies in urological tumors. II. Cytogenetics and molecular genetics of bladder cancer. J Urol 1994;151:545–560.
2. Knowles MA, Williamson M. Mutation of H-ras is infrequent in bladder cancer: confirmation by single-strand conformation polymorphism analysis, designed restriction fragment length polymorphisms, and direct sequencing. Cancer Res 1993;53(1):133–139.
3. Ooi A, Herz F, Ii S, et al. Ha-ras codon 12 mutation in papillary tumors of the urinary bladder: a retrospective study. Int J Oncol 1994;4:85–90.
4. Fitzgerald JM, Ramchurren N, Rieger K, et al. Identification of H-ras mutations in urine sediments complements cytology in the detection of bladder tumors. J Natl Cancer Inst 1995;87:129–133.
5. Cappellen D, De Oliveira C, Ricol D, et al. Frequent activating mutations of FGFR3 in human bladder and cervix carcinomas. Nat Genet 1999;23(1):18–20.
6. Sibley K, Cuthbert-Heavens D, Knowles MA. Loss of heterozygosity at 4p16.3 and mutation of FGFR3 in transitional cell carcinoma. Oncogene 2001;20:686–691.
7. Coombs LM, Pigott DA, Sweeney E, et al. Amplification and over-expression of c-erbB-2 in transitional cell carcinoma of the urinary bladder. Br J Cancer 1991;63(4):601–608.

8. Sauter G, Moch H, Moore D, et al. Heterogeneity of erbB-2 gene amplification in bladder cancer. Cancer Res 1993;53:2199–2203.

9. Sato K, Moriyama M, Mori S, et al. An immunohistologic evaluation of c-erbB-2 gene product in patients with urinary bladder carcinoma. Cancer 1992;70:2493–2498.

10. Proctor AJ, Coombs LM, Cairns JP, Knowles MA. Amplification at chromosome 11q13 in transitional cell tumors of the bladder. Oncogene 1991;6:789–795.

11. Bringuier PP, Tamimi Y, Schuuring E, Schalken J. Expression of cyclin D1 and EMS1 in bladder tumours; relationship with chromosome 11q13 amplification. Oncogene 1996; 12: 1747–1753.

12. Habuchi T, Kinoshita H, Yamada H, et al. Oncogene amplification in urothelial cancers with p53 gene mutation or MDM2 amplification. J Natl Cancer Inst 1994;86:1331–1335.

13. Lianes P, Orlow I, Zhang Z-F, et al. Altered patterns of MDM2 and TP53 expression in human bladder cancer. J Natl Cancer Inst 1994;86:1325–1330.

14. Orlow I, Lacombe L, Hannon GJ, et al. Deletion of the p16 and p15 genes in human bladder tumors. J Natl Cancer Inst 1995;87:1524–1529.

15. Williamson MP, Elder PA, Shaw ME, Devlin J, Knowles MA. p16 (CDKN2) is a major deletion target at 9p21 in bladder cancer. Hum Mol Genet 1995;4:1569–1577.

16. Cairns P, Tokino K, Eby Y, Sidransky D. Homozygous deletions of 9p21 in primary human bladder tumors detected by comparative multiplex polymerase chain reaction. Cancer Res 1994;54:1422–1424.

17. Yeager TR, DeVries S, Jarrard DF, et al. Overcoming cellular senescence in human cancer pathogenesis. Genes Dev 1998;12(2):163–174.

18. Cairns P, Proctor AJ, Knowles MA. Loss of heterozygosity at the RB locus is frequent and correlates with muscle invasion in bladder carcinoma. Oncogene 1991;6:2305–2309.

19. Logothetis CJ, Xu H-J, Ro JY, et al. Altered expression of retinoblastoma protein and known prognostic variables in locally advanced bladder cancer. J Natl Cancer Inst 1992;84:1256–1261.

20. Cordon-Cardo C, Wartinger D, Petrylak D, et al. Altered expression of the retinoblastoma gene product: prognostic indicator in bladder cancer. J Natl Cancer Inst 1992;84:1251–1256.

21. Sidransky D, von Eschenbach A, Tsai YC, et al. Identification of p53 gene mutations in bladder cancers and urine samples. Science 1991;252:706–709.

22. Habuchi T, Takahashi R, Yamada H, et al. Influence of cigarette smoking and schistosomiasis on p53 gene mutation in urothelial cancer. Cancer Res 1993;53:3795–3799.

23. Spruck CH III, Rideout WM III, Olumi AF, et al. Distinct pattern of p53 mutations in bladder cancer: relationship to tobacco usage. Cancer Res 1993;53:1162–1166.

24. Aveyard JS, Skilleter A, Habuchi T, Knowles MA. Somatic mutation of PTEN in bladder carcinoma. Br J Cancer 1999;80(5–6):904–908.

25. Cairns P, Evron E, Okami K, et al. Point mutation and homozygous deletion of PTEN/MMAC1 in primary bladder cancers. Oncogene 1998;16(24):3215–3218.

26. Aboulkassim TO, LaRue H, Lemieux P, Rousseau F, Fradet Y. Alteration of the PATCHED locus in superficial bladder cancer. Oncogene 2003;22(19):2967–2971.

27. McGarvey TW, Maruta Y, Tomaszewski JE, Linnenbach AJ, Malkowicz SB. PTCH gene mutations in invasive transitional cell carcinoma of the bladder. Oncogene 1998;17(9):1167–1172.

28. Knowles MA, Habuchi T, Kennedy W, Cuthbert-Heavens D. Mutation spectrum of the 9q34 tuberous sclerosis gene TSC1 in transitional cell carcinoma of the bladder. Cancer Res 2003;63(22):7652–7656.

29. Hornigold N, Devlin J, Davies AM, Aveyard JS, Habuchi T, Knowles MA. Mutation of the 9q34 gene TSC1 in sporadic bladder cancer. Oncogene 1999;18(16):2657–2661.

30. Adachi H, Igawa M, Shiina H, Urakami S, Shigeno K, Hino O. Human bladder tumors with 2-hit mutations of tumor suppressor gene TSC1 and decreased expression of p27. J Urol 2003;170(2 Pt 1):601–604.

31. Habuchi T, Takahashi T, Kakinuma H, et al. Hypermethylation at 9q32–33 tumor suppressor region is age-related in normal urothelium and an early and frequent alteration in bladder cancer. Oncogene 2001;20(4):531–537.

32. Habuchi T, Yoshida O, Knowles MA. A novel candidate tumor suppressor locus at 9q32–33 in bladder cancer: localisation of the candidate region within a single 840kb YAC. Hum Mol Genet 1997;6:913–919.

33. Brewster SF, Gingell JC, Browne S, Brown KW. Loss of heterozygosity on chromosome 18q is associated with muscle-invasive transitional cell carcinoma of the bladder. Br J Cancer 1994;70:697–700.

34. Malumbres M, Barbacid M. RAS oncogenes: the first 30 years. Nat Rev Cancer 2003;3(6):459–465.

35. Theodorescu D, Cornil I, Fernandez BJ, Kerbel RS. Overexpression of normal and mutated forms of HRAS induces orthotopic bladder invasion in a human transitional cell carcinoma. Proc Natl Acad Sci USA 1990;87(22):9047–9051.

36. Theodorescu D, Cornil I, Sheehan C, Man MS, Kerbel RS. Ha-ras induction of the invasive phenotype results in up-regulation of epidermal growth factor receptors and altered responsiveness to epidermal growth factor in human papillary transitional cell carcinoma cells. Cancer Res 1991;51:4486–4491.

37. Zhang ZT, Pak J, Huang HY, et al. Role of Ha-ras activation in superficial papillary pathway of urothelial tumor formation. Oncogene 2001;20(16):1973–1980.

38. Lipponen P. Expression of c-erbB-2 oncoprotein in transitional cell bladder cancer. Eur J Cancer 1993;29A(5):749–753.

39. Gardiner RA, Samaratunga ML, Walsh MD, Seymour GJ, Lavin MF. An immunohistological demonstration of c-erbB-2 oncoprotein expression in primary urothelial bladder cancer. Urol Res 1992;20(2):117–120.

40. Neal DE, Sharples L, Smith K, Fennelly J, Hall RR, Harris AL. The epidermal growth factor receptor and the prognosis of bladder cancer. Cancer 1990;65(7):1619–1625.

41. Tuna B, Yorukoglu K, Tuzel E, Guray M, Mungan U, Kirkali Z. Expression of p53 and mdm2 and their significance in recurrence of superficial bladder cancer. Pathol Res Pract 2003;199(5):323–328.

42. Schmitz-Drager BJ, Kushima M, Goebell P, et al. p53 and MDM2 in the development and progression of bladder cancer. Eur Urol 1997;32(4):487–493.

43. Pfister C, Moore L, Allard P, et al. Predictive value of cell cycle markers p53, MDM2, p21, and Ki-67 in superficial bladder tumor recurrence. Clin Cancer Res 1999;5(12):4079–4084.

44. Richter J, Jiang F, Gorog JP, et al. Marked genetic differences between stage pTa and stage pT1 papillary bladder cancer detected by comparative genomic hybridization. Cancer Res 1997;57(14):2860–2864.

45. Lee CC, Yamamoto S, Morimura K, et al. Significance of cyclin D1 overexpression in transitional cell carcinomas of the urinary bladder and its correlation with histopathologic features. Cancer 1997;79(4):780–789.

46. Suwa Y, Takano Y, Iki M, et al. Cyclin D1 protein overexpression is related to tumor differentiation, but not to tumor progression or proliferative activity, in transitional cell carcinoma of the bladder. J Urol 1998;160(3 Pt 1):897–900.

47. Wagner U, Suess K, Luginbuhl T, et al. Cyclin D1 overexpression lacks prognostic significance in superficial urinary bladder cancer. J Pathol 1999;188(1):44–50.

48. Shiina H, Igawa M, Shigeno K, et al. Beta-catenin mutations correlate with over expression of c-myc and cyclin D1 genes in bladder cancer. J Urol 2002;168(5):2220–2226.

49. Sauter G, Carroll P, Moch H, et al. c-myc copy number gains in bladder cancer detected by fluorescence in situ hybridization. Am J Pathol 1995;146(5):1131–1139.

50. Bruch J, Wohr G, Hautmann R, et al. Chromosomal changes during progression of transitional cell carcinoma of the bladder and delineation of the amplified interval on chromosome arm 8q. Genes Chromosomes Cancer 1998;23(2):167–174.

51. Masters JR, Vesey SG, Munn CF, Evan GI, Watson JV. c-myc oncoprotein levels in bladder cancer. Urol Res 1988;16(5):341–344.

52. Schmitz-Drager BJ, Schulz WA, Jurgens B, et al. c-myc in bladder cancer. Clinical findings and analysis of mechanism. Urol Res 1997;25(Suppl 1):S45–S49.

53. Billerey C, Chopin D, Aubriot-Lorton MH, et al. Frequent FGFR3 mutations in papillary non-invasive bladder (pTa) tumors. Am J Pathol 2001;158(6):1955–1959.

54. Sibley K, Stern P, Knowles MA. Frequency of fibroblast growth factor receptor 3 mutations in sporadic tumors. Oncogene 2001;20(32):4416–4418.

55. van Rhijn BW, Lurkin I, Radvanyi F, Kirkels WJ, van der Kwast TH, Zwarthoff EC. The fibroblast growth factor receptor 3 (FGFR3) mutation is a strong indicator of superficial bladder cancer with low recurrence rate. Cancer Res 2001;61(4):1265–1268.

56. Elder PA, Bell SM, Knowles MA. Deletion of two regions on chromosome 4 in bladder carcinoma: definition of a critical 750kB region at 4p16.3. Oncogene 1994;9(12):3433–3436.

57. van Rhijn BW, Montironi R, Zwarthoff EC, Jobsis AC, van der Kwast TH. Frequent FGFR3 mutations in urothelial papilloma. J Pathol 2002;198(2):245–251.

58. van Rhijn BW, van der Kwast TH, Vis AN, et al. FGFR3 and P53 characterize alternative genetic pathways in the pathogenesis of urothelial cell carcinoma. Cancer Res 2004;64(6):1911–1914.

59. Bakkar AA, Wallerand H, Radvanyi F, et al. FGFR3 and TP53 gene mutations define two distinct pathways in urothelial cell carcinoma of the bladder. Cancer Res 2003;63(23):8108–8112.

60. Passos-Bueno MR, Wilcox WR, Jabs EW, Sertie AL, Alonso LG, Kitoh H. Clinical spectrum of fibroblast growth factor receptor mutations. Hum Mutat 1999;14(2):115–125.

61. Ornitz DM, Itoh N. Fibroblast growth factors. Genome Biol 2001;2(3):1–12.

62. Karoui M, Hofmann-Radvanyi H, Zimmermann U, et al. No evidence of somatic FGFR3 mutation in various types of carcinoma. Oncogene 2001;20(36):5059–5061.

63. van Rhijn BW, Vis AN, van der Kwast TH, et al. Molecular grading of urothelial cell carcinoma with fibroblast growth factor receptor 3 and MIB-1 is superior to pathologic grade for the prediction of clinical outcome. J Clin Oncol 2003;21(10):1912–1921.

64. Rieger-Christ KM, Mourtzinos A, Lee PJ, et al. Identification of fibroblast growth factor receptor 3 mutations in urine sediment DNA samples complements cytology in bladder tumor detection. Cancer 2003;98(4):737–744.

65. van Rhijn BW, Lurkin I, Chopin DK, et al. Combined microsatellite and FGFR3 mutation analysis enables a highly sensitive detection of urothelial cell carcinoma in voided urine. Clin Cancer Res 2003;9(1):257–263.

66. Tsai YC, Nichols PW, Hiti AL, Williams Z, Skinner DG, Jones PA. Allelic losses of chromosomes 9, 11, and 17 in human bladder cancer. Cancer Res 1990;50:44–47.

67. Cairns P, Shaw ME, Knowles MA. Preliminary mapping of the deleted region of chromosome 9 in bladder cancer. Cancer Res 1993;53:1230–1232.

68. Cairns P, Shaw ME, Knowles MA. Initiation of bladder cancer may involve deletion of a tumor-suppressor gene on chromosome 9. Oncogene 1993;8:1083–1085.

69. Ruppert JM, Tokino K, Sidransky D. Evidence for two bladder cancer suppressor loci on human chromosome 9. Cancer Res 1993;53:5093–5095.

70. Keen AJ, Knowles MA. Definition of two regions of deletion on chromosome 9 in carcinoma of the bladder. Oncogene 1994;9(7):2083–2088.

71. Hartmann A, Moser K, Kriegmair M, Hofstetter A, Hofstaedter F, Knuechel R. Frequent genetic alterations in simple urothelial hyperplasias of the bladder in patients with papillary urothelial carcinoma. Am J Pathol 1999;154(3):721–727.

72. Habuchi T, Luscombe M, Elder PA, Knowles MA. Structure and methylation-based silencing of a gene (DBCCR1) within a candidate bladder cancer tumor suppressor region at 9q32–q33. Genomics 1998;48(3):277–288.

73. Czerniak B, Chaturvedi V, Li L, et al. Superimposed histologic and genetic mapping of chromosome 9 in progression of human urinary bladder neoplasia: implications for a genetic model of multistep urothelial carcinogenesis and early detection of urinary bladder cancer. Oncogene 1999;18(5):1185–1196.

74. Simoneau M, Aboulkassim TO, LaRue H, Rousseau F, Fradet Y. Four tumor suppressor loci on chromosome 9q in bladder cancer: evidence for two novel candidate regions at 9q22.3 and 9q31. Oncogene 1999;18(1):157–163.

75. Wada T, Berggren P, Steineck G, et al. Bladder neoplasms—regions at chromosome 9 with putative tumor suppressor genes. Scand J Urol Nephrol 2003;37(2):106–111.

76. Cairns P, Mao L, Merlo A, et al. Rates of p16 (MTS1) mutations in primary tumors with 9p loss. Science 1994;265(5170):415–417.

77. Devlin J, Keen AJ, Knowles MA. Homozygous deletion mapping at 9p21 in bladder carcinoma defines a critical region within 2cM of IFNA. Oncogene 1994;9:2757–2760.

78. Berggren P, Kumar R, Sakano S, et al. Detecting homozygous deletions in the CDKN2A(p16(INK4a))/ARF(p14(ARF)) gene in urinary bladder cancer using real-time quantitative PCR. Clin Cancer Res 2003;9(1):235–242.

79. Nishiyama H, Takahashi T, Kakehi Y, Habuchi T, Knowles MA. Homozygous deletion at the 9q32–33 candidate tumor suppressor locus in primary human bladder cancer. Genes Chromosomes Cancer 1999;26(2):171–175.

80. Stadler WM, Steinberg G, Yang X, Hagos F, Turner C, Olopade OI. Alterations of the 9p21 and 9q33 chromosomal bands in clinical bladder cancer specimens by fluorescence in situ hybridization. Clin Cancer Res 2001;7(6):1676–1682.

81. Chang LL, Yeh WT, Yang SY, Wu WJ, Huang CH. Genetic alterations of p16INK4a and p14ARF genes in human bladder cancer. J Urol 2003;170(2 Pt 1):595–600.

82. Florl AR, Franke KH, Niederacher D, Gerharz CD, Seifert HH, Schulz WA. DNA methylation and the mechanisms of CDKN2A inactivation in transitional cell carcinoma of the urinary bladder. Lab Invest 2000;80(10):1513–1522.

83. Orlow I, LaRue H, Osman I, et al. Deletions of the INK4A gene in superficial bladder tumors. Association with recurrence. Am J Pathol 1999;155(1):105–113.

84. Serrano M. The INK4a/ARF locus in murine tumorigenesis. Carcinogenesis 2000;21(5):865–869.

85. Carnero A, Hudson JD, Price CM, Beach DH. p16INK4A and p19ARF act in overlapping pathways in cellular immortalization. Nat Cell Biol 2000;2(3):148–155.

86. Wright KO, Messing EM, Reeder JE. DBCCR1 mediates death in cultured bladder tumor cells. Oncogene 2004;23(1):82–90.

87. Nishiyama H, Gill JH, Pitt E, Kennedy W, Knowles MA. Negative regulation of G1/S transition by the candidate bladder tumor suppressor gene DBCCR1. Oncogene 2001;20:2956–2964.

88. Manning BD, Cantley LC. United at last: the tuberous sclerosis complex gene products connect the phosphoinositide 3-kinase/Akt pathway to mammalian target of rapamycin (mTOR) signalling. Biochem Soc Trans 2003;31(Pt 3):573–578.

89. Kagan J, Liu J, Stein JD, et al. Cluster of allele losses within a 2.5 cM region of chromosome 10 in high-grade invasive bladder cancer. Oncogene 1998;16(7):909–913.

90. Cappellen D, Gil Diez de Medina S, Chopin D, Thiery JP, Radvanyi F. Frequent loss of heterozygosity on chromosome 10q in muscle-invasive transitional cell carcinomas of the bladder. Oncogene 1997;14(25):3059–3066.

91. Yamada KM, Araki M. Tumor suppressor PTEN: modulator of cell signaling, growth, migration and apoptosis. J Cell Sci 2001;114(Pt 13):2375–2382.

92. Liu J, Babaian DC, Liebert M, Steck PA, Kagan J. Inactivation of MMAC1 in bladder transitional-cell carcinoma cell lines and specimens. Mol Carcinog 2000;29(3):143–150.

93. Wang DS, Rieger-Christ K, Latini JM, et al. Molecular analysis of PTEN and MXI1 in primary bladder carcinoma. Int J Cancer 2000;88(4):620–625.

94. Tanaka M, Koul D, Davies MA, Liebert M, Steck PA, Grossman HB. MMAC1/PTEN inhibits cell growth and induces chemosensitivity to doxorubicin in human bladder cancer cells. Oncogene 2000;19(47):5406–5412.

95. Fujimoto K, Yamada Y, Okajima E, et al. Frequent association of p53 gene mutation in invasive bladder cancer. Cancer Res 1992;52:1393–1398.

96. Williamson MP, Elder PA, Knowles MA. The spectrum of TP53 mutations in bladder carcinoma. Genes Chromosomes Cancer 1994;9:108–118.

97. Esrig D, Spruck CH 3rd, Nichols PW, et al. p53 nuclear protein accumulation correlates with mutations in the p53 gene, tumor grade, and stage in bladder cancer. Am J Pathol 1993;143(5):1389–1397.

98. Esrig D, Elmajian D, Groshen S, et al. Accumulation of nuclear p53 and tumor progression in bladder cancer. N Engl J Med 1994;331:1259–1264.

99. Sarkis AS, Dalbagni G, Cordon-Cardo C, et al. Association of p53 nuclear overexpression and tumor progression in carcinoma in situ of the bladder. J Urol 1994;152:388–392.

100. Sarkis AS, Dalbagni G, Cordon-Cardo C, et al. Nuclear overexpression of p53 protein in transitional cell bladder carcinoma: a marker for disease progression. J Natl Cancer Inst 1993;85:53–59.

101. Sarkis AS, Zhang Z-F, Cordon-Cardo C, et al. p53 nuclear overexpression and disease progression in Ta bladder carcinoma. Int J Oncol 1993;3:355–360.

102. Xu H-J, Cairns P, Hu S-X, Knowles MA, Benedict WF. Loss of RB protein expression in primary bladder cancer correlates with loss of heterozygosity at the RB locus and tumor progression. Int J Cancer 1993;53:781–784.

103. Cordon-Cardo C, Zhang Z-F, Dalbagni G, et al. Cooperative effects of p53 and pRB alterations in primary superficial bladder tumors. Cancer Res 1997;57:1217–1221.

104. Cote RJ, Dunn MD, Chatterjee SJ, et al. Elevated and absent pRb expression is associated with bladder cancer progression and has cooperative effects with p53. Cancer Res 1998;58(6):1090–1094.

105. Grossman HB, Liebert M, Antelo M, et al. p53 and RB expression predict progression in T1 bladder cancer. Clin Cancer Res 1998;4(4):829–834.

106. Chatterjee SJ, Datar R, Youssefzadeh D, et al. Combined effects of p53, p21, and pRb expression in the progression of bladder transitional cell carcinoma. J Clin Oncol 2004;22(6):1007–1013.

107. Wood RD, Mitchell M, Sgouros J, Lindahl T. Human DNA repair genes. Science 2001;291(5507):1284–1289.

108. Breivik J, Gaudernack G. Genomic instability, DNA methylation, and natural selection in colorectal carcinogenesis. Semin Cancer Biol 1999;9(4):245–254.

109. Gonzalez-Zulueta M, Ruppert JM, Tokino K, et al. Microsatellite instability in bladder cancer. Cancer Res 1993;53:5620–5623.

110. Hartmann A, Zanardo L, Bocker-Edmonston T, et al. Frequent microsatellite instability in sporadic tumors of the upper urinary tract. Cancer Res 2002;62(23):6796–6802.

111. Hartmann A, Dietmaier W, Hofstadter F, Burgart LJ, Cheville JC, Blaszyk H. Urothelial carcinoma of the upper urinary tract: inverted growth pattern is predictive of microsatellite instability. Hum Pathol 2003;34(3):222–227.

112. Lynch HT, Smyrk T. An update on Lynch syndrome. Curr Opin Oncol 1998;10(4):349–356.

113. Ahrendt SA, Decker PA, Doffek K, et al. Microsatellite instability at selected tetranucleotide repeats is associated with p53 mutations in non-small cell lung cancer. Cancer Res 2000;60(9):2488–2491.

114. Stern MC, Umbach DM, Lunn RM, Taylor JA. DNA repair gene XRCC3 codon 241 polymorphism, its interaction with smoking and XRCC1 polymorphisms, and bladder cancer risk. Cancer Epidemiol Biomarkers Prev 2002;11(9):939–943.

115. World Health Organization. WHO Classification of Tumors of the Urinary System and Male Genital Organs. Lyons: IARC Press, 2004.

116. Zhao J, Richter J, Wagner U, et al. Chromosomal imbalances in noninvasive papillary bladder neoplasms (pTa). Cancer Res 1999;59(18):4658–4661.

117. Takahashi T, Habuchi T, Kakehi Y, et al. Clonal and chronological genetic analysis of multifocal cancers of the bladder and upper urinary tract. Cancer Res 1998;58(24):5835–5841.

118. Rosin MP, Cairns P, Epstein JI, Schoenberg MP, Sidransky D. Partial allelotype of carcinoma in situ of the human bladder. Cancer Res 1995;55:5213–5216.

119. Hanahan D, Weinberg RA. The hallmarks of cancer. Cell 2000;100(1):57–70.

# Molecular biology of bladder cancer: cell cycle alterations

10

*Ben George, Ram H Datar, Richard J Cote*

## THE NORMAL CELL CYCLE

The normal cell cycle consists of a series of highly structured and sequential events, culminating in cell growth and eventual division into two daughter cells. The cell's chromatin (chromosomal DNA and associated proteins) is the most important structure that must double in size in preparation for cell division. The active cell cycle is divided into four phases: M, G1, S, and G2; the time spent outside of M (G1, S, and G2) is referred to as interphase. The period of mitosis, termed M phase, usually takes less than an hour and is comprised of a series of events involving breakdown of the nuclear membrane, polarization of two sets of condensed chromosomes to opposite poles of the cell, reformation of two nuclear membranes around the segregated chromosomes, and the breaking off and separation of the two daughter cells. Usually, there is a period of approximately 10–12 hours after M phase during which time the recently divided cell prepares itself for S phase. This long preparation period allows the cell to synthesize a number of macromolecular constituents and increase its mass. The period after M but before S is termed the first gap period, or G1 phase of the cell cycle. The replication of genomic DNA is accomplished during a discrete window of time, termed S (synthetic) phase. S phase in mammalian cells usually takes 6–8 hours, and during this phase the entire complement of chromosomal DNA is replicated. Following successful completion of DNA synthesis and chromosomal replication in S phase, there is a long period (typically 4–5 hours) when the cell prepares itself for mitosis. This period after S phase and before M phase is the second gap phase in the cell cycle, termed G2. Under normal circumstances the process of genomic doubling is carried out with great precision and involves a complex series of checkpoints that ensure fidelity of the newly replicated genome.

The normal cell has several intrinsic checkpoints for interrupting the cell cycle in the event of cellular damage. The different checkpoints include:

- a check on completion of S phase when the cell is believed to monitor the presence of Okazaki fragments on the lagging strand during DNA replication; the cell is not permitted to proceed in the cell cycle until these have disappeared
- DNA damage checkpoints that occur before the cell enters S phase (a G1 checkpoint), during S phase itself, and after DNA replication (a G2 checkpoint)
- spindle checkpoints that act through a variety of mechanisms to: 1) detect any failure of spindle fibers to attach to kinetochores and arrest the cell in metaphase; 2) detect improper alignment of the spindle itself and block cytokinesis; and 3) trigger apoptosis if the damage is irreparable.

Alterations in the normal cell cycle can occur for numerous reasons, and they have been implicated in a variety of cancers. Disruption of the normal cell division cycle has been reported to be crucial in the development and progression of bladder cancer.[1] These disruptions can occur singly or in combination, suggesting the importance of studying the entire pathway of cell cycle regulation in order to understand the molecular mechanisms leading to bladder tumorigenesis. Furthermore, the cell cycle is not an autonomous pathway; it is guided by extraneous signals from apoptotic and signal transduction pathways. Hence, understanding alterations in the cell cycle in the context of other cellular pathways is critical in elucidating mechanisms underlying the development of bladder cancer. Figure 10.1 depicts key regulators of the cell cycle known to be altered during bladder cancer progression.

## MOLECULAR BASIS FOR THE DEVELOPMENT AND PROGRESSION OF BLADDER CANCER

Advances in molecular biology over the last decade have led to the identification of many genetic alterations in bladder cancer and a better understanding of its malignant evolution and progression. Two predominant chromosomes involved in the development and progression of bladder cancer are chromosome 9 and chromosome 17.[2] Approximately 60% to 65% of all transitional cell tumors are characterized by loss of heterozygosity (LOH) on chromosome 9. Chromosomal analysis of various stages of transitional cell carcinoma (TCC) has revealed that allelic loss only on chromosome 9 is found exclusively in early stage, well-differentiated tumors, whereas in more advanced lesions, other genetic changes are frequently observed. LOH on chromosome 9 is considered to be the earliest event in bladder tumorigenesis.[3]

Two main categories of genes are considered to be responsible for malignant transformation: oncogenes and tumor suppressor genes. The critical genetic event that transforms a proto-oncogene into an oncogene might be a mutation, overexpression, gene amplification, or insertion of viral genetic material into the human DNA. Activation of the proto-oncogene results in derangement of cell cycle control, thereby stimulating malignant transformation. Tumor suppressor genes have two alleles, and since they are recessive in function, both

must be inactivated in order to induce tumorigenesis. The proposed mechanisms for this event are via LOH and mutations in the sequence of the remaining allele. Many studies have been conducted to identify the proto-oncogenes and tumor suppressor genes contributing to the development and progression of bladder cancer. The major problems associated with localization of specific target genes in bladder cancer are the high frequency of monosomy of chromosome 9, the rarity of partial chromosome 9 losses, and the sporadic prevalence of bladder cancer with almost no familial form. In contrast to the early events involving chromosome 9,[4] loss of genetic material on chromosome 17 is considered to be a late event in the development of bladder cancer. LOH of chromosome 17, especially on the short arm, has been observed in approximately 40% of bladder tumors. These genetic events were found mainly in high-grade, high-stage tumors. These studies indicate the existence of at least two divergent pathways of bladder tumor progression; furthermore they suggest that the order in which these genetic events take place is important in determining the outcome of the lesion.

## SUPERFICIAL BLADDER CANCER

The term 'superficial bladder cancer' is used to denote pTa and pT1 bladder tumors. pTa tumors are those tumors that are confined to the epithelial layer of the bladder ('non-invasive papillary carcinoma'), whereas pT1 tumors are those that invade into subepithelial connective tissue or lamina propria.

Approximately 70% to 75% of bladder cancers are papillary at their initial clinical presentation. Of these, 70% to 75% are mucosally confined (stage Ta) and 30% are invasive of the lamina propria (stage T1). Only 2%

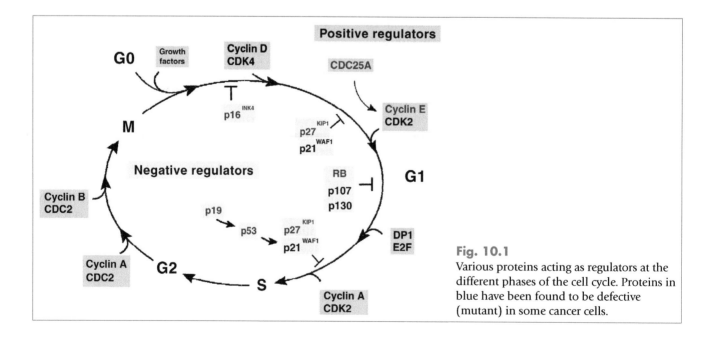

**Fig. 10.1**
Various proteins acting as regulators at the different phases of the cell cycle. Proteins in blue have been found to be defective (mutant) in some cancer cells.

to 4% of the mucosally confined tumors are likely to progress, whereas 30% to 50% of T1 tumors have the potential to progress. However, aggressive behavior is generally limited to those tumors that are high grade, that have penetrated the lamina propria extensively, and that are accompanied by flat carcinoma in situ, either adjacent to the tumor or at distant sites. The majority of bladder cancers (nearly all of those that are mucosally confined, and 50% to 70% of those that have infiltrated the lamina propria) will progress. On the other hand, 70% to 75% of all papillary tumors are likely to recur.

The proposed pathway for development of superficial bladder cancer is quite different from that of invasive bladder tumors. The sequence of events leading to the development of superficial bladder cancer includes urothelial hyperplasia, urothelial atypia, and, eventually, low-grade papillary TCC.[5] Comparative genomic hybridization studies have identified many alterations leading to the development of superficial bladder cancer[6] (Table 10.1).

Several cell cycle alterations have been implicated in the progression of superficial bladder cancer. These markers can be divided broadly into markers that predict recurrence and those that predict progression. Additional markers have been identified that might be predictive of response to treatment. These markers have been dealt with in the context of specific alterations later in the chapter.

## INVASIVE BLADDER CANCER

Most invasive bladder tumors have no known papillary precursor, are solid invasive lesions, and are commonly associated with carcinoma in situ (CIS) elsewhere in the bladder. The proposed pathway for progression of these lesions, in a sequential fashion, includes urothelial atypia, dysplasia, CIS, and, finally, invasive TCC.[5] Molecular analyses have shown that CIS contains a spectrum of genetic alterations similar to those seen in invasive TCC and very distinct from those seen in low-grade papillary TCC. A number of cell cycle alterations have been identified to be of predictive and prognostic value in invasive bladder cancer and they have been dealt with under relevant sections in the chapter.

## ALTERATIONS IN THE RETINOBLASTOMA GENE AND PROTEIN

The Rb gene product is a nuclear phosphoprotein and Rb was the first tumor suppressor gene to be identified.[7] It is localized to band q14 on chromosome 13 (13q14) and its phosphorylation plays a central role in the regulation of the cell cycle. The Rb protein (pRb) interacts with multiple cell cycle regulatory proteins that are involved at the G1/S transition.[1,8] The active nonphosphorylated form of pRb binds to and sequesters the transcription factor E2F. During late G1, pRb is phosphorylated and inactivated by the cyclin D1-CDK4/6 complex and releases E2F. Free E2F can transcribe genes such as thymidylate synthase (TS), which are required for DNA synthesis. Cyclin-dependent kinase (CDK) inhibitors such as p16, p21, and p27 inhibit CDK activity and regulate pRb phosphorylation. Many of these proteins have been well characterized by immunohistochemistry (Figure 10.2).

### Superficial bladder cancer

The role of pRb inactivation in papillary tumors has rarely been addressed. Grossman et al studied p53 accumulation along with Rb expression in 45 patients with T1 bladder cancer. Patients with abnormal expression of either or both proteins had a significant increase in tumor progression (p<0.04 and p=0.005, respectively).[9]

### Invasive bladder cancer

The most common inactivation of Rb in bladder tumors is deletion of chromosome 13q. The reported frequency of Rb inactivation in bladder cancers varies considerably between different investigations. Depending on the method used, frequencies between 14% and 80% have been reported. Miyamoyo et al examined the entire coding region of the RB gene using polymerase chain reaction–single strand conformational polymorphism (PCR–SSCP) analysis. Of 30 samples obtained from

**Table 10.1**  Genomic alterations during development of superficial bladder cancer identified by comparative genomic hybridization studies

| Tumour stage | Losses | Gains | Amplification |
|---|---|---|---|
| Ta | 9p, 9q, Y | 1q, 17 | 11q |
| T1 | 2q, 4p, 4q, 5q, 6q, 8p, 9p, 9q, 10q, 11p, 11q, 13q, 17p, 18q, Y | 1q, 3p, 3q, 5p, 6p, 8q, 10p, 17q, 20q | 1q22–24, 3p24–25, 6p22, 8p12, 8q22, 10p12–14, 10q22–23, 11q13, 12q12–21, 17q21, 20q13 |
| T2–4 | As for T1 + 15q | As for pT1 + 7p, Xq | As for pT1 |

Amended and reproduced from Knowles[6] with permission from BMJ Publishing Group.

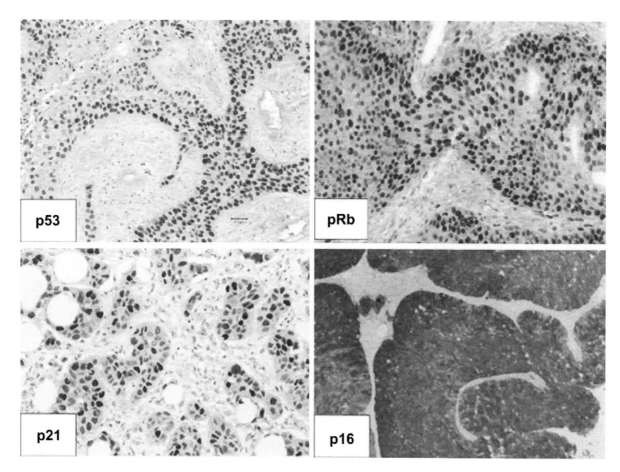

**Fig. 10.2**
Immunohistochemical expression of p53, pRb, p21, and p16 in bladder cancer.

patients with bladder cancer, eight (27%) were found to have RB gene mutations. DNA sequencing of the PCR products revealed five cases with single point mutations and three cases with small deletions. Mutations were detected in 4 (21%) of 19 superficial (pTa and pT1) tumors and 4 (36%) of 11 invasive (pT2 or greater) tumors. These results suggest that RB gene mutations are involved in low-grade and superficial bladder cancers as well as in high-grade and invasive cancers.[10] Acikbas et al have suggested that detection of LOH of the RB1 gene by polymerase chain reaction–restriction fragment length polymorphism (PCR–RFLP) can be a good adjunctive test for evaluation of the bladder cancer.[11]

Loss of expression of Rb tumor suppressor protein has been shown to be important in bladder cancer progression.[12-14] Rb alterations have been thought to take place only at the gene level, resulting in loss of protein expression. However, we have demonstrated that a significant proportion of tumors expressing Rb show clinical consequences of loss of pRb function. Patients with tumors expressing high levels of pRb have clinical outcomes virtually identical to those with no detectable pRb. These patients have significantly lower recurrence-free survival and overall survival rates than patients with tumors expressing moderate levels of pRb.[14]

Furthermore, we have elucidated the biologic basis for constitutive alteration of RB function in human tumors in the presence of an intact, expressed pRb protein; the mechanism of RB inactivation is through hyperphosphorylation which results from loss of p16 expression and/or cyclin D1 overexpression.[15] The high levels of expression of pRb in these tumors were associated with a loss of p16 expression. Thus, elevated pRb expression is associated with pRb hyperphosphorylation, which in turn is associated with loss of p16 expression and/or increased cyclin D1 expression.

## P53 ALTERATIONS

The protein encoded by the p53 tumor suppressor gene, located on chromosome 17p13.1, is a 393 amino acid, 53 kDa nuclear phosphoprotein.[16] The p53 gene (genotype) and protein (phenotype) play a critical role in regulation of the normal cell cycle and apoptotic response. In accordance with the important role of p53 in bladder carcinogenesis, the majority of TCCs display a loss of one allele of 17p. This phenomenon has been described as loss of heterozygosity and is an important mechanism by which tumor suppressor genes can be inactivated. After the initial loss of the first allele, the remaining allele (and thus entire tumor suppressor function) becomes inactivated by mutation. At the cellular level, this functional inactivation can be assessed by nuclear accumulation as seen by immunohistochemistry (see Figure 10.2).

## Superficial bladder cancer

Several trials have addressed the impact of immunohistochemical p53 accumulation in predicting tumor recurrence in patients with papillary bladder cancer. While some of the smaller trials have shown a correlation between p53 accumulation and tumor recurrence by univariate analysis, none of these studies reported p53 accumulation to provide additional information compared to clinical parameters.

The predictive value of alterations of the p53 tumor suppressor gene as a marker of disease progression in papillary bladder cancer has been the subject of many studies. Information from multivariate analysis is available in 16 such studies. In half of these studies, additional prognostic value for p53 protein expression was observed when compared with clinicopathologic parameters; in the remaining eight studies no significant differences were reported. Although the sample size in the positive trials tended to be slightly larger than in the negative studies, the actual question still remains open.

## Invasive bladder cancer

Alterations in the p53 protein, leading to a loss of its tumor suppressor function, have been reported previously by us and by others.[17] The p53 protein plays a key role in mediating growth arrest and repairing DNA damage at the G1/S transition.[18] In response to DNA damage, p53 protein expression is upregulated, which in turn upregulates its downstream target p21Waf1, a CDK inhibitor (CDKI), thereby arresting cell-cycle progression.[19] Once the DNA damage is repaired, accumulated p53 protein levels are abrogated by mdm2, an upstream regulator of p53 expression.[20] Alternatively, in cells where an effective cell-cycle arrest cannot be mediated in response to DNA damage, the p53 protein has been shown to initiate and execute an apoptotic response.[21] The tumor suppressor function of the p53 protein occurs at the G1/S transition as well as the G2/M checkpoint, thereby making it a guardian of the cell cycle.

The wild-type p53 protein (wt p53) has a short half-life of less than 30 minutes. Hence, nuclear accumulation of p53 protein as detected by immunostaining has been hypothesized to correlate with a loss of p53 function. Furthermore, nuclear accumulation of p53 protein has been correlated with a poor clinical outcome in invasive bladder cancer.[17,22,23] Many studies in bladder cancer have concluded that p53 immunohistochemistry (IHC) can provide independent prognostic information, whereas others have failed to

show this relationship as independent from known prognostic factors. Some studies have even failed to find any prognostic value for p53 IHC, regardless of whether or not it is independent. A literature-based meta-analysis on the association of immunohistochemical p53 accumulation and prognosis reports conflicting results.[24] While a correlation between tumor grade and p53 immunostaining was obvious, a correlation between p53 and disease outcome varied greatly between studies on superficial bladder cancer and muscle-invasive tumors. In addition, trials differ considerably with regard to the correlation between p53 staining and progression, as recently reported.[25] There are several inherent problems in comparing these studies. Tissue preparation (frozen or formalin-fixed, paraffin-embedded), antigen-retrieval methods (boiling or microwaving), the type of p53 antibody used (different monoclonal and polyclonal antibodies from various sources), and assessment of p53 positivity (thresholds from 0% to 40% of stained nuclei defined as positive) vary between these studies.[26] The use of standardized thresholds, and clear definitions of 'progression' and 'recurrence' with standard Kaplan–Meier/log-rank and multivariate analysis would make comparison between the conclusions of these studies more meaningful. Furthermore, these studies differ in the stage-wise distribution of patients in the study cohort as well as treatment received.

Mutations in the p53 gene have been thought to be responsible for the nuclear accumulation of p53 (altered p53 phenotype). However, there are reports to suggest that this is not always the case.[27] The absence of nuclear accumulation (wild-type p53 phenotype) of p53 protein, however, does not rule out p53 gene alterations. In fact, nonsense mutations may produce unstable transcripts or truncated proteins that lack the nuclear localization signal, thereby giving negative results on immunostaining. These events have been reported to contribute to approximately 20% of the p53 gene mutations detected in particular tumor types.

Previous reports indicate that not all cases with a nuclear accumulation of p53 have a loss of function of p53 and conversely not all cases with a wild-type phenotype have intact p53 function. Both these findings support the existence of a p53 phenotype which, in a substantial minority of patients, is not completely predictive of p53 function. One of the major reasons for this finding could be the discordance between the p53 phenotype and corresponding genotype. Although previous studies have investigated the relationship between p53 phenotype and genotype in bladder TCC, these studies were limited by either small cohort size and/or lack of specificity of the technology used to investigate mutations in the p53 gene.

We have extensively investigated the p53 phenotype in archival paraffin-embedded tissue specimens by IHC. In the same tissue specimens, we have examined the complete p53 gene (exons 2–11; exon 1 is situated 25 kb upstream of exon 2 and does not contribute to p53 function) for mutations and polymorphisms by multiexon amplification using the Roche Affymetrix p53 gene chip. Thus, we assessed the concordance between p53 phenotype and genotype in a cohort of 160 invasive bladder tumors. We have also evaluated the functional status of p53 in these cases by studying the expression of p21, a downstream target of p53. Furthermore, we have sought to identify specific exonic mutations that have an impact on the p53 phenotype and function. We have observed that while there is significant concordance between the p53 phenotype and genotype, there are a substantial number of discordant cases. Our findings also suggest a role for specific exonic mutations in determining the p53 phenotype and p53 function (unpublished data). The results of our study underscore the significance of determining both p53 genotype and phenotype in predicting clinical outcomes in bladder cancer. Most importantly, we show that examining the p53 genotype along with p53 phenotype renders crucial insight related to the functional status of the p53 protein in addition to providing vital predictive and prognostic information in patients with invasive bladder cancer.

## CDKN2A ALTERATIONS

The CDKN2A locus encodes two proteins, p16$^{INK4a}$ and p19$^{ARF}$ (alternative reading frame), both of which inhibit the cell cycle.[28] These proteins are encoded by two overlapping open reading frames in such a way that p19$^{ARF}$ is entirely distinct from p16$^{INK4a}$. The dual coding capacity of the CDKN2A locus is conserved from mice to humans; the mouse homolog is termed p19$^{ARF}$ while the human homolog is designated as p14$^{ARF}$. The p14$^{ARF}$ protein does not directly bind and inhibit CDKs but appears to function upstream of p53.[29] This arrangement facilitates coordinated regulation of two key cell cycle regulatory pathways, namely the RB and p53 pathways from a single locus.[28] The p16$^{INK4a}$ is a tumor suppressor gene; it acts as a CDK inhibitor and prevents phosphorylation of pRb during cell cycle progression.[30] Reports indicate that p14$^{ARF}$ protein is not only a cell cycle inhibitor but also a tumor suppressor, because mice with disrupted p19ARF expression but intact p16INK4a expression have a susceptibility to develop tumors.[31] Homozygous deletions of the CDKN2A locus in sporadic tumors have been shown to eliminate expression of both p16$^{INK4a}$ and p19$^{ARF}$.[32] However, there is evidence to show that point mutations within shared coding sequences can impair the function of the p16$^{INK4a}$ protein while leaving the activity of p14$^{ARF}$ intact.[33] Alterations in p16INK4a and p14ARF at both the gene and the protein level have elicited great interest because of their key cell cycle regulatory functions, and have been extensively investigated in bladder cancer.

## Superficial bladder cancer

Deletions and methylation of the INK4A gene occur frequently in superficial bladder tumors. Inactivation of the p16 gene through homozygous deletion appears to be a contributing factor for the development and progression of urothelial cancers, whereas point mutations appear to be an uncommon mechanism in inactivating this gene.[34] In most of these studies, however, patient numbers were small, and multivariate analysis was lacking. Orlow et al showed that homozygous deletion of the INK4A gene correlated with a lower recurrence-free survival (p=0.040). Although deletions and methylation of the INK4A gene occur frequently in superficial bladder tumors, only those deletions that affected both p16 and p14$^{ARF}$ correlated with clinicopathologic parameters of worse prognosis.[32]

## Invasive bladder cancer

Alterations of the CDKN2A locus on chromosome 9p21 were investigated by Florl et al in order to elucidate the mechanisms of inactivation of this locus in invasive bladder cancer.[35] In a study of 86 TCCs, 34 tumors (39%) had LOH, and, of those, 17 tumors (20%) carried homozygous deletions of at least one CDKN2A exon and flanking microsatellites. Only three specimens, each with LOH across 9p21, had hypermethylation of the CDKN2A exon 1$\alpha$ CpG-island in the remaining allele. Thus, DNA hypermethylation may be rare in TCC and deletions appear to be the most important mechanism for inactivation of the CDKN2A locus. Berggren et al designed a real-time quantitative PCR (QPCR) application to study homozygous deletion of CDKN2A/ARF (9p21) in 186 urinary bladder cancer patients.[36] No association was established between occurrence of genetic aberrations at 9p21 and tumor stage or grade. Their data support the notion that inactivation, including homozygous deletions of CDKN2A/ARF, is an early event in TCC.

A report from Chang et al indicates that p14ARF is a primary target of homozygous deletion, whereas p16INK4a is the hot spot of hypermethylation on the 9p21 region in bladder cancer.[37] Homozygous deletion of p16INK4a and p14ARF genes was observed in 23% (12 of 53 samples) and 43% (23 of 53 samples), respectively. Most deletions occurred exclusively on the E1$\beta$-p14ARF region, while concomitant deletion of p16INK4a and p14ARF genes was found in only two samples. Aberrant methylation of the p16INK4a gene was found in 60% of tumors. However, no p14ARF gene methylation was detected in any case.

In a study performed on 27 bladder carcinomas, p14ARF showed a higher rate of hypermethylation than p16INK4a as detected by methylation-specific PCR (MS-PCR).[38] Further, p16INK4a and p14ARF aberrant methylation was significantly correlated with poor prognosis and clinicopathologic parameters among three tumor types. Thus, both p16INKa and p14ARF hypermethylation may be involved in bladder carcinogenesis.[38] Recent reports indicate that p14ARF promoter hypermethylation in plasma DNA may be an indicator of disease recurrence in bladder cancer patients. Plasma p14ARF promoter hypermethylation was associated with the presence of multicentric foci, larger tumors, relapse of the disease, and disease recurrence.[39] Thus, p14ARF aberrant promoter methylation could be involved in bladder carcinogenesis, and plasma DNA might be a useful prognostic marker in urinary bladder cancer.

In an effort to determine the utility of genetic detection of bladder cancer by p16[INK4a] microsatellite analysis, Sourvinos et al analyzed a series of 28 cytologic urine specimens from bladder cancer patients; DNA from tumor specimens was also available for 15 of these patients. Allelic losses were found in 18 patients (64%) for the p16 locus, while no microsatellite alterations were found in the normal group without evidence of bladder cancer. In 11 cases, genetic alterations in the cytologic urine specimens were not detectable in the corresponding tumor specimen, suggesting heterogeneity of bladder cancer.[40] The detection of LOH in cytologic urine specimens may be a potentially useful tool for detection and prognostication of bladder cancer.

## ALTERATIONS IN CYCLINS AND CDKS

Transition through G1 to S phase is regulated by cyclin-dependent kinases (CDKs) which, when bound to a cyclin molecule, are activated by CDK-activating kinase.[41] This active CDK/cyclin complex then acts to phosphorylate the tumor suppressor retinoblastoma protein (pRb), which releases bound transcription factors such as the E2F family. The net result is transcription of genes encoding proteins necessary for progression through S phase.[42] The ability of CDK/cyclin to drive the cell cycle forward can be blocked by members of the CIP (p21, p27, p57) or KIP (p15, p16, p18, p19) families of protein inhibitors.[43]

Cyclin D1 is the major cyclin involved in transition from G1/S phase; cyclin D1 is thought to act primarily as a regulatory subunit of CDKs such as CDK4 and CDK6.[44] The cyclin D1 gene (CCND1) is located on chromosome 11q13, and both gene activation (due to amplification or chromosomal rearrangement) and/or protein overexpression of cyclin D1 have been described in a variety of tumor types.[45–48] A splice donor site polymorphism in exon 4 of CCND1 has been described.[49] This adenine/guanine polymorphism at nt870 (A870G) is associated with splice variants coding for two mRNA transcripts: transcript 'a' and transcript 'b'. The A allele is associated with transcript 'b', while the G allele is associated with both transcript 'a' and transcript 'b'.[50] Cells overexpressing transcript 'a' promote entry into the cell cycle, whereas transcript 'b'-expressing cells

are associated with cell-cycle exit. However, high levels of transcript 'a' expression caused inhibition of entry to and completion of the S phase.

In a study conducted to explore the association between the CCND1 exon 4 polymorphism and increased risk for development of TCC of the bladder, the mRNA splicing pattern in TCC cells was evaluated by semiquantitative reverse-transcription PCR. The CCND1 variant 'A' allele was found to be associated with an increased risk of TCC of the bladder, especially in men without a history of smoking.[51] However, no association between the A/A genotype and risk was observed in a population-based case control study conducted by Cortessis et al.[52] The null association was not appreciably modified by bladder cancer risk factors, including lifetime smoking history, or by histopathologic classification.

Although cyclin D1 protein is frequently overexpressed in tumors without CCND1 gene amplification, the mechanism for this is not well defined. Cyclin D1 overexpression has been reported to play an important role in the early stages of urothelial tumorigenesis, driving cell proliferation; however, ectopic expression of cyclin D2 or amplification of CDK4 does not occur at a significant frequency in urothelial carcinomas.[53] In patients with papillary superficial bladder cancer, cyclin D1 protein expression was reported to be an independent predictor of recurrence in a multivariate analysis that also included p27Kip1 expression and tumor stage. The simultaneous presence of low cyclin D1, low p27Kip1, and high Ki67 expression defined a 'high-risk' group of patients who displayed a significantly increased risk of recurrence.[54]

Takagi et al have reported that immunohistochemical detection of cyclin D1 protein expression could be used as an inverse indicator for the level of invasiveness of bladder cancer, but not as an independent prognostic factor. In their study set, which comprised 102 bladder cancer patients, all pTa tumors stained positively for cyclin D1, whereas the positive staining rates of invasive tumors were 47% in pT1, 73% in pT2, 31% in pT3, and 0% in pT4 tumors.[55] Although univariate analysis revealed that patients with positive cyclin D1 expression had more favorable survival rates than those with loss of expression, multivariate analysis showed that cyclin D1 expression was not an independent prognostic factor.

The cyclin E gene (CCNE), coding for a regulatory subunit of CDK2, has been mapped to 19q13. Richter et al investigated the role of cyclin E alterations in bladder cancer, using a high-throughput tissue microarray of 2317 specimens from 1842 bladder cancer patients. CCNE amplification was analyzed by fluorescence in situ hybridization and by immunohistochemistry for cyclin E protein overexpression. The frequency of protein expression increased from stage pTa to pT1 but decreased for stage pT2–4. Low cyclin E expression was associated with poor overall survival in all patients but had no prognostic impact independent of stage.[56] Makiyama et al have reported that cyclin E protein expression may be associated with aggressive tumor growth and may have a relationship with p27Kip1 for the regulation of cell-cycle progression in transitional cell-bladder carcinoma.[57]

CDK4, CDK6, and cyclin D1 are the predominant phosphorylators of the retinoblastoma protein at the G1/S transition. CDK4 gene amplification has been reported in bladder cancer. The frequency of amplification has been observed to increase with stage (pTa to pT1–4) and grade (low grade to high grade).[58]

## ALTERATIONS IN CDKIS

p21Waf1 is a downstream effector of p53 and belongs to the Cip1/Kip1 family of cyclin-dependent kinase inhibitors (CDKIs). Thus, it is a potential tumor-suppressor gene and most likely plays an important role in tumor development. Moreover, reduced expression of p21Waf1 has been reported to have prognostic value in several human malignancies. Loss of p21 expression is thought to be a mechanism by which p53 alterations may influence tumor progression. However, it has been demonstrated that p21 expression may be mediated through p53 independent pathways.[59] This indicates that p21 expression can be maintained despite p53 alterations. p53-altered tumors that were p21-negative demonstrated a significantly increased probability of recurrence and significantly lowered probability of overall survival than in patients that maintained expression of p21.[60] The association between p21 status and prognosis in p53-altered bladder tumors was independent of tumor grade, pathologic stage, and lymph node status. The strongest association between p21 status and tumor progression was demonstrated in patients with organ-confined (Pis, P1, P2, P3A) and extravesical disease (P3B, P4) with no evidence of lymph node metastases. Loss of p21 expression was strongly associated with an increased probability of recurrence and decreased probability of survival in patients with lymph-node-negative organ-confined and lymph-node-negative extravesical disease. In fact, p21 was the only independent predictor of disease progression in p53-altered bladder tumors in a multivariate analysis of p21 status, histologic grade, and pathologic stage. Maintenance of p21 expression appeared to abrogate the deleterious effects of p53 alterations on bladder cancer progression.

Chen et al have reported that polymorphism of p21 codon 31 is associated with development of bladder cancer.[61] Lancombe et al found WAF1 mutations in 2 of 27 primary bladder tumors and concluded that p21/WAF1 gene aberrations are infrequent in bladder cancer.[62]

p27Kip1 is a member of the Cip1/Kip1 family of CDKIs and is a potential tumor-suppressor gene. A significant correlation has been reported between low expression of p27Kip1 and decreased disease-free survival and overall survival. Furthermore, on multivariate analysis, low p27Kip1 protein expression was an independent predictor of reduced disease-free survival second only to tumor stage.[63] Low p27 expression is more common in poorly differentiated muscle-invasive TCCs and is a major player in cell-cycle control in these neoplasms.[64] Loss of expression of p27Kip1 protein has been reported to be associated with the subsequent development of invasive disease; this predictive value was enhanced significantly when combined with overexpression of caspase 3 protein.[65]

## MDM2 ALTERATIONS

The Mdm2 gene is located on chromosome 12q14.3–q15. It is involved in an autoregulatory feedback loop with p53.[66] An increase in the level of p53 leads to transactivation of the Mdm2 promoter, thereby upregulating the expression of Mdm2. Mdm2 in turn binds p53 and transports it to the proteasome for polyubiquitination and subsequent degradation; Mdm2 levels are reduced when p53 levels are lowered. Mdm2 gene amplification has been reported in bladder cancer. The frequency of this amplification increased with stage (pTa to pT1–4) and grade (low grade to high grade).[58] Lianes et al reported a >20% nuclear staining with MDM2 IHC in 30% of 87 bladder tumors (66/87 were T2–4) and found an association with low grade and stage.[67] MDM2 overexpression was also associated with positive p53 nuclear reactivity in 16 tumors in this study. In contrast, there was no correlation between p53 positivity and MDM2 expression in 25 tumors studied by Barbareschi et al.[68] They proposed that a combined MDM2/p53 evaluation might be of prognostic relevance.[68] Multivariate analysis in a set of 21 patients with pT1 disease that had subsequently progressed and 17 patients with pT1 disease that had remained progression-free, showed that both p53 and MDM2 IHC were independent predictors of a reduced progression-free interval.[69] Novel forms of MDM2 with alternatively spliced transcripts have been reported in bladder cancer, and these appear to be more common in muscle-invasive disease.[70] The biologic importance of these alternate forms and their relationship to MDM2 IHC remains to be established. Evaluation of the expression of MDM2 in bladder cancer is likely to be important, and its simultaneous use with p53 IHC for the prediction of prognosis in bladder cancer needs to be pursued further.

## COMBINED ANALYSIS OF MARKERS

Alterations in single cell cycle proteins have limited predictive and prognostic value in bladder cancer. A number of studies have attempted to evaluate the utility of combining data pertaining to alterations in multiple cell cycle regulatory proteins in order to improve the predictive value of such markers in bladder cancer.

Cote et al have demonstrated that alteration in both p53 and pRb may act in cooperative or synergistic ways to promote bladder tumor progression.[14] The combination of p53 and p21 status may provide additional clinical outcome information that is superior to that obtained from a single determinant.[60] However, in a series of 173 patients treated with cystectomy for advanced bladder cancer, Jahnson et al have shown that altered expression for pRb and/or p53 was not correlated with cancer-specific death and hence could not be used as a predictor of treatment outcome after cystectomy.[71]

Loss of expression of p27Kip1 protein has been reported to be associated with the subsequent development of invasive disease; this predictive value was enhanced significantly when combined with overexpression of caspase 3 protein.[65] Low p27 expression is more common in poorly differentiated muscle-invasive TCCs, and is a major player in cell cycle control in these neoplasms. Further, in a multivariate analysis, Ki67/p27 status had the strongest bearing on the overall survival of muscle-invasive TCCs.[64]

Altered expressions of p53, p21, and Rb are independent predictors of bladder cancer progression when examined as individual determinants.[14,15,60] Chatterjee et al have reported that alterations in p53, p21, and Rb act in cooperative or synergistic ways to promote tumor progression in bladder cancer. To examine these determinants in combination, patients were categorized into four groups: group I (no alteration in any marker, 47 patients), group II (alteration in any one marker, 51 patients), group III (alteration in any two markers, 42 patients), and group IV (alteration in all three markers, 24 patients). The 5-year recurrence rates in these groups were 23%, 31%, 60%, and 93%, respectively; 5-year survival rates were 68%, 56%, 28%, and 8%, respectively.[72] Shariat et al evaluated the expression of p53, p21, and pRb/p16 and found that the incremental number of altered markers was independently associated with an increased risk of bladder cancer progression and mortality.[73] These reports suggest that examining markers in combination provides additional information beyond that resulting from the use of a single determinant alone.

## CELL CYCLE ALTERATIONS AND RESPONSE TO CHEMOTHERAPY

A wealth of information is available regarding the molecular pathogenesis, predictors of progression, response to therapy, and clinical outcome in TCC of the bladder. Retrospective studies have demonstrated the importance of cell cycle regulatory proteins in the development and progression of bladder TCC; some of these proteins also have a role in predicting response to therapy in bladder cancer. Numerous studies have been performed to identify molecular markers which are reliable predictors of chemoresponse in bladder cancer. An international randomized p53-targeted therapy trial, led by investigators at the USC Keck School of Medicine, Baylor College of Medicine, and the University of Chicago, is currently underway to study the effects of three cycles of adjuvant MVAC (methotrexate, vinblastine, adriamycin, cisplatin) chemotherapy after radical cystectomy for pathologic T1–2 tumors with negative lymph nodes and expression of mutated p53.

Kielb et al have demonstrated in vitro that p53 mutations are required for paclitaxel to induce cell death in human bladder cell lines although this agent did not affect cells with wild type p53; however, the cytotoxic action of gemcitabine was not modulated by p53 status.[74] This suggests a differential response to cytotoxic agents based on cellular genotype. The clinical significance of p53 mutations modulating chemoresponse in the context of cytotoxic chemotherapy is a controversial issue. Studies from the Memorial Sloan-Kettering Cancer Center have suggested that p53 mutation is associated with resistance to neoadjuvant chemotherapy with the MVAC regimen.[75] However, Cote et al have reported that, in patients with tumors that did not demonstrate p53 alterations, adjuvant chemotherapy conferred no recurrence or survival benefit. In patients with p53-altered tumors, on the other hand, adjuvant chemotherapy resulted in a three-fold decreased risk of recurrence and a 2.6-fold increased chance of surviving.[76] The molecular basis for this observation has been described by Waldman et al.[77] Siu et al have demonstrated in a detailed study on invasive bladder cancer patients treated with MVAC regimen that the immunohistochemical expression of p53 did not predict survival.[78] Thus, the question still remains unanswered and the ongoing p53 targeted therapy trial may provide conclusive evidence in this matter.

There are reports suggesting a role for additional cell-cycle regulators in modulating chemoresponse in bladder cancer. Koga et al have reported that negative p53/positive p21 immunostaining is a predictor of favorable chemotherapeutic response in bladder cancer patients treated with intra-arterial chemotherapy (IAC) comprising 100 mg/m2 of cisplatin (CDDP) and 40 mg/m2 of pirarubicin (THP).[79] Qureshi et al have reported that p53 and/or MDM2 immunopositivity were not predictive of tumor response or patient survival after systemic chemotherapy in bladder cancer; however, patients with p53-positive tumors were observed to derive survival benefit from salvage therapy, and those with concomitant p53 and MDM2 positivity received the most benefit.[80] Jankevicius et al have reported that positive p21 protein expression confers a survival advantage to patients receiving systemic adjuvant chemotherapy for locally advanced bladder cancer.[81]

One of the suggested mechanisms for drug resistance in solid tumors is the phenomenon of multidrug resistance modulated by the MDR gene.[82] The protein responsible for the action is a P-glycoprotein, but a broader family of MDR proteins has been identified, and the expression of proteins in this family is correlated with resistance to the taxanes, vinca alkaloids, and anthracycline antibiotics. Petrylak et al have demonstrated an increased expression of P-glycoprotein in pretreatment and post-treatment biopsies of human tumors that were treated with the MVAC regimen. Interestingly, the highest proportion of tumor cells expressing P-glycoprotein was observed in metastases from patients that were treated with six or more cycles of chemotherapy.[83]

While there is a tremendous amount of information available regarding the existence or nonexistence of predictive value of cell cycle regulatory molecules in modulating chemoresponse in bladder cancer, there are currently no specific molecular targets that are clinically used to determine treatment modalities. Detailed clinical trials are necessary to identify molecular targets which can predict chemoresponse in an efficacious manner. However, the future design of clinical trials needs to incorporate parameters that will take into account the significant differences in drug metabolism systems among individuals (age, sex, etc.) and also among population groups. These differences are likely to account for many of the unexplained inconsistencies in drug response, toxicity, and long-term outcomes of treatment with conventional and novel cytotoxic regimens. The increasing demographic heterogeneity of the population receiving these chemotherapeutic regimens warrants consideration of such variables when designing large-scale clinical trials.

## ASSAYS TO DETECT CELL-CYCLE ALTERATIONS

### IMMUNOHISTOCHEMISTRY AND IMMUNOFLUORESCENCE

Immunohistochemistry is the technique of detecting specific proteins (antigens) in cells or tissues and consists of the following steps: 1) primary antibody directed against the protein (antigen) to be detected binds to specific antigen; 2) antibody–antigen complex is bound by a secondary, enzyme-conjugated, antibody; and 3) in the presence of substrate and chromogen, the enzyme forms a colored deposit at the sites of antibody–antigen binding. Immunofluorescence uses a fluorescent substrate instead of the chromogen. With the expansion and development of immunohistochemical techniques, enzyme labels such as peroxidase[84,85] and alkaline phosphatase[86] have been introduced. Colloidal gold label has also been used to identify immunohistochemical reactions with both light and electron microscopy.[87] Other labels include radioactive elements, and the immunoreaction can be visualized by autoradiography. Since immunohistochemistry involves a specific antigen–antibody reaction, it has a definite advantage over traditionally used enzyme staining techniques that identify only a limited number of proteins, enzymes, and tissue structures.

Immunohistochemistry has found tremendous application in clinical translational research in the last decade. This technique can be used for detection of target proteins in fresh frozen tissue specimens as well as archival paraffin-embedded tissue sections. To ensure the preservation of tissue architecture and cell morphology, prompt and adequate fixation is essential. There is no one universal fixative that is ideal for the demonstration of all antigens. However, in general, many antigens can be successfully demonstrated in formalin-fixed, paraffin-embedded tissue sections. The discovery and development of antigen retrieval techniques further enhanced the use of formalin as a routine fixative for immunohistochemistry in many research laboratories. As certain cellular antigens do not survive routine fixation and paraffin embedding, the use of frozen sections still remains essential for the demonstration of many antigens. However, the disadvantages of frozen sections include poor morphology, poor resolution at higher magnifications, special storage requirements, and difficulty in obtaining sections compared to paraffin-embedded tissue.

Immunohistochemical detection of protein in archival paraffin-embedded tissue sections has improved dramatically since the introduction of the antigen retrieval technique,[88] which optimizes detection of target antigen by removing the formaldehyde cross-linkages and exposing the epitopes necessary for antibody binding. This technique involves the application of heat for varying lengths of time to formalin-fixed, paraffin-embedded tissue sections in an antigen retrieval buffer. The most widely used buffers are citrate buffer (pH 6.0), EDTA (pH 10.0), and acetate buffer (pH 1.0). Microwave oven, pressure cooker, and steamer are the most commonly used heating methods. Proteolytic enzyme methods (e.g. trypsin, chymotrypsin, pepsin, pronase, and various other proteases) have also been reported for restoring immunoreactivity to tissue antigens, with varying degrees of success. Application of immunohistochemistry analyses to archival paraffin-embedded tissue sections has facilitated the optimal use of vast tissue resources, triggering a series of retrospective studies in various fields including bladder cancer.

Immunohistochemical detection of antigens could use either a direct one-step staining method involving a labeled antibody that reacts directly with the antigen in tissue sections, or an indirect method involving an unlabeled primary antibody and a labeled secondary antibody that reacts with the primary antibody. The second-layer antibody may be labeled with an enzyme such as peroxidase, alkaline phosphatase, or glucose oxidase—an indirect immunoenzyme method. In a further development of the indirect method, a third link has been added to the technique using: 1) a very stable peroxidase antiperoxidase complex; and 2) the avidin–biotin complex method (ABC method). This additional link increases the sensitivity of the technique many fold.

Immunohistochemistry uses a chromogen as a substrate, and the tissue section can be visualized under a microscope, whereas immunofluorescence uses a fluorescent dye as the substrate, and the tissue can be visualized using a fluorescence microscope. Use of both immunohistochemistry and immunofluorescence has contributed greatly to our understanding of the cellular localization of proteins as well as their role as predictive and prognostic indicators of clinical outcome in bladder cancer.

## EXPRESSION PROFILING TECHNOLOGIES

Inability of single/multiple markers to provide a comprehensive understanding of the biology of neoplasia has ushered in an era of high-throughput expression profiling. The need for expression profiling has resulted in the development of new techniques and advancement of currently available technologies. Given below is a brief overview of some particularly relevant and useful expression profiling technologies which have been broadly divided into those that deal with transcript-expression profiling and those that deal with protein profiling. A more detailed description of these techniques has been provided by Pagliarulo et al.[89]

### TRANSCRIPTIONAL PROFILING

#### Differential display

Invented in 1992 by Liang and Pardee, mRNA differential display technology works by systematic amplification of the 3′ termini of mRNAs and resolution of those fragments on a DNA sequencing gel.[90] Reverse transcription is carried out using anchored primers designed to anneal to and extend differentially from the 5′ boundary of the poly-A tails for transcripts, and PCR amplification is carried out with upstream arbitrary primers. The mRNA subpopulations are visualized by denaturing polyacrylamide electrophoresis to allow

direct side-by-side comparison of most of the mRNAs between or among related cells. The differential display method permits visualization of all the expressed genes, both known and unknown.

### Microarray for gene expression

Expression microarrays, as used currently, are capable of generating vast databases of information that provide high-resolution snapshots of cellular activity. Either the complementary DNA (cDNA) or oligonucleotides are used as 'probes'.[91] While 20–50-mers are used in oligonucleotide arrays, cDNA arrays are usually 500–1000 nucleotide-long PCR products generated using either vector-specific or gene-specific primers. More than 30,000 cDNAs can be fitted onto the surface of a conventional microscope slide. In a common example, different fluorescent dyes (e.g. Cy3 and Cy5) are used for labeling of mRNA 'targets' from two different cell populations, mixed and hybridized to the same oligonucleotide 'probe' array, and the resulting competitive binding of the targets to the arrayed sequences is measured. A measurement of the ratio of transcript levels for each gene is thus obtained. Target amplification is achieved either by in vitro transcription or by posthybridization; signal amplification is achieved using labeled antibodies or molecules carrying larger numbers of fluorophores, such as branched DNA dendrimers[92] or tyramide derivatives.[93] Despite significant technologic innovations in various array formats, significant impediments must be surmounted before this versatile technology can support routine, reliable, high-throughput assays.

### Standardized RT-PCR

Although high-density array technology has potential for large-scale measurement of all human genes simultaneously, it requires at least 1 μg of RNA for each experiment in its current form.[94] Willey and collaborators at Rochester University have developed a modified quantitative method for competitive reverse transcriptase PCR (RT-PCR) that allows simultaneous measurement of many genes using nanogram amounts of cDNA.[95] The transcript levels are expressed as numerical values per million molecules of β-actin, thus allowing intra- and inter-sample comparisons. Capillary electrophoresis has recently been applied to this technology, making it much more robust.

### PROTEIN PATHWAY PROFILING

Although transcript profiling may provide an idea about gene activity, it may not accurately parallel the activity of the protein product of a gene.[96–99] Apart from cataloging the protein moieties themselves, protein profiling can also yield information about various pivotal post-translational protein modifications, including phosphorylation, acetylation, sulfation, and glycosylation. Although the majority of protein identification still continues to be by two-dimensional (2D) gel electrophoresis,[100-102] many new technologies such as high-throughput protein arrays are being developed for protein characterization and discovery.[103-107] These are expected to replace the tedium and large protein loads typically associated with the 2D gels. Other novel formats include Ciphergen systems based on MALDI-TOF mass spectrometry,[108,109] and Biacore detection systems based upon surface plasmon resonance.[110]

An important requisite for proteomic arrays is specific antibodies with high affinities and low dissociation rates, which permit detection over a wide concentration range. Enzyme-liked immunosorbent assay (ELISA) has been the preferred technology for most clinical and research applications. Array-based technologies have now been adapted to ELISA-like formats for proteomic analysis.[111] This format can detect unique target proteins from a mixture of numerous proteins in a high-throughput manner. An extension to this technology is antibody arrays to detect post-translationally modified ('activated') forms of proteins (e.g. phosphorylated forms), an example of which is the microprinted protein array for kinase activity assay.[112]

Novel technologies are emerging to detect antibody–protein interactions at high sensitivity without the need for a label. One such label-free technology, which utilizes optically detectable deflection of microcantilevers following specific antigen–antibody interaction, has been described by Wu et al.[113] In another technology, atomic force microscopy (AFM) arrays topographically image and map the protein interactions.[114,115] This is achieved by analyzing surface modulation where the increase in 'height' results from the successful capture of the protein within the discrete bait area. Other classes of protein array under development include gel-immobilized arrays,[116] fiberoptic sensing arrays,[117,118] multiplexed capillary-based flow immunosensors, and multiplexed microbead antibody capture technologies.[119-121] These technologies add a third-dimensional space (spherical, cylindrical, or elongated domains), thereby expanding the surface area available for interaction.

## CONCLUSION

Cell-cycle alterations in bladder cancer have been investigated extensively. Alterations have been detected in both tumor suppressor genes and oncogenes, which maintain a delicate balance to ensure the fidelity of the normal cell division cycle. Alterations in a number of crucial regulators of the G1/S transition have been shown to be important in the development and progression of bladder cancer. While alterations in some markers may be more predictive of clinical outcome, none of these molecular markers yet provides a completely reliable and comprehensive understanding of the biology of bladder tumorigenesis. Combining predictive and prognostic information offered by multiple markers has significantly improved our understanding of the development of bladder cancer progression and subsequent clinical behavior, but even this is a far from ideal situation. The lack of predictive potential offered by single markers or a combination of three or four markers arises for the following reasons:

- Bladder cancer has a multifactorial etiology and a complex pathogenesis involving various pathways; hence investigation of alterations of a few markers cannot yield significant information.
- Alterations in these pathways are not necessarily a linear cascade of events, but may be an interrelated series of signals.
- The pattern in which these alterations occur may not be a simple bidirectional (upward/downward) regulation of a few markers.
- Changes in expression of different proteins/genes might have a context-dependent significance; the scaling of expression change might not be directly correlated to impact on its function on a similar scale.
- Lack of availability of tools to combine the expression patterns of proteins/genes, which fall in different pathways, and to generate an algorithm to predict progression, response to therapy, and clinical outcome in bladder cancer.

There are classic clinicopathologic and morphologic correlates which predict the aggressiveness of a tumor. However, these parameters have limited success in defining an aggressive as opposed to an indolent phenotype. The clinical behavior of a tumor is determined by its molecular characteristics, which in turn are influenced by germline changes as well as acquired somatic changes. The molecular characteristics of a tumor can be better understood by studying the 'molecular profile' of the tumor. These molecular profiles may be better indicators of the clonal origin of these tumors as well as their biology. Molecular profiles can be generated at the level of the transcriptome as well as the protein. Protein status is more indicative of function than the transcript; however, using the currently available analytical tools, generation of an expression profile at the transcript level is more feasible and hence attractive. Generation of a molecular profile in an individual tumor offers a number of advantages: 1) it provides an understanding of the deregulation occurring in multiple pathways; 2) it helps identification of gene expression patterns specific to given tumors; 3) it helps detection of novel targets for therapy; and 4) it aids in rational drug design directed against these specific targets.

Bladder tumors are grouped into various clinical stages based on the depth of tumor invasion, lymph node involvement, and presence/absence of distance metastasis. The type of treatment administered to these patients is based on this staging system. Currently bladder-sparing approaches are adopted for superficial bladder cancer while radical cystectomy, along with adjuvant chemotherapy (when necessary), is the norm for invasive bladder cancer. A substantial number of patients with superficial bladder cancer treated with bladder-sparing approaches develop local recurrence; likewise a significant proportion of patients who undergo chemotherapy following radical cystectomy do not benefit from it. These events result in significant morbidity and financial burden to the patient. It is essential to develop a system of staging that can optimize the therapy administered to bladder cancer patients. Molecular profiling can facilitate a molecular staging of bladder tumors based on their transcript profiles. Such molecular class prediction based on transcript expression will make possible better prediction of tumor progression and clinical outcomes. Furthermore, this ultrastaging can lead to identification of specific molecular classes which respond better to specific chemotherapeutic agents. This will eventually lead to targeted, therapy-tailored specific molecular defects, thereby significantly lowering the morbidity associated with bladder cancer. The future goal, therefore, will be to approach each individual tumor as a specific entity and to identify the molecular characteristics that make each tumor unique. In this way, specific management strategies and therapeutic modalities most efficacious for each individual patient can be administered.

## REFERENCES

1. Cordon-Cardo C. Mutations of cell cycle regulators. Biological and clinical implications for human neoplasia. Am J Pathol 1995;147:545–560.

2. Spruck CH III, Ohneseit PF, Gonzales-Zulueta M, et al. Two molecular pathways to transitional cell carcinoma of the bladder. Cancer Res 1994;54:784–788.

3. Ruppert JM, Tokino K, Sidransky D. Evidence for two bladder cancer suppressor loci on human chromosome 9. Cancer Res 1993;53:5093–5095.

4. Simoneau AR, Spruck CH III, Gonzalez-Zulueta M, et al. Evidence for two tumor suppressor loci associated with proximal chromosome 9p to q and distal chromosome 9q in bladder cancer and the initial screening for GAS1 and PTC mutations. Cancer Res 1996;56:5039–5043.

5. Knowles MA. Molecular genetics of bladder cancer: pathways of development and progression. Cancer Surv 1998;31:49–76.

6. Knowles MA. What we could do now: molecular pathology of bladder cancer. Mol Pathol 2001;54:215–221.

7. Knudson AG Jr. Retinoblastoma: a prototypic hereditary neoplasm. Semin Oncol 1978;5:57–60.

8. Cote RJ, Chatterjee SJ. Molecular determinants of outcome in bladder cancer. Cancer J Sci Am 1999;5:2–15.

9. Grossman HB, Liebert M, Antelo M, et al. p53 and RB expression predict progression in T1 bladder cancer. Clin Cancer Res 1998;4:829–834.

10. Miyamoto H, Shuin T, Torigoe S, et al. Retinoblastoma gene mutations in primary human bladder cancer. Br J Cancer 1995;71:831–835.

11. Acikbas I, Keser I, Kilic S, et al. Detection of LOH of the RB1 gene in bladder cancers by PCR-RFLP. Urol Int 2002;68:189–192.

12. Cordon-Cardo C, Wartinger D, Petrylak D, et al. Altered expression of the retinoblastoma gene product: prognostic indicator in bladder cancer. J Natl Cancer Inst 1992;84:1251–1256.

13. Logothetis CJ, Xu HJ, Ro JY, et al. Altered expression of retinoblastoma protein and known prognostic variables in locally advanced bladder. J Natl Cancer Inst 1992;84:1256–1261.

14. Cote RJ, Dunn MD, Chatterjee SJ, et al. Elevated and absent pRb expression is associated with bladder cancer progression and has cooperative effects with p53. Cancer Res 1998;58:1090–1094.

15. Chatterjee SJ, Shi SR, Datar RH, et al. Hyperphosphorylation of pRb: a mechanism for RB tumor suppressor pathway inactivation in bladder cancer. J Pathol 2004;203:762–770.

16. Finlay CA, Hinds PW, Levine AJ. The p53 proto-oncogene can act as a suppressor of transformation. Cell 1989;57:1083–1093.

17. Esrig D, Elmajian D, Groshen S, et al. Accumulation of nuclear p53 and tumor progression in bladder cancer. N Engl J Med 1994;331:1259–1264.

18. Livingstone LR, White A, Sprouse J, et al. Altered cell cycle arrest and gene amplification potential accompany loss of wild-type p53. Cell 1992;70:923–935.

19. Harper JW, Adami GR, Wei N, et al. The p21 Cdk-interacting protein Cip1 is a potent inhibitor of G1 cyclin-dependent kinases. Cell 1993;75:805–816.

20. Schmitz-Drager BJ, Kushima M, Goebell P, et al. p53 and MDM2 in the development and progression of bladder cancer. Eur Urol 1997;32:487–493.

21. Symonds H, Krall L, Remington L, et al. p53-dependent apoptosis suppresses tumor growth and progression in vivo. Cell 1994;78:703–711.

22. Esrig D, Spruck CH, Nichols PW, et al. p53 nuclear protein accumulation correlates with mutations in the p53 gene, tumor grade, and stage in bladder cancer. Am J Pathol 1993;143:1389–1397.

23. Sarkis AS, Dalbagni G, Cordon-Cardo C, et al. Nuclear overexpression of p53 protein in transitional cell bladder carcinoma: a marker for disease progression. J Natl Cancer Inst 1993;85:53–59.

24. Schmitz-Drager BJ, Goebell PJ, Ebert T, et al. p53 immunohistochemistry as a prognostic marker in bladder cancer. Playground for urology scientists? Eur Urol 2000;38:691–699; discussion 700.

25. Goebell PJ, Groshen S, Schmitz-Drager BJ, et al. The International Bladder Cancer Bank: proposal for a new study concept. Urol Oncol 2004;22:277–284.

26. Messing EM, Catalona W. Urothelial tumours of the urinary tract. In Walsh PC, Retik AB, Vaughan EAJW (eds): Campbell's Urology, vol 3, 7th ed. Philadelphia: Saunders, 1997, pp 2327–2410.

27. Cordon-Cardo C, Sheinfeld J, Dalbagni G. Genetic studies and molecular markers of bladder cancer. Semin Surg Oncol 1997;13:319–327.

28. Clurman BE, Groudine M. The CDKN2A tumor-suppressor locus—a tale of two proteins. N Engl J Med 1998;338:910–912.

29. Zhang Y, Xiong Y, Yarbrough WG. ARF promotes MDM2 degradation and stabilizes p53: ARF-INK4a locus deletion impairs both the Rb and p53 tumor suppression pathways. Cell 1998;92:725–734.

30. Rocco JW, Sidransky D. p16(MTS-1/CDKN2/INK4a) in cancer progression. Exp Cell Res 2001;264:42–55.

31. Kamijo T, Zindy F, Roussel MF, et al. Tumor suppression at the mouse INK4a locus mediated by the alternative reading frame product p19ARF. Cell 1997;91:649–659.

32. Orlow I, LaRue H, Osman I, et al. Deletions of the INK4A gene in superficial bladder tumors. Association with recurrence. Am J Pathol 1999;155:105–113.

33. Quelle DE, Cheng M, Ashmun RA, et al. Cancer-associated mutations at the INK4a locus cancel cell cycle arrest by p16INK4a but not by the alternative reading frame protein p19ARF. Proc Natl Acad Sci USA 1997;94:669–673.

34. Wu W-J, Huang C-H, Huang C-N, et al. Homozygous deletion of p16/cdkn2/mts1 gene in human urothelial carcinomas. Br J Urol 1997;80(Suppl 2):67.

35. Florl AR, Franke KH, Niederacher D, et al. DNA methylation and the mechanisms of CDKN2A inactivation in transitional cell carcinoma of the urinary bladder. Lab Invest 2000;80(10):1513–1522.

36. Berggren P, Kumar R, Sakano S, et al. Detecting homozygous deletions in the CDKN2A (p16(INK4a))/ARF(p14(ARF)) gene in urinary bladder cancer using real-time quantitative PCR. Clin Cancer Res 2003;9(1):235–242.

37. Chang L-L, Yeh W-T, Yang S-Y, et al. Genetic alterations of p16INK4a and p14ARF genes in human bladder cancer. J Urol 2003;170:595–600.

38. Dominguez G, Silva J, Garcia JM, et al. Prevalence of aberrant methylation of p14ARF over p16INK4a in some human primary tumors. Mutat Res 2003;530:9–17.

39. Dominguez G, Carballido J, Silva J, et al. p14ARF promoter hypermethylation in plasma DNA as an indicator of disease recurrence in bladder cancer patients. Clin Cancer Res 2002;8:980–985.

40. Sourvinos G, Kazanis I, Delakas D, et al. Genetic detection of bladder cancer by microsatellite analysis of p16, rb1 and p53 tumor suppressor genes. J Urol 2001;165(1):249–252.

41. Morgan DO. Principles of CDK regulation. Nature 1995;374:131–134.

42. Sellers WR, Kaelin WG Jr. Role of the retinoblastoma protein in the pathogenesis of human cancer. J Clin Oncol 1997;15:3301–3312.

43. Grana X, Reddy EP. Cell cycle control in mammalian cells: role of cyclins, cyclin dependent kinases (CDKs), growth suppressor genes and cyclin-dependent kinase inhibitors (CKIs). Oncogene 1995;11:211–219.

44. Sherr CJ. Cancer cell cycles. Science 1996;274:1672–1677.

45. Bartkova J, Lukas J, Muller H, et al. Abnormal patterns of D-type cyclin expression and G1 regulation in human head and neck cancer. Cancer Res 1995;55:949–956.

46. Arber N, Hibshoosh H, Moss SF, et al. Increased expression of cyclin D1 is an early event in multistage colorectal carcinogenesis. Gastroenterology 1996;110:669–674.

47. Musgrove EA, Lee CS, Buckley MF, et al. Cyclin D1 induction in breast cancer cells shortens G1 and is sufficient for cells arrested in G1 to complete the cell cycle. Proc Natl Acad Sci USA 1994;91:8022–8026.

48. Han EK, Lim JT, Arber N, et al. Cyclin D1 expression in human prostate carcinoma cell lines and primary tumors. Prostate 1998;35:95–101.

49. Betticher DC, Thatcher N, Altermatt HJ, et al. Alternate splicing produces a novel cyclin D1 transcript. Oncogene 1995;11:1005–1011.

50. Sawa H, Ohshima TA, Ukita H, et al. Alternatively spliced forms of cyclin D1 modulate entry into the cell cycle in an inverse manner. Oncogene 1998;16:1701–1712.

51. Wang L, Habuchi T, Takahashi T, et al. Cyclin D1 gene polymorphism is associated with an increased risk of urinary bladder cancer. Carcinogenesis 2002;23:257–264.

52. Cortessis VK, Siegmund K, Xue S, et al. A case-control study of cyclin D1 CCND1 870A→G polymorphism and bladder cancer. Carcinogenesis 2003;24:1645–1650.

53. Oya M, Schmidt B, Schmitz-Drager BJ, et al. Expression of G1→S transition regulatory molecules in human urothelial cancer. Jpn J Cancer Res 1995;89:719–726.

54. Sgambato A, Migaldi M, Faraglia B, et al. Cyclin D1 expression in papillary superficial bladder cancer: its association with other cell cycle-associated proteins, cell proliferation and clinical outcome. Int J Cancer 2002;97:671–678.

55. Takagi Y, Takashi M, Koshikawa T, et al. Immunohistochemical demonstration of cyclin D1 in bladder cancers as an inverse indicator of invasiveness but not an independent prognostic factor. Int J Urol 2000;7:366–372.

56. Richter J, Wagner U, Kononen J, et al. High-throughput tissue microarray analysis of cyclin E gene amplification and overexpression in urinary bladder cancer. Am J Pathol 2000;157:787–794.

57. Makiyama K, Masuda M, Takano Y, et al. Cyclin E overexpression in transitional cell carcinoma of the bladder. Cancer Lett 2000;151:193–198.

58. Simon R, Struckmann K, Schraml P, et al. Amplification pattern of 12q13-q15 genes (MDM2, CDK4, GLI) in urinary bladder cancer. Oncogene 2002;21:2476–2483.

59. Li D, Tian Y, Ma Y, et al. p150(Sal2) is a p53-independent regulator of p21(WAF1/CIP). Mol Cell Biol 2004;24:3885–3893.

60. Stein JP, Ginsberg DA, Grossfeld GD, et al. Effect of p21WAF1/CIP1 expression on tumor progression in bladder. J Natl Cancer Inst 1998;90:1072–1079.

61. Chen W-C, Wu H-C, Hsu C-D, et al. p21 gene codon 31 polymorphism is associated with bladder cancer. Urol Oncol 2002;7:63–66.

62. Lacombe L, Orlow I, Silver D, et al. Analysis of p21WAF1/CIP1 in primary bladder tumors. Oncol Res 1996;8:409–414.

63. Sgambato A, Migaldi M, Faraglia B, et al. Loss of P27Kip1 expression correlates with tumor grade and with reduced disease-free survival in primary superficial bladder cancers. Cancer Res 1999;59:3245–3250.

64. Korkolopoulou P, Christodoulou P, Konstantinidou AE, et al. Cell cycle regulators in bladder cancer: a multivariate survival study with emphasis on p27Kip1. Hum Pathol 2000;31:751–760.

65. Burton PB, Anderson CJ, Corbishly CM. Caspase 3 and p27 as predictors of invasive bladder cancer. N Engl J Med 2000;343:1418–1420.

66. Wu X, Bayle JH, Olson D, et al. The p53-mdm-2 autoregulatory feedback loop. Genes Dev 1993;7:1126–1132.

67. Lianes P, Orlow I, Zhang ZF, et al. Altered patterns of MDM2 and TP53 expression in human bladder cancer. J Natl Cancer Inst 1994;86:1325–1330.

68. Barbareschi M, Girlando S, Fellin G, et al. Expression of mdm-2 and p53 protein in transitional cell carcinoma. Urol Res 1995;22:349–352.

69. Keegan PE, Griffiths TRL, Marsh C, et al. MDM2 and p53 immunoreactivity: independent predictors of stage progression in pT1 bladder cancer (TCC). Br J Urol 1998;81:14.

70. Sigalas I, Calvert AH, Anderson JJ, et al. Alternatively spliced mdm2 transcripts with loss of p53 binding domain sequences: transforming ability and frequent detection in human cancer. Nature Med 1996;2:912–917.

71. Jahnson S, Karlsson MG. Predictive value of p53 and pRb immunostaining in locally advanced bladder cancer treated with cystectomy. J Urol 1998;160:1291–1296.

72. Chatterjee SJ, Datar RH, Youssefzadeh D, et al. The combined effects of Rb, p21, and p53 expression in the progression of bladder transitional cell carcinoma. J Clin Oncol 2004;22:1007–1013.

73. Shariat SF, Tokunaga H, Zhou J-H, et al. p53, p21, pRB, and p16 expression predict clinical outcome in cystectomy with bladder cancer. J Clin Oncol 2004;22:1014–1024.

74. Kielb SJ, Shah NS, Rubin MA, Sanda MG. Functional p53 mutation as a molecular determinant of paclitaxel and gemcitabine susceptibility in human bladder cancer. J Urol 2001;166(2):482–487.

75. Sarkis A, Bajorin D, Reuter V, et al. Prognostic value of p53 nuclear overexpression in patients with invasive bladder cancer treated with neoadjuvant MVAC. J Clin Oncol 1995;13:1384–1390.

76. Cote RJ, Esrig D, Groshen S, et al. p53 and treatment of bladder cancer. Nature 1997;385:123–125.

77. Waldman T, Lengauer C, Kinzler KW, et al. Uncoupling of S phase and mitosis induced by anticancer agents in cells lacking p21. Nature 1996;81:713–716.

78. Siu LL, Banerjee D, Khurana RJ, et al. The prognostic role of p53, metallothionein, P-glycoprotein, and MIB-l in muscle invasive urothelial transitional cell carcinoma. Clin Cancer Res 1998;4(3):559–565.

79. Koga F, Kitahara S, Arai K, et al. Negative p53/positive p21 immunostaining is a predictor of favorable response to chemotherapy in patients with locally advanced bladder cancer. Jpn J Cancer Res 2000;91:416–423.

80. Qureshi KN, Griffiths TRL, Robinson MC, et al. TP53 and MDM2 immunoreactivity as predictors of response in muscle-invasive

bladder cancer treated by systemic chemotherapy. BJU Int 1999;84:140–141.

81. Jankevicius F, Goebell P, Kushima M, et al. p21 and p53 immunostaining and survival following systemic chemotherapy for urothelial cancer. Urol Int 2002;69:174–180.

82. Dicato M, Duhem C, Pauly M, et al. Multidrug resistance: molecular and clinical aspects. Cytokines Cell Mol Ther 1997;3:91–99.

83. Petrylak DP, Scher HI, Reuter V, O'Brien JP, Cordon-Cardo C. P-glycoprotein expression in primary and metastatic transitional cell carcinoma of the bladder. Ann Oncol 1994;5(9):835–840.

84. Pierce GB Jr, Nakane PK. Antigens of epithelial basement membranes of mouse, rat, and man. A study utilizing enzyme-labeled antibody. Lab Invest 1967;17:499–514.

85. Avrameas S, Uriel J. Method of antigen and antibody labeling with enzymes and its immunodiffusion application. C R Acad Sci Hebd Seances Acad Sci D 1966;262:2543–2545.

86. Mason DY, Sammons R. Alkaline phosphatase and peroxidase for double immunoenzymatic labelling of cellular constituents. J Clin Pathol 1978;31:454–460.

87. Faulk WP, Taylor GM. An immunocolloid method for the electron microscope. Immunohistochemistry 1971;8:1081–1083.

88. Shi SR, Imam SA, Young L, et al. Antigen retrieval immunohistochemistry under the influence of pH using monoclonal antibodies. J Histochem Cytochem 1995;43:193–201.

89. Pagliarulo V, Datar RH, Cote RJ. Role of genetic and expression profiling in pharmacogenomics: the changing face of patient management. Curr Issues Mol Biol 2002;4:101–110.

90. Liang P, Pardee AB. Differential display of eukaryotic mRNA by means of the polymerase chain reaction. Science 1992;257:967–971.

91. Ekins R, Chu FW. Microarrays: their origins and applications. Trends Biotechnol 1999;17:217–218.

92. Murakami T, Hagiwara T, Yamamoto K, et al. A novel method for detecting HIV-1 by non-radioactive in situ hybridization: application of a peptide nucleic acid probe and catalysed signal amplification. J Pathol 2001;194:130–135.

93. Capaldi S, Getts RC, Jayasena SD. Signal amplification through nucleotide extension and excision on a dendritic DNA platform. Nucleic Acids Res 2000;28:E21.

94. Lockhart DJ, Dong H, Byrne MC. Expression monitoring by hybridization to high-density oligonucleotide arrays. Nat Biotechnol 1996;14:1675–1680.

95. Willey JC, Crawford EL, Jackson CM, et al. Expression measurement of many genes simultaneously by quantitative RT-PCR using standardized mixtures of competitive templates. Am J Respir Cell Mol Biol 1998;19:6–17.

96. Hancock W, Apffel A, Chakel J, et al. Integrated genomic/proteomic analysis. Anal Chem 1999;71:743–748.

97. Luo L, Salunga RC, Guo H, et al. Gene expression profiles of laser-captured adjacent neuronal subtypes. Nature Med 1999;5:117–122.

98. Gygi SP, Rist B, Gerber SA, et al. Quantitative analysis of complex protein mixtures using isotope-coded affinity tags. Nat Biotechnol 1999;17:994–999.

99. Humphery-Smith I, Cordwell SJ, Blackstock WP. Proteome research: complementarity and limitations with respect to the RNA and DNA worlds. Electrophoresis 1997;18:1217–1242.

100. Page MJ, Amess B, Townsend RR, et al. Proteomic definition of normal human luminal and myoepithelial breast cells purified from reduction mammoplasties. Proc Natl Acad Sci USA 1999;96:12589–12594.

101. Banks RE, Dunn MJ, Forbes MA, et al. The potential use of laser capture microdissection to selectively obtain distinct populations of cells for proteomic analysis. Electrophoresis 2000;20:689–700.

102. Emmert-Buck M, Gillespie JW, Paweletz CP, et al. An approach to the proteomic analysis of human tumors. Mol Carcinogen 2000;27:158–165.

103. Ekins R, Chu FW. Multianalyte microspot immunoassay—microanalytical 'compact disk' of the future. Clin Chem 1991;37:1955–1967.

104. Chiem NH, Harrison DJ. Microchip systems for immunoassay: an integrated immunoreactor with electrophoretic separation for serum theophylline determination. Clin Chem 1998;44:591–598.

105. Hancock W, Apffel A, Chakel J, et al. Integrated genomic/proteomic analysis. Anal Chem 1999;71:743–748.

106. Rowe CA, Tender LM, Feldstein MJ, et al. Array biosensor for simultaneous identification of bacterial, viral, and protein analytes. Anal Chem 1999;71:3846–3852.

107. Paweletz CP, Gillespie JW, Ornstein DK, et al. Rapid protein display profiling of cancer progression directly from human tissue using a protein biochip. Drug Dev Res 2000;49:34–42.

108. Davies HA. The protein chip system from Ciphergen: a new technique for rapid, micro-scale protein biology. J Mol Med 2000;78:B29.

109. Boyle MD, Romer TG, Meeker AK, et al. Use of surface-enhanced laser desorption ionization protein chip system to analyze streptococcal exotoxin B activity secreted by Streptococcus pyogenes. J Microbiol Methods 2001;46:87–97.

110. Rich RL, Day YS, Morton TA, et al. High-resolution and high-throughput protocols for measuring drug/human serum albumin interactions using BIACORE. Anal Biochem 2001;296:197–207.

111. Mendoza LG, McQuary P, Mongan A, Gangadharan R, Brignac S, Eggers M. High throughput microarray based enzyme linked immunosorbent assay. BioTechniques 1999;27:778–788.

112. MacBeath G, Schreiber SL. Printing proteins as microarrays for high-throughput function determination. Science 2000;289:1760–1763.

113. Wu G, Datar RH, Hansen KM, et al. Bioassay of prostate-specific antigen (PSA) using microcantilevers. Nat Biotechnol 2001;19:856–860.

114. Jones VW, Kenseth JR, Porter MD, Mosher CL, Henderson E. Microminiaturized immunoassays using atomic force microscopy and compositionally patterned antigen arrays. Anal Chem 1998;70:1233–1241.

115. Silzel JW, Cercek B, Dodson C, Tsay T, Obremski RJ. Mass-sensing multianalyte microarray immunoassay with imaging detection. Clin Chem 1998;44:2036–2043.

116. Vasiliskov V, Timofeev EN, Surzhikov SA, et al. Fabrication of microarray of gel-immobilized compounds on a chip by copolymerization. BioTechniques 1999;27:592–606.

117. Shriver-Lake LC, Ogert RA, Ligler FS. A fiber optic evanescent-wave immunosensor for large molecules. Sensors Actuators 1993;11:239–243.

118. Wadkins RM, Golden JP, Pritsiolas LM, Ligler FS. Biosensors and bioelectronics: detection of multiple toxic agents using a planar array immunosensor. Biosens Bioelectron 1998;13:407–415.

119. Fulton RJ, McDade RL, Smith PL, Kienker LJ, Kettman JR Jr. Advanced multiplexed analysis with the Flow Metrix system. Clin Chem 1997;43:1749–1756.

120. Narang U, Gauger PR, Kusterbeck AW, et al. Multianalyte detection using a capillary-based flow immunosensor. Anal Biochem 1998;255:13–19.

121. Carson RT, Vignali DA. Simultaneous quantitation of 15 cytokines using a multiplexed flow cytometric assay. J Immunol Methods 1999;227:41–52.

# Cytogenetics of urothelial neoplasias

# 11

*Pamela J Russell, Guido Sauter, Tzong-Tyng Hung, Frederick M Waldman*

## INTRODUCTION

### GENETICS OF URINARY BLADDER CANCER DEVELOPMENT AND PROGRESSION

Chromosomal gains or losses may indicate the presence of potential oncogenes or tumor suppressor genes in bladder cancers. Initial studies involved chromosomal analysis by G-banding that looked for clones carrying similar cytogenetic changes (reviewed in Sandberg & Berger[1]). More recent methods have used fluorescence in situ hybridization (FISH) analysis, in which fluorescent probes, such as pericentric or centromeric probes, are allowed to interact with interphase nuclei, and can indicate copy number or alterations for a given chromosome carrying the marker in question (see Waldman et al[2]). DNA isolated from microdissected tumors or from nearby specified tissues, from urinary sediments, blood or serum, has been subjected to the use of the polymerase chain reaction (PCR) for microsatellite markers that exhibit known polymorphisms on known chromosomes. Loss of heterozygosity (LOH) for given markers may be related to inactivation of tumor suppressor genes, which are generally recessive in somatic cells, so loss of function by both alleles is necessary for their effects on growth regulation to be changed. This can occur by deletion of both alleles (homozygous deletion) or by deletion of one allele (LOH), with alteration (e.g. mutation) or inactivation (e.g. by methylation) of the other. In some cases, decreased expression, such as can occur with LOH, can mediate functional change (haplo-insufficiency). Further analysis is by high-density deletion mapping to pinpoint regions of interest, and then by searching for expressed sequences of candidate genes in common regions of deletion.

To study oncogenes, comparative genomic hybridization (CGH) is useful.[3] Genomic DNA from tumor and normal cells is differentially fluorescently labeled, mixed, and hybridized to normal metaphase spreads. This technique has been useful for identifying regions of high level DNA amplification (potential oncogenes) (resolution of CGH is approximately 20 megabases), but fine deletion mapping is not feasible. More recently, array-based CGH, using arrays of thousands of bacterial artificial chromosomes (BACs) mapped throughout the genome, has allowed analysis at the megabase level.[4]

Urinary bladder cancers are most commonly transitional cell carcinomas (TCC), but squamous cell carcinomas (SCC; often associated with bilharzia infection), adenocarcinomas, and carcinoma in situ (CIS) also occur. These have previously been categorized into 'superficial' (pTa, pT1, CIS) or 'invasive' (pT2–4) cancer depending on whether or not tumor infiltration extended to the muscular bladder wall.[5] The available genetic data based on the above techniques now suggest another subdivision of urinary bladder neoplasia (Figure 11.1). Two genetic subtypes with marked difference in their degree of genetic instability correspond to morphologically defined entities. Those that are genetically stable include non-invasive low-grade papillary tumors (pTa G1–2), whereas high-grade (including pTa G3 and CIS) and invasively growing carcinomas (stage pT1–4) are genetically unstable.

Genetically stable tumors—the non-invasive low-grade papillary bladder neoplasms (pTa, G1–2)—exhibit few genomic alterations,[6–9] the most common of which are

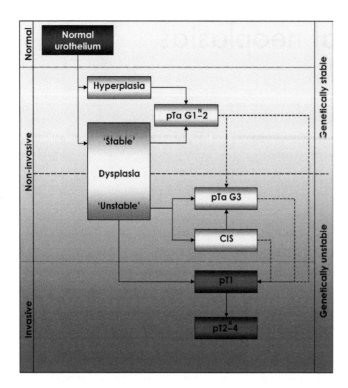

**Fig. 11.1**
Putative model of bladder cancer development and progression based on genetic findings. Thick arrows indicate the most frequent pathways, dotted lines the most rare events. The typical genetic alterations in genetically stable and unstable tumors are described in the text. CIS, carcinoma in situ.

losses of chromosome 9 (often the entire chromosome) and mutations of FGFR3 (on chromosome 4p16.3). Gene amplifications and p53 mutations are rare,[10-15] and less than half show DNA aneuploidy.[16-18]

High-grade neoplasias and invasive carcinomas are genetically unstable, with multiple chromosomal aberrations, including high-level amplifications and p53 mutations,[19-22] and thus differ markedly from non-invasive low-grade papillary tumors. Secondary abnormalities appear to result in an accumulation of changes, rather than a given sequence of events. DNA aneuploidy occurs in most invasive carcinomas.[16,17] In contrast, genetic differences between minimally invasive (pT1) and extensively invasive (pT2-4) carcinomas are minimal.[23,24] Putative roles have been suggested for 5p+, 5q-, and 6q- for further progression from pT1 to pT2-4 cancers.[25-28] Genetic changes in non-invasive high-grade precursor lesions (pTa G3, CIS) show a strong similarity to those in invasively growing cancers.[29,30] Given the frequency of individual genetic alterations in high-grade or invasive tumors compared with pTa G1-2 neoplasias, it is much more likely that high-grade (pTa G3, CIS) cancers rather than non-invasive low-grade papillary tumors are the precursors of invasive cancers. This is consistent with the clinical observation that the vast majority of invasive bladder cancers was not preceded by a pTa G1-2 tumor.[31] Therefore, pT1 cancers and pTa

tumors represent completely different entities, and should not be combined into one group as 'superficial bladder cancer'.[23,24]

A putative model of bladder cancer development and progression is described in Figure 11.1 where invasive urothelial cancers (stage pT1-4) are thought to derive from either papillary (pTa G3) or flat (CIS) neoplasias with little relationship to non invasive low grade papillary tumors (pTa G1-2).

## CHROMOSOMAL ABNORMALITIES

### NON-INVASIVE UROTHELIAL NEOPLASIAS

Non-invasive low-grade papillary neoplasms (pTa, G1-2) that are genetically stable show few cytogenetic changes,[6-9] with total or partial loss of chromosome 9 occurring in some 50% of cases of all grades and stages,[6,7,32] and also in hyperplasia and in morphologically normal appearing urothelium.[33,34] A change that appears to precede loss of chromosome 9, and is a marker of non-invasive cancer, is mutation of the FGFR3 receptor on chromosome 4.[35] Loss of the Y chromosome is the next most frequent cytogenetic alteration in low-grade tumors,[7,36,37] but is also seen in normal urothelium from patients with a history of bladder cancer,[36] making its biologic significance unclear. Non-invasive high-grade precursor lesions (pTa G3, CIS) differ markedly from low-grade neoplasias in presenting with many different cytogenetic changes,[7,29,30,38] resembling invasively growing tumors. Predominant deletions at 2q, 5q, 10q, and 18q, as well as gains at 5p and 20q, were shown by CGH in 18 pTa G3 tumors,[7] while in 31 CIS, LOH were found at 3p, 4q, 5q, 8p, 9p, 9q, 11p, 13q, 14q, 17p, and 18q.[29] A summary of the frequencies of cytogenetic changes found in both low- and high-grade non-invasive urothelial tumors is given in Table 11.1.[2,6,7,9,29,30,34,36,38,42-56]

Alterations in the cellular DNA content are common in bladder cancer.[16-18] Aneuploidy is strongly associated with stage and grade, and differences are most striking between pTa and pT1 tumors.[17] Aneuploidy detection (e.g. by FISH or by cytometry) may be a suitable tool for the early detection of bladder cancer and recurrences. It has been shown that a panel of 4-10 FISH probes is sufficient to detect chromosomal alterations in bladder tumors and tumor cells in voided urines.[16,39-41]

### INVASIVELY GROWING CANCERS

Invasive bladder cancers are characterized by the presence of a high number of genetic alterations (an average of

**Table 11.1** Cytogenetic changes in non-invasive transitional cell carcinoma of the urinary bladder

| Chromosomal location | Frequency of alteration in | | | References |
|---|---|---|---|---|
| | pTa G1–2 | pTa G3 | CIS | |
| 1p– | | | 1 of 2 (F) | 34, 42 |
| 1q+ | 13% (C) | 17% (C) | | 6, 9 |
| 2p+ | | 5% (C) | | 9 |
| 2q– | 4–5% (C) | 39% (C) | | 6, 7, 9 |
| 3p– | 1% (C) 6% (K) | 5% (C) | 31% (L) | 6, 9, 29, 43, 44 |
| 3q+ | 1% (C) | 5% (C) | | 6, 9 |
| 4p– | 2–5% (C) | 22% (C) | 32% (L) | 6, 7, 9, 29 |
| 4q– | 1–10% (C) | 17% (C) | 52% (L) | 6, 7, 9, 29 |
| 5p+ | 2% (C) 3% (K) | 28% (C) | | 6, 9, 45 |
| 5q– | 4–20% (C) 3% (K) | 33% (C) | 20% (L) | 6, 7, 9, 29, 46 |
| 6p+ | 1–5% (C) | 11% (C) | | 6, 7, 9 |
| 6q– | 1–10% (C) 16% (K) | 33% (C) | | 6, 7, 9, 44, 47–49 |
| 7p+ | 5–10% (C) 19% (K) | 5% (C) | | 6, 7, 9, 43, 45, 50, 51 |
| 8p– | 5–15% (C) 19% (K) | 28% (C) | 1 of 2 (F) 65% (L) | 6, 7, 9, 29, 34, 43, 47, 51–53 |
| 8q+ | 5–10% (C) 3% (K) | 22% (C) | | 2, 6, 7, 9 |
| 9p– | 36–45% (C) 28% (K) 15–33% (L) | 45% (C) | 40–77% (F) 61–76% (L) | 6, 7, 9, 29, 30, 38, 43, 44, 47, 48, 51, 53 |
| 9q– | 45% (C) 31% (K) 2 of 7 (L) | 38% (C) | 74% (F) 52–61% (L) | 6, 7, 9, 29, 30, 38, 43, 44, 47, 48, 51, 53 |
| 10p+ | 3% (K) | 5% (C) | | 6, 9 |
| 10q– | 5% (C) 9% (K) | 28% (C) | | 9, 44, 47 |
| 11p– | 10% (C) 16% (K) 1 of 3 (L) | 17% (C) | 54% (L) | 6, 7, 9, 29, 43, 47, 49, 54 |
| 11q– | 6% (C) 3% (K) | 23% (C) | 36% (L) | 6, 9, 29, 49 |
| 11q+ | 5–25% (C) | | 1 of 2 (F) | 6, 7, 9, 34 |
| 12p+ | 1% (C) | 5% (C) | | 6, 9 |
| 12q+ | 1–15% (C) 3% (K) | 5% (C) | | 6, 7, 9, 44 |
| 13q– | 0–20% (C) 19% (L) | 17% (C) | 56% (L) | 6, 7, 9, 29, 55 |
| 14q– | 1% (C) 9% (l) | | 70% (L) | 6, 7, 9, 29, 56 |
| 17p– | 1–5% (C) 6% (K) | 11% (C) | 81% (F) 60–64% (L) | 6–8, 29, 30, 34, 44, 49 |
| 17q+ | 10–30% (C) | 33% (C) | | 6, 7, 9 |
| 18q– | 7–10% (C) 3% (K) | 39% (C) | 29% (L) | 6, 7, 9, 29, 52 |
| 20q+ | 7–15% (C) | 33% (C) | | 6, 7, 9 |
| Y | 10–20% (C) 6% (K) | 28% (C) | 29% (K) | 6, 7, 9, 44, 48 |
| –Y | 40% (K) | | | 6, 36 |

C, comparative genomic hybridization (CGH); F, fluorescence in situ hybridization (FISH) (FISH analyses of carcinoma in situ (CIS) have been included because of the lack of CGH data in this tumor type); K, karyotyping/classic cytogenetics (average of 32 cases from references 44, 52; >100 from reference 36); L, loss of heterozygosity (LOH).

7–10 changes by CGH) involving multiple different chromosomal regions.[6,7,9,23,24] The most frequently observed gains and losses of chromosomal regions are separately summarized for cytogenetic, CGH, and LOH studies in Table 11.2.[2,6,23–25,27,29,36,43,44,47,48,50,53,55,56,58–66] Taken together, the data highlight losses of 2q, 5q, 8p, 9p, 9q, 10q, 11p, 18q, and the Y chromosome, as well as gains of 1q, 5p, 8q, and 17q, as the most important cytogenetic changes in these tumors. However, losses at 6q, 10p, 11q, 12p, and 12q, and gains at 3p, 3q, 6p, 8q, and 20q, are also relatively frequent. Important regions of amplification found in invasive cancers include 1q24–q25,[7] 5p11–p13,[24] 5q21,[7] 7q11–q21, 7q21–q31,[24] 7q36,[7] 8q21–q22,[7] 9p24,[24] 10p12–p14,[7] 10q22.1–q23,[57] 12q12,[7] 12q14,[7] 17q11–q21.3,[57] and 17q24–q25.[24] Isochromosome (5p) has also been associated with aggression.[58]

Aberrations detected by CGH or cytogenetics are usually of a large size, making it difficult to identify the target gene(s) of which an altered function (caused by a gain or loss of chromosomal material) leads to a selective growth advantage. Despite this, high levels of amplification detected by cytogenetic (karyotyping, CGH, FISH) or molecular genetic methods (Southern blotting, PCR) have led to the identification of over 30 different areas of the genome, which can be highly amplified in urinary bladder cancer as summarized in Table 11.3.[4,6,7,11,12,16,24,25,43,44,48,50,53,54,58,62,67–78] It is likely, given the large number of poorly understood or previously unstudied genes located in affected areas, that genes important for bladder cancer development and progression still remain to be discovered.

The gene NM_017774, overexpressed in relation to the amplicon at 6p22.3, is a potential new oncogene that is amplified in four TCC cell lines.[79] Multiple adjacent oncogenes are frequently co-amplified and simultaneously overexpressed in bladder cancers. For example, amplification of CCND1 at 11q13 can be accompanied by amplification of FGF4/FGF3 in 88% (R. Simon, personal communication); amplification of CCNE1 is accompanied by amplification of E2F3 at 6p22.3;[4] MDM2 amplification at 12q15 is accompanied by CDK4 amplification in 11%, and HER2 amplification at 17q23 includes TOP2A in 15%.[11] Similarly, there is a significant correlation between gain of CCND1 and deletion of TP53.[4] Whether this is an epiphenomen, or whether genomic amplification provides a growth advantage when simultaneous overexpression of two or more adjacent genes occurs, is currently unknown.

## SPECIFIC GENE ALTERATIONS

### Chromosome 9

The similarity of frequency of chromosome 9 losses in non-invasive low-grade papillary tumors and in high-grade invasive cancers triggered extensive research to find the suggested one or several tumor suppressor genes on chromosome 9 that appear to play an important role in bladder cancer initiation.[59,80,81] Mapping studies using microsatellite analysis identified multiple common regions of heterozygosity (LOH),[59,62,63,82] two of which have been identified at 9p21, the loci of the cell cycle control genes CDKN2A (p16/p14^{ARF}) and CDKN2B (p15).[82,83] Of 48% of TCC with LOH at the p16/p14^{ARF} site, three had point mutations and three had homozygous deletions.[84,85] Breakpoints at 9p21 deletions were thought to result from nonhomologous recombination or other unknown mechanisms.[86] In some cases (5/17), deletions of CDKN2 have been found in the absence of homozygous interferon-α (IFNα) deletion, whereas in other tumors, both genes tend to be deleted together.[87] Another three putative suppressor gene loci have been mapped to 9q13–q31, 9q32–q33, and 9q34, containing the PTCH, DBCCR1, and TSC1 genes, respectively.[88] Because homozygous deletions are slightly more frequent for CDKN2A than for CDKN2B, it has been postulated that p16/p14^{ARF} might be the primary target of 9p21 deletions.[89] On 9q, the putative cell cycle regulator DBCCR1 (deleted in bladder cancer chromosome region candidate 1), which might be involved in cell cycle regulation,[90,91] seems to be a promising candidate tumor suppressor. Loss of DBCCR1 expression has been found in 50% of bladder tumors,[90] and FISH analysis revealed deletions of 9q33 in 73% of samples.[92] Mutations of DBCCR1 have not yet been reported. Although hemizygous deletions have been seen in rare cases, it is believed that promoter hypomethylation and homozygous deletions are the main mechanisms for DBCCR1 silencing.[90,92,93] The bladder cancer cell line DSH1 (pT1G2) was shown to have a homozygous deletion of DBCCR1,[94] making it useful for functional studies.

### PTCH and TSC1

The roles of the sonic hedgehog receptor PTCH and the tuberous sclerosis gene TSC1 in bladder cancer remain only poorly investigated. Haploid sufficiency of a region encompassing PTCH has been suggested as an early event in bladder cancer development,[95] and both somatic and novel mutations in the TSC1 gene have been detected in TCC and bladder cancer cell lines.[96] Mutations of the ZNF189 and TSC1 genes on 9q[97] have been found in bladder cancer cell lines, suggesting that they could also be putative tumor suppressor genes.

### FGFR3

Mutations of the FGF receptor 3 (FGFR3) gene, located at chromosome 4p16.3, have only recently been suggested as a molecular alteration characteristic for pTa tumors.[35,98–102] The mutations of FGFR3 are more common in pTa than in pT2–4 tumors,[101,102] and appear to be almost mutually exclusive of p53 mutations.[101,102]

**Table 11.2** Cytogenetic changes in muscle-invasive transitional cell carcinoma of the urinary bladder

| Chromosomal location | Frequency of alteration by | | | |
| --- | --- | --- | --- | --- |
| | Karyotyping* | CGH† | LOH | References |
| 1p– | 18% | NA | 20%<br>3% | 58, 59 |
| 1q+ | 7–11% | 33–54% | | 23–25, 58 |
| 2p– | | | 22% | 60 |
| 2p+ | 2% | 8–30% | | 24, 61 |
| 2q– | 13% | 17–36% | 58% | 6, 24, 25, 44, 53 |
| 3p– | 4% | 2–9% | 20%<br>CIS 31% | 6, 29, 53, 59 |
| 3p+ | 27% | 18% | | 6, 48 |
| 3q+ | 7% | 7–24% | | 6, 23, 24, 50 |
| 4p– | 7% | 8–21% | 22%<br>CIS 32% | 6, 29, 48 |
| 4q– | 4% | 10–30%<br>30% | 26% | 24, 43, 61 |
| 5p– | | | 45% | 27, 50 |
| 5p+ | 20% | 18–25% | | 6, 48, 50, 58 |
| 5q– | 9% | 16–30% | 6–50%<br>CIS 20% | 6, 24, 29, 44, 47 |
| 6p+ | 7% | 16–24% | | 6, 24, 25, 47, 61 |
| 6q– | 18%<br>7% | 19% | 27% | 23, 44, 48, 58 |
| 7p+ | 13%<br>trisomy 7: 14% | 20–23% | | 2, 43, 44, 61 |
| 8p– | 16% | 29–42% | 18–83%<br>CIS 65% | 6, 23–25, 29, 43, 60 |
| 8q+ | 11% | 37–54% | | 6, 23–25, 53 |
| 9p– | 22–50% | 31–47% | 38%<br>CIS 61% | 23, 25, 29, 43, 44, 62 |
| 9q– | 27–47% | 23–33% | 55–61%<br>CIS 61% | 6, 24, 25, 29, 44, 59, 63 |
| 10p+ | 4% | 13–19% | | 6, 44 |
| 10q– | 11–25% | 18–28% | 23–45% | 24, 44, 48, 64, 65 |
| 11p– | 11–33% | 24–43% | 9–72%<br>CIS 54% | 6, 23–25, 29, 47, 53, 59 |
| 11q– | 9% | 22–34% | 17–30% | 23–25, 29, 50 |
| 12p+ | 4% | 4–30% | | 6, 24, 48 |
| 12q+ | 9% | 14–30% | | 24, 58 |
| 13q– | 18% | 19–29%<br>19% | 26%<br>CIS 56% | 6, 25, 29, 50, 55, 59 |
| 14q– | | | 24%<br>CIS 70% | 29, 56 |
| 15q– | | | 39% | 66 |
| 17p– | 2%<br>Translocation of 17: 40% | 19–24% | 27–81%<br>CIS 60% | 6, 23, 24, 29, 47, 59, 60 |
| 17q+ | 4% , iso 17q | 29–49% | | 6, 23–25, 44, 47, 53 |
| 18q– | 4% | 13–30% | 36–51%<br>CIS 29% | 6, 23–25, 29, 58 |
| 20q+ | 7% | 28–33% | | 6, 23, 25, 44, 61 |
| Y– | 11–100% | 15–37% | | 25, 36, 44 |

* Average frequency from bladder cancers from references 36, 43, 44, 48, 50, 51.
† Only large studies on invasive tumors (pT1–4; >50 analyzed tumors) included.
CGH, comparative genomic hybridization; CIS, carcinoma in situ; LOH, loss of heterozygosity; NA, not analyzed.

**Table 11.3** Amplification sites

| Amplicon | Putative target gene(s) | Amplification frequency* | References |
|---|---|---|---|
| 1p22–p32 | JUN, TAL1 | 2 of 10 (C) | 44 |
| 1q21–q24 | TRK, SKI, MUC1, CKS1, COAS2, KIAA-1096 | 3–33% (C)<br>2% (K)<br>6% (AC)<br>(RT-PCR) | 4, 6, 7, 24, 25, 43, 48, 50, 53, 58, 67, 68 |
| 2q13 | RADL2A | 2% (K) | 16 |
| 3pter–p23 | RAF1 | 1–4% (C)<br>4% (F) | 12, 24, 54 |
| 5p11–p13 | | 1% (C) | 24 |
| 5p15 | TRIO, SKP2 | 1–2% (C) | 24 |
| 5q21 | EFNA5 | 1% (C) | 7 |
| 6p22 | E2F3, DEK | 3–26% (C)<br>6–10% (AC)<br>64% (C and F)<br>2% (K) | 4, 6, 24, 25, 69, 70 |
| 7p12–p11<br>7q21–q31 | EGFR<br>MET, WNT2 | Case report (K)<br>1% (C) | 48, 58<br>24 |
| 7q36 | | 2% (C) | 7 |
| 8p12–p11 | FGFR1 | 2–3% (C)<br>6% (AC)<br>1–3% (F)<br>2% (K) | 4, 6, 12 |
| 8q21–q22 | MYBL1 | 4–28% (C)<br>10% (AC) | 4, 6, 7, 24, 25, 58 |
| 8q24 | MYC | 1–2% (C)<br>3–8% (F)<br>33% (S) | 4, 24, 71 |
| 9p24 | JAK2 | 1% (C) | 24 |
| 9p21 | – | 4% (F) | 72 |
| 10p11–p12 | MAP3K8 | 2% (C) | 7 |
| 10p13–p15 | STAM, IL15RA | 1–2% (C) | 7, 54 |
| 10q22–q23 | | 33% (C) | 58 |
| 10q25 | CSPG6, FACL5 | 1% (C) | 7 |
| 11p15.5 | Between c-Ha-ras and MUC2 | – | 73 |
| 11q13 | CCND1, EMS1, TAOS1 | 4–9% (C)<br>5–12% (AC)<br>30% (F)<br>21% (S) | 4, 6, 74 |
| 12q13–q21 | MDM2, CDK4, SAS | 3% (C)<br>5% (F)<br>4% (S)<br>6–10% (AC) | 4, 6, 7, 11, 54, 62, 74 |
| 13q34 | ARHGEF7, GAS6, TFDP1, FGF14, | 1% (C) | 6 |
| 17q11–q21 | HER2, TOP2A, KSR, WNT3 | 2–24% (C)<br>3–7% (F)<br>4–14% (S)<br>11% (P) | 4, 7, 24, 58, 75–77 |
| 17q22–q23 | FLJ21316, HS.6649, RPS6KB1, PPM1D | 1 of 14 (C) | 54 |
| 17q24–q25 | MAP2K6, GRB2, BIRC5 | 3% (C) | 24 |
| 18p11 | YES1, MC2R | 1–3% | 24, 54 |
| 19q13 | CCNE | 6% (AC) | 4 |
| 20q11 | CDC9IL1 (PIG-U) | 33% (F) | 78 |
| 20q12–q13 | BCAS1, NCOA3, STK6, MYBL2, CSE1L, TFAP2C | 2–9% (C)<br>50% (F)<br>35% (S) | 24, 58 |
| 22q11–q13 | MAPK1, CECR1, ECGF1 | 1 of 14 (C) | 54 |
| Xp21 | – | 2% | 24 |
| Xq21 | RPS6KA6 | 1% | 6 |

Only studies with >20 patients are included. If one amplicon was detected only in a single study with <20 tumors, the number of amplified cases is given in relation to the total number of analyzed tumors. Method of analysis: AC, array-based comparative genomic hybridization (CGH); C, CGH; F, fluorescence in situ hybridization (FISH); K, karyotyping; P, polymerase chain reaction (PCR); RT-PCR, reverse transcriptase PCR; S, Southern blotting.
* Definition of amplification is not consistent between studies.

No FGFR3 mutations have been found in CIS.[98] All mutations described are missense mutations located in exons 7, 10, or 15 that have been previously described as germline mutations in skeletal dysplasia syndromes.[35,98,103] These mutations are predicted to cause constitutive activation of the receptor. In one study, mutations have been linked to a lower risk of recurrence, indicating that this genetic event may identify a group of patients with favorable disease course.[99]

## Her2/neu

Her2/neu is a transmembrane receptor tyrosine kinase without a known ligand. Its activation occurs through interaction with other members of the epidermal growth factor receptor (EGFR) gene family. HER2 has regained considerable interest because the protein is the molecular target of trastuzumab (Herceptin) therapy in breast cancer. HER2 is amplified in 7% to 20% and overexpressed in 10% to 70% of invasively growing bladder cancers.[3,7,24,58,75–77,104–108] This makes bladder cancer the tumor entity with the highest frequency of HER2 overexpression. In contrast to bladder cancer, where HER2 overexpression is almost always due to gene amplification, the majority of HER2-positive cancers do not seem to be amplified. However, large studies using Food and Drug Administration-approved reagents that yield results which are comparable to breast cancer studies are still lacking. Amplifications or deletions of the adjacent topoisomerase 2 alpha (TOP2A) are present in about 23% of HER2 amplified cases.[77] TOP2A is the target of anthracyclines. Thus, the anatomy of the 17q23 amplicon may also influence the response to cytotoxic therapy regimens.

The epidermal growth factor receptor (EGFR) is another member of the class II receptor family. EGFR is a transmembrane tyrosine kinase acting as a receptor for several ligands including epidermal growth factor (EGF) and transforming growth factor-α (TGFα). EGFR also serves as a therapeutic target for several drugs including small inhibitory molecules and antibodies. EGFR is amplified in 3% to 5% and overexpressed in 30% to 50% of invasively growing bladder cancers.[2,47,58,109,110] It is currently unclear whether exon 18–21 mutations, known to be predictive for response to gefitinib in lung cancer,[111] also occur in bladder carcinomas.[112]

## H-ras

H-ras is the only member of the ras gene family reported to be altered in urinary bladder cancer.[113,114] Whilst the H-ras mutations are usually confined to specific alterations within codons 12, 13, and 61, a single nucleotide polymorphism at nucleoside 81T, a wobble position, is over-represented in patients with poorly differentiated tumors.[115] There are also reports of co-amplification of N- and H-ras in bladder cancer,[116] and rarely of mutated Ki-ras.[117] A recent study has suggested that H-ras has <10% frequency of mutation in bladder cancer (F.M. Waldman, personal communication). However, depending on the method of detection, H-ras mutations have been reported in up to 45% of bladder cancers, without clear-cut associations to tumor stage or grade.[116,118,119]

## CDKs

Cyclin-dependent kinases (CDKs) and their regulatory subunits, the cyclins, are important promoters of the cell cycle. The cyclin D1 gene (CCND1) located at 11q13 is one of the most frequently amplified and overexpressed oncogenes in bladder cancer. About 10% to 20% of bladder cancers show gene amplification,[4,45,47,74,120] and overexpression has been reported in 30% to 50% of tumors.[4,74,120] Some investigators found associations between CCND1 expression and tumor recurrence and progression or patient survival,[4,120] but these data were not confirmed by others.[74]

## MDM2

The MDM2 gene, located at 12q14.3–q15, codes for more than 40 different splice variants, only two of which interact with p53 and thereby inhibit its ability to activate transcription.[11,121] Conversely, the transcription of MDM2 is induced by wild-type p53.[122] In normal cells this autoregulatory feedback loop regulates p53 activity and MDM2 expression. MDM2 also promotes p53 protein degradation, making MDM2 overexpression an alternate mechanism for p53 inactivation.[123] MDM2 amplification is frequent in human sarcomas,[124] but occurs in only 1/87[125] (up to 5%[11,125]) of invasively growing bladder cancers. MDM2 amplification was unrelated to patient prognosis in one study.[125] Detectable MDM2 protein expression has been reported in 10% to 43% of bladder cancers, but there is disagreement about associations to tumor stage and grade between the studies.[125–130]

## p53

The p53 gene, located at 17p13.1, encodes a 53 kDa protein that plays a role in several cellular processes including cell cycle, response to DNA damage, cell death, and neovascularization (reviewed in Slee et al[131]). Its gene product regulates the expression of many different genes (see references in Slee et al[131]). Mutations of the p53 gene, mostly located in the central, DNA-binding portion of the gene, are a hallmark of invasively growing bladder cancers. An online query of the International Agency for Research on Cancer (IARC) database (R7 version, September 2002) at www.iarc.fr/P53/ revealed p53 mutations in 40% to 60%[132,133] of invasive bladder cancers (in studies investigating at least 30 tumors). More than 90% of mutations have been found in exons 4–9, with occasional hotspots such as codon 273.[132] Often p53 mutations can be detected immuno-histochemically since many p53 mutations lead to protein stabilization, resulting in nuclear p53 accumulation. Immunohistochemical p53 analysis has practical utility in surgical pathology. In addition to a postulated role as a prognostic marker, immunohistochemical p53 positivity is a strong argument for the presence of genetically unstable neoplasia in cases with questionable morphology.

## PTEN

The PTEN (phosphatase and tensin homology) gene, also known as MMAC1 (mutated in multiple advanced cancers) and as TEP1 (TGFβ regulated and epithelial cell-enriched phosphatase), is a candidate tumor suppressor gene located at chromosome 10q23.3.[134] The relatively high frequency (20–30%) of LOH at 10q23 in muscle-invasive bladder cancer[65,135] makes PTEN a good tumor suppressor candidate. However, the frequency of PTEN mutations is not clear at present. In three technically well-performed studies that included 35,[136] 63,[135] and 345[65] tumor samples, mutations were detected in 0%, 0.6%, and 17% of cases. A small number of cases of homozygous deletions has been described,[65,135] and it has been suggested that haploinsufficiency may be associated with lack of function. These results leave open the question of the predominant mechanism of inactivation of the second allele, or indicate that PTEN is not the (only) target gene at 10q23.

## RB

The retinoblastoma (RB) gene product was the first tumor suppressor gene to be identified in human cancer. RB, which is localized at 13q14, plays a crucial role in the regulation of the cell cycle. Inactivation of RB occurs in 30% to 80% of bladder cancers,[55,137,138] with altered staining patterns,[137,139–141] most frequently as a consequence of heterozygous 13q deletions in combination with mutation of the remaining allele.[137] A strong association has been found between RB inactivation and muscle invasion.[55,138,141,142] Some investigators reported an association between altered Rb expression and reduced patient survival.[143]

## DNA repair genes

Alterations of DNA repair genes are important for many cancer types. In invasive bladder cancer, alterations of mismatch repair genes (mutator phenotype) are rare. Whilst a study using a panel of six microsatellite markers found microsatellite instability (MSI) to be rare in bladder cancer,[144] other studies suggest that MSI is associated with more primary tumors[145] or invasive bladder cancer,[146,147] including cancers of the upper urothelial tract.[147] Reduced expression of MMR proteins was seen in 23% of 111 tumors but was not associated with MSI.[148] LOH at 16q13–q22.1 is associated with methylation of the promoter region of E-cadherin (47% of 23 TCC and 89% of 16 CIS) in high-grade rather than invasive bladder cancers.[149]

## MULTIFOCAL BLADDER NEOPLASMS

Neoplasias of the urothelium typically are not limited to one single tumor. Multifocality, frequent recurrence, and presence of barely visible, flat accompanying lesions such as hyperplasia or dysplasia are characteristic for these tumors. Morphological, cytogenetic, and immunohistochemical mapping studies of cystectomy specimens demonstrated areas of abnormal cells adjacent to grossly visible tumors.[150,151] The majority (80–90%) of multicentric bladder neoplasias are of monoclonal origin.[8,152–163] It is assumed that neoplastic cells that have originated in one area later spread out to other regions, either by active migration through the urothelium or through the urine by desquamation and reimplantation. Monoclonality seems to be especially frequent in advanced stage neoplasia.[164] However, there are also reports of polyclonal cancers, mainly in early-stage tumors or in premalignant lesions.[154,159,164–169] These observations have given rise to the 'field defect' hypothesis, suggesting that environmental mutagens may cause fields of genetically altered cells that become the source of polyclonal multifocal tumors.[150] It appears possible that selection and overgrowth of the most rapidly growing clone from an initially polyclonal neoplasia might lead to pseudoclonality in some cases of multiple bladder cancer.

Several groups have studied the genetic changes in apparently normal urothelium close to tumor sites. Precursor lesions of either invasive or non-invasive urothelial tumors include hyperplasia since the same changes in chromosomal numbers and significant chromosomal aberrations can be found in these lesions, even in the absence of dysplasia.[33] These include amplifications of 11q, 12q13, and 17, and LOH at 2q, 4, 8p, and 11p.[170] The presence of chromosomal aberrations in histologically 'normal appearing urothelium' in bladders from cancer patients suggests that genetic analysis may be superior to histology for diagnosing early neoplasia.[150–152] Genetic changes in dysplasia[30,34,171,172] are similar to alterations that are typical for CIS, including changes of different regions of chromosome 16,[173] aneuploidy of chromosome 19, and monosomy 9,[174] suggesting that at least a fraction of them can be considered CIS precursors.

## CYTOGENETIC ALTERATIONS IN NON-UROTHELIAL BLADDER CANCER

### SQUAMOUS CELL CARCINOMAS

Among non-urothelial cancers of the urinary bladder, squamous cell carcinomas—often related to schistosoma infection—have been most frequently analyzed genetically. Cytogenetic and classic molecular analyses have revealed that whilst some of the changes that occur overlap between SCC and TCC, others differ.[175] Chromosomal over-representation is seen mostly at 5p, 6p, 7p, 8q, 11q, 17q, and 20q, while deletions were most frequent at 3p, 4q, 5q, 8p, 13q, 17p, and 18q.[175-180] Squamous cell cancers showed more frequent losses of 17p and 18p than transitional cell carcinomas.[181] The rate of p53-positive tumors ranged between 30% and 90% in multiple studies (average 40%; n=135),[182,183] which is not significantly different from the findings in urothelial cancer. However, on the basis of a 73% frequency of mutant p53 expression, one study[184] suggests that schistosomal bladder SCC is an aggressive disease de novo. A separate study has shown that TP53 mutations in schistosoma included more base transitions at CpG dinucleotides than seen in urothelial carcinomas.[182] Of interest is that homozygous p16/p19 deletion, hypermethylation of the p16 promoter, or LOH on 9p21 is associated with early carcinogenesis of SCC of the bladder, and squamous metaplasia of the bladder in cancer patients has already sustained genetic changes found in cancer; genetic mosaicism occurs in cases of TCC with SCC, with the SCC component showing more frequent 9p21 alterations than the TCC component.[185]

Only a few non-schistosoma-associated SCC have been molecularly analyzed. The predominant changes were losses of 3p (2/11), 9p (2/11), and 13q (5/11) as well as gains of 1q (3/11), 8q (4/11), and 20q (4/11) in a CGH study.[180] Circumscribed high-level amplifications were reported at 8q24 (two cases) and 11q13 (one case) in this study.

## ADENOCARCINOMAS

Only a relatively small number of adenocarcinomas have been analyzed genetically, including 93 schistosoma-associated cancers[186] and 155 primary pure adenocarcinomas.[187-190] These studies found a high frequency (>80%) of aneuploidy[186,188] in urachal and non-urachal adenocarcinomas,[188] indicating that prognosis, as with urothelial carcinomas, depends on tumor stage rather than on molecular features. No significant genetic differences between adeno-carcinomas and urothelial cancers were observed in comparative studies.[10-12,77,138,176,191-193]

## SMALL CELL CARCINOMA

CGH data suggest that a small cell carcinoma of the urinary bladder is a genetically unstable tumor, typically exhibiting a high number of cytogenetic changes.[194] The most frequent changes included deletions of 10q, 4q, 5q, and 13q, as well as gains of 8q, 5p, 6p, and 20q. High-level amplifications, potentially pinpointing the location of activated oncogenes, were found at 1p22–p32, 3q26.3, 8q24 (including CMYC), and 12q14–q21 (including MDM2).[194] Only one tumor was analyzed by cytogenetics.[195] Complex and hetero-geneous cytogenetic alterations were found in this tumor, including rearrangements of chromosomes 6, 9, 11, 13, and 18. The same tumor also showed a nuclear p53 accumulation.

## CARCINOMASARCOMA

Both the carcinomatous and sarcomatous components of a carcinosarcoma of the bladder had identical LOH on 9p, 9q, 8p, and 8q, suggesting a common origin of the cancer in both types of cell. Discordant losses were confined to advanced cancer cells and thought to be associated with progression. Loss of E-cadherin expression (also observed) was thought to allow conversion of epithelial cells to a sarcomatous phenotype.[196] CGH of microdissected tissues also showed a high level of homology in the epithelial and stromal tumor components,[196] and indicated that both had some aberrations in only one tissue type, suggesting that the tumor was monoclonal in origin followed by some divergence.[197]

However, when allelic loss of various chromosomes in DNA from microdissected epithelium and stroma was evaluated to see if epithelial–stromal interactions could be involved in the pathogenesis of TCC, stromal cells from high-grade muscle-invasive TCCs showed LOH on 17p13 (29%), 3p25–p26 (61%), and 9q32–q33 (47%), but there was no concordance with LOH in adjacent tumor cells.[198] X-chromosome inactivation, assessed by analysing the methylation status of the androgen receptor, was found to be non-random.

REFERENCES

1. Sandberg AA, Berger CS. Review of chromosome studies in urological tumors. II. Cytogenetics and molecular genetics of bladder cancer. J Urol 1994;151:545–560.
2. Waldman FM, Carroll PR, Kerschmann R, Cohen MB, Field FG, Mayall BH. Centromeric copy number of chromosome 7 is strongly correlated with tumor grade and labeling index in human bladder cancer. Cancer Res 1991;51:3807–3813.
3. Kallioniemi A, Kallioniemi OP, Citro G, et al. Identification of gains and losses of DNA sequences in primary bladder cancer by comparative genomic hybridization. Genes Chromosomes Cancer 1995;12:213–219.
4. Veltman JA, Fridlyand J, Pejavar S, et al. Array-based comparative genomic hybridization for genome-wide screening of DNA copy number in bladder tumors. Cancer Res 2003;63:2872–2880.
5. Raghavan D, Shipley WU, Garnick MB, Russell PJ, Richie JP. Biology and management of bladder cancer. N Engl J Med 1990;322:1129–1138.
6. Richter J, Jiang F, Gorog JP, et al. Marked genetic differences between stage pTa and stage pT1 papillary bladder cancer detected by comparative genomic hybridization. Cancer Res 1997;57:2860–2864.
7. Simon R, Burger H, Brinkschmidt C, Bocker W, Hertle L, Terpe HJ. Chromosomal aberrations associated with invasion in papillary superficial bladder cancer. J Pathol 1998;185:345–351.
8. Takahashi T, Habuchi T, Kakehi Y, et al. Clonal and chronological genetic analysis of multifocal cancers of the bladder and upper urinary tract. Cancer Res 1998;58:5835–5841.

9. Zhao J, Richter J, Wagner U, et al. Chromosomal imbalances in noninvasive papillary bladder neoplasms (pTa). Cancer Res 1999;59:4658–4661.

10. Richter J, Wagner U, Kononen J, et al. High-throughput tissue microarray analysis of cyclin E gene amplification and overexpression in urinary bladder cancer. Am J Pathol 2000;157:787–794.

11. Simon R, Struckmann K, Schraml P, et al. Amplification pattern of 12q13–q15 genes (MDM2, CDK4, GLI) in urinary bladder cancer. Oncogene 2002;21:2476–2483.

12. Simon R, Richter J, Wagner U, et al. High-throughput tissue microarray analysis of 3p25 (RAF1) and 8p12 (FGFR1) copy number alterations in urinary bladder cancer. Cancer Res 2001;61:4514–4519.

13. Fujimoto K, Yamada Y, Okajima E, et al. Frequent association of p53 gene mutation in invasive bladder cancer. Cancer Res 1992;52:1393–1398.

14. Pfister C, Flaman JM, Martin C, Grise P, Frebourg T. Selective detection of inactivating mutations of the tumor suppressor gene p53 in bladder tumors. J Urol 1999;161:1973–1975.

15. Miyamoto H, Kubota Y, Shuin T, et al. Analyses of p53 gene mutations in primary human bladder cancer. Oncol Res 1993;5:245–249.

16. Zhang FF, Arber DA, Wilson TG, Kawachi MH, Slovak ML. Toward the validation of aneusomy detection by fluorescence in situ hybridization in bladder cancer: comparative analysis with cytology, cytogenetics, and clinical features predicts recurrence and defines clinical testing limitations. Clin Cancer Res 1997;3:2317–2328.

17. Sauter G, Gasser TC, Moch H, et al. DNA aberrations in urinary bladder cancer detected by flow cytometry and FISH. Urol Res 1997;25(Suppl 1):S37–43.

18. Tetu B, Allard P, Fradet Y, Roberge N, Bernard P. Prognostic significance of nuclear DNA content and S-phase fraction by flow cytometry in primary papillary superficial bladder cancer. Hum Pathol 1996;27:922–926.

19. Spruck CH 3rd, Rideout WM 3rd, Olumi AF, et al. Distinct pattern of p53 mutations in bladder cancer: relationship to tobacco usage. Cancer Res 1993;53:1162–1166.

20. Cordon-Cardo C, Dalbagni G, Saez GT, et al. p53 mutations in human bladder cancer: genotypic versus phenotypic patterns. Int J Cancer 1994;56:347–353.

21. Nouri AM, Darakhshan F, Cannell H, Paris AM, Oliver RT. The relevance of p53 mutation in urological malignancies: possible clinical implications for bladder cancer. Br J Urol 1996;78:337–344.

22. Kusser WC, Miao X, Glickman BW, et al. p53 mutations in human bladder cancer. Environ Mol Mutagen 1994;24:156–160.

23. Richter J, Beffa L, Wagner U, et al. Patterns of chromosomal imbalances in advanced urinary bladder cancer detected by comparative genomic hybridization. Am J Pathol 1998;153:1615–1621.

24. Simon R, Burger H, Semjonow A, Hertle L, Terpe HJ, Bocker W. Patterns of chromosomal imbalances in muscle invasive bladder cancer. Int J Oncol 2000;17:1025–1029.

25. Richter J, Wagner U, Schraml P, et al. Chromosomal imbalances are associated with a high risk of progression in early invasive (pT1) urinary bladder cancer. Cancer Res 1999;59:5687–5691.

26. Schaffer AA, Simon R, Desper R, Richter J, Sauter G. Tree models for dependent copy number changes in bladder cancer. Int J Oncol 2001;18:349–354.

27. Bohm M, Kleine-Besten R, Wieland I. Loss of heterozygosity analysis on chromosome 5p defines 5p13–12 as the critical region involved in tumor progression of bladder carcinomas. Int J Cancer 2000;89:194–197.

28. Hoglund M, Sall T, Heim S, Mitelman F, Mandahl N, Fadl-Elmula I. Identification of cytogenetic subgroups and karyotypic pathways in transitional cell carcinoma. Cancer Res 2001;61:8241–8246.

29. Rosin MP, Cairns P, Epstein JI, Schoenberg MP, Sidransky D. Partial allelotype of carcinoma in situ of the human bladder. Cancer Res 1995;55:5213–5216.

30. Hartmann A, Schlake G, Zaak D, et al. Occurrence of chromosome 9 and p53 alterations in multifocal dysplasia and carcinoma in situ of human urinary bladder. Cancer Res 2002;62:809–818.

31. Koss LG. Natural history and patterns of invasive cancer of the bladder. Eur Urol 1998;33(Suppl 4):2–4.

32. Higashi S, Habuchi T, Takahashi T, et al. Allelic imbalances on chromosome 20 in human transitional cell carcinoma. Jpn J Cancer Res 2000;91:499–503.

33. Hartmann A, Moser K, Kriegmair M, Hofstetter A, Hofstaedter F, Knuechel R. Frequent genetic alterations in simple urothelial hyperplasias of the bladder in patients with papillary urothelial carcinoma. Am J Pathol 1999;154:721–727.

34. Steidl C, Simon R, Burger H, et al. Patterns of chromosomal aberrations in urinary bladder tumours and adjacent urothelium. J Pathol 2002;198.115–120.

35. Cappellen D, De Oliveira C, Ricol D, et al. Frequent activating mutations of FGFR3 in human bladder and cervix carcinomas. Nat Genet 1999;23:18–20.

36. Powell I, Tyrkus M, Kleer E. Apparent correlation of sex chromosome loss and disease course in urothelial cancer. Cancer Genet Cytogenet 1990;50:97–101.

37. Sauter G, Moch H, Wagner U, et al. Y chromosome loss detected by FISH in bladder cancer. Cancer Genet Cytogenet 1995;82:163–169.

38. Hopman AH, Kamps MA, Speel EJ, Schapers RF, Sauter G, Ramaekers FC. Identification of chromosome 9 alterations and p53 accumulation in isolated carcinoma in situ of the urinary bladder versus carcinoma in situ associated with carcinoma. Am J Pathol 2002;161:1119–1125.

39. Friedrich MG, Toma MI, Hellstern A, et al. Comparison of multitarget fluorescence in situ hybridization in urine with other noninvasive tests for detecting bladder cancer. BJU Int 2003;92:911–914.

40. Veeramachaneni R, Nordberg ML, Shi R, Herrera GA, Turbat-Herrera EA. Evaluation of fluorescence in situ hybridization as an ancillary tool to urine cytology in diagnosing urothelial carcinoma. Diagn Cytopathol 2003;28:301–307.

41. Uchida A, Tachibana M, Miyakawa A, Nakamura K, Murai M. Microsatellite analysis in multiple chromosomal regions as a prognostic indicator of primary bladder cancer. Urol Res 2000;28:297–303.

42. Eleuteri P, Grollino MG, Pomponi D, De Vita R. Chromosome 9 aberrations by fluorescence in situ hybridisation in bladder transitional cell carcinoma. Eur J Cancer 2001;37:1496–1503.

43. Vanni R, Scarpa RM, Nieddu M, Usai E. Cytogenetic investigation on 30 bladder carcinomas. Cancer Genet Cytogenet 1988;30:35–42.

44. Smeets W, Pauwels R, Laarakkers L, Debruyne F, Geraedts J. Chromosomal analysis of bladder cancer. III. Nonrandom alterations. Cancer Genet Cytogenet 1987;29:29–41.

45. Gibas Z, Griffin CA, Emanuel BS. Trisomy 7 and i(5p) in a transitional cell carcinoma of the ureter. Cancer Genet Cytogenet 1987;25:369–370.

46. Atkin NB, Fox MF. 5q deletion. The sole chromosome change in a carcinoma of the bladder. Cancer Genet Cytogenet 1990;46:129–131.

47. Atkin NB, Baker MC. Cytogenetic study of ten carcinomas of the bladder: involvement of chromosomes 1 and 11. Cancer Genet Cytogenet 1985;15:253–268.

48. Babu VR, Lutz MD, Miles BJ, Farah RN, Weiss L, Van Dyke DL. Tumor behavior in transitional cell carcinoma of the bladder in relation to chromosomal markers and histopathology. Cancer Res 1987;47:6800–6805.

49. Atkin NB, Baker MC. Numerical chromosome changes in 165 malignant tumors. Evidence for a nonrandom distribution of normal chromosomes. Cancer Genet Cytogenet 1991;52:113–121.

50. Gibas Z, Prout GR, Pontes JE, Connolly JG, Sandberg AA. A possible specific chromosome change in transitional cell carcinoma of the bladder. Cancer Genet Cytogenet 1986;19:229–238.

51. Pauwels RP, Smeets AW, Schapers RF, Geraedts JP, Debruyne FM. Grading in superficial bladder cancer (2). Cytogenetic classification. Br J Urol 1988;61:135–139.

52. Trent JM, Stanisic T, Olson S. Cytogenetic analysis of urologic malignancies: study of tumor colony forming cells and premature chromosome condensation. J Urol 1984;131:146–151.

53. Gibas Z, Prout GR Jr, Connolly JG, Pontes JE, Sandberg AA. Nonrandom chromosomal changes in transitional cell carcinoma of the bladder. Cancer Res 1984;44:1257–1264.

54. Voorter C, Joos S, Bringuier PP, et al. Detection of chromosomal imbalances in transitional cell carcinoma of the bladder by

comparative genomic hybridization. Am J Pathol 1995;146:1341–1354.

55. Wada T, Louhelainen J, Hemminki K, et al. Bladder cancer: allelic deletions at and around the retinoblastoma tumor suppressor gene in relation to stage and grade. Clin Cancer Res 2000;6:610–615.

56. Chang WY, Cairns P, Schoenberg MP, Polascik TJ, Sidransky D. Novel suppressor loci on chromosome 14q in primary bladder cancer. Cancer Res 1995;55:3246–3249.

57. Hovey RM, Chu L, Balazs M, et al. Genetic alterations in primary bladder cancers and their metastases. Cancer Res 1998;58:3555–3560.

58. Fadl-Elmula I, Kytola S, Pan Y, et al. Characterization of chromosomal abnormalities in uroepithelial carcinomas by G-banding, spectral karyotyping and FISH analysis. Int J Cancer 2001;92:824–831.

59. Cairns P, Shaw ME, Knowles MA. Initiation of bladder cancer may involve deletion of a tumour-suppressor gene on chromosome 9. Oncogene 1993;8:1083–1085.

60. Choi C, Kim MH, Juhng SW, Oh BR. Loss of heterozygosity at chromosome segments 8p22 and 8p11.2–21.1 in transitional-cell carcinoma of the urinary bladder. Int J Cancer 2000;86:501–505.

61. Koo SH, Kwon KC, Ihm CH, Jeon YM, Park JW, Sul CK. Detection of genetic alterations in bladder tumors by comparative genomic hybridization and cytogenetic analysis. Cancer Genet Cytogenet 1999;110:87–93.

62. Habuchi T, Devlin J, Elder PA, Knowles MA. Detailed deletion mapping of chromosome 9q in bladder cancer: evidence for two tumour suppressor loci. Oncogene 1995;11:1671–1674.

63. Simoneau AR, Spruck CH 3rd, Gonzalez-Zulueta M, et al. Evidence for two tumor suppressor loci associated with proximal chromosome 9p to q and distal chromosome 9q in bladder cancer and the initial screening for GAS1 and PTC mutations. Cancer Res 1996;56:5039–5043.

64. Kagan J, Liu J, Stein JD, et al. Cluster of allele losses within a 2.5 cM region of chromosome 10 in high-grade invasive bladder cancer. Oncogene 1998;16:909–913.

65. Cairns P, Evron E, Okami K, et al. Point mutation and homozygous deletion of PTEN/MMAC1 in primary bladder cancers. Oncogene 1998;16:3215–3218.

66. Natrajan R, Louhelainen J, Williams S, Laye J, Knowles MA. High-resolution deletion mapping of 15q13.2–q21.1 in transitional cell carcinoma of the bladder. Cancer Res 2003;63:7657–7662.

67. Meza-Zepeda LA, Forus A, Lygren B, et al. Positional cloning identifies a novel cyclophilin as a candidate amplified oncogene in 1q21. Oncogene 2002;21:2261–2269.

68. Huang WC, Taylor S, Nguyen TB, et al. KIAA1096, a gene on chromosome 1q, is amplified and overexpressed in bladder cancer. DNA Cell Biol 2002;21:707–715.

69. Evans AJ, Gallie BL, Jewett MA, et al. Defining a 0.5-mb region of genomic gain on chromosome 6p22 in bladder cancer by quantitative-multiplex polymerase chain reaction. Am J Pathol 2004;164:285–293.

70. Oeggerli M, Tomovska S, Schraml P, et al. E2F3 amplification and overexpression is associated with invasive tumor growth and rapid tumor cell proliferation in urinary bladder cancer. Oncogene 2004;23(33):5616–5623.

71. Wagner U, Bubendorf L, Gasser TC, et al. Chromosome 8p deletions are associated with invasive tumor growth in urinary bladder cancer. Am J Pathol 1997;151:753–759.

72. Sauter G, Moch H, Carroll P, Kerschmann R, Mihatsch MJ, Waldman FM. Chromosome-9 loss detected by fluorescence in situ hybridization in bladder cancer. Int J Cancer 1995;64:99–103.

73. Paris MJ, Williams BR. Characterization of a 500-kb contig spanning the region between c-Ha-Ras and MUC2 on chromosome 11p15.5. Genomics 2000;69:196–202.

74. Zaharieva BM, Simon R, Diener PA, et al. High-throughput tissue microarray analysis of 11q13 gene amplification (CCND1, FGF3, FGF4, EMS1) in urinary bladder cancer. J Pathol 2003;201:603–608.

75. Ohta JI, Miyoshi Y, Uemura H, et al. Fluorescence in situ hybridization evaluation of c-erbB-2 gene amplification and chromosomal anomalies in bladder cancer. Clin Cancer Res 2001;7:2463–2467.

76. Latif Z, Watters AD, Dunn I, Grigor KM, Underwood MA, Bartlett JM. HER2/neu overexpression in the development of muscle-invasive transitional cell carcinoma of the bladder. Br J Cancer 2003;89:1305–1309.

77. Simon R, Atefy R, Wagner U, et al. HER-2 and TOP2A coamplification in urinary bladder cancer. Int J Cancer 2003;107:764–772.

78. Guo Z, Linn JF, Wu G, et al. CDC91L1 (PIG-U) is a newly discovered oncogene in human bladder cancer. Nat Med 2004;10:374–381.

79. Hurst CD, Fiegler H, Carr P, Williams S, Carter NP, Knowles MA. High-resolution analysis of genomic copy number alterations in bladder cancer by microarray-based comparative genomic hybridization. Oncogene 2004;23:2250–2263.

80. Habuchi T, Ogawa O, Kakehi Y, et al. Accumulated allelic losses in the development of invasive urothelial cancer. Int J Cancer 1993;53:579–584.

81. Tsai YC, Nichols PW, Hiti AL, Williams Z, Skinner DG, Jones PA. Allelic losses of chromosomes 9, 11, and 17 in human bladder cancer. Cancer Res 1990;50:44–47.

82. Keen AJ, Knowles MA. Definition of two regions of deletion on chromosome 9 in carcinoma of the bladder. Oncogene 1994;9:2083–2088.

83. Louhelainen J, Wijkstrom H, Hemminki K. Initiation-development modelling of allelic losses on chromosome 9 in multifocal bladder cancer. Eur J Cancer 2000;36:1441–1451.

84. Cairns JP, Chiang PW, Ramamoorthy S, Kurnit DM, Sidransky D. A comparison between microsatellite and quantitative PCR analyses to detect frequent p16 copy number changes in primary bladder tumors. Clin Cancer Res 1998;4:441–444.

85. Baud E, Catilina P, Bignon YJ. p16 involvement in primary bladder tumors: analysis of deletions and mutations. Int J Oncol 1999;14:441–445.

86. Florl AR, Schulz WA. Peculiar structure and location of 9p21 homozygous deletion breakpoints in human cancer cells. Genes Chromosomes Cancer 2003;37:141–148.

87. Balazs M, Carroll P, Kerschmann R, Sauter G, Waldman FM. Frequent homozygous deletion of cyclin-dependent kinase inhibitor 2 (MTS1, p16) in superficial bladder cancer detected by fluorescence in situ hybridization. Genes Chromosomes Cancer 1997;19:84–89.

88. Habuchi T, Yoshida O, Knowles MA. A novel candidate tumour suppressor locus at 9q32–33 in bladder cancer: localization of the candidate region within a single 840 kb YAC. Hum Mol Genet 1997;6:913–919.

89. Orlow I, Lacombe L, Hannon GJ, et al. Deletion of the p16 and p15 genes in human bladder tumors. J Natl Cancer Inst 1995;87:1524–1529.

90. Habuchi T, Luscombe M, Elder PA, Knowles MA. Structure and methylation-based silencing of a gene (DBCCR1) within a candidate bladder cancer tumor suppressor region at 9q32–q33. Genomics 1998;48:277–288.

91. Nishiyama H, Gill JH, Pitt E, Kennedy W, Knowles MA. Negative regulation of G(1)/S transition by the candidate bladder tumour suppressor gene DBCCR1. Oncogene 2001;20:2956–2964.

92. Stadler WM, Steinberg G, Yang X, Hagos F, Turner C, Olopade OI. Alterations of the 9p21 and 9q33 chromosomal bands in clinical bladder cancer specimens by fluorescence in situ hybridization. Clin Cancer Res 2001;7:1676–1682.

93. Habuchi T, Takahashi T, Kakinuma H, et al. Hypermethylation at 9q32–33 tumour suppressor region is age-related in normal urothelium and an early and frequent alteration in bladder cancer. Oncogene 2001;20:531–537.

94. Williams SV, Sibley KD, Davies AM, et al. Molecular genetic analysis of chromosome 9 candidate tumor-suppressor loci in bladder cancer cell lines. Genes Chromosomes Cancer 2002;34:86–96.

95. Aboulkassim TO, LaRue H, Lemieux P, Rousseau FYF. Alteration of the PATCHED locus in superficial bladder cancer. Oncogene 2003;22:2967–2971.

96. Knowles MA, Habuchi T, Kennedy W, Cuthbert-Heavens D. Mutation spectrum of the 9q34 tuberous sclerosis gene TSC1 in transitional cell carcinoma of the bladder. Cancer Res 2003;63:7652–7656.

97. van Tilborg AA, de Vries A, Zwarthoff EC. The chromosome 9q genes TGFBR1, TSC1, and ZNF189 are rarely mutated in bladder cancer. J Pathol 2001;194:76–80.

98. Sibley K, Cuthbert-Heavens D, Knowles MA. Loss of heterozygosity at 4p16.3 and mutation of FGFR3 in transitional cell carcinoma. Oncogene 2001;20:686–691.

99. van Rhijn BW, Lurkin I, Radvanyi F, Kirkels WJ, van der Kwast TH, Zwarthoff EC. The fibroblast growth factor receptor 3 (FGFR3) mutation is a strong indicator of superficial bladder cancer with low recurrence rate. Cancer Res 2001;61:1265–1268.

100. van Rhijn BW, Montironi R, Zwarthoff EC, Jobsis AC, van der Kwast TH. Frequent FGFR3 mutations in urothelial papilloma. J Pathol 2002;198:245–251.

101. Bakkar AA, Wallerand H, Radvanyi F, et al. FGFR3 and TP53 gene mutations define two distinct pathways in urothelial cell carcinoma of the bladder. Cancer Res 2003;63:8108–8112.

102. van Rhijn BW, van der Kwast TH, Vis AN, et al. FGFR3 and P53 characterize alternative genetic pathways in the pathogenesis of urothelial cell carcinoma. Cancer Res 2004;64:1911–1914.

103. Billerey C, Chopin D, Aubriot-Lorton MH, et al. Frequent FGFR3 mutations in papillary non-invasive bladder (pTa) tumors. Am J Pathol 2001;158:1955–1959.

104. Moch H, Sauter G, Mihatsch MJ, Gudat F, Epper R, Waldman FM. p53 but not erbB-2 expression is associated with rapid tumor proliferation in urinary bladder cancer. Hum Pathol 1994;25:1346–1351.

105. Moch H, Sauter G, Moore D, Mihatsch MJ, Gudat F, Waldman F. p53 and erbB-2 protein overexpression are associated with early invasion and metastasis in bladder cancer. Virchows Archiv 1993;423:329–334.

106. Gorgoulis VG, Barbatis C, Poulias I, Karameris AM. Molecular and immunohistochemical evaluation of epidermal growth factor receptor and c-erb-B-2 gene product in transitional cell carcinomas of the urinary bladder: a study in Greek patients. Mod Pathol 1995;8:758–764.

107. Coombs LM, Pigott DA, Sweeney E, et al. Amplification and over-expression of c-erbB-2 in transitional cell carcinoma of the urinary bladder. Br J Cancer 1991;63:601–608.

108. Sauter G, Moch H, Moore D, et al. Heterogeneity of erbB-2 gene amplification in bladder cancer. Cancer Res 1993;53:2199–2203.

109. Wagner U, Sauter G, Moch H, et al. Patterns of p53, erbB-2, and EGF-r expression in premalignant lesions of the urinary bladder. Hum Pathol 1995;26:970–978.

110. Cardillo MR, Castagna G, Memeo L, De Bernardinis E, Di Silverio F. Epidermal growth factor receptor, MUC-1 and MUC-2 in bladder cancer. J Exp Clin Cancer Res 2000;19:225–233.

111. Lynch TJ, Bell DW, Sordella R, et al. Activating mutations in the epidermal growth factor receptor underlying responsiveness of non-small-cell lung cancer to gefitinib [see comment]. N Engl J Med 2004;350:2129–2139.

112. Nutt JE, Lazarowicz HP, Mellon JK, Lunec J. Gefitinib ('Iressa', ZD1839) inhibits the growth response of bladder tumour cell lines to epidermal growth factor and induces TIMP2. Br J Cancer 2004;90:1679–1685.

113. Viola MV, Fromowitz F, Oravez S, Deb S, Schlom J. ras Oncogene p21 expression is increased in premalignant lesions and high grade bladder carcinoma. J Exp Med 1985;161:1213–1218.

114. Shinohara N, Koyanagi T. Ras signal transduction in carcinogenesis and progression of bladder cancer: molecular target for treatment? Urol Res 2002;30:273–281.

115. Johne A, Roots I, Brockmoller J. A single nucleotide polymorphism in the human H-ras proto-oncogene determines the risk of urinary bladder cancer. Cancer Epidemiol Biomarkers Prev 2003;12:68–70.

116. Vageli D, Kiaris H, Delakas D, Anezinis P, Cranidis A, Spandidos DA. Transcriptional activation of H-ras, K-ras and N-ras proto-oncogenes in human bladder tumors. Cancer Lett 1996;107:241–247.

117. Grimmond SM, Raghavan D, Russell PJ. Detection of a rare point mutation in Ki-ras of a human bladder cancer xenograft by polymerase chain reaction and direct sequencing. Urol Res 1992;20:121–126.

118. Oxford G, Theodorescu D. The role of Ras superfamily proteins in bladder cancer progression. J Urol 2003;170:1987–1993.

119. Bittard H, Descotes F, Billerey C, Lamy B, Adessi GR. A genotype study of the c-Ha-ras-1 locus in human bladder tumors. J Urol 1996;155:1083–1088.

120. Watters AD, Latif Z, Forsyth A, et al. Genetic aberrations of c-myc and CCND1 in the development of invasive bladder cancer. Br J Cancer 2002;87:654–658.

121. Sturzenhofecker B, Schlott T, Quentin T, Kube D, Jung W, Trumper L. Abundant expression of spliced HDM2 in Hodgkin lymphoma cells does not interfere with p14(ARF) and p53 binding. Leukemia Lymphoma 2003;44:1587–1596.

122. Chang CJ, Freeman DJ, Wu H. PTEN regulates Mdm2 expression through the P1 promoter. J Biol Chem 2004;279(28):29841–29848.

123. Stommel JM, Wahl GM. Accelerated MDM2 auto-degradation induced by DNA-damaged kinases is required for p53 activation. EMBO J 2004;23:15547–15556.

124. Oliner JD, Kinzler KW, Meltzer PS, George DL, Vogelstein B. Amplification of a gene encoding a p53-associated protein in human sarcomas [see comment]. Nature 1992;358:80–83.

125. Lianes P, Orlow I, Zhang ZF, et al. Altered patterns of MDM2 and TP53 expression in human bladder cancer. J Natl Cancer Inst 1994;86:1325–1330.

126. Barbareschi M, Girlando S, Fellin G, Graffer U, Luciani L, Dalla Palma P. Expression of mdm-2 and p53 protein in transitional cell carcinoma. Urol Res 1995;22:349–352.

127. Schmitz-Drager BJ, Kushima M, Goebell P, et al. p53 and MDM2 in the development and progression of bladder cancer. Eur Urol 1997;32:487–493.

128. Korkolopoulou P, Christodoulou P, Kapralos P, et al. The role of p53, MDM2 and c-erbB2 oncoproteins, epidermal growth factor receptor and proliferation markers in the prognosis of urinary bladder cancer. Pathol Res Pract 1997;193:767–775.

129. El-Kenawy Ael M, El-Kott AF, Khalil AM. Prognostic value of p53 and MDM2 expression in bilharziasis-associated squamous cell carcinoma of the urinary bladder. Int J Biol Markers 2003;18:284–289.

130. Uchida T, Minei S, Gao JP, Wang C, Satoh T, Baba S. Clinical significance of p53, MDM2 and bcl-2 expression in transitional cell carcinoma of the bladder. Oncol Rep 2002;9:253–259.

131. Slee EA, O'Connor DJ, Lu X. To die or not to die: how does p53 decide? Oncogene 2004;23:2809–2818.

132. Moore LE, Smith AH, Eng C, et al. P53 alterations in bladder tumors from arsenic and tobacco exposed patients. Carcinogenesis 2003;24:1785–1791.

133. Husgafvel-Pursiainen K, Kannio A. Cigarette smoking and p53 mutations in lung cancer and bladder cancer. Environ Health Perspect 1996;104(Suppl 3):553–556.

134. Liu J, Babaian DC, Liebert M, Steck PA, Kagan J. Inactivation of MMAC1 in bladder transitional-cell carcinoma cell lines and specimens. Mol Carcinog 2000;29:143–150.

135. Aveyard JS, Skilleter A, Habuchi T, Knowles MA. Somatic mutation of PTEN in bladder carcinoma. Br J Cancer 1999;80:904–908.

136. Wang DS, Rieger-Christ K, Latini JM, et al. Molecular analysis of PTEN and MXI1 in primary bladder carcinoma. Int J Cancer 2000;88:620–625.

137. Miyamoto H, Shuin T, Torigoe S, Iwasaki Y, Kubota Y. Retinoblastoma gene mutations in primary human bladder cancer. Br J Cancer 1995;71:831–835.

138. Cairns P, Proctor AJ, Knowles MA. Loss of heterozygosity at the RB locus is frequent and correlates with muscle invasion in bladder carcinoma. Oncogene 1991;6:2305–2309.

139. Jahnson S, Karlsson MG. Predictive value of p53 and pRb immunostaining in locally advanced bladder cancer treated with cystectomy. J Urol 1998;160:1291–1296.

140. Pollack A, Wu CS, Czerniak B, Zagars GK, Benedict WF, McDonnell TJ. Abnormal bcl-2 and pRb expression are independent correlates of radiation response in muscle-invasive bladder cancer. Clin Cancer Res 1997;3:1823–1829.

141. Tzai TS, Tsai YS, Chow NH. The prevalence and clinicopathologic correlate of p16INK4a, retinoblastoma and p53 immunoreactivity in locally advanced urinary bladder cancer. Urol Oncol 2004;22:112–118.

142. Chatterjee SJ, Datar R, Youssefzadeh D, et al. Combined effects of p53, p21, and pRb expression in the progression of bladder transitional cell carcinoma. J Clin Oncol 2004;22:1007–1013.

143. Shariat SF, Tokunaga H, Zhou J, et al. p53, p21, pRB and p16 expression predict clinical outcome in cystectomy with bladder cancer. J Clin Oncol 2004;22:1014–1024.

144. Bonnal C, Ravery V, Toublanc M, et al. Absence of microsatellite instability in transitional cell carcinoma of the bladder. Urology 2000;55:287–291.

145. Furihata M, Shuin T, Takeuchi T, et al. Missense mutation of the hMSH6 and p53 genes in sporadic urothelial transitional cell carcinoma. Int J Oncol 2000;16:491–496.

146. Thykjaer T, Christensen M, Clark AB, Hansen LR, Kunkel TA, Orntoft TF. Functional analysis of the mismatch repair system in bladder cancer. Br J Cancer 2001;85:568–575.

147. Amira N, Rivet J, Soliman H, et al. Microsatellite instability in urothelial carcinoma of the upper urinary tract. J Urol 2003;170:1151–1154.

148. Catto JW, Xinarianos G, Burton JL, Meuth M, Hamdy FC. Differential expression of hMLH1 and hMSH2 is related to bladder cancer grade, stage and prognosis but not microsatellite instability. Int J Cancer 2003;105:484–490.

149. Horikawa Y, Sugano K, Shigyo M, et al. Hypermethylation of an E-cadherin (CDH1) promoter region in high grade transitional cell carcinoma of the bladder comprising carcinoma in situ. J Urol 2003;169:1541–1545.

150. Koss LG. Mapping of the urinary bladder: its impact on the concepts of bladder cancer. Hum Pathol 1979;10:533–548.

151. Igawa M, Urakami S, Shirakawa H, et al. A mapping of histology and cell proliferation in human bladder cancer: an immunohistochemical study. Hiroshima J Med Sci 1995;44:93–97.

152. Sidransky D, Frost P, Von Eschenbach A, Oyasu R, Preisinger AC, Vogelstein B. Clonal origin of bladder cancer. N Engl J Med 1992;326:737–740.

153. Habuchi T, Takahashi R, Yamada H, Kakehi Y, Sugiyama T, Yoshida O. Metachronous multifocal development of urothelial cancers by intraluminal seeding. Lancet 1993;342:1087–1088.

154. Miyao N, Tsai YC, Lerner SP, et al. Role of chromosome 9 in human bladder cancer. Cancer Res 1993;53:4066–4070.

155. Xu X, Stower MJ, Reid IN, Garner RC, Burns PA. Molecular screening of multifocal transitional cell carcinoma of the bladder using p53 mutations as biomarkers. Clin Cancer Res 1996;2:1795–1800.

156. Chern HD, Becich MJ, Persad RA, et al. Clonal analysis of human recurrent superficial bladder cancer by immunohistochemistry of P53 and retinoblastoma proteins. J Urol 1996;156:1846–1849.

157. Li M, Cannizzaro LA. Identical clonal origin of synchronous and metachronous low-grade, noninvasive papillary transitional cell carcinomas of the urinary tract. Hum Pathol 1999;30:1197–1200.

158. Fadl-Elmula I, Gorunova L, Mandahl N, et al. Cytogenetic monoclonality in multifocal uroepithelial carcinomas: evidence of intraluminal tumour seeding. Br J Cancer 1999;81:6–12.

159. Hartmann A, Rosner U, Schlake G, et al. Clonality and genetic divergence in multifocal low-grade superficial urothelial carcinoma as determined by chromosome 9 and p53 deletion analysis. Lab Invest 2000;80:709–718.

160. Louhelainen J, Wijkstrom H, Hemminki K. Allelic losses demonstrate monoclonality of multifocal bladder tumors. Int J Cancer 2000;87:522–527.

161. Simon R, Eltze E, Schafer KL, et al. Cytogenetic analysis of multifocal bladder cancer supports a monoclonal origin and intraepithelial spread of tumor cells. Cancer Res 2001;61:355–362.

162. Takahashi T, Habuchi T, Kakehi Y, et al. Molecular diagnosis of metastatic origin in a patient with metachronous multiple cancers of the renal pelvis and bladder. Urology 2000;56:331.

163. Dalbagni G, Ren ZP, Herr H, Cordon-Cardo C, Reuter V. Genetic alterations in tp53 in recurrent urothelial cancer: a longitudinal study. Clin Cancer Res 2001;7:2797–2801.

164. Hafner C, Knuechel R, Stoehr R, Hartmann A. Clonality of multifocal urothelial carcinomas: 10 years of molecular genetic studies. Int J Cancer 2002;101:1–6.

165. Hafner C, Knuechel R, Zanardo L, et al. Evidence for oligoclonality and tumor spread by intraluminal seeding in multifocal urothelial carcinomas of the upper and lower urinary tract. Oncogene 2001;20:4910–4915.

166. Petersen I, Ohgaki H, Ludeke BI, Kleihues P. p53 mutations in phenacetin-associated human urothelial carcinomas. Carcinogenesis 1993;14:2119–2122.

167. Spruck CH 3rd, Ohneseit PF, Gonzalez-Zulueta M, et al. Two molecular pathways to transitional cell carcinoma of the bladder. Cancer Res 1994;54:784–788.

168. Yoshimura I, Kudoh J, Saito S, Tazaki H, Shimizu N. p53 gene mutation in recurrent superficial bladder cancer. J Urol 1995;153:1711–1715.

169. Goto K, Konomoto T, Hayashi K, et al. p53 mutations in multiple urothelial carcinomas: a molecular analysis of the development of multiple carcinomas. Mod Pathol 1997;10:428–437.

170. Obermann EC, Junker K, Stoehr R, et al. Frequent genetic alterations in flat urothelial hyperplasias and concomitant papillary bladder cancer as detected by CGH, LOH, and FISH analyses. J Pathol 2003;199:50–57.

171. Shirahama T. Cyclooxygenase-2 expression is up-regulated in transitional cell carcinoma and its preneoplastic lesions in the human urinary bladder. Clin Cancer Res 2000;6:2424–2430.

172. Li B, Kanamaru H, Noriki S, Yamaguchi T, Fukuda M, Okada K. Reciprocal expression of bcl-2 and p53 oncoproteins in urothelial dysplasia and carcinoma of the urinary bladder. Urol Res 1998;26:235–241.

173. Yoon DS, Li L, Zhang RD, et al. Genetic mapping and DNA sequence-based analysis of deleted regions on chromosome 16 involved in progression of bladder cancer from occult preneoplastic conditions to invasive disease. Oncogene 2001;20:5005–5014.

174. Krause Sfeil G, Beiter T, Pressler H, Schrott KM, Bichler KH. Examination of tumorigenesis of precursor lesions in bladder cancer by in situ hybridisation. Urol Int 2004;72:118–122.

175. Fadl-Elmula I, Gorunova L, Lundgren R, et al. Chromosomal abnormalities in two bladder carcinomas with secondary squamous cell differentiation. Cancer Genet Cytogenet 1998;102:125–130.

176. Shaw ME, Elder PA, Abbas A, Knowles MA. Partial allelotype of schistosomiasis-associated bladder cancer. Int J Cancer 1999;80:656–661.

177. Pycha A, Mian C, Posch B, et al. Numerical chromosomal aberrations in muscle invasive squamous cell and transitional cell cancer of the urinary bladder: an alternative to classic prognostic indicators? Urology 1999;53:1005–1010.

178. Khaled HM, Aly MS, Magrath IT. Loss of Y chromosome in bilharzial bladder cancer. Cancer Genet Cytogenet 2000;117:32–36.

179. Aly MS, Khaled HM. Chromosomal aberrations in early-stage bilharzial bladder cancer. Cancer Genet Cytogenet 2002;132:41–45.

180. El-Rifai W, Kamel D, Larramendy ML, et al. DNA copy number changes in Schistosoma-associated and non-Schistosoma-associated bladder cancer. Am J Pathol 2000;156:871–878.

181. Muscheck M, Abol-Enein H, Chew K, et al. Comparison of genetic changes in schistosome-related transitional and squamous bladder cancers using comparative genomic hybridization. Carcinogenesis 2000;21:1721–1726.

182. Warren W, Biggs PJ, el-Baz M, Ghoneim MA, Stratton MR, Venitt S. Mutations in the p53 gene in schistosomal bladder cancer: a study of 92 tumours from Egyptian patients and a comparison between mutational spectra from schistosomal and non-schistosomal urothelial tumours. Carcinogenesis 1995;16:1181–1189.

183. Habuchi T, Takahashi R, Yamada H, et al. Influence of cigarette smoking and schistosomiasis on p53 gene mutation in urothelial cancer. Cancer Res 1993;53:3795–3799.

184. Badr KM, Nolen JD, Derose PB, Cohen C. Muscle invasive schistosomal squamous cell carcinoma of the urinary bladder: frequency and prognostic significance of p53, BCL-2, HER2/neu, and proliferation (MIB-1). Hum Pathol 2004;35:184–189.

185. Tsutsumi M, Tsai YC, Gonzalgo ML, Nichols PW, Jones PA. Early acquisition of homozygous deletions of p16/p19 during squamous cell carcinogenesis and genetic mosaicism in bladder cancer. Oncogene 1998;17:3021–3027.

186. Shaaban AA, Elbaz MA, Tribukait B. Primary nonurachal adenocarcinoma in the bilharzial urinary bladder: deoxyribonucleic acid flow cytometric and morphologic characterization in 93 cases. Urology 1998;51:469–476.

187. Grignon DJ, Ro JY, Ayala AG, Johnson DE, Ordonez NG. Primary adenocarcinoma of the urinary bladder. A clinicopathologic analysis of 72 cases. Cancer 1991;67:2165–2172.

188. Song J, Farrow GM, Lieber MM. Primary adenocarcinoma of the bladder: favorable prognostic significance of deoxyribonucleic acid diploidy measured by flow cytometry. J Urol 1990;144:1115–1118.

189. Badalament RA, Cibas ES, Reuter VE, Fair WR, Melamed MR. Flow cytometric analysis of primary adenocarcinoma of the bladder. J Urol 1987;137:1159–1162.

190. Nakanishi K, Kawai T, Suzuki M, Torikata C. Prognostic factors in urachal adenocarcinoma. A study in 41 specimens of DNA status, proliferating cell-nuclear antigen immunostaining, and argyrophilic nucleolar-organizer region counts. Hum Pathol 1996;27:240–247.

191. Kocher T, Zheng M, Bolli M, et al. Prognostic relevance of MAGE-A4 tumor antigen expression in transitional cell carcinoma of the urinary bladder: a tissue microarray study. Int J Cancer 2002;100:702–705.

192. Werling RW, Yaziji H, Bacchi CE, Gown AM. CDX2, a highly sensitive and specific marker of adenocarcinomas of intestinal origin: an immunohistochemical survey of 476 primary and metastatic carcinomas. Am J Surg Pathol 2003;27:303–310.

193. Hartmann A, Zanardo L, Bocker-Edmonston T, et al. Frequent microsatellite instability in sporadic tumors of the upper urinary tract. Cancer Res 2002;62:6796–6802.

194. Terracciano L, Richter J, Tornillo L, et al. Chromosomal imbalances in small cell carcinomas of the urinary bladder. J Pathol 1999;189:230–235.

195. Atkin NB, Baker MC, Wilson GD. Chromosome abnormalities and p53 expression in a small cell carcinoma of the bladder. Cancer Genet Cytogenet 1995;79:111–114.

196. Halachmi S, DeMarzo AM, Chow NH, et al. Genetic alterations in urinary bladder carcinosarcoma: evidence of a common clonal origin. Eur Urol 2000;37:350–357.

197. Gronau S, Menz CK, Melzner I, Hautmann R, Moller P, Barth TF. Immunohistomorphologic and molecular cytogenetic analysis of a carcinosarcoma of the urinary bladder. Virchows Archiv 2002;440:436–440.

198. Paterson RF, Ulbright TM, MacLennan GT, et al. Molecular genetic alterations in the laser-capture-microdissected stroma adjacent to bladder carcinoma. Cancer 2003;98:1830–1836.

# Gene microarrays 12

*Torben F Ørntoft*

## INTRODUCTION

Unlike many other malignant diseases, bladder cancer is characterized by recurrence in the majority of the patients, often more than once. The relatively benign tumors such as Ta grade 1 and 2 recur in approximately 50% of patients, some of whom will continue to experience recurrences for as long as 5–10 years. About 20% of these patients will develop an invasive disease. Today it is impossible on the basis of known markers or histology to predict the outcome in an individual patient. Ostensibly homogenous groups of cancers classified by conventional histopathology and clinical parameters (stage, grade, histotype, size, growth patterns, recurrence pattern, concomitant carcinoma in situ, etc.) still show marked variation in disease course from completely benign courses to rapid invasion.

Over many years, great effort has been expended to identify tools or markers that could reveal the properties of individual tumors in terms of their potential to remain benign or become malignant. A large number of markers exist that correlate with disease course and outcome. However, they are correlated at a statistical level when groups of patients are compared, and none of them has sufficient specificity and sensitivity for use in individual cases. A new hope has been raised, however, with the sequencing of the human genome and our entry into the postgenomic era. It is now possible to fabricate DNA microarrays that, for the first time, can analyze the whole genome in one measurement.

During the last few years we have moved from many samples and one or a few parameters, to more than 50,000 parameters and a few samples, the latter partly due to the fact that only fresh material can be used because RNA is degraded rapidly under the conditions traditionally used for storage. Existing files of paraffin-embedded tumors have been difficult to use in the analysis of global gene expression.

DNA microarrays have been tested for different uses. One has been to classify bladder tumors more accurately than by conventional classification methods, such as histopathologic grading and TNM classification. Another has been to try to identify new tumor-specific markers that could be transferred to the protein level and utilized, for example, in urine or in plasma. A further purpose has been to obtain information on the biology of bladder cancer disease, for example:

- Are specific pathways linked to certain disease courses?
- Are aberrant changes in gene transcription in the apoptotic pathway related to a fast recurrence rate and poor survival?
- Can we detect new pathways or complete new signaling networks in the cells on the basis of the information we get now?

Answering these questions is now turning into a new discipline termed 'systems biology', in which a cell is regarded as a complex system rather than as separated pathways having their own individual life and fate.

Analysis of many targets in parallel has been used not only for measuring gene expression but also for analyzing genomic instability by using the natural variations along the genome, named single nucleotide polymorphisms, which are responsible for differences between human beings. Because many of these are heterozygous in a given individual, they can be used to examine loss of heterozygosity, long regarded as one of the basic mechanisms behind neoplastic transformation and progression of tumors. It is now possible (in the year 2004) to screen the genome using up to 500,000 single nucleotide polymorphism (SNP) probes on a commercial array.

Together with the expression data, that means an almost overwhelming amount of data or information load which has to be handled in an intelligent way. New tools and new standards are constantly being created to organize the data into meaningful information without erroneous conclusions based on the existence of multiple evaluations. This area, termed 'bioinformatics', has improved dramatically during the years following the millennium, and quite robust data are now obtained from microarrays.

Finally, microarrays have been used for resequencing of genes such as P450 and p53. At least theoretically, multiple probes should be very fast and very safe. However, the many ways a gene can be altered continue to offer a challenge to array-based sequencing. Some results have been obtained within the area of bladder cancer and, as for the sequencing arrays described above, this chapter will focus on the data acquired by using microarrays on bladder tumors and bladder tumor cell lines, and on the future potential of this technology.

## THE GENE ARRAY TECHNOLOGY

Basically, a gene array consists of a number of gene probes placed next to each other in an ordered fashion on a solid support. The number of probes has been steadily increasing and has now reached around 1 million probes on a square centimeter, as for example with the newest generation of arrays from the California-based company, Affymetrix. Some commercial arrays are made by photolithography—in a similar way to computer chips—and these have the highest density. However, it is only possible to synthesize probes of around 20–25 nucleotides in length. This could mean a problem in terms of specificity as some genes may share regions that have the same sequences. However, using multiple probes per gene has largely eliminated this problem.

Arrays that are simpler to produce are those where a synthetic oligonucleotide of, for example, 60 nucleotides is linked to a conventional pathology glass slide. These arrays can be produced in any laboratory that invests in an array gridder and the time to optimize the rather complex system. Both types of array seem to work well. Those produced with the highest precision can be used for analysis of single targets (the target is the sample from the tumor we wish to analyze), whereas those that are produced in-house at most laboratories need a standard in each experiment to correct for variation in spot size and morphology, and density from spot to spot. Usually these are labeled with different fluorophore molecules such as Cy3 and Cy5, and the ratio between these is the data produced in each spot when analyzing gene expression.

Arrays have to be scanned to detect the fluorescence, and a number of efficient scanners are on the market. The software used to identify the spots and to make background correction has improved considerably, and is now of a standard that makes routine use a possibility.

In general, the arrays are very reproducible with a low array-to-array variation in signal level, and the linearity covers more than three decades. Thus, robust and meaningful data can be obtained for most purposes. Working with very small amounts of starting material, such as laser microdissected tissue, may require additional amplification, but this is of relatively low importance when SNPs and sequencing are analyzed because the measurements are not acutely sensitive to asymmetrical amplification of the different SNP alleles. However, for counting alleles with precision and measuring transcripts with high precision, some performance is lost when the two-round amplification steps are used.

## MEASURING GENE EXPRESSION USING MICROARRAYS

The material to use for measuring gene expression is RNA molecules extracted from bladder tumor tissue. As RNA molecules are subjected to breakdown by ubiquitously existing RNA'ses, much effort must be devoted to the sampling of the tissue: either it should be frozen immediately in liquid nitrogen or a chemical protecting against RNA'ses should be added to the tissue biopsy. These requirements can be met only if there is strong effective collaboration between laboratories and surgeons providing the tissue.

RNA can, if protected or extracted, be stored for long time periods at –80°C or lower, without significant breakdown. Before RNA is labeled, the quality should be assured by measuring the ratio between 28S and 18S ribosomal RNA, and by securing minimal breakdown products (ratio should be above 1 and breakdown less than 10% of total RNA). Several standard protocols exist for labeling the RNA molecules for array analysis. These will work on 1 μg or more of total RNA of good quality, and lead to labeling of mRNA or the corresponding cRNA.

Hybridization is made to an array holding probes for the targets to analyze, be they whole human genomes or subfractions of this. There are several competing producers that can provide oligoarrays from 25 nucleotides in length (photolithography) to around 60 (spotted arrays). Very few use cDNA arrays based on polymerase chain reaction (PCR) products because of crosshybridization problems that arise when hybridizing to 500 bp or longer probe fragments.

After hybridization (usually overnight) and washing, the arrays are scanned in order to detect the fluorescence. From this point, data are produced in terms of signals from the scannings. If a two-color system is used, there is a signal from the reference sample and a signal from the test sample. The ratio between these two is used to generate the level in the test sample. For one-color systems such as Affymetrix, no reference is used. Next, the arrays are normalized and, in the case of one-color systems, scaled to the same level.[1-3] When this process has been completed the data are ready for analysis.

## ANALYSIS OF GENE EXPRESSION DATA

Basically, data analysis can be divided into two separate approaches: unsupervised (class discovery) and supervised (class prediction) methods.[4]

### Unsupervised methods

Unsupervised analysis has no a priori assumption about organization of the samples or data, and aims to identify previously known or unknown relationships between samples. For this purpose, hierarchical cluster analysis has been used extensively to group tumors according to similarity in expression profiles. This technique can also be applied to group genes with similar expression profiles across the tumor samples, and in this way identify possible co-varying and/or functionally related genes. Hierarchical cluster analysis is a powerful tool for visualization of the expression patterns.[5]

Other unsupervised methods used are principal-component analysis (PCA), self-organizing maps (SOM), and relevance networks. The unsupervised methods are suited for finding novel relationships between samples (or genes) based on similarities in the gene expression patterns. However, the possibility of identifying nonrelevant groups exists because of the complexity in large-scale gene expression data. (As an effect of this, at least two groups will always be defined, although the definition of each group may be rather vague.)

### Supervised methods

Supervised analysis techniques are used for identifying differentially expressed genes between groups of samples, for example when the histopathologic stage or clinical outcome (survival, metastasis, recurrence, progression, etc.) is known. Optimal expression signatures for disease classification or outcome prediction are in this way generated from a set of training samples, and the significance of the identified expression signature is tested using independent test samples. Standard statistical tests, such as the student's t-test, are used to identify the genes that show the largest differential expression between the groups. Mathematical methods used for classifying samples based on the optimal gene expression signatures include, among others, maximum-likelihood estimates, k-nearest neighbors, support vector machines, and weighted voting schemes.[6]

The use of supervised methods in the analysis of gene expression data, however, involves the risk of oversimplifying the clinical groups under investigation. A single clinical class (e.g. poor outcome) may contain several molecular subclasses of tumors with distinct expression patterns, making the identification of genes differentially expressed between the clinical groups virtually impossible. In bladder cancer, such groups could be tumors that evolve over many years as papillomas and end up as muscle-invasive carcinomas as opposed to those that are diagnosed as muscle-invasive at first visit. Are they molecularly the same muscle-invasive tumors?

When supervised methods are used for selection of differentially expressed genes, the significance of the selected genes can be determined by permutation analysis. This is usually done with multiple permutations of the sample labels, followed by generation of statistics relating to the ability to select good differentially expressed genes in random classes. Results are then compared to the real data. Such tests determine the likelihood of obtaining the observed expression patterns by chance, a real problem when thousands of statistical tests are performed.

## MICROARRAY-BASED STUDIES OF GENE EXPRESSION IN BLADDER CANCER

Bladder cancers, together with breast and lung cancer and leukemias/lymphomas, are the diseases in which microarrays have been used most intensely to classify the disease. In the first study from 2001, Thykjaer et al described the gene expression patterns that are characteristic of superficial and invasive bladder tumors, based on Affymetrix oligoarrays holding about 5000 probes.[7] At that time the cost of arrays was overwhelming, and, accordingly, the samples were pooled within each stage of disease and hybridized to one array each. Thykjaer et al also first described the correlation between Affymetrix array-based gene expression and Northern blotting in bladder cancer as evidence of reproducibility of the findings. In this paper the 400 transcripts that co-varied best with tumor stage were isolated and used for unsupervised hierarchical clustering. That identified two cluster arms, one holding the superficial and one holding the invasive tumors, thus showing that it might be possible to construct molecular classifiers for bladder cancer. The 400 genes were then subjected to hierarchical cluster analysis, which identified genes with related functions clustering closely together. The functional groups detected were genes related to the cell cycle, oncogenes, and immunology-related genes, all being upregulated in invasive tumors, with cell adhesion-encoding genes as well as transcription factors and proteinases being relatively lower in invasive tumors than in superficial tumors. These findings were subsequently reproduced by other studies.[8-10] Interestingly, the study reported upregulation of all the components in the cell cycle needed to direct the cell through the cell cycle.

The same group demonstrated in a large study of 40 training tumors and 68 validation tumors the ability to identify signatures of genes characteristic for subgroups of bladder cancers.[11] For example, the group of Ta papillomas without recurrence clustered together in an unsupervised clustering as did those that recurred. Furthermore, some Ta tumors surrounded by CIS clustered together with muscle-invasive tumors of stage T2 or higher. The CIS-surrounded Ta tumors showed a very strong signature related to connective tissue remodeling and angiogenesis.

This prompted a recent study of gene expression in CIS patients[12] that examined the gene expression patterns in superficial transitional cell carcinomas (TCCs) with surrounding CIS (13 patients) and without surrounding CIS lesions (15 patients), and in muscle-invasive carcinomas (13 patients). Hierarchical cluster analysis of gene expression in the papillomas separated the superficial TCC samples according to the presence or absence of CIS in the surrounding urothelium. No close relationship between TCC with adjacent CIS and invasive TCC was observed using hierarchical cluster analysis. Expression profiling of a series of biopsies from normal urothelium and urothelium with CIS lesions, from the same urinary bladder, revealed that the gene expression found in superficial Ta papillomas with surrounding CIS is also found in the CIS biopsies, and, remarkably, in histologically normal urothelial samples adjacent to the CIS lesions. This signature could also be found in muscle-invasive tumors and seems to be a signature reflecting malignant properties (Figure 12.1).

Among the genes with elevated expression in the signature were a few genes that highlight the aggressive nature of CIS; for example, the GG2-1 gene, which may encode an antiapoptotic protein (inferred from structural domains), and the VEGF gene, which encodes a protein that is a prognostic marker for stage progression and recurrence in bladder cancer[13,14] and is involved in angiogenesis.[15] Furthermore, the cluster included the TGFBR2 gene, which has been shown to be mutated in colon cancer cell lines with high rates of microsatellite instability. It is believed that the mutations make cancer cells able to escape TGFβ-mediated growth control.[16] Interestingly, the TIEG gene (TGFβ-inducible early gene) encoding a transcription factor that plays an important role in the TGFβ signaling

pathway[17] is also found in this cluster. Most other genes identified in these clusters remain interesting candidates for further studies.

On a different platform, another report demonstrated the possibility of separating bladder tumors into superficial and invasive tumors using unsupervised methods.[9] In this report an array with 17,842 image clones was used together with microdissected tumor cell preparations from frozen sections. Although only 15 samples were included it was possible to identify genes showing a differential expression. Remarkably, the tumors seemed to cluster according to whether or not metastatic disease developed, using a principal-component analysis. The most important genes separating the benign disease courses from the aggressive invasive courses appeared to be ninjurin, p33ING1, and ACE2.

Another approach to analysis of gene expression in bladder cancer was made by Mor et al who used a cDNA library from TCC samples to print an array with 9930 clones.[10] They hybridized the array with RNA from pools of tumors or single tumors and used a common reference extracted from 15 samples (10 TCCs and 5 normal urothelium). Normal urothelium and tumors clustered separately using unsupervised clustering, and defined a set of genes characteristic for non-invasive TCC. Some of these (S100P, keratin7, Cyclophilin A, HAI-2, and Syndecan1) were validated by reverse transcriptase PCR (RT-PCR) and showed a strong increase in papillomas compared to normal urothelium. It is characteristic of these experiments that S100 proteins are upregulated, as well as cathepsin E and claudin-7 to mention a few.

## CLASSIFICATION OF BLADDER CANCER USING GENE EXPRESSION AND DOWNSTREAM METHODS

It is evident from a number of reports that expression microarrays can be used to classify tumors into subgroups. Even minor histologic features are reflected in a specific gene expression pattern, not only making this technique extremely powerful but also setting strict criteria for its use. It is important to group tumors according to their properties and molecular phenotypes before studying, for example, the outcome of the disease, or, alternatively, to reduce the predictive genes set to a minimum, which—hopefully—is independent of the molecular phenotype and related *only* to the outcome.

The most comprehensive report on the classification of bladder cancer using gene expression was based on a training set of 40 bladder tumors and a test set of 68 tumors.[11] These were analyzed by arrays with 5000 genes and led to the identification of a 32-gene classifier

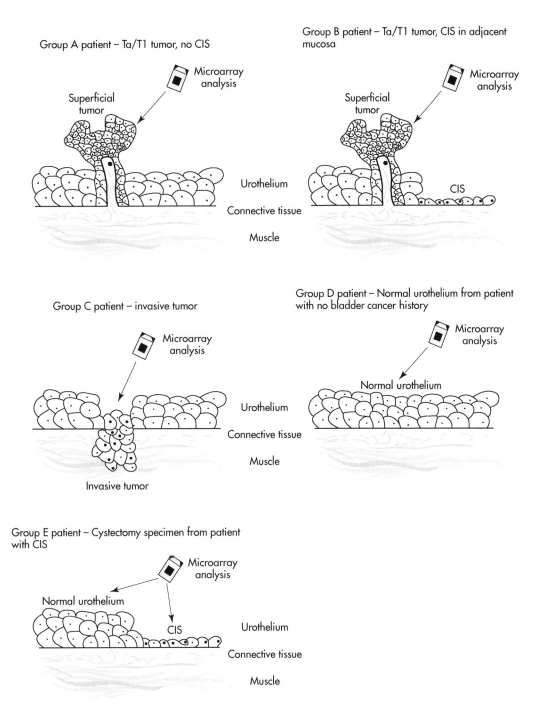

**Fig. 12.1**
The use of microarrays to pinpoint the gene expression signatures that accompany carcinoma in situ (CIS). Group A: a Ta tumor without CIS has no CIS signature. Group B: a Ta tumor with surrounding CIS has a specific CIS signature in the Ta tumor. Group C: an invasive tumor has parts of the CIS signature. Group D: normal urothelium has no CIS signature. Group E: normal urothelium from a patient with CIS has the CIS signature, as does, of course, the CIS itself.

that could classify according to the tumor stages Ta, T1, and T2–4 (Figure 12.2). Remarkably, the classifier named some tumors staged as Ta by histopathology as T1 or even T2. These, and almost only these, tumors progressed from Ta to T1 or T2. Thus it was confirmed that not only breast cancers have a signature that predicts the outcome[18] but also, in very early bladder

papillomas, there is a signature consisting of a few genes that predicts eventual upstaging of the disease.

The biologic explanation for this is not yet understood, but these findings suggest a change in the concept that tumor progression is a gradual increase of more and more malignant properties over time to the present observations, suggesting that is it possible to

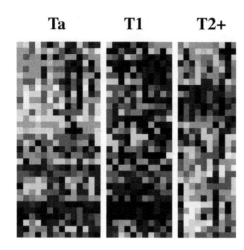

**Ta    T1    T2+**

**Fig. 12.2**
Genes selected for classification of stage Ta, T1 and T2+ bladder tumors. Each line is a gene and each column is a sample. The set of genes was selected by leaving one out crossvalidation. It is evident that the set of genes falls into two groups: those that are highly expressed (yellow) in Ta and low (blue) in T2+, and those that have a reverse pattern. T1 is classified by the fact that all the genes are low in T1.

find signs early in tumor formation that predict a malignant course of the disease. Whether this signature and the genes it contains are a functional set of genes defining the events to come—or whether it is just a way of 'statistically' grouping tumors together that share a common property (same genomic aberrations?)—is unknown. However, our knowledge of the function of the genome is rudimentary. Many genes serve more than one function, especially transcription factors, and their possible role in controlling events during malignant progression will require much attention in the coming years.

Another approach[9] used gene expression to identify genes that characterized an invasive disease course as opposed to a non-invasive disease course. An antibody against the encoded protein was then used to define the relation of the protein to survival on the basis of a tissue microarray having 69 tumors with follow-up data. This clearly showed a relation between the detection of p33ING1 and a poor survival. A similar approach could be used in the future for many other molecules and could lead to a library of antibodies with predictive power. This would make it possible using paraffin sections and immunohistochemistry, which are less technically demanding than using gene expression, to construct an algorithm that will predict the disease course.

A gene expression classifier for CIS has also been published.[12] A supervised learning approach was used to build a 16-gene molecular CIS classifier. The classifier was able to classify stage Ta tumors according to the presence or absence of surrounding CIS with a high accuracy. This study demonstrated that a CIS gene-expression signature is present not only in CIS biopsies but also in superficial Ta tumors, in muscle-invasive T2–4 tumors, and, remarkably, in histologically normal urothelium from bladders with CIS. Identification of this expression signature could provide guidance for the selection of therapy and follow-up regimen in patients with early stage bladder cancer.

A recent, yet unpublished, study has demonstrated the possibility of classifying the grade of Ta tumors on the basis of microarrays. It is well known that grade 3 Ta tumors are much more malignant than grade 1 tumors in terms of likelihood of progression and recurrence. However, it is a subjective task to perform the grading, and the correspondence between pathologists is not very high. In a study of 25 Ta tumors, it was possible to construct a 39-gene grade classifier that objectively could grade the Ta grade 2 tumors into a relatively benign group and a relatively malignant group on the basis of gene expression. The two groups differed in recurrence rates and time to recurrence (M. Aaboe, personal communication). This indicates that it may be an option for objective classification of the grade of tumor cells in the near future.

## RELATION BETWEEN DNA LOSS OR GAIN, TRANSCRIPT LEVEL, AND PROTEIN LEVEL

In one study, 2-dimensional gel electrophoresis was used to detect the expression of several of the genes that were changing their expression according to tumor stage. It is now clear that the correlation between gene transcript and protein level is restricted to certain genes and proteins.[19] Further, the relation between gene dose (gain and loss of genomic material) and gene expression is rather complex, although a statistical relationship exists with genes in gained regions expressed at a higher level and those in lost regions at a reduced level.[19]

## SNP ARRAYS FOR THE ANALYSIS OF LOSS OF HETEROZYGOSITY

One hallmark of cancer is the common genomic instability seen in most tumors. Very few tumors are diploid with an intact 46 chromosome set. Almost all tumors show rearrangements and often unbalanced changes with multiple regions being reduced to homozygosity. This formed the basis for the two-hit hypothesis[20] in which one allele is hit by a mutation or methylation of the promoter and the other allele is lost due to chromosomal instability.

In bladder cancer, as in most other cancers, microsatellites—which are mono- or oligonucleotide repeats of a given length in a given individual—have been used to detect loss of heterozygosity (LOH). They can be selected in chromosomal areas of interest and have been used to pinpoint LOH in, for example, chromosome 9, which has frequent LOH in early bladder tumors. However, the possibility of using SNPs on microarrays has introduced the analysis of the whole genome for LOH in one analysis using 1500, 10,000 and, soon, 500,000 SNPs along the genome. SNPs occur along the genome in vast numbers (>5 million). They are somewhat population restricted, but the most common ones occur with a relatively well-defined heterozygosity frequency in a given population. It is possible to screen the whole genome with SNPs located in the coding regions of the genome, or to select SNPs that are located in a given pathway and lead to amino acid shifts in the encoded proteins belonging to that pathway.

In bladder cancer three studies have used the Affymetrix 1500 SNP array to detect LOH in bladder tumors or in urine sediments.[21-23] In the first study, eight patients—having both a superficial stage T1 tumor and a muscle-invasive tumor—were analyzed, comparing tumor and blood from the same individual. Of the 1500 SNPs, 343 were heterozygous, and these informative SNPs showed LOH to a varying extent from 2/343 to 85/343. The latter is remarkable as it indicates that 25% of the genome was lost in these tumors. A major factor determining the extent of LOH was the presence of homozygous p53 mutations. If these occurred in T1 tumors, they showed very frequent LOH. The LOH rate was significantly related to increasing stage (p<0.001) as T1 tumors showed a median of 8.5 and T2–4 tumors a median of 28 losses. The clonal evolution of bladder cancer was underlined by the fact that 68% of allelic losses in the early tumors were rediscovered in subsequent muscle-invasive tumors. This strongly supports the theory that it is one clone of cells that expands and invades the patient. Some changes occur along the progression, but it is still possible to trace the tumor back to its superficial origin. Common losses were found in chromosomes 6, 8, 9, 11, and 17, which have been identified previously using other techniques. However, with SNP arrays the throughput is increased exponentially, and it was possible to find a new LOH area associated with invasive growth at chromosome 6p.

A later study of 36 tumors also showed a stage-related increase in LOH, increasing from 37 in Ta to 51 in T1 and 68 losses in T2–4 using the same Affymetrix 1500 SNP array.[22] In this study the losses of heterozygosity detected by SNPs were validated by microsatellites and showed similar results. Some new areas of loss were also detected in this study at 1p, 2q, 12q, and 16p. The group that initiated the latter study tried to use the SNP detection of losses on urine from the same set of patients.[23] They found abnormal SNPs in all tumor urines but not in the few control urines examined. This indicates a possible clinical use of the non-invasive SNP array assay in urine DNA. One might, however, fear that,

with examination of more controls, the specificity would be reduced because inflammation is known to be able to lead to micosatellite instability,[24] possibly by oxidative stress mechanisms.

## MICROARRAY-BASED SEQUENCING OF P53 IN BLADDER CANCER

Another area in which microarrays have been used is in sequencing of genes, in particular p53. With the many probes per array it is possible to synthesize all combinations of the four nucleotides along the sequence of a gene. This procedure is very well suited for detection of single nucleotide shifts (missense and nonsense mutations). However, in cancer, all kinds of possible mutations exist. Deletions and insertions of one or more nucleotides may occur as well as mutations in introns that, by unknown mechanisms, lead to reduced transcript amount or altered splicing. In two studies of bladder cancer, a p53 sequencing array from Affymetrix was used to detect mutations in 140 bladder tumors.[25,26] The same samples were previously sequenced by manual dideoxy sequencing. Of 1464 gene chip positions, each of which corresponded to an analyzed nucleotide in the sequence, 251 had background signals that were not attributable to mutations, causing the specificity of mutation identification without mathematical correction to be low. This problem was solved by regarding each chip position as a separate entity with its own noise and threshold characteristics. The use of background plus two standard deviations as the cut-off improved the specificity from 0.34 to 0.86 at the cost of reducing sensitivity from 0.92 to 0.84, but leading to a much better concordance (92%) with results obtained by traditional sequencing. The chip method detected as little as 1% mutated DNA. The latter is important as it is quite demanding to microdissect the tumor tissue to obtain pure tumor cell preparations. The data are promising as chip-based sequencing could be a fast and cost-effective alternative to conventional sequencing, given that insertions and deletions could also be analyzed with precision.

## FUNCTIONAL ANALYSIS OF PATHWAYS IN BLADDER CANCER USING EXPRESSION MICROARRAYS

Experiments based on expression arrays have pinpointed a number of genes whose encoded proteins could be of value in controlling the behavior of bladder cancer. These may be related to a good or a poor outcome of the disease, and form relevant drug targets for therapy based on small molecules. However, to obtain a deeper insight into their function, it is necessary to manipulate these genes in a standard context. This can be done by transfecting them into cell lines and overexpressing them, or by transfecting interfering RNA into cell lines, thereby closing down the genes. These two approaches—up- or downregulation of genes of interest—can be followed by a time course analysis of the gene expression using expression microarrays (Figure 12.3). A number of such experiments have been carried out but are not yet published (T. Thykjaer, personal communication). They clearly identify the pathways activated or controlled by the genes of interest. A significant step ahead for the understanding of the function of the genes has been the possibility of linking the expression data to pathway maps. In that way, using color coding, it is possible to get a simple and clear view of the impact of single genes on cellular metabolism and behavior. The latter can be refined by using simple functional assays on the cells subjected to up- or downregulation, such as measures of cellular proliferation, invasion, apoptosis, peptide phosphorylation, etc.

Such functional use of microarrays will provide us with extremely interesting data on the cellular networks that are active in bladder tumor cells as they progress from benign papillomas to aggressive invasive tumors. A hope for the future is that it will be possible to direct therapy to the most important of these molecules, and thereby improve the outcome of bladder cancer treatment.

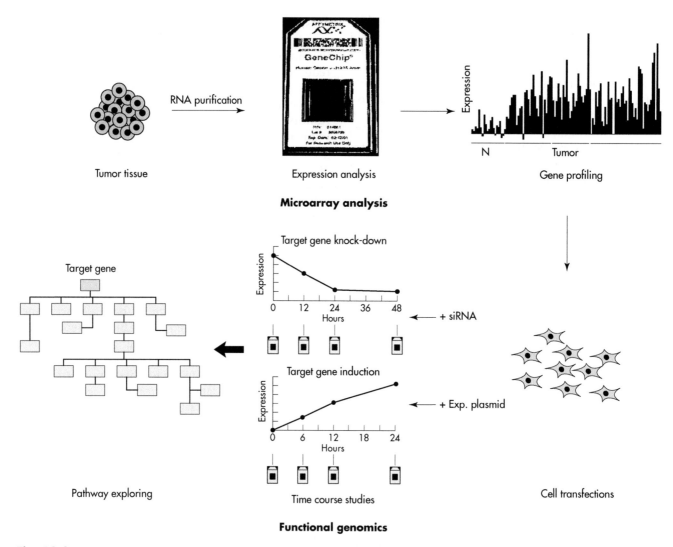

**Fig. 12.3**
The use of microarrays to obtain functional knowledge of genes that show a clear upregulation in bladder cancer. First, bladder tumor tissue from patients is analyzed. Then those genes that show a profile with increased expression in tumors are sorted out. These genes are a) cloned and transfected into cell lines; and b) subjected to downregulation by interfering RNAi in cell lines where they are already expressed. Following a) or b), microarrays are used on a time course basis to detect altered gene expression, which subsequently is coupled to pathway databases to gain insight into which functional pathways are altered because of the change in gene expression.

## FUTURE USE OF MICROARRAYS

As evidenced above, DNA microarrays have come to play a prominent role as a tool for whole genome analysis of bladder tumors. Use of expression signatures for classification of bladder tumors also seems promising, as there appear to be signatures that can identify histotypes such as squamous metaplasia (Figure 12.4), grade of tumor, recurrence rate, and progression to a higher stage. SNP arrays with a high density can pinpoint even minor, commonly lost, areas and may also form a basis for diagnosis and prediction of disease course.

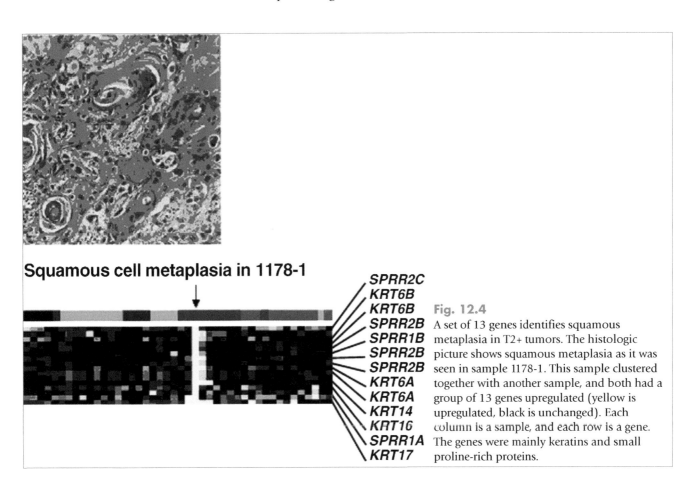

**Fig. 12.4** A set of 13 genes identifies squamous metaplasia in T2+ tumors. The histologic picture shows squamous metaplasia as it was seen in sample 1178-1. This sample clustered together with another sample, and both had a group of 13 genes upregulated (yellow is upregulated, black is unchanged). Each column is a sample, and each row is a gene. The genes were mainly keratins and small proline-rich proteins.

## REFERENCES

1. Schena M, Shalon D, Davis RW, Brown PO. Quantitative monitoring of gene expression patterns with a complementary DNA microarray. Science 1995;270:467–470.
2. Bolstad BM, Irizarry RA, Astrand M, Speed TP. A comparison of normalization methods for high density oligonucleotide array data based on variance and bias. Bioinformatics 2003;19:185–193.
3. Quackenbush J. Microarray data normalization and transformation. Nat Genet 2002;32(Suppl):496–501.
4. Golub TR, Slonim DK, Tamayo P, et al. Molecular classification of cancer: class discovery and class prediction by gene expression monitoring. Science 1999;286:531–537.
5. Eisen MB, Spellman PT, Brown PO, Botstein D. Cluster analysis and display of genome-wide expression patterns. Proc Natl Acad Sci USA 1998;95:14863–14868.
6. Dudoit S, Fridlyand J, Speed TP. Comparison of discrimination methods for the classification of tumors using gene expression data. Technical Report. Berkeley, CA: Berkeley University, 2000.
7. Thykjaer T, Workman C, Kruhoffer M, et al. Identification of gene expression patterns in superficial and invasive human bladder cancer. Cancer Res 2001;61:2492–2499.
8. Sanchez-Carbayo M, Socci ND, Charytonowicz E, et al. Molecular profiling of bladder cancer using cDNA microarrays: defining histogenesis and biological phenotypes. Cancer Res 2002;62:6973–6980.
9. Sanchez-Carbayo M, Socci ND, Lozano JJ, et al. Gene discovery in bladder cancer progression using cDNA microarrays. Am J Pathol 2003;163:505–516.
10. Mor O, Nativ O, Stein A, et al. Molecular analysis of transitional cell carcinoma using cDNA microarray. Oncogene 2003;22(48):7702–7710.
11. Dyrskjot L, Thykjaer T, Kruhoffer M, et al. Identifying distinct classes of bladder carcinoma using microarrays. Nat Genet 2003;33:90–96.
12. Dyrskjot L, Kruhoffer M, Thykjaer T, Marcussen N, Jensen JL, Moller K, Orntoft TF. Gene expression in the urinary bladder: a common carcinoma in situ gene expression signature exists disregarding histopathological classification. Cancer Res 2004;64(11):4040–4048.
13. Crew JP, O'Brien T, Bradburn M, Fuggle S, Bicknell R, Cranston D, Harris AL. Vascular endothelial growth factor is a predictor of relapse and stage progression in superficial bladder cancer. Cancer Res 1997;57:5281–5285.
14. Crew JP, O'Brien T, Bicknell R, Fuggle S, Cranston D, Harris AL. Urinary vascular endothelial growth factor and its correlation with bladder cancer recurrence rates. J Urol 1999;161:99–104.
15. Ferrara N, Gerber HP, LeCouter J. The biology of VEGF and its receptors. Nat Med 2003;9:669–676.

16. Markowitz S, Wang J, Myeroff L, et al. Inactivation of the type II TGF-beta receptor in colon cancer cells with microsatellite instability. Science 1995;268:1336–1338.

17. Hefferan TE, Reinholz GG, Rickard DJ, et al. Overexpression of a nuclear protein, TIEG, mimics transforming growth factor-beta action in human osteoblast cells. J Biol Chem 2000;275:20255–20259.

18. van't Veer LJ, Dai H, van de Vijver MJ, et al. Gene expression profiling predicts clinical outcome of breast cancer. Nature 2000;415:530–536.

19. Orntoft TF, Thykjaer T, Waldman FM, Wolf H, Celis JE. Genome-wide study of gene copy numbers, transcripts, and protein levels in pairs of non-invasive and invasive human transitional cell carcinomas. Mol Cell Proteomics 2002;1:37–45.

20. Knudson A. Alfred Knudson and his two-hit hypothesis. (Interview by Ezzie Hutchinson.) Lancet Oncol 2001;2(10):642–645.

21. Primdahl H, Wikman FP, von der Maase H, Zhou XG, Wolf H, Orntoft TF. Allelic imbalances in human bladder cancer: genome-wide detection with high-density single-nucleotide polymorphism arrays. J Natl Cancer Inst 2002;94(3):216–223.

22. Hoque MO, Lee CC, Cairns P, Schoenberg M, Sidransky D. Genome-wide genetic characterization of bladder cancer: a comparison of high-density single-nucleotide polymorphism arrays and PCR-based microsatellite analysis. Cancer Res 2003;63(9):2216–2222.

23. Hoque MO, Lee J, Begum S, et al. High-throughput molecular analysis of urine sediment for the detection of bladder cancer by high-density single-nucleotide polymorphism array. Cancer Res 2003;63(18):5723–5726.

24. Christensen M, Wolf H, Orntoft TF. Microsatellite alterations in urinary sediments from patients with cystitis and bladder cancer. Int J Cancer 2000;85(5):614–617.

25. Wikman FP, Lu ML, Thykjaer T, Olesen SH, Andersen LD, Cordon-Cardo C, Orntoft TF. Evaluation of the performance of a p53 sequencing microarray chip using 140 previously sequenced bladder tumor samples. Clin Chem 2000;46(10):1555–1561.

26. Lu ML, Wikman F, Orntoft TF, et al. Impact of alterations affecting the p53 pathway in bladder cancer on clinical outcome, assessed by conventional and array-based methods. Clin Cancer Res 2002;8(1):171–179.

# Molecular biology of invasive and metastatic urothelial cancer

13

*Dan Theodorescu*

## INTRODUCTION

Carcinoma of the urinary bladder is the second most common urologic malignancy. In addition, these tumors are one of the best-understood genitourinary neoplasms with well-defined etiology, natural history, tumor biology, treatment options, and outcome. This level of understanding arises as a consequence of multiple factors and represents a convergence of knowledge from diverse scientific disciplines. Insight provided by these disciplines, coupled with unique features of this neoplasm which make it assessable for detection, monitoring, and treatment, combine to make this disease a model system for modern oncology. While not comprehensive, the intent of this chapter is to provide the reader with an overview of our current understanding of this tumor from the standpoint of its molecular biology as related to tumor progression and metastasis. Excellent recent reviews on biomarkers of tumor progression have also been published and would complement the work described in this chapter.[1]

## INVASION AND METASTASIS

The ability of tumors to invade, colonize, and destroy distant organs was first recognized by Jean-Claude Recamier in 1829. He termed this phenomenon metastasis.[2,3] Since it was first described, metastasis has been shown to be a complex, multistep process.[4] One important step is cell migration—a critical component of both cancer cell invasion at the primary site (allowing cells to gain access to the vasculature) and for cells to penetrate the host tissue at distant sites.[5]

The most widely accepted model of mammalian-adherent cell migration is derived from observation of cells on two-dimensional surfaces and classically involves four fundamental processes: lamellipod extension, leading-edge attachment, cell contraction, and trailing-edge detachment.[6-8] At the leading edge of a moving cell, localized remodeling of the actin cytoskeleton results in the extension of a single lamellipodium or, in some cases, multiple smaller filopodia. Dozens of proteins that interact with actin monomers and/or microfilaments, and modulate actin polymerization and organization, have been shown to participate in this process.[9] Other cytoskeletal changes behind the leading edge result in contraction, which pulls the cell body forward. Contraction is driven by changes in actin/myosin interactions, regulated to a large extent by myosin light-chain (MLC) phosphorylation, which is controlled by MLC kinases and phosphatases.[10]

In order for contraction to result in forward cell movement, new contacts between the cell and its substratum must be established at the leading edge. These contacts involve integrins and other trans-membrane receptors for extracellular matrix (ECM) components and must be dynamically altered in composition and/or activity for a cell to continue moving forward.[6] Finally, at the trailing edge, a moving cell detaches by breaking contact with the ECM. This process can involve proteolytic cleavage of adhesion proteins (via calpain or other proteases), mechanical ripping,[11] or possibly local changes in integrin activation state.[12] Although this model of cell migration is based primarily on experiments using fibroblasts, similar processes appear to be important for epithelial cell movement as well, with perhaps some differences in the molecules involved. A second mode of cell migration has been observed for cancer cells and leukocytes moving through three-dimensional matrices, such as collagen gels.[13] This type of migration, termed amoeboid movement, involves weak adhesion and dynamic changes in cell shape that allow cells to move through collagen filament networks.

## MOLECULAR BASIS OF BLADDER CANCER PROGRESSION

While less common than tumor recurrence, progression of superficial tumors to muscle invasion has profound consequences with respect to prognosis and treatment. In fact, tumor progression encompasses a spectrum of clinical and biologic changes in both the tumor and the host,[14] from early invasion of the basement membrane to widely metastatic disease. In this section we will focus on and highlight the changes occurring when superficial bladder cancers become muscle invasive.

In general, organs are composed of a series of tissue compartments separated from each other by two types of extracellular matrix: basement membranes and interstitial stroma.[15] The extracellular matrix determines tissue architecture, has important biologic functions, and is a mechanical barrier to tumor cell invasion. The nuances of what is meant by invasive and superficial bladder cancer are worth mentioning here, since they are somewhat at odds with the pure definition of tumor invasion, which is the penetration of normal tissue barriers such as the basement membrane. In the purest sense, only stage Ta and carcinoma in situ (CIS) tumors are truly 'superficial', thus not penetrating the basement membrane of the bladder wall. Historically, however, urologists have also considered T1 tumors as superficial despite their invasion of the lamina propria. On the other hand, tumors labeled as 'invasive' are those penetrating the true muscle of the bladder wall. As a group, most stage T1 lesions are more prone eventually to invade the detrusor during subsequent recurrences than are Ta tumors. Conversely, despite being truly superficial, CIS is more aggressive and behaves more akin to T1 than Ta tumors. This may be the result of the differing genetic lesions that led to its formation compared to those leading to Ta/T1 cancers.[16] Due to the significant drop in a patient's prognosis with any step in tumor progression, the genetic basis of this phenomenon is therefore a subject of considerable clinical importance. In the current section we will highlight the cytogenetic, molecular genetic and immunohistochemical evidence supporting the role of specific genetic changes in the progression of bladder cancer to muscle invasive disease.

## CYTOGENETIC CHANGES ASSOCIATED WITH TRANSITIONAL CELL CARCINOMA PROGRESSION

Several recent studies have examined the common regions of deletion in human bladder tumors.[16,17] In a recent series, Knowles and associates[17] screened 83 cases of transitional cell carcinoma for loss of heterozygosity (LOH) on all autosomal chromosome arms. The most frequent losses were monosomies of chromosome 9 (57%), and losses on chromosomes 11p (32%), 17p (32%), 8p (23%), 4p (22%), and 13q (15%). This series was composed of a majority of superficial low-grade lesions and thus the incidence of the various losses would be reflective of the genetic alterations specifically present in this cohort of patients. Other groups have focused on identifying the common · deletions specifically associated with tumor progression. In these cases, a somewhat different spectrum of abnormalities was observed, involving alterations at chromosomal locations 3p,[18] 4q,[19] 8p,[20] 18q,[21] 10,[22,23] 15,[24,25] and 17p.[26] Some of these changes have also been observed in a recently characterized highly tumorigenic variant of the T24 human bladder cell line.[27]

Previous studies on predominantly superficial bladder cancer specimens[17] indicated an overall low frequency of chromosome 10 allele losses and deletions in bladder cancer. However, when cohorts with significant proportions of invasive tumors were investigated,[23] the incidence of LOH on this chromosome was found in 40% of tumors for at least one locus. Remarkably, LOH on chromosome 10 was observed mainly in muscle-invasive or high-grade tumors, the latter of which were most likely invasive or had a high chance of future progression to invasive disease. Confirming these findings, Kagan and colleagues[22] found LOH with at least one allele lost on the long arm of chromosome 10 in 9/20 (45%) invasive transitional cell carcinomas (TCCs). Recently, LOH studies have also suggested that human chromosome 15 may harbor a novel putative tumor suppressor gene which appears to play a role during metastasis in breast and bladder[25] cancer. This observation supported other studies where fluorescence in situ hybridization (FISH) for chromosome 15-specific centromeric repeat sequences revealed loss of this chromosome in 67% of specimens from patients with histologically confirmed TCC.[24]

Recently, our laboratory has developed a novel technique which combines information obtained from gene expression array analysis of human cancer cells with that of chromosomal position to allow expression mapping.[28] Comparing the results obtained with this technique to those of comparative genomic hybridization (CGH), has allowed us to focus on areas of the genome which have both altered expression and chromosomal changes, leading to the discovery of a new metastasis suppressor gene (see 'Molecular and immunohistochemical changes associated with transitional cell carcinoma progression' below).

## MOLECULAR AND IMMUNOHISTOCHEMICAL CHANGES ASSOCIATED WITH TRANSITIONAL CELL CARCINOMA PROGRESSION

Studies utilizing immunohistochemical techniques (IHC) have suggested that overexpression of HRAS protein (discussed above),[29] P53,[30] and the epidermal growth factor receptor (EGFR)[31] in bladder tumors may be related to bladder tumor progression. Loss of RB[26] and E-cadherin[32] expression has also been related to this transition. Below, we will discuss the evidence suggesting roles for these genes in bladder cancer progression.

### E-CADHERIN (CDH1)

The disruption of intercellular contacts, which accompanies cell dissociation and acquisition of motility, is correlated with a redistribution of E-cadherin over the entire cell surface and within the cytoplasm. Normal urothelium expresses E-cadherin, a calcium-dependent cell adhesion molecule, located on chromosome 16q22.1 and shown to behave like an invasion suppressor gene in vitro and in vivo in experimental systems.[33] This may explain the inverse relation between expression of E-cadherin and bladder tumor grade.[34]

Several investigators further examined E-cadherin expression in bladder cancer samples and sought a correlation with tumor behavior. In an early study on 49 patient specimens (24 superficial and 25 invasive tumors), decreased E-cadherin expression correlated with both increased grade and stage of bladder cancer. More importantly, abnormal E-cadherin expression correlated with shorter patient survival.[35] These relationships to stage and grade were subsequently confirmed by other groups,[36–39] while those to survival were sometimes[37] but not always[40] shown, despite a correlation with progression[38,39] and distant metastasis.[41] This latter apparent inconsistency may be due to a lack of statistical power in the various analyses to demonstrate an effect.

### EPIDERMAL GROWTH FACTOR RECEPTOR (EGFR)

Similar to HRAS, EGFR expression levels in bladder cancer have been associated with increasing pathologic grade, stage,[42] and higher rates of recurrence,[43] and progression in superficial forms of the disease.[31] As such,

they may be causally related to the transition from superficial to invasive disease. Most importantly, patients with increased EGFR expression on their tumor cells did not survive as long as patients with normal EGFR expression. However, when the comparison of survival was limited to patients with invasive bladder cancer, no significant difference was found between patients with high levels of EGFR expression and those with low EGFR values,[44] suggesting that EGFR overexpression might be associated with the phenotypic transition from superficial to invasive forms of disease. Interestingly, gene amplification and gene rearrangement does not appear to be a common mechanism for EGFR overexpression in bladder cancer.[45] However, superficial human bladder cancer cells, engineered to overexpress either mutated or normal HRAS, also begin overexpressing EGFR at both the mRNA and protein levels; as such, HRAS might also play a role in transcriptional regulation of EGFR besides its role in EGFR signal transduction.[46,47]

Taken together, these data suggest that regulation of EGFR is altered in bladder cancer. In addition, since EGF is present in large quantities in urine,[48] with concentrations up to 10-fold greater per milliliter than those found in blood, this situation is likely to potentiate the consequences of EGFR overexpression since EGFRs in bladder cancer are functional.[49] Supporting the notion that EGFR overexpression is causally related to tumor progression, and not merely an epiphenomenon, are a number of in vitro[47,50] studies that have implicated this molecule in several of the steps involved in tumor invasion, such as cell motility.

### RETINOBLASTOMA (RB)

Deletions of the long arm of chromosome 13, including the RB locus on 13q14, were found in 28 of 94 cases, with 26 of these 28 lesions being present in muscle-invasive tumors.[51] RB alterations in bladder cancer as a function of stage were studied in 48 primary bladder tumors[52] where a spectrum of altered patterns of expression, from undetectable RB levels to heterogeneous expression of RB, was observed in 14 patients. Of the 38 patients diagnosed with muscle-invasive tumors, 13 were categorized as RB altered, while only 1 of the 10 superficial carcinomas had the altered RB phenotype. Patient survival was decreased in RB altered patients compared with those with normal RB expression. In addition, RB changes are associated with proliferative indices.[53]

Two recent studies[54,55] have also shown that RB and P53 alterations can further deregulate cell cycle control at the G1 checkpoint and produce tumor cells with reduced response to programmed cell death. The imbalance produced by an enhanced proliferative activity and a decreased apoptotic rate may further enhance the aggressive clinical course of the bladder tumors harboring both P53 and RB alterations. A study focusing on the clinical progression of T1 tumors has demonstrated that patients with normal expression of both proteins have an excellent outcome, with no patient showing disease progression. Patients with abnormal expression of either or both proteins had a significant increase in progression.[56] However, this is not found in all studies.[57] These data indicate some clinical utility of stratification of T1 bladder cancer patients based on P53 and RB nuclear protein status. Thus patients with normal protein expression for both genes may be managed conservatively, whereas patients with alterations in one gene, and particularly in both genes, may require more aggressive treatment. Conversely, conflicting results have been obtained when RB status has been examined in patients with invasive tumors,[58,59] indicating perhaps that this gene may have its primary role in progression from superficial to muscle-invasive disease rather than further downstream in the metastatic cascade. More recently, two groups reported on cumulative alterations in p53, p21, and Rb/p16 and the effect on outcome after radical cystectomy. Both groups found that alterations of both pathways or cumulative alterations were associated with worse prognosis and that these alterations provided independent prognostic information in addition to pathologic T stage, node status, and lymphovascular invasion.[60,61]

## P53

Genetic alterations of the P53 gene, such as intragenic mutations, homozygous deletions, and structural rearrangements, are frequent events in bladder cancer.[62] Structural alterations of the P53 gene were investigated using single strand conformation polymorphism (SSCP) in 25 bladder tumors and mutations were found in 6 of 12 invasive carcinomas, while only 1 of 13 superficial bladder tumors had such mutations.[63] Moreover, mutations were not identified in any of the 10 grade 1 and 2 lesions, while 8 of 15 grade 3 bladder carcinomas were found to have intragenic mutations. In another study,[64] IHC detectable P53 protein was studied in 42 bladder carcinomas. One out of 11 grade 1 (9%), 12/22 grade 2 (55%) and 8/9 grade 3 (89%) tumors showed positivity for P53. There were significantly more P53 positive cases in grade 2–3 tumors than in grade 1 tumors. There were significantly more P53 positive cases in stage T2–4 tumors than in stage T1 tumors. Another study[65] analyzed 42 specimens of TCC by interphase cytogenetics with a FISH technique, and found that P53 deletion was significantly correlated with grade, stage, S-phase fraction, and DNA ploidy, while P53 overexpression correlated only with grade. Moch et al[66] studied the overexpression of P53 by IHC in 179 patients and found that P53 immunostaining strongly correlated with tumor stage. In addition, this was driven

by a marked difference in P53 expression between pTa (37%) and pT1 (71%) tumors, while there was no difference between pT1 and pT2–4 tumors. Similarly, a strong overall association between P53 expression and grade was driven by a marked difference between grade 1 (28%) and grade 2 (71%) tumors; there was no significant difference between grade 2 and grade 3 tumors.

Several groups[53,67,68] have investigated the possibility that altered patterns of P53 expression correlated with tumor progression in patients with T1 bladder cancer. Patients with T1 tumors were retrospectively stratified into two groups with either <20% tumor cells (group A) with positive nuclear staining or >20% of cells with nuclear immunoreactivity for P53 (group B).[67] Disease progression rates were 20.5% per year for group B and 2.5% for Group A, with patients in group 2 having significantly shorter progression-free intervals. Disease-specific survival was also associated with altered patterns of P53 expression. Another study[68] reported an analysis of T1 tumors using immunohistochemistry and 20% positive nuclear staining as the cut-off value. The mean follow-up time was more than 10 years. Progression and tumor grade were both significantly related to P53 nuclear overexpression. However, in this last study, P53 expression was not an independent predictor of disease progression. The relationship of P53 expression and bacillus Calmette–Guérin (BCG) treatment response in patients with high risk superficial cancer has been evaluated but no clear consensus is yet apparent.[69–72]

Other studies have attempted to clarify the role of P53 as a prognostic marker in muscle-invasive tumors. In one study, P53 was evaluated in 90 bladder tumors from 111 patients treated with neoadjuvant MVAC (methotrexate, vinblastine, adriamycin, cisplatin).[73] Patients with P53 overexpression had a significantly higher proportion of cancer deaths. The long-term survival in the P53 overexpressors was 41% versus 77% in the non-expressors, independent of stage and grade. In another study, histologic specimens of TCC of the bladder, stages pTa to pT4, from 243 patients treated by radical cystectomy were examined for the IHC detection of P53 protein.[74] Nuclear P53 reactivity was then analyzed in relation to time to recurrence and overall survival. In patients with TCC confined to the bladder, an accumulation of P53 in the tumor cell nuclei predicted a significantly increased risk of recurrence and death, independent of tumor grade, stage, and lymph node status. In a third study, IHC P53 protein expression analysis was performed in 90 patients with TCC of the urinary bladder.[75] Positive nuclear staining of tumor cells by the antibody to P53 protein was detected in 32 cases, most of which were invasive and nonpapillary tumors, and in high-grade tumors. In addition, patients with tumors positive for P53 staining had a significantly worse survival rate.

## RHO FAMILY GTPases

Many of the basic mechanisms of cell migration are thought to be largely conserved among most cell types. These processes involve the simultaneous and sequential changes in the activities and/or locations of hundreds of proteins. Such complexity underscores the extensive level of coordinate regulation, in which members of the Rho family of small GTPases play a central role. The larger Ras superfamily in humans comprises over 100 small (20–30 kDa), related monomeric guanine nucleotide-binding proteins including six subfamilies: Ras, Rho, Arf, Rab, Ran, and Rad.[76] The Rho subfamily has been implicated as a nexus for signal transduction pathways that affect the actin and tubulin cytoskeletons, cell migration, cell-cycle progression, membrane recycling, and gene expression.

Underlying the functional diversity in the Rho family is a common guanosine triphosphate (GTP)/guanosine diphosphate (GDP) cycle (Figure 13.1). Small G proteins

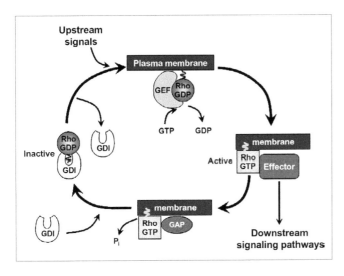

**Fig. 13.1**

The GTPase cycle. GTPases cycle between an active (GTP-bound) and an inactive (GDP-bound) conformation. Rho cycle shown as generic example. Activated GTPases interact with target proteins (effectors). The cycle is regulated by three classes of proteins: nucleotide exchange factors (GEFs) catalyze nucleotide exchange to induce activation; GTPase-activating proteins (GAPs) stimulate GTP hydrolysis, leading to inactivation; and guanine nucleotide exchange inhibitors (GDIs) extract the inactive GTPase from membranes. Twenty mammalian Rho GTPases have been described: Rho (three isoforms: A, B, C); Rac (1, 2, 3); Cdc42; TC10; TCL; Chp (1, 2); RhoG; Rnd (1, 2, 3); RhoBTB (1, 2); RhoD; Rif; and TTF. All Rho GTPases are prenylated at their C terminus, which is required for membrane targeting and function. Rnd proteins are exceptional in that they do not hydrolyse GTP in vitro, which is an unusual property for a regulatory GTPase. Adapted from Takai et al[119] and Etienne-Manneville & Hall.[120]

cycle between a GTP-bound state and a GDP-bound state. In vivo, this cycle is tightly regulated by guanine nucleotide exchange factors (GEFs), which stimulate the exchange of GDP for GTP,[77] and GTPase activator proteins (GAPs), which increase the rate of GTP hydrolysis.[78] Rho family proteins are further regulated by GDP dissociation inhibitors (GDIs).[79,80] These proteins bind to the GTPases and sequester the C-terminal prenyl moieties to confer solubility in the cytoplasm.

The evidence for Rho family member involvement in human cancer has recently been reviewed.[81] Although Rho family gene mutations in tumors are rare, overexpression is fairly common.[82] RhoA, RhoB, and RhoC show approximately 85% amino acid sequence identity, though there is greater sequence divergence in the C-terminal 15 amino acids of each protein.[83] RhoA is overexpressed in head and neck squamous carcinomas,[84] as well as in lung, colon, testicular germ cell,[85] and breast tumors.[86] In breast tumors, increasing RhoA expression has been shown to correlate with increasing tumor grade, suggesting a role for RhoA in tumor progression.[87–89] Significant association of the Rho/ROCK pathway (Figure 13.2) with invasion and metastasis of bladder cancer has been reported by Kamai et al.[90] In this study, surgical specimens of bladder cancer obtained from 107 Japanese patients with newly diagnosed primary TCC of the bladder were examined. By univariate analysis, disease-free survival was influenced significantly by RhoA, RhoC, ROCKI, ROCKII, stage, and grade. By multivariate analysis, RhoC was identified as an independent prognostic factor for disease-free survival. With regard to overall survival, all of the factors analyzed above were statistically significant by univariate analysis, but only RhoC, RhoA, stage, and grade were significant by multivariate analysis. Comparison of Kaplan–Meier survival-rate plots in patients with low versus high expression of RhoA protein indicated that high RhoA expression was associated with shortened disease-free and overall survival. Similarly, high expression of RhoC, ROCKI, and ROCKII was associated with poorer disease-free and overall survival.

As mentioned above, Rho GDP dissociation inhibitors (GDIs) bind to Rho proteins in the cytoplasm, conferring aqueous solubility. They also block dissociation of bound nucleotides and interactions with GEFs, GAPs, and effectors, blocking activation or function. To date, three RhoGDIs have been identified: GDI1, GDI2, and GDI3.[79]

## RHOGDI1

RhoGDI1 was first identified on the basis of its ability to inhibit GDP dissociation from RhoA,[91] CDC42Hs,[92] and Rac1.[93] The functions of RhoGDI1 in cell culture have largely been investigated using transfection and microinjection of mammalian cell lines. These experiments have shown that RhoGDI1 overexpression

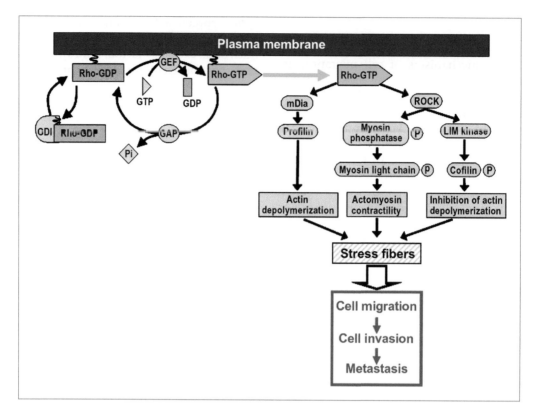

**Fig. 13.2**

Rho biochemistry in cell migration and metastasis. Most Rho GTPases cycle between an active (GTP-bound) and an inactive (GDP-bound) conformation. In the active state, they interact with one or more of over 60 effector molecules. The cycle is highly regulated by three classes of protein: in mammalian cells, around 60 guanine nucleotide exchange factors (GEFs) catalyze nucleotide exchange and mediate activation; more than 70 GTPase-activating proteins (GAPs) stimulate GTP hydrolysis, leading to inactivation; and three guanine nucleotide dissociation inhibitors (GDIs) extract the inactive GTPase from membranes. All Rho GTPases are prenylated at their C terminus, a requirement for proper function. Rnd proteins are exceptional in that they do not hydrolyse GTP in vitro, which is an unusual property for a regulatory GTPase. It has been argued that they are controlled by expression, but it is possible that an as yet unidentified GAP is required for hydrolysis. The interaction of activated Rho proteins with their respective effectors results in downstream effects on actin stress fibers. These changes, in part, ultimately affect global cellular processes, such as motility, invasion, and metastasis. Adapted from Takai et al[119] and Etienne-Manneville & Hall.[120]

inhibits function of the GTPases.[94–96] However, in some settings, interaction of RhoGDI with its target GTPases is required for function,[97] most likely because it is needed for translocation between different compartments. The targeted disruption of RhoGDI1 appears to result in the impairment of function of the kidneys and reproductive organs, with renal disorders mimicking nephrotic syndrome. Knockout mice that were grossly normal in appearance, size, growth, development, and behavior showed increasing malaise and weakness with age.[98] Recently, RhoGDI1 has been shown to increase estrogen receptor transactivation by antagonizing Rho function in mammalian cells.[99] At present, there is little evidence for a role for RhoGDI1 in cancer initiation, invasion, migration, or metastasis.

## RHOGDI2

RhoGDI2 (also known as D4-GDI or Ly-GDI) shares 67% amino acid identity with RhoGDI1[100–102]; however,

in contrast to RhoGDI1, which is ubiquitous, this protein was initially believed to be exclusively expressed in cells of hematopoietic lineage.[100,101] RhoGDI2 knockout mice are ostensibly normal except for deregulation of T- and B-cell interactions, resulting in overexpansion of B lymphocytes under certain conditions. This phenotype is mild, however, since the mice exhibited mostly normal immune responses, including lymphocyte proliferation, interleukin (IL) 2 production, cytotoxic T-lymphocyte activity, antibody production, antigen processing and presentation, immune-cell aggregation and migration, and protection against an intracellular protozoan. These data suggest that these functions may be partially complemented by other Rho regulatory proteins in the absence of RhoGDI2.[103]

More recently, a thorough evaluation of RhoGDI2 mRNA expression as a function of tissue type revealed high expression in a variety of types of epithelial cells. These included transitional epithelium of the bladder;

basal cells of vas, seminal vesicle, and epididymis; fallopian tube; skin (basal layer); renal collecting ducts; and ducts and some acini of breast, sweat, Bartholin's, lacrimal, and salivary glands.[104] By contrast, neural, pancreatic, testicular, and hepatic tissues had very low levels. As previously noted,[100–102] tissues with significant hematopoietic cell components, such as spleen and thymus, had higher than average levels of RhoGDI2 mRNA expression. Interestingly, tissues with significant vasculature, such as heart, lung, and placenta, had high levels of mRNA expression, supporting the notion of a common embryonic precursor of hematopoietic and endothelial cell lineages.

An extensive survey of tumor-derived cell lines revealed an overall decrease in RhoGDI2 expression, with the exception of tumorigenic, immortalized, or normal cells of hematopoietic or endothelial lineages, where levels were higher.[104] Importantly, reduced expression of RhoGDI2 correlated with increasing invasive and metastatic activity in human bladder carcinoma lines.[104,105] Microarray-expression analysis of human prostate tumors revealed that RhoGDI2 expression is also significantly downregulated in prostate tumors compared to normal prostate epithelium.[106] DNA-array analysis of a novel animal model of bladder cancer metastasis identified RhoGDI2 as a metastasis-suppressor gene in human bladder cancer.[107] In human bladder tumors, the RhoGDI2 level inversely correlated with development of metastatic disease, and multivariate analysis revealed that it was an independent prognostic marker of disease relapse following radical cystectomy.[104] Taken together, these data show that, although RhoGDI2 is expressed more widely than originally thought, its loss or reduction in bladder and perhaps other tumors is an independent predictor for the development of metastatic disease and disease-specific death. Thus RhoGDI2 is a putative metastasis-suppressor gene and clinical prognostic marker. It may therefore also represent a potential target for therapy.

## OTHER GENES

### MYC

Early studies in bladder cancer have indicated a strong association of low level MYC (8q24) gains with tumor grade, stage, chromosome polysomy, p53 protein expression, p53 deletion and tumor cell proliferation as assessed by Ki67 labeling index.[108,109] These data were consistent with a role of chromosome 8 alterations in bladder cancer progression.[20] However, subsequent studies have not found statistically significant correlation between the methylation, expression of the MYC gene and clinical–histopathologic parameters,[110] and between the MYC methylation pattern and clinical

stage.[111] Furthermore, MYC overexpression did not correlate with tumor grade or tumor progression.[112] Thus the role of this gene in bladder cancer development or progression is at present unclear.

### ERBB2

Amplification and protein overexpression of the ERBB2 gene, located on 17q11.2–q12, have been suggested as prognostic markers for patients with recurrent progressive bladder tumors.[113,114] However, other studies have failed to link ERBB2 expression levels as an independent variable predicting disease progression.[115] Other studies have indicated a high level of expression of this gene in malignant as compared to benign bladder epithelium.[115] From these studies it would appear that the role of ERBB2 as a diagnostic marker may outweigh its usefulness as a prognostic indicator.

### MDM2

The MDM2 (mouse double minute 2, human homolog of; p53-binding protein) gene is located at 12q13–14 and codes for a 90 Kd nuclear protein which is a negative regulator of P53. In urinary bladder, a strong statistical association between MDM2 and P53 overexpression was found in addition to an association between MDM2 overexpression and low-stage, low-grade bladder tumors.[116] In addition, the simultaneous assessment of MDM2 and P53 was found to be an independent factor for both disease progression and survival.[109,117] However, as with MYC and ERBB2, not all studies have shown assessment of this gene product to be independently related to tumor progression.[118]

## CONCLUSION

We have attempted to highlight our current understanding of the molecular basis of urothelial invasion and metastasis. For those patients with neoplastic disease, this will lead the way toward therapy that can be tailored to the specific biology of the individual tumor and aim to prevent metastatic disease development. The ongoing integration of molecular biology with clinical science promises to bring all of this within our reach.

## REFERENCES

1. Gontero P, Banisadr S, Frea B, Brausi M. Metastasis markers in bladder cancer: a review of the literature and clinical considerations. Eur Urol 2004;46(3):296–311.
2. Beavon IR. Regulation of E-cadherin: does hypoxia initiate the metastatic cascade? Mol Pathol 1999;52(4):179–188.
3. Beavon IR. The E-cadherin-catenin complex in tumour metastasis: structure, function and regulation. Eur J Cancer 2000;36(13 Spec No):1607–1620.

4. Fiddler IJ. Melanoma metastasis. Cancer Control 1995;2(5):398–404.

5. Chambers AF, MacDonald IC, Schmidt EE, et al. Steps in tumor metastasis: new concepts from intravital videomicroscopy. Cancer Metastasis Rev 1995;14(4):279–301.

6. Webb DJ, Parsons JT, Horwitz AF. Adhesion assembly, disassembly and turnover in migrating cells—over and over and over again. Nat Cell Biol 2002;4(4):E97–100.

7. Horwitz AR, Parsons JT. Cell migration—movin' on. Science 1999;286(5442):1102–1103.

8. Wells A, Gupta K, Chang P, Swindle S, Glading A, Shiraha H. Epidermal growth factor receptor-mediated motility in fibroblasts. Microsc Res Tech 1998;43(5):395–411.

9. Feldner JC, Brandt BH. Cancer cell motility—on the road from c-erbB-2 receptor steered signaling to actin reorganization. Exp Cell Res 2002;272(2):93–108.

10. Somlyo AP, Somlyo AV. The sarcoplasmic reticulum: then and now. Novartis Found Symp 2002;246:258–268; discussion 68–71, 72–76.

11. Palecek SP, Huttenlocher A, Horwitz AF, Lauffenburger DA. Physical and biochemical regulation of integrin release during rear detachment of migrating cells. J Cell Sci 1998;111(Pt 7):929–940.

12. Hughes PE, Pfaff M. Integrin affinity modulation. Trends Cell Biol 1998;8(9):359–364.

13. Friedl P, Wolf K. Tumour-cell invasion and migration: diversity and escape mechanisms. Nat Rev Cancer 2003;3(5):362–374.

14. Mahadevan V, Hart IR. Metastasis and angiogenesis. Acta Oncol 1990;29(1):97–103.

15. Bernstein LR, Liotta LA. Molecular mediators of interactions with extracellular matrix components in metastasis and angiogenesis. Curr Opin Oncol 1994;6(1):106–113.

16. Rosin MP, Cairns P, Epstein JI, Schoenberg MP, Sidransky D. Partial allelotype of carcinoma in situ of the human bladder. Cancer Res 1995;55(22):5213–5216.

17. Knowles MA, Elder PA, Williamson M, Cairns JP, Shaw ME, Law MG. Allelotype of human bladder cancer. Cancer Res 1994;54(2):531–538.

18. Li M, Zhang ZF, Reuter VE, Cordon-Cardo C. Chromosome 3 allelic losses and microsatellite alterations in transitional cell carcinoma of the urinary bladder. Am J Pathol 1996;149(1):229–235.

19. Polascik TJ, Cairns P, Chang WY, Schoenberg MP, Sidransky D. Distinct regions of allelic loss on chromosome 4 in human primary bladder carcinoma. Cancer Res 1995;55(22):5396–5399.

20. Wagner U, Bubendorf L, Gasser TC, et al. Chromosome 8p deletions are associated with invasive tumor growth in urinary bladder cancer. Am J Pathol 1997;151(3):753–759.

21. Brewster SF, Gingell JC, Browne S, Brown KW. Loss of heterozygosity on chromosome 18q is associated with muscle-invasive transitional cell carcinoma of the bladder. Br J Cancer 1994;70(4):697–700.

22. Kagan J, Liu J, Stein JD, Wagner SS, et al. Cluster of allele losses within a 2.5 cM region of chromosome 10 in high-grade invasive bladder cancer. Oncogene 1998;16(7):909–913.

23. Cappellen D, Gil Diez de Medina S, Chopin D, Thiery JP, Radvanyi F. Frequent loss of heterozygosity on chromosome 10q in muscle-invasive transitional cell carcinomas of the bladder. Oncogene 1997;14(25):3059–3066.

24. Wheeless LL, Reeder JE, Han R, et al. Bladder irrigation specimens assayed by fluorescence in situ hybridization to interphase nuclei. Cytometry 1994;17(4):319–326.

25. Wick W, Petersen I, Schmutzler RK, et al. Evidence for a novel tumor suppressor gene on chromosome 15 associated with progression to a metastatic stage in breast cancer. Oncogene 1996;12(5):973–978.

26. Reznikoff CA, Belair CD, Yeager TR, et al. A molecular genetic model of human bladder cancer pathogenesis. Semin Oncol 1996;23(5):571–584.

27. Gildea JJ, Golden WL, Harding MA, Theodorescu D. Genetic and phenotypic changes associated with the acquisition of tumorigenicity in human bladder cancer. Genes Chromosomes Cancer 2000;27(3):252–263.

28. Harding MA, Arden KC, Gildea JW, et al. Functional genomic comparison of lineage-related human bladder cancer cell lines with differing tumorigenic and metastatic potentials by spectral karyotyping, comparative genomic hybridization, and a novel method of positional expression profiling. Cancer Res 2002;62(23):6981–6989.

29. Fontana D, Bellina M, Scoffone C, et al. Evaluation of c-ras oncogene product (p21) in superficial bladder cancer. Eur Urol 1996;29(4):470–476.

30. Lacombe L, Dalbagni G, Zhang ZF, et al. Overexpression of p53 protein in a high-risk population of patients with superficial bladder cancer before and after bacillus Calmette–Guérin therapy: correlation to clinical outcome. J Clin Oncol 1996;14(10):2646–2652.

31. Lipponen P, Eskelinen M. Expression of epidermal growth factor receptor in bladder cancer as related to established prognostic factors, oncoprotein (c-erbB-2, p53) expression and long-term prognosis. Br J Cancer 1994;69(6):1120–1125.

32. Schmitz-Drager BJ, Jankevicius F, Ackermann R. Molecular biology of dissemination in bladder cancer—laboratory findings and clinical significance. World J Urol 1996;14(3):190–196.

33. Mareel M, Boterberg T, Noe V, et al. E-cadherin/catenin/cytoskeleton complex: a regulator of cancer invasion. J Cell Physiol 1997;173(2):271–274.

34. Syrigos KN, Krausz T, Waxman J, et al. E-cadherin expression in bladder cancer using formalin-fixed, paraffin-embedded tissues: correlation with histopathological grade, tumour stage and survival. Int J Cancer 1995;64(6):367–370.

35. Bringuier PP, Umbas R, Schaafsma HE, Karthaus HF, Debruyne FM, Schalken JA. Decreased E-cadherin immunoreactivity correlates with poor survival in patients with bladder tumors. Cancer Res 1993;53(14):3241–3245.

36. Griffiths TR, Brotherick I, Bishop RI, et al. Cell adhesion molecules in bladder cancer: soluble serum E-cadherin correlates with predictors of recurrence. Br J Cancer 1996;74(4):579–584.

37. Shimazui T, Schalken JA, Giroldi LA, et al. Prognostic value of cadherin-associated molecules (alpha-, beta-, and gamma-catenins and p120cas) in bladder tumors. Cancer Res 1996;56(18):4154–4158.

38. Shariat SF, Pahlavan S, Baseman AG, et al. E-cadherin expression predicts clinical outcome in carcinoma in situ of the urinary bladder. Urology 2001;57(1):60–65.

39. Byrne RR, Shariat SF, Brown R, et al. E-cadherin immunostaining of bladder transitional cell carcinoma, carcinoma in situ and lymph node metastases with long-term followup. J Urol 2001;165(5):1473–1479.

40. Lipponen PK, Eskelinen MJ. Reduced expression of E-cadherin is related to invasive disease and frequent recurrence in bladder cancer. J Cancer Res Clin Oncol 1995;121(5):303–308.

41. Mialhe A, Louis J, Montlevier S, et al. Expression of E-cadherin and alpha-, beta- and gamma-catenins in human bladder carcinomas: are they good prognostic factors? Invasion Metastasis 1997;17(3):124–137.

42. Gorgoulis VG, Barbatis C, Poulias I, Karameris AM. Molecular and immunohistochemical evaluation of epidermal growth factor receptor and c-erb-B-2 gene product in transitional cell carcinomas of the urinary bladder: a study in Greek patients. Mod Pathol 1995;8(7):758–764.

43. Chow NH, Liu HS, Lee EI, et al. Significance of urinary epidermal growth factor and its receptor expression in human bladder cancer. Anticancer Res 1997;17(2B):1293–1296.

44. Nguyen PL, Swanson PE, Jaszcz W, et al. Expression of epidermal growth factor receptor in invasive transitional cell carcinoma of the urinary bladder. A multivariate survival analysis. Am J Clin Pathol 1994;101(2):166–176.

45. Sauter G, Haley J, Chew K, et al. Epidermal-growth-factor-receptor expression is associated with rapid tumor proliferation in bladder cancer. Int J Cancer 1994;57(4):508–514.

46. Bos JL. All in the family? New insights and questions regarding interconnectivity of Ras, Rap1 and Ral. EMBO J 1998;17(23):6776–6782.

47. Theodorescu D, Cornil I, Sheehan C, Man MS, Kerbel RS. Ha-ras induction of the invasive phenotype results in up-regulation of epidermal growth factor receptors and altered responsiveness to epidermal growth factor in human papillary transitional cell carcinoma cells. Cancer Res 1991;51(16):4486–4491.

48. Chow NH, Tzai TS, Cheng PE, Chang CJ, Lin JS, Tang MJ. An assessment of immunoreactive epidermal growth factor in urine of patients with urological diseases. Urol Res 1994;22(4):221–225.

49. Messing EM, Reznikoff CA. Normal and malignant human urothelium: in vitro effects of epidermal growth factor. Cancer Res 1987;47(9):2230–2235.

50. Theodorescu D, Laderoute KR, Gulding KM. Epidermal growth factor receptor-regulated human bladder cancer motility is in part a phosphatidylinositol 3-kinase-mediated process. Cell Growth Differ 1998;9(11):919–928.

51. Cairns P, Proctor AJ, Knowles MA. Loss of heterozygosity at the RB locus is frequent and correlates with muscle invasion in bladder carcinoma. Oncogene 1991;6(12):2305–2309.

52. Cordon-Cardo C, Wartinger D, Petrylak D, et al. Altered expression of the retinoblastoma gene product: prognostic indicator in bladder cancer [see comments]. J Natl Cancer Inst 1992;84(16):1251–1256.

53. Ioachim E, Charchanti A, Stavropoulos NE, Skopelitou A, Athanassiou ED, Agnantis NJ. Immunohistochemical expression of retinoblastoma gene product (Rb), p53 protein, MDM2, c-erbB-2, HLA-DR and proliferation indices in human urinary bladder carcinoma. Histol Histopathol 2000;15(3):721–727.

54. Cordon-Cardo C, Zhang ZF, Dalbagni G, et al. Cooperative effects of p53 and pRB alterations in primary superficial bladder tumors. Cancer Res 1997;57(7):1217–1221.

55. Cote RJ, Dunn MD, Chatterjee SJ, et al. Elevated and absent pRb expression is associated with bladder cancer progression and has cooperative effects with p53. Cancer Res 1998;58(6):1090–1094.

56. Grossman HB, Liebert M, Antelo M, et al. p53 and RB expression predict progression in T1 bladder cancer. Clin Cancer Res 1998;4(4):829–834.

57. Wada T, Louhelainen J, Hemminki K, et al. Bladder cancer: allelic deletions at and around the retinoblastoma tumor suppressor gene in relation to stage and grade. Clin Cancer Res 2000;6(2):610–615.

58. Jahnson S, Karlsson MG. Predictive value of p53 and pRb immunostaining in locally advanced bladder cancer treated with cystectomy. J Urol 1998;160(4):1291–1296.

59. Logothetis CJ, Xu HJ, Ro JY, et al. Altered expression of retinoblastoma protein and known prognostic variables in locally advanced bladder cancer [see comments]. J Natl Cancer Inst 1992;84(16):1256–1261.

60. Shariat SF, Tokunaga H, Zhou J, et al. p53, p21, pRB, and p16 expression predict clinical outcome in cystectomy with bladder cancer. J Clin Oncol 2004;22(6):1014–1024.

61. Chatterjee SJ, Datar R, Youssefzadeh D, et al. Combined effects of p53, p21, and pRb expression in the progression of bladder transitional cell carcinoma. J Clin Oncol 2004;22(6):1007–1013.

62. Cordon-Cardo C, Sheinfeld J, Dalbagni G. Genetic studies and molecular markers of bladder cancer. Semin Surg Oncol 1997;13(5):319–327.

63. Fujimoto K, Yamada Y, Okajima E, et al. Frequent association of p53 gene mutation in invasive bladder cancer. Cancer Res 1992;52(6):1393–1398.

64. Soini Y, Turpeenniemi-Hujanen T, Kamel D, et al. p53 immunohistochemistry in transitional cell carcinoma and dysplasia of the urinary bladder correlates with disease progression. Br J Cancer 1993;68(5):1029–1035.

65. Matsuyama H, Pan Y, Mahdy EA, et al. p53 deletion as a genetic marker in urothelial tumor by fluorescence in situ hybridization. Cancer Res 1994;54(23):6057–6060.

66. Moch H, Sauter G, Moore D, Mihatsch MJ, Gudat F, Waldman F. p53 and erbB-2 protein overexpression are associated with early invasion and metastasis in bladder cancer. Virchows Arch A Pathol Anat Histopathol 1993;423(5):329–334.

67. Sarkis AS, Dalbagni G, Cordon-Cardo C, et al. Nuclear overexpression of p53 protein in transitional cell bladder carcinoma: a marker for disease progression. J Natl Cancer Inst 1993;85(1):53–59.

68. Lipponen PK. Over-expression of p53 nuclear oncoprotein in transitional-cell bladder cancer and its prognostic value. Int J Cancer 1993;53(3):365–370.

69. Zlotta AR, Noel JC, Fayt I, et al. Correlation and prognostic significance of p53, p21WAF1/CIP1 and Ki-67 expression in patients with superficial bladder tumors treated with bacillus Calmette–Guérin intravesical therapy. J Urol 1999;161(3):792–798.

70. Pfister C, Flaman JM, Dunet F, Grise P, Frebourg T. p53 mutations in bladder tumors inactivate the transactivation of the p21 and Bax genes, and have a predictive value for the clinical outcome after bacillus Calmette–Guérin therapy. J Urol 1999;162(1):69–73.

71. Fontana D, Bellina M, Galietti F, et al. Intravesical bacillus Calmette–Guérin (BCG) as inducer of tumor-suppressing proteins p53 and p21 Waf1-Cip1 during treatment of superficial bladder cancer. J Urol 1999;162(1):225–230.

72. Peyromaure M, Weibing S, Sebe P, et al. Prognostic value of p53 overexpression in T1G3 bladder tumors treated with bacillus Calmette–Guérin therapy. Urology 2002;59(3):409–413.

73. Sarkis AS, Bajorin DF, Reuter VE, et al. Prognostic value of p53 nuclear overexpression in patients with invasive bladder cancer treated with neoadjuvant MVAC. J Clin Oncol 1995;13(6):1384–1390.

74. Esrig D, Elmajian D, Groshen S, et al. Accumulation of nuclear p53 and tumor progression in bladder cancer [see comments]. N Engl J Med 1994;331(19):1259–1264.

75. Furihata M, Inoue K, Ohtsuki Y, Hashimoto H, Terao N, Fujita Y. High-risk human papillomavirus infections and overexpression of p53 protein as prognostic indicators in transitional cell carcinoma of the urinary bladder. Cancer Res 1993;53(20):4823–4827.

76. Oxford G, Theodorescu D. Ras superfamily monomeric G proteins in carcinoma cell motility. Cancer Lett 2003;189(2):117–128.

77. Cherfils J, Chardin P. GEFs: structural basis for their activation of small GTP-binding proteins. Trends Biochem Sci 1999;24(8):306–311.

78. Donovan S, Shannon KM, Bollag G. GTPase activating proteins: critical regulators of intracellular signaling. Biochim Biophys Acta 2002;1602(1):23–45.

79. Olofsson B. Rho guanine dissociation inhibitors: pivotal molecules in cellular signalling. Cell Signal 1999;11(8):545–554.

80. Yamada M, Tachibana T, Imamoto N, Yoneda Y. Nuclear transport factor p10/NTF2 functions as a Ran-GDP dissociation inhibitor (Ran-GDI). Curr Biol 1998;8(24):1339–1342.

81. Ridley AJ. Rho proteins and cancer. Breast Cancer Res Treat 2004;84(1):13–19.

82. Sahai E, Marshall CJ. RHO-GTPases and cancer. Nat Rev Cancer 2002;2(2):133–142.

83. Wheeler AP, Ridley AJ. Why three Rho proteins? RhoA, RhoB, RhoC, and cell motility. Exp Cell Res 2004;301(1):43–49.

84. Abraham MT, Kuriakose MA, Sacks PG, et al. Motility-related proteins as markers for head and neck squamous cell cancer. Laryngoscope 2001;111(7):1285–1289.

85. Kamai T, Arai K, Sumi S, et al. The rho/rho-kinase pathway is involved in the progression of testicular germ cell tumour. BJU Int 2002;89(4):449–453.

86. Fritz G, Just I, Kaina B. Rho GTPases are over-expressed in human tumors. Int J Cancer 1999;81(5):682–687.

87. Adamson P, Paterson HF, Hall A. Intracellular localization of the P21rho proteins. J Cell Biol 1992;119(3):617–627.

88. Michaelson D, Silletti J, Murphy G, D'Eustachio P, Rush M, Philips MR. Differential localization of Rho GTPases in live cells: regulation by hypervariable regions and RhoGDI binding. J Cell Biol 2001;152(1):111–126.

89. Wang HR, Zhang Y, Ozdamar B, et al. Regulation of cell polarity and protrusion formation by targeting RhoA for degradation. Science 2003;302(5651):1775–1779.

90. Kamai T, Tsujii T, Arai K, et al. Significant association of Rho/ROCK pathway with invasion and metastasis of bladder cancer. Clin Cancer Res 2003;9(7):2632–2641.

91. Ueda T, Kikuchi A, Ohga N, Yamamoto J, Takai Y. Purification and characterization from bovine brain cytosol of a novel regulatory protein inhibiting the dissociation of GDP from and the subsequent binding of GTP to rhoB p20, a ras p21-like GTP-binding protein. J Biol Chem 1990;265(16):9373–9380.

92. Leonard D, Hart MJ, Platko JV, et al. The identification and characterization of a GDP-dissociation inhibitor (GDI) for the CDC42Hs protein. J Biol Chem 1992;267(32):22860–22868.

93. Adra CN, Ko J, Leonard D, Wirth LJ, Cerione RA, Lim B. Identification of a novel protein with GDP dissociation inhibitor activity for the ras-like proteins CDC42Hs and rac I. Genes Chromosomes Cancer 1993;8(4):253–261.

94. Miura Y, Kikuchi A, Musha T, et al. Regulation of morphology by rho p21 and its inhibitory GDP/GTP exchange protein (rho GDI) in Swiss 3T3 cells. J Biol Chem 1993;268(1):510–515.

95. Takaishi K, Kikuchi A, Kuroda S, Kotani K, Sasaki T, Takai Y. Involvement of rho p21 and its inhibitory GDP/GTP exchange protein (rho GDI) in cell motility. Mol Cell Biol 1993;13(1):72–79.

96. Takaishi K, Sasaki T, Kato M, et al. Involvement of Rho p21 small GTP-binding protein and its regulator in the HGF-induced cell motility. Oncogene 1994;9(1):273–279.

97. Lin R, Bagrodia S, Cerione R, Manor D. A novel Cdc42Hs mutant induces cellular transformation. Curr Biol 1997;7(10):794–797.

98. Togawa A, Miyoshi J, Ishizaki H, et al. Progressive impairment of kidneys and reproductive organs in mice lacking Rho GDIalpha. Oncogene 1999;18(39):5373–5380.

99. Su LF, Knoblauch R, Garabedian MJ. Rho GTPases as modulators of the estrogen receptor transcriptional response. J Biol Chem 2001;276(5):3231–3237.

100. Scherle P, Behrens T, Staudt LM. Ly-GDI, a GDP-dissociation inhibitor of the RhoA GTP-binding protein, is expressed preferentially in lymphocytes. Proc Natl Acad Sci USA 1993;90(16):7568–7572.

101. Lelias JM, Adra CN, Wulf GM, et al. cDNA cloning of a human mRNA preferentially expressed in hematopoietic cells and with homology to a GDP-dissociation inhibitor for the rho GTP-binding proteins. Proc Natl Acad Sci USA 1993;90(4):1479–1483.

102. Leffers H, Nielsen MS, Andersen AH, et al. Identification of two human Rho GDP dissociation inhibitor proteins whose overexpression leads to disruption of the actin cytoskeleton. Exp Cell Res 1993;209(2):165–174.

103. Yin L, Schwartzberg P, Scharton-Kersten TM, Staudt L, Lenardo M. Immune responses in mice deficient in Ly-GDI, a lymphoid-specific regulator of Rho GTPases. Mol Immunol 1997;34(6):481–491.

104. Theodorescu D, Sapinoso LM, Conaway MR, Oxford G, Hampton GM, Frierson HF Jr. Reduced expression of metastasis suppressor RhoGDI2 is associated with decreased survival for patients with bladder cancer. Clin Cancer Res 2004;10(11):3800–3806.

105. Seraj MJ, Harding MA, Gildea JJ, Welch DR, Theodorescu D. The relationship of BRMS1 and RhoGDI2 gene expression to metastatic potential in lineage related human bladder cancer cell lines. Clin Exp Metastasis 2000;18(6):519–525.

106. Ashida S, Nakagawa H, Katagiri T, et al. Molecular features of the transition from prostatic intraepithelial neoplasia (PIN) to prostate cancer: genome-wide gene-expression profiles of prostate cancers and PINs. Cancer Res 2004;64(17):5963–5972.

107. Gildea JJ, Seraj MJ, Oxford G, et al. RhoGDI2 is an invasion and metastasis suppressor gene in human cancer. Cancer Res 2002;62(22):6418–6423.

108. Sauter G, Moch H, Gasser TC, Mihatsch MJ, Waldman FM. Heterogeneity of chromosome 17 and erbB-2 gene copy number in primary and metastatic bladder cancer. Cytometry 1995;21(1):40–46.

109. Pfister C, Moore L, Allard P, et al. Predictive value of cell cycle markers p53, MDM2, p21, and Ki-67 in superficial bladder tumor recurrence. Clin Cancer Res 1999;5(12):4079–4084.

110. Sardi I, Dal Canto M, Bartoletti R, Guazzelli R, Travaglini F, Montali E. Molecular genetic alterations of c-myc oncogene in superficial and locally advanced bladder cancer. Eur Urol 1998;33(4):424–430.

111. Sardi I, Dal Canto M, Bartoletti R, Montali E. Abnormal c-myc oncogene DNA methylation in human bladder cancer: possible role in tumor progression. Eur Urol 1997;31(2):224–230.

112. Schmitz-Drager BJ, Schulz WA, Jurgens B, et al. c-myc in bladder cancer. Clinical findings and analysis of mechanism. Urol Res 1997;25(Suppl 1):S45–49.

113. Novara R, Coda R, Martone T, Vineis P. Exposure to aromatic amines and ras and c-erbB-2 overexpression in bladder cancer. J Occup Environ Med 1996;38(4):390–393.

114. Ravery V, Grignon D, Angulo J, et al. Evaluation of epidermal growth factor receptor, transforming growth factor alpha, epidermal growth factor and c-erbB2 in the progression of invasive bladder cancer. Urol Res 1997;25(1):9–17.

115. Underwood M, Bartlett J, Reeves J, Gardiner DS, Scott R, Cooke T. C-erbB-2 gene amplification: a molecular marker in recurrent bladder tumors? Cancer Res 1995;55(11):2422–2430.

116. Lianes P, Orlow I, Zhang ZF, et al. Altered patterns of MDM2 and TP53 expression in human bladder cancer [see comments]. J Natl Cancer Inst 1994;86(17):1325–1330.

117. Shiina H, Igawa M, Shigeno K, et al. Clinical significance of mdm2 and p53 expression in bladder cancer. A comparison with cell proliferation and apoptosis. Oncology 1999;56(3):239–247.

118. Schmitz-Drager BJ, Kushima M, Goebell P, et al. p53 and MDM2 in the development and progression of bladder cancer. Eur Urol 1997;32(4):487–493.

119. Takai Y, Sasaki T, Matozaki T. Small GTP-binding proteins. Physiol Rev 2001;81(1):153–208.

120. Etienne-Manneville S, Hall A. Rho GTPases in cell biology. Nature 2002;420(6916):629–635.

# Animal models of bladder cancer 14

*Xue-Ru Wu, Tung-Tien Sun*
*David J McConkey, Marissa Shrader, Angela Papageorgiou*

## INTRODUCTION

Transitional cell carcinoma (TCC) is almost certainly two different diseases, one that is characterized by superficial (papillary) growth and a high frequency of recurrence, and another that is characterized by invasive and metastatic growth that represents the highly lethal form of the disease.[1,2] Work conducted over the past two decades has defined many of the genetic and epigenetic alterations associated with each pathway of tumorigenesis and progression,[2] and it is now fairly well established that Ras pathway activation plays a central role in superficial disease[3,4] whereas loss of p53 and Rb play more important roles in invasive and metastatic TCC.[5,6] Other studies indicate that epigenetic activation of the epidermal growth factor receptor (EGFR)[7-10] and cyclooxygenase-2 (COX2)[11] pathways are associated with disease progression. Epidemiologic studies indicate that, like lung cancer, bladder cancer is associated with tobacco smoking and exposure to certain other environmental carcinogens,[12] and familial markers of disease susceptibility are being identified.[13] Finally, analyses of global patterns of gene and protein expression are beginning to provide a more comprehensive picture of the pathways involved in the transformed phenotype.[14-16] However, precisely how these alterations influence tumor biology, and especially how they might influence treatment outcome, remains unclear.

Fortunately, researchers have access to an unusually large number of excellent rodent models that recapitulate key features of TCC in humans. Although none of the models is perfect, each allows investigators to perform mechanistic studies that currently are not possible in human patients. Carcinogens implicated in

human TCC induce bladder tumors in rats and mice,[17] and these tumors display features (loss of p53, activation of the EGFR pathway) consistent with human disease. Even 'cleaner' mouse models have been developed in which specific transgenes are selectively expressed within the bladder epithelium, allowing investigators using these models to interrogate the biologic mechanisms controlled by the pathways these genes regulate under carefully controlled conditions. Finally, a large number of human cell lines have been established from primary TCCs (and for that matter squamous cell carcinomas and adenocarcinomas), and preliminary analyses indicate that they retain the genetic complexity observed in primary TCCs.[15] These cell lines have been used to establish orthotopic and subcutaneous tumor models that also display many of the crucial features of human cancer. Each of the models has strengths and weaknesses that make them more or less appropriate for a particular experimental question. The purpose of this chapter is to provide an overview of these three major animal model systems and to discuss how they have yielded information that has proven critical to the design of ongoing clinical trials in human patients.

## CARCINOGEN-INDUCED RODENT BLADDER TUMORS

As is true in other forms of human cancer, environmental carcinogens appear to play a major role in the initiation and progression of bladder cancer. Most of the bladder carcinogens identified to date are aromatic amines or nitrosoamines that are found in tobacco smoke or industrial solvents.[16] Early studies linked occupational exposure to naphthylamines to an increased incidence of urinary bladder cancer in German dyestuff workers, and subsequent epidemiologic studies identified 2-naphthylamine, benzidine, and 4-aminobiphenyl (4-ABP) as the causative agents.[18] Tobacco smoke also contains 4-ABP as well as a number of other reactive amines, and epidemiologic evidence has established a strong link between bladder cancer risk and smoking. Therefore, there has been a longstanding interest in developing appropriate animal models to study the effects of these carcinogens on DNA damage, tumorigenicity, and metastasis in vivo.

One of the best studied bladder carcinogens is N-butyl-N-(4-hydroxybutyl) nitrosamine (BBN).[19] BBN is a downstream metabolite of N-nitrosodibutylamine, found in tobacco smoke as well as a variety of different food and industrial products. BBN is a complete carcinogen in mice and rats when administered in the drinking water or via gastric intubation. Typically, BBN is delivered via the drinking water at concentrations of 0.01% to 0.05% for 16–30 weeks. Tumors arise in nearly 100% of animals with consistent timing and display fairly homogeneous morphologies. Tumors arising in BBN-exposed mice exhibit features of transitional cell and squamous morphology and are often muscle-invasive and metastatic, whereas in rats, BBN induces almost exclusively papillary tumors that are not muscle invasive. Consistent with these observations, most BBN-induced murine tumors contain p53 mutations,[20] whereas most of the rat tumors do not.[21-23] Similar to human bladder cancer,[24] H-ras mutations are observed at low frequencies in both rodent models,[25-27] and BBN-induced carcinogenesis occurs more efficiently in H-ras transgenic mice.[28] Finally, mice heterozygous for wild-type p53 are more susceptible to bladder carcinogenesis induced by N,N-dibutylnitrosamine than wild-type mice, and 50% of the tumors that develop display loss of the remaining wild-type allele.[29] BBN-induced tumors display elevated levels of EGFR and require receptor activation for growth in vitro and in vivo,[30] making them an attractive model system in which to study the effects of EGFR inhibitors on tumor growth and metastasis. The tumors also display elevated levels of COX2, and nonsteroidal anti-inflammatory drugs (NSAIDs) inhibit tumor growth in mice and rats.[31] Allelic losses within mouse chromosome 4 (syntenic to human 9p21–p22) are also common, mirroring the loss of 9p21–p22 that occurs in human cancer.[32]

Another carcinogen that has been linked to bladder cancer in humans is 4-aminobiphenyl (4-ABP). Found in tobacco smoke as well as in certain industrial products, 4-ABP forms DNA adducts and induces bladder tumors in mice.[33,34] The compound is administered to animals in their drinking water at concentrations ranging from 50 to 300 parts per million

(ppm), usually for about 4 weeks. A clear dose–response relationship exists between 4-ABP dose, DNA adduct levels, and tumor incidence in these models,[34] providing strong evidence for the relevance of DNA adduct formation to tumorigenesis. There is some concern, however, that the p53 'mutational signature' in 4-ABP-exposed cells may not resemble the spectrum observed in primary human tumors.[18] Therefore, it is possible that the effects of 4-ABP in these models do not strictly mimic the process of carcinogenesis in humans.

A third group of carcinogens that have received a good deal of epidemiologic attention for their possible involvement in human bladder carcinogenesis are the arsenicals. Exposure to inorganic arsenic has been linked to increased incidences of skin, lung, and bladder cancer.[35] For example, a high incidence of bladder cancer has been linked to elevated arsenic levels in a region of southwest Taiwan in which a peripheral vascular disease known as 'black foot disease' is endemic.[36,37] It has been postulated that inorganic arsenicals are typically too cytotoxic to be effective carcinogens, whereas the organic metabolic intermediates that are produced during detoxification may be significantly more so.[38] Although exposure to organic arsenicals may be sufficient to induce bladder tumors in rodent models, tumorigenesis requires very prolonged exposures (2 years) to relatively high concentrations of these agents (up to 100 ppm, delivered via the drinking water).[38] On the other hand, organic arsenicals do appear to be very efficient promoters in tumors initiated by relatively brief (4 weeks) exposure to BBN.[38] Importantly, the molecular genetic analyses performed to date in the bladder tumors that arise in mice exposed to organic arsenicals alone have not identified some of the signature molecular alterations that are thought to be important in human cancer or in the other preclinical carcinogenesis models, including alterations in p53,[38] even though p53 mutations have been detected in bladder tumors arising in the black foot region of Taiwan.[36] It should also be mentioned that recent epidemiologic studies have cast some doubt on the idea that exposure to arsenicals plays a major role in human bladder cancer.[39]

## TRANSGENIC MOUSE MODELS

The conversion of a normal urothelial cell to a malignant one is a multistage process driven by specific genetic alterations. Analyses of frank urothelial carcinomas of human patients have revealed a spectrum of genetic alterations ranging from gene mutation, deletion, and epigenetic silencing to gene amplification and overexpression. While these genetic profiling studies are informative, they do not address the functional role(s) of a specific genetic alteration in tumor onset and progression. Neither do they definitively link a genetic alteration with a particular phenotype. One cannot be certain, therefore, that a given genetic alteration found in advanced human urothelial carcinomas is the cause or the consequence of tumorigenesis. In this regard, it is necessary to verify in experimental animal models the biologic potential of a particular genetic defect in urothelial transformation, and to define the temporal evolution of urothelial carcinomas along different phenotypic pathways. These biologic studies are complementary to human studies and can help elucidate the molecular basis of urothelial carcinomas.

The ability to engineer genetic defects in a living organism has fundamentally changed the way animal models are used to study tumorigenesis.[40–42] Genes suspected to induce tumor formation can now be overexpressed in a tissue of interest in transgenic mice. Conversely, genes suspected to inhibit tumor growth can be ablated in a tissue-specific manner in knockout mice. These transgenic and knockout approaches offer several major advantages over other experimental model systems:

1. The transgenic/knockout approaches allow for an in vivo analysis of well-defined genetic defects in the multistage tumorigenesis. The biologic roles of specific gene defects in tumor initiation, maintenance, and progression can be ascertained and correlated with specific pathologic stages and phenotypic pathways. The critical issue of whether or not a well-defined defect is causally involved in a particular tumor can thus be definitively addressed.[40,43]
2. The cooperative activities among specific oncogenes and tumor suppressor genes can be examined by generating bi- or even tri-transgenic animals that harbor two or more distinct genetic alterations.[44]
3. The transgenic/knockout studies can be carried out in a well-defined genetic background, thus averting the tremendous diversity of genetic background in humans.
4. Transgenic/knockout mice allow for reproducible isolation of fresh materials at all stages of tumor progression, including precursor lesions and normal tissues, for pathologic, biochemical, and genetic analyses.[45]
5. Transgenic/knockout mice have been proven to be excellent preclinical models for assessing novel diagnostic, preventive, and therapeutic strategies.[46]

## UROPLAKIN-BASED UROTHELIAL TRANSGENESIS

The ability to drive urothelium-specific expression of foreign genes relies on a urothelium-specific gene promoter, which has recently been made available through the study of uroplakins. Uroplakins Ia, Ib, II and III are the major protein components of asymmetric unit membrane (AUM)—a hallmark of urothelial differentiation.[47–50] Well conserved across mammalian species, these proteins are expressed in a urothelium-specific fashion, as evidenced by reverse transcriptase polymerase chain reaction (RT-PCR), Northern blotting and immunohistochemistry.[51–56] To explore the utility of uroplakins in transgenesis, Lin et al isolated a mouse uroplakin II (UPII) gene and showed that its 3.6 kb 5'-upstream sequence could direct expression of a bacterial reporter gene (LacZ) specifically within the mouse urothelium.[57] A series of subsequent transgenic studies showed that the UPII promoter possesses several distinct properties that are pivotal for the success of urothelial transgenesis.

1. *The UPII promoter is strictly urothelium specific.* When the UPII promoter was first used to drive the LacZ reporter gene, LacZ activity was detected not only in the urothelium but also in the hypothalamus of the transgenic lines.[57] If this pattern of expression had been observed with other transgenes, it would have severely limited the utility of using the promoter for tumorigenesis studies, because expression of oncogenes in the hypothalamus of the brain would very likely be lethal. Fortunately, subsequent studies proved that the hypothalamic expression was not shared by other transgenes, including an SV40 large T oncogene, an activated Ha-ras, an EGF receptor and a dominant-negative mutant of p53, all of which were expressed in the urothelium but not in the brain or any other tissues.[58,61] Moreover, no tumors were detected in non-urothelial tissues, thus confirming that the 3.6 kb UPII promoter contains all essential elements capable of conferring urothelium specificity, and that the initially observed LacZ activity in the hypothalamus was due to the transgene (LacZ) sequence per se, a phenomenon known to exist in other transgenic systems.[57,62,63]
2. *Transgene expression under the control of the UPII promoter is insertion-site independent and copy-number dependent.* It is well known that transgene insertion into the mouse genome is a random event. For this reason, the tissue specificity and activity of the promoter can sometimes be influenced by the chromosomal enhancer/silencer elements surrounding the transgene insertion site, making it difficult to predict transgene behavior. It was found, however, that the transgene expression driven by the UPII promoter is quite stable and highly predictable. All transgenic lines that have been generated so far faithfully expressed the transgene and did so in a urothelium-specific manner. Moreover, the level of transgene expression and the consequent biologic effects are directly related to the transgene copy

number. Thus, transgenic mice harboring high transgene copy numbers display higher transgene expression and exhibit more profound biologic effects than do mice harboring low transgene copy numbers[58,59] (see below). Such a copy-number dependence and insertion-site independence may reflect the fact that the isolated UPII gene promoter contains long stretches of repetitive sequences at the 5' end that probably serve as an insulator sequence to prevent interference from adjacent chromosomal genetic elements.[57,63,64]

3. *The UPII promoter remains active even after malignant transformation.* Multiple studies show that uroplakin mRNA is persistently expressed in poorly differentiated human bladder cancers.[56,65–68] The continued activity of the UPII promoter in tumor cells explains why there is continued expression of transgenically introduced oncoproteins in well-advanced mouse tumors and why these tumors can not only persist, but also progress (see below).

4. *The UPII promoter has a much earlier onset of gene expression in rodents than in higher mammals.* Unlike the urothelium in humans and other higher mammals, where it is five to seven cell layers thick and where uroplakins are confined to the superficial umbrella cells, the thin rodent urothelium (two to four layers) expresses uroplakins in all cell layers including the basal layer.[58] Indeed, in transgenic mice, oncoproteins—the expression of which is controlled by the UPII promoter—are readily detected in the basal cells.[58,59] Such an expression pattern is important for tumorigenic purposes because the less differentiated urothelial cell layer probably contains stem cells and is thus a more likely target for oncogenic transformation than the well-differentiated layers. Taken together, these features make the UPII promoter ideal for urothelial transgenesis.

During the past few years, the UPII promoter has been used to drive the urothelium-specific expression of oncogenes, growth factor receptors, and mutated tumor suppressor genes, yielding a significant amount of information regarding the in vivo roles of specific genetic alterations in the multistage and multipathway bladder tumorigenic process. The following summarizes several UPII-based mouse models of bladder tumorigenesis.

## UROTHELIAL EXPRESSION OF A CONSTITUTIVELY ACTIVE HA-RAS ONCOGENE INDUCES UROTHELIAL HYPERPLASIA AND LOW-GRADE SUPERFICIAL PAPILLARY TUMORS

In spite of the fact that the Ras pathway mediates signal transduction of many oncogenes and growth factors,[69] and that Ha-ras is one of the more frequently mutated oncogenes in bladder cancer,[70,71] little was known about the role of Ras activation in urothelial transformation and in different phenotypic pathways of bladder tumorigenesis until a few years ago. Transgenic lines expressing a constitutively active Ha-ras under the control of the UPII promoter were therefore generated. Of the three independent lines obtained, two harbored 48 and 30 copies (high copy), respectively, and the third harbored only two copies (low copy) of the UPII/Ha-ras* transgene.[59] The urinary bladders of the low-copy mice exhibited age-dependent urothelial alterations, with newborn mice exhibiting normal morphology, 1- to 5-month-old mice displaying simple urothelial hyperplasia, and 6- to 9-month-old mice presenting with nodular urothelial hyperplasia. Approximately 63% of the transgenic mice over 10 months of age developed low-grade, superficial papillary tumors of the bladder (Figure 14.1). The high-copy mice exhibited similar morphologic changes, but the superficial papillary tumors developed at much earlier ages. These results provide the first in vivo evidence indicating that activation of the Ras pathway plays a significant role in bladder tumorigenesis leading to the formation of superficial papillary tumors. They also indicate that urothelial hyperplasia is an important precursor of the low-grade superficial papillary tumors of the bladder, and that Ha-ras mutation, in conjunction with overexpression, is sufficient to induce the superficial papillary tumors. While the Ha-ras mutation rate in human bladder cancer remains controversial, the Ras signaling pathway is commonly activated by oncogenes and growth factor receptors, many of which are altered in human bladder cancer.[8,69] Therefore, the activation of the Ras pathway (via mutation or not) appears to be responsible for the genesis of a considerable proportion of low-grade superficial papillary tumors.

## TRANSGENIC MICE EXPRESSING AN SV40T ANTIGEN IN UROTHELIUM DEVELOPS CARCINOMA IN SITU AND INVASIVE UROTHELIAL CARCINOMAS

The SV40 large T antigen functionally inactivates p53 and pRb, both of which are frequently dysfunctional in human bladder cancer.[72,73] Transgenic mice harboring the UPII promoter-SV40T transgene were produced, yielding four founder lines, two of which harbored 6 and 10 copies of the transgene, while the other two lines harbored only 1–2 copies per haploid genome.[58] The urothelia of the low-copy mice exhibited a high degree of atypia with pleomorphic nuclei, frequent mitotic figures, and loss of polarity. These alterations were flat in appearance in distended bladders and were confined to the epithelial layer, resembling human carcinoma in situ (CIS) of the bladder[2] (see Figure 14.1). The high-copy mice developed rapidly progressing bladder tumors that were invasive and metastatic, and the mice died between 3 and 5 months of age. The coexistence of CIS and

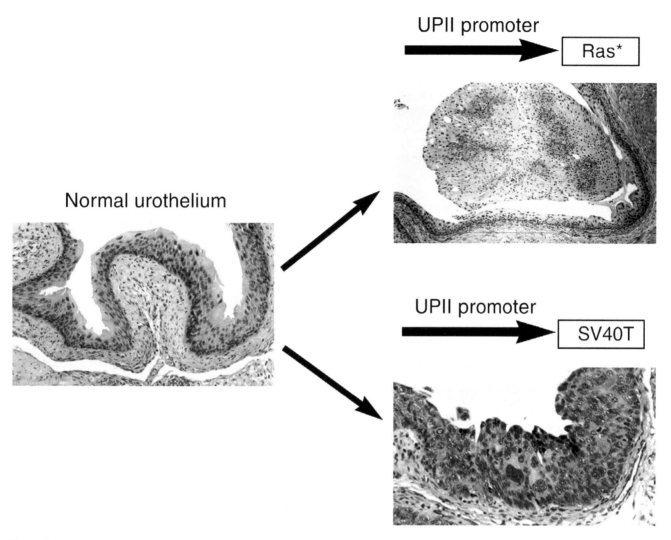

**UPII promoter**

Ras*

**Normal urothelium**

**UPII promoter**

SV40T

**Fig. 14.1**
Urothelial expression of an activated Ha-ras oncogene and SV40 large T antigen under the control of the mouse uroplakin II (UPII) promoter in transgenic mice induces low-grade superficial papillary tumors and high-grade carcinoma in situ of the bladder, respectively.

invasive tumors in the same bladder, and the fact that some of the invasive tumors were preceded by CIS in high-copy mice, suggest that CIS can progress to become invasive/metastatic bladder cancers, at least in high-copy SV40T mice. The formation of CIS and invasive TCCs, but not superficial papillary TCC, in this model directly supports the notion that the inactivation of p53 and pRb is largely responsible for the more aggressive type of bladder cancer.[74-79]

## OVEREXPRESSION OF EGFR INDUCES UROTHELIAL HYPERPLASIA AND SYNERGIZES WITH SV40T ONCOGENE TO ACCELERATE BLADDER TUMOR GROWTH

Previous work demonstrated that the receptor for epidermal growth factor (EGFR) is overexpressed in over half of advanced human bladder cancers and that

human urine contains abundant EGF.[7,80] These observations have prompted considerable research aimed at determining the biologic effects of EGFR activation on bladder cancer progression, and they serve as the rationale for ongoing clinical trials of EGFR antagonists in patients with TCC. However, whether or not EGFR overexpression per se is sufficient to induce urothelial growth and tumorigenesis is not clear. Three independent transgenic lines harboring the UPII/EGFR transgene were recently produced, all expressing higher levels of the EGFR mRNA and protein in the urothelium than the nontransgenic controls.[60] The overexpressed EGFR was autophosphorylated at the tyrosine residues, and its downstream mitogen-activated protein kinases were highly activated. Although urothelia of all transgenic lines exhibited hyperproliferative changes, they failed to evolve into any frank tumors, despite long-term follow-up. Simultaneous expression of EGFR and activated Ha-ras* in bitransgenic mice also failed to promote bladder tumor progression. In contrast, coexpression of EGFR and SV40T resulted in the formation of high-grade bladder carcinomas without triggering tumor invasion. These results indicate that while urothelial overexpression of EGFR can induce urothelial proliferation, it is insufficient to induce frank carcinoma formation. The results also indicate that both EGFR and Ha-ras stimulated urothelial hyperplasia, probably reflecting the fact that they act within the same signaling pathway. Finally, EGFR overexpression did cooperate with loss of p53 and pRb function to promote bladder tumor growth and progression in the SV40 large T antigen transgenics, consistent with the observation that EGFR pathway activation is more closely associated with invasive/metastatic TCC than it is with superficial TCC. The observation that EGFR overexpression did not drive tumor cell invasion and metastasis in this model may indicate that the role of the EGFR pathway in mouse bladder tumorigenesis is distinct from its role in certain preclinical human models, where abundant evidence exists implicating the EGFR in both processes as well as in angiogenesis.[81–87] The differences may be related to distinctions in the specific sequence of epigenetic and genetic events driving tumorigenesis in the models or to the adaptation of human cell lines to EGFR dependency in vitro.

## THE ROLE OF P53 DEFICIENCY IN UROTHELIAL TUMORIGENESIS

p53 is probably the most commonly mutated tumor suppressor gene in bladder cancer.[73] However, p53 mutations occur mainly in advanced bladder cancers, and their effects on urothelial tumor initiation are largely unknown. While the development of p53 knockout mice established p53 as a general tumor suppressor,[88] the knockouts have provided little insight into the potential role(s) p53 plays in urothelial tumorigenesis because the mice die of lymphoma and soft tissue sarcomas before any alteration in the urothelium is observed.[61,88] Transgenic lines were therefore generated that express a dominant-negative mutant of p53[61] that lacks the DNA-binding domain but retains the tetramerization domain.[89] The urothelium-expressed p53 mutant bound to and stabilized the endogenous wild-type p53 and induced nuclear abnormality, hyperplasia, and, occasionally, dysplasia, without eliciting frank carcinomas. Expression of the p53 mutant along with an activated Ha-ras, the latter alone inducing urothelial hyperplasia at early ages, failed to accelerate tumor formation. In contrast, expression of the activated Ha-ras in the absence of p53, as accomplished by crossing the activated Ha-ras transgenic mice with the p53 knockout mice, resulted in early-onset bladder tumors. These results indicate that:

- p53 deficiency predisposes the urothelium to hyperproliferation but is insufficient for bladder tumorigenesis
- the reduction of p53 dosage, as produced in transgenic mice expressing the dominant-negative p53 or in heterozygous p53 knockouts, is incapable of synergizing with Ha-ras to induce bladder tumors
- the complete loss of p53 is a prerequisite for collaborating with activated Ha-ras to promote bladder tumorigenesis.[61]

## TRANSGENIC MOUSE MODELS PROVIDE DIRECT EXPERIMENTAL EVIDENCE FOR THE 'TWO PATHWAY' MODEL OF BLADDER TUMORIGENESIS

An important lesson from the transgenic mouse models is that specific genetic alterations can be introduced into the urothelium in vivo to induce phenotypically different bladder tumors (see Figure 14.1). Thus, urothelial overexpression of either activated Ha-ras or EGFR elicits urothelial hyperplasia. These data define the role of Ha-ras signaling in causing low-grade superficial papillary urothelial tumors—the most common type of bladder tumors.[90,91] While it remains an open question as to how frequently Ha-ras is mutated in human bladder cancer, the Ha-ras signaling pathway, through which many oncogenes and growth factors must act, is frequently activated and therefore plays a significant role in bladder tumor formation.[69] Despite long-term observation, the ras-induced papillary tumors remain low grade and non-invasive, indicating that these tumors lack the potential to progress. In striking contrast, the SV40T antigen, which functionally inactivates p53 and pRb, produces exclusively high-grade bladder cancers, suggesting that the dysfunction of these two key tumor suppressors is responsible for the aggressive forms of bladder cancer[17,58,79,92–95] (see Figure 14.1). These transgenic studies, therefore, provide direct experimental evidence supporting the pathway concept that has been proposed on the basis of the human data.[2,74–79] The fact that bladder cancers in these transgenic mice harboring well-defined genetic defects evolve in a time-dependent manner also raises the important question regarding the possible existence of other genetic and epigenetic factors required for bladder tumors to progress.

## HUMAN TUMOR XENOGRAFTS

While there are clear advantages associated with using transgenic or carcinogen-induced endogenous mouse tumor models to investigate the molecular mechanisms underlying tumor initiation, progression, and immunity, there is valid concern that the tumors that arise in these systems do not necessarily precisely model the molecular mechanisms involved in human bladder cancer, since assumptions must be made in advance concerning which gene(s) and/or chemical(s) are important for tumorigenesis. Fortunately, a large number of human bladder cancer cell lines have been established, some of which have been available for many years,[96,97] and, for a subset of these cell lines, their tumorigenic, angiogenic, and metastatic behaviors have been well characterized. Furthermore, excellent models that recapitulate the two major pathways of bladder cancer presentation (superficial versus invasive) have been established that have proven invaluable in preclinical studies of angiogenesis and experimental therapeutics. Although passage in culture (and in nude mice) has almost certainly imposed selective pressures on these cell lines, there is no doubt as to the relevance of the genetic pathways that gave rise to them (because

they occurred in real patients with bladder cancer), and their cytogenetic, biologic, and molecular phenotypes are surprisingly stable. Another attractive feature of xenografts is that tumors can be established within 1–2 weeks, enabling more rapid (and less costly) experimentation.

As part of The University of Texas M.D. Anderson Cancer Center SPORE in Bladder Cancer, we are characterizing the biologic and molecular characteristics of a panel of 20 human bladder cancer cell lines, most of which were established by Drs Monica Liebert and H. Barton Grossman at the University of Michigan (the so-called 'UM-UC' lines) (Table 14.1).[98] Given their established importance in human cancer progression, we are focusing attention on the mutational status of Ras, p53, and Rb, and on the EGF receptor pathway (H. Barton Grossman, manuscript in preparation). We have also characterized their sensitivities to apoptosis induced by interferon-α (IFNα) and recombinant human tumor necrosis factor-related apoptosis-

**Table 14.1** Biologic characteristics of selected human bladder cancer cell lines

| Cell line | Type | EGFR dependency* | IFN sensitivity† | TRAIL sensitivity‡ |
|---|---|---|---|---|
| 253J-BV | TCC | +++ | – | – |
| KU7 | TCC | – | – | – |
| RT4 | TCC | + | +++ | +++ |
| UM-UC1 | TCC | + | – | +++ |
| UM-UC2 | TCC | – | – | + |
| UM-UC3 | TCC | – | – | – |
| UM-UC4 | Adeno | ++ | ++ | +++ |
| UM-UC5 | Squamous | ++++ | – | ++ |
| UM-UC6 | TCC | ++ | ++ | +++ |
| UM-UC7 | TCC | + | – | – |
| UM-UC9 | TCC | + | – | ++ |
| UM-UC10 | TCC | +++ | ++ | + |
| UM-UC11 | TCC | – | – | + |
| UM-UC12 | TCC | + | +++ | + |
| UM-UC13 | TCC | – | – | ++ |
| UM-UC14 | TCC | + | – | +++ |
| UM-UC15 | Squamous | ++ | – | + |
| UM-UC17 | TCC | ++ | — | + |

* Epidermal growth factor receptor (EGFR) dependency was determined by incubating cells for 24 hours in serum-free medium in the presence of increasing concentrations of the EGFR antagonist, ZD1839 (Iressa) and measuring DNA synthesis by ³H-thymidine incorporation. Cells were determined to be sensitive if they displayed ≥50% inhibition of DNA synthesis at 1 μM drug.
† Interferon (IFN) sensitivity was established by incubating cells in the presence of up to 100,000 units/ml of recombinant human IFNα for 48 hours and measuring apoptosis-associated DNA fragmentation by propidium iodide staining and flow cytometry. Cells displaying a statistically significant (p<0.05) increase in DNA fragmentation (versus controls) were determined to be IFN sensitive.
‡ Tumor necrosis factor-related apoptosis-inducing ligand (TRAIL) sensitivity was established by incubating cells with 10–100 ng/ml recombinant human TRAIL for 48 hours and measuring apoptosis-associated DNA fragmentation by propidium iodide staining and flow cytometry.
Adeno, adenocarcinoma; Squamous, squamous cell carcinoma; TCC, transitional cell carcinoma.

inducing ligand (TRAIL),[99] pathways that appear to mediate the growth inhibitory effects of bacillus Calmette–Guérin (BCG) and are attractive therapeutic modalities in their own right. The vast majority of the cell lines in our panel are TCC in origin, with two adenocarcinomas and one squamous cell carcinoma. The interim results confirm that inactivating mutations in p53 and Rb are quite common. Furthermore, in vitro studies with the EGF receptor antagonist ZD1839 (Iressa) indicate that some of the cell lines (approximately 50%) are dependent on EGFR activation for their growth, consistent with the evidence emerging from other solid tumor models. Preliminary evidence in tumor xenografts strongly suggests that in vitro EGFR dependency correlates with sensitivity to ZD1839-mediated growth inhibition in vivo (W Kassouf et al, Cancer Research, in press). The molecular mechanisms underlying this EGFR dependency are still under investigation. We speculate that once they have been identified they might be used prospectively to identify the subset of patients that will benefit from EGFR-directed therapy.

Many human tumor cell lines are poorly tumorigenic when they are grown in nude mice without Matrigel. We have therefore employed a technique known as 'orthotopic recycling' to isolate variants of human TCC lines that display markedly increased tumorigenicity and metastatic potential.[100] In this approach, human tumor cells are implanted directly into the bladder wall and grown in vivo until tumors of sufficient size are established. Tumors arising in the first passage typically display long latencies (>6 months) with 10% to 30% of animals possessing visible tumors. Tumors and regional and/or distant metastases are then harvested, the tumor cells are isolated and re-expanded in culture, and the cells are used for immediate generation of new orthotopic tumors. This cycle is repeated several times until tumor takes approach 100% and tumor latency is reduced from 6 months to an average of 1–2 months.

# ORTHOTOPIC XENOGRAFT MODELS

## SUPERFICIAL DISEASE

Most human TCCs are superficial. Although these tumors can be resected, there is considerable interest in developing non-surgical strategies to control superficial disease in the interest of preserving bladder function. The fact that therapies can be delivered locally via intravesicular instillation broadens the range of possible therapies that can be employed, including strategies such as gene therapy that are still not feasible within the context of systemic therapy. Therefore, there is a great need to develop models that accurately recapitulate the

biology and architecture of superficial TCC. The Ras transgenic mice described above represent one such model, and a recent xenograft model developed by Benedict's group represents another.[101]

In this model, human tumor cells are instilled directly into the bladders of nude mice to allow for the engraftment of superficial lesions. The bladders are pretreated with a gentle trypsin solution to loosen the glycosaminoglycan (GAG) layer that covers the bladder epithelium. To ensure that the tumor cells are given sufficient time to adhere to the epithelium, the mouse urethra is tied off with a suture (for approximately 3 hours) via a simple surgical procedure. Engraftment rates approaching 100% can be achieved.

Because the superficial lesions generated in this model are not necessarily discrete masses, the major experimental challenge associated with using the model is quantifying tumor burden during and after therapy. One solution to this problem is to use microscale imaging techniques (contrast-enhanced MRI, FdG-glucose PET, various CT methods). However, a more accessible approach is to prelabel the tumor cells with a marker that can be visualized non-invasively without the need of such expensive equipment.[102] One popular method involves transfecting the tumor cells with luciferase, implanting the cells orthotopically or subcutaneously, and injecting animals with intravenous luminol to visualize as few as 1000 tumor cells non-invasively.[102] Alternatively, Benedict's group has stably transfected human bladder cancer cells with green fluorescent protein (GFP), and they directly measure GFP fluorescence to estimate tumor volumes.[103] The advantage of their approach is that it does not require the use of a contrast-enhancing agent that might not penetrate all areas of a tumor equally. However, the major challenge associated with using GFP is that, in order to quantify fluorescence accurately, the mouse abdomen has to be opened at the time of each measurement. Benedict's group has shown that this type of invasive monitoring is highly feasible with low associated morbidity. Furthermore, it is possible to accurately approximate tumor burden by monitoring GFP fluorescence in voided urine by protein cytology.[104]

This model of superficial disease has been used most extensively to develop novel methods for intravesical delivery of viral gene therapy constructs to the urothelium.[105–107] Use of a synthetic detergent (Syn3) in conjunction with an adenoviral vector encoding β-galactosidase resulted in transduction of virtually all urothelial cells in this model, including both the superficial tumor cells and the normal mouse epithelium.[106] In a subsequent study, Syn-3 was used to deliver adenoviral IFNα to superficial GFP-expressing KU-7 tumors, resulting in marked tumor regression.[107] These studies served as the conceptual basis for a clinical trial of intravesical adenoviral IFNα scheduled to open in 2005.

## INVASIVE DISEASE

Dinney and coworkers were the first to employ 'orthotopic recycling' to isolate invasive and metastatic variants of the human 253J TCC cell line.[100] They isolated two variants—253J B-V and 253J lung-IV—because they grew invasively in the bladder or metastasized to the lung, respectively. Tumorigenicity was increased from less than 5% (1/25 mice bearing tumors) at 6 months to almost 100% at 1 month. Cytogenetic analyses confirmed that 253J B-V and 253J lung-IV contained marker chromosomes shared by the parental line,[100] confirming their isogenic background. The invasive and metastatic variants displayed increased growth in soft agar, increased collagenase activity, decreased adhesion to laminin (a basement membrane component), and increased invasion through Matrigel membranes, all of which are consistent with increased metastatic potential. Importantly, the metastatic variants expressed much higher levels of basic fibroblast growth factor (bFGF), a crucial mediator of tumor angiogenesis. Together, these results indicate that the process of orthotopic recycling selected for biologic alterations (increased invasion and angiogenesis) that are known to be associated with tumor metastasis in humans[108] is consistent with the idea that orthotopic tumors are better models of human disease than are ectopic tumors.[109,110] The availability of isogenic nonmetastatic and metastatic variants that differentially express these markers makes the system ideal for hypothesis-based studies as well as expression profiling (i.e. cDNA microarrays and proteomics) to define the molecular mechanisms involved in metastasis.

Since it was first developed, the orthotopic 253J B-V model has been used extensively to study the influence of the bladder microenvironment on tumor angiogenesis and to evaluate the preclinical efficacy of various antiangiogenic therapeutic strategies. In an initial study, Perrotte and colleagues compared the growth of orthotopic 253J B-V tumors to that of tumors growing subcutaneously (ectopically) in nude mice.[111] Primary tumors grew at both sites with no major differences in tumor weights. However, lung and lymph node metastases were observed only in mice bearing the orthotopic tumors. The orthotopic tumors also contained more blood vessels than did the subcutaneous tumors, effects that were associated with higher expression of bFGF, vascular endothelial growth factor (VEGF), and collagenase. These results established the fact that angiogenesis and metastasis in TCC are critically regulated by the organ microenvironment. Independent studies have confirmed that orthotopic RT4 bladder tumors also better recapitulate the features of primary human tumors than do ectopic (subcutaneous) tumors.[109]

In subsequent studies the 253J B-V model was used to study the effects of systemic IFNα[112-114] and inhibitors of the epidermal growth factor receptor,[84,86,87] both of which had displayed antiangiogenic activity in preclinical models (and, in the case of IFN, in clinical trials). In the first study, Dinney and coworkers evaluated the effects of IFNα on angiogenic factor production in vitro and on angiogenesis and tumor growth in vivo.[112] They showed that IFNα selectively downregulated bFGF mRNA and protein levels in vitro and in vivo (without affecting VEGF levels), resulting in marked inhibition of tumor microvessel densities and growth. Subsequent studies showed that the effects of IFNα in this model were schedule- and dose-dependent and were associated within increased apoptosis in tumor-associated endothelial cells. Other studies showed that the effects of IFNα were dose- and schedule-dependent,[113] and that IFNα restored a normal balance between MMP9 and E-cadherin,[114] two proteins implicated in invasion and metastasis.[85,108] Furthermore, the model was the first one used to demonstrate that intravesical administration of IFN was effective in blocking tumor growth and angiogenesis,[115] and it has also been used to demonstrate that systemic therapy with a plasmid-based p53 expression construct is feasible and also leads to tumor regression.[116] These findings served as a major part of the scientific rationale for ongoing clinical trials of systemic neoadjuvant IFNα and intravesical adenoviral IFNα in patients with bladder cancer that are open or will open soon at our institution.

Similar studies were performed in orthotopic 253J B-V tumors treated with clinically relevant inhibitors of the EGFR. The first studies were performed with small molecule inhibitors of the EGFR tyrosine kinase,[87] and were followed by experiments with C225 (cetuximab, or Erbitux), a blocking anti-EGFR antibody.[86] Subsequent experiments have employed chemical inhibitors of the EGFR (ZD1839/Iressa, from Astra-Zeneca) or of the EGFR and HER-2/erbB-2 (CI-1033, from Pfizer) (manuscripts in preparation). In all cases single-agent therapy resulted in inhibition of tumor growth associated with downregulation of angiogenic factor (particularly VEGF) production, increased endothelial cell apoptosis, and reduced tumor microvessel densities. Furthermore, combined therapy with EGFR inhibitors plus conventional chemotherapy (taxanes) resulted in at least additive effects on tumor growth.[84] These preclinical studies provided the conceptual framework for an ongoing clinical trial employing ZD1839 plus docetaxel (Taxotere) in patients who have received conventional combination chemotherapy (methotrexate, vinblastine, adriamycin, cisplatin; MVAC) to maximum benefit. The hypothesis being tested is that the antiangiogenic effects of ZD1839 (and possibly taxanes) will be best exploited within the context of minimal residual disease. Inhibition of VEGF production and tumor angiogenesis may also underlie the synergistic tumor growth inhibition observed in 253J B-V tumors treated with the proteasome inhibitor bortezomib (PS-341, also known as Velcade) plus gemcitabine,[117] and a clinical trial designed to evaluate the effects of bortezomib-based combination therapy will open at our institution in 2005.

Orthotopic 253J B-V tumors have also been used to study the effects of direct VEGF receptor blockade.[118,119] In these studies established tumors were treated with a blocking anti-mouse VEGF receptor 2 (VEGFR2) antibody (DC-101, from ImClone). Initial experiments confirmed that DC-101 was a potent inhibitor of tumor growth and that its effects were associated with increased endothelial cell death and decreased tumor microvessel densities.[118] In subsequent studies we employed highly quantitative methods involving immunofluorescence staining and laser scanning cytometry to show that effective therapy with DC-101 was associated with a 50% decrease in active VEGFR2 levels and that these effects were mostly localized to CD31-positive, CD105-negative cells located in the tumor periphery.[119] Expression of VEGF correlates with poor prognosis in patients with TCC.[108] The observation that VEGFR2 blockade is efficacious in this preclinical model supports the idea that clinical trials should be performed to determine the efficacy of this approach.

More recently we have used orthotopic recycling to isolate highly tumorigenic and metastatic variants of RT4 cells (A. Kamat, manuscript in preparation). The RT4 line is considered the prototypic superficial TCC line, and expression-profiling studies have confirmed that its pattern of gene expression correlates well with those observed in primary superficial tumors.[15] Unlike the 253J parental line, the parental RT4 cells grew fairly well at a reasonable inoculum at the orthotopic site, although tumor latency was significant (about 4 months). The recycled lines display progressively shorter latency, and variants capable of local and distant metastasis have been isolated (A. Kamat, manuscript in preparation).

## PERSPECTIVES AND POTENTIAL APPLICATIONS

The successful generation of a panel of transgenic mice developing urothelial carcinomas that bear strong resemblance to the human counterparts has amply demonstrated the feasibility of the uroplakin-based transgenic approach. The next few years will likely see a significant expansion of the number of mouse models that express a variety of known and novel genes implicated in urothelial growth, differentiation, apoptosis, and tumorigenesis. There will also be a refinement of target gene selection, shifting from

globally acting genes such as the SV40T to more specific signaling molecules such as pathway-specific kinases. In addition, by expressing the cre recombinase under the control of the UPII promoter, it will be possible to delete any genes flanked by the loxP sequences to achieve urothelium-specific gene knockout.[120] Thus, the problem of embryonic lethality resulting from the whole-body knockout of tumor suppressor genes can be circumvented. Our group plans to use the approach to study the roles of genes that are altered at very early stages of clonal expansion in the bladder (the so-called 'forerunner genes').[2,121-123] Moreover, UPII-directed gene expression can be combined with an inducible system so that target gene expression or knockout is not only urothelium specific but also temporally controlled. Finally, more sophisticated compound transgenics can be produced that express oncogenes but simultaneously lack tumor suppressor genes. This will allow systematic dissection of the synergistic effects among different genes. With the completion of the human genome project and near-completion of the mouse genome project, the pace of gene discovery will quicken. There is little doubt that the transgenic and knockout models will play a pivotal role in understanding novel gene functions and help elucidate the molecular mechanisms of bladder cancer formation.

Selected mouse models can also serve as invaluable tools for assessing various chemopreventive strategies for urothelial carcinomas, because the time course of tumor development is highly predictable in most existing models. Not only can the route of delivery, the efficacy, and the toxicity be evaluated, but the mechanisms of action can also be explored in mouse tumors. By the same token, the mouse models can serve as important preclinical models for identifying and validating drug targets, before they are applied to human patients. Finally, genetically altered mice have been proven to be a valuable alternative in assessing the hazardous levels of potential chemical carcinogens.[124] Compared with the classic 2-year mouse bioassay, transgenic and knockout mice may be more sensitive and cost-effective for screening genotoxic and non-genotoxic chemicals and carcinogens.

While there are plenty of reasons to be enthusiastic about the animal models of bladder cancer that are available for molecular research, there is also a tremendous need to validate the molecular and biologic properties of these models by comparing them directly to primary human tumors. Efforts to do so with emerging genomics and proteomics technologies are under-way.[15,16] Even more important is the design and execution of intelligent, biology-based clinical trials in TCC patients that will directly test the hypotheses put forward in the laboratory research efforts. As a relatively accessible tumor, biopsy-based laboratory studies are feasible within the context of these trials, and, with more sophisticated quantitative methods available,[125-127] it is to be expected that new mechanistic information will be gained from these trials which can be translated back into the laboratory.

## REFERENCES

1. Simoneau AR, Jones PA. Bladder cancer: the molecular progression to invasive disease. World J Urol 1994;12:89–95.
2. Dinney CP, McConkey DJ, Millikan RE, et al. Focus on bladder cancer. Cancer Cell 2004;6:111–116.
3. Oxford G, Theodorescu D. The role of Ras superfamily proteins in bladder cancer progression. J Urol 2003;170:1987–1993.
4. Czerniak B, Deitch D, Simmons H, Etkind P, Herz F, Koss LG. Ha-ras gene codon 12 mutation and DNA ploidy in urinary bladder carcinoma. Br J Cancer 1990;62:762–763.
5. Grossfeld GD, Muscheck M, Stein JP, et al. Cellular proliferation and cell–cell cycle regulatory proteins as prognostic markers for transitional cell carcinoma of the bladder. Adv Exp Med Biol 1999;462:425–435.
6. Shariat SF, Tokunaga H, Zhou J, et al. p53, p21, pRB, and p16 expression predict clinical outcome in cystectomy with bladder cancer. J Clin Oncol 2004;22:1014–1024.
7. Messing EM. Clinical implications of the expression of epidermal growth factor receptors in human transitional cell carcinoma. Cancer Res 1990;50:2530–2537.
8. Messing EM. Growth factors and bladder cancer: clinical implications of the interactions between growth factors and their urothelial receptors. Semin Surg Oncol 1992;8:285–292.
9. Liebert M. Growth factors in bladder cancer. World J Urol 1995;13:349–355.
10. Theodorescu D. Molecular pathogenesis of urothelial bladder cancer. Histol Histopathol 2003;18:259–274.
11. Sabichi AL, Lippman SM. COX-2 inhibitors and other nonsteroidal anti-inflammatory drugs in genitourinary cancer. Semin Oncol 2004;31:36–44.
12. Petrovich Z, Baert L, Boyd SD, et al. Management of carcinoma of the bladder. Am J Clin Oncol 1998;21:217–222.
13. Kiemeney LA, Schoenberg M. Familial transitional cell carcinoma. J Urol 1996;156:867–872.
14. Sanchez-Carbayo M, Socci ND, Lozano JJ, et al. Gene discovery in bladder cancer progression using cDNA microarrays. Am J Pathol 2003;163:505–516.
15. Sanchez-Carbayo M, Socci ND, Charytonowicz E, et al. Molecular profiling of bladder cancer using cDNA microarrays: defining histogenesis and biological phenotypes. Cancer Res 2002;62:6973–6980.
16. Hoque MO, Lee CC, Cairns P, Schoenberg M, Sidransky D. Genome-wide genetic characterization of bladder cancer: a comparison of high-density single-nucleotide polymorphism arrays and PCR-based microsatellite analysis. Cancer Res 2003;63:2216–2222.
17. Cohen SM. Urinary bladder carcinogenesis. Toxicol Pathol 1998;26:121–127.
18. Besaratinia A, Bates SE, Pfeifer GP. Mutational signature of the proximate bladder carcinogen N-hydroxy-4-acetylaminobiphenyl: inconsistency with the p53 mutational spectrum in bladder cancer. Cancer Res 2002;62:4331–4338.
19. Cohen SM. Promotion in urinary bladder carcinogenesis. Environ Health Perspect 1983;50:51–59.
20. Ogawa K, Uzvolgyi E, St John MK, de Oliveira ML, Arnold L, Cohen SM. Frequent p53 mutations and occasional loss of chromosome 4 in invasive bladder carcinoma induced by N-butyl-N-(4-hydroxybutyl)nitrosamine in B6D2F1 mice. Mol Carcinog 1998;21:70–79.
21. Asamoto M, Mann AM, Cohen SM. p53 mutation is infrequent and might not give a growth advantage in rat bladder carcinogenesis in vivo. Carcinogenesis 1994;15:455–458.
22. Asamoto M, Mann AM, Macatee TL, Cohen SM. Mutations and expression of the p53 gene in rat bladder carcinomas and cell lines. Mol Carcinog 1994;9:236–244.
23. Jones RF, Matuszyk J, Debiec-Rychter M, Wang CY. Mutation and altered expression of p53 genes in experimental rat bladder tumor cells. Mol Carcinog 1994;9:95–104.
24. Fujita J, Yoshida O, Yuasa Y, Rhim JS, Hatanaka M, Aaronson SA. Ha-ras oncogenes are activated by somatic alterations in human urinary tract tumours. Nature 1984;309:464–466.
25. Fujita J, Ohuchi N, Ito N, et al. Activation of H-ras oncogene in rat bladder tumors induced by N-butyl-N-(4-hydroxybutyl)nitrosamine. J Natl Cancer Inst 1988;80:37–43.
26. Enomoto T, Ward JM, Perantoni AO. H-ras activation and ras p21 expression in bladder tumors induced in F344/NCr rats by N-butyl-N-(4-hydroxybutyl)nitrosamine. Carcinogenesis 1990;11:2233–2238.
27. Yamamoto S, Masui T, Murai T, et al. Frequent mutations of the p53 gene and infrequent H- and K-ras mutations in urinary bladder carcinomas of NON/Shi mice treated with N-butyl-N-(4-hydroxybutyl)nitrosamine. Carcinogenesis 1995;16:2363–2368.
28. Ota T, Asamoto M, Toriyama-Baba H, et al. Transgenic rats carrying copies of the human c-Ha-ras proto-oncogene exhibit enhanced susceptibility to N-butyl-N-(4-hydroxybutyl)nitrosamine bladder carcinogenesis. Carcinogenesis 21:1391–1396.
29. Nishikawa T, Salim EI, Morimura K, et al. High susceptibility of p53 knockout mice to esophageal and urinary bladder carcinogenesis induced by N, N-dibutylnitrosamine. Cancer Lett 2003;194:45–54.
30. el-Marjou A, Delouvee A, Thiery JP, Radvanyi F. Involvement of epidermal growth factor receptor in chemically induced mouse bladder tumour progression. Carcinogenesis 2000;21:2211–2218.
31. Grubbs CJ, Lubet RA, Koki AT, et al. Celecoxib inhibits N-butyl-N-(4-hydroxybutyl)-nitrosamine-induced urinary bladder cancers in male B6D2F1 mice and female Fischer-344 rats. Cancer Res 2000;60:5599–5602.
32. Miyao N, Tsai YC, Lerner SP, et al. Role of chromosome 9 in human bladder cancer. Cancer Res 1993;53:4066–4070.
33. Flammang TJ, Couch LH, Levy GN, Weber WW, Wise CK. DNA adduct levels in congenic rapid and slow acetylator mouse strains following chronic administration of 4-aminobiphenyl. Carcinogenesis 1992;13:1887–1891.
34. Poirier MC, Fullerton NF, Smith BA, Beland FA. DNA adduct formation and tumorigenesis in mice during the chronic administration of 4-aminobiphenyl at multiple dose levels. Carcinogenesis 1995;16:2917–2921.
35. Boffetta P. Epidemiology of environmental and occupational cancer. Oncogene 2004;23:6392–6403.
36. Shibata A, Ohneseit PF, Tsai YC, et al. Mutational spectrum in the p53 gene in bladder tumors from the endemic area of black foot disease in Taiwan. Carcinogenesis 1994;15:1085–1087.
37. Chiang HS, Guo HR, Hong CL, Lin SM, Lee EF. The incidence of bladder cancer in the black foot disease endemic area in Taiwan. Br J Urol 1993;71:274–278.
38. Wanibuchi H, Salim EI, Kinoshita A, et al. Understanding arsenic carcinogenicity by the use of animal models. Toxicol Appl Pharmacol 2004;198:366–376.
39. Lamm SH, Engel A, Kruse MB, et al. Arsenic in drinking water and bladder cancer mortality in the United States: an analysis based on 133 U.S. counties and 30 years of observation. J Occup Environ Med 2004;46:298–306.
40. Wu X, Pandolfi PP. Mouse models for multistep tumorigenesis. Trends Cell Biol 2001;11:S2–9.
41. Jackson-Grusby L. Modeling cancer in mice. Oncogene 2002;21:5504–5514.
42. Van Dyke T, Jacks T. Cancer modeling in the modern era: progress and challenges. Cell 2002;108:135–144.
43. Clarke AR. Manipulating the germline: its impact on the study of carcinogenesis. Carcinogenesis 2000;21:435–441.
44. Hakem R, Mak TW. Animal models of tumor-suppressor genes. Annu Rev Genet 2001;35:209–241.
45. Resor L, Bowen TJ, Wynshaw-Boris A. Unraveling human cancer in the mouse: recent refinements to modeling and analysis. Hum Mol Genet 2001;10:669–675.
46. McCormick F. Cancer gene therapy: fringe or cutting edge? Nat Rev Cancer 2001;1:130–141.

47. Koss LG. The asymmetric unit membranes of the epithelium of the urinary bladder of the rat. An electron microscopic study of a mechanism of epithelial maturation and function. Lab Invest 1969;21:154–168.

48. Hicks RM. The fine structure of the transitional epithelium of rat ureter. J Cell Biol 1965;26:25–48.

49. Wu XR, Lin JH, Walz T, et al. Mammalian uroplakins. A group of highly conserved urothelial differentiation-related membrane proteins. J Biol Chem 1994;269:13716–13724.

50. Wu XR, Manabe M, Yu J, Sun TT. Large scale purification and immunolocalization of bovine uroplakins I, II, and III. Molecular markers of urothelial differentiation. J Biol Chem 1990;265:19170–19179.

51. Lin JH, Wu XR, Kreibich G, Sun TT. Precursor sequence, processing, and urothelium-specific expression of a major 15-kDa protein subunit of asymmetric unit membrane. J Biol Chem 1994;269:1775–1784.

52. Wu XR, Sun TT. Molecular cloning of a 47 kDa tissue-specific and differentiation-dependent urothelial cell surface glycoprotein. J Cell Sci 1993;106:31–43.

53. Yu J, Lin JH, Wu XR, Sun TT. Uroplakins Ia and Ib, two major differentiation products of bladder epithelium, belong to a family of four transmembrane domain (4TM) proteins. J Cell Biol 1994;125:171–182.

54. Yu J, Manabe M, Wu XR, Xu C, Surya B, Sun TT. Uroplakin I: a 27-kD protein associated with the asymmetric unit membrane of mammalian urothelium. J Cell Biol 1990;111:1207–1216.

55. Moll R, Wu XR, Lin JH, Sun TT. Uroplakins, specific membrane proteins of urothelial umbrella cells, as histological markers of metastatic transitional cell carcinomas. Am J Pathol 1995;147:1383–1397.

56. Li SM, Zhang ZT, Chan S, et al. Detection of circulating uroplakin-positive cells in patients with transitional cell carcinoma of the bladder. J Urol 1999;162:931–935.

57. Lin JH, Zhao H, Sun TT. A tissue-specific promoter that can drive a foreign gene to express in the suprabasal urothelial cells of transgenic mice. Proc Natl Acad Sci USA 1995;92:679–683.

58. Zhang ZT, Pak J, Shapiro E, Sun TT, Wu XR. Urothelium-specific expression of an oncogene in transgenic mice induced the formation of carcinoma in situ and invasive transitional cell carcinoma. Cancer Res 1999;59:3512–3517.

59. Zhang ZT, Pak J, Huang HY, et al. Role of Ha-ras activation in superficial papillary pathway of urothelial tumor formation. Oncogene 2001;20:1973–1980.

60. Cheng J, Huang H, Zhang ZT, et al. Overexpression of epidermal growth factor receptor in urothelium elicits urothelial hyperplasia and promotes bladder tumor growth. Cancer Res 2002;62:4157–4163.

61. Gao J, Huang HY, Pak J, et al. p53 deficiency provokes urothelial proliferation and synergizes with activated Ha-ras in promoting urothelial tumorigenesis. Oncogene 2004;23:687–696.

62. Byrne C, Fuchs E. Probing keratinocyte and differentiation specificity of the human K5 promoter in vitro and in transgenic mice. Mol Cell Biol 1993;13:3176–3190.

63. Thorey IS, Cecena G, Reynolds W, Oshima RG. Alu sequence involvement in transcriptional insulation of the keratin 18 gene in transgenic mice. Mol Cell Biol 1993;13:6742–6751.

64. Willoughby DA, Vilalta A, Oshima RG. An Alu element from the K18 gene confers position-independent expression in transgenic mice. J Biol Chem 2000;275:759–768.

65. Seraj MJ, Thomas AR, Chin JL, Theodorescu D. Molecular determination of perivesical and lymph node metastasis after radical cystectomy for urothelial carcinoma of the bladder. Clin Cancer Res 2001;7:1516–1522.

66. Xu X, Sun TT, Gupta PK, Zhang P, Nasuti JF. Uroplakin as a marker for typing metastatic transitional cell carcinoma on fine-needle aspiration specimens. Cancer 2001;93:216–221.

67. Zhang J, Ramesh N, Chen Y, et al. Identification of human uroplakin II promoter and its use in the construction of CG8840, a urothelium-specific adenovirus variant that eliminates established bladder tumors in combination with docetaxel. Cancer Res 2002;62:3743–3750.

68. Olsburgh J, Harnden P, Weeks R, et al. Uroplakin gene expression in normal human tissues and locally advanced bladder cancer. J Pathol 2003;199:41–49.

69. Olson MF, Marais R. Ras protein signalling. Semin Immunol 2000;12:63–73.

70. Rabbani F, Cordon-Cardo C. Mutation of cell cycle regulators and their impact on superficial bladder cancer. Clin Urol North Am 2000;27:83–102.

71. Shinohara N, Koyanagi T. Ras signal transduction in carcinogenesis and progression of bladder cancer: molecular target for treatment? Urol Res 2002;30:273–281.

72. Bryan TM, Reddel RR. SV40-induced immortalization of human cells. Crit Rev Oncog 1994;5:331–357.

73. Cordon-Cardo C, Reuter VE. Alterations of tumor suppressor genes in bladder cancer. Semin Diagn Pathol 1997;14:123–132.

74. Dalbagni G, Presti J, Reuter V, Fair WR, Cordon-Cardo C. Genetic alterations in bladder cancer. Lancet 1993;342:469–471.

75. Spruck CH 3rd, Ohneseit PF, Gonzalez-Zulueta M, et al. Two molecular pathways to transitional cell carcinoma of the bladder. Cancer Res 1994;54:784–788.

76. Rosin MP, Cairns P, Epstein JI, Schoenberg MP, Sidransky D. Partial allelotype of carcinoma in situ of the human bladder. Cancer Res 1995;55:5213–5216.

77. Reznikoff CA, Belair CD, Yeager TR, et al. Molecular genetic model of human bladder cancer pathogenesis. Semin Oncol 1996;23:571–584.

78. Koss LG. Natural history and patterns of invasive cancer of the bladder. Eur Urol 1998;33:2–4.

79. Cordon-Cardo C, Cote RJ, Sauter G. Genetic and molecular markers of urothelial premalignancy and malignancy. Scand J Urol Nephrol 2000;S82–93.

80. Sidransky D, Messing E. Molecular genetics and biochemical mechanisms in bladder cancer. Oncogenes, tumor suppressor genes, and growth factors. Urol Clin North Am 1992;19:629–639.

81. Highshaw RA, McConkey DJ, Dinney CP. Integrating basic science and clinical research in bladder cancer: update from the first bladder Specialized Program of Research Excellence (SPORE). Curr Opin Urol 2004;14:295–300.

82. Bellmunt J, Hussain M, Dinney CP. Novel approaches with targeted therapies in bladder cancer. Therapy of bladder cancer by blockade of the epidermal growth factor receptor family. Crit Rev Oncol Hematol 2003;46:S85–104.

83. Mendelsohn J, Dinney CP. The Willet F. Whitmore, Jr, Lectureship: blockade of epidermal growth factor receptors as anticancer therapy. J Urol 2001;165:1152–1157.

84. Inoue K, Slaton JW, Perrotte P, et al. Paclitaxel enhances the effects of the anti-epidermal growth factor receptor monoclonal antibody ImClone C225 in mice with metastatic human bladder transitional cell carcinoma. Clin Cancer Res 2000;6:4874–4884.

85. Izawa JI, Slaton JW, Kedar D, et al. Differential expression of progression-related genes in the evolution of superficial to invasive transitional cell carcinoma of the bladder. Oncol Rep 2001;8:9–15.

86. Perrotte P, Matsumoto T, Inoue K, et al. Anti-epidermal growth factor receptor antibody C225 inhibits angiogenesis in human transitional cell carcinoma growing orthotopically in nude mice. Clin Cancer Res 1999;5:257–265.

87. Dinney CP, Parker C, Dong Z, et al. Therapy of human transitional cell carcinoma of the bladder by oral administration of the epidermal growth factor receptor protein tyrosine kinase inhibitor 4,5-dianilinophthalimide. Clin Cancer Res 1997;3:161–168.

88. Donehower LA, Harvey M, Slagle BL, et al. Mice deficient for p53 are developmentally normal but susceptible to spontaneous tumours. Nature 1992;356:215–221.

89. Bowman T, Symonds H, Gu L, Yin C, Oren M, Van Dyke T. Tissue-specific inactivation of p53 tumor suppression in the mouse. Genes Dev 1996;10:826–835.

90. Grossman HB. Superficial bladder cancer: decreasing the risk of recurrence. Oncology 1996;10:1617–1624.

91. Liebert M, Gebhardt D, Wood C, et al. Urothelial differentiation and bladder cancer. Adv Exp Med Biol 1999;462:437–448.

92. Grossman HB, Liebert M, Antelo M, et al. p53 and Rb expression predict progression in T1 bladder cancer. Clin Cancer Res 1998;4:829–834.

93. Cote RJ, Dunn MD, Chatterjee SJ, et al. Elevated and absent pRb expression is associated with bladder cancer progression and has cooperative effects with p53. Cancer Res 1998;58:1090–1094.

94. Cheng J, Huang H, Pak J, et al. Allelic loss of p53 gene is associated with genesis and maintenance, but not invasion, of mouse carcinoma in situ of the bladder. Cancer Res 2003;63:179–185.

95. Grippo PJ, Sandgren EP. Highly invasive transitional cell carcinoma of the bladder in a simian virus 40 T-antigen transgenic mouse model. Am J Pathol 2000;157:805–813.

96. Williams RD. Human urologic cancer cell lines. Invest Urol 1980;17:359–363.

97. Raghavan D, Debruyne F, Herr H, et al. Experimental models of bladder cancer: a critical review. Prog Clin Biol Res 1986;221:171–208.

98. Shinohara N, Liebert M, Wedemeyer G, Chang JH, Grossman HB. Evaluation of multiple drug resistance in human bladder cancer cell lines. J Urol 1993;150:505–509.

99. Papageorgiou A, Lashinger L, Millikan RE, et al. Role of tumor necrosis factor-related apoptosis-inducing ligand in interferon-induced apoptosis in human bladder cancer cells. Cancer Res 2004;64(24):8973–8979.

100. Dinney CP, Fishbeck R, Singh RK, et al. Isolation and characterization of metastatic variants from human transitional cell carcinoma passaged by orthotopic implantation in athymic nude mice. J Urol 1995;154:1532–1538.

101. Watanabe T, Shinohara N, Sazawa A, et al. An improved intravesical model using human bladder cancer cell lines to optimize gene and other therapies. Cancer Gene Ther 2000;7:1575–1580.

102. Choy G, Choyke P, Libutti SK. Current advances in molecular imaging: noninvasive in vivo bioluminescent and fluorescent optical imaging in cancer research. Mol Imaging 2003;2:303–312.

103. Zhou JH, Rosser CJ, Tanaka M, et al. Visualizing superficial human bladder cancer cell growth in vivo by green fluorescent protein expression. Cancer Gene Ther 2002;9:681–686.

104. Tanaka M, Gee JR, De La Cerda J, et al. Noninvasive detection of bladder cancer in an orthotopic murine model with green fluorescence protein cytology. J Urol 2003;170:975–978.

105. Rosser CJ, Benedict WF, Dinney CP. Gene therapy for superficial bladder cancer. Expert Rev Anticancer Ther 2001;1:531–539.

106. Yamashita M, Rosser CJ, Zhou JH, et al. Syn3 provides high levels of intravesical adenoviral-mediated gene transfer for gene therapy of genetically altered urothelium and superficial bladder cancer. Cancer Gene Ther 2002;9:687–691.

107. Benedict WF, Tao Z, Kim CS, et al. Intravesical Ad-IFNα causes marked regression of human bladder cancer growing orthotopically in nude mice and overcomes resistance to IFN-alpha protein. Mol Ther 2004;10:525–532.

108. Slaton JW, Millikan R, Inoue K, et al. Correlation of metastasis related gene expression and relapse-free survival in patients with locally advanced bladder cancer treated with cystectomy and chemotherapy. J Urol 2004;171:570–574.

109. Kerbel RS, Cornil I, Theodorescu D. Importance of orthotopic transplantation procedures in assessing the effects of transfected genes on human tumor growth and metastasis. Cancer Metastasis Rev 1991,10.201–215.

110. Killion JJ, Radinsky R, Fidler IJ. Orthotopic models are necessary to predict therapy of transplantable tumors in mice. Cancer Metastasis Rev 1998;17:279–284.

111. Perrotte P, Bielenberg DR, Eve BY, Dinney CP. Organ-specific angiogenesis and metastasis of human bladder carcinoma growing in athymic mice. Mol Urol 1997;1:299–307.

112. Dinney CP, Bielenberg DR, Perrotte P, et al. Inhibition of basic fibroblast growth factor expression, angiogenesis, and growth of human bladder carcinoma in mice by systemic interferon-alpha administration. Cancer Res 1998;58:808–814.

113. Slaton JW, Perrotte P, Inoue K, Dinney CP, Fidler IJ. Interferon-alpha-mediated down-regulation of angiogenesis-related genes and therapy of bladder cancer are dependent on optimization of biological dose and schedule. Clin Cancer Res 1999;5:2726–2734.

114. Slaton JW, Karashima T, Perrotte P, et al. Treatment with low-dose interferon-alpha restores the balance between matrix metalloproteinase-9 and E-cadherin expression in human transitionalcell carcinoma of the bladder. Clin Cancer Res 2001;7:2840–2853.

115. Izawa JI, Sweeney P, Perrotte P, et al. Inhibition of tumorigenicity and metastasis of human bladder cancer growing in athymic mice by interferon-beta gene therapy results partially from various antiangiogenic effects including endothelial cell apoptosis. Clin Cancer Res 2002;8:1258–1270.

116. Sweeney P, Karashima T, Ishikura H, et al. Efficient therapeutic gene delivery after systemic administration of a novel polyethylenimine/DNA vector in an orthotopic bladder cancer model. Cancer Res 2003;63:4017–4020.

117. Kamat AM, Karashima T, Davis DW, et al. The proteasome inhibitor bortezomib synergizes with gemcitabine to block the growth of human 253JB-V bladder tumors in vivo. Mol Cancer Ther 2004;3:279–290.

118. Inoue K, Slaton JW, Davis DW, et al. Treatment of human metastatic transitional cell carcinoma of the bladder in a murine model with the anti-vascular endothelial growth factor receptor monoclonal antibody DC101 and paclitaxel. Clin Cancer Res 2000;6:2635–2643.

119. Davis DW, Inoue K, Dinney CP, Hicklin DJ, Abbruzzese JL, McConkey DJ. Regional effects of an antivascular endothelial growth factor receptor monoclonal antibody on receptor phosphorylation and apoptosis in human 253J B-V bladder cancer xenografts. Cancer Res 2004;64:4601–4610.

120. Jonkers J, Berns A. Conditional mouse models of sporadic cancer. Nat Rev Cancer 2002;2:251–265.

121. Czerniak B, Chaturvedi V, Li L, et al. Superimposed histologic and genetic mapping of chromosome 9 in progression of human urinary bladder neoplasia: implications for a genetic model of multistep urothelial carcinogenesis and early detection of urinary bladder cancer. Oncogene 1999;18:1185–1196.

122. Czerniak B, Li L, Chaturvedi V, et al. Genetic modeling of human urinary bladder carcinogenesis. Genes Chromosomes Cancer 2000;27:392–402.

123. Yoon DS, Li L, Zhang RD, et al. Genetic mapping and DNA sequence-based analysis of deleted regions on chromosome 16 involved in progression of bladder cancer from occult preneoplastic conditions to invasive disease. Oncogene 2001;20:5005–5014.

124. Cohen SM. Alternative models for carcinogenicity testing: weight of evidence evaluations across models. Toxicol Pathol 2001;29:183–190.

125. Herbst RS, Mullani NA, Davis DW, et al. Development of biologic markers of response and assessment of antiangiogenic activity in a clinical trial of human recombinant endostatin. J Clin Oncol 2002;20:3804–3814.

126. Davis DW, Buchholz TA, Hess KR, Sahin AA, Valero V, McConkey DJ. Automated quantification of apoptosis after neoadjuvant chemotherapy for breast cancer: early assessment predicts clinical response. Clin Cancer Res 2003;9:955–960.

127. Davis DW, Shen Y, Mullani NA, et al. Quantitative analysis of biomarkers defines an optimal biological dose for recombinant human endostatin in primary human tumors. Clin Cancer Res 2004;10:33–42.

# Diagnosis

# Animal models: naturally occurring canine urinary bladder cancer

# 15

*Deborah W Knapp*

## INTRODUCTION

There is great need to improve the outlook for patients with transitional cell carcinoma (TCC) of the urinary bladder. Identification of environmental and genetic risk factors, development of effective prevention strategies, elucidation of methods for earlier detection and more accurate staging, and identification of more effective treatment approaches are all areas in which progress must be made. Relevant animal models of TCC are crucially important in these areas of investigation.

Animal models of TCC typically consist of experimentally induced tumors in rodents (described in Chapter 14) and naturally occurring invasive TCC in pet dogs.[1] More than 90% of bladder cancer in pet dogs consists of intermediate to high-grade, invasive TCC.[1,2] Dogs with invasive TCC serve as a useful 'large animal' model of invasive urinary bladder cancer in humans.[1] Similarities and differences between canine and human invasive TCC are summarized in Table 15.1.[1,3,5]

There are several important aspects that make pet dogs with TCC attractive study subjects. One of the most important is the propensity of canine TCC to metastasize (Figure 15.1).[1,2] Metastasis is difficult to reproduce in experimentally induced bladder cancer, yet metastasis is the major cause of death in humans with bladder cancer. Other important aspects of studying pet dogs with TCC include:

- the shared environment, drinking water, and in some instances food, between pet dogs and pet owners, allowing identification of risk factors that may be important to both species
- the intact body processes in pet dogs such as immunologic function and angiogenic activity, allowing studies of host–tumor interactions

- the heterogeneity within canine TCC (such as occurs in human TCC)
- the size of pet dogs which makes specific procedures such as cystoscopy and biopsy possible in an animal model.

In addition, with changes in societal views towards the use of animals in research, studies in animals that already have the disease rather than those in which the disease is induced may be considered more acceptable.

It is estimated that there are more than 65 million pet dogs who receive routine veterinary care in the United States. Of pet dogs that live to be 'old', approximately 25% to 30% will develop some form of cancer. Although TCC comprises only 1.5% to 2% of all canine malignancies,[1,2] thousands of cases are thought to occur each year. Additionally, the hospital prevalence or proportionate morbidity of bladder cancer at university-based veterinary hospitals appears to be increasing.[1] Several studies have been performed in pet dogs with TCC at the Purdue University Veterinary Teaching Hospital and at other institutions in which the pet dogs live at home with their owners and are evaluated and treated at the veterinary hospital at specific time intervals.[1,2,6–10] Such studies are performed with institutional Animal Care and Use Committee approval and informed pet owner consent. Some of the challenges facing veterinary oncologists and comparative oncology researchers are to determine effective means to identify and enroll larger numbers of dogs with TCC in meaningful studies, and strategies to secure funding to cover expenses involved. Complete evaluation and treatment of dogs with invasive TCC may range from less than $1000 to more than $5000 depending on type, length, and outcome of treatment.

**Table 15.1**  Similarities and differences between canine and human invasive transitional cell carcinoma of the urinary bladder

| | Canine invasive TCC[1] | Human invasive TCC[3] |
|---|---|---|
| *I. Similarities* | | |
| Percentage of all cancers | 1.5–2% | 4.4% |
| Age at diagnosis | 11 years (60 human equivalent years)* | 65 years |
| Histopathology | Invasive TCC of intermediate to high grade (>90% grade 2 and 3) | Invasive TCC of intermediate to high grade (70% grade 2 and 3) |
| Other cellular features: | | |
|    DNA ploidy | 79% aneuploid | Aneuploidy correlates with advanced stage and grade |
|    Urine bFGF concentration | Increased in TCC | Increased in TCC |
|    Cyclooxygenase-2 | Expressed in majority of cases, absent in normal bladder epithelium | Expressed in majority of cases, absent in normal bladder epithelium |
| Clinical signs | Hematuria, dysuria, urinary tract infection most common; bone pain infrequent | Hematuria, urinary tract infection most common; bone pain less common |
| Metastasis at diagnosis | 15–20% of cases | 5–20% of cases |
| Develop metastatic disease | 50% of cases | 50% of cases |
| Sites of metastasis | Regional nodes and lung most common | Regional nodes and lung most common |
| Response to single agent chemotherapy†: | | |
|    Cisplatin | 12–20% response (CR+PR) | 17–34% response |
|    Carboplatin | <10% response | 15% response |
| Prognostic factors: | | |
|    TNM stage‡ | Advanced TNM stage associated with decreased survival | Advanced TNM stage associated with decreased survival |
|    Prostate involvement | Associated with distant metastasis at diagnosis and with decreased survival | Associated with decreased survival especially when stroma of gland is involved |
| *II. Differences:* | | |
| Male:female ratio§ | 0.5:1 | 2.8:1 |
| Tumor location within the bladder | Majority trigonal | Lateral wall (37%) Posterior wall (18%) Trigone and neck (23%) Other sites (22%) |

\* Human equivalent years determined as previously reported.[4]
† Comparison between dogs and humans in response to multiagent chemotherapy protocols is not possible as multiagent protocols such as MVAC have not been used in pet dogs due to toxicity.
‡ The T stage in the WHO TNM staging system is defined differently between canine[5] and human TCC. Canine tumors are assigned a T stage of 1–3, rather than a T stage of 1–4 as is the case in human TCC. Regardless of this difference, advanced T stage is associated with a worse prognosis in both species.
§ There are several possible reasons for the difference in male:female ratio between dogs and humans with TCC. Occupational exposures involved in human TCC risk may not apply to canine TCC risk. Male dogs urinate frequently for territorial marking, resulting in less exposure time of the bladder epithelium to carcinogens in urine. Men may not fully void if partial urethral obstruction from prostatic disease is present, increasing exposure to carcinogens in urine. Female dogs have increased body fat compared with male dogs, and therefore increased storage of lipophilic environmental carcinogens. Increased risk of TCC in neutered dogs of both genders has been noted, but the mechanisms involved are not yet understood.

This review focuses on canine invasive bladder cancer. It should be noted that superficial bladder cancer in the dog is infrequent and has not been studied to any extent. Different pathways (different genetic 'hits') are thought to be involved in the development of superficial and invasive bladder cancer in humans.[3] It appears likely that the pathways necessary for superficial bladder cancer development are rarely present or are not functional in the dog. Studies of superficial bladder tumors may be more appropriately performed in rodents. Studies of rodents with experimentally induced bladder tumors also offer advantages of shorter study time, less expense in some cases, and the ability to manipulate the tumors at the cellular and molecular level. Studies in both dogs and rodents will likely be crucial in making the greatest progress against TCC.

## UTILIZATION OF PET DOGS IN TCC RESEARCH

Pet dogs with TCC may contribute to several areas of bladder cancer investigation, including studies of environmental risk factors, genetically related risk factors, chemoprevention, earlier or more accurate detection, and treatment of existing disease. A few examples are included here.

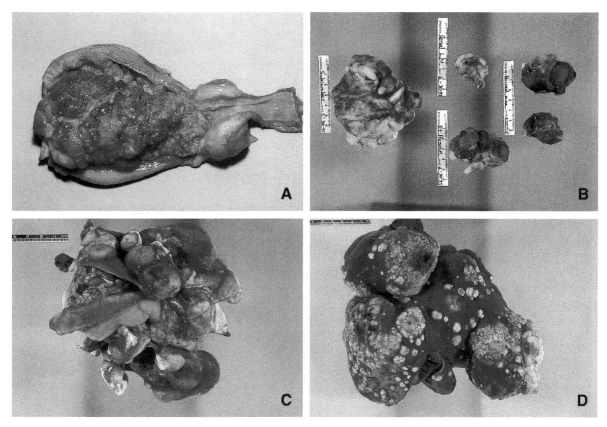

**Fig. 15.1**
**A** Primary, and **B–D** metastatic, naturally occurring canine transitional cell carcinoma (TCC) of the urinary bladder. Approximately 50% of pet dogs with invasive TCC develop metastases. Most frequent sites of metastasis are regional lymph nodes (**B**) and lung (**C**). Metastasis to other internal organs, such as liver (**D**), and to bone also occurs. Photographs courtesy of T. Lin, Purdue University.

## ENVIRONMENTAL RISK FACTORS

Several environmental risk factors for TCC (including smoking and exposure to aniline dyes) have been identified,[3] but it is likely that there are many other risk factors which have not yet been identified. Multiple studies have been performed to help identify environmental risk factors for TCC in dogs,[11–14] in the belief that these factors may be important in human TCC development as well. In one of the earliest studies, a significant positive correlation was found between the proportional morbidity ratios for canine bladder cancer and the overall level of industrial activity in the host county being studied.[11] Bladder cancer mortality in Caucasian men and women in the same counties showed a similar correlation with industrial activity, thus suggesting a role for environmental pollution.[11]

Environmental risk factors identified in a case control study that involved dogs of several different breeds included exposure to topical insecticides for flea and tick control, and exposure to marshes that had been sprayed for mosquito control.[1,12] In obese dogs (which

in theory would have greater storage capacity for lipophilic carcinogens stored in fat) that received more than two flea/tick dips per year, the risk of TCC greatly increased (odds ratio [OR] 24.5, 95% CI: 1.4–43.2) compared to the risk in non-obese dogs receiving no flea/tick dips. Regarding insecticide exposure, several different types of chemicals were identified.[10] The investigators speculated that the 'inert' ingredients, accounting for >95% of the total product, were the likely carcinogens in these products. These 'inert' ingredients included solvents such as benzene, toluene, and xylene, and petroleum distillates. It was of particular concern that, in follow-up contact with dog groomers and veterinary technicians, some of these people reported applying dips to more than 100 dogs per week while using little or no protective clothing.[1,12]

Recently, a case control study in Scottish Terrier dogs (a breed at increased risk for TCC) was performed.[13,14] TCC risk was significantly increased in multivariate analysis for dogs exposed to lawns or gardens treated with herbicides alone (OR=3.62, p=0.002), or herbicides and insecticides in combination (OR=7.19, p=0.001), but not insecticides alone.[13] The increased herbicide risk involved phenoxy herbicides and possibly nonphenoxy herbicides. After controlling for herbicide exposure in a multivariate model, TCC risk was also significantly increased for dogs exposed to flea and/or tick dips, powders, or collars (OR=4.84, p=0.02).[14] TCC risk significantly decreased, however, for dogs exposed to spot-on flea treatments containing fipronil (OR=0.30, p=0.02).[14] Although the cause of the protective effect is not known, the spot-on products are applied to a small area of skin in a minimal volume, and thus have less volume of 'inert' ingredients.

Bladder cancer risk in dogs has not been related to sidestream cigarette smoke.[12] While smoking is a well-known cause of human TCC, the risk of TCC associated with exposure to sidestream smoke is less well defined. The risk of bladder cancer increases linearly (two- to three-fold) for persons who smoke 10 or more cigarettes per day, and then increases substantially in people who smoke 40–60 cigarettes per day.[15,16] It is likely that the dogs' exposure to carcinogens in sidestream cigarette smoke was insufficient to contribute to the development of TCC.

## ELUCIDATION OF GENETICALLY RELATED RISK FACTORS

The observation that approximately half of people who are diagnosed with TCC have no known risk factors[3] raises the issue that important genetic or environmental factors for TCC risk are yet to be identified. Some of the current findings regarding the genetic risks of TCC are included in Chapters 3 and 4. Pet dogs may offer the opportunity to uncover other genetically linked risk factors for TCC.

There is considerable variation in the risk of TCC between different breeds of dogs, with Scottish Terriers having an 18 times greater risk (OR=18.09, 95% CI: 7.30–44.86) than mixed breed dogs.[1] Other breeds of dogs with increased risk for TCC include Beagles, Shetland Sheepdogs, Wire Hair Fox terriers, and West Highland White terriers. The cause of the breed-associated risk for TCC is not known, but could represent genetic predisposition to bladder cancer such as differences in the biochemical pathways that activate and detoxify carcinogens. Work is ongoing to identify specific differences in the Scottish Terrier genome that may be responsible for the increased TCC risk. This work is especially timely given recent efforts mapping the canine and human genomes.[17,18]

## MORE EFFECTIVE TREATMENT

A notable example of the utility of studies of invasive TCC in pet dogs has been the findings of the antitumor activity of cyclooxygenase (COX) inhibitors in dogs followed by promising results in COX inhibitor trials in humans. Our interest in COX inhibitor treatment began when pet dogs with various forms of spontaneous cancer had remission while receiving the nonselective COX inhibitor piroxicam (Feldene) for pain control, and no other therapy.[1] This observation was followed by a phase I clinical study of piroxicam in pet dogs with several types of cancer, and phase II and III clinical studies of piroxicam in pet dogs with TCC.[6,7,19] The chemopreventive effects of COX inhibitors and selective cyclooxygenase-2 (COX2) inhibitors in chemically induced bladder tumors in rodents[20,21] has added further interest to this area of investigation.

COX1 is constitutively expressed in many normal tissues, including the epithelium of the urinary bladder in dogs and humans.[22,23] Although COX2 is expressed in many epithelial malignancies, including canine and human invasive TCC, it is not expressed in the normal bladder epithelium.[22,23] The side effects (gastrointestinal irritation) of nonselective COX inhibitors are most commonly related to inhibition of COX1. Selective COX2 inhibitors are expected to cause fewer side effects.

The phase I clinical study of piroxicam in pet dogs defined an acceptable dosage of the drug for future use and demonstrated antitumor activity against TCC.[19] In the phase II clinical study of single agent piroxicam in 62 dogs with invasive TCC, tumor responses included complete remission (CR) in 2, partial remission in 9, stable disease (SD) in 35, and progressive disease in 16.[6,24] The two dogs with CR lived 2.1 and 3.3 years, respectively, following initiation of treatment, died of unrelated causes, and were tumor-free on postmortem examination. The frequency of SD (SD in 56% of dogs) and the length of SD with piroxicam treatment appeared longer than that observed in other treatment studies in canine TCC, suggesting that piroxicam delayed disease progression. The median survival (195 days, 1.8 human equivalent years) compared favorably with survival of dogs treated with single agent chemotherapy (130 days), and dogs undergoing partial cystectomy alone (109 days).[1,8,9]

Studies of dogs with TCC have also provided insight into the mechanisms involved in COX inhibitor-related tumor regression. In 13 dogs with TCC in which cystoscopy and biopsy were performed before and after 4 weeks of piroxicam treatment, induction of tumor apoptosis and reduction in urine basic fibroblast growth factor (bFGF) concentration were significantly associated with tumor regression.[25] Studies of the antitumor activity and toxicity of combinations of COX inhibitors and chemotherapy are in progress.[7]

The response of canine TCC to piroxicam has led to a phase II clinical trial of piroxicam in humans with carcinoma in situ of the urinary bladder (precursor lesion to invasive bladder cancer[26]). The study is being conducted in patients who have failed to respond to standard intravesical bacillus Calmette–Guérin (BCG) treatment. Although case accrual is early, remission (based on cystoscopic examination, biopsies of previous sites of disease, and biopsies of other areas of the bladder) has been observed in two patients (R. Foster, unpublished data).

Selective COX2 inhibitors are also being studied in TCC. Preliminary results of a study of the COX2 inhibitor, deracoxib, in dogs with TCC suggest activity in delaying tumor progression similar to that observed with piroxicam treatment (D.W. Knapp, P. Boria, unpublished work). Human clinical trials of COX2 inhibitors in TCC are also underway.

## CONCLUSION

Naturally occurring canine invasive TCC is very similar to human invasive TCC in histopathologic characteristics, biologic behavior (including propensity for metastasis), prognostic factors, and response to chemotherapy. Canine TCC provides a useful model for research relating to human invasive bladder cancer. Further characterization of canine TCC at the molecular level is indicated. Canine and rodent bladder tumors are complementary animal models of TCC.

## REFERENCES

1. Knapp DW, Glickman NW, DeNicola DB, et al. Naturally-occurring canine transitional cell carcinoma of the urinary bladder. A relevant model of human invasive bladder cancer. Urol Oncol 2000;5:47–59.
2. Knapp DW. Tumors of the urinary system. In Withrow SJ, MacEwen EG (eds): Small Animal Clinical Oncology, 3rd ed. Philadelphia: WB Saunders, 2001, pp 490–499.
3. Cancers of the genitourinary system. In DeVita VT, Hellman S, Rosenberg SA (eds): Cancer, Principles and Practice of Oncology, 6th ed. Philadelphia: Lippincott Williams & Wilkins, 2001, pp 1343–1490.
4. Patronek GJ, Waters DJ, Glickman LT. Comparative longevity of pet dogs and humans: implications for gerontology research. J Gerentol A Biol Sci Med Sci 1997;52:B171–B178.
5. Owen LN. TNM Classification of Tumours in Domestic Animals, 1st ed. Geneva: World Health Organization, 1980.
6. Knapp DW, Richardson RC, Chan TCK, et al. Piroxicam therapy in 34 dogs with transitional cell carcinoma of the urinary bladder. J Vet Intern Med 1994;8:273–278.
7. Knapp DW, Glickman NW, Widmer WR, et al. Cisplatin versus cisplatin combined with piroxicam in a canine model of human invasive urinary bladder cancer. Cancer Chemother Pharmacol 2000;46:221–226.
8. Chun R, Knapp DW, Widmer WR, et al. Cisplatin treatment of transitional cell carcinoma of the urinary bladder in dogs: 18 cases (1983–1993). J Am Vet Med Assoc 1996;209:1588–1591.
9. Chun R, Knapp DW, Widmer WR, et al. Phase II clinical trial of carboplatin in canine transitional cell carcinoma of the urinary bladder. J Vet Intern Med 1997;11:279–283.
10. Henry CJ, McCaw DL, Turnquist SE, et al. Clinical evaluation of mitoxantrone and piroxicam in a canine model of human invasive urinary bladder carcinoma. Clin Cancer Res 2003;9:906–911.
11. Hayes HM Jr, Hoover R, Tarone R. Bladder cancer in pet dogs: a sentinel for environmental cancer? J Epidemiol 1981;114:229–233.
12. Glickman LT, Schofer FS, McKee LJ. Epidemiology study of insecticide exposures, obesity, and risk of bladder cancer in household dogs. J Toxicol Environ Health 1989;28:407–414.
13. Glickman LT, Raghavan M, Knapp DW, Bonney PL, Dawson MH. Herbicide exposure and the risk of transitional cell carcinoma of the urinary bladder in Scottish Terriers. J Am Vet Med Assoc 2004;224:1290–1297.
14. Raghavan M, Knapp DW, Dawson MH, Bonney PL, Glickman LT. Topical flea and tick pesticides and the risk of transitional cell carcinoma of the urinary bladder in Scottish Terriers. J Am Vet Med Assoc 2004;225(3):389–394.
15. IARC. Overall evaluations of carcinogenicity: an updating of IARC monographs volumes 1 to 42. IARC Monogr Eval Carcinog Risks Hum 1987;Suppl 7:1–440.
16. Hartage P, Silverman D, Hoover R, et al. Changing cigarette habits and bladder cancer risk: a case-control study. J Natl Cancer Inst 1987;78:1119–1125.
17. Ostrander EA, Giniger E. Insights from model systems, Semper Fidelis: What man's best friend can teach us about human biology and disease. Am J Hum Genet 1997;61:475–480.
18. Istrail S, Sutton GG, Florea L, et al. Whole-genome shotgun assembly and comparison of human genome assemblies. Proc Natl Acad Sci USA 2004;101:1916–1921.
19. Knapp DW, Richardson RC, Bottoms GD, Teclaw R, Chan TCK. Phase I trial of piroxicam in 62 dogs bearing naturally occurring tumors. Cancer Chemother Pharmacol 1992;29:214–218.
20. Rao KV, Detrisac CJ, Steele VE, et al. Differential activity of aspirin, ketoprofen and sulindac as cancer chemopreventive agents in the mouse urinary bladder. Carcinogenesis 1996;17:1435–1438.
21. Grubbs CJ, Lubet RA, Koki AT, et al. Celecoxib inhibits N-butyl-n-(4 hydroxybutyl)-nitrosamine-induced urinary bladder cancers in male B6D2F1 mice and female Fischer-344 rats. Cancer Res 2000;60:5599–5602.
22. Khan KNM, Knapp DW, DeNicola DB, Harris K. Expression of cyclooxygenase-2 in transitional cell carcinoma of the urinary bladder in dogs. Am J Vet Res 2000;61:478–481.
23. Mohammed SI, Knapp DW, Bostwick DG, et al. Expression of cyclooxygenase-2 (cox-2) in human invasive transitional cell carcinoma of the urinary bladder. Cancer Res 1999;59:5647–5650.
24. Mutsaers AJ, Widmer WR, Knapp DW. Canine transitional cell carcinoma. J Vet Intern Med 2003;17:136–144.
25. Mohammed SI, Bennett PF, Craig BA, et al. Effects of the cyclooxygenase inhibitor, piroxicam, on tumor response, apoptosis, and angiogenesis in a canine model of human invasive urinary bladder cancer. Cancer Res 2002;62:356–358.
26. Husdon MA, Herr HW. Carcinoma in situ of the bladder. J Urol 1995;153:564–572.

# Cystoscopy 16

Alan M Nieder, Mark S Soloway

## INTRODUCTION

Cystoscopy is an essential procedure in the evaluation of the lower urinary tract. It allows the urologist to visualize the entire lower urinary tract and is a required component of the work-up for hematuria as indicated by the American Urological Association (AUA) Best Practice Guidelines.[1] The first workable cystoscope, created in the 1850s by Desormeaux in Paris, consisted of a hollow tube with a candle as the light source.[2] The technologic advances that have taken place in the cystoscope parallel the modernization of urology as a specialty. Among major advances in the treatment for bladder cancer is the development of fiberoptics and the modern cystoscope.

## FLEXIBLE CYSTOSCOPY

For years, urologists relied upon rigid cystoscopes to fully evaluate the lower urinary tract. However, in the office setting these rigid scopes are uncomfortable. A true revolution in lower urinary tract endoscopy occurred with the introduction of the flexible cystoscope in the early 1970s.[3] The first flexible cystoscopes had only minimal one-way deflection. In 1982, Burchardt described his experience with a 20 Fr. flexible choledochoscope in the urinary bladder.[4] In his original study, air was used as a visual medium. Clayman et al conducted a prospective controlled comparison of rigid and flexible cystoscopes in 1984.[5] They evaluated 80 men with both rigid cystoscopy and a fiberoptic choledochonephroscope. In 94% of the cases, the flexible instrument produced results similar to or more accurate

than the rigid cystoscope. Patients had less pain with the flexible endoscope, preparation and positioning were simplified, and the amount of irrigation fluid was less. Soloway reported on his initial use of flexible cystoscopy for 56 men in 1985.[6] This early report described two flexible scopes: one with a 5 mm (15 Fr.) outer diameter and one with a 6.2 mm (20 Fr.) outer diameter. In this report, it was noted that patients tolerated flexible endoscopy well, and that the cost of the procedure was lower than that of standard rigid endoscopy. Cost reduction was attributed to decreased use of a formal operating room and its expensive equipment, coupled with diminished need for general anesthesia.

Recently, manufacturers have produced smaller flexible endoscopes. Dryhurst and Fowler reported on their experience with a prototype small-caliber cystoscope.[7] This instrument has an outer diameter of 3.7 mm compared to the standard 5.4 mm. They report that the image quality produced by the smaller endoscope compares favorably to that of the larger instrument; in addition, the smaller scope was better tolerated by patients.

Flexible cystoscopy has many advantages over rigid cystoscopy[8]:

- It is easy to perform in the office and thus spares the expense of an operating room facility charge.
- Anesthetic requirements are minimal and the procedure is well tolerated.
- Since the patient is in a supine position when the procedure is performed, the time and expense of positioning and draping the patient are reduced.

In our current practice we utilize a 15.6 Fr. Olympus flexible cystoscope, and use sterile water as an irrigating solution (Figure 16.1).

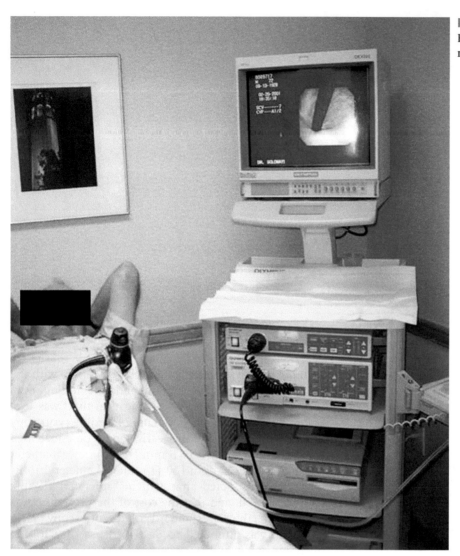

**Fig. 16.1**
Flexible cystoscopy set-up with video monitor.

## PROPHYLACTIC ANTIBIOTICS

Do all patients need to be given prophylactic antibiotics prior to outpatient cystoscopy if their urine does not indicate the presence of infection? Most authors have reported that the risk of urinary tract infection following outpatient cystoscopy is low.[9] Manson conducted a prospective, randomized trial comparing the risk of urinary tract infection in patients following diagnostic cystoscopy.[10] All patients had negative urine cultures prior to cystoscopy. The control group received no antibiotics while the treatment group received a 3-day course of trimethoprim with sulfamethoxazole, nitrofurantoin, or a cephalosporin antibiotic. All patients had a urine culture 2 weeks after the cystoscopy. At follow-up, two asymptomatic patients with bacteriuria were found in the control group, and one symptomatic patient was identified in the prophylaxis group. Manson concluded that the routine use of prophylactic antibiotics in patients undergoing

outpatient cystoscopy is not necessary. A caveat is that all of Manson's patients had documented negative urine cultures prior to cystoscopy.

Almallah et al evaluated the incidence of urinary tract infections in patients following flexible cystoscopy and urodynamic studies.[11] All patients were screened for bacteriuria, and those with a urinary tract infection were excluded. Of 103 patients who underwent flexible cystoscopy, 4.8% were noted to have bacteriuria and 11.6% had irritative lower urinary tract symptoms 48 hours after the procedure. When the authors excluded the 15.5% of the patients who received prophylactic antibiotics, the incidence of bacteriuria was 5.1%. The authors concluded that the risk of bacteriuria following outpatient cystoscopy is low and prophylactic antibiotics are not necessary. Furthermore, post-procedural irritative symptoms are poorly correlated with a urinary tract infection.

Wooster and Krajden prospectively evaluated the incidence of urinary tract infection in 200 patients undergoing either cystoscopy or transurethral resection of the prostate (TURP).[12] At the time of cystoscopy a sterile urine culture was obtained and evaluated for bacteriuria. Positive urine cultures were found in 21% of the patients. Not surprisingly, 64% of the inpatients had positive urine cultures compared with only 8% of the outpatients. Furthermore, positive urine cultures were found in 12% of the patients who had received pre-procedure prophylactic antibiotics compared with 28% of patients that did not. The authors recommended that precystoscopy urine cultures be obtained and specific antibiotic coverage be instituted based on the sensitivities.

We typically give one dose of an antibiotic for prophylaxis (e.g. quinolone or nitrofurantoin) to patients in our office for flexible cystoscopy. We are in agreement with other authors that the risk of postprocedure urinary tract infection is low. All patients should have a urinalysis performed in the clinic prior to cystoscopy. If normal, the risk of postprocedure bacteriuria is very low, and we do not routinely administer prophylactic antibiotics (Box 16.1).

## ANESTHESIA FOR OUTPATIENT CYSTOSCOPY

Most patients, young men in particular, are anxious when told of their need for an outpatient flexible cystoscopy. Even with considerable time spent to discuss the procedure, most first-time patients are apprehensive. Ellerkmann et al asked 87 women to complete a 10-point visual analog pain scale prior to and after cystoscopy.[13] There was a statistically significant difference between the mean anticipated pain score (3.75) and the postprocedure mean pain rating (2.83). A history of previous cystoscopy did not influence the

---

**Box 16.1** University of Miami flexible cystoscopy teaching protocol

- All patients without a documented negative urine culture receive a single dose of prophylactic antibiotics.
- Men are positioned supine, women in lithotomy.
- Men receive 10 ml 1% intraurethral lidocaine which is retained for 10 minutes prior to the procedure with a penile clamp.
- Entire bladder is visualized in a systematic fashion; bladder neck is evaluated by retroflexing the cystoscope.
- Bladder is never overdistended.
- Abnormalities are documented with a digital camera and all images are saved in the patient's chart.
- Small recurrent low-grade papillary lesions are fulgurated with a Bugbee cautery via the working channel of the flexible cystoscope. No further anesthesia is required.
- For patients with a history of carcinoma in situ or a high-grade tumor, a bladder wash is obtained for cytologic examination at the time of cystoscopy.

---

results. Stein et al noted that men who had previously had cystoscopy reported pain that was significantly less than that perceived by men who had never had cystoscopy.[14]

Most urologists use intraurethral lidocaine prior to flexible cystoscopy. Many other agents have been used, including intraurethral cocaine, which was popular in the early 20th century.[15] Goldfischer et al performed a prospective, double-blind, placebo-controlled trial comparing the benefit of 2% intraurethral lidocaine and plain lubricant in men and women.[16] Thirty cubic centimeters of each agent were inserted per urethra and allowed to dwell for 20 minutes prior to rigid cystoscopy. The authors found that pain perception was significantly lower in men who received lidocaine than in those who did not; however, there was no difference in pain perception in women who received lidocaine or plain lubricant. Birch et al reported that 2% lidocaine offers no advantage over plain lubricating gel in providing anesthesia for flexible cystoscopy in men.[17] These authors conducted a randomized, double-blind, placebo-controlled trial comparing intraurethral lidocaine gel with plain gel, and found no statistical difference in pain perception between the two groups.

The volume of intraurethral lidocaine necessary to achieve pain relief has been evaluated by Brekkan et al.[18] These authors conducted a prospective, randomized, double-blind study in both men and women comparing the effects of either 11 ml or 20 ml of 2% lidocaine prior to cystoscopy. There was a statistically significant decrease in the mean visual analog pain scale in men who received the higher volume of intraurethral lidocaine; however, there were no differences between the two groups for women or for men older than 55.

Herr and Schneider conducted a simple, prospective, randomized study to determine whether allowing the lidocaine gel to be retained for at least 10 minutes prior to cystoscopy would improve patient tolerance.[19] Patients randomized to immediate cystoscopy had the lidocaine gel instilled immediately before cystoscopy. In patients randomized to delayed cystoscopy, the lidocaine gel was instilled and retained with a penile clamp for at least 10 minutes prior to the cystoscopy. Following cystoscopy, patients completed a descriptive pain scale and a 10-point visual linear analog self-assessment scale. There were no statistical differences in pain between the two groups as measured by either scale. The authors concluded that there is no advantage to allowing the lidocaine gel to be retained prior to cystoscopy. Choong et al evaluated the optimal time required for 20 ml of 2% intraurethral lidocaine to alleviate cystoscopy discomfort.[20] The authors found that the anesthetic agent produced its greatest beneficial effect if it was administered at least 15 minutes prior to cystoscopy; in addition, these investigators reported that younger patients and those undergoing cystoscopy for the first time reported more pain after the procedure.

In our office, a nurse prepares male patients for cystoscopy and administers 10 cc of 2% intraurethral lidocaine. The lidocaine is then retained with a penile clamp for 5–15 minutes prior to cystoscopy. In our experience, most men have minimal discomfort. However, we agree with those who have reported that older men seem to tolerate the procedure better than younger men.[15,18]

## CYTOLOGY AS ADJUNCT TO CYSTOSCOPY

Carcinoma in situ (CIS) has important prognostic implications for patients with bladder cancer. The diagnosis of CIS requires an experienced eye and even then the changes are subtle. CIS, as typically described with flat erythematous areas, is not always seen. Urine cytology is a helpful adjunct to cystoscopy in detecting CIS and high-grade cancer and is associated with a sensitivity that approaches 90%.[21] Urine cytology is a required component of the work-up for micro-hematuria, as spelled out by the AUA Best Practice Policy Panel on Asymptomatic Microscopic Hematuria.[1] If the findings on cystoscopy or the patient's symptoms are suspicious for CIS, a bladder wash specimen should be sent for cytology. Matzkin et al published a prospective study comparing the diagnostic outcome of voided urine cytology to bladder wash cytology.[22] Of 23 patients with histologically documented bladder cancer, 23 (100%) were diagnosed as having urothelial cancer by the cytologist reading the bladder wash. Only 16 patients (70%) were similarly identified by voided urine cytology. The authors concluded that bladder wash rather than voided urine should be used as an adjunct to cystoscopy to diagnose and follow patients with bladder cancer.

In the office, we obtain urine for cytologic analysis by performing a bladder wash using a 14 Fr. red rubber catheter. The catheter is placed in the urethra and, using a piston syringe, we gently irrigate the bladder with approximately 60 ml of normal saline. Wash specimens can also be obtained via flexible cystoscopy. The use of intraurethral lidocaine prior to cystoscopy, however, may introduce technical difficulties with cytologic preparations.

## CLINICAL AND PATHOLOGIC STAGING

The standard for establishing a diagnosis of carcinoma of the bladder is by pathologic examination of biopsy tissue. For many patients with a history of recurrent low-grade, superficial bladder cancer, repeated transurethral resections of bladder tumors can lead to a reduction in bladder capacity. In addition there is the cost, pain, and psychological burden of repeated operative procedures. Following endoscopic resection, there is a 50% to 70% incidence of a subsequent tumor, either a true recurrence or a new occurrence.[23] Nevertheless, resection or fulguration is the standard treatment for recurrent papillary tumors.[24] Urgent resection of small low-grade papillary lesions may not be necessary, especially for elderly patients or those with comorbidities, since the risk of progression is so low. A caveat is that the urologist must be able to comfortably and reliably confirm that the lesion in question is low grade and confined to the mucosa.

Herr prospectively evaluated 150 consecutive patients with recurrent papillary tumors of the bladder and correlated their cystoscopic appearance with urine cytology and pathologic stage and grade.[25] Outpatient flexible cystoscopy showed disease classified as low grade and non-invasive (Ta G1), high grade and non-invasive (Ta G3), or high grade and invasive (T1 G3). Of 84 patients with a tumor that was identified on endoscopy as Ta G1, 78 (93%) were confirmed as Ta G1 on histology. Only 2 of the 84 were high grade and invasive (T1 G3). Of the 110 tumors considered at cystoscopy as non-invasive (Ta G1 or Ta G3), 9 (8%) were T1. Herr concluded that, for an experienced urologist, lesions appearing to be small (<0.5 cm), low grade, and low stage can be successfully eradicated by outpatient fulguration. Cina et al similarly evaluated 64 non-consecutive patients and prospectively attempted to predict the pathologic diagnosis based upon cystoscopic appearance.[26] Of 57 biopsies which were predicted to show that disease was non-invasive, only three (5%) demonstrated invasion (two were T1 and one was equivocal T1 or T2). The authors concluded that experienced urologists are able to predict accurately whether lesions are benign or malignant by their appearance at cystoscopy. In this article, the authors concede that the urologists contributing to the study could not reliably assess either tumor stage or grade, the conclusion being that urologists know a tumor when they see one, but that is all they know in the absence of histopathologic staging.

If small low-grade superficial lesions can be identified accurately by cystoscopy, then perhaps they can also be managed by observation, since the risk of progression is small.[23] Soloway et al observed 32 patients with recurrent low-grade superficial bladder tumors.[27] The mean observation period was 10 months, during which the mean tumor growth rate was calculated to be 1.7 mm per month. Only 3 of 45 patients (6.7%) had tumor progression from a preobservation, low-grade, non-invasive (Ta G1–2) to a high-grade Ta or T1 tumor. No patient developed a muscle-invasive cancer during the observation period. The authors concluded that small, recurrent, low-grade-appearing lesions are slow growing and carry minimal risk. Therefore, it may not be necessary to remove these tumors immediately upon identification, thus sparing the patients the morbidity and cost of either in-office fulguration or operative resection.

## OFFICE BIOPSY/FULGURATION

Because urologists have become increasingly proficient and comfortable with outpatient flexible cystoscopy, patients do not necessarily have to be brought to the operating room for a biopsy of a small bladder lesion. Procedures using a rigid cystoscope previously performed only under anesthesia can now be accomplished in the office with a flexible cystoscope and minimal anesthetic.

In 1990, Herr reported on his use of outpatient flexible cystoscopy and fulguration of small recurrent superficial bladder tumors in 185 patients using a 15.5 Fr. Olympus flexible cystourethroscope.[28] Women received no anesthetic and men received 1% intraurethral lidocaine gel. Herr noted that no patient experienced significant pain or requested that the procedure be aborted. A 4 Fr. Bugbee electrode was used via the 5 Fr. working channel of the cystoscope. Thirty-seven percent of the subjects required further outpatient fulguration for bladder tumor recurrence during a 24-month observation period.

Grasso et al reported on the use of a flexible cystoscope at the bedside.[29] They performed 55 procedures including dilation of urethral strictures, retrieval of indwelling stents, and biopsy and fulguration of small bladder tumors. They concluded that many procedures previously performed in the operating room can be accomplished at the bedside with minimal anesthesia. In 1994, Beaghler and Grasso reported on the use of a single-step biopsy forceps via a flexible cystoscope.[30] These biopsy forceps not only obtain tissue but are also able to cauterize the tumor base, eliminating the need for exchanging instruments via the flexible cystoscope working port.

Muraishi et al reported on the outpatient use of 'hot' cup biopsy forceps via a flexible cystoscope for biopsy of a small recurrent papillary tumor in a 79-year-old man.[31] Anesthesia consisted of a 50 mg diclofenac suppository 45 minutes prior to biopsy and 20 ml of 2% intraurethral lidocaine allowed to dwell for 15 minutes. Furthermore, 1–2 ml 1% lidocaine was injected into the tumor base with a thin endoscopic needle. They reported that the patient tolerated the 15-minute procedure without complications.

Wedderburn et al treated 103 consecutive patients with flexible cystodiathermy for small recurrent superficial papillary tumors of the bladder.[32] Patients received plain lubricating gel without lidocaine, and 80% of the patients reported no pain or mild pain, and only two patients commented that they would have preferred general anesthesia. The cost savings due to this outpatient procedure were approximately $66,000 per 100 patients. Dryhurst and Fowler similarly reported on their experience with flexible cystodiathermy for the management of small recurrent superficial bladder tumors.[33] These authors administer 60 cc of intravesicular 2% lidocaine, instilled via a 14 Fr. catheter. The patients are asked to retain the lidocaine for 20 minutes prior to the procedure.

## VIRTUAL CYSTOSCOPY

In recent years, with the improvement of radiographic imaging, computed tomographic (CT) virtual endoscopy has emerged as a technique to evaluate the colon for pathologic lesions. Currently, some centers are working to determine whether a similar radiographic study will be able to fully evaluate the bladder. CT virtual cystoscopy typically entails inserting a Foley catheter into the bladder and insufflating the bladder with carbon dioxide. Song et al prospectively evaluated 26 patients with CT virtual cystoscopy and compared the findings with those obtained with conventional cystoscopy.[34] All patients currently had or were previously diagnosed with bladder tumors. Two radiologists evaluated the CT images and were blinded as to the results of the conventional cystoscopy. Of 40 bladder lesions noted on conventional cystoscopy, 36 (90%) were detected by CT virtual cystoscopy. All four of the missed lesions were smaller than 5 mm. After a scout film was obtained, two single-breath hold scans of the bladder were obtained, one with the patient prone and one with the patient supine. The authors reported that the virtual cystoscopy took 30 minutes. Whether patients would prefer a catheter and a potentially time-consuming radiographic imaging study instead of a flexible cystoscopy remains to be seen. Nevertheless, the authors concluded that this is a promising technique. Kim et al conducted a similar prospective study evaluating the sensitivity of CT virtual cystoscopy compared with that of conventional cystoscopy in 73 consecutive patients with gross hematuria.[35] CT virtual cystoscopy correctly identified 56 of 60 lesions (93%) seen on cystoscopy; there were only four false-positive findings on CT virtual cystoscopy.

## USE OF DIGITAL RECORDING/PHOTOS

For years urologists recorded in a patient's chart the location, size, and appearance of all pathologic lesions identified. Usually a picture of the bladder is drawn and all lesions are marked in their location. Over the last decade, the advent of digital imaging has revolutionized the documentation of pathologic lesions. Not only are lesions drawn in a chart, but they are now easily captured via a digital cystoscope and either printed as a digital photograph or saved as a computer file for future reference. This benefits not only the urologist, who is able to review a picture of the pathologic findings at a future time, but also allows patients to view their tumors. Bruno et al reported on the use of a digital image recorder to capture endoscopic images.[36] These authors saved all their images as JPEG files which can be placed in electronic medical records, imported into internet web pages, incorporated in slide presentation, or simply printed and stored.

In our practice, we obtain a digital photograph of all pathologic lesions identified during flexible cystoscopy. These images are shared with the patient and saved in the patient's chart. The images are also reviewed with our house staff to demonstrate and teach the appearance of high- and low-grade lesions.

## TEACHING CYSTOSCOPY

In training to achieve proficiency in cystoscopy, as for most other procedures performed in the practice of medicine and surgery, a learning curve exists. Cystoscopy is a procedure performed by urologists thousands of times during their careers. Since most flexible cystoscopy is performed in the office setting without a video monitor, it behooves teaching urologists to make certain that their novice residents achieve proficiency with this skill, either by directly observing each procedure on a video monitor or by achieving proficiency on a simulator. In 2002, Shah and Darzi validated a flexible cystoscopy simulator, the URO Mentor.[37] The authors compared 10 medical students to 7 senior urologists on the simulator and their time to visualize 10 different sites in a simulated bladder. As expected, the senior urologists were significantly better at flexible cystoscopy and faster in observing the entire simulated bladder than the medical students. However, the medical students significantly improved their time by the 10th attempt. The authors concluded that a flexible cystoscopy simulator can be a useful training tool. Shah et al also evaluated the flexible cystoscopy simulator on 14 urology nurse practitioners with no previous cystoscopy experience.[38]

Wilhelm et al further evaluated the feasibility of teaching cystoscopy and basic endourologic skills with the URO Mentor simulator.[39] The authors prospectively evaluated 21 medical students on the simulator. The subjects were then randomized into either a control group or a training group in which the students underwent five 30-minute training sessions on the simulator. After the training sessions, the subjects had significantly better cystoscopic skills than those of the control (non-training) group. The authors concluded that endourologic training on a simulator may improve performance in the operating room.

## CONCLUSION

The technologic advances in cystoscopy have progressed during the last 150 years to allow urologists to better care for their patients. In male patients, outpatient office-based flexible cystoscopy should be the standard diagnostic tool for men with lower urinary tract signs or symptoms. Anesthetic requirements are minimal and patient comfort is easily obtained with intraurethral lidocaine. All pathologic lesions are digitally photographed and saved in the patient's chart. Further therapeutic procedures are also easily performed in the office via the working channel of the flexible cystoscope. The promising future application of CT virtual cystoscopy has yet to be seen and fully evaluated.

## REFERENCES

1. Grossfeld GD, Litwin MS, Wolf JS Jr, et al. Evaluation of asymptomatic microscopic hematuria in adults: the American Urological Association best practice policy—part II: patient evaluation, cytology, voided markers, imaging, cystoscopy, nephrology evaluation, and follow-up. Urology 2001;57:604–610.
2. Nicholson P. Problems encountered by early endoscopists. Urology 1982;19:114–119.
3. Tsuchida S, Sugawara H. A new flexible fibercystoscope for visualization of the bladder neck. J Urol 1973;109:830–831.
4. Burchardt P. The flexible panendoscope. J Urol 1982;127:479–481.
5. Clayman RV, Reddy P, Lange PH. Flexible fiberoptic and rigid-rod lens endoscopy of the lower urinary tract: a prospective controlled comparison. J Urol 1984;131:715–716.
6. Soloway MS. Flexible cystourethroscopy: alternative to rigid instruments for evaluation of lower urinary tract. Urology 1985;25:472–474.
7. Dryhurst DJ, Fowler CG. A new small-calibre diagnostic flexible cystoscope. BJU Int 2002;89:194–196.
8. Young MJ, Soloway MS. Office evaluation and management of bladder neoplasms. Urol Clin North Am 1998;25:603–611.
9. Kraklau DM, Wolf JS Jr. Review of antibiotic prophylaxis recommendations for office-based urologic procedures. Tech Urol 1999;5:123–128.
10. Manson AL. Is antibiotic administration indicated after outpatient cystoscopy? J Urol 1988;140:316–317.
11. Almallah YZ, Rennie CD, Stone J, Lancashire MJ. Urinary tract infection and patient satisfaction after flexible cystoscopy and urodynamic evaluation. Urology 2000;56:37–39.
12. Wooster DL, Krajden S. Selection of antibiotic coverage in vascular patients undergoing cystoscopy. J Cardiovasc Surg 1990;31:469–473.
13. Ellerkmann RM, Dunn JS, McBride AW, et al. A comparison of anticipated pain before and pain rating after the procedure in patients who undergo cystourethroscopy. Am J Obstet Gynecol 2003;189:66–69.
14. Stein M, Lubetkin D, Taub HC, et al. The effects of intraurethral lidocaine anesthetic and patient anxiety on pain perception during cystoscopy. J Urol 1994;151:1518–1521.
15. Pliskin MJ, Kreder KJ, Desmond PM, Dresner ML. Cocaine and lidocaine as topical urethral anesthetics. J Urol 1989;141:1117–1119.
16. Goldfischer ER, Cromie WJ, Karrison TG, Naszkiewicz L, Gerber GS. Randomized, prospective, double-blind study of the effects on pain

perception of lidocaine jelly versus plain lubricant during outpatient rigid cystoscopy. J Urol 1997;157:90–94.

17. Birch BR, Ratan P, Morley R, et al. Flexible cystoscopy in men: is topical anaesthesia with lignocaine gel worthwhile? Br J Urol 1994;73:155–159.

18. Brekkan E, Ehrnebo M, Malmstrom PU, Norlen BJ, Wirbrant A. A controlled study of low and high volume anesthetic jelly as a lubricant and pain reliever during cystoscopy. J Urol 1991;146:24–27.

19. Herr HW, Schneider M. Outpatient flexible cystoscopy in men: a randomized study of patient tolerance. J Urol 2001;165:1971–1972.

20. Choong S, Whitfield HN, Meganathan V, et al. A prospective, randomized, double-blind study comparing lignocaine gel and plain lubricating gel in relieving pain during flexible cystoscopy. Br J Urol 1997;80:69–71.

21. Wiener HG, Mian C, Haitel A, et al. Can urine bound diagnostic tests replace cystoscopy in the management of bladder cancer? J Urol 1998;159:1876–1880.

22. Matzkin H, Moinuddin SM, Soloway MS. Value of urine cytology versus bladder washing in bladder cancer. Urology 1992;39:201–203.

23. Heney NM, Ahmed S, Flanagan MJ, et al. Superficial bladder cancer: progression and recurrence. J Urol 1983;130:1083–1086.

24. Smith JA Jr, Labasky RF, Cockett AT, et al. Bladder cancer clinical guidelines panel summary report on the management of nonmuscle invasive bladder cancer (stages Ta, T1 and TIS). The American Urological Association. J Urol 1999;162:1697–1701.

25. Herr HW. Does cystoscopy correlate with the histology of recurrent papillary tumours of the bladder? BJU Int 2001;88:683–685.

26. Cina SJ, Epstein JI, Endrizzi JM, et al. Correlation of cystoscopic impression with histologic diagnosis of biopsy specimens of the bladder. Hum Pathol 2001;32:630–637.

27. Soloway MS, Bruck DS, Kim SS. Expectant management of small, recurrent, noninvasive papillary bladder tumors. J Urol 2003;170:438–441.

28. Herr HW. Outpatient flexible cystoscopy and fulguration of recurrent superficial bladder tumors. J Urol 1990;144:1365–1366.

29. Grasso M, Beaghler M, Bagley DH, Strup S. Actively deflectable, flexible cystoscopes: no longer solely a diagnostic instrument. J Endourol 1993;7:527–530.

30. Beaghler M, Grasso M III. Flexible cystoscopic bladder biopsies: a technique for outpatient evaluation of the lower urinary tract urothelium. Urology 1994;44:756–759.

31. Muraishi O, Mitsu S, Suzuki K, Koshimizu T, Tokue A. A technique for resection of small bladder tumors using a flexible cystoscope on an outpatient basis: bladder tumor resection with newly designed hot cup forceps. J Urol 2001;166:1817–1819.

32. Wedderburn AW, Ratan P, Birch BR. A prospective trial of flexible cystodiathermy for recurrent transitional cell carcinoma of the bladder. J Urol 1999;161:812–814.

33. Dryhurst DJ, Fowler CG. Flexible cystodiathermy can be rendered painless by using 2% lignocaine solution to provide intravesical anaesthesia. BJU Int 2001;88:437–438.

34. Song JH, Francis IR, Platt JF, et al. Bladder tumor detection at virtual cystoscopy. Radiology 2001;218:95–100.

35. Kim JK, Ahn JH, Park T, et al. Virtual cystoscopy of the contrast material-filled bladder in patients with gross hematuria. Am J Roentgenol 2002;179:763–768.

36. Bruno D, Delvecchio FC, Preminger GM. Digital still image recording during video endoscopy. J Endourol 1999;13:353–356; discussion 356–357.

37. Shah J, Darzi A. Virtual reality flexible cystoscopy: a validation study. BJU Int 2002;90:828–832.

38. Shah J, Montgomery B, Langley S, Darzi A. Validation of a flexible cystoscopy course. BJU Int 2002;90:833–835.

39. Wilhelm DM, Ogan K, Roehrborn CG, Cadeddu JA, Pearle MS. Assessment of basic endoscopic performance using a virtual reality simulator. J Am Coll Surg 2002;195:675–681.

# Fluorescence endoscopy

17

*Martin Kriegmair*

## INTRODUCTION

### WHITE LIGHT ENDOSCOPY

White light endoscopy of the lower urinary tract is limited in detection of bladder cancer. Flat neoplastic urothelial lesions such as dysplasia and carcinoma in situ (CIS) can be concealed in normal or nonspecific inflamed-appearing mucosa. The value of random biopsies, recommended when flat lesions were suspected, was challenged by Witjes et al[1] who showed in a cooperative study of 1026 unselected patients that biopsies of normal-appearing mucosa were of little value in determining patients' prognoses.

The risk of overlooking even papillary tumors is significant. Grimm et al[2] reported that after transurethral resection of superficial bladder cancer, residual tumor has been identified in 33% of cases at repeat resection. In 28% of the patients with fractional resection of T1 transitional cell carcinoma (TCC), residual tumor was found at the margins of the resected area.[3] Patients with newly diagnosed superficial, moderately or well-differentiated tumors had significantly fewer recurrences when the bladder was free of tumor 3 months after the initial resection.[4]

### 5-ALA PHOTODETECTION

For years, methods of labeling urothelial neoplasms have been sought.[5,6] Fluorescence photodetection of neoplastic urothelial lesions using 5-aminolevulinic acid (5-ALA) was first described in 1994.[7] 5-ALA is a precursor of heme biosynthesis. Following intravesical instillation, 5-ALA induces selective enhancement of protoporphyrin IX (a strongly fluorescent dye) in the mucosa of neoplastic lesions. Protoporphyrin IX is excited with blue light (375–440 nm) and becomes visible using an observation filter in the eyepiece of the endoscope for color contrast enhancement.[8]

Photodetection using 5-ALA has proved to have high sensitivity for detecting early stage bladder cancer—ranging from 87% to 96%. Specificity is lower due to false-positive results caused by inflammatory lesions.[9–14] These lesions are found particularly after intravesical chemotherapy, bacillus Calmette–Guérin (BCG) treatment, and endoscopic resection.[15] Photodetection is recommended primarily for evaluation of the untreated urothelium or if the mucosa has healed after the treatment. Quantification of 5-ALA-induced fluorescence improves the specificity by 30% without affecting the sensitivity.[16]

Detection of flat neoplastic lesions, which can easily be missed during white light endoscopy, was significantly enhanced by using 5-ALA photodetection. In comparison to white light cystoscopy, with the use of 5-ALA up to 53% more patients with CIS were detected[17] (Figure 17.1). Sixty-three patients with cytology positive or suspicious for disease and a negative standard cystoscopy underwent 5-ALA enhanced cystoscopy. In 51 of these cases (80.9%), the cytological findings were verified by fluorescence endoscopy detecting the precise site of malignancy within the bladder. The 12 remaining patients from this group did not show positive fluorescence with 5-ALA photodetection, and no positive histology was found in the random biopsies taken. In all these cases, neoplastic disease of the upper urinary tract was excluded by a retrograde pyelography.[18] In order to improve the diagnostic quality of the

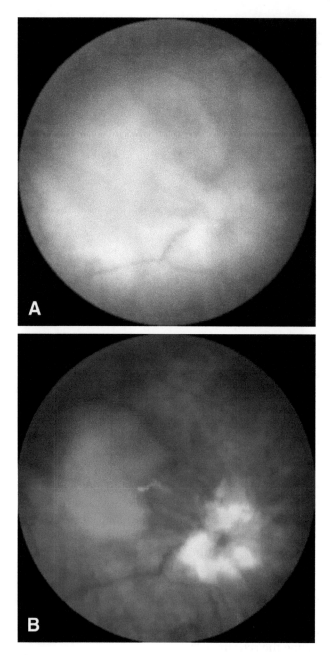

**Fig. 17.1**

Carcinoma in situ (CIS) observed with **A**, standard white light cystoscopy, and **B**, fluorescence enhanced 5-ALA cystoscopy. The red fluorescing lesion (CIS) is not visible with white light cystoscopy. The adjacent scar is visible in both panels.

procedure, an ester of aminolevulinic acid—hexaminolevulinate (HAL)—was investigated in a multicentric study. It was found that photodetection with HAL identified 28% more patients with CIS than standard cystoscopy.[19] Photodetection of neoplasia that was missed under white light cystoscopy resulted in a change in treatment strategy in 9%.[20]

Three prospective randomized studies have clearly shown that the risk of residual tumor after transurethral resection of TCC is significantly decreased by 5-ALA fluorescence endoscopy.[21–23] To date, results of only one

prospective randomized phase III trial have been published. It focused on the risk of recurrent tumor after transurethral resection with 5-ALA photodetection compared with risk after conventional white light endoscopy. Recurrence-free survival in the fluorescence group was 91% after 24 months compared with 70% in the white light group (p=0.0005). The adjusted hazard ratio of photodiagnostic versus white light transurethral resection was 0.29 (95% CI: 0.15–0.56), and photodetection proved to be an independent prognostic factor.[24] Figure 17.2 demonstrates detection of an

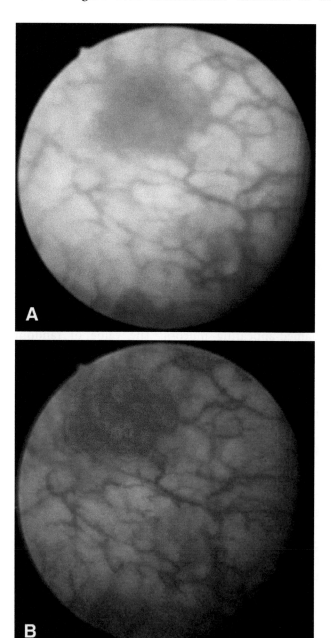

**Fig. 17.2**

Ta papillary lesion (upper left) is visible by both **A**, white light cystoscopy, and **B**, fluorescence enhanced 5-ALA cystoscopy. The smaller lesion (lower right) is prominent with fluorescence enhanced 5-ALA cystoscopy.

additional papillary lesion barely visible with white light cystoscopy.

## CONCLUSION

Fluorescence-enhanced cystoscopy with 5-ALA improves detection of occult papillary lesions and CIS compared to standard white light cystoscopy. This may translate to lower recurrence rates directly attributable to recognition and ablation of these occult lesions. Now approved for use in Europe, a registration trial in the United States is underway.

### REFERENCES

1. Witjes JA, van der Meijden APM, Collette L, et al. Long-term follow-up of an EORTC randomized prospective trial comparing intravesical bacille Calmette-Guérin-Rivm and mitomycin C in superficial bladder cancer. Urology 1998;52(3):403-410.

2. Grimm MO, Steinhoff C, Simon X, Spiegelhalder P, Ackermann R, Vögeli TA. Effect of routine repeat transurethral resection for superficial bladder cancer: a long-term observational study. J Urol 2003;170(2 Pt 1):433-437.

3. Klan R, Loy V, Huland H. Residual tumor discovered in routine second transurethral resection in patients with stage T1 transitional cell carcinoma of the bladder. J Urol 1991;146:316-318.

4. Fitzpatrick JM, West AB, Butler MR, Lane V, O'Flynn JD. Superficial bladder tumors (stage pTa grades 1 and 2): the importance of recurrence pattern following initial resection. J Urol 1986;135:920-922.

5. Whitmore WF Jr, Bush IM. Ultraviolet cystoscopy in patients with bladder cancer. J Urol 1966;95:201.

6. Vicente J, Chéchile G, Algaba F. Value of in vivo mucosa-staining test with methylene blue in the diagnosis of pretumoral and tumoral lesions of the bladder. Eur Urol 1987;13:15-16.

7. Kriegmair M, Baumgartner R, Knuechel R, et al. Fluorescence photodetection of neoplastic urothelial lesions following intravesical instillation of 5-aminolevulinic acid. Urology 1994;44(6):836-841.

8. Kriegmair M, Zaak D, Stepp H, et al. Transurethral resection and surveillance of bladder cancer supported by 5-aminolevulinic acid-induced fluorescence endoscopy. Eur Urol 1999;36:386-392.

9. Kriegmair M, Baumgartner R, Knuechel R, Stepp H, Hofstadter F, Hofstetter A. Detection of early bladder cancer by 5-aminolevulinic acid induced porphyrin fluorescence. J Urol 1996;155:105-110.

10. Jichlinski P, Forrer M, Mizeret J, et al. Clinical evaluation of a method for detecting superficial surgical transitional cell carcinoma of the bladder by light-induced fluorescence of protoporphyrin IX following the topical application of 5-aminolevulinic acid: preliminary results. Lasers Surg Med 1997;20:402-408.

11. König F, McGovern FJ, Larne R, Enquist H, Schomacker KT, Deutsch TF. Diagnosis of bladder carcinoma using protoporphyrin IX fluorescence induced 5-aminolevulinic acid. BJU Int 1999;83:129-135.

12. Filbeck T, Roessler W, Knuechel R, Straub M, Kiel HJ, Wieland WF. Clinical results of the transurethral resection and evaluation of superficial bladder carcinomas by means of fluorescence diagnosis after intravesical instillation of 5-aminolevulinic acid. J Endourol 1999;13:117-121.

13. Riedl C, Plas E, Pfluger H. Fluorescence detection of bladder tumors with 5-aminolevulinic acid. J Endourol 1999;13(10):755-759.

14. De Dominicis C, Liberti M, Perugia G, et al. Role of 5-aminolevulinic acid in the diagnosis and treatment of superficial bladder cancer: improvement in diagnostic sensitivity. Urology 2001;57(6):1059-1062.

15. Filbeck T, Roessler W, Knuechel R, Straub M, Kiel HJ, Wieland WF. 5-aminolevulinic acid-induced fluorescence endoscopy applied at secondary transurethral resection after conventional resection of primary superficial bladder tumors. Urology 1999;53(1):77-81.

16. Zaak D, Kriegmair M, Stepp H, et al. Endoscopic detection of transitional cell carcinoma with 5-aminolevulinic acid—results of 1012 fluorescence endoscopies. Urology 2001;57(4):690-694.

17. Zaak D, Hungerhuber E, Schneede P, et al. Role of 5-aminolevulinic acid in the detection of urothelial premalignant lesions. Cancer 2002;95(6):1234-1238.

18. Zaak D, Frimberger D, Stepp H, et al. Quantification of 5-aminolevulinic acid induced fluorescence improves the specificity of bladder cancer detection. J Urol 2001;166:1665-1669.

19. Schmidbauer J, Witjes F, Schmeller N, et al. Improved detection of urothelial carcinoma in situ with hexaminolevulinate fluorescence cystoscopy. J Urol 2004;171:135-138.

20. Filbeck T, Pichlmeier U, Knuechel R, Wieland WF, Roessler W. Do patients profit from 5-aminolevulinic acid-induced fluorescence diagnosis in transurethral resection of bladder carcinoma? Urology 2002;60(6):1025-1028.

21. Kriegmair M, Zaak D, Rothenberger KH, et al. Transurethral resection for bladder cancer using 5-aminolevulinic acid induced fluorescence endoscopy versus white light endoscopy. J Urol 2002;168:475-478.

22. Riedl CR, Daniltchenko D, Koenig F, Simak R, Loening SA, Pflueger H. Fluorescence endoscopy with 5-aminolevulinic acid reduces early recurrence rate in superficial bladder cancer. J Urol 2001;165:1121-1123.

23. Filbeck T, Pichlmeier U, Knuechel R, Wieland WF, Roessler W. Clinically relevant improvement of recurrence-free survival with 5-aminolevulinic acid induced fluorescence diagnosis in patients with superficial bladder tumors. J Urol 2002;168:67-71.

24. Filbeck T, Pichlmeier U, Knuechel R, Wieland WF, Rößler W. Senkung des Rezidivrisikos oberflächlicher Harnblasenkarzinome mittels 5-Aminolävulinsäure-induzierter Fluoreszenzdiagnostik. Urologe A 2003;42:1366-1373.

# Imaging in the assessment of urinary bladder carcinoma

18

*Barthold PH Schrier, J Alfred Witjes, Yoshifumi Narumi, Jelle Barentsz*

## INTRODUCTION

Bladder cancer is the fourth most common malignancy in men and the eighth most common malignancy in women in Europe and the United States. Each year approximately 20 new cases per 100,000 persons are diagnosed with bladder cancer, resulting in 5 per 100,000 persons dying from this disease annually. It develops more predominantly in males than in females with a sex ratio of 3:1 and has a peak incidence in the seventh decade of life.[1-3]

The majority (90–95%) of these cancers are transitional cell carcinomas (TCC) of various histologic grades (WHO 1–3). Some 70% to 80% of patients with TCC have superficial tumors, and 1% to 3% are associated with an upper urinary tract (UUT) tumor at initial diagnosis.[4,5]

The nonmuscle-invasive lesions appear as papillary tumors limited to the mucosa (Ta) or invading the lamina propria without involving the muscularis propria (T1) or as flat carcinoma in situ (CIS) with diffuse malignant cells confined to the mucosa. The likelihood that nonmuscle-invasive bladder cancer will recur is approximately 70% in 5 years, with a peak incidence in the first year after initial treatment. As many as 30% of these recurrent tumors present with a higher histologic grade and about 10% progress to muscle-invasive tumor, creating a risk for death.[4]

The remaining 20% to 30% of neoplasms are muscle invasive (≥T2) and/or metastatic at the time of initial presentation. Stage T2 tumors extend into the superficial (T2a) or deep (T2b) muscularis propria. Stage T3 tumors extend either microscopically (T3a) or macroscopically (T3b) in the perivesical fat. Stage T4 tumors extend into contiguous organs.[6] Approximately 50% of patients with muscle-invasive bladder cancer already have occult distant metastases, which limits the efficacy of therapy. Most of these patients develop clinical evidence of metastases within 1 year and succumb within 2 years of initial diagnosis.[4]

Invasive bladder cancer initially spreads radially through the inner part of the bladder wall and then circumferentially through the muscular layer. Depending on its point of origin, it may invade perivesical fat, prostate, seminal vesicles, or obturator internus muscle. In women, it rarely invades the uterus or cervix. Invasion of or growth into the ureter or prostatic urethra is common when the tumor originates near one of these structures.[7]

Invasion of tumor cells into superficial lymphatic and vascular vessels just beneath the lamina propria causes metastatic spread of bladder cancer.

The bladder lymphatics drain to perivesical, external iliac, hypogastric, and common iliac lymph nodes. Lymphatic spread is rare in stage T1 tumors and found in 24% of the muscle-invasive tumors. Lymph node (LN) metastases in patients with T2 tumors are confined to the true pelvis in more than 95%. In patients with T3 or T4 tumors, LN metastases are seen more often (15%) outside the common boundaries for standard LN dissection, namely at or above the aortic bifurcation.[8]

Hematogenous spread of bladder carcinoma is infrequent. If they occur, these metastases usually appear in lungs, bones, and liver. Bony metastases are predominantly seen in pelvic bones, upper femora, ribs, and skull in that order of frequency and always osteolytic.[9]

Once the diagnosis has been confirmed by cystoscopy, transurethral surgery, and histologic evaluation, the stage of the cancer according the TNM (tumor, node, metastasis) staging system must be determined (Table 18.1).[6] Staging is important because it indicates the most appropriate treatment, provides a guide to the likely prognosis, and permits assessment of the response to therapy.[10–12]

As clinical staging is not reliable for determining tumor extension into and beyond the bladder wall, imaging techniques are needed.[13] In this chapter the role of imaging in the assessment of urinary bladder cancer will be reviewed.

| Table 18.1 TNM classification | |
|---|---|
| **TNM 2002** | **Histological description** |
| Tis | Carcinoma in situ |
| Ta | Epithelial confined, usually papillary |
| T1 | Invading lamina propria |
| T2a,b | Invasion of the muscularis propria: 2A: superficial invasion 2B: deep invasion |
| T3a,b | Perivesical fat invasion: 3A: microscopically 3B: macroscopically |
| T4a,b | Invasion of contiguous organs: 4A: prostate, vagina, uterus 4B: pelvic sidewall, abdominal wall |
| N0 | No lymph node involvement |
| N1 | Single ≤2 cm |
| N2 | Single >2 cm, ≤5 cm Multiple ≤5 cm |
| N3 | Single or multiple >5 cm |
| M0 | No distant metastases |
| M1 | Distant metastases |

# IMAGING

## INTRAVENOUS UROGRAPHY

Intravenous urography (IVU) is indicated in all patients with signs and symptoms suggestive of bladder cancer. It is not a sensitive tool in detecting bladder cancer because small tumors are easily overlooked. A filling defect of the bladder is present in approximately 60% of cases. IVU can be useful in screening the UUT for associated urothelial tumor, but the incidence of synchronous UUT tumor is low (about 2%), and IVU is effective in diagnosing synchronous UUT tumors in only two-thirds of cases.[14]

If the tumor is located near the ureteral orifice, there may be incomplete or even complete obstruction, subsequent dilation of the urinary tract, or even decreased excretion of the kidney on that side. Ureteral

obstruction at the time of initial diagnosis of bladder cancer usually indicates muscle-invasive cancer.[15]

The development of an UUT tumor during follow-up of patients with superficial bladder carcinoma is very rare and therefore IVU should not be carried out routinely. IVU is recommended in selected patient groups, such as heavy smokers, industrial workers, and those with high-risk tumors (pT1 grade 3 and/or CIS), or in presence of vesicoureteral reflux. IVU should also be carried out when cytology remains positive during follow-up or tumor progression occurs.[16]

## RETROGRADE PYELOGRAPHY

Retrograde pyelography (RP) is indicated if the UUT is inadequately visualized by IVU. RP can also be used to better demarcate a filling defect found on IVU or to delineate suspected renal pelvic and ureteric abnormality. Prior to RP, urine from the UUT can be collected for cytology. Occasionally, RP is performed in patients in whom intravenous contrast material is contraindicated. Although anaphylactoid reactions to contrast material with RP have been described, the incidence is very low.[17,18]

## ULTRASONOGRAPHY

### TRANSABDOMINAL ULTRASOUND

The value of transabdominal ultrasound (TAUS) in detection of bladder tumors is limited. Bladder tumors <0.5 cm in diameter, regardless of location, as well as those of any size located in the bladder neck or dome of the bladder, are difficult to detect. On the other hand, the diagnostic accuracy for tumors >0.5 cm in diameter and situated on the posterior or lateral wall of the bladder is about 95%.[19]

TAUS is inaccurate in the assessment of tumor spread beyond the bladder wall and in evaluating lymph node metastasis. In general, ultrasound visualization is limited in obese patients and patients with air-containing bowel loops. A moderately distended bladder is necessary for complete evaluation of the bladder wall.

Bladder tumors appear on ultrasound as echogenic lesions. The bladder wall has a more intense echo pattern than tumor tissue, thus permitting distinction of early superficial lesions from those invading the deeper layers of the bladder wall. However, tumors involving the superficial muscle cannot be distinguished accurately from tumors involving the deep muscle.

### TRANSURETHRAL ULTRASOUND

Transurethral ultrasound (TUUS) with high frequency (5.5 MHz) endoscopic transducers allows better resolution and better staging. The degree of filling of the bladder can be changed during TUUS so that fixation or muscle infiltration may be studied. It is most valuable in determining the stage of tumor confined to the bladder wall, and appears to be useful in monitoring the completeness of tumor resection. The main limitations are the inabilities to discriminate between Ta and T1 tumors.[20] Additionally, TUUS is an invasive procedure requiring a special transducer.

## POSITRON EMISSION TOMOGRAPHY

Positron emission tomography (PET) is a noninvasive method for recording tissue metabolism with radiopharmaceuticals. The most widely used pharmaceutical in oncology is the radioactive glucose analogue 2-deoxy-2-[$^{18}$F] fluoro-D-glucose (FDG). After intravenous injection, FDG is transported into cells and phosphorylated by hexokinase to FDG-6-phosphate. The following metabolic step is blocked and FDG-6-phosphate therefore accumulates intracellularly. $^{18}$F emits positrons at this site and these undergo annihilation reactions, emitting two photons that escape in opposite directions. These pairs of photons are detected by the PET camera that consists of ring arrays of detectors around the patient. Transversal high-quality images reconstructed from the data obtained show distribution of the radioactive tracer within the registration plane. As malignant cells have an increased glycolysis, growing tumors or metastases may be detected by FDG-PET.[21] However, the clinical experience with FDG-PET in bladder cancer is limited for $^{18}$F because FDG is rapidly excreted in urine, causing an accumulation of activity in the bladder and making visualization of tumor and/or pelvic lymph node metastases more difficult.[22,23] Flushing the bladder with saline during examination can diminish this problem, but does not resolve it completely. More specific PET radiotracers that are not excreted into the bladder would be of use in bladder cancer.

$^{11}$C labeled choline (CHOL) has recently been reported as a new PET radiopharmaceutical for tumor detection with minimal excretion of radioactivity in the urine.[24] Choline is one of the components of phosphatidylcholine, an essential element of phospholipids in the cell membrane. As malignant tumors show a high proliferation and increased metabolism of cell membrane components, which will lead to an increased uptake of choline, the rationale for the use of CHOL-PET in oncology is provided.[25] The experience with CHOL-PET in bladder cancer is limited, and the potential has not yet been defined.

In general, PET may be a valuable diagnostic tool in the staging of pelvic lymph nodes in bladder cancer and useful for identifying uncertain or unknown metastases. It is capable of differentiating tumor recurrence from radiation or necrosis, and can play a role in the evaluation of the efficacy of chemotherapy.[26,27] Further investigations are, however, necessary to determine its definite value in diagnosis, staging, and follow-up of bladder cancer.

## COMPUTED TOMOGRAPHY (CT)

The major role of CT in bladder carcinoma is to stage rather than to detect the primary tumor, since CT appearance of bladder tumors is not specific.[28] This technique is less accurate in low stage tumors, and its reliability increases with more advanced disease.[29,30] However, double contrast techniques with air or carbon dioxide and 30% meglumine diatrizoate can be used to assess small mucosal lesions.[31] On CT, bladder neoplasm appears as sessile pedunculated soft tissue masses projecting into the bladder lumen. The tumors have a density similar to that of the bladder wall on enhanced scans, and occasionally the intraluminal surface is encrusted with calcium. However, due to neovascularization, these tumors may show increased attenuation.[32]

Bladder cancer involving superficial and deep muscles usually produces focal bladder wall thickening and retraction, but CT cannot reliably differentiate between the various layers of the bladder wall and cannot, therefore, distinguish T1 from T2a and T2b tumors (Table 18.2).[31,33] Moreover, evaluation of the bladder wall after transurethral resection (the primary treatment in bladder cancer) is difficult since the reaction of the bladder wall after the resection also appears as thickening on CT scanning.

Tumors of the anterior, posterior, and lateral walls are easily detected and evaluated, but difficulties arise in showing tumors at the dome and trigone because of the axial plane imaging used routinely in body CT.[33]

CT is clinically useful for detecting invasion into perivesical fat (T3a and T3b) as it can distinguish tumors confined to the bladder wall from those spreading into the fat (Table 18.2).[31,33]

Macroscopic extravesical extension (T3b) is characterized by poor definition of the outer aspect of the bladder wall with an increase in density of the perivesical fat. When no distinct fat planes are present between the bladder and the rectum, uterus, prostate, and vagina, early tumor invasion into these neighboring structures may be difficult to exclude.[31]

Tumor invasion of the seminal vesicle should be suspected if a soft tissue mass obliterates the seminal vesicle fat angle. This sign should be interpreted with caution because the normal seminal vesicle angle may be lost if the rectum is overdistended or if the patient is scanned in a prone position.[31,33]

CT can, in addition, evaluate retroperitoneal pelvic lymph nodes. Unfortunately, only nodal size and shape

**Table 18.2** MRI and CT criteria in bladder cancer staging

| TNM | CT criteria | MRI criteria |
|---|---|---|
| Tis | Not applicable | Not applicable |
| T1 T2a | T1–3A stages cannot be differentiated | Stage T1 and T2 are diagnosed when the tumor is confined to bladder wall, with the outer bladder wall being of normal low signal intensity on $T_2$-weighed images |
| T2b, T3a | | Interruption of low signal intensity bladder wall on T2-weighed images |
| T3b | Irregularity, soft tissue mass extending into perivesical fat | Transmural tumor extension into the perivesical fat |
| T4 | Direct invasion of adjacent organs | Direct invasion of adjacent organs |
| N+ | More than 1 cm | More than 1 cm |
| M+ | Distant metastasis | Distant metastasis |

can be evaluated, and sensitivity is 76%. Spherical nodes with a diameter >10 mm, or round nodes with a diameter >8 mm, are suspected of being metastatic (Table 18.2).[12,31]

## MAGNETIC RESONANCE IMAGING

Magnetic resonance imaging (MRI) is superior to CT for staging urinary bladder carcinoma (Table 18.3).[34,35] The multiplanar capabilities and soft tissue characterization capabilities of MRI make it a valuable diagnostic tool for visualizing the urinary bladder.[35,36]

## NORMAL MRI ANATOMY

On $T_1$-weighted images, the urine has low signal intensity, and normal bladder wall has an intermediate signal intensity equal to skeletal muscle (Figure 18.1A).

**Table 18.3** Accuracy of different staging techniques

| Stage | Clinical staging including TURBT | CT | MRI |
|---|---|---|---|
| T0–T+ | ++ | – | + |
| Tis–Ta | ++ | – | – |
| Ta–T1 | ++ | – | – |
| T1–T2a | ++ | – | + |
| T2a–T2b | 0 | – | + |
| T2b–T3a | 0 | – | – |
| T3a–T3b | – | ++ | ++ |
| T3b–T4a | – | + | ++ |
| T4a–T4b | – | + | ++ |
| N0–N+ | – | + | + |
| M0–M+ | – | 0/+ | ++ |

M+, bone marrow infiltration; T0, no malignancy (e.g. scar, fibrosis, granulation tissue, hypertrophy); T+, malignancy; TURBT, transurethral resection of bladder tumor; ++, highly accurate; +, accurate; 0, not accurate; –, not possible.

On these images, perivesical vessels and vas deferens appear as low signal intensity tubular structures surrounding the bladder base interspersing the perivesical fat. On fat-saturated $T_1$-weighted images, the bladder wall has a slightly higher signal intensity than urine or perivesical fat.[35,37,38]

On $T_2$-weighted images, the urine has a very high, and the bladder a low, signal intensity[35,37,38] (Figure 18.1B). The thickness of the bladder wall varies with the degree of the bladder distension. The normal values range from 2.9 to 8.8 mm, with a mean of 5.4 mm. When the bladder is distended, the wall should not exceed 5 mm in thickness.[36]

The perivesical fat has a high signal intensity both on $T_1$- and on fast spin-echo $T_2$-weighted images, and an intermediate signal intensity on spin-echo (SE) $T_2$-weighted images.[35,37,38] On fat-saturated $T_2$-weighted images, the signal intensity of perivesical fat is lower than that of the bladder wall. On these images the bladder wall can only be delineated if there are adjacent higher signal intensity perivesical venous plexus or seminal vesicles.[35,37,38]

Immediately after injection of gadolinium (Gd) contrast intravenously, the urinary bladder wall shows rapid enhancement.[39] Differential enhancement between the inner mucosa and submucosa, and the outer muscular layer, has been reported on early images. The inner layer is more vascular and shows early enhancement whereas the less vascular muscular layer enhances later.[36,39] About 2 minutes after injection, the Gd contrast is excreted into the urine. In order to visualize enhancement within the bladder wall, these images must be acquired before the mixture of contrast and urine reaches the bladder, i.e. within 2 minutes. Patent blood vessels with normal flow can be recognized without intravenous contrast by the typical signal void on turbo or fast SE images.[40]

On $T_1$-weighted images, lymph nodes have an intermediate signal intensity (Figure 18.2). On $T_2$-weighted images, the signal intensity varies (Figure 18.3). It is, however, always higher than that of muscle. $T_1$-weighted images provide the optimal contrast

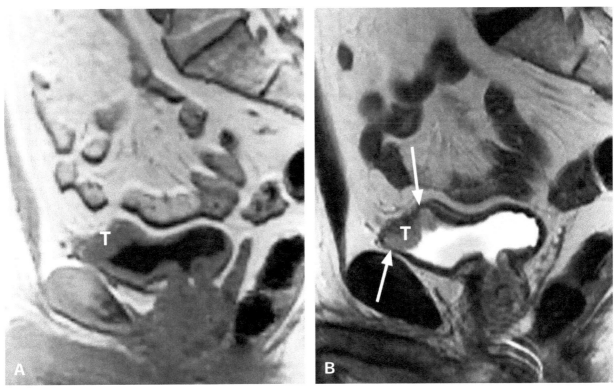

**Fig. 18.1**
T2b bladder cancer (T). **A** On T$_1$-weighted magnetic resonance (MR) image, tumor has signal intensity identical to that of the wall. Urine has lower and perivesical fat has higher signal intensity. **B** On T$_2$-weighted MR image, urinary bladder tumor (T) has signal intensity higher than bladder wall, and lower than urine. At arrows low signal bladder wall is disrupted by tumor, which argues for at least deep muscle invasion (T2b).

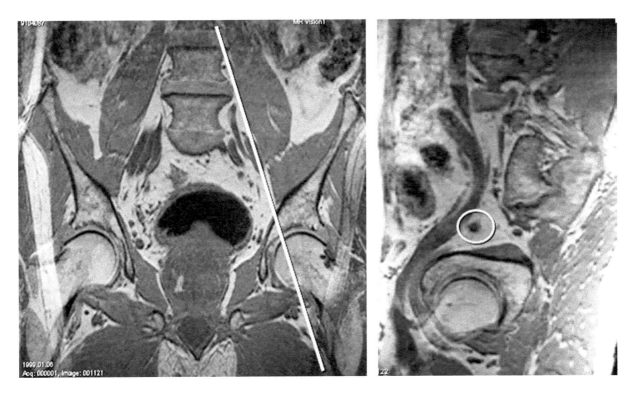

**Fig. 18.2**
Normal node. **A** On coronal T$_1$-weighted image, the imaging plane of **B**, parallel to psoas muscle ('obturator' plane), is indicated by the white line. **B** On T$_1$-weighted 'obturator' plane, a small 3 mm normal node (circle) can easily be separated from longitudinal running vessels. On this T$_1$-weighted image, node has lower signal intensity compared to fat.

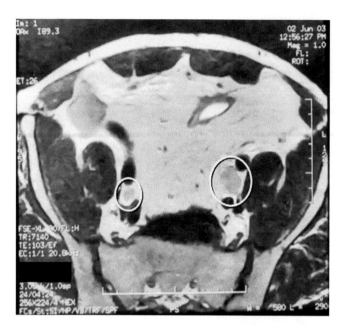

**Fig. 18.3**
Metastatic enlarged nodes (circles). On T$_2$-weighted image, nodes have signal intensity higher than muscle and identical signal to bladder cancer.

between intermediate signal intensity nodes and high signal intensity fat.[12]

## OPTIMIZING MR IMAGING OF URINARY BLADDER

Several factors must be considered when trying to optimize MR images of the urinary bladder. These factors are related both to the patient and the technique. Numerous artifacts are important, in particular motion–artifact reduction[41] and the degree of bladder filling.[38] Bowel motion can be reduced by glucagon or hyoscine butylbromide (Buscopan) intravenously before and during examination. Respiratory movements can be restricted by wrapping an adjustable belt around the patient's abdomen. Optimal distension of the bladder will improve evaluation of the wall and tumor. An empty or scarcely filled bladder can be avoided by asking the patient to drink two glasses of water and refrain from voiding 2 hours before the examination.

Selection of appropriate pulse sequences and use of surface coils and of contrast agent must also be considered in attempting to improve image quality.[10] In general, axial images should be acquired using T$_1$- and T$_2$-weighted sequences followed by imaging in other planes, depending on the site of the tumor.[10,33] Use of multiplanar reconstruction with a three-dimensional (3D) sequence gives the best results. An important plane direction in evaluating lymph nodes is parallel to the psoas muscle. This so called 'obturator' plane allows visualization of nodes along their long axis, and can locate them in relation to the iliac vessels and obturator

nerve (see Figure 18.2). The slice thickness should be 4 mm at the most, with a maximum gap of 1 mm. A thinner slice produces better anatomic details and improved partial volume. Image quality in the pelvis should be improved by using surface coils. Phased array body coils are well suited for pelvic MRI.[38]

Since MRI is a highly flexible and versatile system, many different imaging sequences and imaging planes are used for pelvic scanning. The choice will depend largely on the type of scanner used and its ability to obtain fast images. However, irrespective of the scanner features, T$_1$- and T$_2$-weighted sequences are mandatory.[10,38] T$_1$-weighted images are used to determine tumor infiltration into the perivesical fat; these sequences are most suitable for imaging lymph nodes as well. In addition there is a good contrast between bony metastasis and surrounding fatty bone marrow. For T$_2$-weighting, turbo or fast SE sequences are considered state of the art. These sequences are used for determining depth of tumor infiltration within the bladder wall, for differentiating tumor from fibrosis, for assessment of invasion into the prostate, uterus or vagina, and for confirming bone marrow metastasis seen on T$_1$-weighted images (Figure 18.4A).

Urinary bladder carcinoma develops neo-vascularization.[13,42–48] Therefore, after intravenous administration of Gd, bladder cancer shows earlier and more enhancement than normal bladder wall or other nonmalignant tissues. Urinary bladder cancer starts to enhance 7 seconds after the beginning of arterial enhancement, which is at least 4 seconds earlier than most other structures.[42] Contrast enhancement has many advantages, including improved detection of small bladder tumors, especially those measuring <1 cm that may be missed on T$_2$-weighted images because the high signal tumor can be obscured by urine. Other advantages are improved differentiation of bladder tumors from blood clot and other debris, improved detection of muscular and perivesical fat invasion,[49] and improved visibility of (small) vessels. For contrast-enhanced imaging of bladder cancer, T$_1$-weighted sequences with a time resolution of less than 20 seconds should be used. In the early (first pass) phase, discrimination between cancer and wall or fibrosis is best visible. To enhance tumor visualization in the perivesical fat, either subtraction or fat saturation must be applied.

## BLADDER CANCER STAGING

Local tumor extension, the degree of lymph node and distant metastases, and histologic tumor type largely determine treatment and prognosis. Therefore, exact staging is imperative. To determine local tumor extension (T), presence of lymph node (N), and distant metastases (M), the International Union against Cancer

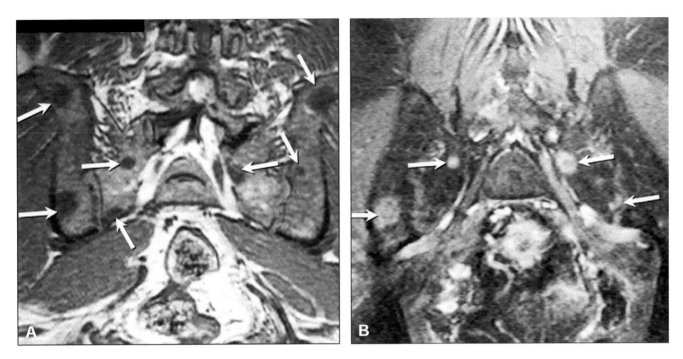

**Fig. 18.4**
Bone marrow metastases (arrows). **A** On $T_1$-weighted magnetic resonance image, metastases can be seen as low signal intensity around lesions. **B** On postgadolinium fat-saturated $T_1$-weighted image, due to enhancement, bone marrow metastases can be recognized as high signal intensity lesions.

proposed a uniform clinical staging method (see Table 18.1).[6]

## TUMOR STAGING

Because conventional clinical staging—bimanual examination under anesthesia, cystoscopy, and transurethral resection of bladder tumor (TURBT)—is not reliable in determining tumor extension beyond the bladder wall, other methods such as CT and MRI are needed. Indeed, CT cannot reliably differentiate between the various layers of the bladder wall and therefore cannot distinguish between nonmuscle-invasive (Ta–T1) and muscle-invasive (T2) disease. CT is clinically useful for detecting invasion into perivesical fat (T3a and T3b) as it can distinguish tumors confined to the bladder wall from those spreading into the fat. Since the introduction of pelvic MR imaging in 1983, several reports have shown the superiority of this technique for staging urinary bladder carcinoma.[50–52]

Bladder tumors demonstrate different patterns of growth: papillary, sessile, infiltrative, or mixed pattern. Papillary tumors are usually superficial (Ta or T1) and are best demonstrated on $T_1$-weighted images in which the intermediate signal intensity of the intraluminal tumor is outlined by surrounding low signal intensity urine. On $T_2$-weighted images, the signal intensity of both bladder tumor and intravesical urine increase, and intraluminal projections of bladder tumors may be less

conspicuous than on $T_1$-weighted images. Papillary TCC of the bladder has a loose connective tissue stalk. The identification of the stalk of a polypoid tumor, which has a lower signal intensity than tumor on $T_2$-weighted images, may be an important observation to exclude muscle wall invasion of the tumor (Figure 18.5).[53] Findings suggestive of superficial (T1) tumors are seen on $T_1$-weighted postcontrast images: smooth muscle layer, tenting of the bladder wall, fern-like vasculature, and uninterrupted submucosal enhancement (Figure 18.6).[54]

Muscle wall infiltrative tumors ($\geq$T2) present as a diffuse or focal thickening of the bladder wall with increased signal intensity on $T_2$-weighted images. This higher signal intensity is in contrast to the low signal intensity of normal bladder wall.[37] Early contrast enhanced images may help to identify muscle wall infiltration. Findings that suggest muscle invasion are irregular wall at the base of the tumor, focal wall enhancement, or wall thickening around the tumor (Figure 18.7).[54]

Muscle wall invasion is separated into superficial (T2a) and deep (T2b). In stage T2b the low signal intensity layer of the bladder wall is disrupted on $T_2$-weighted images by the higher signal tumor (see Figure 18.1B). Stage T2b cannot be separated on MRI from stage T3a (microscopic fat infiltration). Macroscopic tumor extension through the bladder wall into the perivesical fat (stage T3b) will cause a focal irregular decrease of signal intensity of the fat on standard $T_1$- or

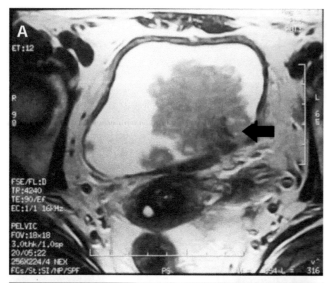

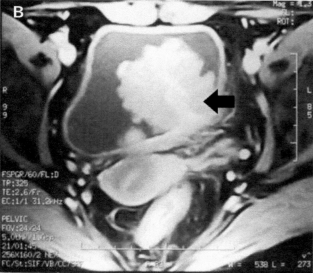

**Fig. 18.5**
Papillary T1 tumor with stalk. **A** On T$_2$-weighted tSE image, low signal intensity muscle is not disrupted by higher signal intensity tumor. In the center of the papillary tumor, a low signal intensity stalk (arrowhead) can be seen. **B** On postgadolinium fat-saturated T$_1$-weighted image, the stalk has more enhancement compared to the rest of the tumor (arrowhead). Images courtesy of E. Abou-Bieh, Mansoura, Egypt.

T$_2$-weighted images. Contrast-enhanced images with fat saturation also show tumor (enhancement) in the perivesical fat. Invasion of adjacent organs may be inferred from the extension of abnormal tumor signal intensity through fat planes into adjacent structures. This is well demonstrated with contrast-enhanced images. Invasion of the seminal vesicles can be demonstrated by an increase in vesicular size, decrease in signal intensity on T$_2$-weighted images, and obliteration of angle between the seminal vesicle and the posterior bladder wall. Invasion of the prostate and rectum is seen as direct tumor extension with an

increase of signal intensity. Obliteration of the angle between bladder and prostate also indicates prostate invasion. Invasion of the pelvic sidewall (T4b) is seen on T$_1$-weighted images as a loss of normal fat plane between bladder wall (tumor) and the vessels or musculature of the sidewall, or on T$_2$-weighted images as invasion of the sidewall musculature by intermediate to high signal intensity tumor.

Multiplanar imaging allows better visualization of the bladder dome, trigone, and adjacent structures such as the prostate and seminal vesicles. The accuracy of MRI in staging bladder cancer varies from 73% to 96%. These values are 10% to 33% higher than those obtained with CT.[51] Recently, several reports have been published on the staging of urinary bladder carcinoma with the use of intravenous Gd contrast. A 9% to 14% increase in local staging accuracy has been reported with use of this agent. Furthermore, when contrast agents are used, visualization of small tumors (>7 mm) improves, and tumor can be differentiated from postbiopsy effects with an accuracy of 90%.[42] The most accurate staging results using Gd contrast material are obtained with very fast T$_1$-weighted sequences.[55] This can be explained by earlier enhancement of tumors compared to surrounding tissues.

A tumor in a bladder diverticulum can be a problem for imaging. TUUS is of value in detecting tumors in a diverticulum, especially if the mouth of the diverticulum is not accessible for cystoscopy. Multiplanar MRI can demonstrate the presence and precise location of the bladder diverticular neck. Also, the intrinsic tissue contrast of both the T$_1$- and T$_2$-weighted images allows differentiation of urine and tumor, showing the intraluminal extent of tumor.[56]

## LYMPH NODE STAGING

Lymph node metastases in patients with nonmuscle-invasive tumors (<T2) are rare, but if the deep muscle layer is involved (T2), or if extravesical invasion is seen (T3–4), the incidence of lymph node metastasis rises to 20% to 30%, and 50% to 60%, respectively. Detection of lymph node metastases has very important clinical consequences. If lymph node metastatic disease is present, an extended lymph node dissection should be performed in order to maximize the curative intent of radical cystectomy. A noninvasive, reliable method for detecting and staging nodal metastasis could allow modification of the extent of the node dissection. Currently, there are five imaging techniques described for nodal staging: lymphangiography, ultrasound (US), CT, MRI, and PET scanning.

### Lymphangiography, US and CT
Bipedal lymphangiography is no longer used as an imaging method, although it has the capacity to show

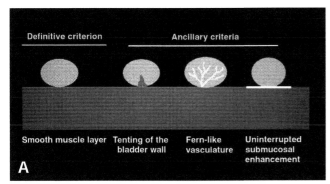

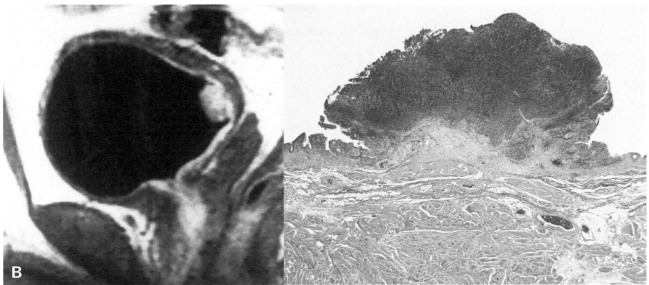

**Fig. 18.6**
Staging bladder cancer (MRI). **A** Findings suggestive of superficial (T1) tumors on $T_1$-weighted postcontrast images. **B** Bladder tumor–wall interface is smooth at the base of the tumor. Histopathology showed the tumor minimally invaded into the submucosal layer, but no invasion into the muscle layer at the tumor base.

micrometastases in normal-sized nodes. Its inability to depict internal iliac nodes and its invasiveness are major drawbacks. The sensitivity of US and CT is too low to reliably detect all lymph node metastases.[57] CT scans fail to detect nodal metastases in more than half of patients with pathologically proven positive nodes.[58]

## MRI

Normal nodes down to a size of 2 mm can be recognized with MRI. With multiplanar imaging, both the size and shape of the nodes can be assessed. The maximal length (long axis) and the minimal axial size of the node can be determined. Round nodes can be distinguished from oval nodes by using an index derived by dividing the axial size by the long axis. Lymph nodes are considered to be rounded when this index is between 1.0 and 0.8 and to be spherical or elongated if this index is less than 0.8. The cut-off value for a pathologic node is a minimal axial diameter of 10 mm for a spherical/elongated node and 8 mm for a rounded node. An asymmetric cluster of small lymph nodes is also considered to be pathologic.[12]

Current imaging techniques can show only nodal size. Different sensitivities and specificities are acquired depending on the selection of cut-off size for lymph nodes.[59] Recently Jager and coworkers showed that with a 3D high-resolution technique, not only nodal size but also nodal shape could be assessed.[12] Using the nodal shape in relation to the cut off size also improved their results with an accuracy of 90% and a positive predictive value of 94%.[11] This is clinically relevant as a high positive predictive value for the detection of nodal metastasis can also support the indication for (MR-guided) biopsy.[60] In cases of positive biopsy this may cause a change of treatment from surgery to initial chemotherapy. Cross-sectional imaging modalities such as CT and (3D) MRI have a low sensitivity (76%) as metastases in normal-sized lymph nodes are still missed, since both modalities use the nonspecific criterion of size to distinguish between normal and malignant nodes.[12,59] Although fast dynamic MRI has been shown to improve sensitivity by showing fast and high enhancement in metastatic nodes, specificity decreases. In addition, application of fast dynamic techniques is further limited by low resolution and pronounced vascular artifacts.[42]

## PET

Although very promising in metastatic lung cancer,[61] the role of FDG-PET scanning is limited in the assessment of pelvic lymph nodes. In a study using PET in 64 patients with urinary bladder cancer, Bachor et al obtained a sensitivity of 67% and a negative predictive value of

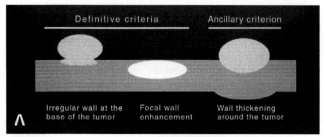

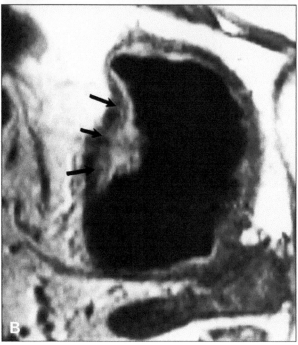

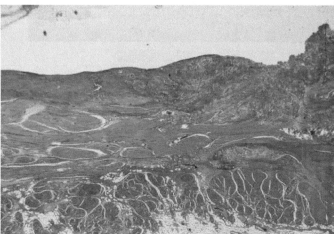

**Fig. 18.7**
Staging bladder cancer (MRI). **A** Findings suggestive of minimal muscle invasion (T2a). **B** Bladder tumor–wall interface is irregular at the base of the tumor without disruption of the bladder wall by the tumor. Histopathology showed invasion of the tumor into the muscle layer less than inner half.

84%. In addition, their reported specificity of 86% is lower than specificity obtained with CT and MRI.[62] Heicappell et al obtained with their data a sensitivity of 65%.[63] Thus the accuracy of FDG-PET scanning is not high enough to replace pelvic lymph node dissection (PLND). The value of PET with other positron-emitting radionuclides needs to be evaluated. Staging PLND still remains the most sensitive method for assessing lymph node metastases, and thus continues to be the first step in the management protocol of patients with muscle-invasive cancer and no visceral metastasis.

## DISTANT METASTASES

Currently, the mainstay for the detection of bone metastases is a radionuclide bone scan. However, MRI is superior to $^{99m}$Tc bone scan in assessment of bone marrow involvement.[64] The high sensitivity of MRI for evaluating bone marrow metastasis makes it an ideal tool for detecting suspected osseous metastatic disease and for determining its extent.[65,66] Osseous metastases generally are hematogenously spread, and the vascular bone marrow is usually the earliest site of involvement. For purposes of screening, $T_1$-weighted images are

adequate to detect foci of abnormal marrow. Therefore, MRI can be useful in the evaluation of patients suspected of having vertebral metastases with equivocal or negative bone scans. Thanks to its high spatial resolution, MRI may also guide needle biopsy procedures. Plain radiographs are the least sensitive in evaluating the axial skeleton for metastases in that 50% of bone mineral content must be altered before evidence of metastasis is visible. The limitation of MRI, however, is the inability to produce 'whole body' images.

## NEW TECHNIQUES

### MULTIDETECTOR ROW CT UROGRAPHY

During the past few years CT has challenged IVU in the evaluation of the urinary tract. Unenhanced helical CT is more sensitive than either IVU or US for the detection of urinary tract stones.[67,68] Contrast-enhanced helical CT is well established as being more sensitive and specific in the detection and characterization of renal masses.[69] Until recently, the only remaining advantage of IVU over CT has been its ability to depict intraluminal filling defects and mucosal abnormalities in the upper urinary tract. Recent improvements in CT hardware have led to the development of the multidetector (MD) row (or multislice) CT scanner. Multidetector row CT urography (MDCTU) offers single breath-hold coverage of the entire urinary tract and high resolution images. Multiple thin overlapping slices provide excellent 2D and 3D reformatted images.

The ability of MDCTU to detect urothelial tumors in the renal collecting system or in the ureter has not been thoroughly evaluated or established in the literature. Caoili and coworkers reported that six of six proven urothelial malignancies in the renal pelvis and ureters were detected by MDCTU.[70] IVU has been reported in the literature to have detection rates for urothelial neoplasms of only two-thirds of cases.[14] MDCTU seems to perform at least as well as IVU in detecting UUT. Moreover, on MDCTU the urinary tract distal to an obstructing lesion is also well demonstrated, thus overcoming the limitations of IVU in a nonfunctioning kidney with obstructive disease.[71] Other advantages of MDCTU over IVU include identification and characterization of the causes of ureteric obstruction, including short segment malignant strictures with associated mural thickening, retroperitoneal masses and lymphadenopathy, retroperitoneal fibrosis, benign ureteric strictures, and iatrogenic causes such as posthysterectomy and postcolectomy injuries.[72,73]

Evaluation of the bladder by MDCTU requires pre- and postcontrast studies. The precontrast study is useful as calcifications within the bladder wall or lumen are easily detected. Focal bladder wall calcification can occur with carcinoma of the bladder. However, bladder masses frequently cannot be detected on noncontrast images. Focal areas of bladder wall thickening or masses that protrude into the bladder lumen suggest bladder carcinoma, particularly when it is associated with greater enhancement than the adjacent bladder wall. Kim et al evaluated the accuracy of MDCTU in the detection and staging of bladder cancer. Bladder cancers show peak enhancement to approximately 106 ± 14 HU (Hounsfield units) with 60-second delayed scanning. A detection rate of 97% (75/77) for all bladder cancers and 85% (11/13) for bladder cancers <1 cm was reported. Sensitivity and specificity in the diagnosis of perivesical invasion in this study were 89% and 95%, respectively.[74] MDCTU seems to be useful in the detection and staging of bladder cancer. Therefore, at most academic medical institutions, MDCTU has replaced IVU as the diagnostic imaging study of choice for the evaluation of patients with hematuria (or suspected urolithiasis).

## USPIO MRI

Previous reports have shown that the information about lymph nodes on MR images can be improved by pharmaceutical manipulation of tissue proton relaxation times. Ultrasmall superparamagnetic iron oxide (USPIO) particles with a long plasma circulation time have been shown to be suitable as an MR contrast agent for intravenous MR lymphangiography.[75,76] After intravenous injection, the USPIO particles are transported to the interstitial space and from there they are transported through the lymph vessels to the lymph nodes. Once within normally functioning nodes the iron particles are taken up by macrophages and reduce the signal intensity of normal lymph node tissue in which they accumulate because of the T2 and susceptibility effect of iron oxide, and this produces a negative enhancement. In areas of lymph nodes that are involved with malignant cells, macrophages are replaced by cancer cells, which lack reticuloendothelial activity and are unable to take up the USPIO particles (Figure 18.8). The uptake may also be decreased in inflammatory nodes. In addition, because of increased vascular permeability and increased diffusion in cancer tissue, there is leakage of USPIO particles into the metastatic areas, which produces a low local concentration and nonclustering of USPIO particles at these metastatic sites.[76] Through their T1 relaxivity, this can induce an increase in signal intensity on $T_1$-weighted images, producing positive enhancement.[77–79]

Thus the ability of post-USPIO MRI to identify metastatic areas in the lymph nodes depends primarily on the degree of uptake of USPIO particles by the macrophages in normal lymph node tissue and the leakage of USPIO particles in the metastatic area itself. Twenty-four hours after intravenous injection of USPIO, normal lymph node and malignant tissue have different signal intensity on MR images (Figure 18.8), and thus this noninvasive technique may result in the detection of metastatic normal-sized nodes.[80]

Papers describing this technique in the evaluation of pelvic malignancies report a sensitivity of 82% to 100%.[79–82] Other papers include lymph node evaluation in other areas, predominantly in the head and neck, and chest. Reported sensitivities (mean 91%, variation 84–100%) are higher than with precontrast MRI.[83–86] As these authors did not use high resolution techniques, they had limited visualization of small (<8 mm) lymph nodes. In a study performed at UMC in Nijmegen and Massachusetts General in Boston,[81] in 80 patients with histologically proven prostate cancer, using high resolution techniques (at 1.5 T using a body phased-array coil), on post-USPIO MRI the rate of detection of small nodal metastases in normal 5–8 mm sized nodes was significantly improved. Sensitivity, accuracy, and negative predictive value showed significant improvement with use of post-USPIO MRI to 100%, 98%, and 100%, respectively. This was due to the detection of small 3–4 mm metastases in normal-sized nodes. In addition, in 9 out of 80 patients, nodes were found outside of the surgical field. During the slow (30-

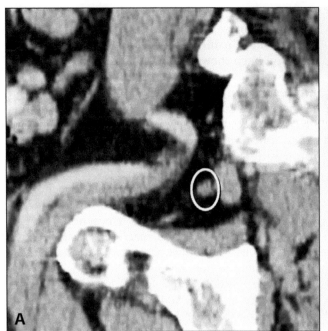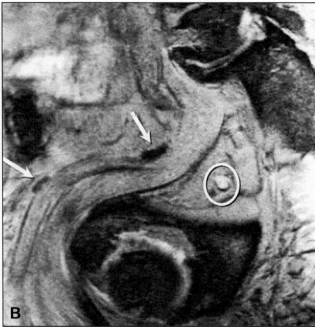

**Fig. 18.8**
Normal size (5 mm) metastatic node in hypogastric region (circle). **A** CT reconstruction in 'obturator' plane shows normal size (5 mm) node (circle). **B** On $T_2$*-weighted MR image (sensitive to iron) in identical plane obtained 24 hours post-USPIO, this node (circle) has high signal intensity which argues for metastasis. Also two small normal nodes (arrows) are visible; they have low signal intensity due to accumulation of iron-loaded macrophages in normal nodal tissue.

minute) infusion of the USPIO contrast, only two patients showed minor side effects (low back pain), which were due to a too rapid infusion. After the infusion rate was slowed, the symptoms decreased, and no further treatment was needed. In a similar study of bladder cancer post-USPIO results, MRI was associated with sensitivity, specificity, accuracy, and negative and positive predictive values of 96%, 95%, 95%, 89%, and 98%, respectively.[87] A proportion of patients with node-positive bladder cancer can be cured with extended pelvic lymphadenectomy.[88] USPIO MRI may provide a reliable map of positive pelvic lymph nodes and guide a radical lymphadenectomy.

## VIRTUAL CYSTOSCOPY

Recent studies reported the feasibility of 3D rendering of the bladder, which provides an imaging format familiar to the urologist.[88–90] Bernhardt et al noted that the findings at MR cystoscopy, as compared with those at cystoscopy for the detection of the tumors, did not reveal a statistically significant difference. Compared with axial images, however, CT or MR cystoscopy showed no significant differences in detection of papillary lesions with a diameter of ≥10 mm, and had almost the same sensitivity and specificity as these modalities.[90–92] The clinical value of virtual cystoscopy requires further study.

## SUMMARY AND RECOMMENDATIONS FOR IMAGING APPROACH

On the basis of published reports and our own experiences,[10,33,35] Table 18.3 offers an overview of the value of the several staging techniques for urinary bladder carcinoma. MRI is superior to CT for staging as CT cannot differentiate between the various layers of the bladder wall and cannot, therefore, distinguish lesions invading the lamina propria from those invading the superficial and deep muscle wall. There are also difficulties in assessing tumors at the dome and trigone. The multiplanar and soft tissue characterization capabilities of MRI make it a valuable diagnostic tool among the noninvasive imaging modalities. Also, MRI is the most promising technique in the detection of nodal and bone marrow metastases. When MRI is available, CT is no longer needed. In addition, recent advances of MRI such as fast imaging, fast dynamic Gd-enhanced techniques, and the use of specific contrast for assessment of lymph nodes improve the imaging quality and diagnostic accuracy for staging urinary bladder carcinoma and detection of positive nodes. However, due to limited resources, this technique should only be used to obtain information in a preselected subset of patients, and only when imaging results directly influence management. To achieve this, both urologists' knowledge of MRI and radiologists' knowledge of clinical management are required. Therefore, continuous education and communication between these two specialties is a necessity.

## INTEGRATION OF IMAGING AND MANAGEMENT

Figure 18.9 outlines the diagnostic management of urinary bladder cancer. Detection of bladder cancer should be performed by cystoscopy. Once bladder cancer is diagnosed, the next step should be staging. For superficial tumors, clinical staging, which includes TUR, is the best technique. If, however, there is muscle invasion, further staging has to be performed with MRI. To avoid postbiopsy overstaging from edema and fibrosis, or the inconvenience of waiting 2–3 weeks after transurethral biopsy, we recommend fast dynamic imaging. Superficial tumors without muscle invasion

(Ta-T1) are treated with TURBT with or without adjuvant intravesical instillations. If cystoscopy reveals large multiple nodular or papillary tumors, an MRI examination can be helpful in providing an overview of the tumor prior to the biopsy.

Patients with muscle invasion (T2a–b) and with perivesical infiltration (stages T3a–b), or with invasion into prostate, vagina, or uterus (T4a), will be treated by radical cystectomy and extended lymphadenectomy. In cases of pelvic sidewall or abdominal wall infiltration (T4b), or metastases in lymph nodes (N3–4) or bone marrow (M+), palliative chemo- or radiotherapy will be considered. Follow-up for these therapies can be best monitored with fast dynamic MRI.[13]

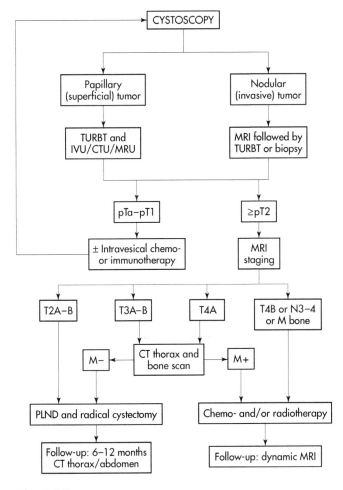

**Fig. 18.9**

The diagnostic management of urinary bladder cancer. CT, computed tomography; CTU, CT urography; IVU, intravenous urography; MRI, magnetic resonance imaging; MRU, magnetic resonance urography; PLND, pelvic lymph node dissection; TURBT, transurethral resection of bladder tumor.

## REFERENCES

1. Greenlee RT, Murray T, Bolden S, Wingo PA. Cancer statistics, 2000. CA Cancer J Clin 2000;50:7–33.

2. Lynch CF, Cohen MB. Urinary system. Cancer 1995;75(Suppl 1):316–329.

3. Jensen OM, Esteve J, Moller H, Renard H. Cancer in the European Community and its member states. Eur J Cancer 1990;26:1167–1256.

4. Heney NM. Natural history of superficial bladder cancer. Prognostic features and long-term disease course. Urol Clin North Am 1992;19:429–433.

5. Shinka T, Uekado Y, Aoshi H, Hirano A, Ohkawa T. Occurrence of uroepithelial tumors of the upper urinary tract after the initial diagnosis of bladder cancer. J Urol 1988;140:745–748.

6. Sobin LH, Wittekind Ch (eds). TNM Classification of Malignant Tumors, 6th ed. Union Internationale Contre le Cancer (UICC). Chichester: Wiley, 2002.

7. Heiken JP, Fofman HP, Brown JJ. Neoplasms of the bladder, prostate and testis. Radiol Clin North Am 1994;32:81–98.

8. Vazina A, Dugi D, Shariat SF, Evans J, Link R, Lerner SP. Stage specific lymph node metastasis mapping in radical cystectomy specimens. J Urol 2004;171:1830–1834.

9. Elkin M (ed). Tumors of urinary tract. In Radiology of the Urinary System, 1st ed. Boston: Little, Brown, 1980, pp 296–426.

10. Barentsz JO, Debruyne FMJ, Ruijs SHJ (eds). Magnetic Resonance Imaging of Carcinoma of the Urinary Bladder. Dordrecht: Kluwer, 1990.

11. Barentsz JO, Jager GJ, Mugler JP, et al. Staging urinary bladder cancer: value of T1-weighted three-dimensional magnetization prepared-rapid gradient-echo and two-dimensional spin-echo sequences. Am J Roentgenol 1995;164:109–115.

12. Jager GJ, Barentsz JO, Oosterhof GO, Witjes JA, Ruijs SHJ. Pelvic adenopathy in prostatic and urinary bladder carcinoma: MR imaging with a three-dimensional T1-weighted magnetization-prepared-rapid gradient-echo sequence. Am J Roentgenol 1996;167:1503–1507.

13. Barentsz JO, Berger-Hartog O, Witjes JA, et al. Evaluation of chemotherapy in advanced urinary bladder cancer with fast dynamic contrast-enhanced MR imaging. Radiology 1998;207:791–797.

14. Herranz-Amo F, Diez-Cordero JM, Verdu-Tartajo F, Bueno-Chomon G, Leal-Hernandez F, Bielsa-Carrillo A. Need for intravenous urography in patients with primary transitional carcinoma of the bladder? Eur Urol 1999;36:221–224.

15. Hatch TR, Barry JM. The value of excretory urography in staging bladder cancer. J Urol 1986;135:49–54.

16. Holmang S, Hedelin H, Anderstrom C, Holmberg E, Johansson SL. Long-term follow-up of a bladder carcinoma cohort: routine followup urography is not necessary. J Urol 1998;160:45–48.

17. Schulam PG, Kawsashima A, Sandler C, et al. Urinary tract imaging—basic principles. In Walsh PC, Retik AB, Vaughan E, Wein AJ (eds): Campbell's Urology, 8th ed. Philadelphia: WB Saunders, 2002, Chapter 5.

18. Johenning PW. Reactions to contrast material during retrograde pyelography. Urology 1980;16:442–444.

19. Itzchak Y, Singer D, Fischelovitch Y. Ultrasonographic assessment of bladder tumors. I. Tumor detection. J Urol 1981;126:31–33.

20. Koraitim M, Kamal B, Metwalli N, Zaky Y. Transurethral ultrasonographic assessment of bladder carcinoma: its value and limitation. J Urol 1995;154:375–378.

21. Harney JV, Barton Grossman H, Hutchins GD, Wahl RL. Positron-emission tomography with FDG in genitourinary cancer. Proceedings of the 86th Annual Meeting of the American Urological Association 1991, Abstract 253A.

22. Effert PJ, Bares R, Handt S, Wolff JM, Bull M, Jakse G. Metabolic imaging of untreated prostate cancer by positron tomography with $^{18}$fluorine-labeled deoxyglucose. J Urol 1996;155:994–998.

23. Kosuda S, Kison PV, Greenough R, Grossman HB, Wahl RL. Preliminary assessment of fluorine-18 fluorodeoxyglucose positron emission tomography in patients with bladder cancer. Eur J Nucl Med 1997;24:615–620.

24. Podo F. Tumour phospholipid metabolism. NMR Biomed 1999;12:413–439.

25. de Jong IJ, Pruim J, Elsinga PH, Vaalburg W, Mensink HJ. 11C-choline positron emission tomography for the evaluation after treatment of localized prostate cancer. Eur Urol 2003;44:32–38.

26. Stephens AW, Gonin R, Hutchins GD, Eihorn LH. Positron emission tomography of residual radiological abnormalities in postchemotherapy germ cell tumour patients. J Clin Oncol 1996;14:1637–1641.

27. Cremerius U, Effert PJ, Adam G, et al. FDG PET for detection and therapy control of metastatic germ cell tumour. J Nucl Med 1998;39:815–822.

28. Sherwood T. Bladder and urethra. In Sherwood T, Davidson AJ, Talner LB (eds): Uro-Radiology, 1st ed. Oxford: Blackwell Scientific, 1980, pp 255–312.

29. Macvicar AD. Bladder cancer staging. BJU Int 2000;86:111–121.

30. Hricak H, White S. Radiological evaluation of the urinary bladder and prostate. In Grainger RG, Allison D (eds): Grainger and Allison's Diagnostic Radiology: A Textbook of Medical Imaging, 3rd ed. New York: Churchill Livingstone, 1997, pp 1427–1438.

31. Barentsz JO, Jager GJ, Witjes JA, Ruijs SHJ. Primary staging of urinary bladder carcinoma: the role of MR imaging and a comparison with CT. Eur Radiol 1996;6:134–139.

32. Tsuda K, Narumi U, Nakamura H, et al. Staging urinary bladder cancer with dynamic MRI [abstract]. Hinyokika kiyo 2000;46:835–859.

33. Barentsz JO. Bladder cancer. In Pollack H, McClennan BL (eds): Clinical Urography, 2nd ed. Philadelphia: WB Saunders, 2000, pp 1642–1668.

34. Lipson SA, Hricak H. The urinary bladder and female urethra. In Higgins CB, Hricak H, Helms CA (eds): Magnetic Resonance Imaging of the Body, 3rd ed. New York: Lippincott-Raven, 1997, pp 875–900.

35. Barentsz JO, Witjes JA, Ruijs SJH. What's new in bladder cancer imaging? Urol Clin North Am 1997;24:583–602.

36. Takeda K, Kawaguhi T, Shiraishi T, et al. Normal bladder wall morphology in Gd-DTPA-enhanced clinical MR imaging using an endo-rectal surface coil and histological assessment of submucosal linear enhancement using Gd- DTPA auto-radiography in an animal model. Eur J Radiol 1998;26:290–296.

37. Barentsz JO. Magnetic resonance imaging of urinary bladder carcinoma. In Jafri SH, Diokno AC, Amendola MA (eds): Lower Genitourinary Radiology, Imaging and Intervention. New York: Springer-Verlag, 1998, pp 138–158.

38. Barentsz JO, Ruijs SHJ, Strijk SP. The role of MR imaging in carcinoma of the urinary bladder. Am J Roentgenol 1993;160:937–947.

39. Siegelman ES, Schnall MD. Contrast-enhanced MR imaging of the bladder and prostate. Magnetic Resonance Imaging Clin North Am 1996;4:153–169.

40. Fisher MR. Pelvis. In Runge VM (ed): Clinical Magnetic Resonance Imaging. Philadelphia: JB Lippincott, 1990, pp 385–401.

41. Farahani K, Lufkin RB. Flow motion and artifacts in MRI. In Lufkin RB (ed): The MRI Manual, Basic Principles, 2nd ed. St Louis: Mosby, 1998, pp 101–151.

42. Barentsz JO, Jager GJ, van Vierzen PB, et al. Staging urinary bladder cancer after transurethral biopsy: value of fast dynamic contrast-enhanced MR imaging. Radiology 1996;201:185–193.

43. El-Diasty T, El-Sobky E, Abou El-Ghar M, et al. Triphasic helical CT of urinary bladder carcinomas correlation with tumour angiogenesis and pathologic types [abstract]. Eur Radol 2002;12:D1–D25.

44. Nicolas V, Spielmann R, Mass R, et al. The diagnostic value of MRI tomography following gadolinium-DTPA compared to computed-tomography in bladder tumors. Fortschr Rontgenstr 1991;154:357–363.

45. Braun RD, Lanzen JL, Dewhirst NW. Fourier analysis of fluctuations of oxygen tension and blood flow in R3230Ac tumors and muscle of rats. Am J Physiol 1999;277:551–568.

46. Dovark HF, Nagy JA, Feng D, et al. Vascular permeability factor/vascular endothelial growth factor and the significance of micro-vascular hyper-permeability in angiogenesis. Curr Top Microbiol Immunol 1999;237:97–132.

47. Dewhirst M. Angiogenesis and blood flow in solid tumors. In Teicher B (ed): Drug Resistance in Oncology. New York: Marcel Dekker, 1993, pp 3–24.

48. Neeman M, Provenzale JP, Dewhirst MW. MRI application in evaluation of tumor angiogenesis. Semin Radiol Oncol 2001;11:70–82.

49. Narumi Y, Kadota T, Inoue E, et al. Bladder tumors: staging with gadolinium-enhanced oblique MR imaging. Radiology 1993;187:145–150.

50. Woolf N (ed). Urinary bladder. In Pathology, Basic and System. Philadelphia: WB Saunders, 1998, pp 713–717.

51. Ross MH, Romrell LJ, Kaye GI. Urinary system. In: Histology: A Text and Atlas, 3rd ed. Philadelphia: William & Wikins, 1995, pp 582–583.

52. Fawcett DW, Jensh RP. Histology of the urinary system. In: Concise Histology. London: Chapman & Hall International/Thomson Publishing, 1998, pp 240–251.

53. Saito W, Amanuma M, Tanaka J, et al. Histopathological analysis of bladder cancer stalk observed on MRI [abstract]. MRI 2000;18:411.

54. Narumi Y, Tsuda K, Takahashi S, et al. Staging of bladder cancer: review of 160 cases [abstract]. Radiology 1996;201.

55. Richards D, Jones S. The bladder and prostate. In Sutton D (ed): Textbook of Radiology and Imaging, 6th ed. London: Churchill Livingstone, 1998, pp 1167–1187.

56. Husband JE. Review of staging bladder cancer. Clin Radiol 1992;46:153–159.

57. Yaman O, Baltaci S, Arikan N, Yilmaz E, Gogus O. Staging with computed tomography, transrectal ultrasonography and transurethral resection of bladder tumour: comparison with final pathological stage in invasive bladder carcinoma. Br J Urol 1996;78:197–200.

58. Paik ML, Scolieri MJ, Brown SL, Spirnak JP, Resnick MI. Limitations of computerized tomography in staging invasive bladder cancer before radical cystectomy. J Urol 2000;163:1693–1696.

59. Wolf JS, Cher M, dalla 'Era M, Presti JC, Hricak H. The use and accuracy of cross-sectional imaging and fine needle aspiration cytology for detection of pelvic lymph node metastases before radical prostatectomy. J Urol 1995;153:993–999.

60. Barentsz JO. MR intervention in the pelvis: an overview and first experiences in MR-guided biopsy in nodal metastases in urinary bladder cancer. Abdom Imaging 1997;22:524–530.

61. Pieterman RM, Van Putten JWG, Meuzelaar JJ, et al. Preoperative staging of non-small-cell lung cancer with positron-emission tomography. N Engl J Med 2000;343:254–261.

62. Bachor R, Kotzerke J, Reske SN, Hautmann R. Lymph node staging of bladder neck carcinoma with positron emission tomography. Urologe 1999;38:46–50.

63. Heicappell R, Muller Mattheis V, Reinhardt M, et al. Staging of pelvic lymph nodes in neoplasms of the bladder and prostate by positron emission tomography with 2-[18F]-2-deoxy-D-glucose. Eur Urol 1999;36:582–587.

64. Manyak MJ, Hinkle GH, Olsen JO, et al. Immunoscintigraphy with indium-111-capromab penetide: evaluation before definitive therapy in patients with prostate cancer. Urology 1999;54:1058–1063.

65. Hinkle GH, Burgers JK, Neal CE, et al. Multicenter radioimmunoscintigraphic evaluation of patients with prostate carcinoma using indium-111 capromab pendetide. Cancer 1998;83:739–747.

66. Vassallo P, Matei C, Heston WDW, et al. AMI-227-enhanced MR lymphography: usefulness for differentiating reactive from tumor bearing lymph nodes. Radiology 1994;193:501–506.

67. Choe KA, Smith RC, Rosenfeld AT. Acute flank pain: comparison of non-contrast-enhanced CT and intravenous urography. Radiology 1995;194:789–794.

68. Freed KS, Sheafor DH, Hertzberg BS. Nonenhanced helical CT and US in the emergency evaluation of patients with renal colic: prospective comparison. Radiology 2000;217:792–797.

69. Street L, Warshauer DM, McCarthy SM. Detection of renal masses: sensitivities and specificities of excretory urography/linear tomography, US and CT. Radiology 1988;169:363–365.

70. Caoili EM, Cohan RH, Korobkin M, et al. Urinary tract abnormalities: initial experience with multi-detector row CT urography. Radiology 2002;222:353–360.

71. Liu W, Esler SJ, Kenny BJ, et al. Low-dose nonenhanced helical CT of renal colic: assessment of ureteric stone detection and measurement of effective dose equivalent. Radiology 2000;215:51–55.

72. Atasoy C, Yagci C, Fitoz S, et al. Cross-sectional imaging in ureter tumors: findings and staging. Clin Imaging 2001;25:197–202.

73. Song JH, Francis IR, Platt JF, et al. Bladder tumor extension at virtual cystoscopy. Radiology 2001;218:95–100.

74. Kim JK, Park SY, Ahn HJ, Kim CS, Cho KS. Bladder cancer: analysis of multi-detector row helical CT enhancement pattern and accuracy in tumor detection and perivesical staging. Radiology 2004;231:725–731.

75. Weissleder R, Elizondo G, Wittenberg J, et al. Ultrasmall paramagnetic iron oxide: an intravenous contrast agent for assessing lymph nodes with MR imaging. Radiology 1990;175:494–498.

76. Gerlowski LE, Jain RK. Microvascular permeability of normal and neoplastic tissues. Microvasc Res 1986;31:288–305.

77. Bellin MF, Roy C, Kinkel K, et al. Lymph node metastases: safety and effectiveness of MRI with ultrasmall superparamagnetic iron oxide particles. Initial clinical experience. Radiology 1998;207:799–808.

78. Chambon C, Clement O, Le Blanche A, Schouman-Claeys, Frija G. Superparamagnetic iron oxides as positive MR contrast agents : in vitro and in vivo evidence. J Magn Res Imaging 1993;11:509–519.

79. Guimares R, Clement O, Bittoun J, Carnot F, Frija G. MR Lymphography with super paramagnetic nanoparticles in rats: pathologic basis for contrast enhancement. Am J Roentgenol 1994;162:201–207.

80. Harisinghani MG, Saini S, Slater GJ, Schnall MD, Rifkin MD. MR imaging of pelvic lymph nodes in primary pelvic carcinoma with ultrasmall superparamagnetic iron oxide (Combidex): preliminary observations. J Magn Res Imaging 1997;7:161–163.

81. Harisinghani MG, Barentsz J (co-first-authors), Hahn PF, et al. Noninvasive detection of clinically occult lymph-node metastases in prostate cancer. N Engl J Med 2003;348:2491–2499.

82. Anzai Y, Prince MR. Iron oxide-enhanced MR lymphography: the evaluation of cervical lymph node metastases in head and neck cancer. J Magn Res Imaging 1997;7:75–81.

83. Kerstine KH, Stanford W, Mullan BF, et al. PET, CT, and MRI with Combidex for mediastinal staging in non-small lung carcinoma. Ann Thorac Surg 1999;68:1022–1028.

84. Hoffman HT, Quets J, Toshiaki T, et al. Functional magnetic resonance imaging using iron oxide particles in characterizing head and neck adenopathy. Laryngoscope 2000;110:1425–1430.

85. Nguyen BC, Stanford W, Thompson BH, et al. Multicenter clinical trial of ultrasmall superparamagnetic iron oxide in the evaluation of mediastinal lymph nodes in patients with primary lung cancer. J Magn Res Imaging 1999;10:468–473.

86. Pannu HK, Wang KP, Borman TL, Bluemke DA. MR imaging of mediastinal lymph nodes: evaluation using superparamagnetic contrast agent. J Magn Res Imaging 2000;12:899–904.

87. Deserno WMLLG, Harisinghani MG, Taupitz M, et al. Urinary bladder cancer: preoperative nodal staging with Ferumoxtran-10-enhanced MR imaging. Radiology 2004;233(2):449456.

88. Herr HW. Extent of surgery and pathology evaluation has an impact on bladder cancer outcomes after radical cystectomy. Urology 2003;61:105–108.

89. Narumi Y, Kumatani T, Sawai Y, et al. The bladder and bladder tumors: imaging with three-dimensional display of helical CT data. Am J Roentgenol 1996;167:1134–1135.

90. Vining DJ, Zagoria RJ, Liu K, Stelts D. CT cystoscopy. An innovation in bladder imaging. Am J Roentgenol 1996;166:409–410.

91. Fenlon HM, Bell TV, Ahari HK, Hussain S. Virtual cystoscopy, early clinical experience. Radiology 1997;205:272–275.

92. Bernhardt TM, Schmidl H, Philipp C, Allhoff EP, Rapp-Bernhadt U. Diagnostic potential of virtual cystoscopy of the bladder: MRI vs CT. Preliminary report. Eur Radiol 2003;13:305–312.

# Cytology and DNA ploidy

19

*Ralph W DeVere White, Arline D Deitch*

## INTRODUCTION

Bladder cancer, the fifth most prevalent cancer worldwide, is a major healthcare problem. Transitional cell carcinoma (TCC) is the most common form of bladder cancer. At the time of presentation, three-fourths of patients with TCC have superficial, stage Ta or T1 disease. The first clinical problem encountered is that half of these patients will experience recurrent disease following resection of their tumors. In order to detect these recurrences as early as possible, such patients are subjected to regular cystoscopic examination. It is evident that both patients and the healthcare system would benefit if the number of repetitive cystoscopic examinations could be reduced. Both cytology and flow cytometric evaluation of DNA ploidy have been evaluated for this role.

Tumors that are multifocal, grade 3, and are accompanied by carcinoma in situ (CIS) will recur in 90% of patients. Therefore, the real issue for these patients is not recurrence, but progression, since progression in this situation results in the death of the patient from TCC in 50% to 78% of cases.[1] Tumor detection after progression is too late. Would either of the tests under consideration predict progression? Much has been made of the fact that Ta cancer in patients with tumors seldom progress (6%), whereas in those with T1 disease progression may occur in as many as 45%. However, most stage Ta TCCs are grade 1–2, whereas most T1 tumors are grade 3. In reality, therefore, progression is much more grade- than stage-dependent. Moreover, observer variability is a less important factor in assigning tumor grade than in assigning tumor stage.

We thus need to evaluate cytology and DNA ploidy as methods both for detecting disease recurrence and for predicting disease progression. In both cases tumor grade will be known from earlier resections. Therefore, for the tests to be routinely employed in a cost-effective manner, they would have to either replace or, at the very least, reduce the need for cystoscopic examinations. While reducing cystoscopic examinations is laudable in terms of reducing the cost of healthcare, it would be the ability of such tests to predict progression that would ultimately save patients' lives.

## CYTOLOGY

The use of cytology for monitoring bladder cancer was discussed in a chapter published by the authors in 2000.[2] Dr Wijkström, one of the world's experts in urinary cytology, was the lead author of that chapter. It is fair to state, as noted in that chapter, that he was far more enthusiastic about the use of cytology than we were. Views of one of the authors of that chapter (RdVW) on the use of cytology was the subject of an editorial comment in the *Journal of Urology* in 2002.[3] This paper noted that three markers—NMP22, BTA stat, and UBC—performed better than urinary or bladder washing cytology during surveillance of bladder cancer patients. Nevertheless, none of these markers was as sensitive as surveillance cystoscopy, missing 45% to 60% of the tumors detected by cystoscopy.[4] While the chapter by Wijkström and the present authors refers to many excellent articles, including an article from the WHO consensus conference of 1998[5] supporting the use of cytology for monitoring bladder cancer patients, we will explain our more limited use of urine cytology.

Urinary cytology has been used since 1856 when Lamb described it as a way of detecting cancer cells.[6] Use of urinary cytology received a huge boost in 1945 when Papanicolaou and Marshall described criteria for interpreting the presence of TCC in voided urine. Nevertheless, the routine use of urinary cytology is still questioned, and we will explore the reasons why.

We might first ask why urinary cytology has gained such popular acceptance. This is easily answered by noting that in 1945 cystoscopy was not what it is today, and, moreover, there was no other way of detecting TCC of the bladder. These circumstances no longer hold true. Flexible office cystoscopy is now much easier for all concerned. There are now also many point-of-care diagnostic tests available. These uniformly require no instrumentation. As point-of-care tests are reviewed in Chapter 20, we will confine ourselves here to general remarks.

It is always pointed out that cytology is the gold standard by which the new diagnostic tests are measured. While this is true, one might ask why this is the case: a pragmatic answer is that the companies presenting these tests know that they can easily beat the gold standard and, therefore, readily gain Food and Drug Administration (FDA) approval. We include data from our chapter with Dr Wijkström to underscore this point (Table 19.1).[7-14] Indeed, if cytology were a new test measured against these markers, we might wonder whether it would receive FDA approval. If cytology were being used to detect all grades of TCC, we believe that the answer would be no.

Seventy-five percent of all cases of TCC are stage Ta or T1 at presentation. Of these, 75% are grade 1 or grade 2. Cytology does not fare well in detecting these cases. These tumors are hard to detect in voided urine because low-grade TCC cells are more adherent than higher grade cells and are therefore are less likely to be shed.[15,16] For the cells that are shed, the cellular characteristics closely resemble those of normal transitional cells, adding further to recognition and diagnostic problems. For these reasons, cytology is a poor test for routine screening of bladder cancer patients.

Cytology clearly is useful in patients who have grade 3 TCC or CIS. However, these are relatively rare tumors. In the Southwest Oncology Group (SWOG) study of 223 high-risk patients, only 17% had grade 3 tumors (see below). In our opinion such numbers do not justify the routine use of screening cytology, either to make diagnoses or to detect recurrences.

In patients who are being followed and are known from previous pathologic studies to have grade 3 disease, it would be reasonable to use cytology because of its high detection rate and specificity. However, in these high-risk patients, we would never substitute cytology for cystoscopy because, even for this group of patients, the sensitivity of cytology is too low. Again, as shown in Table 19.1, detection of grade 3 tumors may range from 38% to 92%.[7-14]

There are also situations in which urinary cytology is positive and cystoscopy negative. Under these circumstances, random bladder biopsies, upper tract washings, and prostatic urethra and prostate biopsies need to be obtained to determine the source of the positive cells. There are also certain other situations in which urinary cytology can be very helpful, for example when a male patient presents with symptoms suggestive of CIS. Another instance would be when patients undergo resection of grade 3 T1 tumors, followed by urinary cytology performed 2 weeks later to check for presence of any unresected tumor. With studies showing that one-third of such cases will still harbor TCC, this is a reasonable use of urinary cytology. However, in most such cases, patients will be receiving intravesical therapy. Under these circumstances, cytology will not be helpful.

Cytology has been used for over 140 years. Clearly, if it is to remain a widely used clinical test, it will have to be improved. One such improvement would be the use of fluorescent markers that help to identify TCC cells.[17,18] This not only improves diagnosis but may also allow use of these cells for subsequent diagnostic studies.

**Table 19.1** Reported diagnostic accuracy of cytology (percentage malignant specimens) in histologically confirmed TCC bladder tumors with regards to grade

| Lead author | Grade 1 (%) | Grade 2 (%) | Grade 3 (%) | Grade 4 (%) |
|---|---|---|---|---|
| Esposti[7] | 3 | 68 | 89* | |
| Kern[8] | 29 | 42 | 70† | |
| Maier[9] | 29 | 77 | 92 | |
| Farrow[10] | 22 | 62 | 84 | 83 |
| Sarosdy[11] | 8 | 18 | 38 | |
| Wiener[12] | 17 | 61 | 90 | |
| Van der Poel[13] | 29 | 30 | 75 | |
| Leyh[14] | 4 | 20 | 69 | |

\* Grade 3 + 4.

† Grade 3 + 4 including 65 carcinoma in situ tumors.

## DNA PLOIDY

The authors have had extensive experience in DNA ploidy analysis as performed by flow cytometry (FCM) and, with others, have shown excellent detection of TCC by FCM. However, in most cases the sources of cells were bladder washings. This has clearly proved unacceptable as a standard clinical tool. Another issue is whether the ploidy analysis of TCC tumors predicts future tumor progression. As noted earlier, Ta and T1 tumors that progress result in a death rate from TCC of approximately 50%. Clearly, the ability to predict progression before it occurs would be extremely beneficial.

In following the pioneering work of Drs Tribukait and Vindelov, among others, we first reported in 1998 on the ability of FCM to predict progression in patients with Ta disease who had been followed without any intravesical therapy for 10 years.[19] Based on this work, SWOG undertook a FCM analysis of Ta and T1 tumors obtained from patients who were believed to be at high risk for recurrence. These patients were registered in a SWOG study comparing intravesical bacillus Calmette–Guérin (BCG) versus mitomycin C. While DNA ploidy (diploid versus nondiploid) was predictive of disease progression, this feature was not additive to information from tumor grade.[20] We, therefore, repeated the analysis, this time dividing the 223 tumors into diploid, tetraploid, and aneuploid. Each of these categories was then divided on the basis of whether they had high or low S-phase fractions. Of the 223 patients, 121 experienced recurrence and 29 experienced progression of disease. Of these 29 patients, 14 died of TCC.

While most diploid tumors were low grade and most aneuploid tumors were high grade, interestingly, in the case of the tetraploid tumors, they tended to be grade 2 although most grade 2 tumors were in fact not tetraploid. This strongly suggests that tumor grade and DNA ploidy do contain different prognostic information.[21] However, considering the small number of events available at the time of that report, ploidy was not additive to grade in determining outcome.

In the case of S-phase analysis, that feature did give prognostic information beyond that of tumor grade. The risk ratio for grade was 4.3 while for S-phase it was 1.9. Tribukait had published similar findings in 1993. His report had been a follow-up of patients for over 10 years at a time before the routine use of intravesical therapy. The SWOG paper[21] showed that S-phase was predictive of outcome even in the face of intravesical therapy.

In the last 3–4 years, single marker analysis has been replaced by high-throughput analysis, tissue arrays, and microarrays. It is unlikely that DNA ploidy will find a place in this new situation. However, S-phase analysis can be readily performed as part of tissue array studies, and may well be helpful in identifying those cancers that will progress. This was the conclusion reached by Popov et al, who used MIB1 to quantify S-phase.[22]

## CONCLUSION

We believe that conventional urinary cytology has only a limited role in the management of patients having TCC, such as those with a history of high-grade disease. DNA ploidy analysis by FCM is probably an investigation of the past while S-phase analysis utilizing immunohistochemical techniques might be profitably incorporated into marker studies. It should help predict patient outcome, giving information beyond that of tumor grade alone.

REFERENCES

1. deVere White RW, Deitch AD, Daneshmand S, et al. The prognostic significance of S-phase analysis in stage Ta/T1 bladder cancer. Eur Urol 2000;37:595–600.
2. Wijkström H, Baker WC, Deitch AD, deVere White RW. Urinary cytology and its role in diagnosis and monitoring of urothelial carcinoma. In Droller MJ (ed): Bladder Cancer: Current Diagnosis and Treatment. Totowa, NJ: Humana Press, 2001, pp 105–132.
3. deVere White RW. Editorial comment. J Urol 2002;167(1):83.
4. Boman H, Hedelin H, Holmang S. Four bladder tumor markers have a disappointingly low sensitivity of small size and low grade recurrence. J Urol 2002;167(1):80–83.
5. Epstein JI, Amin MB, Reuter VR, Mostofi FK. The Bladder Consensus Conference Committee. The World Health Organization/International Society of Urological Pathology consensus classification of urothelial (transitional cell) neoplasms of the urinary bladder. Am J Surg Pathol 1998;22:1435–1448.
6. Koss LG. The cellular and acellular components of the urinary sediment. In Koss LG (ed): Diagnostic Cytology of the Urinary Tract with Histopathologic and Clinical Correlations. Philadelphia: Lippincott-Raven, 1996, p 28.
7. Esposti P-L, Zajiek J. Grading of transitional cell neoplasms of the urinary bladder from smears of bladder washings. A critical review of 326 tumors. Acta Cytol 1972;16:529–537.
8. Kern W. The diagnostic accuracy of sputum and urine cytology. Acta Cytol 1988;32:651–654.
9. Maier U, Simak R, Neuhold N. The clinical value of urinary cytology: 12 years of experience with 615 patients. J Clin Pathol 1995;48:314–317.
10. Farrow GM. Urine cytology of transitional cell carcinoma. In Wied GL, Marluce B, Keeble CM, Koss LG, Patten SF, Rosenthal DL (eds): Compendium on Diagnostic Cytology, 8th ed. Chicago: Tutorials of Cytology, 1997, p 280.
11. Sarosdy MF, Hudson MA, Ellis WJ, et al. Improved detection of recurrent bladder cancer using the bard BTA stat test. Urology 1997;50:349–353.
12. Wiener HG, Mian C, Haitel A, Pycha A, Schatzl G, Marberger M. Can urine bound diagnostic tests replace cystoscopy in the management of bladder cancer? J Urol 1988;159:1876–1880.
13. Van der Poel HG, Van Balken MR, Schamhart DHJ, et al. Bladder wash cytology, quantitative cytology, and qualitative BTA test in patients with superficial bladder cancer. Urology 1998;51:44–50.
14. Leyh H, Marberger M, Conort P, et al. Comparison of the BTA stat test with voided urine cytology and bladder wash cytology in the diagnosis and monitoring of bladder cancer. Eur Urol 1999;35:52–56.
15. Ross JS, del Rosario AD, Figge HL, Sheehan C, Fisher HA., Bui HX. E-cadherin expression in papillary transitional cell carcinoma of the urinary bladder. Hum Pathol 1995;26:940–944.

16. Imao T, Koshida K, Endo Y, Uchibayashi T, Sasaki T, Namiki M. Dominant role of E-cadherin expression in the progression of bladder cancer. J Urol 1999;161:692–698.

17. Tauber S, Schneede P, Liedl B, Liesmann F, Zaak D, Hofstetter A. Fluorescence cytology of the urinary bladder. Urology 2003;61:1067–1071.

18. Pfister C, Chautard D, Devonec M, et al. Immunocyt test improves the diagnostic accuracy of urinary cytology: results of a French multicenter study. J Urol 2003;169:921–924.

19. de Vere White RW, Stapp E. Predicting prognosis in patients with superficial bladder cancer. Oncology 1998;12(12):1717–1723.

20. de Vere White RW, Deitch AD, Tesluk H, et al. Prognostic significance of DNA ploidy in Ta/T1 bladder cancer: a Southwest Oncology Group study. Urol Oncol 1996;2:27–34.

21. de Vere White RW, Deitch AD, Daneshmand S, et al. The prognostic significance of S-phase analysis in stage Ta/T1 bladder cancer: a Southwest Oncology Group Study. Eur Urol 2000;37:595–600.

22. Popov Z, Gil-Diez-de-Medina S, Ravery V, et al. Prognostic value of EGF receptor and tumor cell proliferation in bladder cancer: therapeutic implications. Urol Oncol 2004;22:93–101.

# Voided urine markers 20

*Vinata B Lokeshwar, Robert H Getzenberg*

## INTRODUCTION

The management of bladder cancer patients is challenging because bladder tumors frequently recur and show heterogeneity in their ability to invade and metastasize. Tumor markers with early detection capabilities, recurrence monitoring abilities, and prognostic capabilities should help in detecting bladder tumors before they become muscle invasive (stage ≥T2), improve patients' quality of life by reducing the number of surveillance cystoscopies, individualize treatment regimens, and cut medical cost. The impetus for finding a reliable non-invasive bladder cancer test lies in the current mode of bladder cancer diagnosis. Although cystoscopy is an office procedure, performed under local anesthesia, it is invasive and relatively expensive (Medicare reimbursement cost: $200–300).[1] In fact, because of the life-long need for cystoscopic monitoring for recurrence as well as treatment of recurrent tumors, the cost per bladder cancer patient from diagnosis to death is the highest among all cancer patients: $96,000–187,000 per patient in the United States.[2] In addition to being costly, cystoscopy may also be inconclusive at times. For example, in patients with an indwelling catheter or active inflammation, cystoscopy may not be definitive because of the grossly abnormal appearance of bladder mucosa.[3] Since bladder cancer patients are subjected to cystoscopy every 3–6 months to monitor for recurrence, the procedure also affects patients' quality of life. Therefore, an accurate non-invasive marker/test for bladder cancer diagnosis and surveillance is desirable.

The standard non-invasive test for detecting/ monitoring bladder cancer is voided urine cytology. It is a highly tumor-specific marker with specificity reaching as high as 100%.[3,4] It also has good sensitivity to detect high-grade tumors, particularly carcinoma in situ. However, it has low sensitivity for detection of low-grade tumors, it is not available worldwide, its inferences are subjective, and it is relatively expensive (average cost $50–100).[1,4]

## PHASES OF MARKER DEVELOPMENT[5]

To begin a discussion of tumor markers for bladder cancer, it is important to define terminology. As there is a general lack of consensus regarding biomarker terminology in this field, clinicians and scientists do not have a common vocabulary with which to discuss the development and use of tumor markers in the care of bladder cancer patients. One method for defining markers is to use the phase of development as a benchmark for describing functional characteristics and readiness for clinical deployment.

### PHASE I

Phase I describes preclinical or exploratory studies. This is typically the first analysis that will be performed on the biomarkers and often involves comparison of tumor tissue with normal adjacent tissue and/or normal controls. It is important to utilize normal adjacent tissue for comparisons and also to include truly normal individuals as controls for these studies. In fact, the earliest biomarkers for bladder cancer may be identified based on the approach of comparing normal adjacent tissue from individuals with bladder cancer to the normal tissue found in an individual that does not have the disease. Additionally, many of these studies are done with the use of cell model systems. Finally, many investigators are now examining markers directly in body fluids as a way to diagnose cancer and consider them a signature of the disease. The use of proteomic approaches has facilitated this analysis. This approach has revealed not only novel markers but also patterns of changes that can be used to diagnose cancer. There are therefore a number of ways in which initial markers can be identified and then developed in this preliminary phase. As described, the tests at this stage are often protein based, including immunohistochemical, immunoblotting, and other techniques. Alternatively, nucleic acid-based approaches can be used.

Considering the relative incidence of bladder cancer and the associated mortality, a large number of markers have been identified and evaluated. Part of this relates to the fact that many bodily fluids are accessible for analyzing bladder markers, including urine, serum, and cytologic cells, as well as biopsy samples.

## Urine and cytologic cells

Urine provides the most unique environment in which to study tumor markers. The urine is an environment to which very few organs are exposed, and identifying markers in the urine often leads to higher specificity than those found in serum samples. The urine is also a harsh environment for many proteins, and proteins that are able to survive in this environment allow for the subtraction of many proteases and other kinds of degratory enzymes which often make it difficult to develop assays for markers. While this environment is unfriendly for many proteins, it does provide stability to those that are able to survive in it and, therefore, provides an opportunity to focus on this unique set of proteins.

In addition, exfoliated cells are also often located within the urine and are the basis for cytologic examination and cell-based assays. These cells represent unique looks into the bladder in a non-invasive fashion. Many markers are currently being developed to better examine these cells to determine if they are indeed cancerous.

## Serum

Serum is an environment that has not been extensively explored for bladder cancer, mainly because urine has provided an environment in which it is easier to study unique changes that may be associated with the bladder. Some markers are being identified in the serum of individuals with bladder cancer, but these typically are markers of advanced disease or disease that has spread outside of the bladder.

With this fertile environment for development, a number of tumor markers have been analyzed for this first phase. Unfortunately, many markers are not developed beyond this phase into clinical assays.

## PHASE II

The second phase is development of a clinical test for bladder cancer. This is the step in which the biomarker typically moves from the individual research laboratory to a more clinically related laboratory that has more expertise with clinical assays. The primary goal of this phase of development is to determine important characteristics of the assay. The first is referred to as the sensitivity or the true positive rate. This is the indication related to, for example, the number of bladder cancer cases that the assay is able to detect. If it is able to detect 100% of the cases, then the sensitivity or the true positive rate is 100%. In addition to the true positive rate, the false-positive rate—the specificity of the assay— is also analyzed; in other words, the number of individuals without bladder cancer that are being judged positive on the basis of the individual marker. Finally, if the assay allows, a receiver operating characteristic (ROC) curve for the marker should be performed. These curves allow for identification of both the sensitivity and specificity of the assay.

## PHASES III–V

The third phase of the development is described as a retrospective longitudinal repository study. These are much larger studies done on samples from individuals that may have been collected for other analyses. The ultimate goal here is to see whether the marker being developed can indeed identify an individual with the disease prior to clinical diagnosis as well as to obtain as much data as possible about the characteristics of the marker prior to proceeding with the fourth phase of development, which is a prospective validation study. The fifth (final) phase comprises cancer control studies in which large population-based investigations are performed.

As this chapter will show, there are many markers for bladder cancer that are in various phases of development. Because of many of its properties, as described above, bladder cancer has drawn the attention of a number of leading scientists that have focused on this disease as a template for development of biomarkers. There are now a number of exciting markers that are at different stages of development and moving toward clinical use.

# USES OF BLADDER TUMOR MARKERS

## SCREENING AND/OR DIAGNOSIS

Early detection of bladder tumors using a non-invasive diagnostic test offers the advantage of detecting cancer before it invades the muscle. Such early detection would result in decreased morbidity that is associated with metastasis and improve survival. However, the prevalence of bladder cancer in the general population is low (0.001%; NCI SEER Database 2000; http://seer.cancer.gov). In two studies, Messing et al reported that the prevalence of bladder cancer among asymptomatic men above the age of 50 is about 1.3%.[6,7] Since high-grade tumors account for approximately 20% to 30% of bladder tumors, screening the entire population with the aim of diagnosing high-grade bladder cancer in a few patients is not cost effective. In addition, false-positive results will cause unnecessary anxiety and require expensive and invasive work-up.

Bladder cancer screening may be useful in a population of individuals that are at risk for bladder cancer. Cigarette smoking, occupational exposure to aromatic amines, parasitic infections (e.g. *Schistosoma haematobium*), etc. have been shown to increase the risk for bladder cancer.[8–14] In Western Europe, metal workers, machinists, transport equipment operators, and mine workers are among the major occupations contributing to occupational bladder cancer (4.2–7.4% risk).[15] The risk for bladder cancer is even higher when smoking is combined with other known bladder carcinogens (e.g. >80 μg arsenic per day in drinking water of smokers) or genetic polymorphism.[16] For example, polymorphisms in N-acetyltransferase-2 (NAT2, slow acetylator phenotype), glutathione S-transferase (GSTM1, null phenotype), and manganese superoxide dismutase increase the risk for developing bladder cancer among smokers.[17,18] The mean time for the development of bladder cancer following exposure to bladder carcinogens is about 18 years (range 9 to >20 years).[19] Therefore, early detection of bladder cancer prior to the occurrence of muscle-invasive disease may be possible if a single marker or a panel of bladder tumor markers is used for screening the high-risk population.

Hemstreet et al employed a panel of bladder tumor markers to screen Chinese workers that were exposed to benzidine. In that study, the biomarker profile placed only 21% of the exposed workers in a moderate- to high-risk group. However, 87% of the bladder cancer cases in the entire cohort were found in this group and all of the tumors were clinically organ confined.[20] This study suggests that screening a high-risk population using biomarkers may offer early detection advantage. If such early diagnosis translates into detection of tumors prior to progression, clinicians may be able to manage bladder cancer patients with bladder preservation treatments and prolong the time to cystectomy. Lotan and Roehrborn have suggested that use of bladder tumor markers, together with cystoscopy, could improve prognosis and reduce medical cost, due to fewer individuals needing cystectomy because of an early detection advantage.[1]

Parekattil et al have developed a neural network, using combined urine levels of nuclear matrix protein-22, monocyte chemoattractant protein-1, and urinary intercellular adhesion molecule-1 to identify patients with bladder cancer. This algorithm has 100% sensitivity and 75% specificity to identify patients that will require cystoscopy, patients that have bladder cancer, and those patients with muscle-invasive disease. Interestingly, they suggest that screening of potential bladder cancer patients with this neural network may save 41% of the cost of the conventional bladder cancer diagnosis.[21]

## BLADDER TUMOR MARKERS AND SURVEILLANCE

The management of bladder cancer patients is challenging since bladder tumors frequently recur and often progress to a higher stage. For example, 30% to 80% of bladder tumors recur within 3 years after the treatment of the initial tumor.[22] A simple, non-invasive, highly sensitive and specific method for detecting bladder cancer would decrease the morbidity associated with cystoscopy, improve patients' quality of life, and decrease medical costs, since most non-invasive methods are cheaper than cystoscopy. However, more important than the issues of cost and quality of life are the accuracy and reliability of a marker. Vriesema et al reported that patients are reluctant to replace cystoscopy with a marker/test if it misses >10% of tumor recurrence.[23] Thus, if a marker is to be used for monitoring recurrence, it should have high sensitivity and reasonable specificity in order to detect every single case of tumor recurrence. However, it is noteworthy that several current bladder tumor markers show <90% sensitivity.[3,4] In fact, even the widely used prostate cancer marker PSA shows sensitivity well below 90%.[24]

One way to increase the sensitivity of bladder tumor markers, and to use a panel of bladder tumor markers instead of a single marker, is to use the marker in conjunction with cytology/cystoscopy. Since different bladder tumor markers/tests detect different molecules (e.g. microsatellite DNA analysis detects chromosomal abnormality, the NMP22 test detects a nuclear matrix protein in urine), the likelihood of both tests missing the same patient would be lower than that of each individual marker. For example, Mattioli et al found that combining the inferences of the BTA-TRAK and urine cytology increased the sensitivity of detecting bladder tumor recurrence to 91%.[25] In another study, Hautmann et al showed that although the individual sensitivities of the HA-HAase and ImmunoCyt tests (see below) were 83.3% and 63.3% sensitivity, respectively, the combination had 93.3% sensitivity to detect bladder cancer.[133] However, this increase in sensitivity for the panel of markers may result in decreased specificity, because each marker in the panel will have its own set of false-positive results.

Nonetheless, if the goal of bladder cancer surveillance using biomarkers is to detect each and every episode of recurrence, the panel's high sensitivity may compensate for some decrease in specificity. It should also be noted that tumor markers could be more sensitive than cystoscopy in detecting bladder cancer recurrence since they are capable of detecting even one single bladder tumor cell or measuring different bladder tumor-associated molecules at nano- or picomolar range. In several studies, tumor markers were found to detect recurrence before the tumor could be detected by cystoscopy.[26-28] Overall, monitoring tumor recurrence may be the most economically feasible and clinically useful role for bladder markers.

## TUMOR MARKERS AND PROGNOSIS

Understanding of some of the molecular pathways of bladder cancer development has revealed that superficial papillary, high-grade superficial, and high-grade/high-stage tumors arise from different biochemical and genetic pathways, each requiring distinct clinical management.[19,29] Tumor markers that can distinguish the invasive potential of individual bladder tumors of the same histologic grade and stage, predict the frequency of recurrence for individual tumors, and evaluate treatment response will help in making treatment selections that are suited for each patient's need. Several histologic markers such as p53, Ki67, and mitotic index have been examined for their ability to predict both patients' prognosis and treatment response. For example, Ki67 plus p53 predicts stage progression in Ta/T1 tumors.[30] Higher p53 expression in bladder tumors has been shown to correlate with tumor progression after cystectomy and to indicate high probability of bladder cancer-related death.[31,32] High expression of Ki67 correlates with high risk of recurrence, and high cyclin D1 expression correlates with longer disease-free survival.[33] p53 expression and p53 gene mutations have been well studied for predicting the response of bladder cancer patients to bacillus Calmette–Guérin (BCG) treatment. However, they do not seem to have any independent prognostic value.[34] In addition to histologic markers, newer technologies such as cDNA microarrays and proteomics are increasing our understanding of the molecular pathways that regulate bladder cancer progression and recurrence. Newer markers based on these state-of-the-art technologies may become available to help clinicians in individualizing treatment selections for bladder cancer patients.

## IDEAL TUMOR MARKER

An ideal tumor marker should be assayed in a technically simple and rapid fashion, have low intra-

and interassay variability, and, most importantly, have high accuracy. It is relatively easy to design a bladder cancer test, since many 'molecular determinants' of bladder tumor growth and invasion are released into urine when it comes in contact with the tumor during storage in the bladder. Thus, many bladder cancer tests such as BTA-Stat/TRAK, UBC-Rapid, UBC-IRMA, BLCA-4, HA-HAase, NMP22, and survivin detect soluble markers released in urine. Conversely, UroVysion (multicolor fluorescence in situ hybridization), ImmunoCyt, microsatellite DNA analysis, telomerase, DD23, etc. require the presence of exfoliated tumor cells in voided urine specimens or in bladder wash specimens.

Tests such as the BTA-Stat, NMP22 point-of-care test, and UBC-Rapid can be performed in the urologist's office. Other tests, such as fluorescent in situ hybridization (FISH) and ImmunoCyt, require microscopy and image analysis. Telomerase and microsatellite DNA analysis require polymerase chain reaction (PCR), and tests such as the BLCA-4, BTA-TRAK, HA-HAase, and NMP22 are enzyme-linked immunosorbent assays (ELISA). Performing ELISAs, PCR analysis, and fluorescent microscopy/image analysis requires specialized equipment, and urine specimens therefore have to be shipped to a central laboratory for analysis.[4]

The accuracy of a marker is critical to gaining acceptability among patients and urologists. This is because a false-negative result could lead to disease progression, whereas a false-positive result would cause unnecessary anxiety and expensive work-up. To evaluate a marker's efficacy, $2 \times 2$ analysis or contingency table analysis is performed. The $2 \times 2$ analysis allows the determination of parameters such as sensitivity, specificity, and accuracy. When a marker's accuracy is evaluated, each individual in the study population is placed in one of the four cells in the contingency table.

- True positive (TP) individuals have the tumor and test positive.
- False-negative (FN) individuals have the tumor but have negative test results.
- False-positive (FP) individuals do not have the tumor but are positive on the test.
- True negative (TN) individuals do not have the tumor and are negative on the test.

Sensitivity of a marker/test is defined as the percentage of patients with the disease (e.g. bladder cancer) for whom the test is positive.[4,35] It is calculated from the contingency table as:

$$(TP \div (TP + FN)) \times 100$$

The false-negative rate is defined as the percentage of patients with the disease in whom the test is negative. It is calculated as:

$$(FN \div (TP + FN)) \times 100$$

For an ideal tumor marker/test, the sensitivity and the false-negative rate should approach 100% and 0%, respectively.

The specificity of a marker/test is defined as the percentage of individuals without the disease in whom the test is negative.[35,153] Specificity is calculated from the contingency table as:

$$(TN \div (TN + FP)) \times 100$$

The false-positive rate of a marker/test is defined as the percentage of individuals without the disease in whom the test is positive. The false-positive rate is calculated as:

$$(FP \div (TN + FP)) \times 100$$

For an ideal tumor marker/test, the specificity and false-positive rate should approach 100% and 0%, respectively.

The accuracy of a tumor marker/test is the function of both sensitivity and specificity. It is expressed as a percentage and calculated as:

$$((TP + TN) \div \text{total number of study individuals}) \times 100$$

Since both sensitivity and specificity are valid only for the population in which the marker is tested, accuracy of a marker is also dependent on the study population and the cut-off limit used for calculating the sensitivity and specificity of the marker.

The two parameters that are calculated from the contingency table are positive predictive value (PPV) and negative predictive value (NPV) of a marker, and these values are dependent upon the prevalence of the disease in the population. PPV is defined as the percentage of test-positive individuals that have bladder cancer.[4,35] PPV is calculated as:

$$(TP \div (TP + FP)) \times 100$$

NPV is defined as the percentage of test-negative individuals that do not have bladder cancer.[4,35] NPV is calculated as:

$$(TN \div (TN + FN)) \times 100$$

Since PPV and NPV are dependent on the prevalence of the disease in the population, these values can be either low or high in different study populations, even if a marker/test has the same sensitivity and specificity in those different populations.

## BIOMARKERS AND EARLY DETECTION DILEMMA

Biochemical tests such as NMP22, BLCA-4, HA-HAase, and UBC-Rapid have the capability to detect bladder cancer in the nano- or picomolar range. Similarly,

microscopy (e.g. ImmunoCyt, UroVysion tests) or molecular biology techniques (e.g. telomerase, microsatellite DNA analysis) are capable of detecting a single abnormal cell in urine. Thus, in the absence of clinical evidence of bladder cancer, a positive biomarker test will pose a dilemma for the physician, whether to impose treatment to halt the progression of a tumor that is clinically undetectable or to simply watch and wait, considering the test result as false positive.

The significance of false-positive results in predicting the occurrence/recurrence of a bladder tumor within a specified time can be evaluated by calculating the risk ratio (RR) and the odds ratio (OR). In addition, an accurate knowledge of genitourinary conditions that cause a false-positive result on the test, measuring the quantitative changes in the levels of a marker rather than simply noting its presence or absence, repeat testing, improving the clinical means of confirming malignancy, and testing the marker in large community settings will help clinicians in deciding the best course of action.

Overall, the acceptance of a bladder tumor marker/test will not only depend on its accuracy but will also depend on the willingness of physicians and patients to accept its usefulness.

## BIOMARKERS IN CLINICAL USE TODAY

### HEMATURIA DETECTION

The most common symptom among individuals with urinary tract malignancy is hematuria. Approximately 85% of bladder cancer patients have either grossly visible or microscopic hematuria. The grade of hematuria (gross or microscopic) is independent of tumor grade and stage.[36,37] However, the incidence of bladder cancer and other urologic malignancies among individuals with microhematuria is low (<10%). For example, Messing et al reported about 1.3% bladder cancer prevalence among men above the age 50 years that have asymptomatic microhematuria.[38–40] In a study by Britton et al, the prevalence of bladder cancer in a population of men over 60 years was reported as 0.7%.[41] The prevalence of bladder cancer or other urologic cancers among patients with hematuria is low because hematuria is a symptomatic manifestation in several benign urologic conditions (e.g. inflammation, urinary tract infection, benign prostatic hyperplasia, stones, etc.). The Best Practice Policy Panel on asymptomatic microscopic hematuria, sponsored by the American Urological Association, recommends that finding three or more red blood cells per high-power microscopic field in urinary sediment from two or three properly collected urinalysis specimens constitutes hematuria.[42]

Over-the-counter hemoglobin dipstick (Hemastix) is the most common and inexpensive test ($0.61 per test) available for detecting hematuria. The test can be performed in a physician's office or at home. A sample is recorded as positive when any amount of hemoglobin (i.e. trace, small, moderate or large) is detected. Some studies have reported that hematuria detection has high sensitivity for diagnosing bladder cancer (90–95%). However, some recent studies have reported significantly lower sensitivity for hemoglobin dipstick (46–52%).[71,43,44] To improve the sensitivity and specificity of hematuria test for bladder cancer detection, other tests such as a chemiluminescence hemoglobin detection assay, red cell morphology determination using interference-contrast microscopy, and red cell volume distribution tests are being conducted in many laboratories.[1,44–48]

Overall, hematuria screening should, in theory, have high sensitivity for detecting bladder cancer and other urologic malignancies. However, it has low specificity because of the low prevalence of urologic malignancies among hematuria patients. Newer techniques to improve the specificity of hematuria as a marker for urologic malignancies will be needed to improve its use as a screening marker for bladder and other urologic malignancies.

## BTA-STAT/BTA-TRAK

The BTA (bladder tumor antigen)-Stat and BTA-TRAK tests detect a complement factor, H-related protein, in urine. While BTA-Stat is a point-of-care qualitative test, the BTA-TRAK is a quantitative ELISA.

### BTA-Stat

The BTA-Stat is an immunoassay performed by placing five drops of urine in the sample well of the test device and allowing it to react for exactly 5 minutes. A visible red line in the test window indicates a positive result, whereas a line in the control window indicates that the test is working correctly.

The sensitivity of the BTA-Stat test reported in several studies ranges from as low as 9.3% to as high as 89%.[26,28,43,45,49–58] The sensitivity of the BTA-Stat to detect low-grade tumors is low, ranging between 13% and 55%; for high-grade tumors, it ranges between 63% and 90%. The specificity of the BTA-Stat among healthy individuals is high (>90%). However, it has low specificity (about 50%) among patients with urinary tract infections, urinary calculi, 90% positive results on BTA-Stat,[59] nephritis, renal stones, cystitis, benign prostatic hyperplasia, hematuria and 2+ to 3+ protein on urine dipstick.[28,60–62] The BTA-Stat has lower specificity among patients with any one of the several benign genitourinary conditions because the test detects both a complement factor H-related protein and complement factor H (BTA-Stat product insert). Since complement factor H is present in human serum at high concentrations (0.5 mg/cc), conditions that cause hematuria can potentially cause a false-positive result on

this test. Indeed, Oge et al showed that if urine is spiked with blood, the specificity of the BTA-Stat varies depending upon the severity of hematuria: 80% for microscopic hematuria and 24% for gross hematuria.[62] Therefore, the BTA-Stat product insert includes a list of benign conditions, which, if present, preclude use of the test.

Some studies have explored the usefulness of the BTA-Stat as a prognostic marker. Raitanen et al reported that bladder cancer patients with positive BTA-Stat have shorter disease-free survival.[63] However, the same group in another study reported that while 16% of the false-positive cases on the BTA-Stat had a recurrence, the majority of the false-positive cases were due to intravesical therapy or infection.[53,54] Other studies have shown that false-positive BTA-Stat does not predict disease recurrence.[26,28,64, 65]

## BTA-TRAK

BTA-TRAK is a standard ELISA that quantitatively measures the amounts of a complement factor H-related protein and complement factor H in urine (BTA-TRAK product insert). The list price of the BTA-TRAK test is $650 per microtiter test. In various studies, the sensitivity of BTA-TRAK ranges between 52% and 83%.[25,66–69] However, in a recent study that followed the recommendations of the European Group on tumor markers, the sensitivity of the BTA-TRAK was 8% to 17% to detect both primary tumors and recurrence.[70] As in the case of BTA-Stat, the sensitivity of the BTA-TRAK is higher for detecting high-grade/high-stage tumors.[1,69,71,72] The sensitivity of the BTA-TRAK also varies depending upon the cut-off limit used on the test.[69,71–73]

Among patients with benign conditions, the specificity of the BTA-TRAK is low, about 50%. For example, levels of bladder tumor antigen >72 mU/ml are often obtained among patients with hematuria.[67] The reason for this is that the BTA-TRAK test also detects complement factor H, which is abundant in blood. Considering this possibility, the manufacturer recommends that BTA-TRAK should be used only with information available for the clinical evaluation of the patient and other diagnostic procedures, and that the test should not be used as a screening test (BTA-TRAK product insert).

According to BTA product inserts, the Food and Drug Administration (FDA) has approved both BTA-Stat and BTA-TRAK tests for use as an aid in the management of bladder cancer in combination with cystoscopy.

## NMP22

The original NMP22 test is a sandwich ELISA that uses two monoclonal antibodies which detect a nuclear mitotic apparatus protein, NMP22 (NMP22 product insert). NMP22 is distributed during mitosis.[74,75] In tumor cells, NMP22 levels are elevated and the protein is released in urine, most likely following apoptosis. A single NMP22 kit costs $967.50 and a urine stabilizer kit costs $108. Urologists need to ship urine specimens to reference laboratories for testing. The manufacturer recommends a 10 U/ml cut-off limit on the test to make a diagnosis of bladder cancer. However, different studies have used different cut-off limits (3.6–12 U/ml). In these studies, the sensitivity of NMP22 varied from 18.2% to 100%.[1,44,50,51,63–65,70,77–79] It is expected that lowering the cut-off limit on the NMP22 will increase its sensitivity but decrease the specificity. The sensitivity of NMP22 also varies depending on tumor size, grade, and stage.[45] For example, Miyanaga et al reported 18.6% sensitivity for NMP22 to detect recurrent tumors, which are smaller than the primary tumors, and recommended using 5 U/ml as the cut-off limit when testing for bladder cancer recurrence.[50] Boman et al reported similar observations.[45] They found that the NMP22 has 65% sensitivity to detect primary tumors and 45% sensitivity to detect recurrent tumors.[45] The sensitivity of the NMP22 to detect grade 1 tumors varies between 35% and 82%, and for grade 2 and 3 tumors between 41% to 90% and 63% to 100%, respectively.[1,51,64,73,77,80] The NMP22 also has lower sensitivity to detect low-stage Ta tumors (range 42–76%) than it has to detect muscle-invasive tumors (range 50–98%).[1] Eissa et al reported higher sensitivity for NMP22 to detect bilharzial tumors than to detect nonbilharzial tumors.[76] In addition, some reports have suggested that NMP22 may also predict bladder tumor recurrence.[64,65]

The specificity of NMP22 ranges between 60% and 80% in various studies. The NMP22 test has higher false-positive rates (33–50%) among patients with urolithiasis, inflammation, benign prostatic hyperplasia, and urinary tract infection.[77,81–83] Ponsky et al found six categories of benign urologic conditions that increase urinary NMP22 levels well above 10 U/ml, the cut-off limit suggested by the manufacturer.[84] A possible reason why NMP22 is false positive among patients with inflammatory conditions and/or hematuria is that the presence of leukocytes affects the performance of this test.[50] In addition, Atsu et al reported that the presence of both red blood cells and leukocytes affects NMP22 levels in urine. Furthermore, the effect of leukocytes on urinary NMP22 levels is more than that of red blood cells.[85] Recently, a point-of-care NMP22 assay has become available, which involves the addition of four drops of urine in a point-of-care device and reading the results 30–50 minutes later.[86] At the present time, few studies have been conducted on this point-of-care test. However, in a recent large prospective multicenter study that involved 1331 study individuals, the point-of-care NMP22 test had 55.7% sensitivity and 85.7% specificity to detect bladder cancer. As is the case with NMP22 ELISA, the sensitivity of the point-of-care test also increased with tumor grade and stage.[86] This

study is limited, based upon its study design, and therefore the actual clinical utility of this marker has yet to be defined.

Overall, a consensus among researchers regarding the cut-off limit on the NMP22 is necessary so that the usefulness of this test to detect both primary and recurrent tumors can be established. The knowledge of benign conditions that are present at the time of performing NMP22 will improve the specificity of this test. The FDA has cleared the NMP22 test for use as an aid in the diagnosis of patients at risk for, or with symptoms of, bladder cancer, and for use in conjunction with cystoscopy.

## SURVIVIN

Survivin is a member of the inhibitor of apoptosis gene family.[87,88] It is almost undetectable in normal tissues, but it is elevated in human cancers.[89] The survivin test is a bio-dot test in which urine samples are blotted as dots on nitrocellulose membranes, and survivin present in the samples is detected using a rabbit polyclonal antisurvivin antibody and standard dot-blot detection reagents. In initial studies with relatively small numbers of bladder cancer patients, the survivin dot-blot assay had 100% sensitivity.[89,90] Its specificity among normal individuals and patients with benign genitourinary conditions is 100% and 87%, respectively.[88,89] Recently, Shariat et al showed that higher urinary survivin levels are associated with increased risk of bladder cancer and higher-grade tumors.[91] In that study, which involved 117 bladder cancer patients and 97 controls, the survivin dot-blot assay had 64% sensitivity and 93% specificity. More studies on this marker will establish its utility in the diagnosis of bladder cancer.

## UBC

UBC-Rapid and UBC-ELISA tests detect the presence of cytokeratin 8 and 18 in the urine of bladder cancer patients.[81,82] UBC-Rapid is a point-of-care test, whereas UBC-ELISA (i.e. UBC-IRMA) is a 2-hour sandwich ELISA test. The sensitivity of UBC tests to detect bladder cancer varies between 36% and 79%.[43,45,76,81,82,92–94] The sensitivity of UBC tests also depends on tumor size, grade, and stage.[44] The sensitivity of UBC to detect grade 1, 2, and 3 bladder tumors is 13% to 60%, 42% to 79%, and 35% to 75%, respectively.[43,44,81,82,93,95] Except in two studies reported by Mian et al, UBC tests appear to have less sensitivity than several other bladder tumor markers.[43,45,76,93–96] Schroeder et al and Mungan et al also reported low sensitivity (about 20%) of UBC to detect superficial bladder cancer.[43,95] The specificity of the UBC test varies between 65% and 75%.[43,45,76,81,82,93–96]

Other cytokeratins—such as cytokeratin 20 for detection by reverse transcriptase PCR (RT-PCR) and immunocytology, and cytokeratin 19 fragment

(CYFRA21) for detection by immunoradiometric or electrochemiluminescent immunoassays—have also been studied as bladder tumor markers. However, only a limited number of studies have been conducted on these markers.[92,97–100]

## TELOMERASE

Telomeres are repetitive sequences (e.g. TTAGGG in humans) that cap the 5′ ends of eukaryotic chromosomes. In eukaryotes, the DNA polymerase cannot replicate the 5′ end of the chromosome, and, as a result, there is a gradual loss of about 200 bases during each round of DNA replication. The loss of telomeric repeats during each DNA replication protects the crucial genetic information from being lost. When all of the telomeres are lost, crucial genetic information begins to decrease during successive DNA replications. This results in chromosomal instability, which in turn causes cellular senescence.[101,102] Telomerase is a ribonucleo-protein complex containing an RNA template and a reverse transcriptase. Telomerase adds telomeres at the 5′ ends of the chromosomes, and, therefore, sets the cellular clock to immortality. Germ cells, proliferating cells (e.g. leukocytes), and tumor cells express telomerase. However, because normal somatic cells do not express telomerase, it is a sensitive marker for detecting tumors, including bladder cancer.[101–103]

The standard technique to measure telomerase activity is the telomerase repeat amplification protocol (TRAP) assay. It involves PCR amplification of a telomeric template by telomerase present in exfoliated cells in urine specimens. The PCR products are analyzed by a telomerase PCR ELISA kit or by real-time PCR. These assays need technical expertise and sophisticated instrumentation. Taking into consideration the problems associated with the stability of telomerase in urine, the hTERT RT-PCR assay has been developed. This method amplifies the human telomerase reverse transcriptase (hTERT) from exfoliated cells.

The sensitivity of the TRAP assay usually varies between 70% and 86%,[44,69,101–111] although this can be increased up to 95% if voided urine specimens are combined with bladder wash specimens.[106,111] However, in some studies, the TRAP assay has shown low sensitivity (7–50%) due to the degradation of telomerase in the harsh urine environment.[101,112–115] The sensitivity of the TRAP assay to detect bladder cancer may also depend on tumor grade and stage. For example, the sensitivity to detect grade 1, 2, and 3 tumors is about 61% (range 30–85%), 82% (range 49–95%), and 93% (range 59–99%), respectively.[1,105]

The sensitivity of the hTERT RT-PCR assay varies between 75% and 95%.[116–118] However, some studies have reported very low sensitivity for hTERT in detecting bladder cancer.[117,119–121] The lower sensitivity of hTERT RT-PCR observed in some studies may be due to mRNA degradation following the lysis of exfoliated cells.

The specificity of the telomerase assay (i.e. both TRAP and hTERT RT-PCR) in various studies is often reported to be between 60% and 70% (range 60–96%).[104,116–118] Since telomerase is expressed in proliferating cells, benign conditions—such as urinary tract infections and severe inflammation—can cause a false-positive result on telomerase assay.

Overall, telomerase activity measured by the TRAP assay or detection of hTERT mRNA by RT-PCR has high sensitivity and reasonable specificity to detect bladder cancer. However, variable results may be obtained because of the stability of telomerase and hTERT mRNA, and benign conditions that increase leukocyte counts in urine.

## MULTITARGET FLUORESCENCE IN SITU HYBRIDIZATION (UROVYSION TEST)

Cytogenetic studies reveal frequent alterations in chromosomes 1, 3, 7, 8, 9, 11, 17, etc. in urothelial cancers.[122,123] For example, deletion in chromosome 9p21, i.e. the p16 gene locus, is a common early event in bladder cancer development.[17,70] Chromosomal abnormalities can be detected by fluorescent in situ hybridization (FISH). FISH assay involves binding (i.e. hybridization) of specific fluorescently labeled DNA probes to chromosome centromeres or unique loci on the chromosomes that are altered in tumor cells. This hybridization allows detection of cells under a fluorescent microscope and recording system. For detecting bladder cancer cells, the FISH assay is performed on exfoliated cells. The sensitivity of a multicolored, multiprobe (i.e. different DNA probes labeled with different fluorescent dyes) FISH assay is better than that of a single probe.

The UroVysion test is a multitarget, multicolor FISH assay that uses pericentromeric fluorescent probes for chromosomes 3, 7, and 17, and 9p21 regions (p16 locus specific). The test involves fixing of exfoliated cells from 10 to 50 ml of urine specimens and placing them in wells of 12-well slides. The cells are incubated with denatured chromosome enumeration probe (CEP) 3 (spectrum red), CEP7 (spectrum green), CEP17 (spectrum aqua), and locus specific identifier (LSI) 9p21 (spectrum gold). The slides are counterstained and observed under a fluorescent microscope (UroVysion product insert). The criteria for detecting bladder cancer include finding five or more urinary cells with gains of two or more chromosomes, or 10 or more cells with gain of a single chromosome (e.g. trisomy 7). Homozygous detection of the 9p21 locus in >20% of epithelial cells is considered a positive result.[49,124] However, currently there are no universally accepted criteria for determining the positivity of the FISH test. For example, Friedrich et al discarded specimens with <100 cells/slide, and considered a specimen as positive if 20% of the cells gained two or more chromosomes, or 40% of cells gained or lost (i.e. 9p21) one chromosome.[56] Skacel et al considered a specimen as positive if up to five cells gained one or two chromosomes (i.e. 3, 7, or 17) or ≥10% of cells had trisomy of one of chromosomes 3, 7, or 17, and/or ≥12 cells showed the loss of 9p21 locus.[27] Dalquen et al discarded samples with <25 cells, and considered a sample as positive if up to three cells showed a gain of between one and three copies of chromosomes 3, 7, and 17, and a heterozygous or homozygous loss of 9p21 locus.[125] In various studies, the sensitivity of the UroVysion assay to detect bladder cancer varies between 69% and 87%.[49,55,56,58,125,126]

The sensitivity of the UroVysion test to detect bladder cancer is influenced by tumor grade and stage. For example, although in an initial study the UroVysion test was shown to have high sensitivity to detect low-grade (83%) and low-stage (83%) tumors, recent studies report low sensitivity for this test to detect low-grade (36–57%) and low-stage (62–65%) tumors.[49,55,56,58,125,126] The test has high sensitivity to detect high-grade and high-stage tumors (83–97%) and also carcinoma in situ (about 100%).[49,55,56,58,125,126]

In some studies, the UroVysion test has been shown to predict recurrence. For example, Skacel et al reported that eight out of nine FISH-positive patients with atypical cytology but negative biopsy had biopsy-proven bladder cancer in 12 months.[27] Noting the high sensitivity of FISH to detect chromosomal abnormalities, Veeramachaneni et al concluded that a positive FISH test may indicate urothelial carcinoma or unstable urothelium that is capable of malignant transformation.[127]

Overall, the multicolored, multiprobe UroVysion assay appears to be a promising marker in detecting bladder cancer, and is useful for resolving atypical cytology. However, as yet there is no consensus among researchers regarding the criteria for the evaluation of abnormal cells, and, therefore, bladder cancer. The test may also have low sensitivity to detect low-grade and/or low-stage tumors.

## IMMUNOCYT

The ImmunoCyt test involves immunocytochemistry of exfoliated cells. Three monoclonal antibodies that are used in the ImmunoCyt assay detect three cellular markers for bladder cancer using exfoliated cells (ImmunoCyt product insert). Monoclonal antibody 19A21 labeled with Texas red detects a high molecular form of carcinoma embryonic antigen. Fluorescein-labeled monoclonal antibodies M344 and LDQ10 detect mucins (highly glycosylated cell surface proteins) that are expressed in most bladder cancer cells but not in normal cells.[128,129] The ImmunoCyt test requires urologists to add a fixative to urine specimens and then ship them to a reference cytopathology laboratory.

In an initial study involving 264 consecutive patients, Mian et al evaluated the sensitivity of ImmunoCyt either alone or with cytology.[130] The overall sensitivity of ImmunoCyt in that study was 86%, with 84% to 90% sensitivity for detecting grade 1, 2, and 3 tumors, respectively.[130] Together with cytology, ImmunoCyt had 90% sensitivity and 79% specificity for detecting bladder cancer. These results are in agreement with a recent study by Pfister et al who found that the sensitivity of ImmunoCyt to detect grade 1, 2, and 3 bladder cancer is 61%, 76%, and 77%, respectively.[131] Lodde et al, in a prospective study involving 37 patients, examined the ability of ImmunoCyt to complement voided urine cytology in detecting upper urinary tract transitional cell carcinoma (TCC).[132] In that study, cytology and ImmunoCyt alone had 50% and 75% sensitivity, respectively, whereas both methods combined had 87% sensitivity. However, Feil et al and Hautmann et al reported lower overall sensitivity (39% and 63%, respectively) for ImmunoCyt.[133,134] In some studies, ImmunoCyt is reported to have low sensitivity to detect low-grade and low-stage tumors (e.g. 14.3% in the Feil study, 50% in the Hautmann study, and 33% in the Lodde study).[132-134]

Although the specificity of ImmunoCyt is high among patients with a history of TCC and in healthy individuals, the test shows 15%, 50%, and 40% false-positive rates, respectively, among individuals with microhematuria, benign prostatic hyperplasia (BPH), and cystitis.[130,132] Consistent with these observations, Olsson and Zackrisson reported 100% sensitivity and 68.7% specificity for ImmunoCyt to detect bladder cancer.[135] The false-positive cases in this study had either hematuria or inflammation but normal cystoscopy. In contrast to these studies, Vriesema et al found only 50% sensitivity and 73% specificity for ImmunoCyt to detect bladder cancer recurrence.[136] The authors also noted high interobserver variation, which may explain why the sensitivity of ImmunoCyt varies in different studies.

Overall, the ImmunoCyt test is proposed as a useful aid to improve the sensitivity and specificity of cytology, particularly in detecting low-grade superficial tumors. However, in many studies, the test shows low sensitivity for detecting low-grade tumors. It is possible that proper handling of samples that preserves the integrity of exfoliated cells might improve the performance of this test. Furthermore, reduction in interobserver variability and a better knowledge of benign conditions that cause false-positive results on the test should improve the applicability of ImmunoCyt in bladder cancer detection and recurrence monitoring.

## MICROSATELLITE DNA ANALYSIS

Microsatellites are short highly polymorphic tandem repeats (e.g. [GTGT…]n or [CACA…]n) that are found throughout the human genome.[137] The number of repeats at any chromosome location is different in each person. In addition, the two copies of a chromosome (i.e. paternal and maternal alleles) in somatic cells of an individual will have the same microsatellite sequence, but different numbers of it, at any given locus. As a result, PCR amplification of a chromosomal region (i.e. genomic DNA) that contains a particular microsatellite will generate two PCR products, one representing the maternal and the other representing the paternal allele. In bladder cancer, the type of lesion most frequently detected is loss of heterozygosity (LOH; 74%), followed by length alteration (24%) and additional alleles (2%).[138] In bladder cancer, LOH has been demonstrated in chromosomes 4p, 8p, 9p, 9q, 11p, 13p, 16q, 17p, etc.[139–144]

In various other studies, the sensitivity of the microsatellite DNA analysis varies between 72% and 97% in detecting bladder cancer recurrence.[139–146] Schneider et al reported 79%, 82%, and 96% sensitivity for detecting grade 1, 2, and 3 bladder cancer, respectively.[145] However, in the study by van Rhijn et al, microsatellite analysis missed all 11 Ta grade 1 tumors that were small.[26] Consistent with this study, Berger et al found no DNA alterations in grade 1 tumors, but did find a correlation between microsatellite alterations and tumor grade and stage.[137]

Some studies have explored the prognostic potential of microsatellite DNA analysis. For example, van Rhijn et al reported that 55.5% of the false-positive cases, as opposed to only 12% of the true-negative cases, recurred clinically within 6 months.[26] In a study by Sengelov et al, microsatellite markers for chromosomes 1p, 8p, 10p, 13q, and 17p did not predict response to chemotherapy and outcome.[140] Hafner et al reported that microsatellite analysis found chromosome 9 deletion in 73% of the tumors tested, and deletions in chromosome 9q21 correlated with invasive tumor growth.[147] Furthermore, Uchida et al, in a study involving 45 patients, showed that patients with LOH at 18q21.1 and 9p21–p22 exhibited poor prognosis and higher death rate.[146] Taken together, microsatellite DNA analysis may have prognostic capabilities.

The specificity of the microsatellite DNA analysis in a healthy population is high at >95%. However, Christensen et al observed that patients with benign prostatic hyperplasia and cystitis show both LOH and microsatellite instability.[148] These alterations are more pronounced when both benign conditions are present at the same time. Based on these results, Christensen et al concluded that microsatellite alterations in urine are indicators not only of malignancy but also of inflammatory conditions.[148]

Overall, microsatellite DNA analysis appears to have high sensitivity for detecting bladder cancer. However, different microsatellite markers are used in different studies, making a direct comparison of the results of various studies difficult. In addition, the specificity of microsatellite DNA analysis needs to be tested in various benign urologic conditions, which also show LOH and microsatellite instability. New microsatellite markers that are specific for bladder cancer will improve the specificity of this assay. At this point it is unclear whether there might be technical issues related to sample preparation that could affect the integrity of exfoliated cells, stability of chromosomal DNA, etc. A semiautomated microsatellite analysis of urine sediments, such as that reported by Baron et al, may help to resolve some of the technical issues,[149] and a prospective study led by Dr Schoenberg at Johns Hopkins as part of the Early Detection Research Network (EDRN) is underway.

## HA-HAASE TEST

This test measures urinary levels of hyaluronic acid (HA) and hyaluronidase (HAase) using two very similar ELISA-like assays.[28,150,151] HA is a glycosaminoglycan that regulates cell adhesion, migration, and proliferation.[152,153] HA is known to promote tumor metastasis, and its concentration is elevated in several tumors including colon, esophagus, breast, prostate, and bladder.[150,153,154] Small fragments of HA are angiogenic and are generated when HAase degrades.[155] HA fragments are detected in the urine of high-grade bladder cancer patients and tumor tissues.[151,154,156,157] HYAL1 type HAase has been shown to be the major tumor-derived HAase secreted by tumor cells.[154,157,158]

The HA test is based on the competition binding principle, in which HA present in urine competes with HA coated on microtiter wells to bind to a biotinylated bovine nasal cartilage HA-binding protein. Following incubation, the unbound HA-binding protein is washed off and the HA-binding protein bound to microtiter wells is measured using an avidin-biotin detection system.[150] The HA present in each urine sample (ng/ml) is determined from a standard graph. To account for differences due to the hydration status of individuals, urinary HA levels are normalized to total urinary protein and are expressed as ng HA/mg protein. For the HA test, urinary HA levels ≥500 ng/mg (cut-off limit) constitute a positive test.[150,156]

The HAase test measures HAase activity in urine. HAase present in urine degrades HA that is coated on microtiter well plates. Following incubation, the degraded HA is washed off, and the HA remaining on the microtiter well plates is measured using the same biotinylated HA-binding protein and the avidin-biotin detection system as the HA test. Urinary HAase levels (mU/ml) are determined from a standard graph and normalized to total urinary protein (mg/ml). For the HAase test, urinary HAase levels ≥10 mU/ml constitute a positive test.[150,151,159]

In an initial study, urinary HA, measured using the HA test, was found to be elevated 2.5- to 6.5-fold in patients with bladder cancer, regardless of tumor grade.[156] HAase levels, measured using the HAase test, were preferentially elevated (three- to seven-fold) in the urine of patients with grade 2 and 3 bladder cancer.[159] In a study of 504 individuals that included 261 bladder cancer patients and 243 control individuals, the HA test had 83.1% sensitivity and 90.1% specificity in detecting bladder cancer, regardless of the tumor grade.[150] In the same study, the HAase test had 81.5% sensitivity and 83.8% specificity for detecting grade 2 and 3 bladder cancer. Combining these two tests into the HA-HAase test resulted in bladder cancer detection with higher overall sensitivity (91.9%), with 86.4%, 95.7%, and 93.3% sensitivity in detecting grade 1, 2, and 3 bladder tumors, respectively.[150] The HA-HAase test also detected both superficial (stages Ta, T1, and CIS) and invasive (stages ≥T2) tumors with 87% to 100% sensitivity, respectively. The overall specificity of the HA-HAase test in this study was 84%.[150] The control population included normal healthy individuals, patients with genitourinary conditions (e.g. stone disease, BPH, microhematuria, urinary tract infection, and cystitis), and patients with a history of bladder cancer but no evidence of disease at the time of testing. In a study involving 83 bladder tissues and 34 urine specimens, Hautmann et al demonstrated a close correlation between elevated HA and HYAL1 levels in bladder tumor tissues and a positive HA-HAase urine test. The authors concluded that, in patients with bladder cancer, tumor-associated HA and HYAL1 are secreted in urine, with the result being confirmed in a positive HA-HAase test.[160]

The ability of the HA-HAase test to monitor bladder cancer recurrence was compared with that of the BTA Stat in a study of patients with recurrent bladder cancer.[28] In this cohort, the HA-HAase and BTA-Stat had 94% and 61% sensitivity, 63% and 74% specificity, 87% and 64% accuracy, respectively. A false-positive HA HAase test carried a 10-fold risk (RR=10.2) for tumor recurrence within 5 months, whereas a false-positive BTA-Stat test did not carry any statistically significant risk for tumor recurrence within the same time frame (RR=1.4).[28] The utility of the HA-HAase and BTA-Stat tests in bladder cancer screening was evaluated among 401 Department of Energy workers with possible exposure to 4,4′-methylenedianiline (a known bladder carcinogen). In this study, HA-HAase and BTA-Stat tests had 14% and 16.7% false-positive rates, respectively.[28] Contrary to 63% of the positive cases on the BTA-Stat, only 25% of the positives on the HA-HAase test had benign urologic conditions. None of the biomarker-positive cases with clinical follow-up (n=29) had any evidence of bladder cancer at the time of testing.

The accuracy of the HA-HAase test was recently compared in two studies, side-by-side with that of cytology and biomarkers such as BTA-Stat, hematuria detection, UBC-Rapid, and ImmunoCyt. In the study by Schroeder et al, involving 138 urine specimens, the HA-HAase test, cytology, BTA-Stat, Hemastix, and UBC-Rapid had 88.1%, 70.6%, 52.5%, 50.8%, and 35.6% sensitivity, respectively.[43] The tests had 81% (HA-HAase), 81% (cytology), 76.7% (BTA-Stat), 78.2% (Hemastix), and 75% (UBC-Rapid) specificity, respectively, level 2.[43] Among various tests and cytology, the HA-HAase test had the highest sensitivity in detecting both low-grade/low-stage and high-grade/high-stage tumors. Hautmann et al, in a study of 94 consecutive patients, found that the sensitivity of the HA-HAase urine test (83.3%) was significantly higher than that of the ImmunoCyt (63%).[160] In that study, both tests had comparable specificity (HA-HAase 78.1%, ImmunoCyt 75%). The combination of both the HA-HAase and ImmunoCyt tests had 93.3% sensitivity without a significant decrease in specificity.[160]

Overall, the HA-HAase test appears to be a promising method for detecting the onset of new and recurrent bladder tumors. This test may also be useful in screening a high-risk population for bladder cancer. The accuracy of this test needs to be evaluated in larger multicenter trials.

## BLCA-4 AND BLCA-1

One approach to identifying novel tumor markers relies on trying to understand and utilize some of the hallmarks of the bladder cancer cell in order to develop assays that detect protein components specific for the disease. One of the fundamental changes that occurs in a cancer cell is alteration in both cell and nuclear shape. These alterations are used by the pathologist to identify cancer cells on microscopic examination. All cancer cells undergo these characteristic changes that are considered to be defining aspects of the tumorigenic process. Since changes in nuclear shape are characteristic of the cancer cell, studies have focused on understanding nuclear structure as an underlying framework for the observed changes in nuclear shape. In addition, it is known that a number of processes are altered within the cancer cell that could be traced back to changes within nuclear structure.

In cancer cells, it is common to find rearrangements, translocations, and other chromosomal events that are atypical for normal cells. In addition, genetic instability—in which genes that may be differentiation related may be turned off, and embryonic or other types of genes may be turned on—is commonplace in the cancer cell. The hypothesis being suggested is that changes in nuclear structure not only reflect the characteristic changes in nuclear shape observed by the pathologist in a cancer cell but also reflect changes in nuclear structure that may result in some of the loss of fidelity of these nuclear processes that are known to rely upon nuclear structure for organization and function.

Proteomic analysis of the nuclear structural components, termed the nuclear matrix, has been performed in order to determine differences in these components between cancer and normal cells. A series of nuclear structural alterations characteristic of bladder cancer have been identified, and they are not found in individuals that do not have the disease.[161] One of these markers, BLCA-4, is found throughout the bladder in both tumor and normal regions in people with bladder cancer but not found in the bladder of individuals without the disease. This marker, therefore, may reflect a type of 'field effect' that has been observed at the genetic level by a number of investigators. Recent studies have revealed that this marker appears to be a transcriptional regulator that may play an active role in the regulation of gene expression within bladder cancer.[162]

Utilizing two different forms of ELISA, BLCA-4 has been detected in the urine of patients with bladder cancer. The first assay developed was an indirect assay. Urine samples from patients diagnosed with bladder cancer, along with normal controls, were collected and tested with the indirect ELISA. This assay requires no stabilization. In the initial clinical trial of 106 individuals, using a prospectively defined cut-off based upon the first three tumor and normal samples, a sensitivity of 96.4% and a specificity of 100% were demonstrated.[161] Furthermore, this assay was able to identify almost all of the individuals that were not considered to be positive for bladder cancer by cytology.

In order to examine the expression of this and other markers in a population at high risk for the development of bladder cancer, individuals with spinal cord injuries have been followed. It is known that individuals with spinal cord injuries have an up to 460-fold increased risk for developing bladder cancer, and as many as 1 in 10 individuals with spinal cord injuries actually develop the disease.[163] In addition, this population represents a difficult group in whom to utilize bladder cancer markers since the presence of cystitis and other types of inflammation within the bladder, as well as irritation of the bladder, is common.

While the indirect assay revealed both high sensitivity and specificity, it was necessary to develop a higher throughput test that did not require urine precipitation and which used a sandwich assay taking advantage of monoclonal antibodies. This type of assay would provide for a higher throughput clinical test, while requiring neither urine precipitation nor consideration of the amount of protein found in the sample. Ideal characteristics of a tumor marker begin with possessing high sensitivity and specificity for disease, accuracy, precision, rapid turn-around time, and convenience at a low cost. In order to accomplish the rapid turn-around time, it was necessary to develop the immunoassay on straight voided urine samples rather than concentrating the proteins by ethanol precipitation. In tandem, a sandwich-based immunoassay was developed by utilizing several antibodies (both monoclonal and polyclonal) raised against BLCA-4. The advantage to this assay is that any number of different sources of antibodies can be added to the captured antigen, provided that the species in which it was produced is not the same as the capture antibody. More specifically, the enzyme-conjugated antispecies antibody should not react with the antibodies used to capture the antigen.

In order to test the constructed sandwich-based immunoassay on populations of patients that will reflect specificity and sensitivity issues for the detection of bladder cancer, a large number of samples representing unique patient groups were assayed.[164] This study included patients with biopsy-confirmed bladder cancer (Group A), individuals that have identified benign urologic conditions (Groups B and C), individuals with the most prevalent urologic cancer, prostate cancer (Group D), and normal individuals (Group E). A training set was used to establish a cut-off that was then applied to the sample set being tested. The results from the trial, which examined 168 individuals, demonstrated a sensitivity of 89% and a specificity of 100% in this complex mixture of samples.[163] A large national clinical trial is currently underway to validate these studies and determine the utility of this marker in diagnosing bladder cancer. The urine-based marker BLCA-4 appears to have exciting clinical potential.

BLCA-4 is just one of the six nuclear structural proteins identified that are expressed only in bladder cancer. Most of the proteins have now been sequenced and reagents developed for their detection. Recent data for BLCA-1 reveals that it is a potentially valuable marker for bladder cancer. The expression of BLCA-1 is different from that of BLCA-4 described above. BLCA-1 is expressed only in the tumor areas of the bladder and is not expressed in normal adjacent tissue, nor in normal bladder tissue. An immunoassay which detects BLCA-1 in straight urine samples from individuals with bladder cancer with high sensitivity and specificity has now been developed. The urine levels of this marker also appear to be increased with higher tumor stages, another distinction from BLCA-4.[165]

## MARKERS AT EARLY STAGES OF DEVELOPMENT

Several other markers have been developed and have been studied, although not as extensively as some of the others that have been identified—CD44 is one such marker. The message levels for CD44v6 were examined by RT-PCR and recently shown to impart a sensitivity of 77% and a specificity of 100%. In this same study, CD44v8–10 was examined as a prognostic factor in exfoliated cells.[166] Other potential markers include the matrix metalloproteinases and matrix metalloproteinase inhibitors as well as PAX5.[167]

While the above described markers have been focused principally on the diagnosis of bladder cancer, a couple have been identified with potential prognostic implications. p53 has been studied extensively and its ability to stain tissue samples has been shown in most of these studies, as well as its ability to predict patient outcome. Recently, serum vascular endothelial growth factor (VEGF) levels were shown to be a negative prognostic factor for bladder cancer, resulting in a sensitivity of 88% and a specificity of 98%.[168]

The ability to provide prognostic information to patients with bladder cancer would appear to be of high priority. Nevertheless, few markers currently available provide any information in this regard. It is clear that this is an area that is understudied and requires more attention.

## CONCLUSION

In this chapter, we have attempted to outline a number of the currently available and studied urine-based bladder tumor markers. They have different biologic bases and their clinical utility, in most cases, has yet to be determined. Several of these markers are extremely encouraging and may yet revolutionize the way in which we identify individuals with bladder cancer; they may also provide novel ways in which we apply treatment strategies. Most likely, individual markers will always have some limitation, and combinations of markers may be the most useful.

### REFERENCES

1. Lotan Y, Roehrborn CG. Sensitivity and specificity of commonly available bladder tumor markers versus cytology: results of a comprehensive literature review and meta-analyses. Urology 2003;61:109–118; discussion 118.
2. Botteman MF, Pashos CL, Redaelli A, Laskin B, Hauser R. The health economics of bladder cancer: a comprehensive review of the published literature. Pharmacoeconomics 2003;21:1315–1330.
3. Konety BR, Getzenberg RH. Urine based markers of urological malignancy. J Urol 2001;165:600–611.
4. Lokeshwar VB, Soloway MS. Current bladder tumor tests: does their projected utility fulfill clinical necessity? J Urol 2001;165:1067–1077.
5. Pepe MS, Etzioni R, Feng Z, et al. Phases of biomarker development for early detection of cancer. J Natl Cancer Inst 2001;93(14):1054–1061.
6. Messing EM, Young TB, Hunt VB, et al. Home screening for hematuria: results of a multiclinic study. J Urol 1992;148:289–292.
7. Messing EM, Young TB, Hunt VB, Wehbie JM, Rust P. Urinary tract cancers found by home screening with hematuria dipsticks in healthy men over 50 years of age. Cancer 1989;64:2361–2367.
8. Hodder SL, Mahmoud AA, Sorenson K, et al. Predisposition to urinary tract epithelial metaplasia in Schistosoma haematobium infection. Am J Trop Med Hyg 2000;63:133–138.
9. Zeegers MP, Kellen E, Buntinx F, van den Brandt PA. The association between smoking, beverage consumption, diet and bladder cancer: a systematic literature review. World J Urol 2004;21:392–401.
10. Talaska G. Aromatic amines and human urinary bladder cancer: exposure sources and epidemiology [review]. J Environ Sci Health Part C Environ Carcinog Ecotoxicol Rev 2003;21(1):29–43.
11. Skipper PL, Tannenbaum SR, Ross RK, Yu MC. Nonsmoking-related arylamine exposure and bladder cancer risk. Cancer Epidemiol Biomarkers Prev 2003;12:503–507.
12. Tripathi A, Folsom AR, Anderson KE. Risk factors for urinary bladder carcinoma in postmenopausal women. The Iowa Women's Health Study. Cancer 2002;95:2316–2323.
13. Pashos CL, Botteman MF, Laskin BL, Redaelli A. Bladder cancer: epidemiology, diagnosis, and management. Cancer Pract 2002;10:311–322.
14. Castelao JE, Yuan JM, Skipper PL, et al. Gender- and smoking-related bladder cancer risk. J Natl Cancer Inst 2001;93:538–545.
15. Kogevinas M, 't Mannetje A, Cordier S, et al. Occupation and bladder cancer among men in Western Europe. Cancer Causes Control 2003;14:907–914.
16. Steinmaus C, Yuan Y, Bates MN, Smith AH. Case-control study of bladder cancer and drinking water arsenic in the western United States. Am J Epidemiol 2003;158:1193–1201.
17. Giannakopoulos X, Charalabopoulos K, Baltogiannis D, et al. The role of N-acetyltransferase-2 and glutathione S-transferase on the risk and aggressiveness of bladder cancer. Anticancer Res 2002;22:3801–3804.
18. Hung RJ, Boffetta P, Brennan P, et al. Genetic polymorphisms of MPO, COMT, MnSOD, NQO1, interactions with environmental exposures and bladder cancer risk. Carcinogenesis 2004;25(6):973–978.
19. Lee R, Droller MJ. The natural history of bladder cancer. Implications for therapy. Urol Clin North Am 2000;27:1–13, vii.
20. Hemstreet GP 3rd, Yin S, Ma Z, et al. Biomarker risk assessment and bladder cancer detection in a cohort exposed to benzidine. J Natl Cancer Inst 2001;93:427–436.
21. Parekattil SJ, Fisher HA, Kogan BA. Neural network using combined urine nuclear matrix protein-22, monocyte chemoattractant protein-1 and urinary intercellular adhesion molecule-1 to detect bladder cancer. J Urol 2003;169:917–920.
22. Heney NM. Natural history of superficial bladder cancer. Prognostic features and long-term disease course. Urol Clin North Am 1992;19:429–433.
23. Vriesema JL, Poucki MH, Kiemeney LA, Witjes JA. Patient opinion of urinary tests versus flexible urethrocystoscopy in follow-up examination for superficial bladder cancer: a utility analysis. Urology 2000;56:793–797.
24. Platz EA, De Marzo AM, Giovannucci E. Prostate cancer association studies: pitfalls and solutions to cancer misclassification in the PSA era. J Cell Biochem 2004;91:553–571.
25. Mattioli S, Seregni E, Caperna L, Botti C, Savelli G, Bombardieri E. BTA-TRAK combined with urinary cytology is a reliable urinary indicator of recurrent transitional cell carcinoma (TCC) of the bladder. Int J Biol Markers 2000;15:219–225.
26. van Rhijn BW, Lurkin I, Kirkels WJ, van der Kwast TH, Zwarthoff EC. Microsatellite analysis—DNA test in urine competes with cystoscopy in follow-up of superficial bladder carcinoma: a phase II trial. Cancer 2001;92:768–775.
27. Skacel M, Fahmy M, Brainard JA, et al. Multitarget fluorescence in situ hybridization assay detects transitional cell carcinoma in the majority of patients with bladder cancer and atypical or negative urine cytology. J Urol 2003;169:2101–2105.
28. Lokeshwar VB, Schroeder GL, Selzer MG, et al. Bladder tumor markers for monitoring recurrence and screening comparison of hyaluronic acid-hyaluronidase and BTA-Stat tests. Cancer 2002;95:61–72.
29. Cordon-Cardo C, Cote RJ, Sauter G. Genetic and molecular markers of urothelial premalignancy and malignancy. Scand J Urol Nephrol Suppl 2000;205:82–93.
30. Bol MG, Baak JP, van Diermen B, et al. Proliferation markers and DNA content analysis in urinary bladder TaT1 urothelial cell carcinomas: identification of subgroups with low and high stage progression risks. J Clin Pathol 2003;56:447–452.
31. Rodriguez-Alonso A, Pita-Fernandez S, Gonzalez-Carrero J, Nogueira-March JL. p53 and ki67 expression as prognostic factors for cancer-related survival in stage T1 transitional cell bladder carcinoma. Eur Urol 2002;41:182–188; discussion 188–189.

32. Shariat SF, Tokunaga H, Zhou J, et al. p53, p21, pRB, and p16 expression predict clinical outcome in cystectomy with bladder cancer. J Clin Oncol 2004;22:1014–1024.

33. Sgambato A, Migaldi M, Faraglia B, et al. Cyclin D1 expression in papillary superficial bladder cancer: its association with other cell cycle-associated proteins, cell proliferation and clinical outcome. Int J Cancer 2002;97:671–678.

34. Saint F, Salomon L, Quintela R, et al. Do prognostic parameters of remission versus relapse after Bacillus Calmette–Guérin (BCG) immunotherapy exist? Analysis of a quarter century of literature. Eur Urol 2003;43:351–360; discussion 360–361.

35. Duncan RC, Cnapp RG, Miller MC III. Introductory Biostatistics for the Health Sciences, 2nd ed. New York: Wiley, 1983.

36. Hiatt RA, Ordonez JD. Dipstick urinalysis screening, asymptomatic microhematuria, and subsequent urological cancers in a population-based sample. Cancer Epidemiol Biomarkers Prev 1994;3:439–443.

37. Thompson IM. The evaluation of microscopic hematuria: a population-based study. J Urol 1987;138:1189–1190.

38. Messing EM, Young TB, Hunt VB, et al. Hematuria home screening: repeat testing results. J Urol 1995;154:57–61.

39. Messing EM, Young TB, Hunt VB, Wehbie JM, Rust P. Urinary tract cancers found by home screening with hematuria dipsticks in healthy men over 50 years of age. Cancer 1989;64:2361–2367.

40. Messing EM, Young TB, Hunt VB, Emoto SE, Wehbie JM. The significance of asymptomatic microhematuria in men 50 or more years old: findings of a home screening study using urinary dipsticks. J Urol 1987;137:919–922.

41. Britton JP, Dowell AC, Whelan P, Harris CM. A community study of bladder cancer screening by the detection of occult urinary bleeding. J Urol 1992;148:788–790.

42. Grossfeld GD, Wolf JS Jr, Litwan MS, et al. Asymptomatic microscopic hematuria in adults: summary of the AUA best practice policy recommendations. Am Fam Physician 2001;63:1145–1154.

43. Schroeder GL, Lorenzo-Gomez MF, Hautmann SH, et al. A side-by-side comparison of cytology and biomarkers for bladder cancer detection. J Urol 2004;172(3):1123–1126.

44. Ramakumar S, Bhuiyan J, Besse JA, et al. Comparison of screening methods in the detection of bladder cancer. J Urol 1999;161:388–394.

45. Boman H, Hedelin H, Jacobsson S, Holmang S. Newly diagnosed bladder cancer: the relationship of initial symptoms, degree of microhematuria and tumor marker status. J Urol 2002;168:1955–1959.

46. Wakui M, Shiigai T. Urinary tract cancer screening through analysis of urinary red blood cell volume distribution. Int J Urol 2000;7:248–253.

47. Schramek P, Schuster FX, Georgopoulos M, Porpaczy P, Maier M. Value of urinary erythrocyte morphology in assessment of symptomless microhaematuria. Lancet 1989;2:1316–1319.

48. Georgopoulos M, Schuster FX, Porpaczy P, Schramek P. Evaluation of asymptomatic microscopic haematuria—influence and clinical relevance of osmolality and pH on urinary erythrocyte morphology. Br J Urol 1996;78:192–196.

49. Halling KC, King W, Sokolova IA, et al. A comparison of BTA stat, hemoglobin dipstick, telomerase and Vysis UroVysion assays for the detection of urothelial carcinoma in urine. J Urol 2002;167:2001–2006.

50. Miyanaga N, Akaza H, Tsukamoto S, et al. Usefulness of urinary NMP22 to detect tumor recurrence of superficial bladder cancer after transurethral resection. Int J Clin Oncol 2003;8:369–373.

51. Gutierrez Banos JL, Rebollo Rodrigo MH, Antolin Juarez FM, Martin Garcia B. NMP22, BTA stat test and cytology in the diagnosis of bladder cancer: a comparative study. Urol Int 2001;66:185–190.

52. Walsh IK, Keane PF, Ishak LM, Flessland KA. The BTA stat test: a tumor marker for the detection of upper tract transitional cell carcinoma. Urology 2001;58:532–535.

53. Raitanen MP, Kaasinen E, Lukkarinen O, et al. Analysis of false-positive BTA STAT test results in patients followed up for bladder cancer. Urology 2001;57:680–684.

54. Raitanen MP, Marttila T, Nurmi M, et al. Human complement factor H related protein test for monitoring bladder cancer. J Urol 2001;165:374–377.

55. Toma MI, Friedrich MG, Hautmann SH, et al. Comparison of the ImmunoCyt test and urinary cytology with other urine tests in the detection and surveillance of bladder cancer. World J Urol 2004;22(2):145–149.

56. Friedrich MG, Toma MI, Hellstern A, et al. Comparison of multitarget fluorescence in situ hybridization in urine with other noninvasive tests for detecting bladder cancer. BJU Int 2003;92:911–914.

57. Glas AS, Roos D, Deutekom M, Zwinderman AH, Bossuyt PM, Kurth KH. Tumor markers in the diagnosis of primary bladder cancer. A systematic review. J Urol 2003;169:1975–1982.

58. Sarosdy MF, Schellhammer P, Bokinsky G, et al. Clinical evaluation of a multi-target fluorescent in situ hybridization assay for detection of bladder cancer. J Urol 2002;168:1950–1954.

59. Wald M, Halachmi S, Amiel G, et al. Bladder tumor antigen stat test in non-urothelial malignant urologic conditions. Isr Med Assoc J 2002;4:174–175.

60. Heicappell R, Muller M, Fimmers R, Miller K. Qualitative determination of urinary human complement factor H-related protein (hcfHrp) in patients with bladder cancer, healthy controls, and patients with benign urologic disease. Urol Int 2000;65:181–184.

61. Serretta V, Pomara G, Rizzo I, Esposito E. Urinary BTA-stat, BTA-trak and NMP22 in surveillance after TUR of recurrent superficial transitional cell carcinoma of the bladder. Eur Urol 2000;38:419–425.

62. Oge O, Kozaci D, Gemalmaz H. The BTA stat test is nonspecific for hematuria: an experimental hematuria model. J Urol 2002;167:1318–1319; discussion 1319–1320.

63. Raitanen MP, Kaasinen E, Rintala E, et al. Prognostic utility of human complement factor H related protein test (the BTA-stat test). Br J Cancer 2001;85:552–556.

64. Poulakis V, Witzsch U, De Vries R, Altmannsberger HM, Manyak MJ, Becht E. A comparison of urinary nuclear matrix protein-22 and bladder tumour antigen tests with voided urinary cytology in detecting and following bladder cancer: the prognostic value of false-positive results. BJU Int 2001;88:692–701.

65. Friedrich MG, Hellstern A, Hautmann SH, et al. Clinical use of urinary markers for the detection and prognosis of bladder carcinoma: a comparison of immunocytology with monoclonal antibodies against Lewis X and 486p3/12 with the BTA STAT and NMP22 tests. J Urol 2002;168:470–474.

66. Gibanel R, Ribal MJ, Filella X, et al. BTA TRAK urine test increases the efficacy of cytology in the diagnosis of low-grade transitional cell carcinoma of the bladder. Anticancer Res 2002;22:1157–1160.

67. Priolo G, Gontero P, Martinasso G, et al. Bladder tumor antigen assay as compared to voided urine cytology in the diagnosis of bladder cancer. Clin Chim Acta 2001;305:47–53.

68. Malkowicz SB. The application of human complement factor H-related protein (BTA TRAK) in monitoring patients with bladder cancer. Urol Clin North Am 2000;27:63–73, ix.

69. Mahnert B, Tauber S, Kriegmair M, et al. BTA-TRAK—a useful diagnostic tool in urinary bladder cancer? Anticancer Res 1999;19:2615–2619.

70. Mahnert B, Tauber S, Kriegmair M, et al. Measurements of complement factor H-related protein (BTA TRAK assay) and nuclear matrix protein (NMP22 assay)—useful diagnostic tools in the diagnosis of urinary bladder cancer? Clin Chem Lab Med 2003;41:104–110.

71. Chautard D, Daver A, Bocquillon V, et al. Comparison of the Bard Trak test with voided urine cytology in the diagnosis and follow-up of bladder tumors. Eur Urol 2000;38:686–690.

72. Thomas L, Leyh H, Marberger M, et al. Multicenter trial of the quantitative BTA TRAK assay in the detection of bladder cancer. Clin Chem 1999;45:472–477.

73. Khaled HM, Abdel-Salam I, Abdel-Gawad M, et al. Evaluation of the BTA tests for the detection of bilharzial related bladder cancer: the Cairo experience. BJU Int 2001;39:91–94.

74. Getzenberg RH, Pienta KJ, Ward WS, Coffey DS. Nuclear structure and the three dimensional organization of DNA. J Cell Biochem 1991;47:289–299.

75. Shelfo SW, Soloway MS. The role of nuclear matrix protein 22 in the detection of persistent or recurrent transitional-cell cancer of the bladder. World J Urol 1997;15:107–111.

76. Eissa S, Swellam M, Sadek M, Mourad MS, Ahmady OE, Khalifa A. Comparative evaluation of the nuclear matrix protein, fibronectin, urinary bladder cancer antigen and voided urine cytology in the detection of bladder tumors. J Urol 2002;168:465–469.

77. Lahme S, Bichler KH, Feil G, Krause S. Comparison of cytology and nuclear matrix protein 22 for the detection and follow-up of bladder cancer. Urol Int 2001;66:72–77.

78. Del Nero A, Esposito N, Curro A, et al. Evaluation of urinary level of NMP22 as a diagnostic marker for stage pTa–pT1 bladder cancer: comparison with urinary cytology and BTA test. Eur Urol 1999;35:93–97.

79. Giannopoulos A, Manousakas T, Gounari A, Constantinides C, Choremi-Papadopoulou H, Dimopoulos C. Comparative evaluation of the diagnostic performance of the BTA stat test, NMP22 and urinary bladder cancer antigen for primary and recurrent bladder tumors. J Urol 2001;166:470–475.

80. Casella R, Huber P, Blochlinger A, et al. Urinary level of nuclear matrix protein 22 in the diagnosis of bladder cancer: experience with 130 patients with biopsy confirmed tumor. J Urol 2000;164:1926–1928.

81. Sanchez-Carbayo M, Urrutia M, Gonzalez de Buitrago JM, Navajo JA. Utility of serial urinary tumor markers to individualize intervals between cystoscopies in the monitoring of patients with bladder carcinoma. Cancer 2001;92:2820–2828.

82. Sanchez-Carbayo M, Urrutia M, Silva JM, Romani R, De Buitrago JM, Navajo JA. Comparative predictive values of urinary cytology, urinary bladder cancer antigen, CYFRA 21-1 and NMP22 for evaluating symptomatic patients at risk for bladder cancer. J Urol 2001;165:1462–1467.

83. Oge O, Atsu N, Sahin A, Ozen H. Comparison of BTA stat and NMP22 tests in the detection of bladder cancer. Scand J Urol Nephrol 2000;34:349–351.

84. Ponsky LE, Sharma S, Pandrangi L, Kedia S, Nelson D, Agarwal A, Zippe CD. Screening and monitoring for bladder cancer: refining the use of NMP22. J Urol 2001;166(1):75–78.

85. Atsu N, Ekici S, Oge O, Ergen A, Hascelik G, Ozen H. False-positive results of the NMP22 test due to hematuria. J Urol 2002;167:555–558.

86. Grossman HB, Messing E, Soloway M, Tomera K, Katz G, Berger Y, Shen Y. Detection of bladder cancer using a point-of-care proteomic assay. JAMA 2005;293(7):810–816.

87. Altieri DC. Survivin, versatile modulation of cell division and apoptosis in cancer. Oncogene 2003;22:8581–8589.

88. Altieri DC. The molecular basis and potential role of survivin in cancer diagnosis and therapy. Trends Mol Med 2001;7:542–547.

89. Smith SD, Wheeler MA, Plescia J, Colberg JW, Weiss RM, Altieri DC. Urine detection of survivin and diagnosis of bladder cancer. JAMA 2001;285:324–328.

90. Sharp JD, Hausladen DA, Maher MG, Wheeler MA, Altieri DC, Weiss RM. Bladder cancer detection with urinary survivin, an inhibitor of apoptosis. Front Biosci 2002;7:E36–E41.

91. Shariat SF, Casella R, Khoddami SM, et al. Urine detection of survivin is a sensitive marker for the noninvasive diagnosis of bladder cancer. J Urol 2004;171:626–630.

92. Sanchez-Carbayo M, Herrero E, Megias J, Mira A, Soria F. Comparative sensitivity of urinary CYFRA 21-1, urinary bladder cancer antigen, tissue polypeptide antigen, tissue polypeptide antigen and NMP22 to detect bladder cancer. J Urol 1999;162:1951–1956.

93. Mian C, Lodde M, Haitel A, Vigl EE, Marberger M, Pycha A. Comparison of the monoclonal UBC-ELISA test and the NMP22 ELISA test for the detection of urothelial cell carcinoma of the bladder. Urology 2000;55:23–226.

94. Babjuk M, Kostirova M, Mudra K. Qualitative and quantitative detection of urinary human complement factor H-related protein (BTA stat and BTA TRAK) and fragments of cytokeratins 8, 18 (UBC rapid and UBC IRMA) as markers for transitional cell carcinoma of the bladder. Eur Urol 2002;41:34–39.

95. Mungan NA, Vriesema JL, Thomas CM, Kiemeney LA, Witjes JA. Urinary bladder cancer test: a new urinary tumor marker in the follow-up of superficial bladder cancer. Urology 2000;56:787–792.

96. Mian C, Lodde M, Haitel A, Egarter Vigl E, Marberger M, Pycha A. Comparison of two qualitative assays, the UBC rapid test and the BTA

97. stat test, in the diagnosis of urothelial cell carcinoma of the bladder. Urology 2000;56:228–231.

97. Nisman B, Barak V, Shapiro A, Golijanin D, Peretz T, Pode D. Evaluation of urine CYFRA 21-1 for the detection of primary and recurrent bladder carcinoma. Cancer 2002;94:2914–2922.

98. Pariente JL, Bordenave L, Jacob F. Analytical and prospective evaluation of urinary cytokeratin 19 fragment in bladder cancer. J Urol 2000;163:1116–1119.

99. Lin S, Hirschowitz SL, Williams C, Shintako P, Said J, Rao JY. Cytokeratin 20 as an immunocytochemical marker for detection of urothelial carcinoma in atypical cytology: preliminary retrospective study on archived urine slides. Cancer Detect Prev 2001;25:202–209.

100. Golijanin D, Shapiro A, Pode D. Immunostaining of cytokeratin 20 in cells from voided urine for detection of bladder cancer. J Urol 2000;164:1922–1925.

101. Liu BC, Loughlin KR. Telomerase in human bladder cancer. Urol Clin North Am 2000;27:115–123, x.

102. Muller M. Telomerase: its clinical relevance in the diagnosis of bladder cancer. Oncogene 2000;21:650–655.

103. Hiyama E, Hiyama K. Clinical utility of telomerase in cancer. Oncogene 2002;21:643–649.

104. Eissa S, Swellam M, el-Mosallamy H. Diagnostic value of urinary molecular markers in bladder cancer. Oncogene 2003;23:4347–4355.

105. Saad A, Hanbury DC, McNicholas TA, Boustead GB, Morgan S, Woodman AC. A study comparing various noninvasive methods of detecting bladder cancer in urine. BJU Int 2002;89:369–373.

106. Wu WJ, Liu LT, Huang CN, Huang CH, Chang LL. The clinical implications of telomerase activity in upper tract urothelial cancer and washings. BJU Int 2000;86:213–219.

107. Rahat MA, Lahat N, Gazawi H, et al. Telomerase activity in patients with transitional cell carcinoma: a preliminary study. Cancer 1999;85:919–924.

108. Landman J, Chang Y, Kavaler E, Droller MJ, Liu BC. Sensitivity and specificity of NMP-22, telomerase, and BTA in the detection of human bladder cancer. Urology 1998;52:398–402.

109. Kavaler E, Landman J, Chang Y, Droller MJ, Liu BC. Detecting human bladder carcinoma cells in voided urine samples by assaying for the presence of telomerase activity. Cancer 1998;82:708–714.

110. Kinoshita H, Ogawa O, Kakehi Y. Detection of telomerase activity in exfoliated cells in urine from patients with bladder cancer. J Natl Cancer Inst 1997;89:724–730.

111. Lee DH, Yang SC, Hong SJ, Chung BH, Kim IY. Telomerase: a potential marker of bladder transitional cell carcinoma in bladder washes. Clin Cancer Res 1998;4:535–538.

112. Ito H, Kyo S, Kanaya T. Detection of human telomerase reverse transcriptase messenger RNA in voided urine samples as a useful diagnostic tool for bladder cancer. Clin Cancer Res 1998;4:2807–2810.

113. Ito H, Kyo S, Kanaya T, Takakura M, Inoue M, Namiki M. Expression of human telomerase subunit correlation with telomerase activity in urothelial cancer. Clin Cancer Res 1998;4:1603–1608.

114. Muller M, Krause H, Heicappell R, Tischendorf J, Shay JW, Miller K. Comparison of human telomerase RNA and telomerase activity in urine for diagnosis of bladder cancer. Clin Cancer Res 1998;4:1949–1954.

115. Junker K, Kania K, Fiedler W, Hartmann A, Schubert J, Werner W. Molecular genetic evaluation of fluorescence diagnosis in bladder cancer. Int J Oncol 2002;20:647–653.

116. Melissourgos N, Kastrinakis NG, Davilas I, Foukas P, Farmakis A, Lykourinas M. Detection of human telomerase reverse transcriptase mRNA in urine of patients with bladder cancer: evaluation of an emerging tumor marker. Urology 2003;62:362–367.

117. Isurugi K, Suzuki Y, Tanji S, Fujioka T. Detection of the presence of catalytic subunit mRNA associated with telomerase gene in exfoliated urothelial cells from patients with bladder cancer. J Urol 2002;168:1574–1577.

118. Neves M, Ciofu C, Larousserie F. Prospective evaluation of genetic abnormalities and telomerase expression in exfoliated urinary cells for bladder cancer detection. J Urol 2002;167:1276–1281.

119. de Kok JB, Schalken JA, Aalders TW, Ruers TJ, Willems HL, Swinkels DW. Quantitative measurement of telomerase reverse transcriptase

(hTERT) mRNA in urothelial cell carcinomas. Int J Cancer, 2000;87:217–220.

120. de Kok JB, van Balken MR, Ruers TJ, Swinkels DW, Klein Gunnewiek JM. Detection of telomerase activity in urine as a tool for noninvasive detection of recurrent bladder tumors is poor and cannot be improved by timing of sampling. Clin Chem 2000;46:2014–2015.

121. de Kok JB, van Balken MR, Roelofs RW, et al. Quantification of hTERT mRNA and telomerase activity in bladder washings of patients with recurrent urothelial cell carcinomas. Clin Chem 2000;46:2003–2007.

122. Knowles MA. What we could do now: molecular pathology of bladder cancer. Mol Pathol 2001;54:215–221.

123. Cordon-Cardo C, Cote RJ, Sauter G. Genetic and molecular markers of urothelial premalignancy and malignancy. Scand J Urol Nephrol Suppl 2000;205:82–93.

124. Placer J, Espinet B, Salido M, Sole F, Gelabert-Mas A. Clinical utility of a multiprobe FISH assay in voided urine specimens for the detection of bladder cancer and its recurrences, compared with urinary cytology. Eur Urol 2002;42:547–552.

125. Dalquen P, Kleiber B, Grilli B, Herzog M, Bubendorf L, Oberholzer M. DNA image cytometry and fluorescence in situ hybridization for noninvasive detection of urothelial tumors in voided urine. Cancer 2002;96:374–379.

126. Varella-Garcia M, Akduman B, Sunpaweravong P, Di Maria MV, Crawford ED. The UroVysion fluorescence in situ hybridization assay is an effective tool for monitoring recurrence of bladder cancer. Urol Oncol 2004;22:16–19.

127. Veeramachaneni R, Nordberg ML, Shi R, Herrera GA, Turbat-Herrera EA. Evaluation of fluorescence in situ hybridization as an ancillary tool to urine cytology in diagnosing urothelial carcinoma. Diagn Cytopathol 2003;28:301–307.

128. Bergeron A, LaRue H, Fradet Y. Biochemical analysis of a bladder-cancer-associated mucin: structural features and epitope characterization. Biochem J 1997;321:889–895.

129. Bergeron A, Champetier S, LaRue H, Fradet Y. MAUB is a new mucin antigen associated with bladder cancer. J Biol Chem 1996;271:6933–6940.

130. Mian C, Pycha A, Wiener H, Haitel A, Lodde M, Marberger M. ImmunoCyt: a new tool for detecting transitional cell cancer of the urinary tract. J Urol 1999;161:1486–1489.

131. Pfister C, Chautard D, Devonec M. ImmunoCyt test improves the diagnostic accuracy of urinary cytology: results of a French multicenter study. J Urol 2003;169:921–924.

132. Lodde M, Mian C, Wiener H, Haitel A, Pycha A, Marberger M. Detection of upper urinary tract transitional cell carcinoma with ImmunoCyt: a preliminary report. Urology 2001;58:362–366.

133. Feil G, Zumbragel A, Paulgen-Nelde HJ. Accuracy of the ImmunoCyt assay in the diagnosis of transitional cell carcinoma of the urinary bladder. Anticancer Res 2003;23:963–967.

134. Hautmann SH, Toma M, Lorenzo Gomez MF, et al. ImmunoCyt and the HA-HAase urine tests for the detection of bladder cancer: a side-by-side comparison. Eur Urol 2004;46(4):466–471.

135. Olsson H, Zackrisson B. ImmunoCyt: a useful method in the follow-up protocol for patients with urinary bladder carcinoma. Scand J Urol Nephrol 2001;35:280–282.

136. Vriesema JL, Atsma F, Kiemeney LA, Peelen WP, Witjes JA, Schalken JA. Diagnostic efficacy of the ImmunoCyt test to detect superficial bladder cancer recurrence. Urology 2001;58:367–371.

137. Alberts B, Bray D, Lewis J, Raff M, Roberts K, Watson JD. Molecular Biology of the Cell, 3rd ed. New York: Garland, 1994, pp 338, 364, 365.

138. Berger AP, Parson W, Stenzl A, Steiner H, Bartsch G, Klocker H. Microsatellite alterations in human bladder cancer: detection of tumor cells in urine sediment and tumor tissue. Eur Urol 2002;41:532–539.

139. Sengelov L, Christensen M, von der Maase HD. Loss of heterozygosity at 1p, 8p, 10p, 13q, and 17p in advanced urothelial cancer and lack of relation to chemotherapy response and outcome. Cancer Genet Cytogenet 2000;123:109–113.

140. Sengelov L, Horn T, Steven K. p53 nuclear immunoreactivity as a predictor of response and outcome following chemotherapy for metastatic bladder cancer. J Cancer Res Clin Oncol 1997;23:565–570.

141. Utting M, Werner W, Dahse R, Schubert J, Junker K. Microsatellite analysis of free tumor DNA in urine, serum, and plasma of patients: a minimally invasive method for the detection of bladder cancer. Clin Cancer Res 2002;8:35–40.

142. Seripa D, Parrella P, Gallucci M. Sensitive detection of transitional cell carcinoma of the bladder by microsatellite analysis of cells exfoliated in urine. Int J Cancer 2001;95:364–369.

143. von Knobloch R, Hegele A, Brandt H, Olbert P, Heidenreich A, Hofmann R. Serum DNA and urine DNA alterations of urinary transitional cell bladder carcinoma detected by fluorescent microsatellite analysis. Int J Cancer 2001;94:67–72.

144. Zhang J, Fan Z, Gao Y. Detecting bladder cancer in the Chinese by microsatellite analysis: ethnic and etiologic considerations. J Natl Cancer Inst 2001;93:45–50.

145. Schneider A, Borgnat S, Lang H. Evaluation of microsatellite analysis in urine sediment for diagnosis of bladder cancer. Cancer Res 2000;60:4617–4622.

146. Uchida A, Tachibana M, Miyakawa A, Nakamura K, Murai M. Microsatellite analysis in multiple chromosomal regions as a prognostic indicator of primary bladder cancer. Urol Res 2000;28:297–303.

147. Hafner C, Knuechel R, Zanardo L. Evidence for oligoclonality and tumor spread by intraluminal seeding in multifocal urothelial carcinomas of the upper and lower urinary tract. Oncogene 2001;20:4910–4915.

148. Christensen M, Wolf H, Orntoft TF. Microsatellite alterations in urinary sediments from patients with cystitis and bladder cancer. Int J Cancer 2000;85:614–617.

149. Baron A, Mastroeni F, Moore PS. Detection of bladder cancer by semi-automated microsatellite analysis of urine sediment. Adv Clin Path 2000;4:19–24.

150. Lokeshwar VB, Obek C, Pham HT, et al. Urinary hyaluronic acid and hyaluronidase: markers for bladder cancer detection and evaluation of grade. J Urol 2000;163:348–356.

151. Lokeshwar VB, Block NL. HA-HAase urine test. A sensitive and specific method for detecting bladder cancer and evaluating its grade. Urol Clin North Am 2000;27:53–61.

152. Lee JY, Spicer AP. Hyaluronan: a multifunctional, megaDalton, stealth molecule. Curr Opin Cell Biol 2000;12:581–586.

153. Delpech B, Girard N, Bertrand P, Courel MN, Chauzy C, Delpech A. Hyaluronan: fundamental principles and applications in cancer. J Intern Med 1997;242:41–48.

154. Lokeshwar VB, Rubinowicz D, Schroeder GL, et al. Stromal and epithelial expression of tumor markers hyaluronic acid and HYAL1 hyaluronidase in prostate cancer. J Biol Chem 2001;276:11922–11932.

155. West DC, Kumar S. Hyaluronan and angiogenesis. Ciba Found Symp 1989;143:187–201; discussion 201–207; 281–285.

156. Lokeshwar VB, Obek C, Soloway MS, Block NL. Tumor-associated hyaluronic acid: a new sensitive and specific urine marker for bladder cancer. Cancer Res 1997;57:773–777. Erratum, Cancer Res 1998;58:3191.

157. Franzmann EJ, Schroeder GL, Goodwin WJ, Weed DT, Fisher P, Lokeshwar VB. Expression of tumor markers hyaluronic acid and hyaluronidase (HYAL1) in head and neck tumors. Int J Cancer 2003;106:438–445.

158. Lokeshwar VB, Young MJ, Goudarzi G, et al. Identification of bladder tumor-derived hyaluronidase: its similarity to HYAL1. Cancer Res 1999;59:4464–4470.

159. Pham HT, Block NL, Lokeshwar VB. Tumor-derived hyaluronidase: a diagnostic urine marker for high-grade bladder cancer. Cancer Res 1997;57:778–783. Erratum, Cancer Res 1997;57:1622.

160. Hautmann SH, Lokeshwar VB, Schroeder GL, et al. Elevated tissue expression of hyaluronic acid and hyaluronidase validates the HA-HAase urine test for bladder cancer. J Urol 2001;165:2068–2074.

161. Konety BR, Nguyen T-ST, Dhir R, et al. Detection of bladder cancer using a novel nuclear matrix protein, BLCA-4. Clinical Cancer Res 2000;6:2618–2625.

162. Van Le T-ST, Myers J, Konety BR, et al. Fundamental characterization of the bladder cancer marker, BLCA-4. Clinical Cancer Res 2004;10(4):1384–1391.

163. Konety BR, Nguyen T-ST, Brenes G, et al. Evaluation of the effect of spinal cord injury (SCI) on serum PSA levels. Urology 2000;56:82–86.

164. Van Le T-ST, Miller R, Barder T, Babjuk M, Potter DM, Getzenberg RH. A highly specific urine-based marker of bladder cancer. Urology 2005;(in press)

165. Myers JM, Landsittel D, Getzenberg RH. Use of novel marker, BLCA-1, for the detection of bladder cancer. J Urol 2005;174(1):64–68.

166. Miyake H, Eto H, Arakawa S, et al. Over expression of CD44V8-10 in urinary exfoliated cells as an independent prognostic predictor in patients with urothelial cancer. J Urol 2002;167(3):1282–1287.

167. Adshead JM, Ogden CW, Penny MA, et al. The expression of PAX5 in human transitional cell carcinoma of the bladder: relationship with de-differentiation. BJU Int 1999;83:1039–1044.

168. Bernardini S, Fauconnet S, Chabannes E, et al. Serum levels of vascular endothelial growth factor as a prognostic factor in bladder cancer. J Urol 2001;166(4):1275–1279.

# Staging 21

*Atreya Dash, David P Wood Jr*

## INTRODUCTION

Grade and stage are the most important factors in deciding treatment and outcome for patients with urothelial carcinoma. Low-grade tumors are rarely invasive but tend to recur; high-grade tumors have a proclivity towards invasion. Once a tumor has demonstrated invasion, stage becomes the determining factor in treatment. This observation was made early[1] and was used to develop a staging system. Subsequently it has undergone modifications and now combines the benefits of systems developed by the American Joint Commission and the International Union Against Cancer which currently reflect subtleties within substages.[2–4]

Staging itself is divided into clinical and pathologic staging. The clinical stage is determined by subjective criteria including the findings at transurethral resection (TUR), physical examination, and imaging studies. Pathologic staging is objective, but requires the evaluation of entire bladder and lymph nodes to completely assign a pathologic stage. The need for accuracy of clinical staging cannot be overemphasized for counseling patients about treatment options and prognosis. Growing interest in neoadjuvant therapies and bladder preservation for invasive urothelial carcinoma increases the importance of defining clinical stage in order to identify patients that are most suitable before they are exposed to potentially toxic treatments and in order to follow the response.[5,6] Because neoadjuvant treatments have largely been performed in clinical trials, accurate and uniform clinical staging protocols will allow for appropriate enrollment of patients and better interpretation of outcomes.

All patients suspected of having a bladder cancer require a physical examination, cystoscopy to inspect the bladder, and an imaging study such as excretory intravenous urography (IVU) to evaluate upper tracts. If a bladder tumor is confirmed by cystoscopy, the cystoscopic appearance is an unreliable predictor of depth of invasion.[7,8] A bimanual examination detects muscle-invasive or extravesical disease, and IVU usually is not helpful in diagnosing bladder lesions but may detect concurrent upper tract lesions.[9] Additional findings such as hydronephrosis may have implications regarding prognosis as will be discussed, or provide anatomic information that may affect management. Retrograde urography better images the upper tracts than IVU. It can be performed at the time of TUR, and be useful in cases of obstruction where IVU poorly visualized the upper tracts. In the future, computed tomographic (CT) urography may comprehensively evaluate the upper tracts and stage the bladder simultaneously.[10]

## TRANSURETHRAL RESECTION

The mainstay for providing tissue for diagnosis and staging and possible treatment is the transurethral resection (TUR) of tumors. To obtain staging information from a TUR or biopsy, the urologist must provide adequate tissue, including specimens from multiple resection depths including muscle.[11] Cold-cup resection, of smaller lesions especially, better preserves morphology.[12]

To ensure transmission of relevant information, the College of American Pathologists recommend that clinical history, pertinent cystoscopic or radiographic findings, clinical diagnosis, procedure, and site of specimen information be conveyed.[13] The utility of performing biopsies of adjacent normal-appearing epithelium is controversial,[14-16] but it is worthwhile to biopsy erythematous patches to rule out carcinoma in situ (CIS),[17] or if partial cystectomy is contemplated for treatment.[9,18]

The bimanual examination under anesthesia (EUA) performed just before or after TUR, while the patient is anesthetized, is mandatory.[19] It possibly provides easily obtained additional information.[20,21]

clinical staging are whether the tumor penetrates the lamina propria and the deeper muscularis propria, and, if so, whether it is organ confined. The EUA findings of bladder wall thickening, a mobile mass, or a fixed mass correlate with clinical T3a, T3b, or T4b disease, respectively.[2,21] If the tumor extends beyond the lamina propria, more extensive radiographic studies for staging are warranted.[9] It is essential for the pathologist to provide a standardized and complete pathologic report of the radical cystectomy findings to convey information that could influence further therapy.[22]

## TNM CLASSIFICATION SYSTEM

The tumor–node–metastasis (TNM) classification system currently provides the basis for bladder cancer staging (Table 21.1).[2] Complete pathologic staging is dependent on having bladder and lymph node specimens from a radical cystectomy and pelvic lymphadenectomy, whereas clinical staging relies on multiple and subjective factors to assign clinical stage. As outlined in the 2002 American Joint Committee on Cancer Staging manual, this involves histologic confirmation of tumor by biopsy or transurethral resection biopsy, bimanual examination, and imaging studies.[2] The crucial distinctions that need be made in

## IMAGING AND INVESTIGATIVE TECHNIQUES

Ultrasound, computed tomography (CT), and magnetic resonance imaging (MRI) are the three primary imaging modalities that have been investigated to stage bladder cancer. Although imaging technology has steadily been improving, there are few reports within the last decade contributing to the literature of image-based bladder cancer staging. Furthermore, post-TUR imaging studies may demonstrate postsurgical changes that resemble cancer. These studies are crucially important to diagnose extent of disease. Differences in disease-specific and

**Table 21.1** AJCC 2002 tumor–node–metastasis (TNM) staging system[2]

| Tumor | Stage | Description |
| --- | --- | --- |
| Primary tumor (T) | TX | Primary cannot be assessed |
| | T0 | No evidence of primary tumor |
| | Ta | Non-invasive papillary tumor |
| | Tis | Carcinoma in situ |
| | T1 | Tumor invades subepithelial connective tissue |
| | T2 | Tumor invades muscle |
| | pT2a | Tumor invades superficial muscle (inner half) |
| | pT2b | Tumor invades deep muscle (outer half) |
| | T3 | Tumor invades perivesical tissue |
| | pT3a | Tumor invades perivesical tissue microscopically |
| | pT3b | Tumor invades perivesical tissue macroscopically (extravesical mass) |
| | T4 | Tumor invades any of the following: prostate, uterus, vagina, pelvic wall, abdominal wall |
| | pT4a | Tumor invades prostate, uterus, vagina |
| | pT4b | Tumor invades pelvic wall, abdominal wall |
| Regional lymph nodes (N) | NX | Regional lymph nodes cannot be assessed |
| | N0 | No regional lymph node metastases |
| | N1 | Metastasis in a single lymph node, ≤2 cm in greatest dimension |
| | N2 | Metastasis in a single lymph node, >2 cm but not >5 cm in greatest dimension; or multiple lymph nodes, none >5 cm in greatest dimension |
| | N3 | Metastasis in a lymph node, >5 cm in greatest dimension |
| Distant metastasis (M) | MX | Distant metastasis cannot be assessed |
| | M0 | No distant metastases |
| | M1 | Distant metastasis |

overall survival are markedly worse once muscle-invasive urothelial cancer is no longer organ confined.[23-25] However, discrepancies persist in clinically staging organ confinement that must rely on a combination of physical and radiographic examinations.[26] The overall sensitivity, specificity, and accuracy of the imaging modalities for evaluating invasive disease compared with the histology, usually from cystectomy, from the largest contemporary series are compared in Table 21.2.[27-33]

## TRANSURETHRAL ULTRASOUND

Transurethral ultrasound (TUUS) with a 20 MHz transducer is able to distinguish muscle-invasive disease. However, it is unable to detect deeper penetration, especially if the tumor is >2 cm.[34,35] Koraitim et al reported high accuracy in discriminating Ta and T1 tumors from muscle-invasive, organ-confined tumors.[36] The accuracy in predicting extravesical disease decreased to 70%, similar to the accuracy of bimanual examination. Transrectal ultrasound (TRUS) has been compared to TUR and CT, and TUUS to MRI, and was no worse.[29]

## CT

CT is frequently used as a staging study, but has not provided much more information than an adequate TUR. A series of 65 patients that underwent TUR and EUA for bladder tumors were evaluated by CT and TRUS.[29] Although the reported sensitivity of CT was 95%, the accuracy and specificity were as poor as that with TRUS. Air insufflation of the bladder improved the sensitivity of CT staging; however, the study reporting this finding lacked complete cystectomy specimens to verify the imaging.[37]

Kim et al compared CT to several MRI techniques with contrast enhancement. In distinguishing organ-confined from nonconfined disease, using the 1992 TNM system, the accuracy of CT was 83% versus 89% for overall MRI protocols without a statistically significant difference between techniques.[27] The authors noted that the specificity and positive predictive value were low because of overstaging from postprocedural artifact; therefore, the authors urged caution in interpreting these studies, especially in the analysis of non-organ-confined disease. Additionally, these investigators were able to identify only four of six patients with positive lymph nodes preoperatively by either CT or MRI.

Paik et al recently reviewed a series of 82 patients identified with muscle-invasive cancer that underwent preoperative CT prior to cystectomy to assess the utility of CT as a staging study before surgery.[30] Imaging was obtained prior to TUR in approximately half, and after TUR in the remaining half of patients. Overall, the accuracy was 55%, but depth of bladder invasion was correctly identified in only one case. In the subset of eight patients identified with extravesical disease, the finding was verified by the pathology in only four. The 17 patients with either perivesical fat involvement or invasion of contiguous organs were not identified with extravesical disease on CT. Lymph node metastases were correctly diagnosed in four of six patients, but lymph node metastases were missed in 17 others. The authors contended that preoperative CT altered clinical decision-making in a small minority of patients. This finding was consistent with an earlier study by Herr, in which only 38% of patients with extravesical disease were correctly identified on CT as having lymph node metastases.[38] The authors suggested that the utility of preoperative CT is in those patients with clinical extravesical disease to identify appropriate patients for surgery. It appears that obtaining imaging studies to further stage muscle-invasive bladder cancer is of marginal utility. Herr

| Study | Year | Modality | No. pts | Sensitivity (%) | Specificity (%) | Accuracy (%) |
|---|---|---|---|---|---|---|
| Kim et al*[27] | 1994 | CT | 29 | 93 | 71 | 55 |
| Kim et al[28] | 2004 | MRI | 36 | 100 | 76 | 75 |
| | | CT | 44 | 92 | 98 | 96 |
| Yaman et al[29] | 1996 | CT | 65 | 95 | 28 | 35 |
| | | TRUS | 65 | 95 | 32 | 40 |
| Paik et al[30] | 2000 | CT | 82 | – | – | 55 |
| Barentsz et al[31] | 1996 | MRI | 61 | – | – | 84 |
| | | MRI for LN | 61 | 86 | 95 | 93 |
| Jager et al[32] | 1996 | MRI for LN | 71 | 83 | 98 | 92 |
| Bachor et al[33] | 1999 | PET for LN | 64 | 67 | 86 | 80 |

**Table 21.2** Contemporary series of imaging modalities for evaluating invasive urothelial cancer

*Sensitivity and specificity in comparing Ta–T3a versus T3b–T4.

CT, computed tomography; LN, lymph nodes; MRI, magnetic resonance imaging; PET, positron emission tomography; TRUS, transrectal ultrasound

recommended in cases of clinical muscle-invasive, non-organ-confined disease, defined by induration/mass on EUA or tumor in fat on TUR, that CT may be helpful, but does not add further information when disease is organ confined.[38] In his series of 105 patients, only 5 of the 21 patients with ≥T3 disease had obviously positive lymph nodes on preoperative CT scan. A positive mass on exam, however, implied survival similar to that of patients with pathologically confirmed extravesical disease. Recently, however, Kim et al reported promising results in 44 patients by improving a CT staging protocol to better detect extravesical disease.[28] When CT was obtained at least 1 week after TUR and images were obtained 60 and 180 seconds after injection of contrast, the authors reported a sensitivity of 92%, specificity of 98%, and accuracy of 96%, respectively. As a useful clinical reference, the positive and negative predictive values were 92% and 98%, respectively.

Regardless of the imaging findings in the bladder, the presence or absence of hydronephrosis on preoperative imaging offers prognostic value. In a series of 415 cystectomy patients that underwent intravenous pyelogram (IVP) and CT, those patients with bilateral hydronephrosis, unilateral hydronephrosis, or no hydronephrosis (91%, 67%, and 43%) had either metastatic or extravesical disease.[39] When the investigators stratified by pathologic stage, however, they found no statistically significant difference in survival based on the presence of hydronephrosis.

## MRI

MRI is reportedly better at initial staging than CT.[40] Barentsz et al reported on a series of 61 patients, 57 of whom ultimately underwent cystectomy. They were further evaluated by MRI 1–4 weeks after TUR and by MRI with dynamic fast imaging that accurately detected extravesical disease in 28 patients with pathologic confirmation.[31] The authors believed that the described MRI technique better differentiated malignancy from post-TUR artifact. Furthermore, this same study reported 93% accuracy, 86% sensitivity, and 95% specificity in detecting nodal metastases with the same MRI technique. In a larger series of 71 patients evaluated for nodal metastases, the same group reported that MRI had an accuracy of 92%, sensitivity of 83%, and specificity of 98%, although the number of patients that underwent lymphadenectomy to provide tissue for pathologic conformation was not mentioned.[32]

In a series of 143 patients evaluated with MRI before definitive radiotherapy, multivariate analysis identified factors that were predictive of treatment failure and poor cancer survival. These factors, as expected, included stage, but also included tumor size and the presence of hydronephrosis.[41] The administration of lymphotropic supermagnetic nanoparticles in performing MRI demonstrated promise in detecting positive lymph nodes in prostate cancer patients.[42] Interestingly, this technique was able to detect positive lymph nodes even when the positive lymph nodes were not enlarged. Although not yet studied, the use of this MRI modification may enhance the accuracy of lymph node staging in bladder cancer patients as well.

## POSITRON EMISSION TOMOGRAPHY

Positron emission tomography (PET) has received little study but shows promise in diagnosing lymph node metastases. With regard to local disease, the tracer is excreted in the urine, which could obscure the depth of tumor invasion in the bladder.[43] Bachor et al reported on 64 patients that were imaged preoperatively by PET then subsequently underwent cystectomy and lymphadenectomy to provide pathologic tissue for comparison.[33] The authors found that PET had a sensitivity, specificity, and accuracy of 67%, 86%, and 80%, respectively, in predicting nodal metastases. In a smaller series, Heicappell et al reported accurate lymph node staging in seven of eight cystectomy patients.[44] PET, therefore, may be useful in staging patients suspicious for nodal disease.

## FLUOROSCOPICALLY GUIDED FINE NEEDLE ASPIRATION

To improve prediction of lymph node disease, Chagnon et al reported their experience with fluoroscopically guided fine needle aspiration (FNA) biopsy of obturator and other suspicious lymph nodes on lymphography.[45] Of the 101 bladder cancer patients that subsequently underwent lymphadenectomy, only 25% were reported as having false-negative biopsies with no false positives. Unfortunately, although this report was positive in outlook, no preoperative information was provided, especially regarding the clinical stage of these patients, suggesting that there may have been a selection bias.

Uroplakins are transmembrane proteins on urothelial cells that have been demonstrated to be markers of urothelial cells. Staining FNA specimens with polyclonal antiuroplakin antibodies in the future may enhance the sensitivity and specificity of the biopsy.[46]

## SUBSTAGING

Clinical T1 tumors deserve special attention because they have demonstrated invasive behavior by penetrating the basement membrane, but they are frequently understaged.[47,48] Dutta et al recently reported 40% pT2 stage or greater in patients that initially were classified with clinical T1 disease.[49] The Memorial

Sloan-Kettering group, therefore, advocated a repeat resection before initiating intravesical therapy to eradicate residual disease and/or obtain more and possibly deeper tissue for accurate staging.[50] Some patients with T1 disease may benefit from radical cystectomy rather than TUR and intravesical therapy.[51,52]

To stratify patients with worse disease, investigators substaged T1 disease by the depth of invasion within the lamina propria. Holmäng et al reported that patients with grade 3 tumors had a 58% progression rate versus 36% if the tumor remained deep, rather than above the muscularis mucosa.[53] Several multivariable analyses have predicted that invasion through the muscularis mucosa confers a greater risk of progression,[54–56] and, expectedly, associated CIS was also a significant risk factor for progression.[54,56,57] In an attempt to overcome the subjectivity of histologic interpretation in T1 substaging, Cheng et al proposed that TUR specimens with T1 pathology be characterized by micrometer measurement of depth of invasion to provide greater prognostic information.[58,59] Fifty-five patients resected before the bacillus Calmette–Guérin (BCG) era underwent cystectomy. Using a receiver operator characteristic (ROC) analysis to predict muscle-invasive disease, a threshold of >1.5 mm depth of invasion had 81%, 83%, and 95% sensitivity, specificity, and positive predictive value, respectively.[58] However, the negative predictive value was only 56%. Although staining for the presence of the p53 tumor suppressor gene may stratify the prognosis in T1 disease[60] in the previous studies, positive staining for the p53 tumor suppressor was not a significant independent variable for predicting progression.[54,55,57]

The utility of T1 substaging has been questioned because the muscularis mucosa is not a constant finding, and substaging is a subjective interpretation by the pathologist.[57,61] Herr and Reuter critically stated that cases of T1 disease with progression likely represented understaging of muscle-invasive disease on initial resection.[62] The World Health Organization and the International Society of Urologic Pathologists (WHO/ISUP) committee of pathologists in its recommendations did not advocate universal adoption of T1 substaging because depth of invasion and orientation of TUR specimens could not be accurately determined, and presence of the muscularis mucosa was not consistent.[63]

Alternative methods for obtaining or analyzing biopsy tissue have been investigated. Another technique to obtain diagnostic tissue is to perform a needle biopsy of the entire bladder wall thickness rather than a deep TUR that may be impractical.[64] Hoshi et al described a transurethral needle biopsy technique simultaneously visualizing the depth of needle penetration with ultrasound to obtain biopsies of the muscle layer and perivesical fat in 20 patients. The authors reported the accuracy of their technique when employed between neoadjuvant treatment and cystectomy as 90%. To gain greater diagnostic information, Cheng et al proposed

that the depth of invasion in the TUR specimen could predict the presence of extravesical disease.[65] Depth of invasion was measured by micrometer from the basement membrane to the most deeply invasive cancer cells. Using a 4.0 mm cut-off, the specificity was 90%; however, the sensitivity and positive predictive value were only 54% and 81%, respectively. The utility of this information may be low, but, on the other hand, it is easily acquired from already obtained tissue specimens. The WHO/ISUP committee again, however, cautioned that substaging depth of muscularis propria invasion and diagnosis of extravesical disease by viewing tumor in the fat should be reserved for cystectomy rather than TUR specimens.[63]

## NODAL STATUS

In the TNM system, the nodal status is based only upon the total number of positive lymph nodes. As previously discussed, preoperative imaging studies will not identify all nodal metastases, but an adequate lymphadenectomy by the urologist can provide useful diagnostic information.[66–68] Furthermore, the presence of lymph node metastases greatly decreases survival,[25] although lymphadenectomy has curative potential,[69–71] even in the presence of gross disease.[72] Bochner et al noted that submitting separate pelvic lymph node specimens improved the yield of lymph nodes identified by the pathologist.[66] Herr proposed that an adequate lymphadenectomy for therapy and staging include at least nine lymph nodes.[73] In a larger study using Surveillance, Epidemiology and End Results (SEER) data, Konety et al concurred that 10–14 lymph nodes should be retrieved.[74] Herr also found that, in cases of T2 or T3 disease, a >20% cut-off in the ratio of positive to total number of lymph nodes predicted dismal survival.[73]

Stein et al reported that, in a large series of cystectomy patients that underwent extended lymphadenectomy, 244 patients had positive lymph nodes. Of these, 37 underwent perioperative radiation, and 139 received perioperative chemotherapy. The 5- and 10-year recurrence-free survival rates were 44% and 43%, respectively, if the lymph node density was <20%.[68] In contrast, patients with a lymph node density >20% had 5- and 10-year recurrence-free survival rates of 17%. In the multivariable analysis, not only was lymph node density significant in survival outcome, but so also were number of lymph nodes and treatment with neoadjuvant or adjuvant chemotherapies.

## SPECIFIC STAGING CONSIDERATIONS

Bladder cancer outside the bladder proper itself poses questions for staging because the anatomy in these situations can drastically affect the prognosis. Urothelial carcinoma invading the prostatic stroma is characterized as pT4A disease. Involvement of the prostate arises from extravesical contiguous extension or intraurethral spread.[75,76] Donat et al proposed a third mechanism, tumor extension through the bladder neck, the extent of which is difficult to appreciate prior to cystectomy.[77] Stromal invasion of the prostate confers a markedly worse prognosis than isolated urethral tumor, CIS, or ductal involvement. In a series of 124 patients with urothelial carcinoma arising from the prostate, patients without stromal invasion had 81% 5-year recurrence-free survival versus 48% in those with invasion.[78] Pagano et al, however, reported that patients with ductal involvement had a prognosis similar to that of patients with stromal invasion rather than those with epithelial disease.[76] Prostatic stromal involvement is worse if the origin is contiguous disease extending through the bladder wall rather than primarily arising in the prostate. Therefore, it seems warranted that extent of and mechanism of prostatic involvement alters prognosis and perhaps should be incorporated within the current TNM staging system.

Although bladder cancer is more common in men than women, there are considerations unique to women. Bladder cancer may extend through the posterior wall to involve the vagina, staged clinically as T4 disease.[2] Traditionally, radical cystectomy in women involved removal of all internal gynecologic organs for therapy and complete staging. Now that orthotopic urinary diversions are being performed more frequently on women, preservation of the anterior vaginal wall in particular may decrease the rate of neobladder–vaginal fistulas and preserve urinary control.[79] Chang et al reported no involvement of the posterior bladder or urethral margin in 21 patients in whom the anterior vaginal wall was spared.[79] The Mansoura group evaluated female radical cystectomy patients with predominantly squamous cell carcinoma.[80] Patients had been thoroughly evaluated preoperatively by multiple biopsies of the bladder neck and trigone. Vaginal involvement was excluded by physical examination and transvaginal ultrasound. In 145 women that underwent radical cystectomy with orthotopic diversion, none had disease involvement of the vagina or other gynecologic organs, nor did any patients have recurrence in the vaginal remnant. Thus women that are appropriately staged without vaginal disease may benefit from anterior vaginal sparing during radical cystectomy without losing cancer control.

Cancer within a bladder diverticulum also provides a staging challenge. Because a diverticulum is an outpouching of epithelium and not a true diverticulum, it lacks the muscularis propria. Furthermore, it is difficult to obtain a full thickness TUR specimen within a diverticulum without perforating the bladder. In the largest series to date of 39 patients presenting with bladder tumor within a diverticulum, the 5-year disease-specific survival rates for Ta, T1 and extradiverticular disease were 83%, 67%, and 45%, respectively.[81] Of the 13 patients with Ta disease, 7 underwent TUR and 4 had partial cystectomy. These 11 patients were disease-free at final follow-up. The two remaining patients developed refractory CIS and eventually underwent delayed cystectomy, but subsequently developed extradiverticular disease. From this small study it appears warranted to treat non-invasive diverticular tumors conservatively in the absence of CIS.

## CONCLUSION

Imaging technology will only improve, but to date it will not provide a completely accurate assessment of preoperative tumor depth or lymph node involvement in all patients. At this time, however, we agree with the National Comprehensive Cancer Network 2004 guidelines for bladder cancer.[82] For patients suspected of having muscle-invasive disease, we recommend a bimanual EUA at the time of cystoscopy or TUR, chest x-ray, laboratory studies, and an imaging study such as CT or MRI to assess extravesical disease and evaluate the upper tracts. As stated by Millikan et al, staging is not an exclusively anatomic principle but a method to stratify cancers based on prognosis.[83]

To achieve the goal of accuracy, we encourage an interdisciplinary team approach that integrates the urologic findings on cystoscopy and examination with results of radiographic studies, pathologic interpretation, and, in the future, molecular studies. The urologist must also function as the focal point to ensure that the radiologists and pathologists understand how their consultation will impact clinical decision-making. To optimize patient care, this process can only be achieved through open and rapid communication between clinicians.

## REFERENCES

1. Jewett HSG. Infiltrating carcinoma of the bladder. Relation of depth penetration of the bladder wall to incidence of local extension and metastases. J Urol 1946;55:366–372.
2. Greene FL, American Joint Committee on Cancer, American Cancer Society. AJCC Cancer Staging Manual, 6th ed. New York: Springer-Verlag, 2002.
3. Hermanek P, International Union Against Cancer. TNM Atlas: Illustrated Guide to the TNM/pTNM Classification of Malignant Tumours, 4th ed. Berlin: Springer, 1997.
4. Marshall VF, Whitmore WF Jr. The present position of radical cystectomy in the surgical management of carcinoma of the urinary bladder. J Urol 1956;76(4):387–391.
5. Grossman HB, Natale RB, Tangen CM, et al. Neoadjuvant chemotherapy plus cystectomy compared with cystectomy alone for locally advanced bladder cancer. N Engl J Med 2003;349(9):859–866.
6. Michaelson MD, Shipley WU, Heney NM, Zietman AL, Kaufman DS. Selective bladder preservation for muscle-invasive transitional cell carcinoma of the urinary bladder. Br J Cancer 2004;90(3):578–581.

7. Cina SJ, Epstein JI, Endrizzi JM, Harmon WJ, Seay TM, Schoenberg MP. Correlation of cystoscopic impression with histologic diagnosis of biopsy specimens of the bladder. Hum Pathol 2001;32(6):630–637.

8. Satoh E, Miyao N, Tachiki H, Fujisawa Y. Prediction of muscle invasion of bladder cancer by cystoscopy. Eur Urol 2002;41(2):178–181.

9. Messing EJ. Urothelial tumors of the urinary tract. In Campbell MF, Walsh PC, Retik AB (eds): Campbell's Urology, 8th ed. Philadelphia: Saunders, 2002, pp 2732–2784.

10. Noroozian M, Cohan RH, Caoili EM, Cowan NC, Ellis JH. Multislice CT urography: state of the art. Br J Radiol 2004;77(Spec No 1):S74–86.

11. Lopez-Beltran A, Bassi P, Pavone-Macaluso M, Montironi R. Handling and pathology reporting of specimens with carcinoma of the urinary bladder, ureter, and renal pelvis. Eur Urol 2004;45(3):257–266.

12. Busch CHD, Johannson SL, Cote, RJ. Pathologic assessment of bladder cancer and pitfalls in staging. In: Droller MJ (ed): Bladder Cancer: Current Diagnosis and Treatment. Totowa, NJ: Humana Press, 2001, pp 149–182.

13. Amin MB, Srigley JR, Grignon DJ, et al. Updated protocol for the examination of specimens from patients with carcinoma of the urinary bladder, ureter, and renal pelvis. Arch Pathol Lab Med 2003;127(10):1263–1279.

14. Taguchi I, Gohji K, Hara I, et al. Clinical evaluation of random biopsy of urinary bladder in patients with superficial bladder cancer. Int J Urol 1998;5(1):30–34.

15. Kiemeney LA, Witjes JA, Heijbroek RP, Koper NP, Verbeek AL, Debruyne FM. Should random urothelial biopsies be taken from patients with primary superficial bladder cancer? A decision analysis. Members of the Dutch South-East Co-operative Urological Group. Br J Urol 1994;73(2):164–171.

16. van der Meijden A, Oosterlinck W, Brausi M, Kurth KH, Sylvester R, de Balincourt C. Significance of bladder biopsies in Ta,T1 bladder tumors: a report from the EORTC Genito-Urinary Tract Cancer Cooperative Group. EORTC-GU Group Superficial Bladder Committee. Eur Urol 1999;35(4):267–271.

17. Swinn MJ, Walker MM, Harbin LJ, et al. Biopsy of the red patch at cystoscopy: is it worthwhile? Eur Urol 2004;45(4):471–474; discussion 474.

18. Holzbeierlein JM, Lopez-Corona E, Bochner BH, et al. Partial cystectomy: a contemporary review of the Memorial Sloan-Kettering Cancer Center experience and recommendations for patient selection. J Urol 2004;172(3):878–881.

19. Schoenberg M. Management of invasive and metastatic bladder cancer. In Campbell MF, Walsh PC, Retik AB (eds): Campbell's Urology, 8th ed. Philadelphia: Saunders, 2002, pp 2803–2817.

20. Fossa SD, Ous S, Berner A. Clinical significance of the 'palpable mass' in patients with muscle-infiltrating bladder cancer undergoing cystectomy after pre-operative radiotherapy. Br J Urol 1991;67(1):54–60.

21. Wijkstrom H, Norming U, Lagerkvist M, Nilsson B, Naslund I, Wiklund P. Evaluation of clinical staging before cystectomy in transitional cell bladder carcinoma: a long-term follow-up of 276 consecutive patients. Br J Urol 1998;81(5):686–691.

22. Herr HW, Faulkner JR, Grossman HB, Crawford ED. Pathologic evaluation of radical cystectomy specimens: a cooperative group report. Cancer 2004;100(11):2470–2475.

23. Dalbagni G, Genega E, Hashibe M, et al. Cystectomy for bladder cancer: a contemporary series. J Urol 2001;165(4):1111–1116.

24. Quek ML, Stein JP, Clark PE, et al. Microscopic and gross extravesical extension in pathological staging of bladder cancer. J Urol 2004;171(2 Pt 1):640–645.

25. Stein JP, Lieskovsky G, Cote R, et al. Radical cystectomy in the treatment of invasive bladder cancer: long-term results in 1,054 patients. J Clin Oncol 2001;19(3):666–675.

26. Levy DA, Grossman HB. Staging and prognosis of T3b bladder cancer. Semin Urol Oncol 1996;14(2):56–61.

27. Kim B, Semelka RC, Ascher SM, Chalpin DB, Carroll PR, Hricak H. Bladder tumor staging: comparison of contrast-enhanced CT, T1- and T2-weighted MR imaging, dynamic gadolinium-enhanced imaging, and late gadolinium-enhanced imaging. Radiology 1994;193(1):239–245.

28. Kim JK, Park SY, Ahn HJ, Kim CS, Cho KS. Bladder cancer: analysis of multi-detector row helical CT enhancement pattern and accuracy in tumor detection and perivesical staging. Radiology 2004;231(3):725–731.

29. Yaman O, Baltaci S, Arikan N, Yilmaz E, Gogus O. Staging with computed tomography, transrectal ultrasonography and transurethral resection of bladder tumour: comparison with final pathological stage in invasive bladder carcinoma. Br J Urol 1996;78(2):197–200.

30. Paik ML, Scolieri MJ, Brown SL, Spirnak JP, Resnick MI. Limitations of computerized tomography in staging invasive bladder cancer before radical cystectomy. J Urol 2000;163(6):1693–1696.

31. Barentsz JO, Jager GJ, van Vierzen PB, et al. Staging urinary bladder cancer after transurethral biopsy: value of fast dynamic contrast-enhanced MR imaging. Radiology 1996;201(1):185–193.

32. Jager GJ, Barentsz JO, Oosterhof GO, Witjes JA, Ruijs SJ. Pelvic adenopathy in prostatic and urinary bladder carcinoma: MR imaging with a three-dimensional TI-weighted magnetization-prepared-rapid gradient-echo sequence. AJR Am J Roentgenol 1996;167(6):1503–1507.

33. Bachor R, Kotzerke J, Reske SN, Hautmann R. [Lymph node staging of bladder neck carcinoma with positron emission tomography.] Urologe A 1999;38(1):46–50.

34. Horiuchi K, Tsuboi N, Shimizu H, et al. High-frequency endoluminal ultrasonography for staging transitional cell carcinoma of the bladder. Urology 2000;56(3):404–407.

35. Datta SN, Allen GM, Evans R, Vaughton KC, Lucas MG. Urinary tract ultrasonography in the evaluation of haematuria—a report of over 1,000 cases. Ann R Coll Surg Engl 2002;84(3):203–205.

36. Koraitim M, Kamal B, Metwalli N, Zaky Y. Transurethral ultrasonographic assessment of bladder carcinoma: its value and limitation. J Urol 1995;154(2 Pt 1):375–378.

37. Caterino M, Giunta S, Finocchi V, et al. Primary cancer of the urinary bladder: CT evaluation of the T parameter with different techniques. Abdom Imaging 2001;26(4):433–438.

38. Herr HW. Routine CT scan in cystectomy patients: does it change management? Urology 1996;47(3):324–325.

39. Haleblian GE, Skinner EC, Dickinson MG, Lieskovsky G, Boyd SD, Skinner DG. Hydronephrosis as a prognostic indicator in bladder cancer patients. J Urol 1998;160(6 Pt 1):2011–2014.

40. Barentsz JO, Engelbrecht M, Jager GJ, et al. Fast dynamic gadolinium-enhanced MR imaging of urinary bladder and prostate cancer. J Magn Reson Imaging 1999;10(3):295–304.

41. Robinson P, Collins CD, Ryder WD, et al. Relationship of MRI and clinical staging to outcome in invasive bladder cancer treated by radiotherapy. Clin Radiol 2000;55(4):301–306.

42. Harisinghani MG, Barentsz J, Hahn PF, et al. Noninvasive detection of clinically occult lymph-node metastases in prostate cancer. N Engl J Med 2003;348(25):2491–2499.

43. Hain SF, Maisey MN. Positron emission tomography for urological tumours. BJU Int 2003;92(2):159–164.

44. Heicappell R, Muller-Mattheis V, Reinhardt M, et al. Staging of pelvic lymph nodes in neoplasms of the bladder and prostate by positron emission tomography with 2-[(18)F]-2-deoxy-D-glucose. Eur Urol 1999;36(6):582–587.

45. Chagnon S, Cochand-Priollet B, Gzaeil M, et al. Pelvic cancers: staging of 139 cases with lymphography and fine-needle aspiration biopsy. Radiology 1989;173(1):103–106.

46. Xu X, Sun TT, Gupta PK, Zhang P, Nasuti JF. Uroplakin as a marker for typing metastatic transitional cell carcinoma on fine-needle aspiration specimens. Cancer 2001;93(3):216–221.

47. Freeman JA, Esrig D, Stein JP, et al. Radical cystectomy for high risk patients with superficial bladder cancer in the era of orthotopic urinary reconstruction. Cancer 1995;76(5):833–839.

48. Cheng L, Neumann RM, Weaver AL, et al. Grading and staging of bladder carcinoma in transurethral resection specimens. Correlation with 105 matched cystectomy specimens. Am J Clin Pathol 2000;113(2):275–279.

49. Dutta SC, Smith JA Jr, Shappell SB, Coffey CS, Chang SS, Cookson MS. Clinical understaging of high risk nonmuscle invasive urothelial

carcinoma treated with radical cystectomy. J Urol 2001;166(2):490–493.

50. Dalbagni G, Herr HW, Reuter VE. Impact of a second transurethral resection on the staging of T1 bladder cancer. Urology 2002;60(5):822–824; discussion 824–825.

51. Cookson MS, Herr HW, Zhang ZF, Soloway S, Sogani PC, Fair WR. The treated natural history of high risk superficial bladder cancer: 15-year outcome. J Urol 1997;158(1):62–67.

52. Stein JP. Indications for early cystectomy. Urology 2003;62(4):591–595.

53. Holmäng S, Hedelin H, Anderstrom C, Holmberg E, Johansson SL. The importance of the depth of invasion in stage T1 bladder carcinoma: a prospective cohort study. J Urol 1997;157(3):800–803; discussion 804.

54. Bernardini S, Billerey C, Martin M, Adessi GL, Wallerand H, Bittard H. The predictive value of muscularis mucosae invasion and p53 overexpression on progression of stage T1 bladder carcinoma. J Urol 2001;165(1):42–46; discussion 46.

55. Hermann GG, Horn T, Steven K. The influence of the level of lamina propria invasion and the prevalence of p53 nuclear accumulation on survival in stage T1 transitional cell bladder cancer. J Urol 1998;159(1):91–94.

56. Smits G, Schaafsma E, Kiemeney L, Caris C, Debruyne F, Witjes JA. Microstaging of pT1 transitional cell carcinoma of the bladder: identification of subgroups with distinct risks of progression. Urology 1998;52(6):1009–1013; discussion 1013–1014.

57. Shariat SF, Weizer AZ, Green A, et al. Prognostic value of P53 nuclear accumulation and histopathologic features in T1 transitional cell carcinoma of the urinary bladder. Urology 2000;56(5):735–740.

58. Cheng L, Weaver AL, Neumann RM, Scherer BG, Bostwick DG. Substaging of T1 bladder carcinoma based on the depth of invasion as measured by micrometer: a new proposal. Cancer 1999;86(6):1035–1043.

59. Cheng L, Neumann RM, Weaver AL, Spotts BE, Bostwick DG. Predicting cancer progression in patients with stage T1 bladder carcinoma. J Clin Oncol 1999;17(10):3182–3187.

60. Grossman HB, Liebert M, Antelo M, et al. p53 and RB expression predict progression in T1 bladder cancer. Clin Cancer Res 1998;4(4):829–834.

61. Platz CE, Cohen MB, Jones MP, Olson DB, Lynch CF. Is microstaging of early invasive cancer of the urinary bladder possible or useful? Mod Pathol 1996;9(11):1035–1039.

62. Herr HW, Reuter VE. Progression of T1 bladder tumors: better staging or better biology? Cancer 1999;86(6):908–912.

63. Epstein JI, Amin MB, Reuter VR, Mostofi FK. The World Health Organization/International Society of Urological Pathology consensus classification of urothelial (transitional cell) neoplasms of the urinary bladder. Bladder Consensus Conference Committee. Am J Surg Pathol 1998;22(12):1435–1448.

64. Hoshi S, Ono K, Suzuki K, Ohyama C, Namima T, Orikasa S. Trans-urethral whole layer core biopsy for detection of residual tumor after neoadjuvant therapy in invasive bladder cancer. Urol Oncol 2001;6(3):85–89.

65. Cheng L, Weaver AL, Bostwick DG. Predicting extravesical extension of bladder carcinoma: a novel method based on micrometer measurement of the depth of invasion in transurethral resection specimens. Urology 2000;55(5):668–672.

66. Bochner BH, Herr HW, Reuter VE. Impact of separate versus en bloc pelvic lymph node dissection on the number of lymph nodes retrieved in cystectomy specimens. J Urol 2001;166(6):2295–2296.

67. Frank I, Cheville JC, Blute ML, et al. Transitional cell carcinoma of the urinary bladder with regional lymph node involvement treated by cystectomy: clinicopathologic features associated with outcome. Cancer 2003;97(10):2425–2431.

68. Stein JP, Cai J, Groshen S, Skinner DG. Risk factors for patients with pelvic lymph node metastases following radical cystectomy with en bloc pelvic lymphadenectomy: concept of lymph node density. J Urol 2003;170(1):35–41.

69. Herr HW, Bochner BH, Dalbagni G, Donat SM, Reuter VE, Bajorin DF. Impact of the number of lymph nodes retrieved on outcome in patients with muscle invasive bladder cancer. J Urol 2002;167(3):1295–1298.

70. Poulsen AL, Horn T, Steven K. Radical cystectomy: extending the limits of pelvic lymph node dissection improves survival for patients with bladder cancer confined to the bladder wall. J Urol 1998;160(6 Pt 1):2015–2019; discussion 2020.

71. Vieweg J, Gschwend JE, Herr HW, Fair WR. Pelvic lymph node dissection can be curative in patients with node positive bladder cancer. J Urol 1999;161(2):449–454.

72. Herr HW, Donat SM. Outcome of patients with grossly node positive bladder cancer after pelvic lymph node dissection and radical cystectomy. J Urol 2001;165(1):62–64; discussion 64.

73. Herr HW. Superiority of ratio based lymph node staging for bladder cancer. J Urol 2003;169(3):943–945.

74. Konety BR, Joslyn SA, O'Donnell MA. Extent of pelvic lymphadenectomy and its impact on outcome in patients diagnosed with bladder cancer: analysis of data from the Surveillance, Epidemiology and End Results Program data base. J Urol 2003;169(3):946–950.

75. Njinou Ngninkeu B, Lorge F, Moulin P, Jamart J, Van Cangh PJ. Transitional cell carcinoma involving the prostate: a clinicopathological retrospective study of 76 cases. J Urol 2003;169(1):149–152.

76. Pagano F, Bassi P, Ferrante GL, et al. Is stage pT4a (D1) reliable in assessing transitional cell carcinoma involvement of the prostate in patients with a concurrent bladder cancer? A necessary distinction for contiguous or noncontiguous involvement. J Urol 1996;155(1):244–247.

77. Donat SM, Genega EM, Herr HW, Reuter VE. Mechanisms of prostatic stromal invasion in patients with bladder cancer: clinical significance. J Urol 2001;165(4):1117–1120.

78. Esrig D, Freeman JA, Elmajian DA, et al. Transitional cell carcinoma involving the prostate with a proposed staging classification for stromal invasion. J Urol 1996;156(3):1071–1076.

79. Chang SS, Cole E, Cookson MS, Peterson M, Smith JA, Jr. Preservation of the anterior vaginal wall during female radical cystectomy with orthotopic urinary diversion: technique and results. J Urol 2002;168(4 Pt 1):1442–1445.

80. Ali-El-Dein B, Abdel-Latif M, Mosbah A, et al. Secondary malignant involvement of gynecologic organs in radical cystectomy specimens in women: is it mandatory to remove these organs routinely? J Urol 2004;172(3):885–887.

81. Golijanin D, Yossepowitch O, Beck SD, Sogani P, Dalbagni G. Carcinoma in a bladder diverticulum: presentation and treatment outcome. J Urol 2003;170(5):1761–1764.

82. National Comprehensive Cancer Network clinical practice guidelines in oncology, 2004. Online. Available: www.nccn.org/physician_fls/f_guidelines.html.

83. Millikan R, Siefker-Radtke A, Grossman HB. Neoadjuvant chemotherapy for bladder cancer. Urol Oncol 2003;21(6):464–467.

# Etiology and management of urothelial tumors of the renal pelvis and ureter

## 22

*Guillermo Lima, Thomas Jarrett, Noel Clarke*

## INTRODUCTION

### INCIDENCE

Transitional cell carcinoma (TCC) of the upper urinary tract is a relatively uncommon tumor. It accounts for between 2% and 6% of all presenting TCCs,[1,2] and 10% of all presenting renal tumors in the United States.[3] Tumors occur three to four times more commonly in the renal pelvis than in the ureter,[4,5] but when they arise primarily in the ureter, approximately 70% do so in the lower third, with a further 24% occurring in the mid-ureter.[5,6] As with bladder cancer, there is a gender difference, although this is not as pronounced; in the US the disease is three times more common in men than in women.[7] The incidence of the disease rises with age, being commonest in the fifth to seventh decades, with a mean age of occurrence of 65–67 years,[8] and a peak incidence occurring in the age cohort between 70 and 79 years.[2]

Upper tract TCC may be multifocal, with tumors arising in different locations and at different times. This may be related to factors such as cellular implantation[9] or to widespread dysplastic changes in the urothelium,[10] although the true nature of these changes is incompletely understood.[11] Whatever the etiology, the tendency towards the observed polychronotropism is usually confined to the ipsilateral upper tract. The incidence of contralateral TCC is only 3%.[12,13]

Association of ureteric and renal pelvic TCC with bladder cancer is well documented but the discrepant incidence underlines the deficiencies in our understanding of the nature of the disease. Primary upper tract TCC occurs in association with bladder cancer in about 2% to 4% of patients.[14] However, patients that develop a ureteric or renal pelvic lesion subsequently have a very high rate of bladder cancer: this develops in 30% to 75% of patients in the years following treatment.[4,15] This fact has significant implications for follow-up of patients developing the disease (see below).

### ETIOLOGIC FACTORS

Upper tract TCC is associated with a spectrum of risk factors ranging from those with a genetic basis to those arising in association with a combination of chemical and pharmacologic carcinogens. Such factors contribute singly or in concert to produce the manifold genetic and molecular changes reported in this disease, although the series of events that results in normal urothelium becoming malignant remains unknown.

### GENETIC FACTORS

The genetics of TCC are dealt with fully in Chapters 9 and 10. There has been a presumption that upper tract TCC has the same genetic basis as that seen in the bladder. However, the understanding of this disease, while still sparse, has improved recently with the acquisition of new information.

Transitional tumors of the ureter and kidney have been known for some time to be associated with heredity, most notably in Lynch's syndrome.[16] This condition, predominantly associated with development of heredity colonic tumors, tumors of the endometrium, and tumors in other extracolonic sites,[17-19] is known to be associated with the development of ureteral cancer.[16,20] The incidence of this is relatively low (about 5% of Lynch syndrome patients) but further study has enhanced the understanding of the development of this condition. In a study of 164 patients diagnosed with 'sporadic' upper tract TCC, 27 had high levels of microsatellite instability and, in a proportion of these, there was a specific association with abnormalities of DNA mismatch repair, particularly the MSH2 gene and its protein product hMSH2. The findings are consistent with upper tract TCC being associated with specific germline mutations in a small proportion of cases.[21] Further studies of microsatellite instability and of alterations in microsatellite-specific locations[22] have shown clearly that there are distinct differences in the genetic make-up of upper tract TCC and bladder cancer. In the former, there is an association with increased methylation inactivation, particularly in relation to the MLH1 DNA mismatch repair gene. The authors hypothesize that the difference in upper and lower tract microsatellite instability characteristics may be related to differential exposure of bladder and ureteric epithelium to carcinogenic factors (e.g. due to smoking), although this notion remains to be proven.

## CHEMICAL CARCINOGENS

TCC of the upper urinary tract is associated with a number of chemical carcinogens, the most common of which are those related to smoking, industrial exposure (dyestuffs), rubber and plastics manufacturing, aluminum mining, pesticide use, hairdressing and hair dye, and specific pharmaceutical preparations.[23] Smoking increases the risk of developing upper tract TCC by a factor of 3; in long-term smokers, the risk is greater still.[24] In a study correlating incidence with duration of smoking, McLaughlin et al[25] demonstrated that in men and women that had smoked for more than 45 years, the risk of developing a ureteric tumor was seven times greater than that for a nonsmoker.

Industrial processes are also known to be associated with urothelial cancer and, in particular, ureteric TCC. Industrial exposure to carcinogenic agents such as benzidine and β-naphthylamine, formerly used in the manufacturer of rubber and dyestuffs, can increase the risk of developing upper tract TCC by 8- to 10-fold.[26,27] In long-term studies, the incidence of nonbladder urothelial cancer was also significantly elevated in individuals many years after exposure to benzidine.[28] In other, more modern industrial processes, this potential for risk persists despite the proscription of most of the known carcinogenic agents. For example, in toner ink manufacture in printing using modern ink jet printers, some of the indulin and nigrosine dyes used have been shown to contain the urothelial carcinogen 4-amino-biphenyl.[29]

Pharmaceutical preparations are also associated with the development of upper tract TCC. The main causative agents are analgesics and the cytotoxic drug cyclophosphamide, although certain herbal remedies have produced considerable problems in recent years. The most commonly implicated analgesic in upper tract urothelial cancer is phenacetin. In a classical study correlating renal pelvic and ureteric tumor development with analgesic use in 170 patients, Steffens and Nagel[30] showed that over 21% of patients that had developed renal pelvic tumors had a history of prolonged and heavy analgesic use, particularly with phenacetin, and there was a direct association in over 11% of patients developing ureteric tumors. The mean latency from the onset of analgesic use to tumor development was 24–26 years. In a further study of upper tract TCC in women,[31] the synergistic association of phenacetin use and papillary necrosis in the development of TCC was shown, with a 20-fold increased risk when the two factors were considered together. The reasons for the toxicity of phenacetin are not fully known but may relate to the fact that one of the main metabolites of phenacetin is 4-acetoaminophenol, a compound with structural similarity to known carcinogens.[32]

The cytotoxic anticancer agent cyclophosphamide is also associated with the development of urothelial TCC.[33] This is thought to relate to the production of the metabolite acrolein.[34] The toxic effects of this drug are minimized in modern usage by administration of high hydration and synchronous administration of the cytoprotective agent MESNA and, as a consequence, the incidence of urinary tract toxicity is much lower in current practice.

A more recent cause of upper tract TCC arising from pharmaceutical usage is the use of specific herbal preparations which induce a condition known as 'Chinese herb nephropathy'. This progressive form of fibrosing nephropathy has developed in a number of Western European countries and is associated with the use of slimming pills containing the herb *Aristolochia fangchi*, a potent carcinogen. In a study of 39 Belgian women that had developed the disease, 18 had overt TCC following removal of the upper urinary tract and, in a further 19, dysplastic changes were seen in the upper urinary tract, the severity of which correlated with the total drug intake.[35] The analysis of tissue removed was consistent with the effects of Aristolochia toxins. Young patients presenting with upper tract TCC should therefore prompt urologists to take a careful history relating to herbal medication usage in the past.

Other etiologic factors include excessive coffee drinking (an overall relative risk of 1.3)[36] and Balkan nephropathy. The latter condition is characterized by development of low-grade, multiple and often bilateral upper tract tumors.[37] The disease is not obviously inherited, nor has an obvious etiologic factor been discovered to date. However, its local incidence can be very high, with a rate of presentation 100 to 200 times greater in some villages than that seen in other towns in the same locality,[37] prompting speculation that this may be due to a carcinogenic agent.

## TUMOR SPREAD

The aggressive nature of upper tract TCC is determined on the basis of its stage and grade, with high-grade tumors having the most aggressive locally invasive and metastatic tendencies.[4,38] Local spread of renal pelvic tumors occurs into the renal parenchyma and renal hilar vessels, while tumors arising in the mid and distal ureter spread into the retroperitoneal and adjacent pelvic structures. The process is characterized by direct invasion or lymphatic and vascular infiltration.[39]

Metastases from upper tract TCC are more common than those from bladder cancer, possibly because the ureteric wall is thinner and therefore more easily penetrated. However, there remains the possibility that this phenomenon may arise because of the innate genetic differences and the tumor biology as discussed above.[22] Overall, metastases occur in 11% of cases,[5] but there is a marked gradation related to tumor grade. In a study by Zincke and Neves, the recurrence rate for grade 1–2 tumors was 5%, while that for grade 3 tumors was 50%.[40] In a second study by Huben et al, low grade tumors had an excellent long-term prognosis, while the median survival for high-grade TCC was only 14 months.[4] The distribution of metastases in such cases is to the retroperitoneal nodes (34%), distal lymph nodes (17%), liver (17%), axial skeleton (13%), and lungs (9%), although various other structures may be affected.[5]

There have been a large number of studies of molecular markers of prognosis in upper tract TCC but, on the whole, these have been disappointing. A number have shown correlation with poor outcome, including association with aneuploidy on flow cytometry,[41] high cell cycling rate as determined by S-phase fraction[42,43] or Ki67 labeling,[44] low p27 levels,[45] and overexpression of p53 alone or in combination with MDM2.[46] Disappointingly, none of these markers has proved to be more reliable than tumor grade in predicting prognosis for this disease.[47]

## DIAGNOSIS AND STAGING

The classical presentation of upper tract TCC is with micro/macroscopic hematuria (75%) or flank pain (33%).[48] Subsequent imaging is usually with intravenous urography (IVU) or contrast computed tomography (CT), which may be supplemented by computer assisted three-dimensional reconstruction of the radiologic images (Figure 22.1). IVU will reveal a

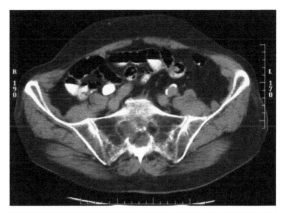

A

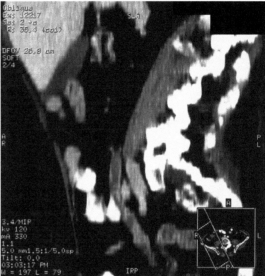

B

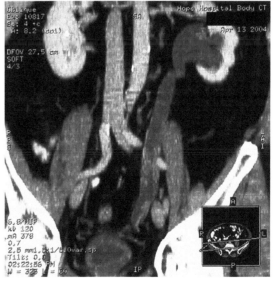

C

**Fig. 22.1**

Three-dimensional reconstruction of upper urinary tract images facilitating diagnosis and treatment planning in ureteric transitional cell carcinoma (TCC). **A, B** Simple lower ureteric TCC, treated by distal ureteric excision and reimplantation. **C** Multiple tumors are visible in the lower and middle thirds of the ureter, in conjunction with hydronephrosis. This patient was treated by nephroureterectomy.

filling defect in 50% to 75% of patients,[49] but this will often need to be distinguished from a benign lesion such as a radiolucent stone, blood clot, ureteritis cystica, or some other benign pathology[50] (Figure 22.2). Supplementary imaging and testing in combination with endoscopy is usually required thereafter to establish the diagnosis definitively. Cystoscopy is essential to exclude a coexistent bladder tumor.

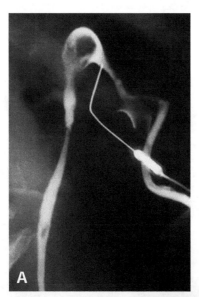

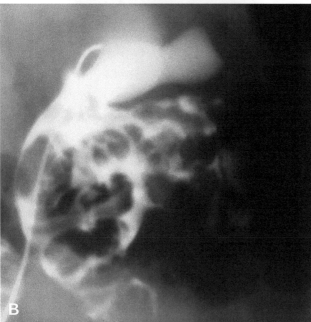

**Fig. 22.2**
The importance of supplementary imaging/cytology/ureteroscopy. **A** Lesion in the renal pelvis on fine needle antegrade contrast imaging. On further investigation, this was proven to be a blood clot. **B** Gross ureteritis cystica mimicking the appearances of a large renal pelvic tumor.

## URINE CYTOLOGY

Notwithstanding the discovery and testing of a variety of novel markers for TCC, none is consistently more reliable than cytology for diagnosis.[51] However, cytology of voided urine in upper urinary tract TCC is also unreliable in low-grade lesions.[52–54] In grade 2 and grade 3 cancers the false-negative rate falls to about 50% and 30%, respectively.[49] However, it is still unreliable to a significant degree, such that, on its own, it is not a sufficiently accurate test on which to base a definitive diagnosis. Bilateral ureteric catheterization and lavage improves accuracy, although this method of urine collection should be stipulated clearly to the cytologist because of errors that can be induced by dislodgement of sheets of cells by the instrumentation.[55] Further specificity is added by the use of brush cytology. In a study of 63% brush cytology specimens from 48 patients with upper tract TCC, the brush technique was more accurate, with a sensitivity of 72% (48% for ureteric lavage) and specificity of 94%.[56] This technique is therefore preferred over and above simple ureteric washing. In the follow-up of patients that have had cystectomy for TCC, urine cytology is a useful diagnostic supplement to imaging in patients with high residual risk of subsequent development of TCC in the upper tract (Figure 22.3).

## DIAGNOSTIC URETEROPYELOSCOPY

Improved technical expertise in instrumentation has enhanced the ability to diagnose upper tract TCC accurately. Although difficulties may be encountered when there is a stricture in the distal ureter, precluding instrumentation, it is often possible using current instrumentation techniques to visualize and biopsy upper tract urothelial lesions directly. In a study that evaluated patients with upper tract TCC investigated by conventional methods (IVU, cystoscopy, ureteric imaging/cytology ± brush sampling), the addition of rigid ureteropyeloscopy increased the diagnostic yield from 58% to 83%.[57] There is an added risk of complications such as ureteric perforation and postoperative stricture formation. Such effects were reported in up to 7% of cases in earlier series using ureteroscopy,[58] although this figure is now much lower following improvements in technique and instrumentation.

Biopsy is possible when lesions are visible and, in a series of 51 patients, there was good correlation (90% in grade 1–2, 92% in grade 3) between the obtained biopsy and the final pathology, although these results only relate to patients in which it was actually possible to obtain tissue from the lesion endoscopically.[59] Perforation of the ureter (or insertion of a nephrostomy tract) does carry a risk of tumor implantation.[60]

In circumstances where there has been previous ureteric surgery, particularly following cystectomy, it

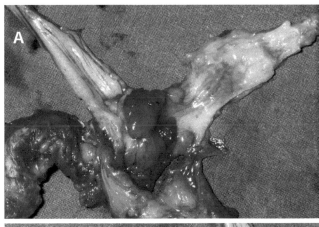

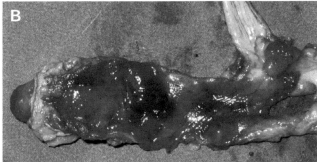

**Fig. 22.3**
**A, B** Ileal loop, ureteroileal anastomosis and distal ureters with recurrent transitional cell carcinoma (TCC) at the urothelial/enteric junction. This patient had multifocal TCC and carcinoma in situ in the bladder, necessitating cystectomy. Her high upper tract risk was monitored with serial urine cytology, with subsequent endoscopy and contrast imaging when the cytology became positive. Treatment was by excision and reconstruction.

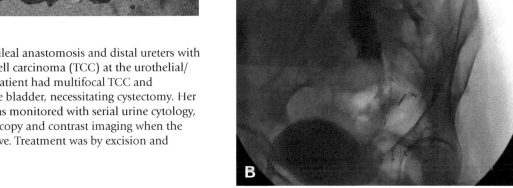

**Fig. 22.4 (opposite)**
Upper tract preservation by conservative strategies in a 70-year-old patient with a lesion in the left upper tract, confirmed as a transitional cell carcinoma (TCC). **A** An incidentally discovered staghorn calculus in a nonfunctioning right kidney. The patient had extensive comorbidity manifest as severe chronic obstructive airways disease. Initial treatment was by local excision and reconstruction of the renal pelvis. Five years later she re-presented with a distal ureteric tumour (**B**) which was managed by distal ureteric excision and reimplantation. Four years later, multifocal TCC obstructed her mid ureter and induced renal failure. Initial treatment by nephrostomy drainage (**C**) enabled serial infusions of BCG via the nephrostomy tube. At 18 months afterwards, ureteric patency is maintained and the TCC remains under control.

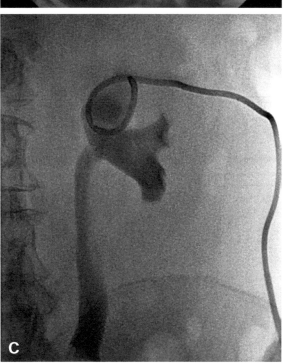

may be possible to pass a flexible ureteroscope over a guide wire in retrograde fashion, enabling diagnosis and treatment of upper tract lesions endoscopically (Figure 22.4). However, approaches involving ureteric instrumentation may be difficult. In circumstances where this is not possible, percutaneous approaches have been reported.[61]

# SURGICAL APPROACH TO UROTHELIAL TUMORS OF THE RENAL PELVIS AND URETER

## RADICAL NEPHROURETERECTOMY

Historically, the standard surgical management of upper urinary tract TCC is total nephroureterectomy with bladder cuff excision.

Although open radical nephroureterectomy with complete ipsilateral ureterectomy has been established and withstood the test of time, in many centers minimally invasive techniques have recently gained in popularity. In the last decade, a laparoscopic approach has been successfully used for the management of such tumors[62,63]; however, an open approach can still be useful in situations where there are complicating factors such as advanced stage or previous surgery.

## OPEN RADICAL NEPHROURETERECTOMY

### Indications
Radical nephroureterectomy with excision of a bladder cuff should be considered for large, high-grade, invasive tumors of the renal pelvis and proximal ureter.[6,47,49,64–70] Radical surgery may also be used for the treatment of medium-grade, noninvasive tumors of the renal pelvis and upper ureter when they are large, multifocal or recurrent.

### Choice of incision
In the open procedure, either two separate incisions—a flank incision and a lower abdominal incision—or one long abdominal incision are required to achieve an intact specimen removal of the affected kidney and ureter. The choice of incision depends on surgeon preference, patient body habitus, medical comorbidities, and the size of the kidney.

### Radical nephrectomy
The kidney should be fully mobilized along with all the perinephric fat and Gerota's fascia. An ipsilateral adrenalectomy may be performed at the same time, but only for parenchyma-invasive tumor. Routine resection is not necessary since this organ is an infrequent site of metastasis for urothelial tumors.[71]

### Distal ureterectomy
The ureter may be kept in continuity with the kidney to avoid the risk of tumor spillage from the lumen or divided if it offers better exposure, provided it is not divided across tumor. The entire distal ureter, including the intramural portion and the ureteral orifice, is removed. This may be done via transvesical, extravesical or combined approaches. The bladder mucosa around the ureteric orifice is incised circumferentially and the intramural ureter is mobilized. The muscle and epithelial defect are closed in two layers with an absorbable suture. The anterior cystotomy (if present) should be closed in a standard manner, and a ureteral catheter maintained for 5–7 days. A drain is left in the perivesical space postoperatively.

Complete endoscopic, transvesical, distal ureterectomy may also be performed and the dissected ureter intussuscepted into the bladder.[72,73] This approach may be useful when it is combined with laparoscopic removal of the kidney, but is of less value for open nephroureterectomy.

### Lymphadenectomy
The exact role of lymphadenectomy is not established but should be included, especially with high-grade lesions. For tumors of the renal pelvis and upper ureter, ipsilateral renal hilar nodes and the adjacent para-aortic or paracaval nodes are resected; for tumors of the distal ureter, an ipsilateral pelvic node dissection should be included. Some limited early studies have shown a survival benefit but other studies show a limited therapeutic value. It may, however, be important for staging and for consideration of chemotherapeutic agents. Extensive retroperitoneal dissections are time consuming and may add to the morbidity, and should be avoided.

### Results
Several studies have shown that final outcome correlates with tumor stage and grade. Because of the high rate of ureteral stump recurrences observed after simple nephrectomy, nephroureterectomy with bladder cuff excision has been the mainstay of treatment of upper urothelial tumors.[74] TCC of the renal pelvis and ureter has a predisposition to recur distal to the site of the original lesion.[74] The risk of tumor recurrence in a remaining ureteral stump is 30% to 75%.[6,68,75–79] This demonstrates that the transvesical dissection of intramural ureter must be done thoroughly to avoid an error. Complete ureterectomy with a bowel cuff should follow nephroureterectomy of a renal unit draining into a urinary diversion. Heney et al[80] reported a tumor recurrence rate of 37.5% when the ureteroenteric anastomosis was not removed.

Radical nephroureterectomy is the gold standard therapy obtaining the best survival results.[68,77,81–83] The rationale for this kind of treatment is the frequency of multifocality, significant ipsilateral recurrences, and relatively low incidence of contralateral involvement.[84]

Batata and Grabstald[64] reported that radical nephroureterectomy provided a 5-year survival rate of 23% among patients with locally advanced disease (stage T3–4, N1–2). Johansson and Wahlqvist[77] reported a survival advantage at 5 years for radical versus simple nephrectomy of 48% versus 51%, respectively, and of 74% versus 37%, respectively, for high-stage patients only. McCarron and associates[68] reported that the subgroup of patients with large, high-grade, but organ-confined disease obtained the most benefit from radical versus conservative surgery. The death rate owing to tumor was 29% versus 89% for the radical and conservative surgery groups, respectively. Murphy et al[49] reported that radical surgery conferred a survival advantage over conservative surgery at 5 years of 88% versus 75% for grade 1 tumors and 90% versus 46% for grade 2 tumors, respectively.

Regional lymphadenectomy at the same time as radical nephroureterectomy is recommended in many reports.[6,47,64–66,68–70,77,80,81,85] However, the authors did not find any great therapeutic value from this, and almost every patient with node-positive disease developed early distant metastases. It serves most importantly as a staging procedure of prognostic significance.

## LAPAROSCOPIC AND RETROPERITONEOSCOPIC RADICAL NEPHROURETERECTOMY

Laparoscopic surgery in urology has been evolving in the last decade, and has been largely employed for ablative procedures involving the kidney and adrenal, and for certain reconstructive procedures such as pyeloplasty.

Nephroureterectomy can be performed transperitoneally, retroperitoneally or hand assisted. The indications for laparoscopic nephroureterectomy are the same as those for open nephroureterectomy. Since Clayman and associates[86] reported the first case of laparoscopic nephroureterectomy in 1991, laparoscopic management of upper tract TCC has gained in popularity, as it is a minimally invasive procedure that does not require a flank incision.

With a laparoscopic-assisted approach, the incision is strategically placed so that the distal ureteral dissection can be done in conjunction with intact specimen removal. Shalhav and coworkers[87] described the transperitoneal approach in 2000; Gill and coworkers[88] first reported retroperitoneoscopic nephroureterectomy for symptomatic end-stage vesicoureteral reflux in 1995; thereafter, they performed retroperitoneoscopic nephroureterectomy for TCC by the retroperitoneal approach.[89] Nakada and associates[90] described the first two clinical cases of hand-assisted laparoscopic

nephrectomy, while Keeley et al[91] described hand-assisted laparoscopic nephroureterectomy in 1999.

Laparoscopic nephroureterectomy, as compared with open nephroureterectomy, has been shown to result in a decrease in blood loss, postoperative pain, and hospitalization.[92–96] In addition, laparoscopic nephroureterectomy is associated with a more rapid recovery time and return to normal activities. Oncologic efficacy, in terms of tumor-free margins and short- to intermediate-term recurrence rates, parallels that of the open approach.[92,93]

All of these approaches have been described, with no clear-cut advantages for any one technique (Matin SF, unpublished). The technique depends on patient factors as well as on surgeon preference.

## TECHNIQUES

### LAPAROSCOPIC-ASSISTED RADICAL NEPHROURETERECTOMY

With laparoscopic-assisted nephroureterectomy, the kidney and proximal ureter are dissected laparoscopically, but a lower abdominal incision is made for continued dissection of the distal ureter and intact specimen removal. The incision decreases both technical complexity and operative times. The incision should be placed so that it can be used for better specimen extraction and distal ureteral dissection.

#### Patient position

The patient is placed supine with the ipsilateral hip and shoulder rotated approximately 15°. The patient is secured to the table and can be easily moved from the flank (nephrectomy portion) to the modified supine position (open portion) by rotating the operating table. A bladder catheter and a nasogastric tube are placed before insufflation of the abdomen for decompression of the bladder and stomach during insufflation, trocar placement, and dissection.

#### Port insertion and configuration

Once a pneumoperitoneum is established, the first 10 or 12 mm port is placed lateral to the rectus muscle at the level of the umbilicus using a visual obturator to allow entry into the abdomen under direct vision. Once in the peritoneal cavity, the visual trocar is removed and the abdomen is then inspected for any injury due to insufflation and to identify adhesions in areas where the secondary ports will be placed. The other trocars (two or three) are placed under direct vision. A 12 mm trocar is placed lateral to the rectus at the level of the umbilicus on the opposite side to the first port. A 10 mm trocar is placed at the umbilicus and a 5 mm port inserted in the midline between the umbilicus and the xiphoid process. With this configuration, the camera is kept at the umbilicus for the entire procedure. The upper midline and lateral trocars are used by the surgeon for the dissection of the kidney and the proximal ureter, while the lower midline, if needed, and lateral trocars are used for dissection of the distal ureter. Sometimes it is necessary to put another trocar (3 mm) just below the xiphoid to help retract the spleen and liver for left and right, respectively.

## Mobilization of the colon

The table should be rotated sufficiently in order to place the patient in the flank position. The peritoneum is incised along the white line of Toldt from the level of the iliac vessels to the hepatic flexure on the right and the splenic flexure on the left. The colon is moved medially.

## Proximal ureteronephrectomy

The proximal ureter is identified, just medial to the lower pole of kidney, and dissected toward the renal pelvis. Distally, the ureter should be dissected as low to the bladder as possible. The renal artery is ligated and divided using a gastrointestinal stapling device. The renal vein is then divided in the same way. With vascular control ensured, the kidney can be dissected free, either inside or outside Gerota's fascia, depending on the tumor location and stage. For upper pole lesions where there is concern that parenchymal invasion may be present, the ipsilateral adrenal should be removed. In the area of primary pathology, surrounding tissue should be removed with the kidney to provide an adequate tumor margin.

## Open distal ureterectomy with excision of bladder cuff

The patient should be rotated back to the horizontal position. Three types of incisions can be used: low midline, Pfanenstiel, or Gibson. Usually, a lower abdominal incision (midline or Pfanenstiel) with anterior cystotomy and bladder cuff excision is used if the ureteral dissection can be carried below the iliac vessels. If, however, the ureteral dissection does not extend into the pelvis, a Gibson incision provides better exposure of the lower half of the ureter. The choice of incision also depends on location of the tumor, the body habitus of the patient, and surgeon preference. Distal ureterectomy is described in the open technique section.

## Approach to the distal ureter

This is one of the bigger controversies in nephroureterectomy performed totally laparoscopically. Currently, there are five different approaches to the lower ureter.[97] One of them, the open technique, is described in laparoscopic-assisted radical nephroureterectomy; the others combine features of laparoscopic and endoscopic management, and include the following.

*Laparoscopic stapling of the distal ureter and bladder cuff*
This technique is often combined with flexible cystoscopy, as described by Shalhav and collaborators.[87] Flexible cystoscopy is performed before the laparoscopic portion of the case begins, and involves placement of a balloon catheter in the intraluminal ureter. The ureter tunnel is incised at the 12 o'clock position. The balloon is removed and the exposed intraluminal ureter, with adjacent bladder mucosa, is fulgurated. This step is important for identification of the distal limits during the laparoscopic portion of the procedure.

*Transvesical laparoscopic detachment and ligation technique*
This approach is described by Gill and collaborators[98] to try to mimic the open technique, with complete excision of the distal ureter and bladder cuff. With a full bladder and the cystoscope in place, two 5 mm balloon-tipped ports are inserted suprapubically into the bladder. A 5 mm Endoloop is placed around the ipsilateral orifice to grasp the ureter. A ureteral catheter is advanced through the Endoloop and up the ureter. A Collings knife is used to incise the bladder cuff circumferentially. A grasper, placed through the contralateral port, serves to retract the orifice. The incision is carried down through the full thickness of the bladder until extraperitoneal fat is seen. The bladder cuff is fulgurated and the Endoloop tail is incised. All instruments are removed, and a Foley catheter is left in place for bladder drainage.

*Transurethral resection of the ureteral orifice and ureteral intussusception*
The resection is carried down to the perivesical fat, facilitating the subsequent approach of the distal ureter during the laparoscopic procedure. Using this technique, McNeill and associates[82] reported similar results between open nephroureterectomy and laparoscopic nephroureterectomy with respect to local tumor control and long-term outcome.

*Ureteral intussusception*
McDonald[72] first described the intussusception ureterectomy in 1953 as a method of removing the ureteral stump at the time of the nephrectomy without an additional incision. It requires extensive transurethral manipulation and does not ensure adequate excision of the intraluminal ureter and bladder cuff. The long-term laparoscopic results using this method are not reported.

The authors prefer the laparoscopic stapling of the distal ureter and bladder cuff approach. After management of the distal ureter, the laparoscopic portion begins, and dissection of the kidney and ureter is performed. The initial approach for the kidney, the proximal ureter, and the midureter is as previously described. Here, however, the dissection of the ureter is continued below the iliac vessels to the intramural ureter and ureteral orifice. The patient should be positioned in Trendelenburg to move the bowel contents out of the pelvis. The bladder is mobilized by transection of the superior vesicle artery and lateral pedicle. The peritoneal incision is extended from the level of the iliac vessels into the pelvis lateral to the bladder and medial to the medial umbilical ligaments. The vas deferens in male patients and the round ligament in female patients is clipped and divided. The detrusor muscle is split and the ureter retracted cephalad. An Endo-GIA stapler then secures the bladder cuff and the distal ureter. The previously created burn in the ureter should be evident, indicating the distal limit of the dissection.

This approach is attractive because the urinary tract is not opened and tumor spillage is minimized. Concerns regarding this approach include the potential for leaving viable urothelial tissue within the staple line[99] which may not be visible with cystoscopic evaluation. Furthermore, the stapled margin cannot be evaluated pathologically. Laparoscopic stapling, with or without unroofing, should not be performed in patients with distal or intramural ureteral tumors, or with perimeatal bladder tumors. The specimen can be removed intact by a small lower abdominal incision.

## Results

Clayman and associates[86] performed the first laparoscopic nephroureterectomy in 1991. Since then, the technical aspects and safety of laparoscopic procedures have been well established. There are several published series of laparoscopic nephro-ureterectomy[87,93,97,100–103]; each varies with regard to approach (transperitoneal versus retroperitoneal) and management of the distal ureter. There is no clear-cut benefit of any one approach with regard to morbidity, cosmesis, or return to activity.

Laparoscopic nephroureterectomy provides some advantages in relation to the open procedure, including fewer pulmonary complications, less postoperative discomfort, a shorter hospital stay, better cosmetic results, and a brief convalescence.

The overall bladder recurrence rate of the combined studies is 16%, which is comparable to that of open nephroureterectomy. In the largest series, Shalhav and colleagues[87] found that, although the laparoscopic procedure requires twice the operating time of open nephroureterectomy, patients had a much shorter recovery time and equivalent outcomes with regard to bladder recurrence, metastatic disease, and cancer-specific survival. Shalhav et al did not describe any case of trocar site or peritoneal seeding after laparoscopy.

In a recent report by Klingler et al,[93] 19 patients treated by laparoscopy presented significantly less postoperative pain and complications, while their final oncologic outcome after 2 years of follow-up was similar to that of patients treated by the open approach.

Historical data have demonstrated the critical importance of distal ureteral excision. Incomplete ureterectomy is associated with a high incidence of recurrence in the ureteral stump and perimeatal bladder mucosa.[76,78,104]

The principles of surgical oncology, such as complete en-bloc resection with avoidance of tumor seeding, dictate the preferred treatment of urothelial cancers.

Oncologically, the open technique remains one of the most reliable and sound procedures. On the other hand, the laparoscopic stapling method keeps the urinary system sealed at all times. Although some ureteral tissue may remain as a result of the staple line, this technique does not appear to present with a high recurrence rate.

Local recurrence and port site seeding are major concerns. There have been three reported instances of port site seeding involving TCC of the upper urinary tract. Two of these cases were discovered after simple nephrectomy for presumed benign disease in which the principles of surgical oncology were inadvertently not followed.[105]

## NEPHRON-SPARING SURGERY

The concept of conservative excision for upper tract urothelial tumors was first introduced by Vest.[106] However, this concept was generally ignored until the early 1970s, when favorable results of conservative surgery were reported in patients with Balkan nephropathy.

Open conservative surgery may be done in select cases where nephron sparing for preservation of renal function is required and they are not candidates for endoscopic management.[6,40,47,66,68,107–115]

Direct endoscopic visualization with cup forceps or brush biopsy of the lesion may establish a definitive diagnosis of the tumor and its grade.[116] However, a preoperative diagnosis of the stage of the renal pelvis tumor remains difficult. Large size, broad base, and nonpapillary pattern favor tumor invasiveness.

Meng and collaborators[117] recently reported two cases of laparoscopic nephrectomy, ex vivo excision, and auto-transplantation for complex renal tumors. This novel approach is feasible when the principles of laparoscopic donor nephrectomy are applied and there is experience with renal transplantation.

### Pyelotomy with tumor ablation

The kidney is exposed via a retro- or transperitoneal approach. After the incision, Gerota's fascia may be opened posteriorly, and the entire kidney is mobilized. For pyelotomy and tumor excision, the renal pelvis and the major calyceal infundibulae are exposed by dissecting the hilar and renal sinus fat as for an extended pyelolithotomy. A curvilinear incision is made in the renal pelvis, and the tumor is excised and the base cauterized with electrocautery, laser, or argon beam coagulator. If an invasive lesion is suspected, the full thickness should be excised if possible. The defect is closed with absorbable sutures and a drain left in place.

## Partial nephrectomy

The technique for renal pelvis tumor is essentially the same as for renal cell carcinoma partial nephrectomy, with the added provision of taking care to minimize the risk of tumor spillage. The involved segment of the intrarenal collecting system should be clamped before removal of the tumor-bearing portion of the kidney is begun. Additional follow-up is necessary to evaluate the effectiveness of this procedure. This should be reserved only for those patients at high risk for dialysis following total nephrectomy.

## Results

Most evidence suggests that, for low-grade, low-stage tumors, equivalent results are achieved with nephron-sparing surgery or nephroureterectomy.[53,118,119]

The reported overall risk of tumor recurrence in the ipsilateral renal pelvis after initial pyelotomy or partial nephrectomy varies from 7% to 60%.[40,47,49,53,109,112] The recurrence rates following conservative resection of a renal pelvis tumor are higher than those following conservative resection of ureteral tumors.[40,109]

Recurrence rates after conservative surgery increase with tumor stage from 10% for grade 1 tumors to 28% for grade 2 tumors and 60% for grade 3 tumors. The moderate to high risk of recurrence primarily reflects the inherent multifocal atypia and the field alteration that occurs in the renal pelvis.[67,68,80,120] Several studies have suggested a good correlation between the grade of TCC and the stage of the tumor.[80] Estimates of overall and cancer-specific survival after conservative surgery of renal pelvis tumors are hampered by the lack of prospective, controlled, randomized trials and the small number of affected patients. Murphy and colleagues reported 5-year survival of 75% and 2-year survival of 46% after conservative surgery in patients with grade 1 and grade 2 renal pelvis tumors, respectively.[53]

Radical nephroureterectomy and dialysis still offer the best chance of cure and survival in patients with a large, invasive, high-grade, organ-confined renal pelvis tumor (T2 N0 M0) in a solitary kidney.[68,111]

## OPEN SEGMENTAL URETERECTOMY

## SEGMENTAL URETERECTOMY WITH URETEROURETEROSTOMY

This approach is indicated for noninvasive low-grade tumors of the proximal ureter or midureter tumors that are too large for complete endoscopic ablation.

Alternatively, it may be used for high-grade or invasive tumors when renal preservation is necessary.

## Technique

A transperitoneal or extraperitoneal approach may be used. The tumor is located and ligated 1–2 cm proximal and distal to the tumor. The involved ureteral segment should be sent for frozen section to confirm the diagnosis and to verify the absence of tumor at the margins. The ureteral ends are spatulated and anastomosed with interrupted absorbable sutures. A ureteral stent and a periureteral drain are placed for 4 weeks.

## DISTAL URETERECTOMY WITH DIRECT NEOCYSTOSTOMY OR URETERONEOCYSTOSTOMY WITH A BLADDER PSOAS MUSCLE HITCH OR A BOARI FLAP

This approach is recommended for appropriate tumors located in the distal ureter that cannot be removed completely by endoscopic means.[6,8,47,70,75,110,121]

## Technique

A lower midline incision is used to approach the distal ureter and bladder for the ureteral excision and the repair. The distal ureterectomy is performed as described in the section on radical nephroureterectomy. Direct ureteroneocystostomy may be possible if only a short segment of the juxtavesical and intramural ureter is removed. Additional techniques are required when the entire distal ureter is removed. A nonrefluxing anastomosis is not necessary.

### Bladder psoas muscle hitch

The contralateral superior vesical attachments are freed and an anterior cystotomy is created. The bladder is then mobilized upward over the iliac vessels to the psoas muscle at the level of the iliac crest. The bladder is secured to the psoas muscle and tendon using nonabsorbable sutures. The ureteral end is spatulated and brought through an opening in the uppermost portion of the bladder. A refluxing or nonrefluxing anastomosis is performed by placing the ureter in a mucosal trough or tunnel if there is sufficient ureteral length. An indwelling ureteral stent, Foley catheter, and a drain in the perivesical space are placed in all cases. Insertion of a suprapubic catheter is optional.

### Boari flap

This may be indicated in cases where the anastomosis is significantly above the iliac vessels and a psoas hitch approach is insufficient to perform an anastomosis. If the need for a Boari flap is anticipated, the incisions for the flap should be marked before making the cystotomy and psoas hitch. The spatulated end of the ureter is anastomosed to the cephalad end of the bladder flap, the bladder tube is folded and closed in two layers.

These techniques may be more difficult with prior bladder surgery, radiation or in those with limited bladder capacity.

## URETERECTOMY WITH ILEAL SUBSTITUTION

This approach is rarely indicated but may be useful for tumors that involve long ureteral segments where renal preservation is necessary and when neither uretero-ureterostomy nor bladder mobilization is feasible

### Technique

A suitable length of ileum to bridge the gap is selected. The proximal ileal segment is anastomosed to the renal pelvis, and the distal ileum is connected to the bladder. The vermiform appendix has also been used for segmental ureteral substitution.[122]

### Results

In the past, some authors recommended radical nephroureterectomy for all patients with upper tract urothelial tumors; others suggested segmental ureterectomy only for patients with low-grade, noninvasive tumors of the distal ureter.[6]

The overall survival for only ureteral tumors is related to stage and grade regardless of the extent of surgical treatment. Overall 5-year survival is excellent for patients with grade 1 and 2 noninvasive ureteral tumors. Three large series correlate stage and grade with survival. Five-year survival remains approximately 50% for patients with stage T2 disease but falls dramatically for stage T3. Anderstrom et al reported no tumor-related deaths and only one recurrence among 21 patients treated with segmental ureterectomy for low-grade, noninvasive ureteral tumors who were followed for a median of 83 months.[8]

The risk of ipsilateral recurrence after conservative treatment of ureteral tumors is 33% to 55%.[6,68,70,109,110] Most recurrences are distal to the original lesion, but proximal recurrences are also seen.[82] The risk for recurrence and the need for follow-up are lifelong.[123] Grossman reported a stage T2 local recurrence in a patient 16 years after segmental ureterectomy and ureteroureterostomy for a grade 1, stage Ta, midureteral tumor.[124]

### Final recommendations

Segmental ureterectomy is offered for low-grade, low-stage tumors of the proximal ureter or midureter that are not amenable to complete ablation by endoscopic means owing to size or multiplicity. Segmental excision of the distal or mid ureter should be considered, provided this conservative approach does not compromise the tumor resection margin and provided that functional reconstruction can be carried out. It may be considered for higher grade, higher stage lesions if renal failure and dialysis are a consideration with removal of the entire renal unit.

## ENDOSCOPIC TREATMENT

Hugh Hampton Young described the first endoscopic evaluation of the upper urinary tract in 1912. Subsequent advances in endoscopic technology with the development of better optics, flexible instruments, actively deflecting telescopes, and adjunctive instrumentation allowed us to reach all parts of the urinary tract with minimal morbidity, either by antegrade or retrograde approaches, permitting us to diagnose and stage more accurately those patients with upper urinary TCC.

Both ureteroscopic (retrograde) and percutaneous (antegrade) tumor resection are possible and are used in selected centers for up to 15% of patients with upper urinary TCC.[125] The approach selected depends largely on the tumor location and size. In general, a retrograde ureteroscopic approach is used for low volume ureteral and renal tumors, whereas the antegrade percutaneous approach is chosen for larger tumors located proximally in the renal pelvis and/or upper ureter, and those that cannot be adequately manipulated in a retrograde approach owing to difficult location.

## URETEROSCOPIC RESECTION

The first ureteroscopic approach for the management of urothelial tumors was described in the early 1980s. The main advantages of this management are lower morbidity and maintenance of a closed system, without the risk of tumor seeding. However, the disadvantages, related to the need for small instruments and a small field of view and working channels, limit the size of tumor that can be approached in a retrograde fashion. For this reason, this approach is generally favored for small-sized tumors.

Another limiting factor for this approach is the difficulty in accurately assessing the entire urothelium and being able to perform the same type of endoscopic resection commonly performed in the bladder. Perhaps, with the recent improvements in instrumentation, the indications for therapeutic ureteropyeloscopy can be broadened to include treatment of select, complex patients with upper urinary tract urothelial tumors.[126]

### Instrumentation

A large variety of ureteroscopic instruments are available, each with its own distinct advantages and disadvantages. Generally, rigid ureteroscopes are used primarily for the distal ureter and mid ureter, while flexible ureteropyeloscopes are preferred in the upper ureter and kidney where the rigid ureteroscope cannot be reliably passed, especially in the male patient. Larger, rigid ureteroscopes provide better visualization because of their larger field of view and better irrigation. Smaller rigid ureteroscopes (8 Fr.) generally do not require active dilation of the ureteral orifice. Modern flexible ureteropyeloscopes are available in sizes smaller than 8 Fr. to allow for simple and reliable passage to most portions of the urinary tract.[127,128] Otherwise, flexible ureteroscopes have technical limitations, such as a small working channel, which limits irrigant flow and impairs the facility to insert working instruments along the telescope.

## Energy source

Endoscopic resection of ureteral tumors is based on either electrocautery or laser energy.

### Electrocautery

If this energy source is employed, sorbitol or glycine irrigant should be used, and the cutting current maintained at the lowest setting that will produce adequate resection of tumor. The variable depth of penetration can make its use in the ureter quite dangerous, and circumferential fulguration should be avoided owing to the high risk of stricture formation. Pure cut without blend and no coagulation during the tumor resection may help minimize postoperative stricture. Electrocautery is used via a small Bugbee electrode (2 or 3 Fr.).

### Laser

More recently, laser energy with either neo-dymium:yttrium–argon–garnet (Nd:YAG)[129,130] or holmium:YAG[131,132] sources have become popular. Each has characteristic advantages and can be delivered through small, flexible fibers (200 or 365 μm) that fit through small, flexible ureteroscopes without significantly altering irrigant flow or scope deflection. The holmium:YAG laser is well suited for use in the ureter. The tissue penetration is less than 0.5 mm, which allows for tumor ablation with excellent hemostasis and minimal risk of full-thickness injury to the ureter. Its shallow penetration may, however, make its use cumbersome with larger tumors, especially in the renal pelvis. Settings most commonly used for holmium:YAG are energy of 0.6–1 joule with a frequency of 10 Hz. The Nd:YAG laser has a tissue penetration of up to 5–6 mm depending on laser settings and duration of treatment. In contrast to the holmium:YAG laser, which ablates tumor, the Nd:YAG laser works by coagulative necrosis with subsequent sloughing of the necrotic tumor. The safety margin is significantly lower and this can limit its use in the ureter, where the ureteral wall is quite thin. Settings most commonly used for the Nd:YAG laser are 15 watts for 2 seconds for ablating tumor and 5–10 watts for 2 seconds for coagulation.

## Steps

First, the bladder should be inspected with a standard rigid cystoscope for concomitant bladder pathology, and a sample of urine sent for cytologic analysis. The ureteral orifice is identified and inspected for lateralizing hematuria. A small diameter ureteroscope (6.9 or 7.5 Fr.) is carefully passed directly into the ureteral orifice, and the distal ureter is inspected for any trauma from a previously placed guide wire or dilation. A guide wire is then placed through the ureteroscope and up the ureter to the level of the renal pelvis under fluoroscopic guidance. The flexible instrument is used to inspect the more proximal ureter and intrarenal collecting system. The urothelium is then mapped, and, if a lesion or suspicious area is seen, a normal saline washing of the area is performed before biopsy or intervention.[133] If the ureter does not accept the smaller ureteroscope, active dilation of the ureter is necessary.

## Biopsy and stage

Tumor sampling and biopsies are then performed with either a 2.5 flat wire basket or a 3 Fr. cup biopsy forceps. Regardless of the technique used, special attention to biopsy specimens is essential. Specimens are frequently minute; they should be placed in fixative at once and specially labeled for either histologic or cytologic evaluation.[134] Tumor grading in this setting is very accurate and is 90% in conformity with the grade of the final pathologic specimen.

Unfortunately, ureteroscopic biopsy is unreliable in determining stage.[135] However, several studies have suggested an excellent correlation between the grade of TCC and the stage of the tumor,[80,136] and high accuracy of the CT scan in detecting evidence of tumor extending beyond the wall of the ureter or renal pelvis.[137] Therefore, the combination of low grade on biopsy and absence of frank extension outside the urinary tract on CT scan strongly suggests that the disease is superficial.[138,139] Retrospective reviews of patients that underwent ureteroscopic biopsy followed by nephro-ureterectomy found the accuracy of ureteroscopic diagnosis to be 89% to 94%,[140,141] and the pathologic grading to match the open surgical technique in 78% to 92%.[142,143] This information supports the notion that tumor grade is the most important prognostic factor and that, although stage cannot be directly assessed, noninvasive disease can be expected in most low-grade tumors. These criteria create a new subset of patients with small, low-grade tumors that can potentially be managed by endoscopic management only, even in the presence of a healthy contralateral kidney.[140]

## Definitive treatment (ureteroscopic technique)

Generally three approaches can be used for tumor ablation: bulk excision with ablation of the base, resection of the tumor to its base, or diagnostic biopsy followed by ablation with electrocautery or laser energy sources. The tumor is debulked using either grasping forceps or a flat wire basket engaged adjacent to the tumor. Next, the tumor base is treated with either electrocautery or laser energy sources. This technique is especially useful for low-grade papillary tumors on a narrow stalk. The specimen is sent for pathologic evaluation.

A ureteroscopic resectoscope is used to remove the tumor. Only the intraluminal tumor is resected, and no attempt is made to resect deep (beyond the lamina propria). Extra care is necessary in the mid and upper ureter, where the wall is quite thin and prone to perforation. Ureteral resectoscopes are approximately 12 Fr. and require more extensive dilation of the ureteral orifice. With larger volume disease of the distal ureter, Jarrett and associates[141] described extensive dilation of the ureter followed by resection with a long standard resectoscope. The tumor is adequately biopsied with forceps and sent to the pathology laboratory for diagnostic evaluation. The tumor bulk is then ablated to its base using laser or electrosurgical energy, as described above.

## Results

### Tumor control

Multiple series have shown the safety and efficacy of ureteroscopic treatment of upper tract TCC. Martinez-Pineiro and colleagues[125] determined that the success rate of ureteroscopic therapy for grade 1–2 tumor is similar to bladder lesions of the same grade treated endoscopically, while no deep tumor invasion was seen in any of the patients with low-grade lesions. Tumor recurrence rates ranged from 27% for grade 1 tumors to 40% for grade 2 tumors. Similarly, Keeley and associates[59] showed a recurrence rate of 26% for grade 1 tumors and 44% for grade 2 tumors, which roughly correlated with previously established recurrence rates for open conservative surgery.

In a literature review of 205 patients,[139] the overall recurrence rates for ureteral and renal pelvic lesions were 33% and 31.2%, respectively, and the risk of bladder recurrence was 43%.

In a recent review by Chen and Bagley,[144] 15 of 23 patients with contralateral normal kidneys, treated ureteroscopically for upper TCC, had multiple recurrences. All were retreated ureteroscopically, and all were alive without evidence of progression. Elliott et al[126] only defined subsequent tumor progression in those patients with higher grade lesions.

A final oncologic concern is whether ureteroscopy promotes progression or spread of disease to other urothelial surfaces or metastatic sites. Kulp et al[145] reported on 13 patients that underwent multiple ureteroscopic treatments followed by nephro-ureterectomy. They found no unusual propagation of TCC in the specimens. Similarly, Hendin and colleagues[146] reported no increased risk of metastatic disease in a group of patients that underwent ureteroscopy before nephroureterectomy when compared to the group undergoing nephroureterectomy alone.

### Complications

Complications associated with retrograde ureteroscopic treatment are uncommon and have decreased with improved instrumentation and refined technique.[147] Complications specific to ureteroscopic therapy include ureteral perforation and stricture. The major long-term sequela of vigorous endoscopic therapy is postoperative ureteral stricture. This is frequently not secondary to ureteroscopic exploration but due to the type of energy used—Nd:YAG laser energy creates a deep coagulative effect (1 cm or greater). Schmeller and Hofstetter[130] published a series of upper tract urothelial tumors treated with Nd:YAG laser and found a significant ureteral stricture rate of 25%. Razvi et al[132] published the initial experience with holmium:YAG laser energy in treating upper urinary tract urothelial lesions and defined a lower stricture rate than with Nd:YAG laser energy.

## PERCUTANEOUS RESECTION

Tomera et al described the first percutaneous approach for the management of urothelial tumors in 1982.[113] The main advantage of the percutaneous approach is the ability to remove a larger tumor volume from any portion of the collecting system due to the use of instruments with larger working channels, which allow better visualization and faster resection. For this reason, percutaneous access is preferred for larger tumors located proximally in the renal pelvis and/or upper ureter. Deeper biopsies can be obtained when compared to those taken with ureteroscopy, while the percutaneous approach may avoid the limitations encountered even by flexible ureteroscopy, especially in complicated calyceal systems or areas difficult to access, such as the lower pole calyx or the upper urinary tract of patients with urinary diversion. Finally, with a percutaneous approach, the established nephrostomy tract can be maintained for immediate postoperative nephroscopy and administration of topical adjuvant therapy.

The main disadvantage with antegrade access is the increased morbidity compared with ureteroscopy. Nephrostomy tube placement has inherent risks and therefore requires inpatient admission. In addition, loss of urothelial integrity and exposure of nonurothelial surfaces to tumor cells carries the risk for tumor seeding along the nephrostomy tract.[60]

### Patient positioning, stent placement

After induction of general anesthesia the patient should be flipped and placed in the prone position on the operating table where flexible cystoscopy is performed and a ureteral catheter placed up to the renal pelvis. The use of the flexible cystoscope allows the surgeon to evaluate the bladder and catheterize the ureter even after the patient has been moved in the prone position. Alternatively, the ureteral catheter may be placed while the patient is in the supine position immediately after anesthesia. Finally, the patient is prepped and draped in the standard sterile fashion.

## Establishment of the nephrostomy tract

To define the calyceal anatomy and tumor location, injection of contrast through the ureteral catheter is necessary. A percutaneous nephrostomy tract is performed through the desired calyx. In some cases additional percutaneous accesses are required for complete resection of the tumor. Access under the 12th rib is usually preferred. Supracostal approaches may be used if necessary but at the risk of pleural injury. Tumors in peripheral calyces are best approached with direct puncture distal to the tumor. Disease in the renal pelvis and upper ureter is best approached through an upper or middle pole access to allow scope maneuvering through the collecting system and down the ureteropelvic junction. After a needle is passed through the desirable calyx and a guide wire is manipulated preferably down the ureter, the tract is then dilated using either sequential (Amplatz) or balloon dilation so as to accommodate a 30 Fr. sheath. Access to the desired calyx and correct positioning of the nephrostomy tract are key determinants of success of this procedure.

Once the 30 Fr. sheath is in place, the nephroscope is inserted, and the ureteral catheter is grasped, brought out of the tract, and exchanged for a stiff guide wire, thus providing both antegrade and retrograde control. This is the second safety guide wire and helps maintain access, should the original wire be inadvertently removed.

## Biopsy and definitive therapy

Through the 30 Fr. inner diameter nephrostomy sheath, which is used to maintain a low-pressure system, the collecting system is evaluated thoroughly using rigid and flexible endoscopes when necessary. After identification, the tumors can be removed by one of the following techniques.

### Biopsy with cold-cup forceps

Cold-cup biopsies of the tumor and surrounding mucosa can be performed to evaluate the extent of the disease and to rule out the possibility of carcinoma in situ (CIS). This can be done through a standard nephroscope. The bulk of the tumor is grasped using forceps and removed in piecemeal fashion until the base is reached. A separate biopsy of the base is performed for staging purposes and the base is cauterized using a Bugbee electrode and cautery. Low-grade papillary lesions on a thin stalk are easily treated in this manner with minimal bleeding.

### Biopsy with cut loop

Alternatively, a cutting loop from a standard resectoscope is used to remove the tumor to its base. Because of the relatively small capacity of the renal pelvis, the specimen must be removed after each loop and irrigation drained in order to keep visualization optimal and prevent migration of the specimen. Once again, the base should be resected and sent separately for staging purposes. This approach is more effective for larger, broad-based tumors for which simple debulking to a stalk is not possible. The resection should be done carefully since the pelvicalyceal system lacks a thick muscle layer and, therefore, perforation with parenchymal and vascular injury is always possible.

### Biopsy with laser

For the third technique, a holmium:YAG or Nd:YAG laser (at settings of 25–30 and 15–20 watts, respectively, for 3-second exposures) can be used to biopsy and ablate the tumor.

Other means of tumor resection have been used but in a smaller number of patients. Nakada and Clayman[148] reported the use of electrovaporization using high levels of pure cut energy for ablation of relatively large tumors. Electrovaporization was found to be effective, safe, fast, and simple in use, but cold-cup biopsies were necessary before the treatment in order to establish a diagnosis.

Finally, at the end of the procedure, a 24 Fr. nephrostomy tube is always left in place. This access can be used for second look follow-up nephroscopy to ensure complete tumor removal.

## Second look nephroscopy

Follow-up nephroscopy is performed 4–14 days later to allow for adequate healing. The tumor site is identified and any residual tumor is removed. If no tumor is identified, the base should be biopsied and treated using cautery or the holmium:YAG laser (15–20 watts and 3-second exposures) because of its very superficial effect. The nephrostomy tube can be removed several days later if all tumors have been resected. Some authors advocate a third look with random biopsies before the nephrostomy tube is finally removed.[149] If the patient is being considered for adjuvant topical therapy, then a small 8 Fr. nephrostomy tube is left to provide access for instillations. The nephrostomy tube is removed after the patient successfully tolerates clamping of the tube for several hours. A nephrostogram can be performed to rule out extravasation but is not routinely performed in our institution.

## Results

### Tumor control

Conservative management of upper urinary tract urothelial tumors requires life-long vigilant follow-up for recurrence in the site of primary resection or elsewhere in the upper urinary tract. Recurrence in the bladder is seen in 30% to 50% of patients and requires cystoscopic surveillance.

Local control can be achieved with the percutaneous approach but long-term results vary from study to study due to the diversity of patient characteristics, follow-up patterns, and the small number of patients in these cohorts. Comparisons are tampered from the viewpoint of selection bias since some studies treat all patients, whereas others treat only patients with a bad prognosis and a history of highly recurrent disease. When comparing results to the gold standard nephro-ureterectomy, the possibility of understaging of conservatively treated patients should be borne in mind since pathologic staging is not available in all cases.

What has been shown invariably is that tumor grade is the strongest prognostic indicator of recurrence and cancer-related deaths. Recurrence rates increased with increasing grade and the only cancer-related deaths were in patients with grade 3 disease. In a study by Jarrett et al,[149] grade 1, 2, and 3 tumors recurred in 18%, 33%, and 50% of patients, respectively. Similarly, time of recurrence depends on tumor grade, with high-grade tumors recurring faster than low grade ones.

Grade 1 tumors generally have a good prognosis. Recurrence rates after percutaneous management are relatively low and comparable to those presented with nephroureterectomy. Excellent results for grade 1 tumors with recurrence rates of 0% to 29% and a disease-specific survival of 100% have been reported by many authors.[143,149,150]

Results with grade 2 tumors are variable, and although progression of grade 2 tumors does not exceed 11% according to the National Bladder Cancer Group, ipsilateral recurrence[49] is frequent after open conservative surgery. It is for this reason that percutaneous management of these tumors is still controversial. Local recurrence rates for grade 2 tumors after percutaneous management vary from 6% to 40%, while disease-specific survival ranges from 80% to 100%. Stage for this subset of tumors can further distinguish prognosis. Ta grade 2 tumors progress in 6% to 20% of cases, while similar grade T1 tumors progress in 21% to 40%.[61,125,126,139,149,151–153] The disease-specific survival is similarly affected, with Ta and T1 grade 2 tumors having 100% and 80% rates, respectively. With Ta tumors, all recurrences are superficial and easily treatable, and only 5% progress to invasive and metastatic disease. Previous history of TCC in the upper urinary tract or bladder is also an important factor and might account for higher recurrence rates.[154]

Grade 3 tumors have a bad prognosis, which is independent of the approach followed. The recurrence rate is as high as 56%, with 5-year survival rates near 60%.[153] These patients are best served by nephroureterectomy unless medically contraindicated.

Tumor stage overall is not as reliable in predicting outcome since disease progression and death from metastasis was also seen in a patient with T1 grade 3 disease. Existing data show that survival can also be directly related to DNA ploidy status,[41] but this is not used in everyday practice.

Resection modality does not influence success of conservative management. Nd:YAG laser success rates are comparable to those obtained after electro-resection,[126,149,155] although some authors had higher recurrence rates when lasers were used and, therefore, are less enthusiastic about this option.[125]

In conclusion, percutaneous management is acceptable in patients with low-grade disease regardless of the status of the contralateral kidney, provided the patient is committed to life-long endoscopic follow-up. Patients with grade 3 disease do poorly regardless, and should probably undergo nephroureterectomy in order to maximize cancer cure. The largest area of controversy is in percutaneous management of patients with grade 2 disease and a normal contralateral kidney. Some studies present acceptable results for the conservative treatment of noninvasive grade 2 disease, others do not.

## Complications

The percutaneous approach is more invasive than ureteroscopy and several complications may occur. In most cases they are similar to those induced during percutaneous surgery for benign reasons.

Bleeding was the most commonly reported complication in a series of 34 patients with upper TCC treated percutaneously[149]: 52.9% required transfusion, 11.7% needed further embolization, and 5.8% finally underwent salvage nephroureterectomy after interventional radiology failed. Blood loss was seen to be directly related to tumor grade. This seems reasonable, since higher grade tumors are usually of higher stage and require more extensive resection.

Usually the percutaneous approach is used for relatively large tumors, where deeper resection is often necessary. Deeper resection carries the risk of perforation and vascular injury. Although the latter can usually be managed conservatively by leaving the nephrostomy tube in place, with perforation, the risk for potential extraluminal seeding, particularly alongside the nephrostomy tract, theoretically exists. Tomera et al[113] first reported local recurrence after open pyeloscopy for filling defects of unclear etiology despite the fact that nephroureterectomy was performed immediately after the diagnosis of TCC was made. The fact that recurrence occurred even for low-grade tumors suggested that pyeloscopy led to seeding of the tumor. Although there are several more reports of nephrostomy tract infiltration with high-grade tumors,[60,156] there was no tract seeding reported in large contemporary series,[61,149,150,156] implying that this event is possible but very rare. Some authors use sterile water as the irrigant for its cytolytic effect[157] in an attempt to prevent seeding of the tract. Alternatively, irradiation of the access tract with an iridium wire or a commercial high-dose rate radiation delivery system has been used[158,159] with good results and acceptable morbidity. A potential but rare complication is the development of a urinary cutaneous fistula that can lead to a nephroureterectomy.[150]

Complications such as hemothorax and hydrothorax have been reported. Avoiding intercostal punctures by using the triangulation or renal displacement technique allows us to avoid entering the pleural space.[149,150] Stricture formation is a long-term complication of percutaneous management. The risk is probably greater for extensive tumors, particularly if they are located near the ureteropelvic junction or the entire circumference of the ureter. The overall incidence of stricture formation with percutaneous management is lower compared to the ureteroscopic approach.

Injury of adjacent solid or hollow viscera can occur but is very rare. For example, only one case of colonic perforation exists in the literature, and was managed conservatively.[125] Water absorption and dilutional hyponatremia can occur and are treated as usual with furosemide and saline infusion.

Overall complications increase in number and severity with higher tumor grade. This finding is likely due to the more extensive pathology and treatments necessary to eradicate the tumor. However, when compared to open or laparoscopic procedures, overall endoscopic management was superior in terms of morbidity.[119]

## TOPICAL CHEMO- AND IMMUNOTHERAPY FOR UPPER TRACT TCC

The adoption of ablative endourologic surgery for upper tract TCC has also been accompanied by the development of experience with the use of topical chemo- or immunotherapy in the management of these tumors. This therapeutic modality has been used both as monotherapy and in combination as adjuvant treatment with percutaneous or ureteroscopic resection.[160] Therapy of this type may be appropriate in situations where there is multifocality (particularly where there is bilateral disease or in multifocal tumor in a single nephron unit), where there is multifocal CIS in the upper tract, or where the degree of comorbidity precludes a more aggressive surgical approach in the first instance. A variety of agents have been used in this approach, including mitomycin C, thiotepa, adriamycin, and interferon; however, the most commonly used therapy has been bacillus Calmette–Guérin (BCG).[161]

Administration of the active agents may be via antegrade or retrograde routes. The antegrade route involves the placement of a nephrostomy tube and use of a volumetric pump or gravity fed infusion. Some authors have advocated the use of manometric control: in a study using mitomycin C, Eastham and Huffman[162] maintained the infusion pressure at a level below 25 cm of water on the hypothetical basis that this would keep the pressure below that in the renal pelvis. While this seems a sensible precaution to minimize the risk of extravasation, it is probably not necessary if modern infusion pumps are used, since these are pressure controlled. The retrograde administrative route involves placement of a ureteric catheter and direct infusion (a particularly useful technique in patients with superficial upper tract TCC following ileal conduit diversion), or instillation of the therapeutic drug into the bladder with a ureteric stent in place and the patient in the Trendelenburg position. This relies on vesicoureteral reflux to get the agent into the appropriate location.[163]

Evaluating the true efficacy of this therapy is difficult, as the data relating to this modality of treatment are drawn from case series with small numbers of patients. There is no class 1 evidence from randomized controlled trials. In an early report, Herr reported the use of BCG in a single patient with multifocal tumor, including a pT2 grade 3 lesion in the renal pelvis. Removal of the renal pelvic tumor and autotransplantation was followed by six weekly courses of intravesical BCG without clinical incident. The patient was tumor-free 13 months after surgery.[164] In a subsequent study using BCG as monotherapy, Studer et al treated eight patients with upper tract CIS with percutaneous administration via a nephrostomy tube: in seven patients the urine cytology became negative,[165] but the long-term effect of treatment was not reported. In a further study, Nishino et al[166] treated six patients via a 6 Fr. indwelling ureteral catheter or an 8 Fr. indwelling J stent. All had CIS diagnosed cytologically and all had 4–8 weeks' treatment without early adverse side effects. Five of the six remained clear cytologically although two went on to develop ureteral strictures. Another study of similar design treated 11 patients with weekly BCG for 6 weeks after placement of a 6 Fr. ureteral stent[167]; nine patients had normalization of the urine cytology although two subsequently failed. The mean recurrence-free time was 19.6 months. Eight of the patients (72%) exhibited bladder irritability and four had a fever of 38°C following instillation, although none required antituberculous treatment.

A number of reports have also documented the use of BCG as an adjunct to percutaneous resection. In a study of 10 patients with TCC arising in solitary kidneys,[155] treatment was by initial percutaneous resection followed by adjuvant intravesical BCG via an indwelling nephrostomy tube. Six of the 10 patients treated in this way showed no evidence of disease recurrence at 19 months. Further studies of adjuvant therapy following initial resection have reported recurrence rates varying between 12.5% and 28%; however, details of tumor type are variable in some of these reports, making interpretation difficult.[161] In one of the largest series,[160] 34 patients were treated with percutaneous resection followed by topical chemotherapy or immunotherapy, following which they were monitored by a combination of ureteroscopy, intravenous urography, and cross-sectional imaging. Recurrence developed in 41% over a median follow-up of 51 months with a median time to recurrence of 24 months. Overall, however, the kidney preservation rate was 73%. Multifocality, the presence of CIS in the bladder, and the presence of tumor in the renal pelvis were associated with a significant increase in the risk of recurrence. The authors concluded that percutaneous surgery in combination with adjuvant chemo/immunotherapy is a valid option, but that post-treatment surveillance must be long term and must be observed strictly.

The question of whether BCG is superior to standard cytotoxic chemotherapy in the upper tract remains unresolved. Both modalities seem to be effective in some patients and the side effect profile is acceptable. In a study of 42 patients with upper tract TCC treated endourologically, the recurrence rate was 24%. Although this was reduced by the addition of adjuvant treatment, mitomycin C and BCG seemed to be equally efficacious. The recurrence rate was reduced to 12.5% in those patients receiving BCG, whereas in those receiving mitomycin C, the recurrence rate was 14%.[125]

In conclusion, topical therapy for upper tract TCC can be administered safely and effectively. It may be administered by the antegrade or retrograde route, and although BCG has been used most widely, it is not clear whether it confers an advantage over standard chemotherapy. If topical chemo- or immunotherapy is used, long-term follow-up by cytology, imaging, and repeated ureteroscopy is necessary as the tumors have a tendency to recur in a significant number of patients.

## REFERENCES

1. Petersen RO. Renal pelvis. In Biello LA (ed): Urologic Pathology. Philadelphia: Lippincott, 1986, pp 181–228.
2. The British Association of Urological Surgeons Cancer Registry. Analyses of Minimum Dataset, September–October 2001. London: BAUS Cancer Registry, 2001.
3. Fraley E. Cancer of the renal pelvis. In Skinner DG, De Kernion JB (eds): Genitourinary Cancer. Philadelphia: WB Saunders, 1978, p 134.
4. Huben RP, Mounzer AM, Murphy GP. Tumor grade and stage as prognostic variables in upper tract urothelial tumors. Cancer 1988;62(9):2016–2020.
5. Khan AN, Chandramohan H. Transitional cell carcinoma. 2005. Online. Available: www.eMedicine.com.
6. Babaian RJ, Johnson DE. Primary carcinoma of the ureter. J Urol 1980;123(3):357–359.
7. National Cancer Institute (US). Division of Cancer Prevention and Control, et al. Annual cancer statistics review. Washington, DC: National Cancer Advisory Board, 1987, p 2789.
8. Anderstrom C, Johansson SL, Pettersson S, Wahlqvist L. Carcinoma of the ureter: a clinicopathologic study of 49 cases. J Urol 1989;142(2 Pt 1):280–283.
9. Harris AL, Neal DE. Bladder cancer—field versus clonal origin. N Engl J Med 1992;326(11):759–761.
10. McCarron JP Jr, Chasko SB, Gray GF Jr. Systematic mapping of nephroureterectomy specimens removed for urothelial cancer: pathological findings and clinical correlations. J Urol 1982;128(2):243–246.
11. Murphy WM, Busch C, Algaba F. Intraepithelial lesions of urinary bladder: morphologic considerations. Scand J Urol Nephrol Suppl 2000;205:67–81.
12. Charbit L, Cendearu MC, Mee S, Cukier J. Tumors of the upper urinary tract: 10 years of experience. J Urol 1991;146(5):1243–1246.
13. Shinka T, Uekado Y, Aoshi H, et al. Occurrence of uroepithelial tumors of the upper urinary tract after the initial diagnosis of bladder cancer. J Urol 1988;140(4):745–748.
14. Oldbring J, Glifberg I, Mikulowski P, et al. Carcinoma of the renal pelvis and ureter following bladder carcinoma: frequency, risk factors and clinicopathological findings. J Urol 1989;141(6):1311–1313.
15. Abercrombie GF, Earley I, Payne SR, Walmsley BH, Vinnicombe J. Modified nephro-ureterectomy. Long-term follow-up with particular reference to subsequent bladder tumours. Br J Urol 1988;61(3):198–200.
16. Lynch HT, Ens JA, Lynch JF. The Lynch syndrome II and urological malignancies. J Urol 1990;143(1):24–28.
17. Watson P, Lynch HT. Extracolonic cancer in hereditary nonpolyposis colorectal cancer. Cancer 1993;71(3):677–685.
18. Watson P, Lynch HT. The tumor spectrum in HNPCC. Anticancer Res 1994;14(4B):1635–1639.
19. Vasen HF, Watson P, Mecklin JP, Lynch HT. New clinical criteria for hereditary nonpolyposis colorectal cancer (HNPCC, Lynch syndrome) proposed by the International Collaborative Group on HNPCC. Gastroenterology 1999;116(6):1453–1456.
20. Greenland JE, Weston PM, Wallace DM. Familial transitional cell carcinoma and the Lynch syndrome II. Br J Urol 1993;72(2):177–180.
21. Roupret M, Catto J, Coulet F, et al. Microsatellite instability as indicator of MSH2 gene mutation in patients with upper urinary tract transitional cell carcinoma. J Med Genet 2004;41(7):e91.
22. Catto JW, Azzouzi AR, Amira N, et al. Distinct patterns of microsatellite instability are seen in tumours of the urinary tract. Oncogene 2003;22(54):8699–8706.
23. Zhang ZF, Sarkis AS, Cardon-Carlo C, et al. Tobacco smoking, occupation, and p53 nuclear overexpression in early stage bladder cancer. Cancer Epidemiol Biomarkers Prev 1994;3(1):19–24.
24. Jensen OM, Knudsen JB, McLaughlin JK, Sorensen BL. The Copenhagen case-control study of renal pelvis and ureter cancer: role of smoking and occupational exposures. Int J Cancer 1988;41(4):557–561.
25. McLaughlin JK, Silverman DT, Hsing AW, et al. Cigarette smoking and cancers of the renal pelvis and ureter. Cancer Res 1992;52(2):254–257.
26. Poole WDS. Occupational tumors of the renal pelvis and ureter arising in the dye making industry. Proc Roy Soc Med 1969;62(1):93–94.
27. Shinka T, Miyai M, Sawada Y, Inagaki T, Okawa T. Factors affecting the occurrence of urothelial tumors in dye workers exposed to aromatic amines. Int J Urol 1995;2(4):243–248.
28. Naito S, Tanaka K, Koga H, Kotoh S, Hirohata T, Kumazawa J. Cancer occurrence among dyestuff workers exposed to aromatic amines. A long term follow-up study. Cancer 1995;76(8):1445–1452.
29. GPMU Health & Safety. Carcinogens 2004. 2005. Online. Available: www.gpmu.org.uk/hs/hsbladcanc.html.
30. Steffens J, Nagel R. Tumours of the renal pelvis and ureter. Observations in 170 patients. Br J Urol 1988;61(4):277–283.
31. McCredie M, Stewart JH, Carter JJ, Turner J, Mahony JF. Phenacetin and papillary necrosis: independent risk factors for renal pelvic cancer. Kidney Int 1986;30(1):81–84.
32. Johansson S, Angervall L, Bengtsson U, Wahlqvist L. Uroepithelial tumors of the renal pelvis associated with abuse of phenacetin-containing analgesics. Cancer 1974;33(3):743–753.

33. Brenner DW, Schellhammer PF. Upper tract urothelial malignancy after cyclophosphamide therapy: a case report and literature review. J Urol 1987;137(6):1226–1227.

34. Cohen SM, Garland EM, St John M, Okamura T, Smith RA. Acrolein initiates rat urinary bladder carcinogenesis. Cancer Res 1992;52(13):3577–3581.

35. Nortier JL, Martinez MC, Schmeiser HH, et al. Urothelial carcinoma associated with the use of a Chinese herb (Aristolochia fangchi). N Engl J Med 2000;342(23):1686–1692.

36. Ross RK, Paganini-Hill A, Landolph J, et al. Analgesics, cigarette smoking, and other risk factors for cancer of the renal pelvis and ureter. Cancer Res 1989;49(4):1045–1048.

37. Petkovic SD. Epidemiology and treatment of renal pelvic and ureteral tumors. J Urol 1975;114(6):858–865.

38. Guinan P, Vogelzang NJ, Randazzo R, et al. Renal pelvic cancer: a review of 611 patients treated in Illinois 1975-1985. Cancer Incidence and End Results Committee. Urology 1992;40(5):393–399.

39. Jitsukawa S, Nakamura K, Nakayama H, Osawa A, Matsji K. Transitional cell carcinoma of kidney extending into renal vein and inferior vena cava. Urology 1985;25(3):310–312.

40. Zincke H, Neves RJ. Feasibility of conservative surgery for transitional cell cancer of the upper urinary tract. Urol Clin North Am 1984;11(4):717–724.

41. Blute ML, Tsushima K, Farrow GM, Therneau TM, Lieber MM. Transitional cell carcinoma of the renal pelvis: nuclear deoxyribonucleic acid ploidy studied by flow cytometry. J Urol 1988;140(5):944–949.

42. Nemoto R, Hattori K, Sasaki A, Miyanaga N, Koiso K, Harada M. Estimations of the S phase fraction in situ in transitional cell carcinoma of the renal pelvis and ureter with bromodeoxyuridine labelling. Br J Urol 1989;64(4):339–344.

43. Miyakawa A, Tachibana M, Nakashima J, Deguchi N, Baba S, Tazaki H. Flow cytometric bromodeoxyuridine/deoxyribonucleic acid bivariate analysis for predicting tumor invasiveness of upper tract urothelial cancer. J Urol 1994;152(1):76–80.

44. Masuda M, Iki M, Takano Y, et al. Prognostic significance of Ki-67 labeling index in urothelial tumors of the renal pelvis and ureter. J Urol 1996;155(6):1877–1880; discussion 1880–1881.

45. Kamai T, Takagi K, Asami H, Ito Y, Arai K, Yoshida KI. Prognostic significance of p27Kip1 and Ki-67 expression in carcinoma of the renal pelvis and ureter. BJU Int 2000;86(1):14–19.

46. Hashimoto H, Sue Y, Saga Y, Tokumitsu M, Yachiku S. Roles of p53 and MDM2 in tumor proliferation and determination of the prognosis of transitional cell carcinoma of the renal pelvis and ureter. Int J Urol 2000;7(12):457–463.

47. Messing EM, Catalona W. Urothelial tumours of the renal pelvis and ureter. In Campbell MF, Walsh PC, Retik AB (eds): Campbell's Urology, 8th ed. Philadelphia: WB Saunders, 2002, pp 2383–2410.

48. Bloom HJ, Hendry WF, Wallace DM, Skeet RG. Treatment of T3 bladder cancer: controlled trial of pre-operative radiotherapy and radical cystectomy versus radical radiotherapy. Br J Urol 1982;54(2):136–151.

49. Murphy DM, Zincke H, Furlow WL. Management of high grade transitional cell cancer of the upper urinary tract. J Urol 1981;125(1):25–29.

50. Malek RS, Aguilo JJ, Hattery RR. Radiolucent filling defects of the renal pelvis: classification and report of unusual cases. J Urol 1975;114(4):508–513.

51. Wijkstrom H, Cohen SM, Gardiner RA, et al. Prevention and treatment of urothelial premalignant and malignant lesions. Scand J Urol Nephrol Suppl 2000;205:116–135.

52. Zincke H, Aguilo JJ, Farrow GM, Utz DC, Khan AU. Significance of urinary cytology in the early detection of transitional cell cancer of the upper urinary tract. J Urol 1976;116(6):781–783.

53. Murphy DM, Zincke H, Furlow WL. Primary grade 1 transitional cell carcinoma of the renal pelvis and ureter. J Urol 1980;123(5):629–631.

54. Sarnacki CT, McCormack LJ, Kiser WS, Hazard JB, McLaughlin TC, Belovich DM. Urinary cytology and the clinical diagnosis of urinary tract malignancy: a clinicopathologic study of 1,400 patients. J Urol 1971;106(5):761–764.

55. Murphy WM, Miller A. Cytology in the detection and follow up of urothelial tumors. In Javadpour N (ed): Bladder Cancer. Baltimore: Williams & Wilkins, 1984, pp 100–122.

56. Dodd LG, Johnston WW, Robertson CN, Layfield LJ. Endoscopic brush cytology of the upper urinary tract. Evaluation of its efficacy and potential limitations in diagnosis. Acta Cytol 1997;41(2):377–384.

57. Streem SB, Pontes JE, Novick AC, Montie JE. Ureteropyeloscopy in the evaluation of upper tract filling defects. J Urol 1986;136(2):383–385.

58. Blute ML, Segura J, Patterson D, et al. Impact of endourology on diagnosis and management of upper urinary tract urothelial cancer. J Urol 1989;141(6):1298–1301.

59. Keeley FX, Bibbo M, Bagley DH. Diagnostic accuracy of ureteroscopic biopsy in upper tract transitional cell carcinoma. J Urol 1997;157(1):33–37.

60. Huang A, Low RK, deVere White R. Nephrostomy tract tumor seeding following percutaneous manipulation of a ureteral carcinoma. J Urol 1995;153(3 Pt 2):1041–1042.

61. Clark PE, Streem SB. Endourologic management of upper tract transitional cell carcinoma. Sci World J 2004;4(Suppl 1):62–75.

62. Eraky I, El-Kappany H, Shamaa M, et al. Laparoscopic nephrectomy: an established routine procedure. J Endourol 1994;8(4):275–278.

63. Gill IS, Clayman RV, McDougall EM. Advances in urological laparoscopy. J Urol 1995;154(4):1275–1294.

64. Batata M, Grabstald H. Upper urinary tract urothelial tumors. Urol Clin North Am 1976;3(1):79–86.

65. Skinner DG. Technique of nephroureterectomy with regional lymph node dissection. Urol Clin North Am 1978;5(1):252–260.

66. Cummings KB. Nephroureterectomy: rationale in the management of transitional cell carcinoma of the upper urinary tract. Urol Clin North Am 1980;7(3):569–578.

67. Nocks BN, Heney NM, Daly JJ, et al. Transitional cell carcinoma of renal pelvis. Urology 1982;19(5):472–477.

68. McCarron JP, Mills C, Vaughn ED Jr. Tumors of the renal pelvis and ureter: current concepts and management. Semin Urol 1983;1(1):75–81.

69. Richie JP. Carcinoma of the renal pelvis and ureter. In Skinner DG, Lieskovsky G (eds): Diagnosis and Management of Genitourinary Cancer. Philadelphia: WB Saunders, 1988, pp 323–336.

70. Williams RD. Renal, perirenal, and ureteral neoplasms. In Gillenwater JY (ed): Adult and Pediatric Urology. Philadelphia: Lippincott Williams & Wilkins, 1991, p 3 v. (xii 2760, 68).

71. Yokoyama H, Tanaka M. Incidence of adrenal involvement and assessing adrenal function in patients with renal cell carcinoma: is ipsilateral adrenalectomy indispensable during radical nephrectomy? BJU Int 2005;95(4):526–529.

72. McDonald D. Intussusception ureterectomy: a method of removal of the ureteral stump at time of nephrectomy without an additional incision. Surg Gynecol Obstet 1953;97(5):565–568.

73. Clayman RV, Garske GL, Lange PH. Total nephroureterectomy with ureteral intussusception and transurethral ureteral detachment and pull-through. Urology 1983;21(5):482–486.

74. Seaman EK, Slawin KM, Benson MC. Treatment options for upper tract transitional-cell carcinoma. Urol Clin North Am 1993;20(2):349–354.

75. Bloom NA, Vidone RA, Lytton B. Primary carcinoma of the ureter: a report of 102 new cases. J Urol 1970;103(5):590–598.

76. Strong DW, Pearse HD, Tank ES Jr, Hodges CV. The ureteral stump after nephroureterectomy. J Urol 1976;115(6):654–655.

77. Johansson S, Wahlqvist L. A prognostic study of urothelial renal pelvic tumors: comparison between the prognosis of patients treated with intrafascial nephrectomy and perifascial nephroureterectomy. Cancer 1979;43(6):2525–2531.

78. Kakizoe T, Fujita J, Murase T, Matsumoto K, Kishi K. Transitional cell carcinoma of the bladder in patients with renal pelvic and ureteral cancer. J Urol 1980;124(1):17–19.

79. Mullen JB, Kovacs K. Primary carcinoma of the ureteral stump: a case report and a review of the literature. J Urol 1980;123(1):113–115.

80. Heney NM, Nocks BN, Daly JJ, Blitzer PH, Parkhurst EC. Prognostic factors in carcinoma of the ureter. J Urol 1981;125(5):632–636.

81. Batata MA, Whitmore WF, Hilaris BS, Tokita N, Grabstald H. Primary carcinoma of the ureter: a prognostic study. Cancer 1975;35(6):1626–1632.

82. McNeill SA, Chrisofos M, Tolley DA. The long-term outcome after laparoscopic nephroureterectomy: a comparison with open nephroureterectomy. BJU Int 2000;86(6):619–623.

83. Zungri E, Chechile G, Algaba F, Diaz I, Vila F, Castro C. Treatment of transitional cell carcinoma of the ureter: is the controversy justified? Eur Urol 1990;17(4):276–280.

84. Pohar KS, Sheinfeld J. When is partial ureterectomy acceptable for transitional-cell carcinoma of the ureter? J Endourol 2001;15(4):405–408; discussion 409.

85. Grabstald H, Whitmore WF, Melamed MR. Renal pelvic tumors. JAMA 1971;218(6):845–854.

86. Clayman RV, Kavoussi LR, Figenshau RS, Chandhoke PS, Albala DM. Laparoscopic nephroureterectomy: initial clinical case report. J Laparoendosc Surg 1991;1(6):343–349.

87. Shalhav AL, Dunn MD, Portis AJ, et al. Laparoscopic nephroureterectomy for upper tract transitional cell cancer: the Washington University experience. J Urol 2000;163(4):1100–1104.

88. Gill IS, Munch LC, Lucas BA, Das S. Initial experience with retroperitoneoscopic nephroureterectomy: use of a double-balloon technique. Urology 1995;46(5):747–750.

89. Gill IS, Sung GT, Hobart MG, et al. Laparoscopic radical nephroureterectomy for upper tract transitional cell carcinoma: the Cleveland Clinic experience. J Urol 2000;164(5):1513–1522.

90. Nakada SY, Moon TD, Gist M, Mahvi D. Use of the pneumo sleeve as an adjunct in laparoscopic nephrectomy. Urology 1997;49(4):612–613.

91. Keeley FX, Sharma NK, Tolley DA. Hand-assisted laparoscopic nephroureterectomy. BJU Int 1999;83(4):504–505.

92. Apul G, Hemal AK, Gupta NP. Retroperitoneal laparoscopic radical nephrectomy and nephroureterectomy and comparison with open surgery. World J Urol 2002;20:219–223.

93. Klingler HC, Lodde M, Pycha A, Remzi M, Janetschek G, Marberger M. Modified laparoscopic nephroureterectomy for treatment of upper urinary tract transitional cell cancer is not associated with an increased risk of tumour recurrence. Eur Urol 2003;44(4):442–447.

94. McDougall EM, Clayman RV, Elashry O. Laparoscopic nephroureterectomy for upper tract transitional cell cancer: the Washington University experience. J Urol 1995;154(3):975–979; discussion 979–980.

95. Kawauchi A, Fujito A, Ukimura O, Yoneda K, Mizutani Y, Miki T. Hand assisted retroperitoneoscopic nephroureterectomy: comparison with the open procedure. J Urol 2003;169(3):890–894; discussion 894.

96. Stifelman MD, Hyman MJ, Shichman S, Sosa RE. Hand-assisted laparoscopic nephroureterectomy versus open nephroureterectomy for the treatment of transitional-cell carcinoma of the upper urinary tract. J Endourol 2001;15(4):391–395; discussion 397.

97. Steinberg JR, Matin SF. Laparoscopic radical nephroureterectomy: dilemma of the distal ureter. Curr Opin Urol 2004;14(2):61–65.

98. Gill IS, Soble JJ, Miller SD, Sung GT. A novel technique for management of the en bloc bladder cuff and distal ureter during laparoscopic nephroureterectomy. J Urol 1999;161(2):430–434.

99. Venkatesh R, Rehman J, Lee D, et al. Cell viability within the stapled tissue following laparoscopic tissue stapling in a porcine model [abstract]. J Urol 2003;169(3):150.

100. Uozumi J, Fujiyama C, Meiri H, et al. Hand-assisted retroperitoneoscopic nephroureterectomy for upper urinary-tract urothelial tumors. J Endourol 2002;16(10):743–747.

101. Chung HJ, Chiu AW, Chen KK. Retroperitoneoscopic assisted nephroureterectomy for management of upper tract transitional cell carcinoma. Minim Invasive Ther 1996;5:266–271.

102. Keeley FX Jr, Tolley DA. Laparoscopic nephroureterectomy: making management of upper-tract transitional-cell carcinoma entirely minimally invasive. J Endourol 1998;12(2):139–141.

103. Salomon L, Hoznek A, Cicco A, et al. Retroperitoneoscopic nephroureterectomy for renal pelvic tumors with a single iliac incision. J Urol 1999;161(2):541–544.

104. Strong DW, Pearse HD. Recurrent urothelial tumors following surgery for transitional cell carcinoma of the upper urinary tract. Cancer 1976;38(5):2173–2183.

105. Ahmed I, Shaikh NA, Kapadia CR. Track recurrence of renal pelvic transitional cell carcinoma after laparoscopic nephrectomy. Br J Urol 1998;81(2):319.

106. Vest SA. Conservative surgery in certain benign tumors of the ureter. J Urol 1945;53:97–121.

107. Gittes RF. Operative nephroscopy. J Urol 1966;116:148–152.

108. Petkovic SD. A plea for conservative operation for ureteral tumors. J Urol 1972;107(2):220–223.

109. Mazeman E. [Tumors of the upper excretory urinary tract, calices, renal pelvis and ureter.] J Urol Nephrol (Paris) 1972;78(Suppl 9):1–219.

110. Johnson DE, Babaian RJ. Conservative surgical management for noninvasive distal ureteral carcinoma. Urology 1979;13(4):365–367.

111. Gittes RF. Management of transitional cell carcinoma of the upper tract: case for conservative local excision. Urol Clin North Am 1980;7(3):559–568.

112. Wallace DM, et al. The late results of conservative surgery for upper tract urothelial carcinomas. Br J Urol 1981;53(6):537–541.

113. Tomera KM, Leary FJ, Zincke H. Pyeloscopy in urothelial tumors. J Urol 1982;127(6):1088–1089.

114. Bazeed MA, Scharfe T, Becht E, et al. Local excision of urothelial cancer of the upper urinary tract. Eur Urol 1986;12(2):89–95.

115. Ziegelbaum M, Novick AC, Streem SB, et al. Conservative surgery for transitional cell carcinoma of the renal pelvis. J Urol 1987;138(5):1146–1149.

116. Gill WB, Lu CT, Thomsen S. Retrograde brushing: a new technique for obtaining histologic and cytologic material from ureteral, renal pelvic and renal caliceal lesions. J Urol 1973;109(4):573–578.

117. Meng MV, Freise CE, Stoller ML. Laparoscopic nephrectomy, ex vivo excision and autotransplantation for complex renal tumors. J Urol 2004;172(2):461–464.

118. Zoretic S, Gonzales J. Primary carcinoma of ureters. Urology 1983;21(4):354–356.

119. Murphy DP, Gill IS, Streem SB. Evolving management of upper-tract transitional-cell carcinoma at a tertiary-care center. J Endourol 2002;16(7):483–487.

120. Mahadevia PS, Karwa GL, Koss LG. Mapping of urothelium in carcinomas of the renal pelvis and ureter. A report of nine cases. Cancer 1983;51(5):890–897.

121. Pagano F. Conservative treatment of lower ureteral tumor: modified ureteroneocystostomy for upper urinary tract endoscopic control. J Urol 1984;132(3):555–557.

122. Goldwasser B, Leibovitch I, Avigad I. Ureteral substitution using the isolated interposed vermiform appendix in a patient with a single kidney and transitional cell carcinoma of the ureter. Urology 1994;44(3):437–440.

123. Herr HW. Long-term results of BCG therapy: concern about upper tract tumors. Semin Urol Oncol 1998;16(1):13–16.

124. Grossman HB. The late recurrence of grade I transitional cell carcinoma of the ureter after conservative therapy. J Urol 1978;120(2):251–252.

125. Martinez-Pineiro JA, Garcia Matres MJ, Martinez-Pineiro L. Endourological treatment of upper tract urothelial carcinomas: analysis of a series of 59 tumors. J Urol 1996;156(2 Pt 1):377–385.

126. Elliott DS, Blute ML, Patterson DE, et al. Long-term follow-up of endoscopically treated upper urinary tract transitional cell carcinoma. Urology 1996;47(6):819–825.

127. Abdel-Razzak O, Bagley DH. The 6.9 F semirigid ureteroscope in clinical use. Urology 1993;41(1):45–48.

128. Grasso M, Bagley D. A 7.5/8.2 F actively deflectable, flexible ureteroscope: a new device for both diagnostic and therapeutic upper urinary tract endoscopy. Urology 1994;43(4):435–441.

129. Smith JA Jr, Lee RG, Dixon JA. Tissue effects of neodymium:YAG laser photoradiation of canine ureters. J Surg Oncol 1984;27(3):168–711.

130. Schmeller NT, Hofstetter AG. Laser treatment of ureteral tumors. J Urol 1989;141(4):840–843.

131. Bagley D, Erhard M. Use of the holmium laser in the upper urinary tract. Tech Urol 1995;1(1):25–30.

132. Razvi HA, Chun SS, Denstedt JD, Sales J. Soft-tissue applications of the holmium:YAG laser in urology. J Endourol 1995;9(5):387–390.

133. Bian Y, Ehya H, Bagley DH. Cytologic diagnosis of upper urinary tract neoplasms by ureteroscopic sampling. Acta Cytol 1995;39(4):733–740.

134. Tawfiek E, Bibbo M, Bagley DH. Ureteroscopic biopsy: technique and specimen preparation. Urology 1997;50(1):117–119.

135. Daneshmand S, Quek ML, Huffman JL. Endoscopic management of upper urinary tract transitional cell carcinoma: long-term experience. Cancer 2003;98(1):55–60.

136. Chesko SB, Gray GF, McCarron JP. Urothelial neoplasia of the upper urinary tract. In Sommers SC, Rosen PP (eds): Pathology Annual. New York: Appleton-Century-Crofts, 1981, pp 127–153.

137. Badalament RA, Bennett WF, Bova JG, et al. Computed tomography of primary transitional cell carcinoma of upper urinary tracts. Urology 1992;40(1):71–75.

138. Gerber GS, Lyon ES. Endourological management of upper tract urothelial tumors. J Urol 1993;150(1):2–7.

139. Tawfiek ER, Bagley DH. Upper-tract transitional cell carcinoma. Urology 1997;50(3):321–329.

140. Huffman JL. Management of upper transitional cell carcinomas. In Vogelzang N, Scardino PT, Shipley WU, Coffey DS (eds): Comprehensive Textbook of Genitourinary Oncology. Philadelphia: Lippincott Williams & Wilkins, 2000, pp 367–383.

141. Jarrett TW, Lee CK, Pardalidis NP, Smith AD. Extensive dilation of distal ureter for endoscopic treatment of large volume ureteral disease. J Urol 1995;153(4):1214–1217.

142. Guarnizo E, Pavlovich CP, Seiba M, et al. Ureteroscopic biopsy of upper tract urothelial carcinoma: improved diagnostic accuracy and histopathological considerations using a multi-biopsy approach. J Urol 2000;163(1):52–55.

143. Keeley FX Jr, Bibbo M, Bagley DH. Ureteroscopic treatment and surveillance of upper urinary tract transitional cell carcinoma. J Urol 1997;157(5):1560–1565.

144. Chen GL, Bagley DH. Ureteroscopic management of upper tract transitional cell carcinoma in patients with normal contralateral kidneys. J Urol 2000;164(4):1173–1176.

145. Kulp DA, Bagley DH. Does flexible ureteropyeloscopy promote local recurrence of transitional cell carcinoma? J Endourol 1994;8(2):111–113.

146. Hendin BN, Streem SB, Levin HS, Klein EA, Novick AC. Impact of diagnostic ureteroscopy on long-term survival in patients with upper tract transitional cell carcinoma. J Urol 1999;161(3):783–785.

147. Grasso M, Bagley D. Small diameter, actively deflectable, flexible ureteropyeloscopy. J Urol 1998;160(5):1648–1653; discussion 1653–1654.

148. Nakada SY, Clayman RV. Percutaneous electrovaporization of upper tract transitional cell carcinoma in patients with functionally solitary kidneys. Urology 1995;46(5):751–755.

149. Jarrett TW, Sweetser PM, Weiss GH, Smith AD. Percutaneous management of transitional cell carcinoma of the renal collecting system: 9-year experience. J Urol 1995;154(5):1629–1635.

150. Patel A, Soonawalla P, Shepherd SF, et al. Long-term outcome after percutaneous treatment of transitional cell carcinoma of the renal pelvis. J Urol 1996;155(3):868–874.

151. Plancke HR, Strijbos WE, Delaere KP. Percutaneous endoscopic treatment of urothelial tumours of the renal pelvis. Br J Urol 1995;75(6):736–739.

152. Heney NM. Natural history of superficial bladder cancer. Prognostic features and long-term disease course. Urol Clin North Am 1992;19(3):429–433.

153. Jabbour ME, Desgrandchamps F, Cazin S, Teillac P, Le Duc A, Smith AD. Percutaneous management of grade II upper urinary tract transitional cell carcinoma: the long-term outcome. J Urol 2000;163(4):1105–1107; quiz 1295.

154. Vasavada SP, Streem SB, Novick AC. Definitive tumor resection and percutaneous bacille Calmette–Guérin for management of renal pelvic transitional cell carcinoma in solitary kidneys. Urology 1995;45(3):381–386.

155. Schoenberg MP, Van Arsdalen KN, Wein AJ. The management of transitional cell carcinoma in solitary renal units. J Urol 1991;146(3):700–702; discussion 702–703.

156. Slywotzky C, Maya M. Needle tract seeding of transitional cell carcinoma following fine-needle aspiration of a renal mass. Abdom Imaging 1994;19(2):174–176.

157. Carson CC 3rd. Endoscopic treatment of upper and lower urinary tract lesions using lasers. Semin Urol 1991;9(3):185–191.

158. Shepherd SF, Patel A, Bidmead AM, et al. Nephrostomy track brachytherapy following percutaneous resection of transitional cell carcinoma of the renal pelvis. Clin Oncol (R Coll Radiol) 1995;7(6):385–387.

159. Nolan RL, Nickel JC, Froud PJ. Percutaneous endourologic approach for transitional cell carcinoma of the renal pelvis. Urol Radiol 1988;9(4):217–219.

160. Palou J, Piovesan LF, Huguet J, Salvador J, Vicente J, Villavicencio H. Percutaneous nephroscopic management of upper urinary tract transitional cell carcinoma: recurrence and long-term followup. J Urol 2004;172(1):66–69.

161. O'Donoghue JP, Crew JP. Adjuvant topical treatment of upper urinary tract urothelial tumours. BJU Int 2004;94(4):483–485.

162. Eastham JA, Huffman JL. Technique of mitomycin C instillation in the treatment of upper urinary tract urothelial tumors. J Urol 1993;150(2 Pt 1):324–325.

163. Jabbour ME, Smith AD. Primary percutaneous approach to upper urinary tract transitional cell carcinoma. Urol Clin North Am 2000;27(4):739–750.

164. Herr HW. Durable response of a carcinoma in situ of the renal pelvis to topical bacillus Calmette-Guérin. J Urol 1985;134(3):531–532.

165. Studer UE, Casanova G, Kraft R, Zingg EJ. Percutaneous bacillus Calmette–Guérin perfusion of the upper urinary tract for carcinoma in situ. J Urol 1989;142(4):975–977.

166. Nishino Y, Yamamoto N, Komeda H, Takahashi Y, Deguchi T. Bacillus Calmette–Guérin instillation treatment for carcinoma in situ of the upper urinary tract. BJU Int 2000;85(7):799–801.

167. Nonomura N, Ono Y, Nozawa M, et al. Bacillus Calmette–Guérin perfusion therapy for the treatment of transitional cell carcinoma in situ of the upper urinary tract. Eur Urol 2000;38(6):701–704; discussion 705.

# Early detection for bladder cancer  23

*George P Hemstreet III, Edward M Messing*

## INTRODUCTION

The rationale for screening for common morbid diseases with minimally invasive, accurate techniques is that detection in the early stages should result in a more efficacious outcome than symptomatic detection of patients with a more advanced stage. Bladder cancer is no exception (see below). Recent exciting advances in diagnostic molecular medicine, improved high-throughput technologies, and translational research provide renewed hope for patients diagnosed early with bladder cancer. Success is further enhanced by an appreciation of the basic concepts of biochemical field disease or field effect with rare event detection of premalignant or neoplastic cells.[1–5]

Accurate detection of bladder cancer has been further confounded by the presence of high- and low-grade carcinogenic pathways requiring a multipronged approach because of early tumor heterogeneity attributable to divergent pathways.[6] This heterogeneity is in contrast to cervical cancer, a disease with an incidence of 10,520 cases and a current mortality of 3700 deaths per year in 2004 compared to an incidence of 60,240 and 12,710 deaths for bladder cancer.[7–9] Cervical cancer death rates decreased by more than 110% during the years 1950–1995, while the deaths from bladder cancer have been reduced by only 2.39%, based on the SEER joinpoint regression program (http://srab.cancer.gov/joinpoint). Thus the mortality of cervical cancer has been reduced markedly compared to bladder cancer because of discreet morphometric features identifiable by Papanicolaou (Pap) cytology screening. These distinct morphologic features have led to the effective automation of cervical cancer detection based primarily on identifiable morphometric features.

The fundamental pathologic concepts for detecting cervical cancer can now be applied to identifying the molecular 'fingerprints' that herald bladder cancer.

This early detection can take the form of an organized screening endeavor, focusing on 'at-risk' populations (including large segments of the general population), employing specific diagnostic tools, a prescribed evaluation triggered by the results of the initial intervention (test), and regularly scheduled test repetitions for participants with an initial negative test. Alternatively, ad lib early detection efforts aimed at large general population segments often enter standard medical care without fully demonstrating improved outcome from the disease. An example of the latter would be the cervical Pap test that has reduced cervical cancer deaths in this country by 50% and now incorporates automated slide preparation, SurePrep, and automated image analysis detection, TriPath, Burlington, NC. This chapter will deal exclusively with screening, an organized effort to detect bladder cancer earlier than it would normally be diagnosed in a defined population.

The rationale for screening for bladder cancer is based upon several principles concerning the disease's behavior:

1. Bladder cancers arise in the uroepithelium. Thus, even with superficial cancers, malignant cells, and their abnormal molecular products, are shed into urine, and are detectable in this fluid.
2. It is very rare that a urothelial cancer metastasizes until it invades the muscularis propria (stage T2+).[10] Therefore, there is a window of time between when the tumor arises and is detectable through examination of urine or cystoscopy, before it invades the muscularis propria.

3. Treatments for superficial (stage Ta and T1) urothelial cancers are far more successful and less morbid than those for muscle-invading or more advanced (stage T2+) tumors.[11]

4. Those tumors destined to become muscle invading had they not been detected at earlier stages demonstrate enough aggressive histologic and molecular characteristics to identify their malignant potential and permit them to be distinguished from the more indolent, low-grade, superficial, papillary cancers.

5. The majority of patients with stage T2+ urothelial cancer have that level of invasion at their initial bladder cancer diagnosis and do *not* primarily come from the 'pool' of patients with prior histories of superficial cancers.[12-15]

6. Bladder cancer is very rarely found incidentally at autopsy, indicating that early detection efforts would not be a disadvantage for those in whom the disease is detected (since it would eventually be diagnosed and treated).[16-19]

The above characteristics of bladder cancer potentially make it ideal for early detection efforts. Further complimenting this rationale is that both general and particularly high-risk populations have been defined.[11,20] Knowing these demographics, a screening program could be designed to test middle-aged and elderly individuals, particularly men with a significant cigarette smoking history, since this is an at-risk population that may have sufficient disease prevalence to test the feasibility of screening. Additional populations at even higher risk will also be described. It is of interest to note that, as opposed to the wide use of prostate-specific antigen (PSA) testing in an asymptomatic population, earlier detection of bladder cancer has not been considered a top priority of most primary care givers, healthcare systems, and the general population. This contention is substantiated by the report that over 72% of patients taking part in a large (n=1106), contemporary (May 1999 to January 2001), intravesical therapy study had macroscopic hematuria as their presenting finding when they were initially diagnosed with bladder cancer.[20]

To be worth undertaking, screening must not only enable earlier diagnosis and treatment, but must also reduce bladder cancer-specific mortality, or overall mortality in screenees that have bladder cancer. The ideal way to determine this is to conduct a randomized prospective study of screened individuals and unscreened controls with outcome from bladder cancer as the major endpoint. Only in this way can biases such as lead time (in which, because screening permits an earlier diagnosis, an individual with a screening-detected cancer will appear to have a longer survival from time of diagnosis than an individual with a cancer detected through standard medical care, although actual outcome from disease is not affected), or length bias sampling (in which, for a given grade and stage, screening-detected cancers will generally have a more indolent course than cancers detected because of symptoms which become clinically evident in the interval between repeat screenings) be controlled for. Such randomized prospective studies have not been completed for prostate cancer or the highly effective cervical cancer screening paradigm.

For bladder cancer, the ideal screening modality would have exquisite sensitivity for high-grade cancer, good sensitivity for lower-grade cancer (so that missed tumors would not undermine the confidence of physicians and participants in the screening endeavor), and a low enough false-positive rate (high specificity and high positive predictive value) to make screening economically acceptable. Performance characteristics of currently available markers and those under intense investigation are promising in these regards (see Chapter 20), but few have been fully tested in the early detection setting and none has been well tested in true screening. Of concern, is that, for almost all available markers, the size of the tumor greatly affects sensitivity. Smaller tumors (the ones that would be tested in screening or in monitoring superficial bladder cancer patients for recurrence), even high-grade ones, have false-negative results far more often than larger ones.[21]

## STRATEGY FOR SCREENING HIGH RISK POPULATIONS

The low incidence of bladder cancer in the general population compared to PSA screening for prostate cancer places stringent requirements on the screening test if it is to have a high positive predictive value (PPV). Epidemiologic studies of occupationally exposed populations resulted in the National Institute for Occupational Safety and Health (NIOSH) and its European counterpart to recommend screening for high-risk, occupationally exposed cohorts. However, to date, such a recommendation has not been forthcoming for screening the general population because of the much lower disease prevalence. Approaches available to improve bladder cancer screening's feasibility are to develop a test with a very high sensitivity and specificity to enrich the population being screened for bladder cancer based on age and smoking history, and/or to incorporate a two-tier (or multi-tier) screening test.

Epidemiologic studies indicate that bladder cancer has an overall incidence of approximately 2–3/10,000 in the United States but up to 15/10,000 in Greece. It is estimated that 1.89% of men over the age of 60 in the US have bladder cancer, based on SEER data.[9] In men between the ages 40 and 50 who smoke, there will be 97 cases per 100,000 patient years. Screening this population with a test that has a sensitivity of 75% with a specificity of 95% will result in approximately 495 screening evaluations to detect 50% of the bladder cancers, with a reduction in death rates of approximately 50% (assuming Ta and T1 cancers have higher cure ratios than T2+ cancers).

## STRATEGY FOR IMPROVING BIOMARKERS FOR SCREENING

The work of Messing and Briton and their respective coworkers (described later) clearly demonstrated that the multiday dipstick test detected bladder cancer in over 1% of the men over 50 years of age (most of whom had significant smoking histories) that were screened, confirming the epidemiologic calculations just described. Although repetitive Hemastix testing is easy to perform and may provide an excellent test in some populations, even if it is assumed that its sensitivity approaches 100% of cystoscopically detectable cancers, its false-positive rate in the entire population is 10% to 20%, leading to many unnecessary evaluations. Indeed, in populations where bicycle riding is prevalent there was no difference in the results of the test between the at-risk individuals and the controls (unpublished data). The major purpose of screening is not to miss high-grade cancers and almost all of the biomarkers identified to date detect high-grade disease, with a higher sensitivity than low grade disease. In the Messing study (see below) the high-grade tumors appeared to be detected early in the disease prior to invasion.[22,23] These results are similar to the reports by Hemstreet et al for screening high-risk occupational cohorts.[24]

A major limitation with urinary biomarker screening for the epidemiologic-enriched population (males, older age, and smokers) is the lack of test specificity. One explanation for the poor specificity is the association of the biomarker with other benign conditions, or the marker is expressed so early that a large proportion of patients do not progress to the disease endpoint.[25] A second alternative is to improve the specificity by quantitating biomarkers in single cells associated with the transformational event and not associated with a clastogenic response such as that observed with the DNA ploidy, 5c-exceeding rate (5CER). Several potential biomarkers hold promise in this regard—for example, telomerase, survivin, and BLCA4. Another potential biomarker is hyaluronic acid-hyaluronidase as described by Lokeshwar and colleagues.[26,27] Rare event detection of these markers in exfoliated uroepithelial cells is likely to be a very powerful approach.

## GENERAL POPULATIONS

The few studies that have been conducted have used cytology or repetitive hematuria tests for case detection, and have reported disease discovery rates.[22,23,28-32] Perhaps the two best studies are ones carried out in the late 1980s and early 1990s in Wisconsin (USA) and Leeds (UK). In each, middle-aged and elderly men, solicited from patient care registries, used repetitive hematuria reagent strip testing to detect hematuria, with a single positive test leading to a urologic evaluation. The two studies had very similar findings. In each, between 10% and 20% of participants had micro-hematuria detected by reagent strip testings and were evaluated. All participants were requested to undergo cystoscopy if they had even a single episode of hematuria, and, of those participants with hematuria that were evaluated, between 6% and 10% were found to have urothelial cancer.[22,23,28-32] In all but one of the 45 men with bladder cancer detected, the disease was confined to the lamina propria or was less invasive. While the outcomes of those participants in the UK study have not been published, in the Wisconsin trial, at between 3 and 10 years follow-up, no subject with bladder cancer detected by screening had succumbed to that disease.[11]

Because the main value of screening is to improve the outcome from the disease being screened for, it should be acknowledged that this is the only bladder cancer screening study in a general population that has been reported with disease outcome as the endpoint.[33] Although the study was not randomized, it did compare the outcome in a screened population with a separate (although contemporary) group of unscreened individuals.

In the screened population, roughly 53% of those with bladder cancer had low-grade tumors, all of which were nonmuscle invasive (stage Ta or T1), and 47% had high-grade tumors. In a contemporary snapshot of all men aged 50 and over that had bladder cancer diagnosed in the state of Wisconsin in 1988, the same low-grade/high-grade proportion of cancers was found. However, in the Wisconsin general population, over half of the high-grade tumors were already muscle invading upon diagnosis, whereas only 10% in the screened population were muscle invasive. This led to a significantly better outcome from bladder cancer in the screened compared to the unscreened populations with a 3–10-year follow-up in the screened population and 2-year follow-up in the unscreened one.[33] Using this study's data, bladder cancer screening using this testing regime was estimated to be more cost effective than breast cancer or hypertension screening.[34]

In a recent follow-up of the hematuria screening study from Wisconsin, at 12 years median follow-up, 57% of the screening participants with bladder cancer diagnosed through screening were still alive and 43% had died of causes other than urothelial cancer, with a median survival of 8.8 years in those that had died. This compares with the 12-year outcome in unscreened men diagnosed with bladder cancer in Wisconsin in 1988, of whom 20% had died of bladder cancer and 51% had died from nonbladder cancer causes. Although they represented less than 24% of newly diagnosed unscreened bladder cancer patients, men with muscle-invading cancers accounted for 57% of all bladder cancer deaths with a median survival of 1.05 years from the date of diagnosis. Those with superficial (Ta, T1) cancers (76% of newly diagnosed unscreened bladder cancer cases) accounted for 43% of bladder cancer deaths, with a median time to death of 3.89 years. The similarity of these long-term findings with those of the original study indicate that lead time bias did not explain the differences in survival between men with screening-detected cancers and those diagnosed with clinical presentation.[33] Additionally, although demographics between the general Wisconsin over age 50 male population and those that took part in screening were similar,[33] in the absence of a prospective randomized design, inequities may have existed.

## BLADDER CANCER SCREENING OF OCCUPATIONALLY EXPOSED HIGH-RISK COHORTS

### HISTORICAL PERSPECTIVE OF OCCUPATIONAL BLADDER CANCER

The original realization that bladder cancer was associated with occupational bladder cancer dates back to Rehn's observation in 1895 that bladder cancer was associated with aniline dye exposures.[35] Because of this sentinel observation, aniline dye manufacturing was prohibited in Germany, but continued in the United States until 1974 when NIOSH mandated the cessation of aniline dye derivative production.[36] Even with the recognized association, manufacturing continued in other countries such as China and India until the 1980s.[37,38] Cohorts have been identified from these exposed workers and also from other exposed groups in Canada and the United Kingdom.[39–41]

In spite of these programs, exposures continue in rural areas in cottage industries immune to government regulation throughout the world. Other occupational exposures are much more diffuse in the population, and in many instances bladder cancer today is the result of incidental exposures at young ages or to groups such as hairdressers or mechanics who are not easily organized into cohorts for large-scale screening programs.

## CONVENTIONAL CYTOLOGIC AND HEMATURIA SCREENING OF OCCUPATIONAL COHORTS

Staining of exfoliated urothelial cells using the method developed by Papanicolaou for cervical cancer was applied to the analysis of the uroepithelial sediment, and served as the primary mode for the bladder screening and surveillance of transitional cell carcinoma (TCC).[42] Pap cytology has proved beneficial for cervical cancer screening, with an over 50% reduction in cervical cancer deaths because sampled cells were abundant and cytologic grade progression was reflected by well-defined progressive nuclear changes. These morphometric changes are now captured by highly automated technologies such as image analysis. DNA ploidy and morphometry have also served to further define the risk of premalignant lesions.[43] It is generally recognized that urine cytology is inadequate for screening high-risk groups as reflected by a poor sensitivity (low-grade tumors) but excellent specificity. A treatise addressing this issue has clearly been elucidated by Brown and is summarized in an important chapter 'Urine Cytology: Is it Still the Gold Standard for Screening?'[44]

In a summary table published from the NIOSH consensus conference in 1989, Farrow correlated the lack of sensitivity with tumor grade, stage, and size, providing a clear explanation for the poor sensitivity of this test for low-grade lesions,[45] albeit of questionable biologic significance. Since this conference was held, innumerable studies comparing routine Pap cytology, including those in occupational cohorts, have confirmed these salient observations. Although Pap cytology with its high PPV for high-grade disease remains a contributor to disease detection in occupational cohorts, many tumors remain undetected until too late. Part of the decreased sensitivity may be related to the requirement for a sophisticated pathologist experienced in the art of sample collection and processing, a major point emphasized by Golden and colleagues in the 1970s that later led to liquid-based preparation for cervical cancer specimens (ThinPrep), and, more recently, automated processing of specimens for bladder cancer detection.[46]

Several studies in occupational cohorts clearly demonstrate that tumors detected by conventional bladder cancer Pap screening are inadequate to detect the cancer early enough to reduce cancer mortality. For example, screening studies by Case et al in 1954 found that nearly 50% of those individuals being screened eventually died of bladder cancer.[47] More recent studies by the groups of Bi[37] and Cartwright[48] in the early 1990s further support the view that bladder cancer screening by cytology does not detect early stage disease. As a result of these studies and the advances in biomarker research, a number of screening programs have been initiated worldwide. These studies evaluate biomarkers on exfoliated urothelial cells as an adjunct to conventional urinary cytology. Occupational cohorts at high risk for bladder cancer have provided a rare opportunity to monitor the process of carcinogenesis.

## BIOMARKER-BASED SCREENING OF HIGH-RISK COHORTS

The integration of biomarkers as an adjunct to urinary cytology has been paralleled by an increased comprehension of bladder cancer carcinogenesis, classification of biomarkers, and their integration into clinical practice. Many of these concepts are discussed early in this chapter and elsewhere in the text. The major issues impacting the use of biomarkers into occupational studies include not only the defined sensitivity of the biomarker, but also when it is expressed in the carcinogenesis pathway, whether it is associated with high- or low-grade disease, and the technical platform for performing the test. An exciting innuendo of these concepts is that all of the parameters contributing to the optimization of these tests have not been reached, and additional opportunities exist to improve biomarker results when tested in the general population.[39,48] A refined strategic approach may well incorporate the multiplexing of cellular and soluble urine and serum biomarkers for bladder cancer risk assessment, screening, diagnosis, and defining signaling pathways relevant to cancer prevention and therapy.

Several occupational screening programs for bladder cancer in the US have incorporated biomarkers into the study design. One of the first of these was a notification and screening program, organized by NIOSH and the Workers Institute of Health in Augusta, Georgia (1981).[49-52] The program was highly relevant because it followed legislation of the right of workers to be notified of their exposures to carcinogens, representing a historical landmark in occupational medicine. This study confirmed that samples for biomarker analysis could be collected at a distant site and shipped for high technology biomarker analysis.[50,51] The Augusta bladder cancer screening program incorporated Pap cytology, urinalysis and single Hemastix hematuria testing on site, and DNA ploidy (5CER). This study identified a high-risk subgroup in which the biomarker(s) correlated with duration of exposure to beta-naphthylamine [OR = 7.6 (95% CI, 3.4, 16.7) p = 0.001].[50-52] Additionally, there was a synergistic risk effect between the two exposures. The paradigm developed in Augusta was used to target exposed workers for cytoscopic intervention to assure early detection.

A second program following the paradigm of the Augusta study involved the Drake Health Registry Study

consisting of 399 persons at high risk for bladder cancer secondary to beta-naphthylamine exposure.[53-58] Three screening tests were included in this study design and included urinalysis, Pap cytology, and quantitative fluorescence image analysis. DNA ploidy expressed as the DNA 5CER was included as the original biomarker and later the p300 and G-actin antigens (detected by immunofluorescence) were incorporated in the biomarker profile. Patients with a positive screen were offered cystoscopy with random biopsies as clinically indicated. In this study, 40 of 51 persons (80%) eligible for diagnostic evaluation underwent cystoscopy: 25 of the 40 had non-bladder cancer abnormalities, such as chronic inflammation, chronic cystitis, urothelial atypia, hyperplasia, or papillary clusters. Twelve had dysplasia only and three had cancer. Of those three, two had previously diagnosed dysplasia and one had cancer as an initial diagnosis. This cohort reflected a young population that continues to be at risk as evidenced by the positive biomarkers and presence of dysplasia. Because of the power of the biomarkers, not all patients were required to undergo cystoscopy.

Hemastix dipstick testing, as defined by Messing, was used to screen workers for bladder cancer in a 3-year case control study at the Dupont Chambers Works.[59] Workers (1725) were exposed to a mixture of bladder cancer carcinogens and were followed at 3-month intervals. In this study participants tested their urine on 14 consecutive days every other quarter. Cytologies were performed on alternating quarters during the first seven periods of screening. Two new cases and one recurrence of TCC of the bladder were detected during the course of the screening.

A Canadian program screened aluminum workers with Pap cytology.[41] This program for screening aluminum workers exposed to benzene-soluble coal tar pitch volatiles has been operational since the 1970s. During this interval there has been a stage shift from 61% invasive to only 37% invasive tumors in the 1980s without any alteration in tumor grade. These results support the notion that an effective screening program is in place for these workers. More recently, biomarkers have been integrated into this screening program and the results of these studies remain pending. A limitation of this cohort and the others reviewed was the few individuals detected with bladder cancer.

## PROSPECTIVE STUDIES IN HIGH-RISK OCCUPATIONAL COHORTS EXPOSED TO BENZIDINE

Cancer screening of occupationally exposed cohorts with sensitive and specific biomarkers that reflect molecular phenotypic alterations is one potential strategy for cancer control. A study by Hemstreet et al incorporating a biomarker profile was used for initial risk stratification and subsequent longitudinal screening of an occupational cohort of Chinese workers located in three different cities who were exposed to benzidine and at known risk for bladder cancer.[24] Prior to the initiation of the biomarker screening program, the cohort had been well characterized and was undergoing routine Pap cytology and urinalysis on a yearly basis. The standardized incidence rate of bladder cancer in this group was very high (25.0), and there was a detrimental multiplicative effect between cigarette smoking and occupational exposure.[37]

Based on the concept of molecular phenotypic alteration in voided urothelial cells, and the notion that biochemical alterations precede morphologic changes, the workers were assigned to a low-, medium- or high-risk group following the initial screen. To confirm the hypothesis that biomarkers can serve as a basis for risk stratification, a longitudinal study was initiated in the benzidine-exposed cohort previously identified by Bi et al.[38] Markers were incorporated into the study based on their performance in studies of symptomatic patients and their clustering in association with their biochemical field expression.[2,60-62] The biomarker panel included DNA ploidy (5CER), a bladder cancer-associated antigen (p300), and a cytoskeletal marker associated with cytoskeletal remodeling (G-actin).

This study attempted to determine whether carcinogenesis-related alterations in urothelial cells shed into urine could be used to stratify individuals for their risk of developing/harboring bladder cancer. The same biomarkers were tested for their ability to detect bladder cancer in a prospective 6-year longitudinal study, the schema for which is shown in Figure 23.1. In this study, 1693 male workers from the exposed group and 373 randomly selected, age-matched male workers from the

non-exposed group were incorporated into the study design. Both groups were screened initially and were then screened a second time, 3 years later. Those at higher risk, depending on their biomarker profile, were either screened at 6-month intervals and recommended for cystoscopy or screened annually. Between 150 and 200 cc of voided urine were equally split for Pap cytology and urinalysis, and the second aliquot was fixed for subsequent biomarker analysis utilizing quantitative fluorescence imaging. The threshold for each of the biomarkers was established in symptomatic patients prior to the initiation of the trial.

A total of 30 cases of bladder cancer were identified in this study, with 2 in the control group and 28 in the exposed group. The incidence in the exposed group was 263.3 per 100,000/year. Of the cases in the exposed group, 20 were low or intermediate grade and 8 were high grade; only 4 cancers had invaded the muscularis propria at the time of diagnosis. Using the risk stratification biomarker schema, only 10.8% of the exposed and non-exposed workers required continuous longitudinal surveillance, avoiding the need to rescreen the entire cohort on an annual or biannual basis. Individuals in whom the p300 biomarker was positive were 31 times more likely to have bladder cancer than individuals with negative markers. In a time-dependent covariate analysis, individuals with p300 positive and DNA ploidy positive were 81.7 times more likely to be at risk for bladder cancer. Based on these studies, workers were recommended for biomarkers, cystoscopy, and bladder biopsy as clinically indicated. The screening program detected 90% of the tumors that developed in this cohort and individuals were targeted for intense surveillance. In some cases individuals were defined as being at high risk 3–5 years prior to clinically detected (cystoscopy) disease. This study confirmed the concept that the molecular fingerprints in the 'normal' cells predict carcinogenesis in an organ at risk for cancer. These same biomarkers were subsequently utilized to monitor symptomatic patients for the response to immunotherapy and the differentiating agent DMSO.[63]

## RELEVANCE FOR FUTURE RESEARCH

While the Wisconsin screening project represented only a single study, its results are sufficiently intriguing to justify further work.

### Smoking

In future screening of the general population, perhaps the prevalence of disease can be increased by including only current cigarette smokers and men with recent smoking histories.[11,20,64] Additionally, various genetic factors in smokers, such as specific polymorphisms of enzymes believed to be important in activation (cytochrome P450 1A2) or deactivation (N-acetyltransferase [NAT] 1) of

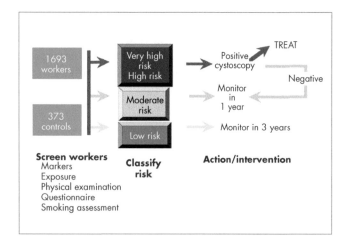

**Fig. 23.1**
Screening study design indicating that subjects were stratified based on biomarker results into three monitoring groups with their associated course of action.

smoking-associated carcinogens, may be able to predict an increased risk for smoking-induced bladder cancer, and justify more focused screening.[11] Other genetic markers of susceptibility may predict a decreased risk depending on the metabolic pathway of the carcinogen. For example, a protective association was noted for the slow NAT2 genotype after adjustment for cumulative benzidine exposure and lifetime smoking (OR = 0.3, 95% CI: 0.1–1.0).[65]

### Testing regime

Men in the Wisconsin study with initially all-negative testing repeated multiple self-testing 9 months later. Of those with hematuria only on this second round of testing, 0.82% were found to have bladder cancer.[22] This indicates that repeat rounds of testing (in those that test negatively for hematuria initially) probably have to be done annually. Whether a biomarker profile of risk (as was utilized in the Chinese benzidine-exposed worker study described above) can be applied to the general population in order to determine the method and intensity of follow-up screening based on risk stratification has not been studied.

### Hematuria

Hematuria, while present in almost all patients diagnosed with bladder cancer if one tests frequently enough,[66] remains a relatively nonspecific sign of the disease. Despite its very high sensitivity with the frequent testing regime, its PPV in the Wisconsin screening study was less than 10%, indicating that over 90% of participants that were worked up did not have bladder cancer. It would seem reasonable to take advantage of hematuria reagent strips' great sensitivity, low cost, and ease of performing at home, by using multiple hematuria reagent strips as an initial screen and then having all subjects with a positive test undergo one or a series of additional marker studies, only requesting those subjects who are also positive on the second tier screens to undergo cystoscopy.

Those with microhematuria detected by reagent strip testing, and at least one positive bladder cancer marker test with a negative cystoscopy, should have thorough upper tract imaging (e.g. computer tomographic urography or intravenous or retrograde urography). If these studies are negative, they should undergo repeat marker tests in 3–6 months, and repeat cystoscopy if any test is positive, depending on the specificity of the individual marker test that was positive (see Chapter 20).

While such an approach might miss significant hematuria-producing diseases that were not due to urothelial malignancy, and may overlook the diagnosis of small, low-grade superficial urothelial cancers (for which none of the currently available marker tests is exquisitely sensitive),[21,67] it is likely that a combination of markers could be developed that would be nearly 100% sensitive for the high-grade cancers, and have an acceptable sensitivity for the low-grade ones. In such a protocol, all subjects with symptoms, including gross hematuria and irritable voiding symptoms, would be cystoscoped as well, regardless of marker test results. With this combination, it is likely that individuals with low-grade tumors missed by the marker tests would ultimately have their cancers diagnosed before invasive disease developed.

## CONCLUSION

The benefits of bladder cancer screening using biomarker tests alone or in combination, with or without repetitive hematuria testing, have yet to be demonstrated. However, based on the biology of urothelial cancer, there is undeniable evidence that the efficacy, the morbidity, and the expense of therapy are directly related to the stage of the disease. The ability to target at-risk and very high-risk populations, and the accessibility of urine to quantitate biomarkers in shed tumor cells, molecules, and related substances in the urine, all provide evidence suggesting that screening is feasible. Furthermore, the efficacy and cost effectiveness of several approaches, and biomarker combinations with evolving technologies, are worth testing.

### REFERENCES

1. Bonner RB, Hurst RE, Rao J, et al. Instrumentation, accuracy and quality control in development of quantitative fluorescence image analysis. In Hanausek M, Walaszek Z (eds): Tumor Marker Protocols, vol 14. Totowa, NJ: Humana Press, 1998, p 181.

2. Rao JY, Hemstreet GP, Hurst RE, et al. Alterations in phenotypic biochemical markers in bladder epithelium during tumorigenesis. Proc Natl Acad Sci USA 1993;90:8287–8291.

3. Koss LG, Tiamson E M, Robbins MA. Mapping cancerous and precancerous bladder changes. A study of the urothelium in ten surgically removed bladders. JAMA 1974;227:281–286.

4. Koss LG. Mapping of the urinary bladder: its impact on the concepts of bladder cancer. Hum Pathol 1979;10:533–548.

5. Slaughter DP, Southwick HW, Smejkal W. 'Field cancerization' in oral stratified squamous epithelium: clinical implications of multicentric origin. Cancer 1953;6:963–968.

6. Rao JY, Hemstreet GP, Hurst RE. Molecular pathology and biomarkers of bladder cancer. In Srivastava S, Henson DE, Gazdar A (eds): Molecular Pathology of Early Cancer. Amsterdam: IOS Press, 1999, p 53.

7. Jemal A, Tiwari RC, Murray T, et al. Cancer statistics, 2004. CA Cancer J Clin 2004;54:8–29.

8. Greenlee RT, Hill-Harmon MB, Murray T, et al. Cancer statistics, 2001. CA Cancer J Clin 2001;51(1):15–36.

9. Ries LA, Kosary CL, Hankey BF, et al. SEER Cancer Statistics Review 1973–1995. Bethesda, MD: National Cancer Institute, 1998.

10. Jewett HJ, Strong GH. Infiltrating carcinoma of the bladder: Relation of depth of penetration of bladder wall with incidence of local extension and metastases. J Urol 1946;55:366–372.

11. Messing EM. Urothelial tumors of the urinary tract. In Walsh PC, Vaughan E, Retik AB, et al (eds): Campbell's Urology, 8th ed. Philadelphia: WB Saunders, 2002, p 2732.

12. Kaye KW, Lange PH. Mode of presentation of invasive bladder cancer: reassessment of the problem. J Urol 1982;128:31–33.

13. Vaidya A, Soloway MS, Hawke C, et al. De novo muscle invasive bladder cancer: is there a change in trend? J Urol 2001;165:47–50.

14. Hopkins SC, Ford KS, Soloway MS. Invasive bladder cancer: support for screening. J Urol 1983;130:61–64.

15. Messing EM. De novo muscle invasive bladder cancer: is there a change in trend? J Urol 2001;165:47–50.

16. Resseguie LJ, Nobrega FT, Farrow GM, Timmons JW, Worobec TG. Epidemiology of renal and ureteral cancer in Rochester, Minnesota, 1950–1974, with special reference to clinical and pathologic features. Mayo Clin Proc 1978;53:503–510.

17. Kishi K, Hirota T, Matsumoto K, et al. Carcinoma of the bladder: a clinical and pathological analysis of 87 autopsy cases. J Urol 1981;125:36–39.

18. Marshall VF. Current clinical problems regarding bladder tumors. Cancer 1956;9:543–550.

19. Oldbring J, Glifberg I, Mikulowski P, et al. Carcinoma of the renal pelvis and ureter following bladder carcinoma: frequency, risk factors and clinicopathological findings. J Urol 1989;141:1311–1313.

20. O'Donnell M, Lilli K, Leopold C. Contemporary profile of superficial bladder cancer as revealed from an open-entry national multi center study. J Urol 2004;171(4):283a.

21. Boman H, Hedelin H, Holmang S. Four bladder tumor markers have a disappointingly low sensitivity for small size and low grade recurrence. J Urol 2002;167:80–83.

22. Messing EM, Young TB, Hunt VB, et al. Hematuria home screening: repeat testing results. J Urol 1995;154:57–61.

23. Messing EM, Young TB, Hunt VB, et al. Home screening for hematuria: results of a multiclinic study. J Urol 1992;148:289–292.

24. Hemstreet GP III, Yin S, Ma Z, et al. Biomarker risk assessment and bladder cancer detection in a cohort exposed to benzidine. J Natl Cancer Inst 2001;93:427–436.

25. Hemstreet GP, Hurst RE, Bonner RB. Selection and development of biomarkers for bladder cancer. In Hanausek M, Walaszek Z (eds): Tumor Marker Protocols, vol 14. Totowa, NJ: Humana Press, 1998, p 37.

26. Lokeshwar VB, Öbek C, Soloway MS, et al. Tumor-associated hyaluronic acid: a new sensitive and specific urine marker for bladder cancer. Cancer Res 1997;57:773–777.

27. Pham HT, Block NL, Lokeshwar VB. Tumor-derived hyaluronidase: a diagnostic urine marker for high-grade bladder cancer. Cancer Res 1997;57:778–783.

28. Britton JP, Dowell AC, Whelan P. Dipstick hematuria and bladder cancer in men over 60: results of a community study. Br Med J 1989;299(6706):1010–1012.

29. Farrow GM, Utz DC and Rife CC. Morphological and clinical observations of patients with early bladder cancer treated with total cystectomy. Cancer Res 1976;36:2495–3002.

30. Britton JP, Dowell AC, Whelan P, et al. A community study of bladder cancer screening by the detection of occult urinary bleeding. J Urol 1992;148:788–790.

31. Messing EM, Young TB, Hunt VB, et al. Urinary tract cancers found by home screening with hematuria dipsticks in healthy men over 50 years of age. Cancer 1989;4:2361–2367.

32. Britton JP, Dowell AC, Whelan P, et al. A community study of bladder cancer screening by the detection of occult urinary bleeding. J Urol 1992;148:788–790.

33. Messing EM, Young TB, Hunt VB, et al. Comparison of bladder cancer outcome in men undergoing hematuria home screening versus those with standard clinical presentations. Urology 1995;45:387–397.

34. Lawrence WF, Messing E, Bram LL, et al. The cost-effectiveness of screening men for bladder cancer using chemical reagent strips to detect microscopic hematuria. J Urol 1995;53:477A.

35. Rehn L. Blasengeschwulste bei fuchsin-arbeitern. Arch Klin Chir 1895;50:588–600.

36. Schulte PA, Ringen K. Notification of workers at high risk: an emerging public health problem. Am J Public Health 1984;74:485–491.

37. Bi WF, Hayes R, Feng P, et al. Mortality and incidence of bladder cancer in benzidine-exposed workers in China. Am J Ind Med 1992;21:481–489.

38. Bi W, Rao J, Hemstreet GP, et al. Field molecular epidemiology. Feasibility of monitoring for the malignant bladder cell phenotype in a benzidine-exposed occupational cohort. J Occup Med 1993;35(1):20–27.

39. Cartwright RA. Bladder cancer screening in the United Kingdom. J Occup Med 1990;32:878–880.

40. Cartwright RA. Historical and modern epidemiological studies on populations exposed to N-substituted aryl compounds. Environ Health Perspect 1983;49:13–19.

41. Theriault G, Tremblay C, Armstrong B. Bladder cancer screening among primary aluminum production workers in Quebec. J Occup Med 1990;32(9):869–872.

42. Koss LG, Deitch D, Ramanathan R, et al. Diagnostic value of cytology of voided urine. Acta Cytol 1985;29:810–814.

43. Smith JJ, Cowan L, Hemstreet GP. Automated quantitative fluorescence image analysis in symptomatic bladder cancer patients. Gynecol Oncol 1987;28:241–254.

44. Brown FM. Urine Cytology: Is it still the gold standard for screening? Urol Clin North Am 2000;1:25–37.

45. Farrow GM. Urine cytology in the detection of bladder cancer: a critical approach. J Occup Med 1990;32:817–821.

46. Golden JF, West SS, Shingleton HM, et al. A screening system for cervical cancer cytology. J Histochem Cytochem 1979;27:522–528.

47. Case R, Hosker M, McDonald D, et al. Tumours of the urinary bladder in workmen engaged in the manufacture and use of certain dyestuff intermediates in the British chemical industry. Br J Ind Med 1954;11:75–104.

48. Cartwright RA, Gadian T, Garland JB, et al. The influence of malignant cell cytology screening on the survival of industrial bladder cancer cases. J Epidemiol Community Health 1981;35:35–38.

49. Crosby JH, Allsbrook WC, Koss LG, et al. Cytologic detection of urothelial cancer and other abnormalities in a cohort of workers exposed to aromatic amines. Acta Cytol 1991;35:263–268.

50. Hemstreet GP, Schulte PA, Ringen K, et al. DNA hyperploidy as a marker for biological response to bladder to carcinogen exposure. Int J Cancer 1988;42:817–820.

51. Hemstreet GP, Schulte PA, Ringen K, Stringer W, Alterkruse EB. DNA hyperploidy as a marker for biological response to bladder carcinogen exposure. Int J Cancer 1988;42:817–820.

52. Schulte PA, Ringen K, Altekruse EB, et al. Notification of a cohort of workers at risk of bladder cancer. J Occup Med 1985;16:529–27(1):19–28.

53. Leviton LC, Marsh GM, Talbott EO, et al. Drake Chemical Workers' Health Registry: coping with community tension over toxic exposures. Am J Public Health 1991;81(6):689–693.

54. Leviton LC, Chen HT, Marsh GM, et al. Evaluation issues in the Drake Chemical Workers Notification and Health Registry Study. Am J Ind Med 1993;23:197–204.

55. Marsh GM, Callahan C, Pavlock D, et al. A protocol for bladder cancer screening and medical surveillance among high-risk groups: the Drake Health Registry experience. J Occup Med 1990;32(9):881–886.

56. Marsh GM, Leviton LC, Talbott EO, et al. Drake chemical workers health registry study: I. Notification and medical surveillance of a group of workers at a high risk of developing bladder cancer. Am J Ind Med 1991;19:291–301.

57. Marsh GM, Cassidy LD. The Drake Health Registry Study: findings from fifteen years of continuous bladder screening. Am J Ind Med 2003;43:142–148.

58. Mason TJ, Walsh WP, Lee K, Vogler W. New opportunities for screening and early detection of bladder cancer. J Cell Biochem Suppl 1992;161:13–22.

59. Mason T, Vogler W. Bladder cancer screening at the Dupont Chambers Works: a new initiative. J Occup Med 1990;32(9):874–877.

60. Bonner RB, Hemstreet GP, Fradet Y, et al. Bladder cancer risk assessment with quantitative fluorescence image analysis of tumor markers in exfoliated bladder cells. Cancer 1993;72:2461–2469.

61. Hemstreet GP, Bonner RB, Hurst RE, et al. Cytology of bladder cancer. In Vogelzang NJ, Scardino PT, Shipley WU, et al (eds): Comprehensive Textbook of Genitourinary Oncology, 2nd ed. Baltimore: Lippincott Williams & Wilkins, 2000, p 322.

62. Hemstreet GP, Rao JY, Hurst RE, et al. G-actin as a risk factor and modulatable endpoint for cancer chemoprevention trials. J Cell Biochem 1996;25(Suppl):197–204.

63. Hemstreet GP, Rao JY, Hurst RE, et al. Biomarkers in monitoring for efficacy of immunotherapy and chemoprevention of bladder cancer with dimethylsulfoxide. Cancer Detec Prev 1999;23:163–171.

64. Paz A, Cytron S, Lobik L, et al. Passive smoking—a risk factor for transitional cell carcinoma of the bladder in patients with hematuria. J Urol 2002;167(4):648A.

65. Carréon T, Ruder A, Schulte PA, et al. NAT2 slow acetylation and bladder cancer in workers exposed to benzidine. Int J Cancer 2005 (in press).**[AU6]**

66. Messing EM, Vaillancourt A. Hematuria screening for bladder cancer. J Occup Med 1990;32:838–845.

67. Messing EM, Korman H, Teot L, et al. Performance of ImmunoCyt® urine test for patients monitored for recurrence of bladder cancer: a multi-center study in the United States. J Urol 2005;174:1238–1241.

# Natural history of stages Ta, T1, and Tis urothelial cancer in the urinary bladder

## 24

*Michael J Droller*

## INTRODUCTION

The 64,000 new cases of urothelial cancer of the urinary bladder that are diagnosed annually in North America represent an age-standardized incidence rate of approximately 24/100,000 person years among men and approximately 5.5/100,000 person years in women.[1,2] This makes urinary bladder cancer the fourth most common noncutaneous malignancy in men (approximately 44,000 estimated new cases annually) and the eighth most common in women (approximately 16,000 cases annually).[1] The mortality rate of >12,000 deaths annually in North America places bladder cancer as the seventh leading cause of cancer death in men and the tenth leading cause of cancer death in women.[2] Worldwide, bladder cancer accounts for approximately 250,000 new diagnoses annually and approximately 120,000 cancer deaths.[3]

Clearly, most patients with bladder cancer do not die of their disease. However, a major proportion is likely to experience recurrence, which may take place multiple times. Therefore, when considering the true prevalence of bladder cancer, the costs of conservative treatment, and the surveillance required to monitor for recurrence and potential progression, make bladder cancer an even greater public health issue than these generally quoted demographic figures might suggest (see Chapter 1).

Of all the new cases of bladder cancer diagnosed annually, 70% to 75% are considered 'superficial', or not invasive of the bladder muscularis propria.[4,5] Among these, 50% to 75% are likely to recur, and the ongoing prevalence of bladder cancer, therefore, far exceeds its annual incidence. Even though only 15% to 25% of bladder cancers that present at initial diagnosis as 'superficial' are likely to progress to muscle invasion,[4,5] these compound the concern and efforts of physicians in their attempts to prevent recurrence of superficial disease and identify and possibly prevent recurrence with progression.

Individuals that present initially with muscle-invasive disease are likely to have developed occult metastases in more than 50% of instances.[6] It is assumed that those who develop muscle-invasive disease, after having been treated and monitored for recurrence of superficial disease, might have had a lesser chance of having occult metastasis if they had been diagnosed just as muscle invasion had occurred. However, the biologic capabilities of these lesions likely determine their metastatic potential, the expression of which may have occurred before the diagnosis of muscle invasion was made. With this in mind, attention to the characteristics of the different forms of 'superficial' disease and the 'early' signals that a particular tumor diathesis provides is of utmost importance in selecting a treatment approach and in identifying patients at risk who might benefit from a more intensive surveillance, and, in some instances, an initially more aggressive treatment approach.

The purpose of this chapter is to describe the different forms of 'superficial' urothelial cancer, characterize their natural history, identify those features both histologically and on a molecular basis that may predict intrinsic biologic potential of a particular form of superficial disease, and suggest a treatment approach in the context of a tumor's biologic potential.

## OVERVIEW OF 'SUPERFICIAL' UROTHELIAL CANCER

The 70% to 75% of newly diagnosed urothelial cancers described as 'superficial' are either confined to the lining (mucosa) of the bladder or extend into the lamina propria (but not to the muscularis propria). Nearly 70% to 75% of these are mucosally confined,[7] and appear to be of low/moderate grade. These generally do not have a life-threatening course, and have therefore been characterized as 'disease of low malignant potential' (see below). Only 2% to 4% present as high-grade tumors,[8] and it is these that may behave in a highly aggressive manner.

Approximately 20% to 25% of newly diagnosed 'superficial' urothelial cancers are found to have penetrated across the epithelial basement membrane into the underlying connective tissue (lamina propria).[7] A thin muscle layer (the muscularis mucosae) has been suggested to assist in demarcating the depth of penetration of urothelial cancers when they extend into the lamina propria.[9] Clinical correlations between depth of invasion in relation to this landmark, disease progression and survival have also been suggested.[10,11] Whether the depth of invasion is indicative of the intrinsic biologic potential for invasiveness (and implied aggressiveness) of a particular cancer, or simply the time at which it happened to have been diagnosed, however, is unclear.

Most lamina propria-invasive tumors are of moderate/high grade, in contrast to the lower grades that characterize mucosally confined tumors.[7,8] Correspondingly, they tend to have a more aggressive biologic potential. If we exclude the 10% to 20% of such tumors that are found on repeat resection to have penetrated the muscularis propria,[12] and consider only the moderate-grade tumors that have penetrated the lamina propria only superficially, such tumors are largely amenable to control by transurethral resection with preservation of the bladder. These require only continued surveillance for possible recurrence. On the other hand, those lamina propria-invasive tumors that are more extensively invasive and of high grade have an at least 50% risk of progression.[13,14] At a minimum these require intensive surveillance and may actually offer only a narrow window of opportunity to avoid missing tumor progression and compromising an opportunity to obtain a cure with more aggressive initial therapy.

These considerations need to be placed in the context of multiplicity of disease that can increase the risk of recurrence,[15] and failure to respond to adjunctive intravesical therapies, which may suggest an increased risk for introduction of additional chromosomal defects and development of more aggressive tumors.[16]

However, these concerns need to be placed in perspective in viewing the general issue of superficial disease. If 50% of high-grade, lamina propria-invasive tumors are likely to progress (50% occur as stage T1 grade 3, and 50% of these are likely to respond to resection and intravesical therapy),[17] then only 7.5% to 10% overall are likely to be at risk for progression, a majority therefore not creating a life-threatening risk.

A third type of superficial disease presents in a form known as 'carcinoma in situ' (CIS). This form of urothelial cancer involves the proliferation of transformed urothelial cells that migrate along the plane of the lining of the bladder, either replacing or undermining the normal urothelium.[18] Characteristically, cells comprising this entity are high grade. They do not demonstrate the degree of cohesiveness that characterizes papillary lesions (either mucosally confined or penetrative of the lamina propria). The cells in CIS also lack adhesiveness to the epithelial basement membrane and, therefore, readily slough into the urine, leaving behind denuded regions of the mucosa.

Although generally assumed to be confined to the lining of the bladder, these lesions appear in 30% of biopsies to demonstrate penetration of cells through the basement membrane into the lamina propria.[19] Carcinoma in situ is diagnosed as the sole neoplastic lesion in only 3% to 5% of all patients biopsied for evaluation of microscopic hematuria in the presence of irritative symptoms (frequency and urgency) and positive urinary cytology but with no concomitant exophytic tumor.[20] More commonly, CIS is diagnosed in the presence of concomitant high-grade exophytic lesions (either papillary or nodular), the majority of which are already infiltrative of the bladder wall. This may involve the lamina propria in most instances but may often extend into the muscularis.[21,22] Those patients presenting with both lamina propria-invasive tumors (especially if extensively invasive) and CIS are at risk for rapid progression.[23]

# NONMUSCLE INVASIVE BLADDER CANCER

## STAGING

The development of a staging system is based upon correlations between the classification of various forms of urothelial cancer and prognosis of the particular cancer diathesis. Classification of bladder cancer has generally been based upon the histologic appearance of pathologic specimens (biopsies, resections, or full-thickness bladder wall) regarding the depth to which the cancer may have penetrated the concentric layers of the bladder wall (Figure 24.1, Box 24.1).[24] Systems based upon the degree of differentiation of the malignant cells (grade) are less commonly used.[25] Prognosis in the context of this classification is based upon an interpretation of the tumor's histologic appearance in association with what is known of the natural history of the disease, its intrinsic biologic potential, and its expected response to various treatments.

Staging of urothelial cancer of the bladder is based upon the pioneering observations of Jewett, who

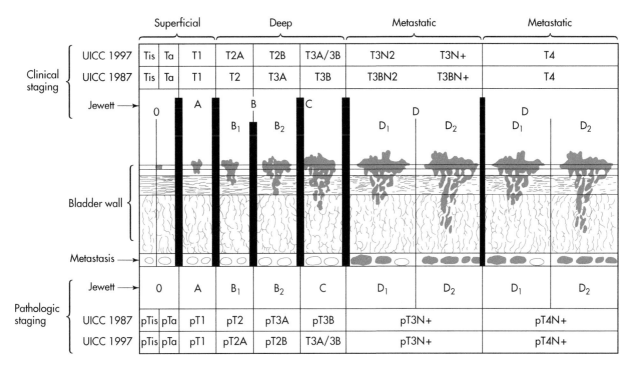

**Fig. 24.1**
Staging system for bladder cancer (see also Box 24.1). Modified after Koss[28] and WF Whitmore, personal communication; by permission of Michael J Droller, 2004.

**Box 24.1** Staging system for bladder cancer

Staging systems facilitate an understanding of the association between different histologic appearances of a cancer and prognosis. Staging systems also facilitate analysis of treatment results for cancers of a given stage, allowing comparisons of different treatments and between multiple treating physicians to be made. Traditionally, staging systems for bladder cancer have correlated prognosis with the depth of invasion of a cancer into and through the different layers of the bladder wall.

Importantly, the staging system is not intended as a depiction of the natural history of the disease. Rather, it represents the histologic presentation of a cancer as a 'snapshot' of its appearance at a particular time and as an indication of its potential activity in a historical context. Through this, decisions in selecting a particular treatment can be made on the basis of what previous applications of such treatments have achieved in terms of disease recurrence, disease progression, and disease-free survival. Thus, the staging system does not depict the pathogenesis of disease or the variations in pathogenesis that can occur with time. Rather, the staging system classifies the disease so that particular treatments can be selected and the results of these treatments assessed.

The original staging system developed by Jewett and Strong in 1946 suggested distinctions between 'superficial' and 'muscle-invasive' disease.[26] The 'superficial' category was subsequently divided into those tumors confined to the urothelium (mucosa) (stage Ta) and those tumors that had penetrated the submucosal connective tissue (lamina propria) (stage T1).[28] Many years later, CIS (stage Tis) was recognized as a separate, albeit superficial, form of disease comprised of neoplastic cells that had replaced the normal urothelium or had undermined it, extending along the normal plane of the urothelium.[18,22]

Muscle-invasive bladder tumors were those that had penetrated the muscularis propria, either superficially (stage T2a) or deeply (stage T2b), or had penetrated through the muscularis propria into the perivesical soft tissue, either microscopically (stage T3a) or extensively (stage T3b). Distinctions between the different types of muscle-invasive disease were adjusted by the World Health Organization (WHO) classification system, which combined all muscle-invasive tumors into one category (stage T2). Correspondingly, those tumors that were found to penetrate through the muscularis propria into the perivesical soft tissues were now classified as stage T3 (instead of the previous classification of deep muscle invasion as T3a).[53,55] Involvement of adjacent structures (most notably the prostate or vaginal wall) were categorized as stage T4, while involvement of lymph nodes was assigned to the N category (with numbers of lymph nodes designated by a numerical subscript); those that had metastasized to distant sites were categorized as M or 'metastatic'.[53,55]

Recent observations have suggested additional categories in accordance with differences in prognosis of particular forms of bladder cancer. For example, the occasional presence of a thin smooth muscle layer in the lamina propria (the 'muscularis mucosae') has been used to distinguish between those lamina propria-invasive tumors that have penetrated the lamina propria only superficially (stage T1a) from those that have penetrated more extensively and deep to the muscularis mucosae (stage T1b).[10–12] Although distinctions in tumor recurrence and disease-free survival have been correlated with these anatomical distinctions, they have not as yet been validated and have therefore not been incorporated into the formal staging system. Similarly, distinctions have been made amongst those urothelial tumors that have involved only the urothelial lining of the prostatic ducts from those that have penetrated into the prostatic stroma, the latter indicating a far more ominous prognosis.[52,54]

Observations of genetic and molecular changes in association with tumor behavior have been suggested to be of value in further categorizing different types of urothelial cancer within the various traditional histologic stages of disease.[91,93] Advances in our understanding of the genetic and biochemical pathways in determining the pathogenesis of different forms of bladder cancer will undoubtedly be incorporated into future staging systems. To date, however, validation of these distinctions in association with a particular form of bladder cancer and its prognosis has not been accomplished, and formal incorporation of such findings into the accepted staging system for bladder cancer has not been possible.

classified cancers as noninvasive and invasive over a half century ago.[26,27] The schematic presentation of tumors that increasingly penetrate the bladder wall suggests a continuum whereby tumors invade progressively more deeply. According to this system, initial neoplastic transformation by definition results in CIS, which then produces papillary mucosally confined lesions that then progress to invade the lamina propria.[78] Such tumors then penetrate more deeply into the muscularis propria, producing a bulkier, more solid nodular mass. Each stage is progressively associated with an increased likelihood of metastasizing, which probably represents the result of an intermixing of new blood vessels and lymphatics that are induced by the growing mass of cells, the growth factors they produce, and their invasive capabilities.[29,30]

## PATHOGENESIS

An awareness that the various forms of superficial cancer manifested different clinical patterns suggested that the linear sequence indicated by this staging schema did not accurately portray the distinct behavioral patterns that the different types of superficial cancers expressed. This prompted suggestions that neoplastic transformation led to tumor diatheses with different intrinsic biologic potentials and varying but still predictable forms of clinical expression (Figure 24.2, Box 24.2).[31,32] One form of diathesis (represented as stage Ta, or mucosally confined papillary disease) (Figure 24.3, Box 24.3) appeared to be solely 'proliferative' and, therefore, likely to recur but not to progress to invasion. The predominant process in these cases could be termed 'atypical hyperplasia', with such tumors often appearing to multiply in the bladder at various sites and recurring frequently over time (so-called 'polychronotropism'). Another form might be more likely to progress by invading the bladder wall, expressing a more aggressive intrinsic biologic potential. In these, as represented by stage T1 in which papillary tumors invaded the lamina propria (Figure 24.4, Box 24.4), a higher grade of cell appears more characteristic, and the predominant process might be termed 'dysplasia' as superimposed on atypical hyperplasia in the formation of a papillary configuration. A third manifestation of these pathogenic processes, as represented by carcinoma in situ (Tis) (Figure 24.5, Box 24.5), produces a dysplastic diathesis in which highly aggressive behavior may lead to the development of deeply invasive nodular cancers, often with vascular invasion, before clinical expression is diagnosed. Observations that adjunctive intravesical therapies might effect recurrence and progression in the short term, but often make little difference in ultimate

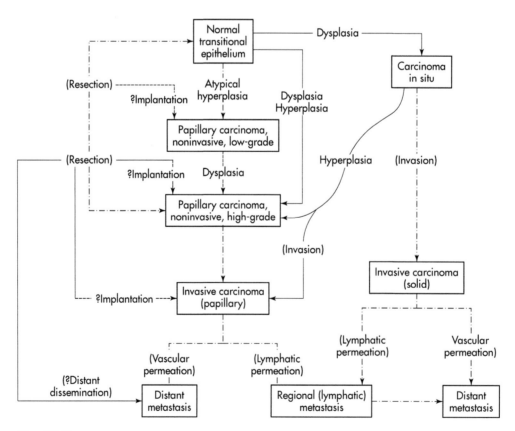

**Fig. 24.2**
The pathogenesis of bladder cancer (see also Box 24.2). With permission of Michael J Droller, 2004.

The staging schema depicted in Figure 24.1 attempts to place the 'snapshot' of a particular tumor's histologic appearance in the context of what its prognosis may be in attempts to design appropriate therapeutic approaches and in attempts to compare results of various therapies for a particular form of malignancy. In contrast, the schema proposed in Figure 24.2 suggests different pathways that a particular neoplastic diathesis may have followed until symptoms (largely hematuria) led to its diagnosis at a particular stage, and what course might be expected as it continued to pursue a particular developmental pathway (as determined by mutational events that had led initially to neoplastic transformation). Biologically, the presumption is that genetic changes produce a particular type of cancer and dictate the cancer's intrinsic biologic potential either to recur or to progress, notwithstanding therapies selected (which for most practical purposes are applied relatively 'late' in the developmental lifetime of a particular cancer diathesis).

The majority of tumors present with a papillary configuration and are generally confined to the urothelial mucosa.[7] Schematically, this is taken to represent a proliferative diathesis which can be termed 'atypical hyperplasia'. With resection, the normal urothelium is presumably restored. The likelihood of recurrence may reflect subvisual neoplastic changes elsewhere in the bladder that are undetectable at the time of resection or tumor cell implantation that may account for recurrence of genetically and histologically identical tumors. Although recurrence of low-grade mucosally confined tumors is common (as often as 70%), progression is rare.[7,8]

Further genetic changes may induce the development of higher grade papillary lesions.[29,30] Although these may account for the transformation of initially low-grade to higher grade lesions (a process designated in this schema as 'dysplasia'), it is equally likely that these events occur at initial neoplastic transformation, the different genetic changes producing histologically less differentiated appearances in either a papillary or more flattened nonpapillary form of disease (so-called CIS).[16,36] High-grade papillary lesions, which manifest the processes of proliferation with dedifferentiation, appear to have the intrinsic ability to penetrate into the submucosal connective tissue (lamina propria), either superficially or more deeply and extensively, and represent a greater risk of cancer progression with ultimate invasion of the muscularis propria with possible dissemination to regional lymph nodes and distant sites.[4,5]

Flat CIS, initially replacing or undermining the normal urothelium, does not lead to the development of papillary structures.[18,20] Instead, it may infiltrate the lamina propria in a micronodular form,[19] ultimately leading to the development of invasive cancers without ever protruding into the lumen of the bladder until much later in their development.[20,21] This may account for the diagnosis of muscle-invasive cancers as their initial clinical presentation,[6] and indicates why the finding of CIS in the setting of high-grade papillary lamina propria-invasive disease signals a highly ominous prognosis.[13,14,17,23] Solid or nodular tumors (in contrast to papillary tumors) appear more commonly to be associated with lymphatic and/or vascular penetration and the development of distant metastases.[83,84] The likelihood that any of these pathways are followed is depicted schematically in Figure 24.2 by the size of the arrows.

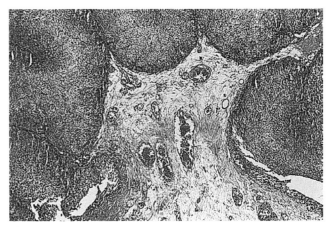

**Fig. 24.3**
Mucosally confined (stage Ta) transitional cell cancer (see also Box 24.3). With permission of Michael J Droller, 2004.

Mucosally confined papillary tumors represent the so-called proliferative pathway of bladder cancer development. In this, transformed cells produce clusters of cells that project into the lumen of the bladder in the form of papillary fronds of cells surrounding a central fibrovascular stalk. The majority of these are low/moderate grade and may occur singly or multiply. The urothelial mucosa adjacent to and between multiple tumors preserves a normal histologic appearance.[52] These papillary lesions can be distinguished from so-called 'papillomas', which are delicate papillary lesions comprised of fibrovascular cores lined by cytologically and architecturally normal urothelium.[52,55]

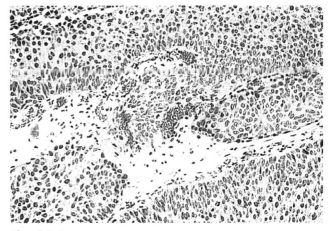

**Fig. 24.4**
Lamina propria-invasive transitional cell cancer (see also Box 24.4). With permission of Michael J Droller, 2004.

Lamina propria-invasive papillary urothelial cancers have the ability to penetrate through the mucosal basement membrane into the underlying connective tissue. They are generally comprised of moderate/high-grade cells. They may penetrate either superficially or more deeply across an inconsistent smooth muscle layer known as the 'muscularis mucosae'.[9–11] They may occur singly or multiply, and are not uncommonly associated with adjacent or distant flat CIS.[61,62] This represents a cancer diathesis that is potentially highly aggressive.[13,14,17]

outcomes, support the concept of an apparently inexorable pathogenesis of these differing forms of superficial malignancy.[33,34]

The recent application of new techniques to study the molecular biology and genetics of bladder cancer correlated the different histologic appearances of specific types of 'superficial' tumors with particular chromosomal defects.[35,36] These were suggested, in fact, to determine the specific biologic and clinical course of

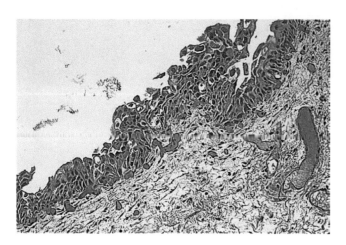

**Fig. 24.5**
Carcinoma in situ (see also Box 24.5). With permission of Michael J Droller, 2004.

---

**Box 24.5** Carcinoma in situ

Occasionally, neoplastic transformation results in the generation of high-grade cells that undermine the normal urothelium and replace it while maintaining the normal contour of the mucosal lining of the bladder.[18,22] These cells are less cohesive than either normal urothelial cells or cells that comprise the papillary superficial tumors depicted in Figures 24.3 and 24.4. As a consequence, cells from these lesions often slough into the urine, leaving behind denuded areas and exposing the lamina propria to the bladder's urine contents. This may account for the irritative symptoms that often accompany this entity. Carcinoma in situ appears to give rise to micronodular disease that penetrates into the wall of the bladder,[19] leading to muscle-invasive cancers of a nodular form[20,21] that are usually diagnosed at this stage at their initial presentation.[6]

---

the various types of superficial cancer (Figure 24.6, Box 24.6).[32,37,38]

An increasing use of cytogenetic and molecular genetic markers may ultimately allow greater precision in determining the prognosis of a particular tumor diathesis as initially defined by pathologic assessment. The development of probes for specific chromosomal defects using fluorescent in situ hybridization (FISH) and amino acid sequencing with polymerase chain reaction (PCR) for DNA sequence analysis, may possibly enhance our ability to create a molecular profile in characterizing these varying tumor diatheses.[39,40] This has been applied in using immunohistochemistry and analysis by DNA single-strand conformational polymorphism (SSCP) to assess the molecular nature of superficial urothelial cancers.

For example, mutations of chromosome 17 with altered expression of p53 have been reported in up to 50% of primary CIS lesions, correlating with the dysplastic nature of this entity.[32,36,37] Similarly, positive staining of stage T1 tumors for p53 (representing the altered protein with a longer half life) and confirmation of mutational abnormalities by SSCP analysis have been proposed as significant prognostic factors in

progression.[35,41,42] In those few patients with stage Ta disease found to be p53 positive, the issue is less clear. Some may be high-grade lesions or represent micropapillary disease, with a histologic appearance unlike the prototypical low-grade papillary stage Ta lesions with normal adjacent mucosa that are p53 negative.

Changes in chromosome 9 may be an early event in the genesis of transitional cell cancer (TCC) (Figure 24.7, Box 24.7).[43,44] The tumor suppressor gene CDKN2A:p16 has been identified in the 9p21 region that is commonly altered in bladder cancer.[45] This gene encodes for a protein that is part of a group of cell cycle inhibitory molecules known as cyclin-dependent kinases. Loss of these genes may result in uncontrolled growth, cell proliferation, and consequent tumor formation (see Figure 24.7).

Loss of heterozygosity (LOH) of chromosome 17p has been associated with a potentially more aggressive urothelial cancer because of the occurrence of this lesion in association with higher stage lesions.[42,46] Several functional consequences have been characterized with this change. Thus, the p53 gene normally encodes for a 53 kD phosphoprotein that binds to DNA and is involved in gene transcription, monitoring of DNA synthesis, and the genesis of programmed cell death (apoptosis).[47] Defects are thought to allow poorly differentiated transformed cells to proliferate and remain viable as the normal pathway of suppression and elimination of abnormal cells with damaged (mutated) DNA by programmed cell death is disrupted. This can then lead to perpetuation of unrepaired mutations in other regulatory genes. Depending upon the biochemical changes that may then occur, the stage may then be set for the development of a diathesis that has the ability to infiltrate the connective tissue stroma, penetrate blood vessels and lymphatics, and metastasize. Overall, however, the various means by which particular genetic changes predispose to the development of cancers with specific epigenetic characteristics remain to be determined.

Incorporation of molecular and genetic profiles into current clinicopathologic staging systems has been proposed as a means to allow a more accurate characterization of the potential biologic activity and prognosis of a particular tumor diathesis. This will require further validation of these presumably predictive associations between specific chromosomal defects and their determination of a particular tumor's intrinsic biologic potential.

## TUMOR GRADE AND CLINICAL ACTIVITY

The grade of a tumor (the degree of differentiation or loss of differentiation) has been important in clinically characterizing its potential biologic behavior.[48,49] Early on, grade of disease was the primary feature used to

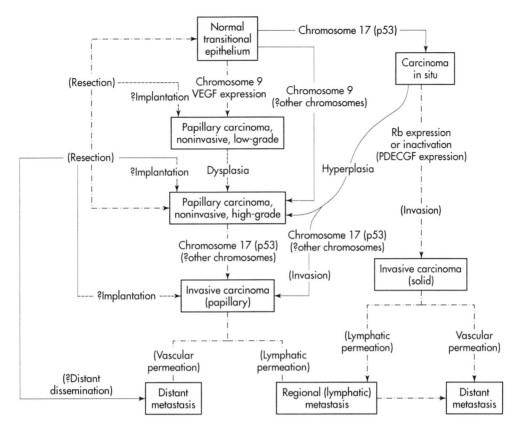

**Fig. 24.6**

Genetic changes in the pathogenesis of bladder cancer (see also Box 24.6). With permission of Michael J Droller, 2004.

---

**Box 24.6** Genetic changes in the pathogenesis of bladder cancer

The schema outlined in Figure 24.6 superimposes various genetic changes on the schema of pathogenesis of the different types of bladder cancer and their developmental pathways as presented in Figure 24.2. This schema is based on studies demonstrating different genetic changes found in association with different histologic patterns of bladder cancer.[30,32,38] Low-grade, mucosally confined papillary transitional cell cancers have commonly demonstrated defects in chromosome 9.[35,43,44] In contrast, high-grade papillary lamina propria-invasive cancers have been more commonly shown to have defects in chromosome 17 with expression of p53.[37,41] While the latter may also commonly be found to have defects in chromosome 9, it appears that chromosome 17 may confer a more dysplastic appearance to the cancer cells in association with activation of factors required for these cells to infiltrate the bladder wall and possibly metastasize.[41,42] Defects in chromosome 17 are also found in CIS, correlating with their potential to become invasive, often with a more nodular appearance.[36,37]

Correlations between specific genetic changes and histologic appearances remain to be defined more precisely. Furthermore, correlations between these changes, particular stages of disease, and their intrinsic biologic potential remain to be validated in order for genetic profiles to be incorporated into standard staging systems for bladder cancer.

---

characterize the aggressiveness of a particular cancer.[50,51] This was supplanted 30 years later by staging systems based upon depth of invasion into the bladder wall.[26,27] However, correlations between grade and stage remained important in the clinical assessment of a particular tumor diathesis, in characterizing the natural history and prognosis of a superficial tumor, in determining what type of therapy was likely to be effective, and in assessing therapeutic efficacy for a particular type (grade) of malignancy.[48,52] Mostofi et al introduced a classification system of grades 1, 2, and 3 based on the degree of cellular differentiation, and this was adopted by the World Health Organization (WHO)

in 1973.[53] Attempts to simplify the system 20 years later by Murphy et al incorporated the proposal of two categories based upon the cytologic features of the malignancy.[54] Low-grade carcinoma, corresponding to WHO grade 1, was used to describe a well-differentiated tumor that was predominantly papillary in architecture and confined to the mucosa. High-grade cancer corresponded to WHO grades 2 and 3 and was used to describe a poorly differentiated tumor. However, the occasional variability of grade within a particular tumor sometimes confounded the use of this system. Generally, the highest grade will be what is reported by the pathologist. More recently, some have suggested that

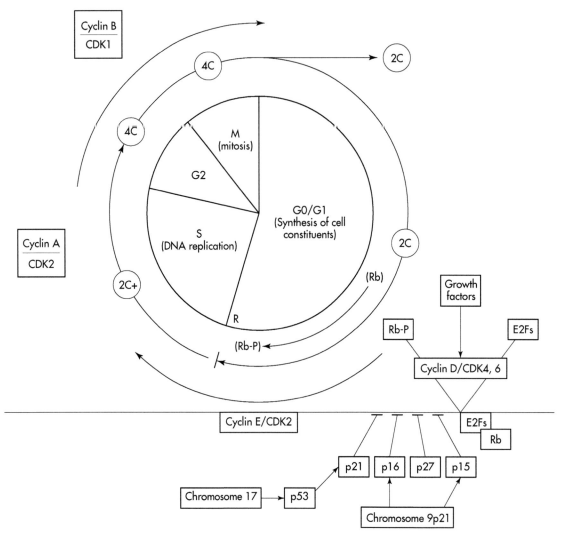

**Fig. 24.7**
The cell cycle and its regulation (see also Box 24.7). With permission of Michael J Droller, 2004.

---

**Box 24.7** The cell cycle and its regulation

Figure 24.7 presents the different phases of the cell cycle through which a cell progresses in the process of replication. Transit through the different phases of the cycle is regulated by stimulatory and inhibitory molecules controlled by a number of loci on various chromosomes. In bladder cancer (and presumably in other cancers), defects in a number of these figure prominently in the development of particular forms of cancer that exhibit specific intrinsic biologic potentials. Growth factors induce the formation of cyclins and cyclin-dependent kinases, which are involved in the phosphorylation of proteins that then allow transit of the cell through a specific checkpoint on its path through the cycle, for example, cyclin D and cyclin D kinase 4/6 (CD/CDK4,6) phosphorylate retinoblastoma tumor suppressor protein (Rb), allowing it to separate from E2F transcriptional regulatory proteins. This permits the cell to proceed through the restriction (R) checkpoint from the G0/G1 phase to the S (DNA synthesis) phase of the cycle. This process can be inhibited by the suppression of CDK activity by p16, p21, and p27 inhibitor proteins, themselves the products of tumor suppressor genes (p16, for example, is the product of the tumor suppressor gene INK4a located on chromosome 9p). Further control can be generated through the p53 protein product of the tumor suppressor gene p53 on chromosome 17, which can induce activity of p21 to inhibit CDK phosphorylation of Rb, preventing a cell from proceeding through the first checkpoint.

Other stimulatory and inhibitory molecules confer a vast complexity of checks on this process. Chromosomal defects lead to deficiencies in these balances and underlie the development of a malignancy and the potential patterns of its biological expression.[106,107]

---

a solitary papillary tumor with no more than seven or eight normal-appearing cell layers be classified as a papilloma (a nonmalignant entity), whereas others have suggested that these be classified as grade 1 papillary carcinomas 'of low malignant potential'.[55,56]

The WHO grading system assesses the degree of dysplasia by determining the presence of increased cellularity, nuclear crowding, disturbance of cellular polarity, the absence of differentiation from base to surface, pleomorphism, variations in nuclear shape and chromatin pattern, number of mitoses, and the presence of giant cells.[52,57] Although the determination of patterns is apparently reproducible for grades 1 and 3 disease, grade 2 remains a heterogeneous intermediate group and difficult in allowing a definitive diagnosis.[58,59]

More recently, an association between grade of disease, specific chromosomal defects, and the number of these defects has also become important in characterizing the malignant potential of a particular cancer.[35,38,41,42,60] It is in this context that the natural history of the different forms of superficial urothelial cancer and their pathogenic pathways can be more profitably explored.

# TRANSITIONAL CELL CANCER (TCC)

## MUCOSALLY CONFINED (STAGE TA) PAPILLARY TCC

Mucosally confined papillary TCC is the most common form of 'superficial' urothelial cancer (see Figure 24.3). Of all superficial lesions, 70% are diagnosed with this stage (Ta), and the majority of these are solitary lesions.[5,7] Most are characterized as being grade 1–2, and only 2% to 4% are characterized as being poorly differentiated (grade 3) cancers.[4,5,15]

It is rare to diagnose concomitant flat CIS (see below) in the context of low/moderate grade, stage Ta papillary TCC. Although some pathologists describe mucosally confined papillary TCC as a form of CIS, the biologic implications of this term versus the more conventionally recognized form of flat high-grade CIS (as discussed below) are dramatically different.[18] From the clinician's perspective, it is therefore better not to use this designation in describing the pathology of mucosally confined papillary low/moderate grade disease.

The types of chromosomal defects that characterize low/moderate grade mucosally confined papillary (stage Ta) tumors support these clinical distinctions as defects in chromosome 9 are common and often the only defects seen.[35,43,44] In contrast, defects in chromosomes 9, 13, 17, and others have been the ones found to characterize the more aggressive tumor diatheses of flat CIS and high-grade mucosally confined papillary lesions (see Figure 24.6).[35,36,38]

Although multiple (2–4) mucosally confined papillary tumors may be observed in as many as 20% to 30% of cases (and often in the same area of the bladder rather than dispersed throughout), the intervening mucosa is generally not histopathologically involved.[4,5,52] The same is not the case in higher grade lamina propria-invasive tumors (see below) in which it

is not uncommon to find CIS at the tumor margin, at intervening sites between adjacent lesions, and at distant sites in the bladder.[4,8,21,61,62]

Mucosally confined papillary tumors need to be distinguished from papillomas, which appear to be the manifestation of a proliferative response to an inflammatory process and have no malignant potential.[52,63,64] Although pathologists have reached a consensus in assigning the term 'tumor of low malignant potential' to grade 1 mucosally confined papillary tumors,[52,55,56,65] this designation, based upon what pathologists have inferred on the biologic behavior of this diathesis, should not lull the clinician into thinking that the subsequent development of aggressive behavior in recurrences, either in the bladder or in the upper tracts, cannot occur. Though admittedly rare, the fact that these particular diatheses reflect a proliferative abnormality that is more than just a response to an irritative process, and actually is the manifestation of a specific chromosomal defect, suggests the possibility that additional genetic defects may be introduced during continued cell proliferation. This could potentially lead to the development of a more aggressive diathesis. Indeed, several studies have reported a change in grade as heralding a change in the potential behavior of mucosally confined tumors, signaling the need for careful monitoring and possibly a change in therapy.[66,67]

Although not formally part of the standard staging system, tumor size and multiplicity have been associated with an increased likelihood of recurrence.[5,15,67] The use of adjunctive intravesical chemotherapy in this setting has been found to increase the interval between recurrences and even to decrease their frequency and multiplicity altogether.[33,34,68–70] In the long term, however, recurrence is only marginally affected, and patients benefit by such treatment in completely eliminating recurrence in only 5% to 10% of cases overall.[33,34,71]

The presence of multiple mucosally confined low/moderate grade papillary transitional cell tumors should not be confused with an entity that has been described as 'micropapillary' disease.[72,73] The latter generally appears endoscopically as an erythematous carpet of small papillary excrescences that histologically are comprised of high-grade malignant cells, which may actually be more akin to a form of flat CIS. This type of diathesis also appears to have a more aggressive intrinsic biologic potential, having been associated with a greater likelihood of progression than might ordinarily be ascribed to mucosally confined single or multiple tumor, moderate-grade papillary disease.

In those rare instances in which mucosally confined papillary tumors are poorly differentiated (2–4%), CIS may be present at the margin of these lesions, and progression may be more likely to occur.[61] Several studies have raised concern regarding the accuracy of pathologic interpretation in diagnosing mucosally confined lesions that have actually penetrated into the lamina propria.[74-76] Indeed, some studies have reported a 50% inaccuracy rate. Other reports have suggested that a small proportion of papillary lesions may actually undergo a higher degree of malignant transformation and then may assume the behavior of a more aggressive diathesis. This probably represents a very small proportion of mucosally confined lesions, or represents the introduction of additional chromosomal defects in the course of cancer cell proliferation and tumor recurrence.

## LAMINA PROPRIA-INVASIVE (STAGE T1) PAPILLARY TCC

The number of superficial cancers diagnosed as invasive of the lamina propria (stage T1) at their initial presentation comprises only 25% to 30% of all superficial cancers (see Figure 24.4).[4,5] Approximately half of these are diagnosed as high grade and deeply invasive of the lamina propria.[7,8,14,17] These present the greatest risk for progression (see below). Those that are of only moderate grade and less deeply infiltrative of the lamina propria are generally successfully treated by standard conservative means (resection with or without adjunctive intravesical therapies), depending upon multiplicity, rapidity of recurrence, and/or concomitant 'flat' CIS.[7,8,10,11,21,23,61]

Accuracy of staging of these lesions is imperative in predicting their biologic potential, characterizing their prognosis, and assigning appropriate therapy. For example, when initial resection specimens have failed to include the muscularis propria for pathologic evaluation, re-resection has documented that what was thought to be stage T1 cancer actually involved the muscularis propria in 10% to 20% of these instances.[12,77] The consequences of such understaging could be manifest in undertreatment. Although some have suggested that re-resection should be required in any patient diagnosed with lamina propria-invasive disease,[78,79] it may be more appropriate to consider particular features that can be used to indicate the need for such an approach. For example, any lamina propria-invasive cancer that appears to involve the lamina propria extensively might benefit from re-resection, particularly if the presence of muscularis propria in the original histologic specimen is questionable or its involvement difficult to characterize.[80-82] Otherwise, if a particular tumor appears to have a more nodular than papillary appearance, or there are multiple aggregated lesions, a thorough resection is important in evaluating the extent of disease.[83,84]

Several studies have suggested that the depth of lamina propria penetration, as demarcated by the muscularis mucosae (a thin muscle layer that is only inconsistently found in the lamina propria), may be an indication of the likelihood of progression.[9-11,80,85] Several studies have indicated that those tumors that invade the lamina propria superficial to the muscularis mucosae have a progression rate of 20% and a 5-year survival rate of 70%. Those tumors that invade deep to the muscularis mucosae, but remain confined to the lamina propria, have a progression rate of 40% and a 5-year survival rate of 50%. These observations have led to the suggestion that stage T1 tumors should be subdivided depending upon whether they have invaded to or through the muscularis mucosae. However, pathologists have not accepted this suggestion, since the inconsistency of this layer has not permitted them to agree on this being a practical landmark upon which such a staging subdivision could be based.

Multiplicity of disease and size of a presenting lesion seem to be less consequential for progression of this diathesis than do grade of disease and extent of penetration into the lamina propria. However, both factors may figure prominently in the likelihood of recurrence.[57,59,62,86] Also of importance is the presence of CIS at the margin of a papillary lesion, in the flat mucosa between adjacent papillary lesions, or at distant sites in the bladder.[8,21,61] Generally, this finding has prompted the use of intravesical treatments as adjuncts to resection. However, failure to completely eradicate the cancer, notwithstanding an initial aggressive intravesical approach, is a signal that the cancer diathesis may be more likely to progress.[20,23,87] Rapidity of recurrence, reflecting either occult persistent disease or active proliferation with recurrent seeding of the lamina propria, may also be associated with a high risk of progression. It is not unusual in such instances to find that residual cancer cells have actually progressed to muscle invasion in the short interval used for treatment and surveillance.[19,21,88-90]

Molecular and genetic aspects of these tumors have been correlated with their intrinsically aggressive or nonaggressive behavior. Defects in chromosome 17, as manifested by the altered expression of p53, and in the retinoblastoma (Rb) gene, appear to indicate a more aggressive behavior.[30,35,37,46] Other genetic defects, and the increasing multiplicity of such defects, have also been associated with a greater likelihood of progression.[91-93] Although such observations have not as yet been incorporated into a staging system for these types of superficial cancer, it seems reasonable to consider determining the molecular profile of a given diathesis in helping to decide an appropriate treatment approach for those patients that appear to be at greatest risk for the development of progressive disease.

At the same time, it is important to keep these issues in perspective in considering the overall magnitude of this problem. Only 25% to 30% of all superficial tumors present with lamina propria invasion, and only half of these (12–15%) are high grade and more likely to progress. If we exclude the 10% to 20% of these that are actually found to be muscle invasive on repeat resection following initial diagnosis (leaving 8–12% of all superficial tumors), and then consider that only half of these are likely to progress after appropriate intravesical treatments, only 4% to 6% of all superficial cancers remain that ultimately will express their intrinsic biologic potential to become muscle invasive. Therefore, notwithstanding an inability to consistently characterize the molecular profile of a given lesion, an indication of those tumor diatheses that are most likely to become life threatening are their extensiveness of penetration into the lamina propria, their degree of differentiation, and the presence of CIS in conjunction with single or multiple exophytic papillary or papillonodular lesions. The presence of these features suggests that a more aggressive treatment plan might be considered early on, particularly when initially conservative treatments fail to completely, definitively, and durably eradicate the tumor.

## CARCINOMA IN SITU (STAGE Tcis) TCC

Carcinoma in situ (CIS) is a term generally reserved for those forms of urothelial cancer that are high grade and that replace the normal urothelium but maintain the contour of the normal urothelial lining of the bladder (see Figure 24.5).[18–22] This entity rarely appears in the absence of concomitant papillary or solid disease, either superficial or muscle invasive. When it does, its diagnosis is prompted by the occurrence of hematuria (generally microscopic) and irritative symptoms, findings of a positive urinary cytology, and confirmed by biopsy of velvety erythematous areas in the bladder, or of random areas at endoscopically normal sites.

Carcinoma in situ may appear either as diffuse areas of erythema involving extensive portions of the bladder, or as smaller 'spot' foci. Occasionally, no abnormal areas are visually present, and random biopsies of the urothelium (including possible sanctuary sites) in the setting of a positive urinary cytology allow the diagnosis to be made.[94,95] Carcinoma in situ, whether diffuse or focal, may involve the prostatic urethra (extending into the prostatic ducts) or the lower ureters. As such, the presence of malignant cells at these sanctuary sites may account for persistence of positive urinary cytology notwithstanding apparently successful eradication of disease by intensive intravesical therapies in the bladder.

Although the response rate of CIS to intravesical treatment—usually with bacillus Calmette–Guérin (BCG)—is reported to be as high as 70%,[33,34] all patients with CIS are at risk for the eventual development of progressive disease, particularly if the initial response to treatment is not complete or maintained.[96–98] Progression may occur not only through the persistence of cancer cells that are not detected by cystoscopy and cytology, but also through involvement of sanctuary sites in which persistence of cancer cells is not affected by intravesical treatments. Progression may also be seen when malignant cells in invaginated or cystic portions of cystitis cystica, cystitis glandularis, or nests of Von Brunn remain, having been inaccessible to resection or intravesical treatments, and having been covered over by normal urothelium following instillations.

Progression appears more likely to occur when there is diffuse involvement of the urothelium by CIS. This may be related to the reported 30% incidence of microscopic penetration of the lamina propria by CIS in cases in which disease had initially been thought to be confined to the bladder mucosa.[19]

The occurrence of progression from initial diagnosis can range from 6 months to as long as 5–7 years.[89,90,96,97] Continued surveillance with monitoring both cytologically and endoscopically is therefore necessary to ensure that the tumor diathesis is under control and is neither recurring nor progressing surreptitiously.

The molecular changes associated with CIS have not been found to be particularly helpful in determining the varying intrinsic biologic potential of the different forms of this diathesis or the likelihood of its response (either initially or in maintenance) to intravesical therapy. At least 50% of cases of flat CIS have defects in chromosome 17, with corresponding nuclear expression of altered p53 protein.[36–38] Those that are not found to have this defect appear to behave in the same potentially aggressive way as do those that express the defect.

Carcinoma in situ may present a particularly ominous prognosis for progression to invasion when it appears in the context of papillary lamina propria-invasive cancers, and particularly when these cancers, after initial resection, recur rapidly despite intensive intravesical therapy (generally with BCG).[61,62,99,100] Moreover, when such patients are explored at cystectomy (some having undergone a second 6-week course of BCG therapy and having had clear documentation that the muscularis propria was not involved initially), 20% to 30% of the cancers are found not only to have penetrated into the muscularis propria, but to have metastasized to regional lymph nodes.[101–103] Thus, if a definitive response to initial resection and intravesical therapy cannot be documented, consideration for aggressive surgical treatment is an appropriate (and many would say imperative) consideration during the apparently limited window of opportunity in which the cancer is still organ confined and curable.[104,105]

Several features of CIS (either at initial diagnosis or during follow-up) therefore indicate that a particular form may be or have become more aggressive:

1. Disease sufficiently diffuse (with involvement of the bladder base, bladder neck, and possibly proximal urethra) to result in severe irritative symptoms.

2. Failure to demonstrate *any* response (and in some instances a truly definitive response) to intensive intravesical therapy.
3. Concomitant papillary lamina propria-invasive cancer that extensively penetrates into the lamina propria.
4. Rapid recurrence of papillary lamina propria-invasive cancer with failure of the CIS to respond to initial intensive intravesical treatments.
5. Involvement of cystitis cystica, cystitis glandularis, and nests of von Brunn by diffuse CIS.
6. Documentation of involvement of sanctuary sites (urethra, distal/intramural ureters).

Some of these findings may be obscured by the presence at initial diagnosis of muscle-invasive disease in which the presence of CIS and lamina propria-invasive disease may have been understaged. However, rapid recurrence (or more likely persistence), particularly when there is extensive penetration of the lamina propria by papillary/nodular disease and failure to respond promptly to intravesical therapy, is a signal that progression may be imminent and aggressive surgical therapy needed if a cure is to be achieved.

Several studies have suggested that flat CIS may be the direct antecedent of nodular tumors, which are more deeply invasive when they become clinically apparent.[19,21,83,84] That solid or nodular tumors, rather than papillary tumors, may arise from foci of flat CIS is in itself suggestive that the presence of this entity, particularly when symptomatic or diffuse, or at sanctuary sites and with foci of basement membrane penetration, may indicate a particularly ominous prognosis unless treated in a surgically definitive manner. In view of observations that 50% of cases of CIS demonstrate abnormalities of chromosome 17 (p53), a defect commonly seen in aggressive lamina propria and muscle-invasive cancers, this may explain why 25% of patients present with muscle-invasive disease at initial diagnosis without ever having had any clinical indication that a malignancy was present at a more superficial phase in its evolution.

## CONCLUSION

We currently have a fundamental clinical appreciation of different pathogenic pathways that appear to characterize the biologic behavior of the various forms of 'superficial' TCC. These can be used to advantage to understand the potential risk a bladder cancer may imply for its host when we obtain its initial 'snapshot' at diagnosis (tumor grade and stage). This should assist us to determine an initial approach to treatment. Depending upon response and recurrence, it may also then be used in characterizing its potential clinical course, and modifying treatment approaches as new

outcomes information is gathered. Additional information at the molecular level may permit further precision and refinement of our understanding of a particular tumor diathesis and more effective application of appropriate treatments.

## REFERENCES

1. Jemal A, Tiwari RC, Murray T, et al. Cancer statistics, 2004. CA Cancer J Clin 2004;54:8–21.
2. Fleshner N, Kondylis F. Demographics and epidemiology of urothelial cancer of the urinary bladder. In Droller MJ (ed): Urothelial Tumors. Hamilton, Ontario: BC Decker, 2004, pp 1–16.
3. Parkin DM, Pisari P, Ferlay G. Estimates of the worldwide incidence of 25 major cancers in 1990. Int J Cancer 1999;80:827–841.
4. Heney NM, Nocks BN, Daley JJ, et al. Ta and T1 bladder cancer: location, recurrence, and progression. Br J Urol 1982;54:152–157.
5. Holmang S, Hedelin H, Anderstrom C, et al. The relationship among multiple recurrences, progression, and prognosis of patients with stages Ta and T1 transitional cell carcinoma of the bladder followed for at least 20 years. J Urol 1995;153:18–23.
6. Kaye RW, Lange PH. Mode of presentation of invasive bladder cancer: reassessment of the problem. J Urol 1982;128:31–34.
7. Heney NM, Ahmed S, Flanagan MJ, et al. Superficial bladder cancer: progression and recurrence. J Urol 1983;130:1083–1086.
8. Pagano F, Garbeglio A, Milani C, et al. Prognosis of bladder cancer I: risk factors in superficial transitional cell carcinoma. Eur Urol 1987;13:145–149.
9. Engel P, Anagnostaki L, Braendstrup O. The muscularis mucosae of the urinary bladder: implications for tumor staging on biopsies. Scand J Urol Nephrol 1992;26(Suppl):249–256.
10. Younes M, Sussman J, True LD. The usefulness of the level of muscularis mucosa in the staging of invasive transitional cell carcinoma of the urinary bladder. Cancer 1990;66:543–547.
11. Hassui Y, Osada Y, Kitada S, et al. Significance of invasion to the muscularis mucosa on the progression of superficial bladder cancer. Urology 1994;43:782–787.
12. Klan R, Loy V, Huland H. Residual tumor discovered in routine second TUR in patients with T1 transitional cell carcinoma of the bladder. J Urol 1991;146:316–319.
13. Abel PO, Hall RR, Williams G. Should pT1 transitional cell carcinoma of the bladder still be classified as superficial? Br J Urol 1988;62:235–240.
14. Birch BRP, Harland SJ. The pT1G3 bladder tumor. Br J Urol 1989;64:109–113.
15. Fitzpatrick JM, West AB, Butler MR, et al. Superficial bladder tumors (stage I pTa grades 1 and 2): the importance of recurrence pattern following initial resection. J Urol 1986;135:920–924.
16. Gildea JJ, Golden WL, Harding MA, et al. Genetic and phenotypic changes associated with the acquisition of tumorigenicity in human bladder cancer. Genes Chromosomes Cancer 2000;27:25–63.
17. Jakse G, Loidle W, Seeber G. Stage T1 grade 3 transitional cell carcinoma of the bladder: an unfavorable tumor. J Urol 1987;137:39–43.
18. Weinstein R, Miller AW III, Pauli BV. Carcinoma in situ: comments on the pathology of a paradox. Urol Clin North Am 1980;18:523–533.
19. Farrow GM, Utz OC. Observations on microinvasive transitional cell carcinoma of the urinary bladder. Clin Oncol 1982;1:609–614.
20. Hudson MA, Herr HW. Carcinoma in situ of the bladder. J Urol 1995;153:564–572.
21. Kakizoe T, Matumoto K, Nishio Y, et al. Significance of carcinoma in situ in association with bladder cancer. J Urol 1985;133:395–399.
22. Melicow M. Histologic study of vesical epithelium intervening between gross neoplasms in total cystectomy. J Urol 1952;68:261–267.
23. Herr HW. When is a cystectomy necessary in carcinoma in situ? In Murphy GP, Khoury S (eds): Therapeutic Progress in Urologic Cancers. New York: Liss, 1989, pp 511–521.

24. Kotake T, Flanigan RC, Kirkels W, et al. The current TNM classification of bladder carcinoma: is it as good as we need it to be? Int J Urol 1995;2:36–41.

25. Jordan AM, Weingarten J, Murphy WM. Transitional cell neoplasms of the urinary bladder. Can biological potential be predicted from histologic grading? Cancer 1987;60:2761–2768.

26. Jewett HJ, Strong GH. Infiltrating carcinoma of the bladder: relation of depth I of penetration of the bladder wall to incidence of local extension and metastases. J Urol 1946;55:366–371.

27. Jewett HJ, Lewis E. Infiltrating carcinoma of bladder: curability by total cystectomy. J Urol 1948;60:107–111.

28. Koss LG. Tumors of the urinary bladder. In Atlas of Tumor Pathology, Series 2, Fascicle II. Washington, DC: Armed Forces Institute of Pathology, 1975.

29. Sweeney P, Dinney CPN. Molecular pathogenesis of proliferative and progressive (invasive) urothelial cancer development. In Droller MJ (ed): Urothelial Tumors. Hamilton, Ontario: BC Decker, 2004, pp 44–58.

30. Theodorescu D. Molecular carcinogenesis of proliferative and progressive (invasive) urothelial cancer. In Droller MJ (ed): Urothelial Tumors. Hamilton, Ontario: BC Decker, 2004, pp 28–43.

31. Droller MJ. Bladder cancer. Curr Prob Surg 1981;18:205–279.

32. Jones PA, Droller MJ. Pathways of development and progression in bladder cancer: new correlations between clinical observations and molecular mechanisms. Semin Urol 1993;11:177–192.

33. Lamm DL. Long-term results of intravesical therapy for superficial bladder cancer. Urol Clin North Am 1992;19:573–580.

34. Lamm DL, van der Meyden AP, Akaza H, et al. Intravesical chemotherapy and immunotherapy: how do we assess their effectiveness and what are their limitations and usefulness? Int J Urol 1995;2(Suppl):23–35.

35. Tsai VC, Nichols PW, Hiti AI, et al. Allelic losses of chromosome 9, 11 and 17 in human bladder cancer. Cancer Res 1990;50:44–52.

36. Hartmann A, Schlake G, Zack D, et al. Occurrence of chromosome 9 and p53 alterations in multifocal dysplasia and carcinoma in situ of human urinary bladder. Cancer Res 2002;62:809–818.

37. Sarkis AS, Dalbagni G, Cordon-Cardo C, et al. Nuclear overexpression of p53 protein in transitional cell bladder carcinoma: a marker for disease progression. J Natl Can Inst 1993;85:53–60.

38. Spruck CH, Ohneseit PF, Gonzalez Zulueta M, et al. Two molecular pathways of transitional carcinoma of the bladder. Cancer Res 1994;54:784–792.

39. Bubendorf L, Grilli B, Sauter G, et al. Multiprobe FISH for enhanced detection of bladder cancer in voided urine specimens and bladder washings. Am J Clin Pathol 2001;116:79–86.

40. Ishiwata S, Takahaski S, Hovima V, et al. Non-invasive detection and prediction of bladder cancer by fluorescence in situ hybridization analysis of exfoliated cells in voided urine. Urology 2001;57:811–815.

41. Gardiner RA, Walsh MD, Allen S, et al. Immunohistological expression of p53 in urinary pT1 transitional cell cancer in relation to tumor progression. Br J Urol 1994;73:526–532.

42. Esrig D, Spruck C, Nichols P, et al. p53 nuclear protein accumulation correlates with mutations in the p53 gene, tumor grade, and stage in bladder cancer. Am J Pathol 1993;143:1389–1396.

43. Miyao N, Tsai VC, Lerner SP, et al. The role of chromosome 9 in human bladder cancer. Cancer Res 1993;53:4066–4072.

44. Knowles MA, Elder PA, Williamson M, et al. Allelotype of human bladder cancer. Cancer Res 1994;54:531–538.

45. Cairns P, Shaw ME, Knowles MA. Initiation of bladder cancer may involve deletion of a tumor suppressor gene on chromosome 9. Oncogene 1993;8:1083–1085.

46. Cote RJ, Dunn MD, Chaterjee SJ, et al. Elevated and absent pRb expression is associated with bladder cancer progression and has cooperative effects with p53. Cancer Res 1998;58:1090–1094.

47. Choissy-Rossi C, Reisdorf P, Yonish-Rouach E. The p53 tumor suppressor gene: structure, function and mechanism of action. Results Prob Cell Differ 1999;23:145–172.

48. Jordan AM, Weingarten J, Murphy WM. Transitional cell neoplasms of the urinary bladder: can biologic potential be predicted from histological gradings? Cancer 1987;60:2766–2774.

49. Kaubisch S, Lum BL, Reese J, et al. Stage T1 bladder cancer: grade is the primary determination for risk of muscle invasion. J Urol 1991;146:28–34.

50. Aschner PW. The pathology of vesical neoplasms. Its evaluation in diagnosis and prognosis. JAMA 1928;91:1697–1702.

51. Broders AC. Epithelioma of the genitourinary organs. Ann Surg 1922;75:574–586.

52. Bostwick DG, Montironi R, Lopez-Beltran A, et al. Pathology of urothelial tumors of the bladder. In Droller MJ (ed): Urothelial Tumors. Hamilton, Ontario: BC Decker, 2004, pp 92–111.

53. Mostofi FK, Sobin LH, Torlini H. Histological typing of urinary bladder tumors. International Histological Classification of Tumors No. 10. Geneva: WHO, 1973.

54. Murphy WM, Beckwith JB, Farrow G. Tumors of the kidney, bladder and related urinary structures. Washington, DC: Armed Forces Institute of Pathology, 1994, pp 298–335.

55. Epstein JJ, Amin MB, Reuter VR, Mostofi FK. The World Health Organization/International Society of Urothelial Pathology consensus classification of urothelial (transitional cell) neoplasms of the urinary bladder. Bladder Consensus Conference Committee. Am J Surg Pathol 1998;22:1435–1448.

56. Reuter VE, Epstein JI, Amin MB, Mostofi FK. The WHO/ISUP consensus classification of urothelial (transitional cell) neoplasm: continued discussion. Hum Pathol 1999;30:879–880.

57. Holmang S, Andrus P, Hedelin H, et al. Stage progression in Ta papillary urothelial tumors: relationship to grade, immunohistochemical expression of tumor markers, mitotic frequency and DNA ploidy. J Urol 2001;165:1124–1130.

58. Carbin BE, Ekman P, Gustafson H, et al. Grading of human urothelial carcinoma based on nuclear atypia and mitotic frequency. I. Histological description. J Urol 1991;145:968–971.

59. Schapers RF, Pauwel RP, Wignen JT, et al. A simplified grading method of transitional cell carcinoma of the urinary bladder: reproducible, clinical significance and comparison with other prognostic parameters. Br J Urol 1994;73:625–631.

60. Kausch I, Bohle A. Molecular aspects of bladder cancer. III. Prognostic markers of bladder cancer. Eur Urol 2002;41:15–29.

61. Althausen AF, Prout GR, Daly JJ. Non-invasive papillary carcinoma of the bladder associated with carcinoma in situ. J Urol 1976;116:575–580.

62. Lutzeyer W, Rubben H, Damin H. Prognostic parameters in superficial bladder cancer: an analysis of 315 cases. J Urol 1982;127:250–256.

63. Lerman RI, Hulter RVP, Whitmore WF. Papilloma of the urinary bladder. Cancer 1970;25:333–338.

64. Cheng L, Darson M, Cheville JC, et al. Urothelial papilloma of the bladder: clinical and biologic implications. Cancer 1999;86:2098–2101.

65. Eble IN, Young RH. Benign and low-grade papillary lesions of the urinary bladder: a review of the papilloma–papillary carcinoma controversy, and a report of five typical papillomas. Semin Diag Pathol 1989;6:351–371.

66. Carbin BE, Eman P, Gustafson H, et al. Grading of human urothelial neoplasms based on nuclear atypia and mitotic frequency. II. Prognostic importance. J Urol 1991;145:972–977.

67. Parmar MKB, Friedman LS, Hargreave TB, et al. Prognostic factors for recurrence follow-up policies in the treatment of superficial bladder cancer: report from the British Medical Research Council Subgroup on superficial bladder cancer. J Urol 1989;142:284–290.

68. Soloway MS, Jordan AM, Murphy WM. Rationale for intravesical chemotherapy in the treatment and prophylaxis of superficial transitional cell carcinoma. Prog Clin Biol Res 1989;310:215–221.

69. Maier U, Hobarth K. Long-term observation after intravesical instillation with mitomycin C in patients with superficial bladder tumors. Urology 1991;37:481–488.

70. Solsona E, Iborra I, Ricos JV, et al. Effectiveness of a single immediate mitomycin C instillation in patients with low-risk superficial bladder cancer: short- and long-term follow-up. J Urol 1999;161:1120–1123.

71. Tolley DA, Parmar MK, Grigor KM, et al. The effects of intravesical mitomycin C on recurrence of newly diagnosed superficial bladder cancer: a further report with 7 years of follow-up. J Urol 1996;155:1233–1238.

72. Amin MB, Ro JY, el-Sharkawy T, et al. Micropapillary variant of transitional papillary cell carcinoma of the urinary bladder. Histologic pattern resembling ovarian papillary serous carcinoma. Am J Surg Pathol 1994;18:1124–1132.

73. Johansson SL, Borghede G, Holmang S. Micropapillary bladder cancer: clinicopathological study of 20 cases. J Urol 1999;161:1798–1802.

74. Abel PB, Henderson D, Bennett MK, et al. Differing interpretations by pathologists of the pT category and grade of transitional cell carcinoma of the bladder. Br J Urol 1988;62:339–348.

75. Olsen LH, Overgaard S, Fredericksen P, et al. The reliability of staging and grading of bladder tumors: impact of misinformation of the pathologists' diagnosis. Scand J Urol Nephol 1993;27:349–357.

76. Witjes JA, Kiemeney LALM, Schaafsma HE, et al. The influence of review; pathology on study outcome of a randomized multicenter superficial bladder cancer trial. Br J Urol 1994;73:172–178.

77. Langenstroer P, See W. The role of a second transurethral resection for high grade bladder cancer. Curr Urol Rep 2000;1:204–207.

78. Herr HW. The value of a second transurethral resection in evaluating patients with bladder tumors. J Urol 1999;162:74–76.

79. Schips L, Augustin H, Zigeuner RE, et al. Is repeated transurethral resection justified in patients with newly diagnosed superficial bladder cancer? Urology 2002;59:220–223.

80. Smits G, Schaafsma E, Kiemeney L, et al. Microstaging of pT1 transitional cell carcinoma of the bladder: identification of subgroups with distinct risks of progression. Urology 1998;52:1009–1013.

81. Soloway MS, Sofer M, Vaidya A. Contemporary management of stage T1 transitional cell carcinoma of the bladder. J Urol 2002;167:1573–1583.

82. Koloszy Z. Histopathological 'self-control' in transurethral resection of bladder tumors. Br J Urol 1991;67:162–166.

83. Kakizoe T, Tobisu K, Takai K, et al. Relationship between papillary and nodular transitional cell carcinoma in the human urinary bladder. Cancer Res 1988;48:2299–2303.

84. Friedell GN, Parija GC, Nagy K, et al. The pathology of human bladder cancer. Cancer 1980;45:1823–1832.

85. Angulo JC, Lopez JI, Grignon DJ, et al. Muscularis mucosa differentiates two populations with different prognosis in stage T1 bladder cancer. Urology 1995;45:47–53.

86. Bostwick DG. Natural history of early bladder cancer. J Cell Biochem Suppl 1992;161:31–38.

87. Cheng L, Cheville JC, Neumann RM, et al. Natural history of urothelial dysplasia of the bladder. Am J Surg Pathol 1999;23:443–447.

88. Zincke N, Utz DC, Farrow GM. Review of Mayo Clinic experience with carcinoma in situ. Urology 1985;26(Suppl):39–46.

89. Nadler RB, Catalona WJ, Hudson MA, et al. Durability of the tumor-free response for intravesical bacillus Calmette–Guérin therapy. J Urol 1994;156:367–373.

90. Herr HW, Wartinger DD, Fair WR, et al. Bacillus Calmette–Guérin therapy for superficial bladder cancer: a 10-year follow-up. J Urol 1992;147:1020–1023.

91. Czerniak B, Hertz F. Molecular biology of common tumors of the urinary tract. In Koss LG (ed): Diagnostic Cytology of the Urinary Tract. Philadelphia: Lippincott-Raven, 1995, pp 345–364.

92. Grossman HB, Liebert M, Antelo M, et al. p53 and RB expression predict progression in T1 bladder cancer. Clin Cancer Res 1998;4:829–834.

93. Cordon-Cardo C, Sheinfeld J, Dalbagni G. Genetic studies and molecular markers of bladder cancer. Semin Surg Oncol 1997;13:319–327.

94. Kiemeney LALM, Witjes JA, Heijbrock RP, et al. Should random urothelial biopsies be taken from patients with primary superficial bladder cancer? A decision analysis. Br J Urol 1994;73:164–169.

95. Richards B, Parmar MKB, Anderson CK, et al. Interpretation of biopsies of 'normal' urothelium in patients with superficial bladder cancer. Br J Urol 1991;67:369–374.

96. Solsona E, Iborra I, Dumont R, et al. The 3-month clinical response to intravesical therapy as a predictive factor for progression in patients with high risk superficial bladder cancer. J Urol 2000;164:685–689.

97. Cookson MA, Herr HW, Zhang ZF, et al. The treated natural history of high risk superficial bladder cancer: 15-year outcome. J Urol 1997;158:62–67.

98. Herr HW, Badalament RA, Amato DA, et al. Superficial bladder cancer treated with bacillus Calmette–Guérin: a multivariate analysis of factors affecting tumor progression. J Urol 1989;141:22–29.

99. Esrig D, Freeman JA, Stein JP, et al. Early cystectomy for clinical stage T1 transitional cell carcinoma of the bladder. Semin Urol Oncol 1997;15:154–160.

100. Vicente J, Laguna MP, Duarte D, et al. Carcinoma in situ as a prognostic factor for G3pT1 bladder tumors. Br J Urol 1991;68:380–385.

101. Stoekle M, Alken P, Engelmann U, et al. Radical cystectomy—often too late? Eur Urol 1987;13:361–367.

102. Hudson MA, Ratliff TL, Gillen DP, et al. Single course versus maintenance bacillus Calmette–Guérin therapy for superficial bladder tumors: a prospective randomized trial. J Urol 1987;138:295–298.

103. Coplen DE, Marcus MD, Myers JA, et al. Long-term follow-up of patients treated with 1 or 2, 6-week courses of intravesical bacillus Calmette–Guérin: analysis of possible predictors of response free of tumor. J Urol 1990;14:1:652–657.

104. Nadler RB, Catalona WJ, Hudson MA, et al. Durability of the tumor-free response for intravesical bacillus Calmette–Guérin therapy. J Urol 1994;12:367–373.

105. O'Donnell MA, Burns JA. Intravesical bacille Calmette–Guérin in the treatment and prophylaxis of urothelial bladder cancer. In Droller MJ (ed): Urothelial Tumors. Hamilton, Ontario: BC Decker, 2004, pp 219–247.

106. Park BH, Vogelstein B. Tumor-suppressor genes. In Holland JF, Frei E III (eds): Cancer 6 Medicine. Hamilton, Ontario: BC Decker, 2003, pp 87–105.

107. Reeder JE, Messing EM. Cell-cycle aberrations in human bladder cancer. In Droller MJ (ed): Urothelial Tumors. Hamilton, Ontario: BC Decker, 2004, pp 17–27.

# Risk stratification of Ta, Tis, T1 cancer

25

*Paula MJ Moonen, Johannes A Witjes*

## INTRODUCTION

The term 'superficial bladder carcinoma' encompasses a spectrum of disease that ranges from the innocuous Ta grade 1 tumor, limited to the mucosa, to the life-threatening T1 grade 3 tumor, invading into the submucosa or lamina propria. Within the spectrum lie grade 2 tumors and carcinoma in situ, the latter being high grade, flat, and confined to the epithelium. Superficial transitional cell carcinoma of the bladder is characterized by a high risk of recurrence (30–85%), with a maximal incidence in the first years.[1-3] Of patients with superficial tumors, 10% to 15% develop subsequent invasive or metastatic cancer.[4] Currently, the standard clinical management consists of routine periodic control cystoscopies to resect recurrent tumors as early as possible and thus decrease the risk of progression to muscle-invasive disease. However, the benefits of maintaining a fixed schedule of routine cystoscopy for all patients, irrespective of their individual risk, are questionable.[5]

There is a low-risk group of patients that are clinically cured after a few transurethral resections, and could be spared the intravesical therapy and radical operations. However, despite the advent of improved intravesical therapies, there remains a group of patients at risk of disease progression, metastases, and death from their disease. It would be ideal if the prognosis of the individual patient could be predicted early in the course of the disease so that patients with potentially progressive cancer could be treated earlier and more aggressively. Risk stratification of patients based on clinical parameters provides new opportunities for adapting monitoring strategies as well as providing a rationale for the use of intravesical chemotherapy and immunotherapy, or a radical operation.

In summary, collection and classification of prognostic factors in superficial bladder cancer enable us to develop a stratification of risk in this heterogeneous patient group. This brings us a step forward in minimizing the burden of unnecessary investigations and treatments while safely identifying those patients with high-risk disease that should receive aggressive treatment.

A great deal has been published about prognostic factors in primary superficial bladder cancer.[6-8] As extensive information about these factors can be found in Chapter 13, they will not be discussed here. However, a few authors have proposed classification of risk groups on the basis of these prognostic factors,[3,9-13] and they will be discussed in this chapter.

## RISK STRATIFICATION

In 1987, Takashi et al[9] clarified the relative importance of factors affecting the survival of patients with bladder cancer. Unfortunately, this study included both superficial and invasive bladder cancer patients. A multivariate analysis by Cox's proportional hazards model was performed on 264 patients. Clinicopathologic data included in the analysis were sex, age, irritative bladder symptoms, interval from onset of symptoms to first consultation, smoking history, and tumor characteristics (location, size, number, shape, histologic stage, and grade). Selection of factors to be studied was based on their contribution to survival. The selected factors were stage (T2–4 versus Ta–T1), size, symptoms, age, and grade, in order of statistical significance, with the last—grade—having the limiting level of significance (p=0.05). According to the presence of these five factors, the patients were categorized into six groups, and their survival was further evaluated (Table 25.1).[9] The six groups clearly demonstrated different survival status, indicating that these five characteristics are definite determinants of survival in bladder cancer patients. Regrettably, no follow-up advice was given for these six risk groups by the authors.

In 1989, Parmar et al[10] used data from two large randomized British Medical Research Council studies to identify several factors influencing the recurrence of newly diagnosed stage Ta or T1 tumors. The factors evaluated were the result of the 3-month cystoscopy study, the number of tumors (multiple or single) at initial diagnosis, the maximum diameter of the largest tumor, the pathology grade, posterior wall involvement, and tumor category (pTa or pT1). Multivariate analysis identified the result of the 3-month cystoscopy study as the single most important prognostic factor. Nearly as important, and the next factor to be chosen, was the number of tumors (multiple or single) at initial diagnosis. The analysis also suggested that the factors grade, category, and maximum diameter are strongly associated with the result of the 3-month cystoscopy study and number of tumors at presentation. Based on the two selected factors, three prognostic groups with regard to the risk of recurrence were formed (Table 25.2):[12]

- Group 1 defined a set of patients that had a particularly good prognosis and, therefore, the follow-up schedule could be less stringent (follow-up at 3 months and then yearly).
- The patients in group 2 had an intermediate prognosis and should undergo an intermediate follow-up schedule (every 3 months for 1 year, every 6 months for 1 year and then yearly).
- The patients in group 3 had the worst prognosis and are likely to have recurrence within 1 year after the 3-month cystoscopy study. Thus, they should be followed intensively (every 3 months for 2 years and then yearly).

According to Parmar and associates, adoption of their proposed system could reduce the number of cystoscopies for the large proportion of patients that have a low risk of recurrence. This should lead to considerable savings in cystoscopy studies that would benefit both clinicians and patients. Modifications of the policy are possible once a tumor has recurred, so a patient could start in group 1 and after recurrence might be reclassified in group 2 or 3. Such modification could provide a more personalized approach to patient management.

In 1993, Kiemeney et al[3] not only wanted to discriminate between low-risk and high-risk patient groups, but also tried to optimize prediction of disease outcome in individual patients. Patient and tumor characteristics of 2705 cases of primary pTa or pT1 bladder cancer were used to identify prognostic factors for recurrence and progression. After analysis, tumor stage, extent (the number of bladder areas in which tumor tissue was found), and multicentricity (multiple tumors versus one solitary tumor) appeared to have predictive ability for the risk of first recurrence. For the risk of progression, the most important prognostic factors were tumor stage, grade, multicentricity, and dysplasia or carcinoma in situ in random biopsy specimens. By summing the regression coefficients (β values) of the multivariate Cox models on recurrence and progression, investigators constructed a prognostic index. A high score indicated that a patient had a poor prognostic profile (Table 25.3).[3] Three risk groups were then defined, based on the distribution of the prognostic index scores, so that the low- and high-risk groups each represented at least 20% of all patients (Table 25.4).[3] Subsequently, they evaluated the reliability of the prognostic index by comparing the observed and predicted actuarial risks of tumor recurrence and progression. Although the reliability appeared to be good, the authors commented that, even if a prognostic factor does have such ability to differentiate in subgroups, this is no guarantee that prediction of disease outcome for individual patients will be accurate.

Two years later, Kurth et al[11] followed and analyzed 576 patients with Ta or T1 tumors to examine the

**Table 25.1** Risk groups (percentage of a total of 264 patients) according to Takashi et al[9]

| Group | Number of characteristics* | No. pts (%) |
|---|---|---|
| 1 | None of the characteristics | 97 (36.7) |
| 2 | Any one of the characteristics | 53 (20.1) |
| 3 | Any two of the characteristics | 41 (15.5) |
| 4 | Any three of the characteristics | 39 (14.8) |
| 5 | Any four of the characteristics | 24 (9.1) |
| 6 | All of the characteristics | 10 (3.9) |

*Characteristics: High-stage tumor; tumor >3 cm; irritative symptoms; age >70 years; high-grade tumor.
Based on data from Takashi et al.[9]

**Table 25.2** Risk groups according to Parmar et al[10]

| Group | Prognostic factors for recurrence | Recurrence-free rate after 2 years (%) |
|---|---|---|
| 1 | Cystoscopy negative at 3 months *and* single tumor at presentation | 74 |
| 2 | Cystoscopy positive at 3 months *or* multiple tumors at presentation | 44 |
| 3 | Cystoscopy positive at 3 months *and* multiple tumors at presentation | 21 |

Based on data from Parmar et al.[10]

**Table 25.3** Prognostic factors according to Kiemeney et al[3]

| Prognostic factor | Recurrence β value | Progression β value |
|---|---|---|
| *Tumor stage* | | |
| pTa | 0 | 0 |
| pT1 | 0.40 | 0.56 |
| *Tumor grade* | | |
| 1 | – | 0 |
| 2 | – | 0.53 |
| 3 | – | 0.98 |
| *Multicentricity* | | |
| Solitary | 0 | 0 |
| Multiple | 0.27 | 0.95 |
| *No. of areas involved* | | |
| 1 | 0 | – |
| 2 | 0.17 | – |
| 3 or more | 0.52 | – |
| *Therapy* | | |
| Transurethral resection alone | 0 | – |
| Instillations | –0.43 | – |
| *Result of random biopsies* | | |
| Normal | – | 0 |
| Not performed | – | 0.37 |
| Dysplasia/carcinoma in situ | – | 0.64 |

β value, regression coefficient of the final multivariate Cox model (high number = poor prognostic risk).

Reproduced from Kiemeney LA, Witjes JA, Heijbroek RP, Verbeek AL, Debruyne FM. 1993 Predictability of recurrent and progressive disease in individual patients with primary superficial bladder cancer. Journal of Urology 150(1):60–64, with permission from Lippincott Williams & Wilkins.

**Table 25.4** Risk groups according to Kiemeney et al[3]

| Risk group | Prognostic index range* Recurrent disease | Progressive disease |
|---|---|---|
| Low | 0 | 0–0.53 |
| Intermediate | 0.17–0.57 | 0.56–1.73 |
| High | 0.67–1.19 | 1.85–3.13 |

*Based on total β scores.

Reproduced from Kiemeney LA, Witjes JA, Heijbroek RP, Verbeek AL, Debruyne FM. 1993 Predictability of recurrent and progressive disease in individual patients with primary superficial bladder cancer. Journal of Urology 150(1):60–64, with permission from Lippincott Williams & Wilkins.

relative importance of prognostic factors in superficial bladder tumors and suggested grouping of patients in three different prognostic groups. The following factors contributing to recurrence, invasion, and survival were investigated: age, sex, size of largest tumor, number of tumors, T category, grade, time from diagnosis (years), prior recurrence rate/year, and site of involvement. A multivariate analysis based on Cox's proportional hazards regression model indicated that three main factors determined patients' prognoses: tumor size, grade, and prior recurrence rate/year. On the basis of these three factors and their association with invasion and death due to malignant disease, an index was computed, reflecting the risk of both early invasion and death due to malignant disease. Risk groups suggested were based on the index (Table 25.5). In the analyzed patient group, the observed rates of tumor progression and death due to malignant disease were 7.1% and 4.3%, respectively, in group 1, and 41.6% and 36.1%, respectively, in group 3. According to Kurth et al, it is easy to assign a given patient to one of the three risk groups, because the prognostic factors used are available in daily practice. Obviously, more aggressive treatment (e.g. cystectomy and urinary diversion) should be considered only for those patients that have failed conservative therapy and those that are assigned to risk group 3 (Table 25.5).[11] Patients possessing the criteria for the best profile might be spared adjuvant chemo- or immunotherapy until a worsening of one of these prognostic factors occurs.

In 1998, Allard et al[12] proposed a simple prognostic index for anticipating more precisely the early clinical

**Table 25.5** Risk groups according to Kurth et al[11]

| Grade | RR <1 <1.5 cm | RR <1 1.5–3 cm | RR <1 >3 cm | RR 1–3 <1.5 cm | RR 1–3 1.5–3 cm | RR 1–3 >3 cm | RR >3 <1.5 cm | RR >3 1.5–3 cm | RR >3 >3 cm |
|---|---|---|---|---|---|---|---|---|---|
| G1 | 1 | 1 | 1 | 1 | 2 | 2 | 2 | 2 | 3 |
| G2 | 1 | 2 | 2 | 2 | 2 | 3 | 3 | 3 | 3 |
| G3 | 2 | 2 | 2 | 2 | 3 | 3 | 3 | 3 | 3 |

Based on three main factors that determine the patient's prognosis:

1. Tumor size: <1.5 cm, 1.5–3 cm, and >3 cm.

2. Prior recurrence rate (RR) per year: RR <1, RR 1–3, and RR >3.

3. Grade: grade 1 (G1), grade 2 (G2), and grade 3 (G3).

Risk groups (1, 2, or 3) are made, reflecting the risk of early invasion and death due to malignant disease.

Reprinted from the European Journal of Cancer, Vol. 31A(11), Kurth KH, Denis L, Bouffioux C, et al. Factors affecting recurrence and progression in superficial bladder tumours, pp 1840–1846. Copyright ©1995, with permission from Elsevier.

course of primary Ta and T1 bladder cancer, based on individual and tumor characteristics of 333 patients. Patients with pure carcinoma in situ (Tis) were systematically excluded. Prognostic factors analyzed were: age, sex, smoking status, number of tumors (single or multiple), largest tumor diameter, stage, grade, mucosal biopsy, and tumor site. Four factors were significant predictors of earlier recurrence in a multivariate Cox regression model. These predictors were: 1) primary tumor multiplicity; 2) diameter >3 cm; 3) stage T1; and 4) grade 2 or 3. Thus, a four-category prognostic index was created in which each category was solely defined by the number of adverse tumor characteristics (ATCs) at initial resection (Box 25.1).[12] According to analysis of the clinical course of the patients (recurrence-free probability at 12 and 24 months, recurrence and tumor rates and progression) in these risk groups, a prognostic index based on the number of ATCs initially present seemed a strong indicator of the clinical course within 3 years of the first endoscopic resection. In the group free of ATCs, the recurrence-free probability at 12 and 24 months was 86% and 69%, respectively, and none experienced progression. Recurrence-free probability was 30% and 19%, respectively, and 7% with progression within 35 months of follow-up in the patient group with three or four ATCs. This four-category prognostic index presented by Allard et al appears easy to apply in urologic practice, as the information needed is routinely available. Although this simple prognostic index could greatly help to identify indicators for adjuvant intravesical therapy, and to determine the optimal periodicity of control cystoscopy regimens, it is their own opinion that it is premature to recommend its use in routine urologic practice, and that further validation in future studies is needed.

Recently, Millán-Rodríguez et al[13] identified risk groups according to progression, mortality, and recurrence rate by a multivariate analysis in a cohort of 1529 patients with primary superficial bladder cancer. Possible prognostic factors including stage, grade, multiplicity, tumor size >3 cm, carcinoma in situ, and treatment with bacillus Calmette–Guérin (BCG) instillation were studied. On the basis of analysis of these factors, a risk group classification was made (Box 25.2).[13] The rates of recurrence, progression, and mortality were 37%, 0%, and 0% in the low-risk group; 45%, 1.8%, and 0.73% in the intermediate risk group; and 54%, 15%, and 9.5% in the high-risk group, respectively. According to Millán-Rodríguez et al, this classification achieves good differentiation of recurrence, and particularly good differentiation of progression and mortality. Moreover, these are the main variables that determine the prognosis and management of superficial bladder cancer, so the classification may be useful for designing treatment and follow-up strategies.

## DISCUSSION AND CONCLUSION

Some factors appear to play a significant role in the majority of the risk stratification schemes we have described, although none of the studies discussed has included all categories of superficial bladder cancer patients. These factors may indeed have prognostic value and thus can be used in daily practice to separate low-risk from high-risk patients. Stage, grade, and multiplicity are factors mentioned in the majority of the studies, whereas size of tumor, recurrence rate, carcinoma in situ association, symptoms, and age are mentioned in only the minority of studies. Additional potentially prognostic clinical factors not used in these schemes are prostatic urethral involvement and response to intravesical therapy; additional histopathologic factors are the level of infiltration into the subepithelial connective tissue, growth pattern (solid versus papillary), and urothelial abnormalities in normal-appearing mucosa. During the last decade, many host and tumor characteristics have been explored for their prognostic ability. Some examples are urinary

---

**Box 25.1**   Risk groups according to Allard et al[12]

Group 1: no adverse tumor characteristics

Group 2: one adverse tumor characteristic

Group 3: two adverse tumor characteristics

Group 4: three or four adverse tumor characteristics

Adverse tumor characteristics: primary tumor multiplicity; diameter >3 cm; stage T1; grade 2 or 3.
Based on data from Allard et al.[12] with permission from Blackwell Publishing Ltd.

---

**Box 25.2**   Risk group according to Millán-Rodríguez et al[13]

1. Low risk
   - Grade 1, stage Ta
   - Grade 1, stage T1, single tumor
2. Intermediate risk
   - Grade 1, stage T1, multiple tumors
   - Grade 2, stage Ta
   - Grade 2, stage T1, single tumor
3. High risk
   - Grade 2, stage T1, multiple tumors
   - Grade 3, stage Ta
   - Grade 3, stage T1
   - Carcinoma in situ association

Reproduced from Millán-Rodríguez F, Chechile-Toniolo G, Salvador-Bayarri J, Palou J, Algaba F, Vicente-Rodríguez J. 2000 Primary superficial bladder cancer risk groups according to progression, mortality and recurrence. Journal of Urology 164(3 Pt 1):680–684, with permission from Lippincott Williams & Wilkins.

markers like BTA-TRAK, BTA-Stat, ImmunoCyt, urinary bladder cancer test, NMP22, and fluorescent in situ hybridization (FISH).

Quek et al[14] recently reviewed the available literature on molecular diagnostic and prognostic factors. As they conclude, ideally the optimal management of bladder cancer patients depends on the assessment of the tumor's biologic potential. They reviewed several categories of molecular changes with potential diagnostic and prognostic value. One group are the chromosomal alterations such as the balance between oncogenes and tumor suppressor genes. With respect to tumor suppressor genes, chromosomes 9, 13, and 17 (the p53 gene) have been studied extensively. A second group of potential markers deals with cellular proliferation in relation to dysregulation of cell cycle control, such as p53, p27, and RB.

Last, but not least, there are factors involved in growth control processes such as angiogenesis (microvessel density), numerous growth factors and their receptors, and loss of cellular adhesion. Accumulation and possibly combination of these changes could ultimately determine the tumor's clinical behavior and response to therapy more accurately than clinical and histologic factors. In the future, a panel of markers will probably be needed rather than one specific marker for, for example, recurrence or progression of superficial tumors. Research in this area is ongoing, and technical developments such as microarray techniques will speed up the application. However, at this moment few, if any, of these factors have found their way from the research laboratory to the clinical setting, and, as the authors conclude, 'Accurate predictions of tumor behaviour based on molecular markers are yet to be realised.'

The most studied nonclinical/nonhistologic factor is p53. Schmitz-Dräger et al[15] reviewed all published literature concerning the association of p53 accumulation and prognosis of patients with bladder cancer. In the results of 43 trials that included 3764 patients, they found that, although comparison between the trials yielded considerable differences, a vast majority of studies demonstrate a correlation between p53 immunohistochemistry on the one hand and tumor stage and grade on the other. Since these parameters are well-established predictors of prognosis, this finding is not surprising, and thus it remains crucial to determine whether this marker provides independent additional information. This question can be answered only by prospective multicenter trials comparing p53 status, preferably even p53 mutation analysis with disease outcome, stratified by tumor stage and grade.

Finally, there are some general limitations in the use of prognostic factors and stratification schemes, as follows:

1. It is difficult to compare the different stratification schemes because of different definitions of start and end points. Most literature deals with Ta and T1 tumors, whereas carcinoma in situ is systematically excluded from the study, or carcinoma in situ association is a bad prognostic factor, as is also the case in some of the aforementioned schemes. Recurrence-free survival, recurrence rate per year, invasion, and mortality are commonly used end points.

2. As Kiemeney et al[3] noted in their own study, even if a prognostic factor seems to have the ability to differentiate between subgroups, this is no guarantee that prediction of disease outcome for individual patients (the ultimate goal of prognostic models) will be accurate.

3. These stratification schemes are hardly ever used in daily practice.

Nevertheless, an important application has been inclusion of these factors in guidelines developed by the American Urological Association (AUA)[16] and European Association of Urology (EAU)[17] guidelines. In the EAU guideline, for example, patients are divided into:

- low risk: single Ta, grade 1, $\leq 3$ cm diameter
- high risk: T1, grade 3, multifocal or highly recurrent, CIS
- intermediate risk: all other tumors, Ta–T1, grade 1–2, multifocal, >3 cm diameter.

Apparently it is impossible to make risk stratification for every tumor and predict its possible evolution. Therefore, further validation of the known risk stratification classifications and development of molecular markers are needed as a basis for designing treatment and follow-up strategies.

REFERENCES

1. Fitzpatrick JM, West AB, Butler MR, Lane V, O'Flynn JD. Superficial bladder tumors (stage pTa, grades 1 and 2): the importance of recurrence pattern following initial resection. J Urol 1986;135(5):920–922.

2. Heney NM, Ahmed S, Flanagan MJ, et al. Superficial bladder cancer: progression and recurrence. J Urol 1983;130(6):1083–1086.

3. Kiemeney LA, Witjes JA, Heijbroek RP, Verbeek AL, Debruyne FM. Predictability of recurrent and progressive disease in individual patients with primary superficial bladder cancer. J Urol 1993;150(1):60–64.

4. Lutzeyer W, Rubben H, Dahm H. Prognostic parameters in superficial bladder cancer: an analysis of 315 cases. J Urol 1982;127(2):250–252.

5. Kirk D. Improving the management of superficial bladder cancer. BMJ 1993;306(6884):1014–1015.

6. Chopin DK, Popov Z, Ravery V, et al. Prognostic factors in superficial bladder cancer. World J Urol 1993;11(3):148–152.

7. Millán-Rodríguez F, Chechile-Toniolo G, Salvador-Bayarri J, Palou J, Vicente-Rodriguez J. Multivariate analysis of the prognostic factors of primary superficial bladder cancer. J Urol 2000;163(1):73–78.

8. Witjes JA, Kiemeney LA, Oosterhof GO, Debruyne FM. Prognostic factors in superficial bladder cancer. A review. Eur Urol 1992;21(2):89–97.

9. Takashi M, Murase T, Mizuno S, Hamajima N, Ohno Y. Multivariate evaluation of prognostic determinants in bladder cancer patients. Urol Int 1987;42(5):368–374.

10. Parmar MK, Freedman LS, Hargreave TB, Tolley DA. Prognostic factors for recurrence and followup policies in the treatment of superficial

bladder cancer: report from the British Medical Research Council Subgroup on Superficial Bladder Cancer (Urological Cancer Working Party). J Urol 1989;142(2 Pt 1):284–288.

11. Kurth KH, Denis L, Bouffioux C, et al. Factors affecting recurrence and progression in superficial bladder tumours. Eur J Cancer 1995;31A(11):1840–1846.

12. Allard P, Bernard P, Fradet Y, Tetu B. The early clinical course of primary Ta and T1 bladder cancer: a proposed prognostic index. Br J Urol 1998;81(5):692–698.

13. Millan-Rodriguez F, Chechile-Toniolo G, Salvador-Bayarri J, Palou J, Algaba F, Vicente-Rodriguez J. Primary superficial bladder cancer risk groups according to progression, mortality and recurrence. J Urol 2000;164(3 Pt 1):680–684.

14. Quek ML, Quinn DI, Daneshmand S, Stein JP. Molecular prognostication in bladder cancer—a current perspective. Eur J Cancer 2003;39(11):1501–1510.

15. Schmitz-Dräger BJ, Goebell PJ, Ebert T, Fradet Y. p53 immunohistochemistry as a prognostic marker in bladder cancer. Playground for urology scientists? Eur Urol 2000;38(6):691–699.

16. Smith JA Jr, Labasky RF, Cockett AT, Fracchia JA, Montie JE, Rowland RG. Bladder cancer clinical guidelines panel summary report on the management of nonmuscle invasive bladder cancer (stages Ta, T1 and TIS). The American Urological Association. J Urol 1999;162(5):1697–1701.

17. Oosterlinck W, Lobel B, Jakse G, Malmstrom PU, Stockle M, Sternberg C. Guidelines on bladder cancer. Eur Urol 2002;41(2):105–112.

# Treatment

SECTION 5

# Issues in staging of Ta, Tis, and T1 bladder cancers

# 26

*Sharon Sharir, Andrew J Evans, Mary K Gospodarowicz,
Michael AS Jewett*

## INTRODUCTION

The primary purpose of staging is to enable clear communication between clinicians regarding their experiences with malignancies by attempting to define disease extent.[1] Accurate staging of cancer is also important for facilitating treatment planning, providing prognostic information, and aiding treatment evaluation.[1] Miscommunication about staging impacts negatively on all of these functions.

Approximately 70% of all bladder malignancies are nonmuscle-invasive Ta, Tis, and T1 cancers.[2-4] These tumors not only behave differently from muscle-invasive cancers, but also from one another.[5-9] Because of these differences in natural history, treatment decisions and prognosis can vary significantly, depending on the tumor stage. It is, therefore, important to ensure that these bladder cancers are accurately staged, and correctly distinguished from one another and from muscle-invasive tumors.

Accurate staging of nonmuscle-invasive bladder cancers may be difficult. This chapter addresses difficulties that may be encountered during staging, and is organized into issues associated with the TNM classification system, those applicable to the surgeon, those encountered during pathologic examination, and those resulting from imaging. Understanding these potential problems is important for ensuring that the intended goals of staging—clear communication, accurate prognostication, and correct treatment selection and assessment—are achieved.

## ISSUES IN STAGING

### TNM CLASSIFICATION SYSTEM ISSUES

The TNM cancer staging classification published by the UICC (Union Internationale Contre le Cancer/ International Union Against Cancer) and the AJCC (American Joint Committee on Cancer) is used worldwide to record the anatomic disease extent of cancer. The sixth edition of the UICC TNM classification published in 2002[1] is the most current version, and it is identical to that published in the 2002 sixth edition of the *AJCC Cancer Staging Manual*.[10]

One of the most common problems encountered with reporting of cancer stage results from changes that have occurred in the TNM classification over time. As our understanding of the disease process changes, TNM classification undergoes change. As a consequence, different editions of the TNM classification describe tumor extent differently (Table 26.1). Moreover, some editions[11-13] have undergone revisions, sometimes with nomenclature changes between the original and revised versions. Furthermore, although the AJCC currently uses the same TNM classification as the UICC, this has not always been the case. The fifth[14,15] and sixth[1,10] editions of the UICC and AJCC classifications are identical, but the AJCC third edition[16] corresponds to the UICC fourth edition,[13] and the AJCC fourth edition[17] corresponds to the revised UICC fourth edition.[18] The first (1977, revised 1978) and second (1983) AJCC manuals are not

**Table 26.1** UICC TNM classifications of urinary bladder carcinomas

| Tumor extent (using TNM 2002 terminology) | 1st edition (1968)[11] (revised 1973)[60] | 2nd edition (1974)[61] | 3rd edition (1978)[12] (revised 1982) | 4th edition (1987)[13] (revised 1992)[18] | 5th edition (1997)[14] | 6th edition (2002)[1] |
|---|---|---|---|---|---|---|
| Primary tumor cannot be assessed | – | TX | TX | TX | TX | TX |
| No evidence of primary tumor | T0 | T0 | T0 | T0 | T0 | T0 |
| Non-invasive papillary carcinoma | Tis | – | Ta | Ta | Ta | Ta |
| Carcinoma in situ: 'flat tumor' | Tis | Tis | Tis | Tis | Tis | Tis |
| Tumor invades subepithelial connective tissue | T1 | T1 | T1 | T1 | T1 | T1 |
| Tumor invades muscle | – | – | – | – | T2 | T2 |
|   Tumor invades superficial muscle (inner half) | T2 | T2 | T2 | T2 | T2a | T2a |
|   Tumor invades deep muscle (outer half) | T3 | T3a | T3a | T3a | T2b | T2b |
| Tumor invades perivesical tissue | T3 | T3b | T3b | T3b | T3 | T3 |
|   Microscopically | – | – | – | 1987: – 1992: T3b | T3a | T3a |
|   Macroscopically (extravesical mass) | – | – | – | 1987: – 1992: T3b | T3b | T3b |
| Tumor invades any of the following: prostate, uterus, vagina, pelvic wall, abdominal wall | T4 | T4 | T4 | T4 | T4 | T4 |
|   Tumor invades prostate, uterus, or vagina | – | T4a | T4a | 1987: – 1992: T4a | T4a | T4a |
|   Tumor invades pelvic wall or abdominal wall | – | T4b | T4b | 1987: – 1992: T4b | T4b | T4b |

identical to the UICC system.[16] It is important to note that although T, N, and M categories usually maintain the same nomenclature (e.g. Ta, T3a, N1) in different editions, their definitions may change over time. For example, the entity now referred to as Ta was referred to as Tis in the first edition of the UICC classification. In the second edition, this entity was not specified at all, so it might have been classified as Tis or as T1 (see Table 26.1). This problem is exacerbated by the fact that many authors do not specify the TNM edition used when reporting the outcomes of treatment in bladder cancer. This practice is in contrast to that of the International Classification of Diseases, for example, where the version being referred to (e.g. ICD9, ICD10) is part of the system name.[19] Readers are therefore cautioned to clarify what organization and edition or year is being referred to for TNM classification, and authors are encouraged to unambiguously specify it, to avoid the possibility of miscommunication. Furthermore, researchers must be aware of the different editions of TNM classification when attempting to make longitudinal comparisons based on recorded stage.

One of the advantages of the TNM system is the broadness of the staging criteria, which permits international consensus and applicability within a wide range of practice patterns and available resources. For example, in T category assessment, physical examination (including examination under anesthesia), imaging, and endoscopy are used, in addition to cytologic or pathologic confirmation of disease. Yet the use of imaging tests is not mandated, and physical examination can be broadly interpreted. This broadness, therefore, also imparts a weakness to TNM classification, in that there is a lack of uniformity in staging methods. This may result in variability of reported outcomes. Investigators should, therefore, report details of the modalities used for staging to permit assessment of differences that may be due to staging practices alone.

It is important to understand what constitutes clinical TNM (designated cTNM or TNM) and pathologic TNM (designated pTNM) staging. The two classifications have different purposes: the cTNM classification is applicable prior to surgical treatment and is used to choose therapy; pTNM is a postsurgical histopathologic classification used to determine prognosis and select adjuvant treatment.[20] To permit accurate communication and comparison, the requirements for correctly assigning cTNM and pTNM staging must be understood. In particular, it is important to dispel the common misconception that obtaining a pathologic specimen necessarily yields a pathologic T (pT) category. For a tumor to be classifiable in terms of pT category, the pathologic specimen must permit evaluation of the highest pT category. Thus, for bladder tumors removed by transurethral resection (TUR), a pT category can only be assigned if all gross tumor is resected and then the deep and lateral margins are resected and sent for pathologic examination separately from the main tumor specimen, and these margins are all found to be tumor-free, thus indicating a complete resection.[20] If this is not done, only a clinical T category can be assigned, as there remains doubt as to the extent of disease.

Clinicians must recognize that determination of the pT category does not imply pathologic staging of the N and M categories as well. The pathologic N (pN) category requires nodal biopsy/resection that is adequate for validating the absence of lymph node metastases and permits evaluation of the highest pN category. A pathologic M (pM) category requires microscopic examination of the metastasis.[1] For nonmuscle-invasive bladder cancers, complete resection yields a pathologic classification for the T category only and the N and M categories usually remain clinical unless these are examined histologically as well. For example, a patient will often be pT1cN0cM0 (also designated pT1N0M0).

Synchronous multiple bladder tumors present some additional challenges. Importantly, the definition of synchronous tumors considers cancers diagnosed within 2 months of one another as a single tumor event.[20] This definition is used to be consistent with the Surveillance, Epidemiology, and End Results (SEER) program of the National Cancer Institute in the United States.[21] Multiplicity of tumors is indicated with an '(m)' after the T category, or alternatively with the number of tumors instead of the 'm', for example, T1 (m) or T1 (3).[1] When carcinoma in situ (CIS) is one of the bladder tumor pathologies but not the highest stage, the suffix 'is' may be used to indicate this, for example T1 (m, is) or T1 (3, is) or T1 (is).[20] If there are multiple synchronous tumors of different T stages, the highest T category must be assigned, and multiplicity should be indicated.[1] However, knowledge regarding the prognostic significance of different T categories has evolved with time; consequently, the hierarchy of T categories has changed with different editions of the TNM classification (Table 26.2). This means that with synchronous Ta and Tis tumors (using the 2002 definitions), a patient would have been classified as Tis (2) from 1968 to 1973, Tis (2) or T1 (2, is) from 1974 to 1977, Ta (2, is) from 1978 to 1991, and Tis (2) from 1992 to the present (see Tables 26.1 and 26.2). To improve consistency in the face of changes in TNM, a better method of recording the T category might be to indicate all tumors, with a separate T category for each, for example Tis (1), Ta (1).

Another potential pitfall is related to staging in the presence of CIS. If there is a primary bladder cancer, but there is CIS in the prostatic urethra, ducts and/or glands, the highest T category for bladder is used, but the 'is' suffix may be appended.[20] It is not classified as T4a, which would be applicable if the primary bladder tumor invades the prostate or prostatic urethra beyond the basement membrane. Thus, a T1 bladder tumor with associated CIS in the prostatic urethra or ducts would be T1 (is), T1 (is pu), or T1 (is pd), where 'pu' signifies extension into prostatic urethra and 'pd' indicates extension into prostatic ducts. Similarly, invasion of the wall of the seminal vesicle or ureter by bladder cancer is designated as T4a, but if there is only CIS in the seminal vesicle or ureter, it should be classified as the bladder component would be, with addition of the 'is' suffix if desired.[20] It should also be noted that if there is a primary prostatic urothelial cancer, the bladder staging system should not be used—there is a prostatic urethral transitional cell carcinoma staging classification that is delineated in the urethral cancer classification.[1]

If the TNM category is unclear, the lowest category should be used.[1] This rule must be kept in mind when the pathologic diagnosis holds some uncertainty, or when imaging and physical examination yield nondefinitive information. Not using the lowest category would result in treatment outcomes appearing better than they really are.

## SURGICAL ISSUES

Inaccurate staging may occur if the presence of tumor is not recognized due to inadequate visualization of the entire urothelium endoscopically. A systematic approach to inspection of the bladder should be used to ensure that no areas are missed. The bladder must not be overly distended, to permit an adequate view of the bladder dome; pressing on the suprapubic region of the abdominal wall can also help to bring this area into view. For rigid cystoscopy, a 70° lens should be used in order to ensure that the entire bladder is adequately surveyed. When the area around the bladder neck cannot be adequately visualized, particularly in a patient with a large prostatic median lobe, a 120° lens may be

**Table 26.2** UICC T category hierarchy for classification of nonmuscle-invasive urinary bladder carcinomas

| Stage hierarchy | 1st edition (1968)[11] (revised 1973)[60] | 2nd edition (1974)[61] | 3rd edition (1978)[12] (revised 1982) | 4th edition (1987)[13] (revised 1992)[18] | 5th edition (1997)[14] | 6th edition (2002)[1] |
|---|---|---|---|---|---|---|
| Lower T category | Tis | Tis | Tis | 1987: Tis 1992: Ta | Ta | Ta |
| Middle T category | – | – | Ta | 1987: Ta 1992: Tis | Tis | Tis |
| Higher T category | T1 | T1 | T1 | T1 | T1 | T1 |

helpful. Increasingly, men are examined with flexible cystoscopes. During flexible cystoscopy, retroflexion of the cystoscope should be performed to allow for visualization of the region around the bladder neck.

Nonvisualization of bladder cancer may also occur because bladder tumors, particularly CIS, may not be visible endoscopically. Studies have demonstrated that when random biopsies are performed, otherwise unrecognized urothelial cancer may be found.[22-24] A proportion of these cases will be upstaged due to the random biopsies.[22] Because of this, some urologists routinely perform random biopsies of normal-looking urothelium. Others do not because of a concern that doing so could result in implantation of carcinoma in otherwise normal tissue, or because the benefits of performing random biopsies are thought to be small.[25,26] This difference in practice patterns means that centers that do not perform random biopsies may not detect occult CIS as often as those that do. Investigators have also explored another strategy to reduce the likelihood of missing invisible tumor. Fluorescence cystoscopy in addition to white light endoscopy may improve the visibility of bladder cancers.[27-30] Differing practice in the use of such adjunctive strategies for finding otherwise invisible CIS means that different centers may stage bladder cancers differently.

Another surgeon-specific pitfall in staging of nonmuscle-invasive bladder tumors results from performing tumor resection incorrectly. If only part of the tumor is resected, it is not possible to know if the tumor is actually of a higher stage. For T1 cancers, for example, there must be muscle in the specimen to exclude the possibility that the tumor is, in fact, T2. It is known that the risk of understaging T1 tumors, when compared with the pT category, is higher if there is no muscle in the pathology specimen (62% versus 30%).[31] However, as discussed above, even if all gross tumor is resected, the deep and lateral margins must be resected and sent separately.[20] Thus, incorrect surgical technique may understage nonmuscle-invasive bladder tumors.

Another area of differing surgical practice is in re-resection of nonmuscle-invasive tumors within a few weeks of the first resection. Particularly if the TNM-required separate resection of the deep and lateral margins is not sent separately during the first resection, a second resection will ensure more accurate pathologic T categorization. Whether a second resection is necessary in cases where the TNM resection guideline was followed during the initial resection is unclear. The likelihood of finding residual tumor on re-resection is approximately 33% to 75%, with upstaging reported to be 5% to 29%.[32-35] Differences in re-resection practice may result in differing T category assignments.

Surgeons must be cognizant that the quality of the resection specimens submitted is critical to accurate staging.[36] Pathologists may have difficulty assigning the T category or even providing a histopathologic diagnosis

when too little material is submitted. Pathologists may also experience difficulty if the specimen demonstrates significant cautery or crush artifact.[37] Thermal artifact can make it impossible to recognize a given specimen as a neoplasm, create 'pseudoinvasion' in papillary non-invasive tumors, and make it difficult to reliably assess involvement of the muscularis propria (Figure 26.1). To avoid this, surgeons must be conversant with the biophysics of electrocautery and the optimal technique for resecting bladder tumors. Some authors suggest using a blended current to resect most tumors, and reserve the pure cut current of the resectoscope for tumors near the ureteric orifices.[38,39] However, we prefer to obtain all specimens with a pure cut current when using the resectoscope to decrease the likelihood of cautery artifact. Additionally, the loop should be moved through the tissue quickly, and only once, to avoid charring; ideally, the current should be turned on before the loop touches the urothelium. Use of cold-cup biopsy forceps for small tumors is another way to avoid thermal artifact. In order to prevent crush artifact, care must be taken when handling the specimen. If an instrument is used, it is best to keep the tips closed, to avoid compressing the specimen between them.

## PATHOLOGY ISSUES

The first issue for pathologists during assessment of nonmuscle-invasive bladder cancer is in deciding whether a given lesion is neoplastic or rather some reactive, inflammatory, or metaplastic process. Once it has been determined that a lesion is neoplastic, the next step is to decide whether it is benign or malignant. The current 1998 World Health Organization/International Society of Urological Pathology (WHO/ISUP) consensus classification of urothelial neoplasms of the urinary bladder recognizes benign entities such as hyperplasia, atypia, dysplasia, papilloma, and inverted papilloma, in addition to malignant neoplasms.[40] The TNM system applies only to malignancies, which include papillary urothelial neoplasm of low malignant potential (PUNLMP), low-grade papillary carcinoma, high-grade papillary carcinoma, CIS, neoplasms invading the lamina propria, and neoplasms invading the muscularis propria.[20,40] While discriminating benign from malignant processes is often straightforward, this distinction may be difficult in certain cases. For example, benign inverted papillomas can potentially be misinterpreted as papillary cancers with stromal invasion.[41]

Problems with interobserver reliability and difficulties with definitions have also been reported when attempting to distinguish dysplasia (low-grade intraurothelial neoplasia), which is classified as a benign lesion, from CIS (high-grade intraurothelial neoplasia).[40] Interobserver variability has similarly

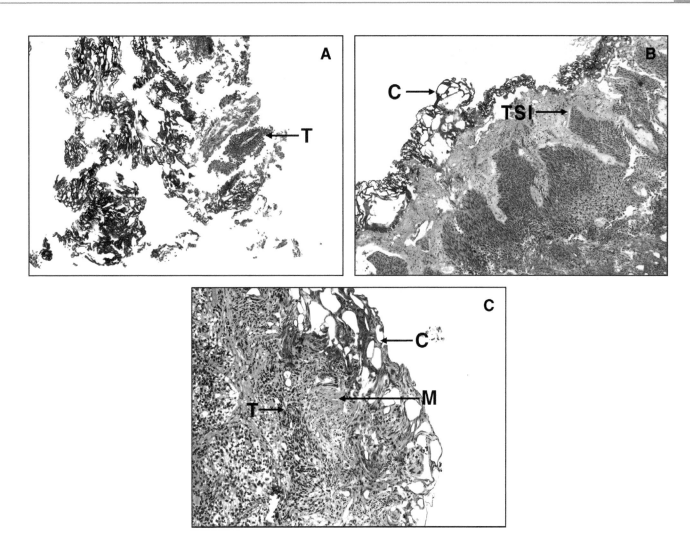

**Fig. 26.1**
Cautery artifact in transurethral resection specimens. **A** Extensive cautery artifact that virtually precludes interpretation of the specimen. A small fragment of viable papillary tumor (T) is visible. In such cases, no reliable comment on grade or stage can be made. **B** Cautery artifact (C) along the edge of a transurethral specimen chip. The thermal effect has tracked into the tissue, causing distortion of the tumor–stroma interface (TSI). Such areas can be mistaken for superficial lamina propria invasion; however, close examination of the TSI reveals a lack of the typical stromal reaction usually associated with such invasion. **C** There is invasive tumor (T) in close apposition to muscle (M). Cautery artifact (C) has distorted the fragment of smooth muscle in this chip of tissue. In this situation, it is not possible to make a definitive statement about whether the muscle is muscularis mucosa or muscularis propria.

occurred when attempting to distinguish benign papillomas from the malignant entity PUNLMP.[42] However, problems with interobserver variability are not limited to issues of distinguishing benign from malignant entities; there can be difficulties in interpreting stage with Ta and T1 tumors.[43] It is hoped that the new WHO/ISUP classification system, with its more detailed histologic descriptors, may result in more uniform use of terminology and greater interobserver reproducibility.[44]

Urothelial denudation represents another problem encountered by pathologists, since a diagnosis of urothelial carcinoma is not possible without urothelium. Shedding of the superficial cell layers of the bladder may occur with CIS (Figure 26.2). When faced with a specimen containing epithelial denudation and no definitive evidence of malignancy, the clinician should consider the possibility that CIS is the cause, particularly in a patient with a history of CIS or in the case of a specimen obtained by cold-cup biopsy.[45] In some instances, scattered malignant cells may remain attached to the mucosal surface, creating so-called 'clinging CIS' that may or may not be recognized as CIS, depending on the pathologist's level of comfort and experience (see Figure 26.2).[46]

Another phenomenon that can create problems in correctly assigning a T category is the presence of inflammation that obscures the tumor–stroma interface. This inflammatory reaction, which can occur with papillary tumors, may obscure small nests of cells that

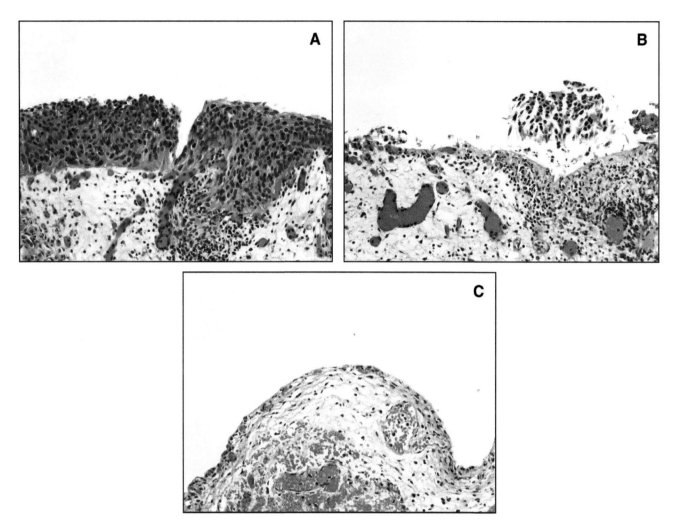

**Fig. 26.2**
Urothelial denudation and carcinoma in situ (CIS). **A** Intact CIS characterized by numerous small, congested superficial blood vessels in the lamina propria. **B** Partially denuded, or 'clinging', CIS. **C** A non-diagnostic area with complete urothelial denudation. Congested superficial vessels are seen that are like those associated with the CIS in **A** and **B**.

are present in the lamina propria, thus resulting in understaging of the tumor.[37]

To avoid some other common pitfalls, an understanding of the anatomic landmarks used during staging is essential (Figure 26.3). Upwards of 50% of bladder specimens contain a discontinuous layer of wispy smooth muscle in the lamina propria known as the muscularis mucosa.[47-49] When identifying tumor cells within muscle fibers, it is therefore necessary for pathologists to determine whether the layer is muscularis mucosa (categorized as T1), or muscularis propria (categorized as T2). Another staging pitfall with TUR specimens may occur with the presumption that the presence of tumor in fat is evidence of perivesical fat involvement (categorized as T3). In fact, adipose tissue has been found within the lamina propria in over 50% of cystectomy specimens and within the muscularis propria in 100% of cases (see Figure 26.3).[50,51] For this reason, the presence of tumor in fat within TUR specimens cannot be used as evidence of perivesical fat invasion.

Problems with pathologic interpretation of TUR specimens are often exacerbated by the presence of tangential sectioning of TUR chips. The lack of clear orientation of the specimens can make it difficult to determine the true depth of tumor cells within the bladder. For example, tangential sectioning of a Ta tumor may result in the presence of nests of tumor cells within the lamina propria, giving the appearance of a T1 cancer.[37]

## IMAGING ISSUES

In the TNM classification of bladder tumors, imaging may be used in assignment of the T, N, and M categories.[1] However, imaging has suboptimal accuracy for determining local tumor extent, particularly for

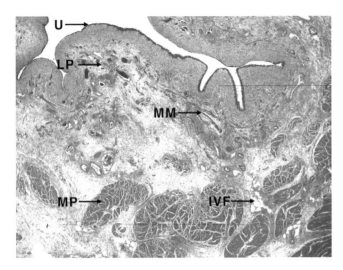

**Fig. 26.3**
Histologic landmarks used for staging of bladder cancer. A full thickness section of the bladder showing the urothelium (U), lamina propria (LP), a discontinuous muscularis mucosa (MM) within the lamina propria, and the thick smooth muscle bundles of the muscularis propria (MP). Intravesical fat (IVF) is present within the muscularis propria.

lower stage cancers without muscle invasion or extravesical spread.[52,53] Computed tomography (CT) can show mural thickening, extravesical extension, and other organ involvement. However, it cannot determine extent of disease in nonmuscle-invasive disease.[54] Magnetic resonance imaging (MRI) may show depth of mural penetration, because tumor gives off a slightly different signal compared to normal bladder wall and enhances with gadolinium contrast. Yet, because the superficial layers of the bladder enhance as well, assigning an accurate T category for nonmuscle-invasive disease is difficult.[55]

Imaging is of benefit in clinical staging of the N and M categories. However, while imaging can show lymph node enlargement, it cannot reliably detect replacement of normal nodes by tumor with no change in nodal size, nor distinguish reactive enlargement of nodes from that due to metastatic disease.[52,56] Furthermore, since nonmuscle-invasive bladder cancers rarely metastasize to the lymph nodes or to more distant sites, radiologic assessment is of limited importance in nonmuscle-invasive disease.

One of the problems that occurs in bladder imaging is that distension of the bladder can be variable. Insufficient bladder distension may give the appearance of increased mural thickening. With CT scan assessments of the bladder, there have been attempts to improve radiologic accuracy in determining the T category with the use of air insufflation of the bladder, rather than the use of urine or contrast.[57] It is thought that the tendency to overstage due to poor bladder distension may be minimized with air distension of the bladder.

Timing of the CT scan relative to contrast administration can also result in variable imaging interpretation. As contrast in the bladder starts to mix with the urine, the urine jets may sometimes take on the appearance of bladder tumors.[58] Performing delayed imaging will permit these 'pseudolesions' to be differentiated from true bladder tumors.

Another potential pitfall relates to the timing of imaging relative to TUR. With nonmuscle-invasive disease in particular, imaging of the bladder may be delayed until after TUR is performed, and histologic confirmation of a bladder tumor diagnosis is obtained. However, if imaging is performed within 6 weeks of resection, alterations in the appearance of the resected area may occur on CT.[54,55] This may give a false impression of significant mural thickening or even extravesical extension of tumor (Figure 26.4). With MRI, a period of up to 3 months may be required to avoid false positives secondary to inflammatory changes that occur after TUR. Modifications in MRI technique may improve the ability to distinguish inflammatory changes from neoplastic growth.[59]

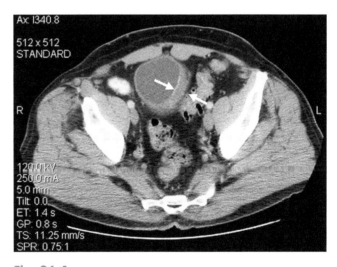

**Fig. 26.4**
CT changes after transurethral resection of bladder tumor. Bladder wall thickening is present, as indicated by arrows. Streaky changes are evident in the perivesical fat, mimicking extravesical disease extension. However, this patient's bladder tumor was confined to the lamina propria (pT1).

## CONCLUSION

Clinicians need to be aware of problems encountered during staging of nonmuscle-invasive bladder cancers. Understanding these difficulties can help to avoid potential problems, or at least facilitate a more nuanced understanding of a patient's assigned stage in situations where uncertainty remains.

TNM classification is an effective tool for communication and prognostication regarding patients with cancer. A good understanding of TNM classification and its requirements is critical for assigning stage accurately. Changes in the classification over time in response to new information on determinants of prognosis, or to improvements in diagnostic modalities, pose a challenge to clinicians. Similarly, ensuring relevance of TNM to differing practice patterns worldwide creates difficulties in ensuring uniformity of staging. Ongoing assessment and improvements to the current shortcomings of the TNM classification will render it even more powerful in the future.

To ensure proper stage classification, surgeons must use meticulous surgical techniques to enable accurate tumor visualization and resection. An understanding of the requirements for TNM pathologic classification is also critical for ensuring correct stage assignment. Differences in surgical practice patterns with respect to adjunctive methods of finding invisible bladder lesions and re-resection of high-risk bladder tumors may result in staging differences between centers.

Pathologists need to be aware of the various pitfalls that may be encountered when examining bladder tumor specimens. The anatomy of the bladder wall must be understood to avoid some of these problems. Further clarifications of stage and grade assignment criteria will hopefully produce better interobserver reliability in the future.

Currently, imaging has a limited role in staging of nonmuscle-invasive bladder tumors. Findings in the bladder may be due to artifact rather than neoplasms. In particular, care must be taken when interpreting imaging shortly after transurethral bladder resection.

## REFERENCES

1. Sobin LH, Wittekind C (eds). International Union Against Cancer (UICC): TNM Classification of Malignant Tumours, 6th ed. New York: Wiley-Liss, 2002.

2. Crow P, Ritchie AW. National and international variation in the registration of bladder cancer. BJU Int 2003;92:563–566.

3. Larsson P, Wijkstrom H, Thorstenson A, et al. A population-based study of 538 patients with newly detected urinary bladder neoplasms followed during 5 years. Scand J Urol Nephrol 2003;37:195–201.

4. Messing EM, Young TB, Hunt VB, et al. Comparison of bladder cancer outcome in men undergoing hematuria home screening versus those with standard clinical presentations. Urology 1995;45:387–396.

5. Holmang S, Hedelin H, Anderstrom C, Johansson SL. The relationship among multiple recurrences, progression and prognosis of patients with stages Ta and T1 transitional cell cancer of the bladder followed for at least 20 years. J Urol 1995;153:1823–1826.

6. Haukaas S, Daehlin L, Maartmann-Moe H, Ulvik NM. The long-term outcome in patients with superficial transitional cell carcinoma of the bladder: a single-institutional experience. BJU Int 1999;83:957–963.

7. Heney NM. Natural history of superficial bladder cancer. Prognostic features and long-term disease course. Urol Clin North Am 1992;19:429–433.

8. Lamm DL. Carcinoma in situ. Urol Clin North Am 1992;19:499–508.

9. Gschwend JE, Dahm P, Fair WR. Disease specific survival as endpoint of outcome for bladder cancer patients following radical cystectomy. Eur Urol 2002;41:440–448.

10. Greene FL, Page DL, Fleming ID, et al (eds). AJCC Cancer Staging Manual, 6th ed. New York: Springer, 2002.

11. International Union Against Cancer (UICC): TNM Classification of Malignant Tumours. Geneva: UICC, 1968.

12. Harmer MH (ed). International Union Against Cancer (UICC): TNM Classification of Malignant Tumours, 3rd ed. Geneva: UICC, 1978.

13. Hermanek P, Sobin LH (eds). International Union Against Cancer (UICC): TNM Classification of Malignant Tumours, 4th ed. Berlin: Springer-Verlag, 1987.

14. Sobin LH, Wittekind C (eds). International Union Against Cancer (UICC): TNM Classification of Malignant Tumours, 5th ed. New York: Wiley-Liss, 1997.

15. Fleming ID, Cooper JS, Henson DE, et al (eds). AJCC Cancer Staging Manual, 5th ed. Philadelphia: Lippincott-Raven, 1997.

16. Beahrs OH, Henson DE, Hutter RVP, Myers MH (eds). Manual for Staging of Cancer, 3rd ed. Philadelphia: Lippincott, 1988.

17. Beahrs OH, Henson DE, Hutter RVP, Kennedy BJ (eds). Manual for Staging of Cancer, 4th ed. Philadelphia: Lippincott, 1992.

18. Hermanek P, Sobin LH (eds). International Union Against Cancer (UICC): TNM Classification of Malignant Tumours, 4th ed, 2nd revision. Berlin: Springer-Verlag, 1992.

19. ICD10: The International Statistical Classification of Diseases and Related Health Problems, 10th revision. Online. Available: www.who.int/classifications/icd/en/.

20. Wittekind C, Henson DE, Hutter RVP, Sobin LH (eds). International Union Against Cancer (UICC): TNM Supplement. A Commentary on Uniform Use, 2nd ed. New York: Wiley-Liss, 2001.

21. National Cancer Institute SEER website. Available: http://seer.cancer.gov.

22. May F, Treiber U, Hartung R, Schwaibold H. Significance of random bladder biopsies in superficial bladder cancer. Eur Urol 2003;44:47–50.

23. Smith G, Elton RA, Beynon LL, Newsam JE, Chisholm GD, Hargreave TB. Prognostic significance of biopsy results of normal-looking mucosa in cases of superficial bladder cancer. Br J Urol 1983;55:665–669.

24. Kiemeney LA, Witjes JA, Heijbroek RP, Verbeek AL, Debruyne FM. Predictability of recurrent and progressive disease in individual patients with primary superficial bladder cancer. J Urol 1993;150:60–64.

25. Soloway MS, Masters S. Urothelial susceptibility to tumor cell implantation: influence of cauterization. Cancer 1980;46:1158–1163.

26. Kiemeney LA, Witjes JA, Heijbroek RP, et al. Should random urothelial biopsies be taken from patients with primary superficial bladder cancer? A decision analysis. Br J Urol 1994;73:164–171.

27. Zaak D, Hungerhuber E, Schneede P, et al. Role of 5-aminolevulinic acid in the detection of urothelial premalignant lesions. Cancer 2002;95:1234–8.

28. Filbeck T, Pichlmeier U, Knuechel R, Wieland WF, Roessler W. Do patients profit from 5-aminolevulinic acid-induced fluorescence diagnosis in transurethral resection of bladder carcinoma? Urology 2002;60:1025–1028.

29. De Dominicis C, Liberti M, Perugia G, et al. Role of 5-aminolevulinic acid in the diagnosis and treatment of superficial bladder cancer: improvement in diagnostic sensitivity. Urology 2001;57:1059–1062.

30. Jichlinski P, Guillou L, Karlsen SJ, et al. Hexyl aminolevulinate fluorescence cystoscopy: new diagnostic tool for photodiagnosis of superficial bladder cancer—a multicenter study. J Urol 2003;170:226–229.

31. Dutta SC, Smith JA Jr, Shappell SB, Coffey CS, Chang SS, Cookson MS. Clinical under staging of high risk nonmuscle invasive urothelial carcinoma treated with radical cystectomy. J Urol 2001;166:490–493.

32. Grimm MO, Steinhoff C, Simon X, Spiegelhalder P, Ackermann R, Vogeli TA. Effect of routine repeat transurethral resection for superficial bladder cancer: a long-term observational study. J Urol 2003;170(2 Pt 1):433–437.

33. Schips L, Augustin H, Zigeuner RE, et al. Is repeated transurethral resection justified in patients with newly diagnosed superficial bladder cancer? Urology 2002;59:220–223.

34. Herr HW. The value of a second transurethral resection in evaluating patients with bladder tumors. J Urol 1999;162:74–76.

35. Brauers A, Buettner R, Jakse G. Second resection and prognosis of primary high risk superficial bladder cancer: is cystectomy often too early? J Urol 2001;165:808–810.

36. Maruniak NA, Takezawa K, Murphy WM. Accurate pathological staging of urothelial neoplasms requires better cystoscopic sampling. J Urol 2002;167:2404–2407.

37. Lopez-Beltran A, Cheng L. Stage pT1 bladder carcinoma: diagnostic criteria, pitfalls and prognostic significance. Pathology 2003;35:484–491.

38. Malkowicz SB. Management of superficial bladder cancer. In Walsh PC, Retik AB, Vaughan ED Jr, Wein AJ (eds): Campbell's Urology, 8th ed. Philadelphia: Elsevier, 2002, pp 2785–2802.

39. Holzbeierlein JM, Smith JA Jr. Surgical management of noninvasive bladder cancer (stages Ta/T1/CIS). Urol Clin North Am 2000;27:15–24.

40. Epstein JI, Amin MB, Reuter VR, Mostofi FK, and The Bladder Consensus Conference Committee. The World Health Organization/International Society of Urological Pathology consensus classification of urothelial (transitional cell) neoplasms of the urinary bladder. Am J Surg Pathol 1998;22:1435–1448.

41. Epstein JI, Amin MB, Reuter VR. Bladder Biopsy Interpretation. Philadelphia: Lippincott, 2004.

42. Cotran RS, Kumar V, Collins T. The lower urinary tract. In Cotran RS, Kumar V, Collins T (eds): Robbins Pathologic Basis of Disease, 6th ed. Philadelphia: WB Saunders, 1999, pp 997–1010.

43. Tosoni I, Wagner U, Sauter G, et al. Clinical significance of interobserver differences in the staging and grading of superficial bladder cancer. BJU Int 2000;85:48–53.

44. Epstein JI. The new World Health Organization/International Society of Urological Pathology (WHO/ISUP) classification for Ta, T1 bladder tumors: is it an improvement? Crit Rev Oncol Hematol 2003;47:83–89.

45. Levi AW, Potter SR, Schoenberg MP, Epstein JI. Clinical significance of denuded urothelium in bladder biopsy. J Urol 2001;166:457–460.

46. McKenney JK, Gomez JA, Desai S, Lee MW, Amin MB. Morphologic expressions of urothelial carcinoma in situ: a detailed evaluation of its histologic patterns with emphasis on carcinoma in situ with microinvasion. Am J Surg Pathol 2001;25:356–362.

47. Younes M, Sussman J, True LD. The usefulness of the level of the muscularis mucosae in the staging of invasive transitional cell carcinoma of the urinary bladder. Cancer 1990;66:543–548.

48. Bernardini S, Billerey C, Martin M, Adessi GL, Wallerand H, Bittard H. The predictive value of muscularis mucosae invasion and p53 over expression on progression of stage T1 bladder carcinoma. J Urol 2001;165:42–46.

49. Keep JC, Piehl M, Miller A, Oyasu R. Invasive carcinomas of the urinary bladder. Evaluation of tunica muscularis mucosae involvement. Am J Clin Pathol 1989;91:575–579.

50. Philip AT, Amin MB, Tamboli P, Lee TJ, Hill CE, Ro JY. Intravesical adipose tissue: a quantitative study of its presence and location with implications for therapy and prognosis. Am J Surg Pathol 2000;24:1286–1290.

51. Bochner BH, Nichols PW, Skinner DG. Overstaging of transitional cell carcinoma: clinical significance of lamina propria fat within the urinary bladder. Urology 1995;45:528–531.

52. Lawler LP. MR imaging of the bladder. Radiol Clin North Am 2003;41:161–177.

53. See WA, Fuller JR. Staging of advanced bladder cancer. Current concepts and pitfalls. Urol Clin North Am 1992;19:663–683.

54. Husband JE. Staging bladder cancer. Clin Radiol 1992;46:153–159.

55. MacVicar AD. Bladder cancer staging. BJU Int 2000;86(Suppl 1):111–122.

56. Roy C, Le Bras Y, Mangold L, et al. Small pelvic lymph node metastases: evaluation with MR imaging. Clin Radiol 1997;52:437–440.

57. Caterino M, Giunta S, Finocchi V, et al. Primary cancer of the urinary bladder: CT evaluation of the T parameter with different techniques. Abdom Imaging 2001;26:433–438.

58. Olcott EW, Nino-Murcia M, Rhee JS. Urinary bladder pseudolesions on contrast-enhanced helical CT: frequency and clinical implications. Am J Roentgenol 1998;171:1349–1354.

59. Barentsz JO, Jager GJ, van Vierzen PB, et al. Staging urinary bladder cancer after transurethral biopsy: value of fast dynamic contrast-enhanced MR imaging. Radiology 1996;201:185–193.

60. International Union Against Cancer (UICC): TNM Classification of Malignant Tumours, revised 1st ed. Geneva: UICC, 1973.

61. International Union Against Cancer (UICC): TNM Classification of Malignant Tumours, 2nd ed. Geneva: UICC, 1974.

# Transurethral resection of bladder tumors

27

*Harry W Herr*

## INTRODUCTION

More than 60,000 new cases of bladder cancer are diagnosed each year in the United States.[1] Another 600,000 men and women are under surveillance for recurrent bladder tumors.[2] About 70% of bladder tumors are superficial, i.e. nonmuscle invasive (stage Ta, Tis, T1), and 30% invade the bladder muscle (stage T2) or perivesical fat (stage T3). Transurethral resection (TUR) is the essential surgical procedure used to diagnose, stage, and treat the majority of primary and recurrent bladder tumors.

TUR of bladder tumors is both a diagnostic and a therapeutic procedure. The initial TUR of a bladder tumor has three main goals:

1. to provide pathologic material to determine the histologic type and grade of bladder tumor
2. to determine the presence, depth, and type of tumor invasion (broad front or tentacular); such information is critical because tumor stage, grade, extent, and pattern of tumor growth direct additional therapy, determine the frequency of follow-up examinations and influence prognosis
3. to remove all visible and microscopic superficial and invasive tumor(s).

This chapter discusses the surgical technique, staging accuracy, and therapeutic efficacy of transurethral resection of bladder tumors.

## SURGICAL TECHNIQUE

A TUR coupled with bimanual examination is best performed under general anesthesia. Anesthesia is induced with propathol (sedative) and fentanyl (narcotic) and maintained during the procedure using inhalational sevofluorane delivered through a laryngeal mask airway (LMA). The LMA is used for both spontaneous and controlled ventilation, and avoids the trauma and discomfort of endotracheal intubation. Such anesthesia is rapid, provides excellent general relaxation for procedures lasting up to an hour, and permits full recovery within 30 minutes.

When fully relaxed, the patient is placed in a low lithotomy position using adjustable stirrups. A bimanual examination is performed both before and after resection. A 24 Fr. resectoscope sheath is introduced into the bladder using the visual obturator, facilitated by a video camera. Urine is collected for cytology. An Iglesias resectoscope is inserted with the video camera attached to a 30° lens. All regions of the bladder are easily visualized using this one lens. Changing the angle of the scope and position of the table facilitates resection. Glycine 1.5% (3000 cc bag) serves as irrigation. A pure monopolar point electrocautery current is used. The cutting current is set at 120 watts and the coagulation current at 60 watts. An Ellik evacuator filled with sterile water retrieves bladder and tumor specimens. The entire procedure is visually performed on a magnified screen using the video camera. Resection of tumors is best performed with the bladder half full.

Box 27.1 illustrates the information desired from a TUR of bladder tumor. Tumors involving the bladder, bladder neck, urethra and prostate should be noted as to their individual characteristics. All visible tumors are systematically resected and submitted separately for histology. It is helpful to record the type, size and location of each tumor on a bladder map, including areas of carcinoma in situ (CIS). At the end of the

**Box 27.1** Transurethral resection of bladder tumor

1. Clinical data
   - Evaluation under anesthesia
     a. Mass versus no mass
     b. Mobile versus nonmobile
   - Tumor
     a. Configuration (papillary versus solid)
     b. Location in bladder
     c. Number of tumors
     d. Size of tumor(s)
     e. Carcinoma in situ (focal versus diffuse)
     f. Bladder neck/urethra
   - Resection
     a. Complete versus incomplete

2. Pathological data
   - Tumor grade (low versus high)
   - Invasion
     a. Depth
     b. Muscle in specimen
     c. Type (broad front versus tentacular)
     d. Carcinoma in situ (focal versus diffuse)
   - Resection of bladder neck/prostate
     a. Urethra/ducts
     b. Stroma

3. Clinical (T) stage

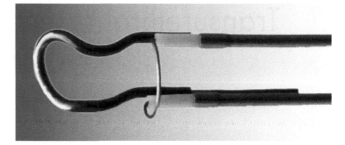

**Fig. 27.1**
Resectoscope loop.

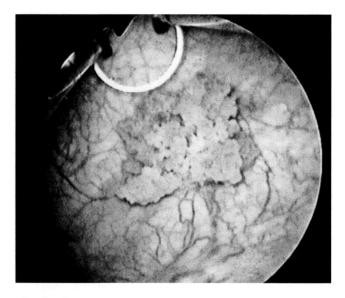

**Fig. 27.2**
Transurethral resection of a papillary tumor.

procedure, the urologist should state whether the TUR is complete or incomplete. The urologist (not the pathologist) is responsible for assigning a primary tumor stage based on assessment of the tumor during cystoscopy and resection coupled with the pathologic findings.

At the initial evaluation, a complete resection of all gross and suspected tumor(s) is attempted, including all areas involved with CIS. This may take more than one procedure, but with due diligence and patience, it is rare that a bladder cannot be cleared of all visible tumors. The bladder neck and prostate are biopsied to detect tumor spread within the bladder neck musculature, prostatic urethra, ducts, and stroma. Biopsies at 4- and 8-o'clock are obtained, extending from the bladder neck to the verumontanum. Selected site loop or cold-cup biopsies of suspicious mucosal lesions are performed,[3] but random biopsies of normal-appearing mucosa rarely show tumor, and urine cytology is more accurate in detecting diffuse mucosal abnormalities. A variety of resectoscope loops are available, but finer diameter loops project a more concentrated current and cut more easily. Figure 27.1 illustrates the loop preferred by the author. The attached 'runner' projecting in front of the right-angled loop allows resection of tumors on a flat surface, even in concave regions of the bladder, reduces cautery artifact, and helps to control a uniform and safe depth of resection.[4] The loop has a cross-width of 8 mm, permitting most tumors 1.0–1.5 cm in size to be resected completely as one specimen (Figure 27.2). Others have also developed innovative methods for en bloc removal of bladder tumors using flat loop, knife, or needle electrodes.[5–7]

Each tumor should be resected completely, if possible, and delivered to pathology as one contiguous specimen oriented so that a longitudinal histologic section through the tumor shows intact overlying and surrounding mucosa, and underlying lamina propria and deep muscle. Figure 27.2 shows the position of the loop prepared to resect a 1.5 cm papillary tumor toward the operator, removing the tumor as one specimen with a single broad sweep of the loop. Larger tumors are resected in multiple pieces, progressing in an orderly fashion from one side of the tumor to the other, until the entire base is reached and excised. The muscle fibers of the detrusor should be readily distinguished from the granular appearance of tumor. Figures 27.3 and 27.4, respectively, show complete resections of solid and papillary tumors. In each case, muscle deep to the tumor bed appears normal, indicating a complete visible resection. In cases of multiple, low-grade papillary tumors, it is not necessary to obtain muscle in each individual specimen if contiguous normal-appearing lamina propria beneath the tumor is provided. For bulky, invasive tumors likely to require cystectomy,

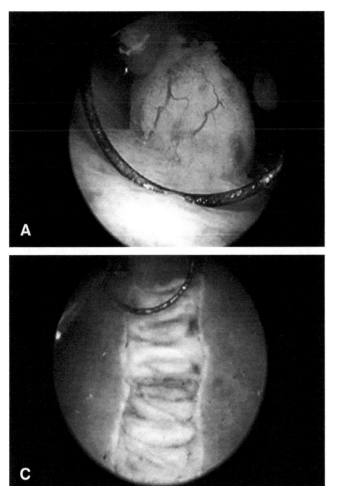

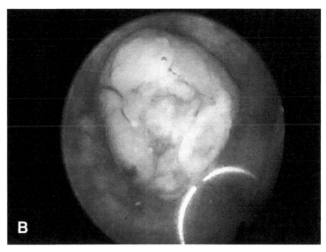

**Fig. 27.3**
Complete transurethral resection of a solid bladder tumor.

biopsies of the margin of the lesion containing muscle suffice. Biopsy of the central portion of such tumors may reveal only necrotic tissue and risks unnecessary bleeding that may prove difficult to control.

Tumors located in the dome or anterior wall can be difficult to reach and resect, especially if the prostate is enlarged. Placing the patient in Trendelenburg position, avoiding overdistension of the bladder, and applying gentle suprapubic pressure brings upper regions of the bladder into sharp focus and permits resection of anterior tumors on a flat surface. An extra long resectoscope sheath can also be used to resect difficult-to-reach tumors. An inferior lateral wall tumor can be difficult to resect because of the stimulated 'obturator nerve reflex' and the risk of bladder wall perforation. Reducing the cutting current and repeatedly tapping the cut peddle during resection of tumors from the lateral walls of the bladder greatly facilitates a controlled and complete resection of even deeply invasive tumors. Moving the entire sheath during resection (in a fashion similar to scooping ice cream with a spoon), rather than using the Iglesias working element, permits a more controlled, smoother, and better resection. Tumor and bladder wall specimens should be at least 1–2 cm in length or longer.

Retrograde resection is usually avoided because it may cause a perforation, but this method may be preferred to separate a papillary tumor from the mucosa if a narrow stalk is clearly visible rather than extending the loop behind a bulky tumor and resecting blindly in the usual manner with the spring-loaded working element. The ureteral orifice can be resected, if necessary, to completely remove a tumor overlying this structure.

In cases of multiple papillary tumors, the larger tumors are resected completely for histology, but smaller tumors (≤5 mm) and adjacent mucosa that may harbor CIS can be fulgurated using a roller ball electrode. An experienced urologist can usually distinguish low-grade papillary tumors from high-grade invasive tumors to permit fulguration of multiple, especially recurrent, tumors.[8] To ensure adequate visibility, bleeding is controlled at each resection site before moving on to another lesion. After all tumors have been resected, the margins and base of each tumor site are fulgurated using a roller ball electrode (see Figure 27.4).

Bladder tumors arising within a bladder diverticulum pose a unique diagnostic and therapeutic challenge. The paucity of muscle in a diverticulum renders TUR of

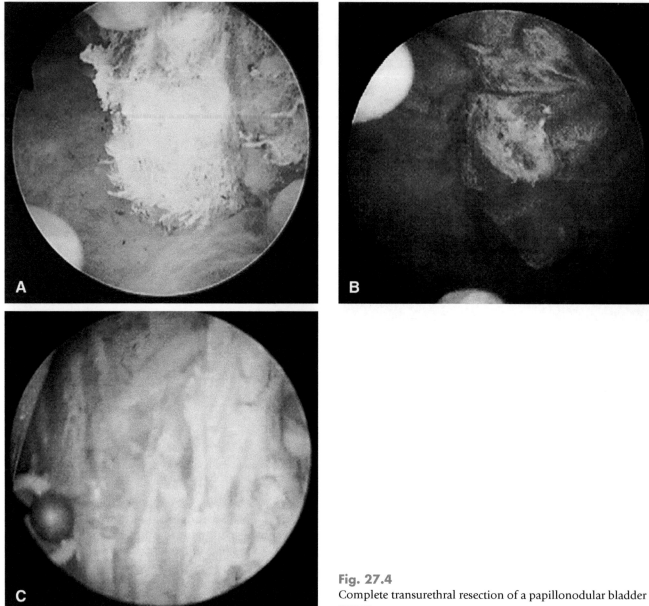

**Fig. 27.4**
Complete transurethral resection of a papillonodular bladder tumor.

diverticular tumors difficult, entailing an increased risk of incomplete resection and bladder perforation. Cystoscopic access and complete visualization of the entire diverticular mucosa is necessary to resect tumors safely and completely within a diverticulum. A narrow-mouthed ostium may be resected to gain access to a capacious diverticulum. A careful TUR of tumors confined to a diverticulum in 39 patients controlled 83% of non-invasive (Ta, Tis) or minimally invasive (T1) diverticular tumors. Our data support a conservative approach for superficial tumors confined to a bladder diverticulum, provided a complete trans-urethral resection is feasible.[9]

Sessile, nodular, and papillonodular tumors are more likely than papillary tumors to be high grade and invasive. In order to remove and accurately stage such tumors, they must be resected wide and deep. How wide

and how deep has practical implications for tumor staging and treatment, and requires considerable judgment, experience, and skill. For example, Figure 27.5 shows a sessile tumor resected at its peripheral margin A. The resection is then extended laterally into normal mucosa for 2 cm to margin B, to ensure complete wide excision of the lesion and to detect adjacent CIS. Figure 27.6 shows how different patterns of invasion of T1 tumors affect margins of resection. Tumor A has broad-front invasion and tumor B displays tentacular invasion. Resection of tumor A around its A margins results in complete resection of all exophytic and invasive components of the tumor. Resecting out to margin B verifies complete resection and may detect adjacent CIS. For tumor B, resection from margin A to A or margin B leaves tumor behind because of finger-like submucosal invasion extending laterally beyond the

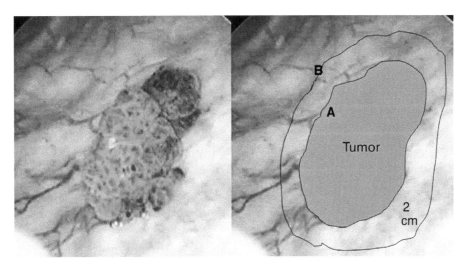

**Fig. 27.5**
Transurethral resection of bladder tumor: margins of resection.

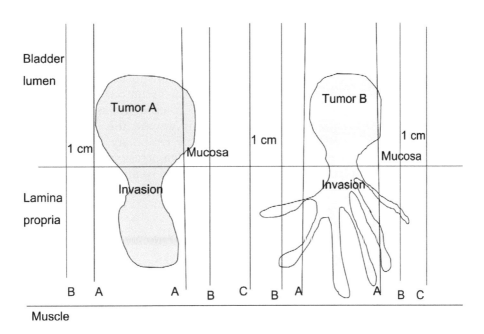

**Fig. 27.6**
Transurethral resection of T1 bladder tumors.

visible limits of the tumor. Complete resection of tumor B requires extending the resection another 1 or 2 cm out to margin C. Figure 27.7 shows a sagittal view of a tumor invading the deep lamina propria. The tumor is resected at margin A, to include much or all of the lamina propria with the tumor. Lateral resection out to margin B includes an ample portion of bladder muscle (that may not be included in the resection margins A to A) to verify complete tumor resection. Transurethral resection performed in this manner is more likely to remove the tumor completely and provides sufficient material to pathology to determine depth of invasion and centripetal extension of bladder tumor. Proof of this concept is illustrated by a study in which 35% of 462

TURs had residual tumor on extended deep resection of the tumor base and at least 2 cm lateral to visible tumor.[10] The extended TUR found incomplete initial resections of 13% of Ta, 36% of T1, 56% of T2, and 83% of T3 tumors.

In cases of muscle-invasive tumors considered for bladder-sparing, a maximum, aggressive transurethral resection is required and is an integral component of multimodality therapy of locally advanced tumors. Deep resection of the detrusor is commenced only after all exophytic tumor has been removed. Tumor deep in the bladder wall is resected one layer at a time, avoiding deep excavation in one place, to maintain a clear view of the whole resection area. Deep resection is considered

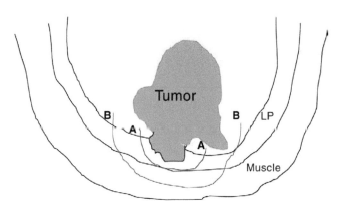

**Fig. 27.7**

Transurethral resection of invasive bladder tumor. (LP, lamina propria.)

complete when normal glistening yellow fat is seen between the deep muscle bundles or perivesical tissues. Invasive tumor is usually firm and easy to resect whereas uninvolved 'normal' fat is difficult to cut or cauterize with the resectoscope. This is a useful finding indicating a complete tumor resection when corroborated by negative histologic examination of separate deep muscle specimens.

At the end of the procedure, a belladonna and opium (B&O) rectal suppository is inserted (may be repeated in 4–6 hours as needed) to reduce bladder spasms. Intravenous diazepam (2.5 mg) also relaxes the bladder and helps to stem bleeding caused by bladder spasms. Intravenous fentanyl (25 mcg) effectively controls postoperative discomfort. Rarely, continuous bladder irrigation through a three-way catheter is necessary to control postoperative hemorrhage. The patient may be safely discharged with or without a Foley catheter (depending on the extent of resection) an hour or two after the operation. In cases of an enlarged prostate, or after vigorous resection of tumor, especially around the bladder neck or prostatic urethra, it is best to leave a catheter overnight to prevent delayed acute urinary retention owing to edema or blood clots.

## COMPLICATIONS OF TUR OF BLADDER TUMORS

Transurethral resection of bladder tumors is associated with a low (5%) overall complication rate.[11] The frequency of complications is higher with large (>5 cm) tumors, multiple tumors, and tumors located in the dome of the bladder. The most common complication, occurring in 1% to 3% of cases, is postresection bleeding, requiring return to the operating room to evacuate retained blood clots and fulgurate bleeders. On occasion, although the urine is crystal clear at the end of

the procedure, bleeding may erupt in the recovery room if the patient coughs or suffers postanesthetic rigors. Vigilant nursing care to maintain a patent catheter (and a collapsed bladder) by gentle bladder irrigation may avert this problem. It is also not uncommon for patients to report passing blood clots and pieces of tissue 7–10 days after the procedure when necrotic tissue sloughs from resection sites. Such blood clots usually pass spontaneously and do not require intervention.

The second most serious complication, occurring in 1% of cases of TUR of bladder tumors, is bladder perforation. The majority (80%) are extraperitoneal perforations (managed with catheter drainage); in 20% of cases they are intraperitoneal (requiring open surgical repair if gaping and associated with significant extravasation of fluid and urine despite bladder drainage). Although tumor seeding is of concern when the bladder is perforated, documented cases of extravesical pelvic disease after resection of invasive tumors have not been reported. TUR of invasive tumors does not appear to disseminate urothelial cells in the peripheral circulation.[12] Clinically silent extravasation probably occurs during many procedures.

Ureteral obstruction owing to resection of a ureteral orifice may occur, but it is unlikely if only the cutting current is used across the orifice. Cautery is used sparingly around the orifices. Obstruction usually is caused by temporary edema and will resolve without stenting. On occasion, a scarred ureteral orifice requires operative intervention to relieve hydronephrosis.

## STAGING ACCURACY AND RESTAGING TUR

Incomplete resection and understaging of bladder tumors is well known owing to the stochastic nature of transurethral resection. Tumors recur at the same site of resection in 20% to 40% of cases and they may progress to invade the muscle layers of the bladder.[13,14] Among patients undergoing cystectomy for nonmuscle-invasive bladder cancer, 25% to 40% are upstaged to muscle invasion,[15] and about half of muscle-invasive tumors are found to have tumor spread outside the bladder or positive pelvic lymph nodes.[16] Accuracy in determining pathologic stage is largely related to the completeness of TUR.

Although most urologists agree that ideally initial TUR of bladder tumors should be thorough and complete, many factors confound the adequacy of resection, including multiplicity and extent of disease, capability and perseverance of the resectionist, quality of specimens provided, and pathologic analysis. The fact that local tumor control and accurate tumor staging depend on a complete TUR suggests that a second, restaging TUR may be of value in evaluating patients with bladder tumors. Another TUR reduces the uncertainty of depth of tumor invasion, better controls the primary tumor, and provides additional pathologic information that may help select appropriate treatment.[17]

Table 27.1 shows results of a second TUR performed 2–6 weeks after an initial TUR in 150 consecutive patients evaluated with localized bladder tumor.[18] A significant proportion (76%) was found on a second TUR to have residual tumor. Of 96 patients with superficial (stage Ta, Tis, T1) tumors, only 25% had no tumor left; 31% had residual non-invasive tumor; 15% had persistent submucosal invasion; and 29% were upstaged to muscle invasion. An incomplete initial resection (and clinical understaging) was observed in 49% of stage T1 tumors with no muscle submitted in the first TUR specimen compared to 14% when muscle was identified. Of 54 patients with muscle-invasive tumors (confirmed by review of initial pathology), 22% had no residual tumor found on a restaging TUR, leading to changes in treatment.

A recent pathology review found that muscularis propria was missing in up to 51% of TUR specimens submitted by urologists.[19] Many of these were papillary low-grade tumors and the absence of muscle can be justified, but in 26% of invasive tumors, a muscle specimen was not submitted. Proper execution of TUR is critical for primary tumor staging and definitive treatment. The pathologist can only evaluate what the urologist submits!

Table 27.2[18-26] shows recently reported series of repeat TUR of stage T1 bladder tumors. Residual invasive T1 tumor was present in 15% to 53% of cases, and another 4% to 29% were upstaged to muscle invasion. The collective data suggest that a restaging TUR improves staging, but can it improve local control of T1 bladder tumors? We addressed this question in a recent cohort of 71 patients with T1 bladder tumors that underwent immediate cystectomy after we performed two sequential resections (same surgeon for both TURs) inclusive of muscle in the specimen.[27] Thirteen percent of the patients had muscle-invasive tumor in the cystectomy specimen, 24% had residual T1 tumor, and the others had either no or non-invasive tumors. All but two of these tumors were correctly identified and staged by the restaging TUR. We concluded from this small study that a restaging TUR of our own previously resected patients markedly improves both staging accuracy and local control of T1 bladder tumors.

**Table 27.1** Comparison of bladder tumor stage after first and second transurethral resections

| Stage at first TUR | No. pts | No. stage at second TUR (%) | | | | |
|---|---|---|---|---|---|---|
| | | T0 | Ta/Tis | T1 | T2 | T3–4 |
| Tis | 20 | 6 (30) | 8 (40) | 4 (20) | 2 (10) | |
| Ta | 18 | 5 (28) | 7 (39) | 5 (28) | 1 (5) | |
| T1 | 58 | 13 (22) | 15 (26) | 14 (24) | 16 (28) | |
| Muscle | 35 | 9 (26) | 11 (31) | 10 (29) | 5 (14) | |
| No muscle | 23 | 4 (17) | 4 (17) | 4 (17) | 11 (49) | |
| T2 | 54 | 12 (22) | 7 (13) | 3 (6) | 30 (55) | 2 (4) |
| Totals | 150 | | | 114 (76) | | |

**Table 27.2** Bladder tumor stage after second transurethral resection of T1 tumors

| Series | Year | No. pts | Stage at second TUR (%) | | | |
|---|---|---|---|---|---|---|
| | | | T0 | Ta/Tis | T1 | T2 |
| Klan et al[20] | 1991 | 46 | | 15 | 26 | 2 |
| Herr[18] | 1999 | 58 | 22 | 26 | 24 | 28 |
| Schwaibold et al[21] | 2000 | 60 | | 17 | 24 | 5 |
| Brauers et al[22] | 2001 | 42 | 35 | 17 | 24 | 24 |
| Ozen et al[23] | 2001 | 28 | | 18 | 53 | 29 |
| Schips et al[24] | 2002 | 76 | 67 | 11 | 15 | 8 |
| Rigaud et al[25] | 2002 | 52 | | 16 | 17 | 4 |
| Grimm et al[26] | 2003 | 19 | | 37 | 43 | 19 |

## CAN A SECOND TUR IMPROVE THE OUTCOME OF PATIENTS WITH SUPERFICIAL BLADDER CANCER?

A recent long-term observational study[26] showed that among a cohort of 124 consecutive patients, a restaging TUR found residual tumor in 33% of cases, including 27% of those with Ta and 53% of those with T1 disease. Residual tumor was found at the original resection site in 81% of cases. After 5 years follow-up, 63% of the patients undergoing a second TUR had disease-free bladders compared to 40% after one TUR. Progression to muscle invasion was observed in only two (3%) patients undergoing a restaging TUR. A second therapeutic TUR also appears to improve the short-term response to bacillus Calmette–Guérin (BCG) therapy.[28] Of 250 consecutive cases of nonmuscle-invasive bladder tumors treated with BCG (with or without maintenance BCG), 96 had one initial TUR before BCG and 154 had two TURs 2–6 weeks apart before starting BCG therapy. Table 27.3 shows that response rates were better after two TURs, and responses improved over time. Further, tumor progression to muscle invasion was more common in patients having only one TUR before BCG therapy. A second TUR appears to provide better local control of superficial bladder tumors and, by reducing tumor volume, contributes to earlier and more complete responses to intravesical therapy against minimal residual disease.

## TUR OF SUPERFICIAL BLADDER TUMORS

Although a thorough TUR is capable of ablating all visible nonmuscle-invasive tumors, subsequent tumor recurrence is common. Many studies show that the presence of tumor within 3 or 6 months after initial TUR is a significant predictor of tumor recurrence and progression, suggesting that an inadequate first resection is partly to blame for the high recurrence rate.[29,30] The 5- and 10-year recurrence rates after TUR exceed 70% and 85%, respectively. The 10-year survival rate after TUR for Ta tumors is 85% and is 70% for T1 tumors. These data argue persuasively for a restaging TUR, especially in high-risk tumors, for which TUR

(with and without intravesical therapy) to preserve the bladder is the mainstay of treatment.

A review of the literature reporting more than 600 cases of T1 bladder tumors treated only by TUR shows that 75% to 90% recurred during follow-up of 5–10 years. In a third of patients disease progressed to muscle invasion in 5 years, and in 39% to 53% it had progressed by 10 years.[31] T1 tumors most likely to be cured by TUR are solitary low-grade papillary T1 tumors, superficially invading the lamina propria (stage T1a) and unassociated with diffuse CIS. Such tumors represent only 10% of all T1 bladder tumors. Tumor recurrence and increased risk of tumor progression are significantly associated with high-grade, multiple, solid T1 tumors displaying vascular invasion, surrounding CIS, and invading the deep portion of the lamina propria (T1b).

Whether subdividing T1 tumors according to depth of invasion, above (T1a) or below (T1b), the muscularis mucosa truly distinguishes different outcomes of T1 tumors is problematic owing to a discontinuous muscularis mucosa layer within the bladder wall and the difficulty pathologists face in evaluating tumor invasion in multiple fragmented pieces of tissue.[32] Most studies are based only on single TURs.[33] Common problems in T1 staging evaluation include tangential sectioning, due to an inability to orient the specimens, crush and cautery artifacts, and a streaking inflammatory infiltrate. All of these inherent pathologic difficulties can be largely eliminated if the urologist resects and submits suspected T1 tumors in a single specimen containing contiguous deep muscle. In one study,[34] substaging T1 tumors did not affect response to BCG therapy in regard to recurrence or progression, suggesting that completeness of the TUR was more important than distinguishing histologic subtypes of T1 tumor.

## RADICAL TUR OF INVASIVE BLADDER CANCER

A radical TUR may cure some muscle-invasive bladder cancers. Evidence for this is two-fold. From the early 1950s until 1977, before the widespread use of radical cystectomy, several series reported 5-year survival rates of 40% to 60% following TUR alone for stage T2

**Table 27.3** Recurrent bladder tumors after one versus two TURs and BCG therapy

| TUR | No. cases | No. recurrent tumor present at | | | |
| | | 3 months | 6 months | 12 months | Progression |
|---|---|---|---|---|---|
| Initial TUR | 96 | 57 (59%) | 58 (60%) | 57 (59%) | 31 (32%) |
| Repeat TUR | 154 | 45 (29%) | 34 (22%) | 25 (16%) | 11 (7%) |

All differences are p=0.000 by Pearson's chi-square and Fisher's exact test.

bladder tumors.[35-38] About 10% to 15% of patients having cystectomy for stage T2 bladder tumors will have no tumor (P0) found within the cystectomy specimen, indicating that the initial 'diagnostic' TUR had completely removed the invasive cancer.[29]

Several recent prospective studies confirm these results. In the first study,[39] of 432 evaluated patients with locally advanced bladder cancer, 99 (23%) were treated by definitive TUR if a restaging TUR of the primary tumor site showed no residual muscle invasion. The 10-year disease-specific survival was 76% (57% with bladder preserved). Of the 99 patients treated by TUR, 82% of 73 that had no tumor on restaging TUR survived, versus 57% of 26 that had residual T1 tumor on restaging TUR. Of the 34 patients (34%) that had recurrence in the bladder with a new invasive cancer, 18 (53%) were successfully treated by salvage cystectomy, and 16 patients (16%) died of disease. In a second study,[40] 133 patients with invasive bladder cancer were treated by radical TUR if they had negative biopsies of the periphery and muscle layer of the tumor bed. At 5 and 10 years follow-up, the cause-specific survival rates were 80% and 75%, respectively. Both of these mature prospective studies justify radical TUR as a successful bladder-sparing therapeutic strategy in selected patients that have their primary muscle-invasive cancers completely and verifiably removed by negative re-resection biopsies of the primary tumor site.

Muscle-invasive bladder neoplasms successfully treated by radical TUR are usually solitary papillary tumors, <5 cm in size, that invade only the superficial layer of muscularis propria (stage T2a). A TUR may be curative only if the margins and base of the tumor site show no residual disease. Radical TUR cures only 20% or fewer bladder tumors that invade the deep muscle (stage T2b) or perivesical fat (stage T3a).

A radical TUR is also the essential first step in any combined modality strategy designed to spare the bladder.[41-45] Debulking the primary tumor, and indeed a visibly complete TUR, is required to select patients with invasive cancers for bladder preservation. In all such cases, biopsies of the tumor base, periphery of the tumor, and adjacent mucosa should verify a microscopically complete (R0) resection. Complete TUR of invasive bladder cancer is the most significant predictor of local control and survival after combined modality therapy. Response to chemotherapy, radiation, bladder preservation, and survival is improved after a maximum TUR. In one study, patients that had a radical TUR (R0) before chemotherapy and radiation had a 69% survival rate at 10 years, with 85% preserving their bladders, compared with only a 40% survival rate with incomplete tumor resection.[46] Cure and survival rates after conservative therapy decline substantially when the primary invasive tumor is incompletely resected.

A TUR also determines the response to induction chemotherapy. Neoadjuvant chemotherapy induces significant responses of invasive bladder cancer. A recently published randomized study showed that compared to radical cystectomy alone, neoadjuvant chemotherapy increases the likelihood of eliminating residual cancer in the cystectomy specimen and improved survival among patients with locally advanced bladder cancer.[47] Significantly more patients in the combination-therapy group had no residual disease (38%) than patients in the cystectomy group (15%). At 5 years, 85% of the patients with a pT0 surgical specimen were alive. This suggests that clinically 'complete responders' that have no tumor (P0) on a postchemotherapy TUR may be candidates for bladder preservation. Such approaches depend entirely on the accuracy of repeat TUR staging.[48] After chemotherapy, the tumor site often shows only a scar. This scar must be re-resected wide and deep in a determined effort to detect residual tumor. Successful bladder preservation requires an initial, visibly complete TUR of invasive tumor, response to chemotherapy, and a skillful re-resection of the primary tumor site.

We evaluated the 10-year outcome of patients with invasive (T2–3N0M0) bladder cancer that responded completely to neoadjuvant chemotherapy followed by bladder-sparing surgery.[49] All patients had residual muscle invasion on a restaging TUR. Of 111 surgical candidates, 60 (54%) achieved a complete clinical response (T0) on postchemotherapy TUR of the primary tumor site. Of 43 patients that elected treatment by chemotherapy plus TUR alone, 32 (74%) survived from 8 to 13 years, including 25 (58%) with an intact functioning bladder. Thirteen patients required salvage cystectomy. A similar study in 87 patients reported that 40 (51%) were T0 on TUR after neoadjuvant chemotherapy.[50] Thirty patients (71%) that had chemotherapy and TUR alone were alive after median follow-up of 54+ months, and 24 (57%) maintained an intact bladder. These two studies suggest that the majority of patients with invasive bladder cancer that achieve T0 status after neoadjuvant chemotherapy may preserve their bladders. Selection of such patients requires an aggressive, radical, postchemotherapy TUR of the primary tumor site to document absence of residual bladder cancer. The retained bladder remains at risk for new tumors, mandating frequent cystoscopies and repeated TURs to detect any sign of recurrent disease.

## CONCLUSION

Transurethral resection of bladder tumor is both diagnostic and therapeutic for nonmuscle-invasive bladder tumors. A restaging TUR improves staging accuracy and improves local control of superficial and minimally invasive bladder tumors. A restaging TUR is recommended for all T1 tumors, multiple high-grade Ta tumors, and in all cases in which an initial TUR fails to clear the bladder of visible tumor. It is not necessary for TaG1 tumors. A radical TUR is curative for some patients with minimal muscle-invasive cancers if a verifiably complete resection is performed, and is an essential component of multimodality bladder-sparing strategies. Such cases usually require a restaging TUR.

Although TUR of bladder tumors is an essential procedure familiar to most urologists, it is difficult to perform well and may not achieve its desired goals. Although treatment outcome is often determined by tumor biology, a complete TUR identifies characteristics and extent of bladder tumors, providing the best method currently available to define individual tumor biology. In the present era of molecular medicine, high tech imaging, better drugs, and advanced surgical techniques, TUR has become a 'lost art'. However, a properly performed and aggressive TUR is one of the most successful and powerful procedures available to the urologist if it is appropriately applied with full knowledge of its inherent limitations. The TUR alone is the most important diagnostic, staging, and treatment modality for the vast majority of bladder tumors. Its success or failure, as well as that of subsequent treatments of non-invasive and invasive tumors localized to the bladder, are directly dependent on the information provided by a well-executed transurethral resection providing quality tumor specimens to permit accurate pathologic evaluation.

## REFERENCES

1. Jemal A, Tiwari RC, Murray T, et al. Cancer statistics, 2004. CA Cancer J Clin 2004;54(1):8–29.

2. Schrag D, Rabbani F, Herr HW, et al. Adherence to surveillance among patients with superficial bladder cancer. J Natl Cancer Inst 2003;95:588–597.

3. May F, Treibor U, Hartung R, et al. Significance of random bladder biopsies in superficial bladder cancer. Eur Urol 2003;44:47–50.

4. Herr HW, Reuter VE. Evaluation of new resectoscope loop for transurethral resection of bladder tumors. J Urol 1998;159:2067.

5. Ukai R, Kawashita E, Ikeda H. A new technique for transurethral resection of superficial bladder tumor in 1 piece. J Urol 2000;163:878–879.

6. Lodde M, Lusuardi L, Palermo S, et al. En bloc transurethral resection of bladder tumors: use and limits. Urology 2003;62:1089–1091.

7. Saito S. Transurethral en bloc resection of bladder tumors. J Urol 2001;166:2148–2150.

8. Herr HW, Donat SM, Dalbagni G. Correlation of cystoscopy with histology of papillary bladder tumors. J Urol 2002;168:978–980.

9. Golijanin D, Yossepowitch O, Beck S, et al. Carcinoma in a bladder diverticulum: presentation and treatment outcome. J Urol 2003;170:1761–1764.

10. Kolozsy Z. Histopathological 'self-control' in TUR of bladder tumors. Br J Urol 1991;67:162–164.

11. Collado A, Chechile GE, Salvador J, et al. Early complications of endoscopic treatment for bladder tumors. J Urol 2000;164:1529–1532.

12. Desgrandchamps F, Teren M, Dal Cortivo L, et al. The effects of transurethral resection on dissemination of epithelial cells in the circulation of patients with bladder cancer. Br J Cancer 1999;81:832–834.

13. Wolf H. Transurethral surgery in the treatment of invasive bladder cancer (stage T1 and T2). Scand J Urol Nephrol 1982;104:127–132.

14. Herr HW, Badalament RA. Superficial bladder cancer treated with BCG: a multivariate analysis of factors affecting tumor progression. J Urol 1989;141:22–29.

15. Dutta SC, Smith JA, Cookson MS, et al. Clinical understaging of high risk nonmuscle invasive urothelial carcinoma treated with radical cystectomy. J Urol 2001;166:490–493.

16. Dalbagni G, Genega E, Herr HW. Cystectomy for bladder cancer: a contemporary series. J Urol 2001;165:1111–1115.

17. Herr HW. Uncertainty and outcome of invasive bladder tumors. Urol Oncol 1996;2:92–94.

18. Herr HW. The value of a second transurethral resection in evaluating patients with bladder tumors. J Urol 1999;162:74–76.

19. Maruniak NA, Takezawa K, Murphy WM. Accurate pathological staging of urothelial neoplasms requires better cystoscopic sampling. J Urol 2002;167:2404–2407.

20. Klan R, Lou V, Huland H. Residual tumor discovered in routine second transurethral resection in patients with stage T1 transitional cell carcinoma of the bladder. J Urol 1991;146:316–318.

21. Schwaibold H, Treibor U, Kubler H, et al. Significance of second TUR for T1 bladder cancer. Eur Urol 2000;37:101–104.

22. Brauers A, Buettner R, Jakse G. Second resection and prognosis of high risk superficial bladder cancer: is cystectomy often too early? J Urol 2001;165:808–810.

23. Ozen H, Ekici S, Uygur MC, et al. Repeated transurethral resection and intravesical BCG for extensive superficial bladder tumors. J Endourol 2001;15:863–867.

24. Schips L, Augustin H, Zigeuner RE, et al. Is repeated transurethral resection justified in patients with newly diagnosed superficial bladder cancer. Urology 2002;59:220–223.

25. Rigaud J, Karam G, Braud G, et al. Value of second endoscopic resection in stage T1 bladder tumor. Prog Urol 2002;12:27–30.

26. Grimm M-C, Ackermann R, Vogeli TA. Effect of routine repeat transurethral resection for superficial bladder cancer: a long-term observational study. J Urol 2003;170:433–437.

27. Dalbagni G, Herr HW, Reuter VE. Impact of a second transurethral resection on staging of T1 bladder cancer. Urology 2002;60:822–825.

28. Herr HW. Tumor recurrence and progression after one versus two transurethral resections and BCG therapy (unpublished data).

29. Lee SE, Jeong IG, Ku H, et al. Impact of transurethral resection of bladder tumor: analysis of cystectomy specimens to evaluate for residual tumor. Urology 2004;63:873–877.

30. Holmang S, Johansson SL. Stage TA–T1 bladder cancer: the relationship between findings at first followup cystoscopy and subsequent recurrence and progression. J Urol 2002;167:1634–1637.

31. Herr HW. High-risk superficial bladder cancer: transurethral resection alone in selected patients with T1 tumor. Semin Urol Oncol 1997;15:142–147.

32. Lopez-Betran A, Cheng L. Stage pT1 bladder carcinoma: diagnostic criteria, pitfalls and prognostic significance. Pathology 2003;35:484–491.

33. Cheng L, Weaver AL, Neumann RM, et al. Substaging of T1 bladder carcinoma based on depth of invasion as measured by micrometer: a new proposal. Cancer 1999;86:1035–1043.

34. Kondylis FI, Demirci S, Schellhammer PF. Outcomes after intravesical BCG are affected by substaging high grade T1 transitional cell carcinoma. J Urol 2000;163:1120–1123.

35. Flocks RH. Treatment of patients with carcinoma of the bladder. JAMA 1951;145:295–299.

36. Milner WA. The role of conservative surgery in the treatment of bladder tumors. Br J Urol 1954;26:375–377.

37. O'Flynn JD, Smith JD, Hanson JS. Transurethral resection for the assessment and treatment of vesical neoplasms. A review of 800 consecutive cases. Eur Urol 1975;1:38–41.

38. Barnes RW, Dick AL, Hadley HL. Survival following transurethral resection of bladder carcinoma. Cancer Res 1977;37:2895–2898.

39. Herr HW. Transurethral resection of muscle-invasive bladder cancer: 10-year outcome. J Clin Oncol 2001;19:89–93.

40. Solsona E, Iborra I, Ricos JV, et al. Feasibility of transurethral resection for muscle infiltrating carcinoma of the bladder: long-term followup of a prospective study. J Urol 1998;159:95–98.

41. Shipley WU, Prout GR, Kaufman D, et al. Invasive bladder carcinoma: the importance of initial transurethral surgery for improved survival with irradiation. Cancer 1987;60:514–519.

42. Kaufman DS, Shipley WU, Griffin PP, et al. Selective bladder preservation by combination treatment of invasive bladder cancer. N Engl J Med 1993;329:1377–1381.

43. Kachnic LA, Kaufman DS, Griffin PP, et al. Bladder preservation by combined modality therapy for invasive bladder cancer. J Clin Oncol 1997;15:1022–1025.

44. Zietman AL, Shipley WU, Kaufman DS, et al. A phase I/II trial of transurethral surgery combined with concurrent cisplatin, 5-fluorouracil and twice daily radiation followed by selective bladder preservation in operable patients with muscle invading bladder cancer. J Urol 1998;160:1673–1677.

45. Michaelson MD, Shipley WU, Heney NM, et al. Selective bladder preservation for muscle-invasive transitional cell carcinoma of the urinary bladder. Br J Cancer 2004;90:578–581.

46. Rodel C, Grabenbauer GG, Kuhn R, et al. Combined-modality treatment and selective organ preservation in invasive bladder cancer: long-term results. J Clin Oncol 2002;20:3061–3071.

47. Grossman HB, Natale RB, Tangen CM, et al. Neoadjuvant chemotherapy plus cystectomy compared with cystectomy alone for locally advanced bladder cancer. N Engl J Med 2003;349:859–866.

48. Kuczk M, Machtens S, Jonas U. Surgical bladder preserving strategies in the treatment of muscle-invasive bladder cancer. World J Urol 2002;20:183–189.

49. Herr HW, Bajorin DF, Scher HI. Neoadjuvant chemotherapy and bladder-sparing surgery for invasive bladder cancer: ten-year outcome. J Clin Oncol 1998;16:1298–1301.

50. Sternberg CN, Pansadoro V, Calabro F, et al. Neo-adjuvant chemotherapy and bladder preservation in locally advanced transitional cell carcinoma of the bladder. Ann Oncol 1999;10:1269–1270.

# Laser ablation and other technology 28

*Jeffrey A Jones*

## INTRODUCTION

### LASER FUNDAMENTALS

LASER is an acronym standing for light amplification by stimulated emission of radiation. Lasers typically make use of electromagnetic energy sources from 150 to 10,000 nanometers ($1.5 \times 10^{-7}$ to $1.0 \times 10^{-3}$ meters) (Figure 28.1) for the radiation emission source.

## LASER DESIGN

There are three basic components of each laser: 1) pump source; 2) lasing material (such as diode, gem or crystal, and gases); and 3) optical reflectors and collimators (Figure 28.2). The pump source adds energy to the lasing system, which allows the amplification necessary to cause the atoms in the lasing material to be excited, thereby pushing electrons from a resting state. The pump source can be optical, electrical, or chemical in nature. The lasing material is a source of atoms whose

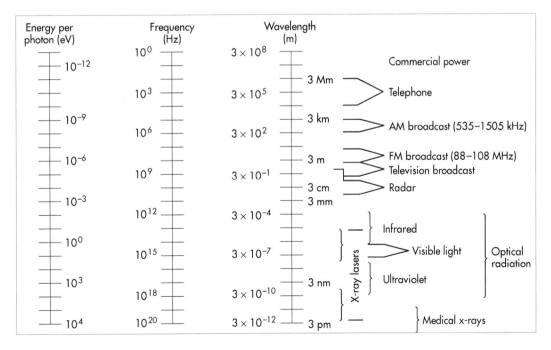

**Fig. 28.1**
Electromagnetic spectrum and relationship between energy, frequency, and wavelength.

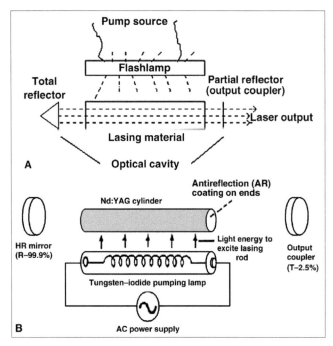

**Fig. 28.2**
A Diagram of generic laser working anatomy. B Specific components of a Nd:YAG laser.

electrons can be driven to different energy states. A typical lasing crystal is a ruby and typical lasing gases are carbon dioxide and helium/neon. The optical reflectors, consisting of totally and partially reflecting mirrors, allow a build up of emitted photons within a chamber containing the lasing material, called the lasing cavity.

## LASER PHYSICS

The smallest particle of light energy is described by quantum mechanics as a photon. The energy, E, of a photon is determined by its frequency, $v$, and Planck's constant, $h$: $E = h \bullet v$. The velocity of light in a vacuum, $c$, is 300 million meters per second. The wavelength, $\lambda$, of light is related to $v$ from the equation: $\lambda = c/v$. The difference in energy levels across which an excited electron drops determines the wavelength of the emitted light.

Electrons within the atomic component of the lasing material normally reside in a steady-state, lower energy level. When radiant energy is added, the majority of the electrons are excited to a higher energy level, a phenomenon called 'population inversion'. The electrons are unstable in this condition. They will only remain in this excited state for a brief period of time before they fall back to their original energy state, called decay. This decay occurs in one of two ways:

- spontaneous decay, i.e. the electrons simply fall to their ground state while emitting randomly directed photons

- stimulated decay, i.e. the photons from spontaneously decaying electrons encounter other excited electrons which induces them to fall to their ground state.

Lasing can be accomplished with media possessing two energy levels; however, most lasers in use today employ media with four or more energy levels, with the intermediate short-lived levels called metastable states. The metastable energy levels must allow the electrons to dwell long enough to produce a population inversion, usually micro- to milliseconds in duration.

## LIGHT AMPLIFICATION

The stimulated transmission will release photon energy that travels in phase at the same wavelength and in the same direction as the incident photon. If the direction is parallel to the optical axis, the emitted photons travel back and forth in the optical cavity through the lasing material between the totally reflecting mirror on one end of the laser cavity and the partially reflecting mirror on the other. (This is also known as an oscillating cavity or resonating chamber.) The light energy is amplified in this manner until sufficient energy is built up for a burst of laser light to be transmitted through the partially reflecting mirror. Thus the laser produces light energy that is monochromatic (one color) and coherent (in-phase). Preventing the release of light other than that directed parallel to the aperture in the partially reflecting mirror collimates the light as well, meaning that the emitted light has minimal divergence (see Figure 28.2).

The output of a laser may be a continuous, constant-amplitude output (known as c.w. or continuous wave), or pulsed (p.w. or pulsed wave) by using the techniques of Q-switching, mode-locking or gain-switching. A Q-switch is a very rapid shutter between the active medium and the partially reflective mirror (see Figure 28.2). A continuous wave laser has a pulse duration >0.25 second, while a pulsed laser has a pulse duration <0.25 second. Pulsing the laser output allows for energy peaks that are typically higher than with continuous wave.

## LASER ENERGY ACCUMULATION

A description of the concepts of laser energy characteristics is found under laser safety (see below), where these characteristics are used to classify lasers according to the risk for human injury. The parameters of energy accumulation and delivery are important in understanding the effects of lasers on tissue.

Tips can be applied to the ends of fiberoptic cables or other transfer instruments that allow concentration of energy density, and therefore more substantial 'cutting' effects on the tissue where the tip is placed in contact with the tissue.[1-3]

## ENERGY TRANSFER

The energy output of the laser can be through air, water, or a delivery system, such as fiberoptic cable to the surgical site. The laser energy, as it strikes the target tissue, is converted to heat.

The beam divergence exiting from the tip of a standard optical fiber is typically 10–15°. Thus, the farther away from the tip, the more the beam is defocused. Within a 1 inch (2.5 cm) working distance, laser intensity can change from making incisions, at the nearest, most concentrated spot size, to vaporizing tissue, when the beam is minimally defocused, to coagulating proteins when the beam is farther away still, and therefore more defocused.

The energy density is inversely proportional to the square of the radius of the spot size, according to the equation $ED=E/\pi r^2$. So, halving the spot size, while maintaining constant energy applied, increases the energy density by a factor of 4.[4]

## TISSUE ABSORPTION

The interaction of the laser with the tissue is affected by properties of the local tissue and, as mentioned above, the wavelength (and thus frequency) of laser used. Relevant tissue properties include its density, water content, opacity (e.g. degree of pigmentation), and blood supply: the greater the tissue density or opacity, the more absorption of laser energy, and thus the more intense the thermal effect.

The absorption of light energy by cellular constituents is dependent on the molecular properties of that component. Lipids absorb maximally at different wavelengths from proteins, which are different from pigments, etc. In fact, specific proteins may absorb light only in a specific range of wavelengths, and that range differs from other proteins; for example:

- Hemoglobin absorbs maximally at wavelengths from 500 to 600 nm, and is translucent to light beyond this range.
- Argon lasers emit 458–515 nm light and, therefore, it is heavily absorbed by hemoglobin.
- Water does not absorb light below 300 nm, and absorbs only small amounts from 300 to 2000 nm. Water does, however, absorb heavily between 2000 and 20,000 nm.
- $CO_2$ lasers emit in the far infrared spectrum, at 10,600 nm. Thus $CO_2$ laser energy is highly absorbed by tissue rich in water. As a result, $CO_2$ laser energy does not penetrate deeply into tissues.

The depth of penetration into tissues is significantly affected by the wavelength of laser light employed: the longer the wavelength, the deeper the expected penetration. Tissue composition and molecular absorption are among several factors that play into the laser end effect. The neodymium:yttrium–aluminum–garnet (Nd:YAG) laser, for example, produces light in the near infrared region (1060 nm) and penetrates to a depth of approximately 5–10 mm in most tissues (at its wavelength, Nd:YAG is not absorbed by hemoglobin or water in any significant quantity). The $CO_2$ laser with a wavelength of 10,600 nm (longer wavelength, thus should penetrate more deeply) only penetrates to a depth of <0.1 mm because its wavelength is very highly absorbed by tissue water. Ultimately, laser energy and tissue characteristics interact in a complex manner that determines the degree of absorption, penetration, reflection, and scattering of laser energy.

## OTHER FACTORS AFFECTING TISSUE ABSORPTION

The degree of laser energy absorption is also affected by local and regional blood circulation via two mechanisms:

1. Circulating blood draws heat away from the laser application site, thereby producing a 'heat sink' effect by carrying the absorbed thermal energy away from the site. Thus, by diverging its local thermal effects, a robust microcirculation to some degree counteracts laser power.
2. The ability of the individual blood components (e.g. hemoglobin and water) to absorb the laser energy, depending on the specific wavelength range of the incident energy. Blood is obviously different in its molecular composition from that of fibrous tissue, matrix, etc.

An important determinant of laser effects on tissue, and its subsequent application and safety of use, concerns scattering of the light energy.[5] As laser light strikes a tissue surface it can be: 1) reflected (back-scatter); 2) absorbed, or 3) transmitted with divergence (forward-scatter) (Figure 28.3). The fraction of extinction of the applied energy will be determined by the relative degree of each of the three possibilities. In addition to the wavelength of the laser light and the tissue composition, the amount of scatter is also dependent on the thermal effect of the laser energy on the tissue itself (Figure 28.4).

For the surgeon, a laser is a device that can produce the thermal effects of cutting, vaporizing, or coagulating tissue. Lasers utilize photons to accomplish this task, rather than the electrons that electrocautery uses. Lasers can also produce photochemical reactions, mechanical (shock wave) effects, and tissue-welding effects. Treating tumors will utilize only thermal or photochemical laser reactions. Mechanical effects—induced by high power densities producing cavitation 'plasma bubbles' at the surface and therefore mini-sonic booms—are used to break up urinary calculi. Tissue-welding effects are

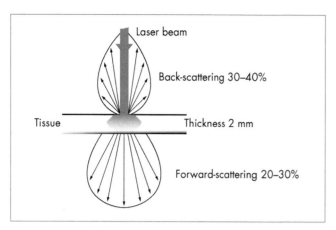

**Fig. 28.3**
Example of a laser light scatter profile for Nd:YAG.
Reproduced with permission from Hoffstetter & Frank.[5]

derived by collagen crosslinking added proteins (e.g. albumin, also known as tissue solder) to the tissue edges. The weld occurs due to the selected thermal effect of the specific laser wavelength on the selected protein. The resulting tensile strength of the welded tissue can exceed that of other reparative means.

The laser effects used for the therapy of neoplasia, i.e. thermal and photochemical effects are as follows:

- The *thermal effect* occurs when light energy is absorbed and converted into heat. As the temperature rises to 40–65°C, proteins are denatured. When the temperature reaches 70°C, arteries and veins show wall contraction as the chemical bonds in the collagen and elastin are altered. At temperatures of 100°C, the cell dehydrates. If the laser energy application continues, the temperature rapidly rises after all the water is evaporated, due to the loss of the heat sink characteristic of water with its high specific heat index. After the temperature reaches 250°C, carbonization ensues. Carbonized tissue can reflect

some of the applied laser energy, without immediate temperature elevation. If the energy application is intense and the temperature rise is rapid, vaporization occurs at a temperature of 300°C.[4] A summary of the thermal tissue alterations can be found in Figure 28.4.[5]

- The *photochemical effect* is discussed in the laser sensitizer section (see below).

Only the laser property of collimation is highly important for its surgical use. The wavelength/color is of minor significance in that mainly it will affect tissue-specific reactivity. Coherence is not especially important for clinical use, as the energy is often dephased during transmission through the waveguide, typically a fiberoptic cable.

Collimation is important because it allows precise delivery of energy to exact tissue locations, and allows transfer of high levels of energy to the selected tissue location.

The laser is a nonthermal energy source and, therefore, the local temperature levels at the point of application are far greater than its own. As per the law of the conservation of energy, the energy density (measure of energy per unit of area) of the laser beam increases as the spot size decreases.

## HISTORY OF LASER AND ITS USE

Albert Einstein originally described lasers as a theoretical concept in 1917, but it was not until 1954 that the first 'stimulated' emissions of radiation, in this case microwaves, were generated by J.P. Gordon and C.H. Townes at Bell Laboratories—a MASER. The invention of the LASER can be dated to 1958 with the publication of the scientific paper, *Infrared and Optical Masers*, by Arthur L. Schawlow, then a Bell Laboratories researcher, and Charles H. Townes, a consultant to Bell Laboratories. In

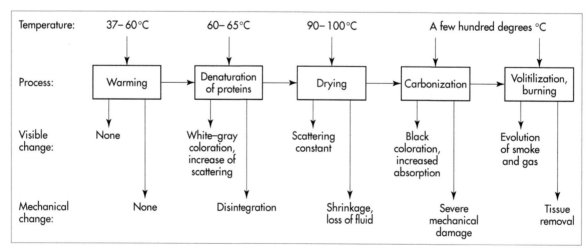

**Fig. 28.4**
Thermal effects of applied laser energy. Reproduced with permission from Hoffstetter & Frank.[5]

1960, Schawlow and Townes received a patent for the invention of the laser and subsequently the Nobel Prize.

The first working laser, using a synthesized ruby rod for the lasing media and generating 694 nm wavelength, red light, was built later that year by the American physicist Theodore Maiman at Hughes Aircraft Company. Shortly thereafter, in 1961, a helium-neon gas laser was produced by Javan, Bennet, and Herriot. In the same year, a 1060 nm (near-infrared) laser light was generated by stimulating glass rods doped with neodymium (Nd:glass laser) by Johnson and Nassan. Gordon devised the argon, krypton, and xenon gas lasers in 1964, while Patel produced the first working $CO_2$ laser in 1965.[6,7]

Interestingly, Townes and Schawlow were actually interested in the field of microwave spectroscopy and the characteristics of molecules, but neither had planned to invent the laser. What they sought was to develop a device to help them study molecular structures. Townes brought the idea of using stimulated emissions to amplify waves, while Schawlow generated the concept of using mirrors to reflect the light to create a pure frequency and highly directed beam.

## LASERS IN MEDICINE

The first medical application of a laser was in 1962 by Goldman who used a ruby laser for dermatologic treatment. He is generally regarded as the 'father of lasers' in surgery and medicine.[7] Campbell first applied a laser to weld together a detached retina, later the same year.

Application of lasers to surgery was almost immediately envisioned by the inventors because of several laser properties: 1) precise control of localized tissue destruction; 2) touch-free delivery of energy ensures sterility; and 3) conductance through fiberoptics could allow delivery via various types of flexible instruments and scopes.[6]

Two very important added components that allowed laser application for medical uses are:

- a switching mechanism that allows the laser to build energy to peak powers above continuous energy delivery, and thus achieve profound tissue effects (e.g. shock waves and cavitation)
- the adaptation of the output to a fiberoptic cable, which allows transmission of certain wavelength lasers through working ports in a variety of medical and surgical scopes and instruments, and allows for some diffusing of the laser beam as the light exits from the tip of the cable.[1,8-11]

## LASERS IN UROLOGY

The first reported application of laser energy in urology was in 1973 by Krylov and Kagan in Russia.[12] The first urologic use for lasers was reported in Western literature in 1976 by Hofstetter and colleagues at the University of Munich.[13] In this landmark publication, Hofstetter described multiple urologic applications for laser energy, including neoplastic disease of the lower urinary system. A summary of the progression of urologic applications of different laser energies can be found in reviews by Sacknoff.[14,15]

## LASERS IN BLADDER LESIONS/CANCER

Using lasers to treat bladder lesions was first described in 1976 by Hofstetter et al, and the first reported case series using Nd:YAG was in 1977, when 15 patients with papillary bladder tumors were successfully treated without complication.[13,16] In later reports, Hofstetter described the treatment of 302 patients with small- to medium-sized bladder tumors treated with Nd:YAG with or without transurethral resection of bladder tumor (TURBT) over a 3-year period. The tumors were stage Ta through T3a and the local recurrence rate was 9%.[5,17-24]

## EFFECTS OF LASERS ON TISSUE BY TYPE, SIDE EFFECTS, AND COMPLICATIONS

A complete listing of the wavelengths and crystals used in the various types of laser for medical application are shown in Table 28.1.[25]

Only lasers useful in the treatment of urothelial and meatal lesions are discussed in this chapter.

## CO2

### Lasing media
Gas tube containing carbon dioxide.

### Wavelength
Invisible region of the infrared spectrum at 10,600 nm, and therefore is usually coupled with a helium-neon targeting laser. It is an older laser and typically employs articulating arms with reflecting mirrors as the waveguide, with a hand unit that can focus/defocus the beam. Since the advent of laparoscopic surgery, wavetubes, which carry the beam through the working port, have been available. However, they cannot be used through water (e.g. via a cystoscope with irrigating fluid).

### Tissue effect
Due to high absorbance by water, minimal tissue penetration occurs, from 0.5 to 1.0 mm. Its main effect, depending on the tissue composition, is cutting, which is unlikely to produce scarring, as the largest

**Table 28.1** Lasing media and associated wavelengths for each type of laser

| Laser type | Media | Wavelengths | Nanometers |
|---|---|---|---|
| Excimer gas lasers | Argon fluoride | UV | 193 |
| | Krypton chloride | UV | 222 |
| | Krypton fluoride | UV | 248 |
| | Xenon chloride | UV | 308 |
| | Xenon fluoride | UV | 351 |
| Gas lasers | Nitrogen | UV | 337 |
| | Helium cadmium | UV | 325 |
| | Helium cadmium | Violet | 441 |
| | Argon | Blue | 488 |
| | Argon | Green | 514 |
| | Krypton | Blue | 476 |
| | Krypton | Green | 528 |
| | Krypton | Yellow | 568 |
| | Krypton | Red | 647 |
| | Xenon | White | Multiple |
| | Helium-neon | Green | 543 |
| | Helium-neon | Yellow | 594 |
| | Helium-neon | Orange | 612 |
| | Helium-neon | Red | 633 |
| | Helium-neon | NIR | 1152 |
| | Helium-neon | MIR | 3390 |
| | Hydrogen fluoride | MIR | 2700 |
| | Carbon monoxide | IR | 5000–6000 |
| | Carbon dioxide | FIR | 10,600 |
| Metal vapor lasers | Copper vapor | Green | 510 |
| | Copper vapor | Yellow | 570 |
| | Gold vapor | Red | 627 |
| | Doubled Nd:YAG | Green | 532 |
| | Neodymium:YAG | NIR | 1064 |
| | Erbium: glass | MIR | 1540 |
| | Erbium: YAG | MIR | 2940 |
| | Holmium: YLF | MIR | 2060 |
| | Holmium: YAG | MIR | 2100 |
| | Chromium sapphire (ruby) | Red | 694 |
| | Titanium sapphire | NIR | 840–1100 |
| | Alexandrite | NIR | 700–815 |
| Dye lasers | Rhodamine 6G | VIS | 570–650 |
| | Coumarin C30 | Green | 504 |
| Semiconductor lasers | Galium arsenide (GaAs) | NIR | 840 |
| | Galium aluminum arsenide | VIS/NIR | 670–830 |
| Laser diodes/solid state | Ruby | VIS (red) | 694.3 |
| | Laser diodes (visible) | VIS (red) to NIR | 630–950 |

FIR, far-infrared; IR, infrared; MIR, mid-infrared; NIR, near-infrared; UV, ultraviolet; VIS, visible light; YLF, yttrium lithium fluoride.
Reproduced with permission from Hoffstetter.[24]

vessel that can be coagulated with $CO_2$ lasers is 0.5 mm diameter.

## Complications

Using lasers on vessels that are too large to be coagulated can easily result in bleeding, especially when used during laparoscopy; also eye injuries can occur when the laser is used externally with the handpiece.

## NEODYMIUM (ND:YAG)

### Lasing media

Yttrium aluminum garnet ($Y_3Al_5O_{12}$ doped with neodymium ($Nd^{3+}$)).

## Wavelength

In the near infrared region (IR-A) at 1064 nm, it is transparent to the cornea and lens of the eye. It can be used in the continuous, pulsed, or Q-switched modes. It uses optical fiber for delivery to the patient, and the fibers can be small enough to pass through the working port of almost all endoscopes.

### Tissue effect

Since the wavelength is outside the peak absorption for both water and hemoglobin, Nd:YAG lasers penetrate most deeply into tissues, as much as 1 cm. It has good hemostatic properties, with the ability to coagulate vessels up to 0.5 cm in diameter.

At lower energy, especially with diffusion, the primary effect is tissue coagulation. At higher energy, especially with an undiffused beam, the primary effect is cutting, and—if used away from the tissue—vaporization, with coagulation effect at depth below. The cutting effect of the Nd:YAG is enhanced with the use of direct contact pointed tips made from sapphire or other gems.

## Complications

Penetration below target tissue and cutting or coagulation of unintended tissues. The largest risk in using the Nd:YAG in the bladder is adjacent organ injury, including bowel injury/perforation, especially if used for posterior wall lesions or tumors near the dome. Placing the patient in the Trendelenburg position may lower the risk of bowel energy, by dropping the bowel mostly below the bladder level.

## KTP-ND:YAG

### Lasing media
Nd:YAG passed through a potassium titanyl phosphate crystal.

### Wavelength
The Nd:YAG output frequency is doubled and therefore its wavelength is halved to 532 nm, in the visible, green range. Since this wavelength is heavily absorbed by hemoglobin, penetration is much less than YAG, limited to 3–4 mm. It is delivered via optical fiber, at sizes passing through all endoscopes. The characteristics of this laser wavelength are similar to the argon laser, which is also heavily absorbed by hemoglobin (80 times greater than Nd:YAG). When interacting with tissue surfaces, the argon and KTP have roughly equal, but minimal penetration via forward and back scatter.

### Tissue effect
Primarily cutting at lower energy; however, as energy and proximity are increased, it is also used for resection and ablation. KTP has a propensity to produce carbonization when held away from the tissue and continuously applied. It coagulates better than $CO_2$ but not as well as Nd:YAG.

### Complication
Incomplete ablation of lesion treated.

## HOLMIUM (HO:YAG)

### Lasing media
YAG crystal doped with holmium, a rare earth metal.

### Wavelength
In the mid-infrared (IR-B) region at 2150 nm.

### Tissue effect
For soft tissue, its penetration is limited to 1–2 mm, if the tissue is water saturated. If the pulsed frequency is kept low at a pulse duration of approximately 250 milliseconds, the holmium laser can induce hemostasis. At more rapid pulse frequencies, it tends to induce cutting. With the addition of increased power, the holmium laser has the added property of inducing a vaporization bubble at the tip of the delivery fiber. This vaporization bubble can be rapidly expanded with repeated pulses, leading to destabilization of surrounding molecules, a property valuable to the creation of cavitation (mini-explosions) at the interface for lithotripsy applications.[4,26]

In the pulsed mode (high peak power density) it can superheat water, causing cavitation (vaporization bubble at the tip of the silica or quartz fiber) to generate a local shock wave, useful for fragmenting calcium-containing material.

### Complications
Incomplete lesion ablation/coagulation; caution is required not to hit other instruments with laser fiber when active, as this could break off a fragment.

In general, laser cutting tends to produce less scarring and fibrosis because of the precise control of energy delivery. Pulsed modes tend to reduce heat conduction away from the site of energy delivery. Using a laser endoscopically has the advantage of readily available cooling via the irrigation fluid, to reduce local thermal build-up.

# LASER APPLICATION IN UROTHELIAL NEOPLASIA

There are advantages and disadvantages of employing lasers rather than electrocautery resection and other surgical means to treat urothelial malignancies.

## ADVANTAGES
- Can be done without general or regional anesthesia; no obturator reflex induction.
- Lower incidence of stricture formation, especially useful when employed near the ureteral orifices and bladder neck.
- Less bleeding, therefore less likelihood of needing a urinary drainage catheter or continuous bladder irrigation.
- 'No touch technique': probable lower likelihood of recurrence or risk of dissemination/implantation resulting from surgical manipulation or tumor.[27]
- Less mucosal irritation; therefore less postoperative morbidity.
- Early postoperative return to full activity.

## DISADVANTAGES

- No accurate means of determining depth of tumor penetration into the bladder wall.
- No tissue for pathologic analysis
- Possible complications associated with adjacent organ injury, e.g. bowel perforation.

Urologists and urologic oncologists have varying philosophies of transitional cell carcinoma (TCC) management, but in general most agree that initially diagnosed lesions need to be appropriately staged and graded with a relatively unperturbed pathologic specimen. The specimen should be obtained with either the resection loop applying pure cutting current or cold biopsy forceps, ensuring that muscularis muscle fibers are obtained in order to assess depth of invasion.

Typically, laser therapy is not employed for new bladder lesions or sessile lesions that are suspicious for invasion, unless the treatment is for palliation or for a patient not undergoing cystectomy because of medical contraindication, patient refusal, experimental protocol, etc.

## ANATOMIC LOCATION: LASER CHOICE, ANESTHESIA, INSTRUMENTS

- *Delivery devices*: Reflective system for $CO_2$ lasers.
- *Fiberoptics*: Angle of energy exit: fiberoptic cables can have no termination device or have a termination reflector/refractor which changes the direction of the beam delivery for tissue application. Most lasers employ a coaxial low-energy helium-neon aiming beam, to ensure precise location of energy delivery.
- *End fire*: When used in the bare cable mode, the laser beam will emanate from the end of the fiber, with a controlled angle of diffusion, depending on the cut angle and state of the fiber's cut surface. This is a common means of delivery for KTP and YAG energy to treat bladder tumors.
- *Power*: Can be further concentrated at the fiber end by employing a tip attachment, most commonly made of cut sapphire, shaped for specific applications (e.g. semicircular, conical, etc.).[2,8,11,28,29]
- *Side fire*: When laser energy is applied to the prostatic parenchyma or onto the anterior wall or dome of the bladder, the energy delivery may be facilitated by the use of a beam reflector attached to the end of the fiber. The reflectors are made in a variety of reflection and beam diffusion angles.
- *Size*: The size of the fiber will determine the amount of energy that can be delivered to the tissue and the size of the working port required in the endoscope to visualize and deliver the beam, with or without an open-ended plastic catheter guide. The larger diameter fibers are less flexible and pose greater difficulty in treating lesions requiring flexible scopes with high degrees of flexion. Typical fiber diameters range from 200 to 600 microns.

## ANATOMIC LOCATION

Lesions in the urethral meatus and fossa navicularis are best treated by direct visualization and hand-held lasers such as the $CO_2$ or KTP if they are superficial. Deeper lesions require the use of Nd:YAG, with appropriate handpiece. Anesthesia is either topical EMLA cream or local injectable lidocaine at the lesion base and surrounding 4–5 mm using small gauge (27 or 30 G) needles. Alternatively, a field block can be carried out, targeting the cutaneous nerves. Larger lesions may necessitate intravenous sedation, or, rarely, regional anesthesia.

Anterior urethral lesions are best treated by flexible cystoscopy and the KTP laser, which has low probability of stricture, delivered by fiberoptic scope. Anesthesia can be achieved with a topical lidocaine jelly, with or without intravenous sedation.

Posterior urethral lesions are best treated by rigid cystoscopy, so that anatomic landmarks can be easily maintained. A cystoscope with a laser bridge (modified Albarron) working port is mandatory. The modified laser bridge includes a fiber entry port with water-tight connectivity and a moveable tip to allow fiber deflection, thereby precisely controlling the direction of the laser light. The KTP is again the laser of choice, unless deeper penetration into the prostate is required, in which case the Nd:YAG is preferred.

Bladder lesions can be managed by both rigid and flexible cystoscopy, depending on the size and location of the tumor(s). Small, superficial tumors can be treated with Ho:YAG or KTP via flexible cystoscopy. The same is true for lesions near the bladder neck or ureteral orifices, although rigid cystoscopy is preferred for those lesions. Larger or deeper tumors are best managed with Nd:YAG. Anesthesia is topical lidocaine jelly, with or without intravenous sedation. Rare cases may require regional or laryngeal mask airway (LMA) general anesthesia.

Other bladder applications for laser energy include control of bleeding associated with radiation cystitis or chemotherapy-induced chemical cystitis. There have been anecdotal reports of successful application of Nd:YAG for focal bleeding, argon for more diffuse bleeding, and even for epithelial lesions due to interstitial cystitis and cystitis glandularis. However, in general, laser energy provides discreet treatment capability and is not applicable for diffuse conditions such as cystitis regardless of etiology.[30]

Ureteral lesions can be managed with rigid, semirigid, or flexible ureteroscopes. Usually the miniureteroscope (e.g. 7.2 Fr.) can be employed to visualize and treat ureteral tumors, and therefore the ureterovesical junction (UVJ) does not require dilation.[31]

Renal pelvic lesions can be managed via an antegrade approach through percutaneous access and a rigid or flexible nephroscope, or via a retrograde approach with a rigid or flexible ureteroscope.

Due to the discomfort associated with dilation of the UVJ and ureter, these cases typically require regional or general anesthesia.[32]

Caliceal lesions, depending on the location, can be managed via an antegrade approach using percutaneous access and either a rigid or flexible nephroscope, or via a retrograde approach employing a flexible ureteroscope. As in the bladder and renal pelvis, smaller superficial lesions are best managed by KTP or Ho:YAG, whereas larger deeper lesions require the Nd:YAG.[33]

Fourteen selected patients with TCCs in the upper tracts were managed by Orihuela and Smith using a percutaneous, antegrade approach, including resection of the tumor with cold-cup biopsy forceps for pathologic submission, and then fulguration of the tumor bed.[33]

Fulguration was accomplished with the Nd:YAG, pulse mode, 15–20 watts for 20 seconds in eight patients. Seven patients overall also received adjuvant intracavitary treatment with mitomycin C or bacillus Calmette–Guérin (BCG) via a nephrostomy tube, after a second-look nephroscopy, with or without biopsy. Six patients were rendered free of disease with this approach, despite having a mixed population of patients, including those with multifocal and superficially invasive disease. Both application of laser energy to the tumor bed and adjuvant BCG therapy lowered the rate of tumor recurrence.[34]

# TUMOR TYPE

## TRANSITIONAL CELL CARCINOMA (TCC)

### SUPERFICIAL DISEASE

Over 50% of patients with superficial TCC (T0, Ta, T1) will develop recurrences after TURBT using standard electrocautery. The rate of recurrence in the bladder is multifactorial, mainly due to the field nature of TCC; however, at least one factor may be local implantation of viable tumor cells liberated during TURBT. There have been several studies attempting to compare recurrence rates between TUR and laser management of superficial disease. The results have been mixed, with some small studies showing an advantage for laser treatment, whereas some large studies, >100 patients, show recurrence rates similar to those with TURBT, ranging from 18% to 38%. Since a large randomized phase III trial to convincingly show an improvement in recurrence rate with laser management has yet to be conducted, it must be stated that the 'no contact' approach to superficial tumors has only a theoretical advantage.

### Ta: LOW GRADE

Endoscopic photographs of a superficial, papillary TCC, both pre- and post-laser treatment, are shown in Figure 28.5.[1,30]

Previously defined low-grade Ta disease is perhaps the most amenable to laser treatment for recurrent disease, since the likelihood of progression is low and since the lesions can be treated with nothing more than topical anesthesia (lidocaine-impregnated urethral lubricant).

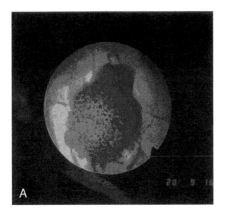 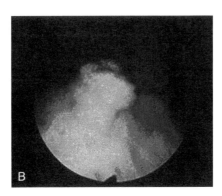 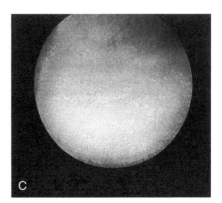

**Fig. 28.5**
**A** Pretreatment papillary bladder tumor. **B** Post Nd:YAG laser energy application produces some tissue volume shrinkage and coloration change from pink to white. **C** 6 months after treatment, shows sloughed tumor and only a residual scar in the bladder wall.

The smallest lesions are easily treated with KTP laser at a power setting of 10–15 watts in continuous mode with 0.5 second bursts using a 1 mm spot size, with the lesion 1–2 mm from the probe tip. However, Nd:YAG is the preferred energy for lesions larger than 2 mm, at a power setting of 15–35 watts, depending on the size of the lesion. Power is applied sparingly as the entire exophytic tumor is painted with energy until it blanches to white.

Since there is usually no bleeding and, with careful application, perforation is unlikely, it is not necessary to leave an indwelling catheter. Both bladder spasms and patient discomfort are quite uncommon. Reflex contraction of the obturator muscle does not occur, due to the lack of electrical stimulation, even with laterally located tumors.

The remnant-coagulated tumor will slough small fragments, beginning 3–5 days after treatment and is usually complete 7–14 days afterwards, depending on the tumor volume. The fragments are small and pliable enough to produce minimal concern for bladder outlet or urethral obstruction.

## Ta: HIGH GRADE

As with low-grade disease, KTP can be used to treat small lesions. Power settings should be at the higher end and energy delivery time should be slightly longer to allow more depth of penetration.

Nd:YAG is set at 20–40 watts to allow penetration of 2–4 mm (approximately 1 mm/10 watts). This can be increased to 50–60 watts for larger lesions. Laser energy is applied in 1–3 second bursts, beginning at the tumor periphery, including a 1 mm rim of normal-appearing urothelium at the base, then proceed radially and centrally until the entire tumor is brushed with laser energy and turns from the usual pink–orange to white in coloration.[3]

## T1 DISEASE

One of the largest concerns in using laser treatment for invasive TCC of the bladder is possible clinical understaging. Therefore it is essential that the treatment for suspected T1 disease extend deeper than the lamina propria. Use of the YAG or Nd:Ho laser is recommended for T1 disease, due to the deeper energy penetration resulting from the forward scatter of these wavelengths. Commonly used YAG power settings for T1 tumors are 35–45 watts, with 2–3 second pulse duration.

## T2–4 INVASIVE DISEASE

Patients with invasive disease are not good candidates for laser treatment of their cancer, and should undergo cystectomy with or without neoadjuvant chemotherapy, except in a limited number of circumstances, for example, T2 (B1) disease as part of a bladder-sparing

study protocol, or for T3–4 disease for palliation of symptoms or bleeding. As mentioned above, clinical understaging is a well-recognized problem with treating invasive TCC. The exact depth of penetration is not precisely controlled using either Nd:YAG or Nd:Ho; however, with power and pulse duration manipulation, it is possible to treat nearly transmural lesions. Even though there are reports of local elimination of T3a (B2) and even T3b in the literature, the treating physician must be wary of regional or even systemic dissemination with muscular invasive disease. As stated in previous chapters, the overall 5-year survival rate for invasive TCC is <50%, even for those undergoing radical surgery.

Laser treatment of invasive disease is best performed after complete TURBT with electrocautery and a 3–10 day waiting period, when the bleeding has stopped and the clot has been lysed by urokinase. This staged method allows the usual pathologic tumor assessment of grade and depth. However, it is possible to treat the tumor de novo, in order to minimize patient morbidity, especially if complete local control is not the treatment objective. The power setting for the Nd:YAG is 45–50 watts and the application of laser energy should include a 1 cm margin of normal-appearing urothelium.[27,30,35] The treatment plan includes an anticipated forward energy scatter into the bladder wall. Most invasive lesions occur in the extraperitoneal part of the bladder, so the risk of energy scatter into the bowel wall is low; however, the patient should be placed in the Trendelenburg position to reduce the risk. Gerber et al described a combined laparoscopic and transurethral laser treatment of invasive cancer to ensure safe delivery of deeply applied laser energy. The authors reported on five patients with extensive T3 TCC, in whom the bowel was mobilized and packed away from the bladder and the serosal surface monitored via the laparoscope while a second surgeon applied laser energy via the cystoscope. The mean energy applied was 58,600 J, while two patients had an additional 8000–10,000 J applied via the laparoscope towards the bladder. No patient suffered a bowel perforation but local recurrence was observed in four patients, although the one patient without local recurrence received the concomitant laparoscopic laser energy.[36] Laparoscopy also allows simultaneous lymph node staging.

Reports of local recurrence after laser treatment for invasive TCC vary from 16% to 68% depending on initial tumor depth (T2–4) and laser energy delivered (3600–26,000 J, mean 13,700 J).[8,11,37–42] After deep laser treatment, it may take 2–3 months for healing and re-epithelialization to occur.

Early in the definition phase of the role of lasers in bladder cancer management, Hofstetter reported on 47 patients with infiltrating bladder carcinomas treated with the Nd:YAG laser alone or in combination with TUR. The mean follow-up was 3.5 years (range 19–133 months), and 39/47 patients (83%) were still alive. Two had developed metastatic disease in the pelvic lymph nodes; 13/47 (27.7%) had no evidence of recurrent disease; 23/47 (48.9%) had recurrences at different sites, without stage progression; 6/47 (12.8%) developed recurrences with progression; and 5/47 (10.6%) died of their cancer.[43] The remaining three patients died of nonbladder cancer causes or were lost to follow-up.

Beisland et al reported on 15 patients with solitary T2 cancers (9 WHO grade 2 and 6 WHO grade 3) who had TUR followed by Nd:YAG irradiation at 45–50 watts, by overlapping single pulses of 4 seconds duration. With minimal 2-year follow-up, 10 patients were alive with no evidence of disease at 56–78 months, but three cases had remote site local recurrences without stage progression. One patient died of cardiovascular disease 24 months after treatment, with no evidence of disease at autopsy. Four patients had local recurrence 4–12 months after treatment, and were treated with either radical cystectomy or external beam radiotherapy. One died from metastatic disease at 1 year after cystectomy; the other three were alive at 2 years. Five-year survival was 67% in this small series. There were no cases of laser-associated complications.[38]

Table 28.2 shows recommendations for energy and frequency settings for a number of fiber types and urologic applications of the Lumenis VersaPulse™ laser instrument using holmium laser energy.

## ADENOCARCINOMA

Bladder adenocarcinomas are typically uncommon, accounting for <2% of all primary bladder carcinomas. Urachal adenocarcinomas are typically extravesical and have a predisposition to wide and deep tumor infiltration, making them less amenable to laser therapy. Care must be taken in treating cancer arising in urachal remnants, because of the location of bladder entry at the dome, and proximity to the peritoneal contents. Early stage primary vesical adenocarcinomas can be managed with the Nd:YAG laser, using settings similar to those for minimally invasive TCC, 30–40 watts in short bursts, due to the concerns of adjacent organ injury. Advanced pelvic adenocarcinoma requires major extirpative surgery, as discussed in Chapter 66, and may include a multimodality approach, including chemotherapy. The role of lasers in managing advanced adenocarcinoma of the bladder is not currently defined, except in the case of palliation in the nonoperative candidate.

Squamous carcinomas often arise from sites of chronic inflammation, as is also the case with exstrophic bladder and schistosomatic adenocarcinomas, and can be focal or diffuse depending on the etiology. The vast majority of cases of squamous bladder cancer occur in association with infection of *Schistosoma haematobium* in the Nile River regions. These tumors are commonly exophytic, fungating, and well differentiated, making them amenable to treatment with laser energy. World experience with the use of lasers to manage squamous cancers is not extensively documented in the literature.[44,45]

Often in the US, squamous carcinomas arise from sites of previous squamous metaplasia, as is seen with chronic indwelling catheters and untreated bladder calculi or other foreign bodies. These patients often have advanced disease at the time of diagnosis, and are less likely to be candidates for laser treatment, except for palliation.

## VASCULAR LESIONS

Vascular lesions, such as cavernous hemangiomas, arteriovenous malformations, and other vascular

| Application | 200-micron SlimLine fiber | 365-micron SlimLine fiber | 550-micron SlimLine fiber | 1000-micron SlimLine fiber | 550-micron DuoTome (side-firing fiber) | Holmium | Nd:YAG | Recommended energy guideline | Recommended repetition rate |
|---|---|---|---|---|---|---|---|---|---|
| **Bladder**<br>Superficial or recurrent TCC | | X | X | X | X | X | | 1.0–1.4 joules | 10–14 Hertz |
| Multifocal (invasive) tumors | | X | X | X | X | X | X | Ho: 1.0–1.4 joules<br>Nd:YAG: 20–30 watts | 10–14 Hertz<br>**2–4 seconds** |
| Soft tissue | X | X | X | X | X | X | X | Ho: 1.0–1.4 joules<br>Nd:YAG: 20–30 watts | 10–14 Hertz<br>**2–4 seconds** |
| **Urethra**<br>Condyloma, carbuncles, or tumors | | X | X | | X | X | | 0.6–1.0 joules | 10 Hertz<br>**(do *not* exceed 15 Hz in air)** |
| **Coagulation**<br>Holmium | | X | X | X | X | X | | 0.6–0.8 joules | 10 Hertz |
| Nd:YAG | | X | X | | | | X | 5–10 watts | **1–2 seconds** |

**Table 28.2** Recommendations for energy settings of several fiber types for Holmium and YAG lasers by lesion application

tumors, due to the high absorption of approximately 500 nm light by hemoglobin and melanin, can be treated with argon lasers 488–524 nm if very superficial, but otherwise are best treated with the KTP-Nd:YAG laser. If the vascular lesion is deep, Nd:YAG can be used, because of the penetrative thermal effects of the laser.[46–50]

## LASER SENSITIZERS

Substances can be given to the patient, either locally or systemically, to enhance the tissue sensitivity to laser energy. If the target tissue (e.g. tumor) selectively uptakes or retains the sensitizer, then its detection and/or destruction can be selectively carried out via exposure to monochromatic laser light. The photochemical effect, as mentioned above, is the selective activation of a specific drug or molecule by a specific wavelength of light. The sensitizing molecule will be transformed into a toxic compound (or compounds) by the effects on chemical bonds induced by absorbing the light energy. It is not uncommon for the toxicity of the generated compounds to be mediated through oxygen-free radicals. Free radicals can produce cellular death by lipid peroxidation and DNA crosslink production or destruction. This is a novel approach to specifically target tissue containing, concentrating, and/or metabolically processing the sensitizer, such as premalignant and in situ carcinomatous lesions. The effect is dependent on an energy source that selectively produces the molecular activation, and lasers can provide that monochromatic, specific wavelength of light. Photodynamic therapy (PDT) will be discussed in more detail in Chapter 36.

For laser surgeons, it is important to remember that some medications have laser light-sensitizing effects, most importantly antibiotics and fungicidal/fungistatic agents that are commonly given perioperatively and to cancer patients receiving multimodal therapy.

## AUTOFLUORESCENCE

Lasers can also be used to detect subclinical lesions via the process of autofluorescence, whereby the tissue of interest, usually neoplastic, will selectively fluoresce under monochromatic light stimulation, thereby allowing its detection. Nitrogen lasers in the ultraviolet (UV-A) range at 337 nm produce optimal auto-fluorescence of TCCs and other urothelial lesions.

## LASER SAFETY

Although, as stated in the laser history section, lasers were not originally intended to be destructive in nature,

refinements in design have allowed them to become a very effective means of destroying matter. Just as any therapy—surgical or medical—laser use carries inherent risks to both the patient, as discussed above, and to the operating team. The American National Standards Institute (ANSI) classifies lasers into one of four classes, based on their characteristics of laser output energy or power, wavelength, exposure duration, and cross-sectional area of the laser beam at the point of interest.[51,52] Further breakdown of these characteristics includes the parameters used for classification purposes: energy, power, fluence, and irradiance.

- *Energy*: The amount of work accomplished; unit = joules (J).
- *Power*: The rate of energy expenditure, i.e. energy per unit time; unit = joules per second (J/s), otherwise known as watts (W), such that 1 J/s = 1 W. The total energy applied to a surface is determined by multiplying the power by the duration of time the surface is exposed.
- *Fluence* (also known as power density): The amount of energy per unit area, unit = joules per $cm^2$ ($J/cm^2$), and is more important in determining a laser's effect on tissues than total energy delivered.
- *Irradiance*: The intensity of a laser beam; unit = watts per $cm^2$ ($W/cm^2$). Irradiance is inversely proportional to the spot size radius. Lenses or optical fibers can manipulate the power density of a laser. Lenses focus or defocus a beam to change spot size, even though the laser may be kept at a constant distance from the surface.

## HAZARD CLASSIFICATION

Lasers are classified according to their potential to cause biologic damage. The pertinent parameters, as described above, are laser output energy or power, radiation wavelengths, exposure duration, and cross-sectional area of the laser beam at the point of interest.

In addition to these general parameters, lasers are classified in accordance with the accessible emission limit (AEL), which is the maximum accessible level of laser radiation permitted within a particular laser class. The ANSI standard laser hazard classifications are used to signify the level of hazard inherent in a laser system, and the extent of safety controls required to utilize that system.

### ANSI LASER CLASSIFICATION SCHEME

- *Class I*: Inherently safe; no possibility of eye damage. This can be either because of a low output power (in which case eye damage is impossible even after hours of exposure), or due to an enclosure that cannot be opened in normal operation without the laser being switched off automatically. Examples include commercial tag readers, laser printers, and CD players. These lasers are exempt from laser safety program requirements.

- *Class II*: The blinking reflex of the human eye will prevent eye damage. Most laser pointers are in this category, with output powers of around 1 milliwatt (mW).
- *Class IIIa*: Similar to IIIb, but with large beam diameters, such that the pupil will only allow a 'class-II'-amount of light to enter the eye. Lasers in this class are mostly dangerous in combination with optical instruments which change the beam diameter. The visible continuous wave helium-neon laser above 1 mW, but not exceeding 5 mW radiant power, is an example of this class.
- *Class IIIb*: Can cause retinal injury if the beam enters the eye directly via either intrabeam viewing or spectral reflections. This applies to laser powers up to a few milliwatts.
- *Class IV*: Highly dangerous; even nondirect scattering of light from the beam can lead to eye or skin damage. This applies to laser powers of more than a few milliwatts.

Laser use safety is monitored by the Occupational Safety and Health Administration (OSHA) and the standards for acceptable exposure limits (AELs) are contained in ANSI Z136 published by the Laser Institute of America.[51,52] The threshold limit values (TLVs) and biologic exposure indices (BEI) for lasers are found in the American Conference of Government Industrial Hygienists (ACGIH) manual.[53,54] Concepts such as the maximum permissible exposure (MPE), accessible emission level (AEL), and nominal hazard zone (NHZ) are important for the laser operator to understand and implement. The MPE is the maximum level of laser radiation to which a person may be exposed without hazardous effects or biologic changes in the eye or skin. The MPE is determined by the wavelength of the laser, the energy involved, and the duration of the exposure. The type of protective hardware (e.g. ocular protection) is dependent on the laser's rated optical density requirements. Tables of optical density of eyewear by type of laser, its AEL rating, and the exposure duration can be found in the ANSI 136.1 standard document. The NHZ is the environment within which the level of direct, reflected, or scattered radiation during normal operation exceeds the appropriate MPE. Exposure levels beyond the NHZ are below the appropriate MPE level; thus no control measures are needed outside the NHZ.

## OCULAR PROTECTION

The eye structure is transparent to light in the visible and near-infrared region, 400–1400 nm; hence these wavelengths pose the greatest risk to the retina itself. The energy of a laser beam can be intensified 10,000–100,000 times by the focusing action of the eye (cornea and lens). If the irradiance entering the eye is 1 mW/cm$^2$, the irradiance at the retina will be 100 W/cm$^2$. Thus, even a low power laser in the milliwatt range can cause a burn if focused directly onto the retina. Due to the natural focusing pattern of the cornea and lens, the most vulnerable region of the eye to laser energy is the macula lutea or fovea. Bottom line: *never* allow a laser to be pointed at a person's eyes no matter how low the power of the laser.

## OTHER PROTECTION FOR SURGEON, ASSISTANTS, OR PERSONNEL AND THE PATIENT

A complete discussion of all laser hazards (electrical, fire, compressed gas cylinders, cryogenic and toxic materials, etc.) is beyond the scope of this text, but is readily available in a number of the listed references. However, surgeons operating lasers must be compliant with the laser safety program at their hospital, surgicenter, or institution in order to prevent inadvertent exposures and subsequent injury.

The main control elements of any laser safety policy include two broad categories: *administrative controls*—for example, staff education and certification requirements for safe laser operation; posted placards to prevent unnecessary, untrained, and unsuspecting personnel from entering the laser environment; procedures for standardized safe laser operations—and *engineering controls*—for example, beam housings and shutters; interlocks for 1) pulsed systems to prevent firing of the laser by dumping the stored energy into a dummy load; and 2) continuous wave systems to turn off the power supply or interrupt the beam by means of shutters; all of which limit inadvertent release of laser energy. Other engineering controls include keeping the beam path free of specularly reflective surfaces and combustible objects, and the beam terminated in a noncombustible, nonreflective barrier or beam stop. This may include laser-safe, fire-retardant draping of nonsurgical external areas, with no metal objects near field, and away from compressed gas sources—oxygen, nitrogen, etc.[55]

One other hazard from laser use that deserves mention is the plume emanating from tissue destruction. The plume is a smoke 'cloud' containing fumes, dust, and aerosols, with possible biologic contaminants. Typically, when lasing lesions in the bladder, the plume will be dissolved into the irrigation fluid filling the bladder, and will not pose risk to the OR team. However, lesions being lased in the urethra, meatus, and external genitalia can produce plumes that escape into the free air of the operating theater. Certain lesions (e.g. condyloma accuminata and squamous carcinomas) can contain virus elements that survive intact into the plume and pose a threat of infection to the mucous membranes of the OR personnel. Other possible contents of plume, especially if the laser energy is exposed to drapes, towels, etc., include polycyclic aromatic hydrocarbons from polymers (e.g. methyl methacrylate); hydrogen cyanide and benzene from aromatic polyamide fibers; fused silica from quartz; heavy metals from etching; benzene from polyvinyl chloride; and cyanide and formaldehyde from synthetic and natural fibers.

For this reason, when any lesion is being destroyed via laser in the urethra or on the skin of the external genitalia, there should be a negative pressure aspiration system (vacuum hose) to capture and contain the plume.

## OTHER (NON-LASER) GENITOURINARY LESION TREATMENT TECHNOLOGY

### THERMAL

Local application of microwave energy to the bladder with and without combined chemotherapy has been used to manage TCC of the bladder in patients who were not surgical candidates, refused cystectomy, or had low-grade lesions. The theory of combination modality treatment is that, in addition to the direct cytotoxic effect of hyperthermia, hyperthermia is felt to have immunomodulatory activity and to be sensitizing for both radio- and chemotherapy, thereby potentiating the effect of the traditional modality.[56-61] Hyperthermia may also enhance the action of other cytotoxics (e.g. tumor necrosis factor).[62] There are three categories of thermotherapy delivery—local, regional, and body part hyperthermia—with the last reserved mainly for the treatment of metastatic disease.[56]

External or endocavitary microwave energy can produce heating of the bladder wall via electromagnetic or dielectric radiation to the target tissue.[63] Another approach is to use a radiofrequency antenna connected to an intravesical catheter to produce bladder hyperthermia which, in combination with mitomycin C, can produce reliable superficial bladder epithelial desquamation without permanent submucosal or muscular scarring.[64] Combining hyperthermia with intravesical chemotherapy increases systemic absorption of the chemotherapeutic agent, but plasma levels typically stay well below the myelosuppressive or toxic range.[65-67] Colombo et al reported on 19 patients who received up to eight sessions of endovesical hyperthermia to 42.5–46°C for 40 minutes via the SB-TS 101 915 MHz radiofrequency generation system simultaneously with mitomycin C at 40 mg/40 ml over a maximum of 2 months; 16/19 (84%) subsequently underwent TURBT. All cases showed tumor necrosis,

with 9/19 (47%) having a complete remission and 7/19 (37%) a partial remission. Three patients had extensive residual disease and later received cystectomy. Irritative bladder symptoms were common during the hyperthermia and for 2–4 days following the treatment.[66] A similar side effect symptom pattern was observed combining 50 minutes of 42–43°C radiofrequency thermotherapy with both 3.0 Gy external beam radiotherapy and intravesical pirarubicin (30 mg THP-ADM).[58]

Postradiation high temperature (>41.5°C) regional thermotherapy resulted in a higher rate of tumor downstaging, lower local recurrence rate, and nonsignificant increase in survival of 28 patients, versus 21 who received radiation alone prior to surgical tumor resection.[68] Complications with the thermotherapy included increased discomfort, but no grade 3–4 toxicities.[69] Achieving tumor temperatures of 42.5°C seems to be universally lethal, but also increases the likelihood of symptoms and possible surrounding tissue injury.[70-77] Several authors have tested hyperthermic saline bladder irrigations from 63–80°C from 10 to 70 minutes of dwell time, as an alternative to cystectomy in poor surgical candidates.[78-82] While coagulation of bleeding vessels and partial bladder wall necrosis was achievable without producing adjacent visceral injury, potentially viable tumor could be left in T3-4 disease due to in vivo tumor heat resistance, while posing hazards to pelvic and intraperitoneal structures when the dwell time and temperature were high.

The need for target tissue monitoring via endoluminal thermistry/thermometry is controversial. Some authors feel improved efficacy in tumor destruction and reduced risk to adjacent structures can be obtained by knowing accurate tissue temperature; others feel the technique is expensive and time consuming, while the benefit is marginal.[64,83]

### HIFU

High-intensity focused ultrasound (HIFU) has been used with and without combined intravesical chemotherapy to treat bladder cancer.[84-88] The combination of mitomycin C and HIFU was felt to be synergistic in inducing tumor necrosis, compared with HIFU alone in BT T739 tumor-bearing mice.[85] The mechanism of destruction with HIFU is felt to be mainly thermal, although conventional cavitation and vaporization of tissue water may also play a role.[87]

Synergy has also been observed with piezoelectric ultrasonic hyperthermia to 44°C applied within 30 minutes to 1 hour prior to injections of either thiotepa, 2 mg/kg intraperitoneally, or cyclophosphamide (Cytoxan) 50 mg/kg intraperitoneally into Fischer rats. Studies indicated that the synergy was due, not to increased uptake or activation of agent, but to a rapid and marked inhibition of DNA synthesis by the alkylating agent–thermotherapy combination.[89,90] The authors hypothesize that the heat may inhibit the enzymes responsible for DNA repair and recovery after alkylation.

## SHOCK WAVE ENERGY

High energy shock waves (HESW), akin to those used to treat urinary calculi, have been applied to grafted tumors in mice. Temporary cytotoxic effects on tumor cells were observed with application of 800 impulses at 15 kV from a Dornier HM3 in nude mice. The effects are thought to be due to direct mechanical damage to cellular membranes/organelles, as well as to disruption of blood supply.[91]

## CYBERKNIFE

Radiosurgical treatment is now being advocated as an alternative for open surgical treatment for genitourinary tumors in patients not considered to be surgical candidates or who refuse surgery.[92] The radiosurgical (CyberKnife) approach divides the high-dose radiotherapy required to ablate the tumor into many (up to 1200) individual beams, such that each one has a significantly reduced dose and produces minimal injury to the tissue traversed. Traditional radiotherapy has been combined with chemotherapy to treat bladder TCC in nonoperative patients with reasonable success.[93]

## FUTURE TREATMENT

The future of therapy for both superficial and invasive bladder cancer will move towards less invasive alternatives that will require the synergistic effects of multimodality therapy. Research efforts in the 21st century will be focused on finding the most efficacious blend of cytotoxic drugs with minimally destructive or non-invasive surgical modalities, while determining how to minimize injury to surrounding structures. The results may be augmented by the addition of computerized refinements in adjuvant radiotherapy.

Patients have already driven urologic surgeons to develop bladder replacement alternatives following cystectomy, and the drive will continue to push for bladder-sparing surgical alternatives. Improvements in technology that allow selective destruction of neoplastic tissue without injury to normal tissue is paramount to this effort.

## CONCLUSION

Lasers provide the urologist with another weapon in the treatment armamentarium for urologic disease. The role of lasers in the management of urothelial neoplasia has been established, with realization that treatment alternatives exist for all urothelial tumors, and that individual patient and tumor factors, as well as surgeon preference, will sway the treatment plan to or from laser therapy.[18,19,30,94,95] Lasers offer a noncontact, low-morbidity, often minimally invasive, means of destroying urothelial malignancy with high confidence. When used with other adjuvant therapies, lasers can provide patients possessing comorbidities with a means of controlling their local disease without major surgery. Lasers can also allow delivery of definitive treatment for low-grade/stage lesions in an outpatient/office setting. However, laser technology, at least in its current form, has limitations, and cannot be advocated as first line therapy for the patient with invasive bladder cancer who has no or minimal comorbidities, and who is otherwise a surgical candidate.

Lasers are only one of several technological developments that are shaping modern surgical extirpation of neoplastic disease. Under scientific evaluation are a host of newer technologies that are being employed as single modalities and in combination with more traditional therapies. The role of technologies such as focused ultrasound, thermotherapy, and cyberknives for urologic malignancy has yet to be defined. Patient demand is pushing the trend towards development of multimodality, non- or minimally invasive treatment approaches, with the goal of controlling disease with minimal morbidity and cost. The future management of bladder neoplasia will certainly include combination therapies that will allow elimination of malignancy while sparing at least a component of the primary organ.

### REFERENCES

1. Dixon JA. Lasers in surgery. Curr Probl Surg 1984;21:1–65.
2. Smith JA Jr. Current concepts in laser treatment of bladder cancer. Prog Clin Biol Res 1989;303:463–469.
3. Smith JA Jr. Lasers in urologic surgery. Current status, Lesson 13. Chicago: Yearbook Medical, 1989, pp 98–103.
4. Grasso M, Beaghler M, Bagley DH, Strup S. Actively deflectable, flexible cystoscopes: no longer solely a diagnostic instrument. J Endourol 1993;7:527–530.
5. Hofstetter A, Frank, F. [Neodymium:YAG laser in urology. Application and results in the treatment of tumors.] Arch Esp Urol 1986;39(Suppl 1):23–32.
6. Bromberg JL. The laser in America: 1950–1970. Cambridge, MA: MIT Press, 1991.
7. Choy DS. History of lasers in medicine. Thorac Cardiovasc Surg 1988;36(Suppl 2):114–117.
8. Smith JA Jr. Treatment of invasive bladder cancer with a neodymium:YAG laser. J Urol 1986;135:55–57.
9. Smith JA Jr, Lundergan D, Lewis CA. Treatment of bladder tumors with an Nd:YAG laser. Aorn J 1985;42:586, 588, 590.
10. Smith JA Jr. Laser treatment of bladder cancer. Semin Urol 1985;3:2–9.
11. Smith JA Jr. Endoscopic applications of laser energy. Urol Clin North Am 1986;13:405–419.

12. Krylov VS, Kagan EM. [Lasers and the prospects for their use in urology.] Urol Nefrol (Mosk) 1973;38:62–66.

13. Hofstetter A, Staehler G, Keiditsch E, Siepe W. [Morpholgical changes in the rabbit's bladder after argon laser irradiation.] Fortschr Med 1976;94:1679–1682.

14. Sacknoff EJ. Instrumentation for urologic laser surgery. Med Instrum 1983;17:404–406.

15. Sacknoff EJ. Laser advances in urology. J Clin Laser Med Surg 1993;11:173–176.

16. Hofstetter A, Frank F. [A new laser endoscope for irradiation of bladder tumors.] Fortschr Med 1979;97:232–234.

17. Hofstetter A, Bowering R, Keiditsch E, Wachutka H. Interferometric laser holography for determination of the localization and extent of bladder tumor. Eur Urol 1979;5:120–127.

18. Hofstetter A. [Endoscopic obliteration of tumors of the bladder using laser (author's transl).] Urologe A 1981;20(Suppl):317–322.

19. Hofstetter A, Frank F, Keiditsch E, Bowering R. Endoscopic neodymium–YAG laser application for destroying bladder tumors. Eur Urol 1981;7:278–282.

20. Hofstetter A, Papo Z, Bowering R, Rothenberger K, Keiditsch E. [Must indications for cystectomy in bladder carcinoma be reconsidered?] Fortschr Med 1982;100:1798–1804.

21. Hofstetter A, Schmiedt E, Staehler G. [Endovesical destruction of bladder tumors with neodymium-YAG laser (author's transl).] Urologe A 1982;21:9–11.

22. Hofstetter AG, Keiditsch E, Schmiedt E, Frank F. [Neodymium YAG laser in clinical urology. Current status and clinical experiences.] Fortschr Med 1984;102:885–890.

23. Hofstetter AG. Application of lasers in bladder cancer. Semin Surg Oncol 1992;8:214–216.

24. Hofstetter A. [Applications for lasers in carcinoma of the urinary bladder.] Urologe A 1994;33:288–290.

25. Office S (ed). Laser Fundamentals. Waterloo, Ontario: University of Waterloo, 2004.

26. Grasso M, Caruso RP. Lasers in urology. eMedicine. Online. Available: www.emedicine.com/med/topic3037.htm

27. See WA, Chapman WH. Tumor cell implantation following neodymium–YAG bladder injury: a comparison to electrocautery injury. J Urol 1987;137:1266–1269.

28. Smith JA Jr, Landau S. Neodymium:YAG laser specifications for safe intravesical therapy. J Urol 1989;141:1238–1239.

29. Smith J, Middleton RG. In Smith J (ed). Lasers in Urologic Surgery. Chicago: Yearbook Medical, 1989, pp. 52–62.

30. Smith JA Jr. Lasers in clinical urologic surgery. In Dixon JA (ed). Surgical Application of Lasers. Chicago: Yearbook Medical, 1987, pp 218–237.

31. Sosa RE. Laserscope KTP/YAG Clinical Updates in Urology. San Jose, CA: Laserscope Surgical Systems, 1990, p 16.

32. Carson CC 3rd. Endoscopic treatment of upper and lower urinary tract lesions using lasers. Semin Urol 1991;9:185–191.

33. Orihuela E, Smith AD. Laser treatment of transitional cell cancer of the bladder and upper urinary tract. Cancer Treat Res 1989;46:123–142.

34. Orihuela E, Smith AD. Percutaneous treatment of transitional cell carcinoma of the upper urinary tract. Urol Clin North Am 1988;15(3):425–431.

35. Malloy TR, Wein AJ. Laser treatment of bladder carcinoma and genital condylomata. Urol Clin North Am 1987;14:121–126.

36. Gerber GS, Chodak GW, Rukstalis DB. Combined laparoscopic and transurethral neodymium:yttrium–aluminum–garnet laser treatment of invasive bladder cancer. Urology 1995;45:230–233.

37. Beisland HO. A contribution to the special discussion on YAG laser irradiation of superficial bladder cancer. Acta Urol Belg 1989;57:693–695.

38. Beisland HO, Sander S. Neodymium–YAG laser irradiation of stage T2 muscle-invasive bladder cancer. Long-term results. Br J Urol 1990;65:24–26.

39. Beisland HO. Possibilities of laser in the treatment of urinary bladder cancer. Ann Chir Gynaecol 1990;79:197–199.

40. Beisland HO. [Laser in urology.] Tidsskr Nor Laegeforen 1991;111:2852–2854.

41. Tarantino AE, Aretz HT, Libertino JA, Bihrle W 3rd, Dowd JB. Is the neodymium:YAG laser effective therapy for invasive bladder cancer? Urology 1991;38:514–518.

42. McPhee MS, Arnfield MR, Tulip J, Lakey WH. Neodymium:YAG laser therapy for infiltrating bladder cancer. J Urol 1988;140:44–46.

43. Spitzenpfeil E, Hofstetter A, Reis M, Muschter R. [The neodymium:YAG laser in infiltrating bladder tumors.] Fortschr Med 1989;107:548–551.

44. Staehler G, Hofstetter A, Schmiedt E, Rother W, Keiditsch, E. [Endoscopic laser therapy of bladder tumors in man.] Fortschr Med 1977;95:3–7.

45. Staehler G, Hofstetter A. Transurethral laser irradiation of urinary bladder tumors. Eur Urol 1979;5:64–69.

46. Hockley NM, Bihrle R, Bennett RM 3rd, Curry JM. Congenital genitourinary hemangiomas in a patient with the Klippel–Trenaunay syndrome: management with the neodymium:YAG laser. J Urol 1989;141:940–941.

47. Kato M, Chiba Y, Sakai K, Orikasa S. Endoscopic neodymium:yttrium aluminium garnet (Nd:YAG) laser irradiation of a bladder hemangioma associated with Klippel–Weber syndrome. Int J Urol 2000;7:145–148.

48. Smith JA Jr, Dixon JA. Neodymium:YAG laser irradiation of bladder hemangioma. Urology 1984;24:134–136.

49. Smith JA Jr. Laser treatment of bladder hemangioma. J Urol 1990;143:282–284.

50. Vicente J, Salvador J. Neodymium:YAG laser treatment of bladder hemangiomas. Urology 1990;36:305–308.

51. American National Standards Institute (ANSI). American National Standard for the Safe Use of Lasers in Health Care Facilities: ANSI Z136.3 1996 Orlando, FL: Laser Institute of America, 2000.

52. American National Standards Institute (ANSI). American National Standard for the Safe Use of Lasers: ANSI Z136.1 Orlando, FLL Laser Institute of America, 2001 (last revised January 8, 2001).

53. American Conference of Governmental Industrial Hygienists (ACGIH). TLVs (threshold limit values) for physical agents adopted by ACGIH for 1973. J Occup Med 1974;16:49–58.

54. American Conference of Industrial Hygienists (ACGIH). TLVs and BEIs. Cincinatti, OH: ACGIH Worldwide, 2004.

55. Laser Safety Guide. Section 2, Laser hazards. Princeton, NJ: Princeton University. Online. Available: http://web.princeton.edu/sites/ehs/laserguide/sec2.htm

56. Schlemmer M, Lindner LH, Abdel-Rahman S, Issels RD. [Principles, technology and indication of hyperthermia and part body hyperthermia.] Radiologe 2004;44:301–309.

57. Mauroy B, Bonnal JL, Prevost B, et al. [Study of the synergy of microwave hyperthermia/intravesical chemotherapy in the prevention of recurrences of superficial tumors of the bladder.] Prog Urol 1999;9:69–80.

58. Takechi T, Kawamura M, Nakagawa H, et al. [Combined treatment in patients with carcinoma in situ of the urinary bladder using intravesical pirarubicin, irradiation and hyperthermia.] Nippon Gan Chiryo Gakkai Shi 1990;25:2724–2727.

59. Kakehi M, Ueda K, Mukojima T, Hiraoka M, Seto O, Akanuma A, Nakatsugawa S. Multi-institutional clinical studies on hyperthermia combined with radiotherapy or chemotherapy in advanced cancer of deep-seated organs. Int J Hyperthermia 1990;6:719–740.

60. Hisazumi H, Nakajima K. [Eight-MHz RF-hyperthermia for advanced urological malignancies..] Gan To Kagaku Ryoho 1986;13:1381–1386.

61. Hisazumi H, Nakajima K. [Eight-MHZ RF hyperthermia in urological malignancies.] Gan To Kagaku Ryoho 1988;15:1382–1386.

62. Iizumi T, Yazaki T, Waku M, Soma G. Immunochemotherapy for murine bladder tumor with a new human recombinant tumor necrosis factor (rTNF-S), VP-16 and hyperthermia. J Urol 1989;142:386–389.

63. Dietsch A, Camart JC, Sozanski JP, Prevost B, Mauroy B, Chive M. Microwave thermochemotherapy in the treatment of the bladder carcinoma—electromagnetic and dielectric studies—clinical protocol. IEEE Trans Biomed Eng 2000;47:633–641.

64. Rath-Wolfson L, Moskovitz B, Dekel Y, Kugel V, Koren R. Combined intravesical hyperthermia and mitomycin chemotherapy: a preliminary in vivo study. Int J Exp Pathol 2003;84:145–152.

65. Paroni R, Salonia A, Lev A, et al. Effect of local hyperthermia of the bladder on mitomycin C pharmacokinetics during intravesical chemotherapy for the treatment of superficial transitional cell carcinoma. Br J Clin Pharmacol 2001;52:273–278.

66. Colombo R, Da Pozzo LF, Lev A, Freschi M, Gallus G, Rigatti P. Neoadjuvant combined microwave induced local hyperthermia and topical chemotherapy versus chemotherapy alone for superficial bladder cancer. J Urol 1996;155:1227–1232.

67. Colombo R, Da Pozzo LF, Lev A, et al. Local microwave hyperthermia and intravesical chemotherapy as bladder sparing treatment for select multifocal and unresectable superficial bladder tumors. J Urol 1998;159:783–787.

68. Hiraoka M, Masunaga S, Nishimura Y, et al. [Clinical assessment of thermoradiotherapy of breast cancer and cancer of the urinary bladder.] Gan No Rinsho 1990;36:2267–2271.

69. Masunaga SI, Hiraoka M, Akuta K, et al. Phase I/II trial of preoperative thermoradiotherapy in the treatment of urinary bladder cancer. Int J Hyperthermia 1994;10:31–40.

70. Yang XH. [Transurethral microwave radiation for bladder neoplasm.] Zhonghua Yi Xue Za Zhi 1992;72:531–533, 572–573.

71. Uchibayashi T, Nakajima K, Hisazumi H, Mihara S, Yamamoto H, Koshida K. Studies of temperature rise in bladder cancer and surrounding tissues during radiofrequency hyperthermia. Eur Urol 1992;21:299–303.

72. Kubota Y, Nishimura R, Takai S, Fukushima S. [Hyperthermic treatment of the bladder cancer: combined hyperthermic treatment with bleomycin and/or radiation (author's transl).] Nippon Gan Chiryo Gakkai Shi 1978;13:394–405.

73. Kubota Y. [Hyperthermic therapy of the bladder cancer. I. Effect of the hyperthermia on the cultured bladder cancer cell lines (author's transl).] Nippon Hinyokika Gakkai Zasshi 1981;72:730–734.

74. Kubota Y. [Hyperthermic therapy of the bladder cancer. III. Clinical studies (author's transl).] Nippon Hinyokika Gakkai Zasshi 1981;72:742–751.

75. Kubota Y. [Hyperthermic therapy of the bladder cancer. II. The kinetics of cell killing by hyperthermia plus bleomycin (author's transl).] Nippon Hinyokika Gakkai Zasshi 1981;72:735–741.

76. Kubota Y, Takebayashi S, Asakura K, Oshima H. [Application of radiofrequency hyperthermia for treating advanced urinary bladder cancer—a case report.] Gan No Rinsho 1984;30:215–219.

77. Kubota Y, Shuin T, Miura T, Nishimura R, Fukushima S, Takai S. Treatment of bladder cancer with a combination of hyperthermia, radiation and bleomycin. Cancer 1984;53:199–202.

78. England HR, Anderson JD, Minasian H, Marshall VR, Molland EA, Blandy JP. The therapeutic application of hyperthermia in the bladder. Br J Urol 1975;47:849–852.

79. Hall RR, Schade RO, Swinney J. Effects of hyperthermia on bladder cancer. Br Med J 1974;2:593–594.

80. Hall RR, Wadehra V, Towler JM, Hindmarsh JR, Byrne PO. Hyperthermia in the treatment of bladder tumours. Br J Urol 1976;48:603–608.

81. Ludgate CM, McLean N, Carswell GF, Newsam JE, Pettigrew RT, Tulloch WS. Hyperthermic perfusion of the distended urinary bladder in the management of recurrent transitional cell carcinoma. Br J Urol 1975;47:841–848.

82. Ludgate CM, McLean N, Tulloch WS. Hyperthermic irrigation of bladder in treatment of transitional cell carcinoma: its effectiveness in controlling persistent haematuria. J R Soc Med 1979;72:336–340.

83. Wust P, Gellermann J, Harder C, et al. Rationale for using invasive thermometry for regional hyperthermia of pelvic tumors. Int J Radiat Oncol Biol Phys 1998;41:1129–1137.

84. Madersbacher S, Marberger M. High-energy shockwaves and extracorporeal high-intensity focused ultrasound. J Endourol 2003;17:667–672.

85. Wang GM, Yang YF, Sun LA, Xu ZB, Xu YQ. [An experimental study on high intensity focused ultrasound combined with mitomycin treatment of bladder tumor.] Zhonghua Wai Ke Za Zhi 2003;41:897–900.

86. Uchida T, Ohori M, Egawa S. [Minimally invasive therapy for bladder and prostate cancer.] Gan To Kagaku Ryoho 2001;28:1094–1098.

87. Hill CR, ter Haar GR. High intensity focused ultrasound—potential for cancer treatment [review]. Br J Radiol 1995;68:1296–1303.

88. Kennedy JE, ter Haar GR, Cranston D. High intensity focused ultrasound: surgery of the future? Br J Radiol 2003;76:590–599.

89. Longo FW, Tomashefsky P, Rivin BD, Tannenbaum M. Interaction of ultrasonic hyperthermia with two alkylating agents in a murine bladder tumor. Cancer Res 1983;43:3231–3235.

90. Rivin BD, Longo FW, Tomashefsky P. Ultrasonic hyperthermia system for tumor irradiation. Med Instrum 1980;14:325–328.

91. Zhou L, Guo Y. In vivo effect of high energy shock waves on growth and metastasis of the heterografted tumors of nude mice. Chin Med J (Engl) 1996;109:157–161.

92. Ponsky L, Crownover M, Rosen M, et al. Initial evaluation of cyberknife technology for extracorporeal renal tissue ablation. Urology 2003;61:498–501.

93. Hussain M, Glass T, Forman J, et al. Combination cisplatin, 5-fluorouracil and radiation therapy in locally advanced unresectable or medically unfit bladder cancer patients: a Southwest Oncology Group Study. J Urol 2001;165:56–60.

94. Stein BS, Kendall AR. Lasers in urology. I. Laser physics and safety. Urology 1984;23:405–410.

95. Stein BS, Kendall AR. Lasers in urology. II. Laser therapy. Urology 1984;23:411–416.

# Perioperative instillation of chemotherapeutic drugs

29

*Willem Oosterlinck, Richard Sylvester*

## INTRODUCTION

### HISTORY

The instillation of a chemotherapeutic drug immediately after transurethral resection (TUR) is an old idea that was tested in the 1970s,[1,2] when thiotepa was used. Later, adriamycin and epodyl were also evaluated.[3,4] These first nonrandomized clinical trials suggested a reduction in the rate of tumor recurrence when a perioperative instillation was given. After these preliminary results, the need for properly conducted, large scale, randomized controlled studies became evident. The first important study of this kind came from the British Medical Research Council. Four hundred and seventeen patients with newly diagnosed superficial bladder tumors were treated with a complete TUR and then randomized into one of three groups.[5] Groups 1 and 2 received an instillation of 30 mg thiotepa at the time of TUR; thereafter patients in group 2 also received instillations of thiotepa every 3 months for a year, and group 3 was a control group that received no instillations at all. Neither the first publication of the MRC in 1985,[5] nor the second publication of the results in 1994[6] with a longer follow-up was able to show any differences in the recurrence rate in the three groups. However, subsequent randomized studies[7-14] have shown impressive improvements in the recurrence-free rate.

Despite the scientific evidence provided by these trials, a single immediate postoperative instillation has not become routine procedure in the urological world. The European Association of Urology guidelines were the first guidelines that advocated one single immediate instillation after TUR in all patients with superficial bladder tumors.[15] As one single instillation has been tested mainly in low-risk tumors, there was still doubt regarding the value of one immediate instillation in patients with multiple tumors at a higher risk for recurrence. There was also no consensus that all patients with a single, low-risk tumor should receive intravesical chemotherapy after the initial TUR. This was the reason for performing a meta-analysis of the published results of randomized clinical trials with one single immediate postoperative instillation of chemotherapy in patients with stage Ta–T1 bladder cancer.

## META-ANALYSIS OF EFFICACY

In their meta-analysis, Sylvester et al[16] included seven randomized trials (Table 29.1) with recurrence information on 1476 patients. After a median follow-up of 3.4 years and a maximum of 14.5 years, 267 of 728 patients (36.7%) receiving one postoperative instillation of epirubicin, mitomycin C, thiotepa, or pirarubicin had recurrences as compared with 362 of 748 patients (48.4%) with TUR alone (odds ratio [OR] = 0.61, p<0.0001). This meta-analysis has thus shown that one immediate instillation of chemotherapy after TUR decreases the relative risk of recurrence by 39% in patients with Ta–T1 bladder cancer (Figure 29.1).

Although the majority of the patients included in these randomized trials had a single tumor, both patients with a single tumor (OR = 0.61) and those with multiple tumors (OR = 0.44) benefited from a single instillation. However, after one instillation, 65.2% of the patients with multiple tumors had a recurrence compared with 35.8% of the patients with a single tumor, showing that one instillation alone is suboptimal treatment in patients

**Table 29.1** Meta-analysis of randomized trials

| First author | Year | Drug | Dosage | Duration (min) | Timing | Study arms | Eligible patients |
|---|---|---|---|---|---|---|---|
| Oosterlinck[9] | 1993 | Epirubicin | 80 mg/50 ml | 60 | Within 6 hours | 2 arms TUR + water | 402 |
| Ali-el-Dein[10] | 1997 | Epirubicin | 50 mg/50 ml | 120 | Immediately | 3 arms TUR alone, + 8 weekly epirubicin + monthly 1 year | 181 |
| Rajala[13] | 2002 | Epirubicin | 100 mg/100 ml | 120 | Immediately | 3 arms TUR alone, TUR + interferon-α2b | 200 |
| Tolley[8] | 1996 | Mitomycin C | 40 mg/40 ml | 60 | Within 24 hours | 3 arms TUR alone + mitomycin every 3 months, 1 year | 452 |
| Solsona[11] | 1999 | Mitomycin C | 30 mg/50 ml | 60 | Within 6 hours | 2 arms TUR alone | 131 |
| MRC[5] | 1995 | Thiotepa | 30 mg/50 ml | Unknown | Immediately | 3 arms TUR alone + 4 additional instillations | 379 |
| Okamura[14] | 2002 | Pirarubicin | 30 mg/30 ml | 60 | Within 6 hours | 2 arms TUR alone | 160 |

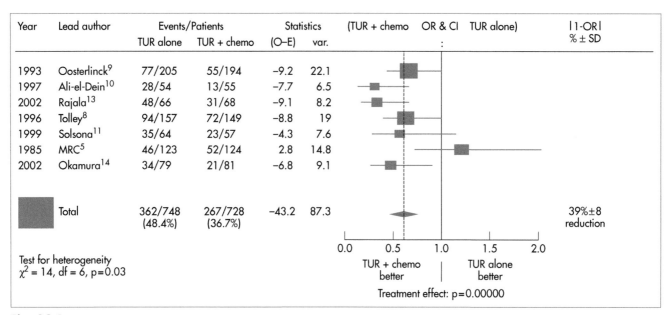

**Fig. 29.1**

Forest plot of the different studies used in the meta-analysis of Sylvester et al[16] on one single postoperative instillation of chemotherapy. (Chemo, chemotherapy; CI, confidence interval; O–E, observed minus expected number of recurrences; OR, odds ratio; SD, standard deviation; TUR, transurethral resection; Var, variation.) Reproduced from Sylvester R, Oosterlinck W, van der Meijden A. A single immediate postoperative instillation of chemotherapy decreases the risk of recurrence in patients with stage Ta T1 bladder cancer: a meta-analysis of published results of randomized clinical trials. Journal of Urology 2004;171:2181–2186, with permission from Lippincott Williams & Wilkins.

with multiple tumors. In a trial excluded from the meta-analysis because some patients received additional instillations before recurrence, Zincke et al also found that patients with multiple tumors benefited from an immediate instillation of thiotepa or adriamycin.[17] Defining risk groups according to whether the tumor was single or multiple, and incorporating the result of the first follow-up cystoscopy, Tolley et al found that the benefit of mitomycin C, in both treatment groups combined, was similar in low-, medium-, and high-risk cases.[8] Other subgroup analyses could not be done in the meta-analysis because of the absence of individual patient data, but the two other studies[9,13] in which they were performed suggest that the treatment is beneficial across all categories of patients.

## WORKING MECHANISM

The effect of one instillation may be explained either by the chemoresection of tumor left behind after an incomplete TUR or by destruction of circulating tumor cells that could implant at the site of the resection. Incomplete TUR may be an issue even in patients with solitary tumors as shown by the great variability between institutions in the recurrence rates at the first follow-up cystoscopy after TUR.[18] Oosterlinck et al[9] found that only one of the 10 patients that had residual tumors 1 month after TUR was in the group that received one instillation. Masters et al[19] found a 44% complete response rate in a marker lesion

3 months after one instillation of epirubicin. Thus one instillation can in fact eradicate tumor left behind during TUR.

Supporting the hypothesis of implantation of circulating tumor cells,[20] Whelan et al[21] found that postoperative irrigation with saline or glycine during 18 hours significantly prolonged the time to first recurrence, with a reduction of 17% in the relative risk of recurrence. Several animal experiments also support the hypothesis of tumor implantation at traumatized places in the bladder.[22,23]

## DURATION OF THE EFFECT

When reported, Kaplan–Meier time to first recurrence curves showed that the time point at which the treatment benefit starts varied somewhat between the studies: in three studies[9,11,13] there was a reduction in the percentage of patients with residual tumors at 1 month or with recurrence already at 3 months. In one study, the benefit appeared to start at 6 months[14]; however, in the remaining study,[8] the treatment effect appeared to start at 1 year. As suggested by Solsona et al,[11] the effect of one instillation appears to occur early on, mainly during the first 2 years, with a possible dilution of the treatment effect with longer-term follow-up. Use of the percentage of patients with recurrence, rather than considering the time to first recurrence, may, in fact, underestimate the size of the treatment effect. However, with long-term follow-up, it is clear that the use of one immediate instillation can prevent rather than simply delay recurrences.

## TIMING OF THE INSTILLATION

In all studies the instillation was given within 24 hours, generally either immediately after TUR or within 6 hours. Kaasinen et al[24] found a doubling in the risk of recurrence if the first of 5-weekly mitomycin C instillations was not given on the same day as the TUR in frequently recurring patients. In two European Organisation for Research and Treatment of Cancer (EORTC) trials,[25] in which patients received nine instillations of epirubicin or mitomycin C over 6 months, starting treatment on the day of TUR was more effective than starting 7–15 days later in patients who did not receive further maintenance after 6 months. In another study,[26] in which patients received 15 instillations of adriamycin or mitomycin C over 1 year, fewer patients randomized to start treatment within 6 hours had recurrence as compared with patients randomized to start treatment after 7–14 days, especially those on the mitomycin C arm. There is thus some evidence that the instillation should be given on the same day as the TUR and not later.

## INTRAVESICAL DRUGS

With the possible exception of the one study with thiotepa in which no difference was found,[5,6] the meta-analysis[16] suggests that no large differences in efficacy between the different chemotherapies exist. However, the study by Burnand et al,[1] which used 90 mg thiotepa in 100 ml rather than 30 mg in 50 ml as in the MRC study, found that one instillation of thiotepa significantly reduced the percentage of patients that had recurrence, as did Zincke et al[17] who used 60 mg thiotepa in 60 ml. This suggests that a lower concentration of thiotepa may be responsible for the lack of efficacy. However, the results from these two studies should be interpreted with caution.

The ideal drug or dosage of the other tested drugs cannot be derived from these studies. Epirubicin in concentrations from 1 to 2 mg/ml has been used with no obvious differences in the results. The same is observed for mitomycin C where concentrations between 0.6 and 1.0 mg/ml have been tested. Experts advise 40 mg over lower dosages because the concentration of the product is less influenced at a higher dose by the urine production which continues during bladder instillation. For epirubicin, 50 mg is considered to be sufficient, as higher doses have failed to show a better outcome in the perioperative setting as well as in other clinical trial designs with this drug.

## COST EFFECTIVENESS

One can expect that this early instillation gives protection against recurrence, especially in the first year, with a diminishing effect thereafter. Evaluating the first recurrence, 11.7 TURs were saved for every 100 patients treated. Thus the number needed to treat (NNT) to prevent one recurrence is $1/0.117 = 8.5$. Since the cost of a TUR, anesthesia, and hospitalization is probably more than 8.5 times that of one instillation in most countries, one instillation should be cost effective.

## TOXICITY

Despite the fact that no serious adverse effects have been mentioned in the reports published on immediate, adjuvant chemotherapy instillations, several reports have appeared on severe and prolonged complications due to leakage of the drug after an early intravesical instillation. Doherty at al[27] reported the local effects of an immediate instillation of chemotherapy (mainly epirubicin) in cystectomy specimens. It was associated with a more extensive necrosis of the bladder wall and fat necrosis of extravesical tissue than the usual muscle necrosis seen after TUR alone. An area of thin muscularis propria may undergo necrosis and result in secondary perforation. None of the 12 patients described by Doherty, however, reported local symptoms. In contrast, the effect of extravasation after intravenously administered chemotherapeutic drugs is well documented. It induces long-lasting necrosis, provoking pain and slowing the healing process. In 2003, a case of severe and long-lasting pain in the pelvic region due to extravasation of mitomycin C was reported.[28] A distal ureteral stenosis that was probably due to intravesical mitomycin C has also been described.[29,30] Undoubtedly, there is certainly an under-reporting of these complications as not every urologist that has seen such a complication is eager to report it. In any event, urologists should be aware of the potential risk of extravasation of chemotherapeutic drugs and its consequences.

Bacillus Calmette–Guérin (BCG) must *never* be used in the perioperative setting as the open wounds of the mucosa can provoke BCG septicemia, and for this reason it has never been tested in these circumstances.

## PRECAUTIONS

If there is a possibility of perforation or after an extended TUR, an immediate instillation should not be given. In cases where there is the possibility of intraperitoneal leakage or important resorption from the extravesical space, it seems advisable not to use a dose greater than the dose that is acceptable as one single intravenous injection. Indeed, one case of myelosuppression has been described when 80 mg of mitomycin C was retained for 2 hours after TUR of a large tumor.[31] It seems prudent to advise a 1-hour retention time and to rinse the bladder actively to ascertain a good free flow of the urine afterwards, and to avoid any overdistension during or immediately after the chemotherapy instillation. Nevertheless, it is clear from the review of the literature that one immediate instillation after TUR is an adjuvant treatment that adds hardly any morbidity to the operation itself. Nearly all patients already have a catheter after TUR and, if local regional anesthesia is used, patients will not suffer from any additional discomfort. The reluctance to use this treatment strategy should be reconsidered since the potential benefits clearly outweigh the possible risks and costs.

## CONCLUSIVE RECOMMENDATIONS ON PERIOPERATIVE INSTILLATIONS

- One instillation with mitomycin C or epirubicin can reduce the recurrence rate by about 40% in single as well as in multiple Ta–T1 bladder tumors, and is thus recommended for all types of papillary superficial bladder cancer. It is *not* indicated in invasive tumors.

- Doses of 40 mg mitomycin C and 50 mg epirubicin are advocated. Higher doses increase the risk of side effects and cost without increasing efficacy.
- After an extensive resection, and in cases of obvious or suspected perforation of the bladder, it is prudent not to instill the bladder as extravasation can provoke annoying and even dangerous complications (expert opinion, a few case reports).
- It is advocated to give the instillation the same day as the TUR as it is probably insufficient the day afterwards.
- Further adjuvant intravesical therapy is indicated in multiple tumors, as one single instillation is insufficient treatment in these patients.

## REFERENCES

1. Burnand K, Boyd P, Mayo M, Shuttleworth K, Lloyd-Davies R. Single dose intravesical thiotepa as an adjuvant to cystodiathermy in the treatment of transitional cell bladder carcinoma. Br J Urol 1976;48:55–59.
2. Garrett J, Lewis R, Meehan W, Leblanc G. Intravesical thiotepa in the immediate post-operative period in patients with recurrent transitional cell carcinoma of the bladder. J Urol 1978;120:410–411.
3. Abrams P, Choa R, Gaches C, Ashken M, Green N. A controlled trial of single dose intravesical adriamycin in superficial bladder tumours. Br J Urol 1981;53:585–587.
4. Kurth K, Maksimovic P, Hop W, Schroder F, Bakker N. Single dose intravesical epodyl after TUR of Ta TCC bladder carcinoma. World J Urol 1983;1:89.
5. MRC Working Party on Urological Cancer. The effect of intravesical thiotepa on the recurrence rate of newly diagnosed superficial bladder cancer. An MRC Study. Br J Urol 1985;57:680–685.
6. Medical Research Council Working Party on Urological Cancer, Subgroup on Superficial Bladder Cancer. The effect of intravesical thiotepa on tumor recurrence after endoscopic treatment of newly diagnosed superficial bladder cancer. A further report with long-term follow-up of a Medical Research Council randomized trial. Br J Urol 1994;73:632–638.
7. Tolley D, Hargreave T, Smith P, et al. Effect of intravesical mitomycin C on recurrence of newly diagnosed superficial bladder cancer: interim report from the Medical Research Council Subgroup on Superficial Bladder Cancer (Urological Cancer Working Party). Br Med J 1988;296:1759–1761.
8. Tolley D, Parmar M, Grigor K, Lallemand G, and the Medical Research Council Superficial Bladder Cancer Working Party. The effect of intravesical mitomycin C on recurrence of newly diagnosed superficial bladder cancer: a further report with 7 years of follow-up. J Urol 1996;155:1233–1238.
9. Oosterlinck W, Kurth K, Schröder F, Bultinck J, Hammond B, Sylvester R. A prospective European Organisation for Research and Treatment of Cancer Genitourinary Group randomized trial comparing transurethral resection followed by a single intravesical instillation of epirubicin or water in single stage Ta, T1 papillary carcinoma of the bladder. J Urol 1993;149:749–752.
10. Ali-el-Dein B, Nabeeh A, el-Baz M, Shamaa S, Ashamallah A. Single dose versus multiple instillations of epirubicin as prophylaxis for recurrence after transurethral resection of pTa and pT1 transitional cell bladder tumors: a prospective randomized controlled study. Br J Urol 1997;79:731–735.
11. Solsona E, Iborra I, Ricos J, Monros J, Casanova J, Dumont R. Effectiveness of a single immediate mitomycin C instillation in patients with low risk superficial bladder cancer: short and long-term follow-up. J Urol 1999;161:1120–1123.
12. Rajala P, Liukkonen T, Raitanen M, et al. Transurethral resection with perioperative instillation of interferon-alpha or epirubicin for the prophylaxis of recurrent primary superficial bladder cancer: a

prospective randomized multicenter study—FinnBladder III. J Urol 1999;161:1133–1135; discussion 1135–1136.

13. Rajala P, Kaasinen E, Raitanen M, Liukkonen T, Rintala E, the FinnBladder Group. Perioperative single dose instillation of epirubicin or interferon-alpha after transurethral resection for the prophylaxis of primary superficial bladder cancer recurrence: a prospective randomized multicenter study—FinnBladder III long-term results. J Urol 2002;168:981–985.

14. Okamura K, Ono Y, Kinukawa T, et al. Randomized study of single early instillation of (2″R)-4′-O-tetrahydropyranyl-doxorubicin for a single superficial bladder carcinoma. Cancer 2002;94:2363–2368.

15. Oosterlinck W, Lobel B, Jakse G, Malmstrom P, Stockle M, Sternberg C. The EAU Working Group on Oncological Urology. Guidelines on bladder cancer. Eur Urol 2002;41:105–112.

16. Sylvester R, Oosterlinck W, van der Meijden A. A single immediate postoperative instillation of chemotherapy decreases the risk of recurrence in patients with stage Ta T1 bladder cancer: a meta-analysis of published results of randomized clinical trials. J Urol 2004;171:2181–2186.

17. Zincke H, Utz D, Taylor W, Myers R, Leary F. Influence of thiotepa and doxorubicin instillation at time of transurethral surgical treatment of bladder cancer on tumor recurrence: a prospective, randomized, double-blind, controlled trial. J Urol 1983;129:505–509.

18. Brausi M, Collette L, Kurth K, et al. Variability in the recurrence rate at first follow-up cystoscopy after TUR in stage Ta T1 transitional cell carcinoma of the bladder: a combined analysis of seven EORTC studies. Eur Urol 2002;41:523–531.

19. Masters J, Popert M, Thompson P, Gibson D, Coptcoat M, Parmar M. Intravesical chemotherapy with epirubicin: a dose–response study. J Urol 1999;161:1490–1493.

20. Soloway M, Masters S. Urothelial susceptibility to tumor cell implantation: influence of cauterization. Cancer 1980;46:1158–1163.

21. Whelan P, Griffiths G, Stower M, et al. Preliminary results of a MRC randomised controlled trial of post-operative irrigation of superficial bladder cancer. Proceedings of the American Society of Clinical Oncology 2001;20:Abstract 708.

22. Weldon T, Soloway M. Susceptibility of urothelium to neoplastic cellular implantation. Urology 1975;5:824–826.

23. Pan J, Slocum H, Rustum Y, Greco W, Gaeta J, Huben R. Inhibition of implantation of murine bladder tumor by thiotepa in cauterized bladder. J Urol 1989;142:1589–1593.

24. Kaasinen E, Rintala E, Hellstrom P, et al. Factors explaining recurrence in patients undergoing chemoimmunotherapy regimens for frequently recurring superficial bladder carcinoma. Eur Urol 2002;42:167–174.

25. Bouffioux C, Kurth K, Bono A, et al. Intravesical adjuvant chemotherapy for superficial transitional cell bladder carcinoma: results of 2 European Organisation for Research and Treatment of Cancer randomized trials with mitomycin C and doxorubicin comparing early versus delayed instillations and short-term versus long-term treatment. J Urol 1995;153:934–941.

26. Iborra J, Ricos J, Monros J, et al. Resultados de un estudio de quimioprofilaxis intravesical, prospectivo, doble aleatorio, entre dos drogas: la adriamicina y el mitomycin; y dos modos de iniciar las instilaciones: precoz y tardio. Efecto sobre la recidiva y la progression, Arch Esp de Urol 1992;45:1001.

27. Doherty A, Trendell Smith N, Stirling R, Rogers H, Bellringer J. Perivesical fat necrosis after adjuvant intravesical chemotherapy. BJU Int 1999;83:420–423.

28. Nieuwenhuijzen J, Bex A, Horenblas S. Unusual complication after immediate postoperative intravesical mitomycin C instillation. Eur Urol 2003;43:711–712.

29. Oehlschlager S, Loessnitzer A, Froehner M, et al. Distal urethral stenosis after early adjuvant intravesical mitomycin C application for superficial bladder cancer. J Urol Int 2003;70:74–76.

30. Oddens J, van der Meyden A, Sylvester R. One immediate postoperative instillation of chemotherapy in low risk Ta, T1 bladder cancer patients. Is it always safe? Eur Urol 2004;46:336–338.

31. Tawkif A, Neal F, Hong K. Bone marrow suppression after intravesical mitomycin C treatment. J Urol 1986;13:459–460.

# The role of intravesical chemotherapy in the treatment of bladder cancer

# 30

*S Bruce Malkowicz*

## INTRODUCTION

Intravesical chemotherapy has been a classic approach to the treatment of nonmuscle-invasive superficial bladder cancer for several decades. Early investigations confirmed the impression that recurrence rates were decreased by this method of therapy, yet aggregate data from many trials were necessary in order to better quantitate this effect and evaluate the potential of such treatment to affect tumor progression. Although multiple agents have been employed over time, there has been a general collapse of the treatment menu over the past several years with the introduction of bacillus Calmette–Guérin (BCG) therapy. During this time, efforts to decrease tumor recurrence in an optimal fashion using immediate postoperative instillation of these agents have been validated, and further techniques to optimize administration and drug delivery have been under development. As our understanding of the appropriate role for intravesical chemotherapy has emerged, newer agents, which have demonstrated activity in advanced disease, are being tested for their applicability in this area.

## PRINCIPLES OF PRACTICE

The theoretical goals of intravesical chemotherapy are threefold: 1) the eradication of residual disease; 2) prophylaxis against tumor recurrence; and 3) the delay or abrogation of tumor progression. The eradication of residual disease is a desirable attribute of an intravesical agent. Recent studies evaluating small marker tumors demonstrate this attribute in principle, yet larger volume and higher stage disease is less susceptible to drug mechanisms of action. Intravesical chemotherapy is not particularly suitable to the treatment of unresected disease.[1]

The goal of reducing tumor recurrence with intravesical chemotherapy has been documented by multiple, well-conducted clinical trials and several meta-analyses. Short-term impact is demonstrated as a 14% to 17% decrease in tumor recurrence, yet over 3–5 years this reduced to approximately 7%.[2,3] The instillation of chemotherapeutic agents shortly after transurethral resection may be the most effective method of capitalizing on the prophylactic effect. Several studies and a recent meta-analysis suggest an up to 37% decrease in tumor recurrence with this practice.[4] This topic is discussed in the previous chapter.

The value of maintenance therapy with chemo-therapeutic agents is negligible. Although some impact on early recurrence may be suggested in some studies, a long-term impact is not demonstrated, especially in carcinoma in situ or larger lesions.[5,6]

The impact of intravesical chemotherapy on tumor progression can unfortunately be stated rather tersely—the current available data demonstrate no advantage with regard to tumor progression survival with the use of this modality.[3] In an evaluation of six large European trials, involving a total of 2535 patients with a median survival follow-up of 7.8 years, no long-term effect of prophylactic therapy was noted.

## PHARMACOLOGIC CONSIDERATIONS

The principal aspect of intravesical chemotherapy is the physical diffusion of the agent into the layers of the bladder. The efficiency of this process is affected by many attributes of the bladder wall, the urine environment, and the nature of the agent. Chemotherapeutic agents must first cross the glycosaminoglycan layer of bladder mucosa and then diffuse through the urothelial cells. Once the lamina propria is reached and then the muscularis propria, there is rich vascularity which results in a decline in drug concentration in a semilogarithmic fashion.[7]

Urine volume affects drug concentration, which has an influence on the diffusion factors mentioned above. Drug concentration can be manipulated by controlling the state of dehydration. Additionally, the chemical nature of these agents can affect their ability to attain maximal contact with a lesion such as the lipophilic properties or overall molecular weight of the agent.

## GENERAL AGENTS

### MITOMYCIN C

Mitomycin C (MMC) is an alkylating agent which, through crosslinking, inhibits DNA synthesis. It is felt to be cell cycle nonspecific, although it is most sensitive in the late G1 phase. It has a molecular weight of 334 kD and has negligible systemic absorption. The average benefit in decreasing tumor recurrence in the prophylactic setting is approximately 15%.[2] There are no data to indicate that it has any impact on tumor progression over a 5-year period.[3] It has been used over a wide range of doses, and an attempt at optimization of therapy is described below.

The most frequent side effects of MMC include palmar rash or other cutaneous symptoms in up to 10%

of patients, and chemical cystitis in up to 40% of patients. Myelosuppression occurs in less than 0.5% of patients and bladder contracture is rare. Most symptoms abate with the cessation of drug use.

Mitomycin therapy has emerged as a standard agent in intravesical therapy because of its equivalent effect in tumor prophylaxis and its slightly increased activity in patients treated with BCG. Efforts to increase its clinical effectiveness have been evaluated by an attempt to optimize conditions of drug stability and drug concentration.[8] An optimization protocol by the international mitomycin C consortium restricted patients from fluid intake for 8 hours prior to and during treatment. They also received 1.3 g sodium bicarbonate the evening before, morning of, and 30 minutes prior to drug administration. The bladder was drained before drug administration and then evaluated with transabdominal ultrasound in order to reduce residual urine to ≤10 cc. It was demonstrated that bladder emptying by catheter was not uniformly efficient for all patients. The dwell time was 2 hours.

Optimized patients (119) were treated with 40 mg mitomycin diluted in 20 cc, while standard therapy patients (111) received 20 mg mitomycin diluted in 20 cc, thereby doubling the concentration in the optimized arm (Figure 30.1). Dysuria occurred more frequently in the optimization group but did not lead to a greater number of treatment discontinuations. There was an increased median time to recurrence of 29.1 months (95% CI: 14–44 months) versus 11.8 months (95% CI: 7.2–16 months), p=0.005, as well as a greater percentage of recurrence-free patients: 41% (95% CI: 30.9–51.1%) versus 24.6% (95% CI: 14.9–34.3%), p=0.002 in the optimization arm. While it is not possible to say if the optimization of a single variable

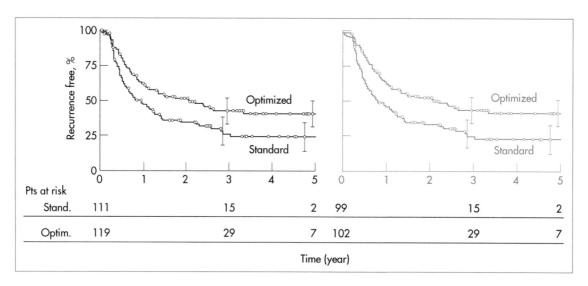

**Fig. 30.1**
Kaplan–Meier curves of (*left*) intent-to-treat and (*right*) evaluable groups for those patients treated with an optimized or standard course of mitomycin C. At 5 years, approximately 43% of optimized patients and 24% of standard patients were recurrence free in either analysis. Reproduced with permission from Au et al.[8]

(drug dose) might be sufficient to lead to overall optimization of outcomes, such a protocol demonstrates an attempt to achieve the best results possible with intravesical chemotherapeutic agents. More elaborate methods to increase drug effectiveness will be discussed later.

## DOXORUBICIN

Doxorubicin is an anthracycline antibiotic that binds DNA base pairs and inhibits topoisomerase II as well as protein synthesis. It has a high molecular weight (580 kD) and virtually no systemic absorption. Chemical cystitis can occur in 25% to 50% of patients, and less common side effects include gastrointestinal reactions, allergic reactions, and reduced bladder capacity.[9] Multiple studies demonstrate prophylaxis in reducing the recurrence probability by 15% but no impact on progression.[2,10] The usual dosage is 30–100 mg given weekly for several weeks.

## EPIRUBICIN

Epirubicin is an anthracycline derivative of doxorubicin with a similar mechanism of action. It has a molecular weight of 579.8 kD, and has been administered in different treatment schedules at a dosage of 30–80 mg. The advantage over transurethral resection (TUR) alone for tumor prophylaxis is in the expected range of 12% to 15%.[11] It is effective as a single dose agent immediately after TUR and may be more effective with a higher cumulative dose.[12,13] It can be effective in intermediate risk patients.[14] There are few systemic side effects (<5% in most series), and chemical cystitis, which is dose dependent, occurs in approximately 15% of patients.

## VALRUBICIN

Valrubicin is a semisynthetic analog of doxorubicin. It has a rapid uptake in cancer cells due to its lipophilic structure. This agent inhibits topoisomerase II and causes cell-cycle arrest in G2. The general dosage is 800 mg, and, in a mixed population of superficial lesions, a 40% initial response rate was noted.[15] In a population of BCG-refractory patients, a 21% response rate was noted with a median time to recurrence greater than 18 months.[16] This agent is currently approved for those patients that are BCG refractory and cannot tolerate a cystectomy.

## THIOTEPA (TRIETHYLENE THIOPHOSPHORAMIDE)

Thiotepa is the classic intravesical agent, which acts as an alkylating agent and is not cell cycle specific. In multiple trials it has demonstrated its effectiveness for tumor prophylaxis (mean decrease over TUR, 16%) and no capacity to affect progression. It has a molecular weight of 189 kD. Because of its low molecular weight it clearly demonstrates a significant level of systemic absorption, which can result in hematologic side effects. Therefore, weekly monitoring of the complete blood count and platelet count is necessary during a treatment course. Local irritation can occur in 12% to 69% of patients. Thrombocytopenia is seen in 3% to 13% of patients and leukopenia in 8% to 55% of patients. The usual dose is 30 mg in 15 ml of sterile water.

## GEMCITABINE

Gemcitabine is a novel deoxycytidine analog (2′,2′-difluoro-2′deoxycytidine), which has demonstrated significant activity in advanced bladder cancer as a single agent and in combination.[17] It has a molecular weight of 299.66 kD, and its active metabolite is incorporated into DNA, thus inhibiting synthesis. It may also inhibit cytidine deaminase and ribonucleotide reductase as a component of its anticancer mechanism. Preclinical studies have suggested its value for intravesical therapy, and several phase I and phase II studies suggest its safety and general efficacy.[18–21]

Preclinical studies demonstrated no systemic absorption, immunosuppression, or histologic damage to normal urothelium.[22] In a phase I study of patients with low-grade, low-stage disease, a dose range of 1000–2000 mg gemcitabine demonstrated low or absent systemic absorption and the presence of the inactive metabolite difluorodeoxyuridine in very low levels as well, suggesting minimal accumulation of drug in the systemic circulation. Dysuria, headache, and fatigue were reported, but there was no dose-limiting toxicity (DLT).[22] Fifty percent of patients experienced no recurrences over a short period of follow-up (12 months). A similar lack of DLT at 2000 mg was noted in another phase I trial.

In a cohort of BCG-refractory patients, gemcitabine was administered twice weekly from 500 to 2000 mg. Of 18 patients, 7 had a complete response, 4 patients had a mixed response (persistent positive cytology), 3 patients demonstrated a skin reaction, and 1 patient had grade 3 thrombocytopenia and neutropenia without infection or DLT at 2000 mg.[20] In another phase I trial of 15 patients treated with between 500 and 2000 mg, gemcitabine was undetectable in the plasma of patients until the 2000 mg dose level, and then it was present (≤1 mcg/ml) only transiently. Plasma difluoro-deoxyuridine (dFdU) levels implied absorption of 0.5% to 5.5% of the instilled dose. At 12 weeks, 9 of 13 evaluable patients were recurrence-free.[21] These studies have suggested that gemcitabine at 40 mg/ml (2000 mg in 50 ml saline solution) weekly for 6 weeks is a reasonable dose for further phase II testing.

In one phase II study of 39 superficial disease patients (30 previously treated with intravesical therapy), 56% of patients demonstrated a complete response to a marker tumor, and no progression was noted among the nonresponders.[23] The majority of toxicity was grade I with dysuria as the most common finding (33% grade I, 5% grade II). Grade I hematologic complications were noted in 5% to 15% of patients.

The clinical evaluation of gemcitabine as an intravesical agent is ongoing in other phase II and phase III trials, and the above data suggest the validity of these endeavors. It remains to be seen if this agent provides any clinical advantage over the already available agents with respect to prophylaxis or tumor progression in general patients or in the refractory/salvage situation.

The molecular weight, dosage, mechanism of action, and side effects of these intravesical chemotherapy agents are summarized in Table 30.1.

## OTHER AGENTS

Additional agents studied in superficial bladder cancer include mitoxantrone, suramin, and paclitaxel.

### Mitoxantrone

Mitoxantrone is an anthracycline derivative similar to doxorubicin. It has been studied in several small trials at doses of 10–20 mg where its tolerability has been demonstrated.[24-26] In comparison to doxorubicin, there was no difference in general efficacy or time to recurrence.[27] It has had limited evaluation in the United States.

### Suramin

Suramin is a polysulfonated naphthylurea that inhibits DNA synthesis by various mechanisms, including growth factor inhibition. It is a very large molecule with minimal systemic absorption, and in phase I trials has been used in doses of up to 153 mg/ml with minimal side effects.[28,29] Recent in vivo studies suggest that this agent in low doses may act as a chemosensitizer for mitomycin C.[30]

### Paclitaxel

At present, taxanes are in early study for their potential use in superficial bladder cancer based on their activity in combination chemotherapy for advanced disease.[31]

## IMPROVED DRUG DELIVERY

Just as attempts to improve drug activity by avoiding dilution and increasing dwell time may have positive effects on overall outcomes, other techniques to augment drug delivery may allow for optimal outcomes with intravesical therapy for bladder cancer. Significant efforts are underway at this time to evaluate combined hyperthermia and chemotherapy, as well as studies to increase drug penetration with electromotive administration (EMDA).

The ability to enhance drug delivery to bladder tissue by the means of electric current has been demonstrated in vitro,[32,33] and tested clinically by several investigators.[32-35] Electromotive administration employs iontophoresis and electrophoresis to improve transportation of the principal agent to the tissue. In this case the sodium chloride solute provides positive sodium ions, which are iontophoresed toward the tissue. Additionally, hydration shells containing the neutral MMC molecules are electrophorized, leading to a net accumulation of drug in the tissue. Phase II data (n=27) employing MMC demonstrated a similar marker tumor response rate (40%), and a longer disease-free interval (14.5 months versus 10 months) in those patients treated with EMDA.[34] The recurrence rate in those treated with EMDA was also lower (33% versus 66% without EMDA). In a recent study of 108 patients, those with multifocal carcinoma in situ, including 98 with T1 lesions, were randomized into groups receiving passive MMC, electromotive MMC, or BCG weekly for 6 weeks with a maintenance schedule.[33] The complete response rate at 3 months was 56% for BCG, 53% for electromotive MMC, and 28% for passive MMC. At 6

**Table 30.1** Intravesical chemotherapy agents

| Agent | Molecular weight (kD) | Dosage | Mechanism of action | Side effects |
|---|---|---|---|---|
| Thiotepa | 189 | 30 mg | Alkylating agent, cell cycle nonspecific | Thrombocytopenia, leukopenia, chemical cystitis |
| Mitomycin C | 334 | 20–40 mg | Alkylating agent, cell cycle nonspecific | Palmar rash, contact dermatitis, chemical cystitis |
| Doxorubicin | 580 | 30–100 mg | DNA base pair binding, topoisomerase II inhibition, protein synthesis inhibition | Chemical cystitis |
| Valrubicin | 585 | 800 mg | Similar to doxorubicin but more lipophilic | Chemical cystitis |
| Epirubicin | 579 | 30–80 mg | Doxycycline derivative | Chemical cystitis |
| Gemcitabine | 299.6 | 2000 mg | Deoxycytidine analog, inhibits DNA synthesis, inhibits cytidine deaminase | Chemical cystitis |

months the complete response rate for these three groups was 64%, 58%, and 31%, respectively. The median time to recurrence was 26 months for BCG, 35 months for electromotive MMC, and 19.5 months for passive MMC. With regard to kinetics, the peak plasma level was higher in the electromotive MMC (43 versus 8 ng/ml), and modeling demonstrated that approximately 50% of the dose was absorbed passively at 60 minutes, whereas with EMDA, more than 80% was absorbed by 30 minutes. No statistical difference was noted in toxicity between the MMC arms, yet there was a trend toward increased numbers and severity in the EMDA arm.

Another approach to enhance intravesical chemotherapy administration is the use of thermo-chemotherapy in which an endocavitary microwave applicator with thermocouples delivers hyperthermia (42.5°C) to the bladder wall, as the intravesical agent is in the bladder. The feasibility of such a system has been demonstrated, and early studies confirmed a significantly improved immediate response rate with this technology.[35] Pharmacokinetic studies demonstrate an increased yet safe plasma concentration of MMC with this technology.[36]

Clinical studies have shown that prophylaxis with MMC and microwave thermotherapy in Ta and T1 patients was superior to MMC alone at 24 months of follow-up.[37] All patients underwent a complete TUR, and approximately 40% of the patients in each group had received prior intravesical therapy. Eight weekly treatments and four monthly maintenance treatments were scheduled. Six (17.1%) versus 23 (57.5%) recurrences were noted among 75 of 83 patients divided into each treatment group (p= 0.002), hazard ratio 4.82 (95% CI: 1.95–11.9). In this study, 20 mg MMC was administered in 50 cc saline. In the passive arm, dwell time was 1 hour, whereas in the thermotherapy arm the instillation was for at least 40 minutes with the solution changed at 3 minutes.

Side effects were more common in the thermotherapy arm, with pelvic pain and posterior wall thermal reaction as the major differences. No patients terminated treatment because of pain. Additionally, one case of reduced bladder capacity with urge incontinence was noted in the thermotherapy group. While this study did not compare optimal MMC therapy to thermo-intravesical therapy, a clear improvement in prophylactic parameters was noted in the thermotherapy arm compared to the intravesical arm treated under similar parameters.

In another study of 52 patients with predominantly higher stage (40 T1) lesions, in an ablative protocol 21 of 28 patients had a complete response (CR). Four of these CR patients (19%) recurred during follow-up. At 15 months no stage progression to T2 was encountered in the entire cohort.[38] In a further study of higher risk superficial patients (n=90), no progression in stage or grade was noted at 24 months, and at 1 and 2 years the recurrence rate was 14.3% and 24.6%, respectively.[39] Smaller studies demonstrate similar results.[40]

Other methods investigated for improving drug delivery include the use of agents to increase bladder wall permeability such as hyaluronidase and dimethylsulfoxide (DMSO).[41,42] More recently, magnetically targeted carriers have been studied for their ability to effect local targeting of chemotherapy to specific bladder locations.[43]

## COMBINATION CHEMOTHERAPY

Although combination chemotherapy is regularly employed in the treatment of advanced transitional cell carcinoma, there is relatively scant literature regarding its use in the treatment of nonmuscle-invasive cancer. The rationale for novel combinations such as gemcitabine and doxorubicin are being studied in vitro.[44] In one study looking at a successive schedule of mitomycin (day 1) and doxorubicin (day 2) given weekly for 6 weeks, the initial complete response rate was 50%, and those patients on maintenance therapy had fewer recurrences in the short term.[45] Other studies demonstrate similar good initial responses but with an increase in local side effects.[46,47]

### REFERENCES

1. Bono AV, Hall RR, Denis JA, et al. Chemoresection in Ta–T1 bladder cancer. Members of the EORTC Genito-urinary group. Euro Urol 1996;29:35–39.
2. Lamm DL, Riggs DR, Traynelis CL, et al. Apparent failure of current intravesical chemotherapy prophylaxis to influence the long term course of superficial transitional cell carcinoma of the bladder. J Urol 1995;153:1444–1450.
3. Pawinski A, Sylvester R, Kurth KH, et al. A combined analysis of European Organization for Research and Treatment of Cancer and Medical Research Council randomized clinical trials for the prophylactic treatment of stage TaT1 bladder cancer. J Urol 1996;156:1934–1941.
4. Sylvester RJ, Oosterlinck W, van der Meijden APM. A single immediate postoperative instillation of chemotherapy decreases the risk of recurrence in patients with stage Ta T1 bladder cancer: a meta-analysis of published results of randomized clinical trials. J Urol 2004;171:2186–2190.
5. Bouffioux C, Kurth KH, Bono A, et al. Intravesical adjuvant chemotherapy for superficial transitional cell bladder carcinoma: results of 2 EORTC randomized trials with MMC and doxorubicin comparing early versus delayed instillations and short-term versus long-term treatment. J Urol 1995;153:934–941.
6. Hamdy FC, Hastie KJ, Kerry R, Williams JL. Mitomycin-C in superficial bladder cancer. Is long-term maintenance therapy worthwhile after initial treatment? Br J Urol 1993;71:183–186.
7. Dedrick RL, Flessier MF, Collin JM, Schultz D. Is the peritoneum a membrane? ASAIO J 1982;5:1–8.
8. Au L-S J, Badalament RA, Wientjes MG, Young DC, Warner JA. Methods to improve efficacy of intravesical Mitomycin C: results of a randomized phase III trial. J Natl Cancer Inst 2001;93(8):597–604.
9. Thrasher JV, Crawford ED. Complications of intravesical chemotherapy. Urol Clin North Am 1992;19:529–536.
10. Lamm DL, Blumenstein BA, Crawford ED, et al. A randomized trial of intravesical doxorubicin and immunotherapy with bacille

Calmette–Guérin for transitional cell carcinoma of the bladder. N Engl J Med 1991;325:1205–1209.

11. Onrust SV, Wiseman LR, Goa KL. Epirubicin: a review of its intravesical use in superficial bladder cancer. Drugs Aging 1999;15(4):307–333.

12. Rajala P, Kaasinen E, Raitanen M, et al. Perioperative single dose instillation of epirubicin or interferon-alpha after transurethral resection for the prophylaxis of primary superficial bladder cancer recurrence: a prospective randomized multicenter study—FinnBladder III long-term results. J Urol 2002;168(3):981–985.

13. Mitsumori K, Tsuchiya N, Habuchi T, et al. Early and large-dose intravesical instillation of epirubicin to prevent superficial bladder carcinoma recurrence after transurethral resection. BJU Int 2004;94(3):317–321.

14. Bassi P, Soinadin R, Longo F, et al. Delayed high-dose intravesical epirubicin therapy of superficial bladder cancer. A way to reduce the side effects and increase the efficacy—a phase 2 trial. Urol Int 2002;68(4):216–219.

15. Greenberg RE, Bahnson RR, Wood D, et al. Initial report on intravesical administration of N-triflouracetyladriamycin-14-valerate (AD-32) to patients with refractory superficial transitional cell carcinoma of the urinary bladder. Urology 1997;49:471–475.

16. Steinberg G, Bahnson R, Brosman S, et al. Efficacy and safety of valrubicin for the treatment of BCG refractory CIS of the bladder. J Urol 2000;163:761–767.

17. Von der Masse H, Hansen SE, Roberts JT, et al. Gemcitabine and cisplatin versus methotrexate, vinblastine, doxorubicin, and cisplatin in advanced or metastatic bladder cancer: results of a large randomized, multinational, multicenter, phase III study. J Clin Oncol 2000;19:2638–2646.

18. Nativ O, Dalal E, Laufer M, Sabo E, Aronson M. Antineoplastic effect of gemcitabine in an animal model of superficial bladder cancer. Urology 2004;64(4):845–848.

19. Cozzi PJ, Bajorin DF, Tong W, et al. Toxicology and pharmacokinetics of intravesical gemcitabine: a preclinical study in dogs. Clin Cancer Res 1999;(9):2629–2637.

20. Dalbagni G, Russo P, Sheinfeld J, et al. Phase I trial of intravesical gemcitabine in bacillus Calmette–Guérin-refractory transitional-cell carcinoma of the bladder. J Clin Oncol 2002;20(15):3193–3198.

21. Laufer M, Ramalingam S, Schoenberg MP, et al. Intravesical gemcitabine therapy for superficial transitional cell carcinoma of the bladder: a phase I and pharmacokinetic study. J Clin Oncol 2003;21(4):697–703.

22. Witjes JA, van der Heijen AG, Vriesema JL, et al. Intravesical gemcitabine: a phase I and pharmacokinetic study. Eur Urol 2004;45(2):182–186.

23. Gontero P, Casetta G, Maso G, et al. Phase II study to investigate the ablative efficacy of intravesical administration of gemcitabine in intermediate-risk superficial bladder cancer (SBC). Eur Urol 2004;46(3):339–343.

24. Flamm J, Donner G, Oberleitner S, Hausmann R, Havelec L. Adjuvant intravesical mitoxantrone after transurethral resection of primary superficial transitional cell carcinoma of the bladder. A prospective randomised study. Eur J Cancer 1995;31A(2):143–146.

25. Namasivayam S, Whelan P. Intravesical mitozantrone in recurrent superficial bladder cancer: a phase II study. Br J Urol 1995;75(6):740–743.

26. Yaman LS, Yardakul T, Zissis NP, Arikan N, Yasar B. Intravesical mitoxantrone for superficial bladder tumors. Anticancer Drugs 1994;5(1):95–98.

27. Huang JS, Chen WH, Lin CC, et al. A randomized trial comparing intravesical instillations of mitoxantrone and doxorubicin in patients with superficial bladder cancer. Chang Gung Med J 2003;26(2):91–97.

28. Ord JJ, Streeter E, Nones A, et al. Phase I trial of intravesical suramin in recurrent superficial transitional cell bladder carcinoma. Br J Cancer 2005;92(12):2140–2147.

29. Uchio EM, Linehan WM, Figg WD, Walther MM. A phase I study of intravesical suramin for the treatment of superficial transitional cell carcinoma of the bladder. J Urol 2003;169(1):357–360.

30. Xin Y, Lyness G, Chen D, et al. Low dose suramin as a chemosensitizer of bladder cancer to mitomycin C. J Urol 2005;174(1):322–327.

31. Vaughn DJ, Malkowicz SB, Zoltick B, et al. Paclitaxel plus carboplatin in advanced carcinoma of the urothelium: an active and tolerable outpatient regimen. J Clin Oncol 1998;16:255–260.

32. Di Stasi SM, Vespasiani G, Giannantoni A, et al. Electromotive delivery of mitomycin C into human bladder wall. Cancer Res 1997;57(5):875–880.

33. Di Stasi SM, Giannantoni A, Stephen RL, et al. Intravesical electromotive mitomycin C versus passive transport mitomycin C for high risk superficial bladder cancer: a prospective randomized study. J Urol 2003;170:777–782.

34. Brausi M, Campo B, Pizzocaro G, et al. Intravesical electromotive administration of drugs for treatment of superficial bladder cancer: a comparative phase II study. Urology 1998;1(3):506–509.

35. Colombo R, Brausi M, Da Pozzo LF, et al. Thermo-chemotherapy and electromotive drug administration of mitomycin C in superficial bladder cancer eradication. Eur Urol 2001;39:95–100.

36. Paroni R, Salonia A, Lev A, et al. Effect of local hyperthermia of the bladder on mitomycin C pharmacokinetics during intravesical chemotherapy for the treatment of superficial transitional cell carcinoma. Br J Clin Pharmacol 2001;52:273–278.

37. Colombo R, Da Pozzo LF, Salania A, et al. Multicentric study comparing intravesical chemotherapy alone and with local microwave hyperthermia for prophylaxis of recurrence of superficial transitional cell carcinoma. J Clin Oncol 2003;21(23):4270–4276.

38. Gofrit ON, Shapiro A, Pode D, et al. Combined local bladder hyperthermia and intravesical chemotherapy for the treatment of high-grade superficial bladder cancer. J Urol 2004;3(3):466–471.

39. Van der Heijden AG, Kiemeney LA, Gofrit ON, et al. Preliminary European results of local microwave hyperthermia and chemotherapy treatment in intermediate or high risk superficial transitional cell carcinoma of the bladder. Eur Urol 2004;46:65–72.

40. Moskovitz B, Meyer G, Kravtzov A, et al. Thermo-chemotherapy for intermediate or high-risk recurrent superficial bladder cancer patients. Ann Oncol 2005;16:585–589.

41. Hashimoto H, Tokunaka S, Sasaki M, et al. Dimethylsulfoxide enhances the absolution of chemotherapeutic drug instillation into the bladder. Urologic Res 20:233–36, 1992.

42. Maier U, Baumgartner G. Metaphylactic effect of mitomycin C with and without hyaluronidase after transurethral resection of bladder cancer. J Urol 1989;141:529–530.

43. Leakakos T, Ji C, Lawson G, Peterson C, Goodwin S. Intravesical administration of doxorubicin to swine bladder using magnetically targeted carriers. Cancer Chemother Pharmacol 2003;51:445–450.

44. Zoli W, Ricotti L, Tesei A, et al. Schedule-dependent cytotoxic interaction between epidoxorubicin and gemcitabine in human bladder cancer cells in vitro. Clin Cancer Res 2004;10(4):1500–1507.

45. Fukui I, Kihara K, Sekine H, et al. Intravesical combination chemotherapy with mitomycin C and doxorubicin for superficial bladder cancer: a randomized trial of maintenance versus no maintenance following a complete response. Cancer Chemother Pharmacol 1992;30(Suppl):37–40.

46. Sekine H, Fukui I, Yamada T, et al. Intravesical mitomycin C and doxorubicin sequential therapy for carcinoma in situ of the bladder: a longer follow-up result. J Urol 1994;151:27–30.

47. Isaka S, Okano T, Abe K, et al. Sequential instillation therapy with mitomycin C and adriamycin for superficial bladder cancer. Cancer Chemother Pharmacol 1992;30(Suppl):S41–44.

# Intravesical chemotherapy of superficial bladder cancer: optimization and novel agents

# 31

*Jessie L-S Au, M Guillaume Wientjes*

## INTRODUCTION

In evaluating treatment of superficial bladder cancer using intravesical chemotherapy, this chapter will explore the pharmacological basis of intravesical chemotherapy, the mathematics of drug transport in bladder tissues, the optimization of intravesical therapy using a computational approach to compare drug exposure in different parts of bladder tissues, current additional investigational and novel agents, and perspectives on future research.

## PHARMACOLOGIC BASIS OF INTRAVESICAL THERAPY

### CURRENT STATUS OF INTRAVESICAL CHEMOTHERAPY

The rationale for regional therapy is to expose tumors to high drug concentrations while minimizing the systemic exposure, thereby enhancing the treatment effect and reducing the host toxicity. The bladder is an ideal organ for regional chemotherapy.[1] The urethra provides easy and relatively noninvasive access for the introduction of therapeutic agents. The intact ureterovesical junction prevents reflux of these agents into the upper urinary tracts. The voluntary control of the external urinary sphincter provides the opportunity to control the dwell time, and the agents can be readily removed from the bladder during micturition.

The goals of intravesical chemo- or immunotherapy, used to treat nonmuscle-invasive bladder cancer since 1950s,[2] are to eradicate existing/residual tumor, prevent tumor recurrence, and prevent disease progression. Intravesical therapy is most effective when tumor burden is minimized by transurethral resection, and is most often used in high-risk patients (i.e. patients with large, multiple, poorly differentiated or recurrent tumors, Tis tumors, or tumors with nuclear p53 overexpression). Bacillus Calmette–Guérin (BCG) represents the agent of choice for immunotherapy (see Chapter 33). For chemotherapy, multiple agents, including thiotepa, mitomycin C (MMC),[3] doxorubicin, epodyl, tenoposide (VM-16), and cisplatin, have been evaluated. Of the 23 reported clinical trials involving more than 4000 patients, 13 showed statistically significant reduction in tumor recurrence (14% at 1–3 years benefit over transurethral resection alone), but not for disease progression.[4,5] Patient response to intravesical chemotherapy is highly variable, ranging from 2% to more than 50%.[6] The common adverse effect of these drugs is local cystitis and reduced bladder capacity. Thiotepa also produces bone marrow suppression in 10% of patients.

The Southwest Oncology Group showed that BCG produces a higher recurrence-free rate than MMC (e.g. 49% for BCG versus 34% for MMC after a 39-month median follow-up), but does not improve the reduction of disease progression rate, and shows a five-fold higher incidence of severe toxicities (cystitis, dysuria, hematuria, low-grade pyrexia).[7] About 10% of patients cannot tolerate BCG because of immunologic reactions.[8] BCG maintenance therapy for 3 years, while more effective than the 6-week induction therapy, is also more toxic.[9] In comparison, chemotherapy with MMC or doxorubicin, usually given as weekly treatments for 6 weeks, is equally effective when given for short or long durations (<5 months versus >3 years).[10] Intravesical chemotherapy has been and remains a popular treatment option.

## DETERMINANTS OF EFFICACY OF INTRAVESICAL CHEMOTHERAPY

In intravesical therapy, the bladder is emptied via catheterization and the drug is instilled and maintained, usually for 2 hours, after which time the patient is allowed to void. The treatment goal is to eliminate the malignant and premalignant cells located in the urine, on the luminal bladder surface, and/or in the bladder wall. As a very small fraction of the intravesical dose is absorbed from the bladder into the systemic circulation (with the exception of thiotepa),[11] systemic toxicity is usually not a concern. Hence, the delivery of drug to tumor cells and the response of tumor cells to the drug together determine the therapeutic outcome.

## PROCESSES GOVERNING THE DRUG DELIVERY TO DIFFERENT PARTS OF THE BLADDER

Our laboratory has established the pharmacokinetic models describing the drug concentration profiles, as a function of time and/or tissue depth, in different parts of the urinary bladder. These models, developed for several drugs (MMC, doxorubicin, 5-fluorouridine), have been validated in animals and/or human patients.[1,3,12–17]

Figure 31.1 shows the cross-section of a human urinary bladder, which consists of urothelium that lines the bladder cavity, lamina propria, and superficial and deep muscle layers. In the bladder cavity, the drug concentration changes as a function of time and urine volume (Equation 1).

$$\text{Urine pharmacokinetics: } C_u = \frac{\text{Dose}}{V_u} \cdot e^{-(k_a + k_d) \cdot t}$$

$$\text{where } V_u = V_0 + k_0 \cdot t + V_{res} \qquad \text{Equation 1}$$

$C_u$ depends on $V_u$ or the urine volume at time t, which in turn is determined by the volume of the dosing solution ($V_0$), residual urine volume $V_{res}$ at the time of drug instillation, and urine production during therapy ($k_0$ is production rate constant). $C_u$ also depends on drug absorption and degradation ($k_a$ and $k_d$ are the respective apparent rate constants). In patients, $V_{res}$ and $k_0$ are the major determinants of the drug exposure responsible for >90% of the intra- and interpatient variability, whereas drug absorption from the bladder and drug degradation are relatively minor determinants.[13]

The parameters in the urine pharmacokinetic model are determined by the treatment conditions such as patient dehydration status and urinary pH. For example, MMC is unstable at pH >8 and pH <5,[18,19] with a 10-times faster degradation in human urine at pH 5 than at pH 7.[13] Both thiotepa and its active metabolite tepa are stable in alkaline medium (pH 8.4), but are completely degraded in 30 minutes at acidic pH of 4.2.[20,21] Urinary pH also affects the ionization status and thereby affects the passive diffusion of acidic and basic drugs across the urothelium.[22] Additionally, abnormalities of the mucosal surface that occur with widespread tumor formation, inflammation, or mucosal denudation may increase drug absorption.[23] Damage to the bladder by acute cystitis or experimental procedures such as electrocoagulation enhance the absorption of doxorubicin and cisplatin in rats,[24,25] and increased extent of tumor involvement enhances the absorption of thiotepa in patients.[11] Administration of MMC within 6 days after transurethral resection also enhances the systemic absorption compared to later administration.[26] An increased urine volume unfolds the bladder, increases the surface area and reduces the thickness of the distendable bladder wall, resulting in increases of drug partition across the urothelium and systemic absorption of doxorubicin in rats.[25] In patients, the instillation volume may affect the drug contact to the lower half of the posterior wall of the bladder adjoining the trigone, which is usually folded by abdominal pressure.[27]

Drug penetration from urine into bladder tissues consists of two processes. The first process is partitioning

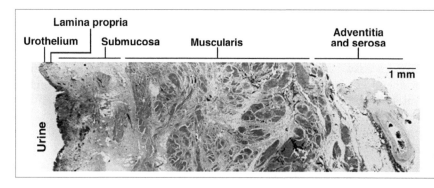

**Fig. 31.1**

Cross-section of a human urinary bladder. Adapted with permission from Wientjes et al.[1]

from urine, presumably by diffusion, across the bladder urothelium, which is not perfused by blood and is the absorption barrier.[28,29] Fick's first law describes the effect of physicochemical and physiologic variables on drug absorption across a single homogeneous diffusion barrier (Equation 2).

$$\text{Across the urothelium: Diffusion rate} = \frac{DKA(C_u - C_{uro})}{h} = k_a V_u C_u \qquad \text{Equation 2}$$

$C_{uro}$ is the concentration at the interface between the urothelium and the deep tissues; D is the drug diffusion coefficient (dependent on the ionization and lipophilicity of the drug); K is the drug partition coefficient; and h and A are the thickness and surface area of the urothelium. The decline in drug concentration across the urothelium is linear with depth. The $C_{uro}:C_u$ ratio indicates the extent of partitioning.

After crossing the urothelium, the drug is transported through the deeper tissues that are perfused by capillaries, a process described by the distributed model.[1,14,15,17] The concentration in tissue declines from $C_{uro}$ to the averaged free drug concentration in blood ($C_b$). $C_{depth}$ is the concentration at a particular tissue depth. A fraction of the drug proportional to ($C_{depth} - C_b$) is removed via absorption into the blood each time the drug encounters a capillary. As the number of capillaries increases with the distance traveled, $C_{depth}$ declines exponentially with respect to tissue depth at a rate equal to half-width ($w_{1/2}$), which is the tissue thickness over which the concentration declines by 50% (Equation 3). Note that a smaller $w_2$ indicates a steeper concentration decline across the tissue and that $C_u$ determines $C_{uro}$ and, therefore, $C_{depth}$

$$\text{Beyond the urothelium: } C_{depth} = (C_{uro} - C_b) \cdot e^{-(0.693/w_{1/2})(\text{depth} - \text{urothelial thickness})} + C_b \qquad \text{Equation 3}$$

Equations 2 and 3 provide the basis to identify the drugs that will show favorable bladder tissue delivery. This is illustrated by computer simulations that compare the tissue concentration–depth profiles of drugs with different parameters. Thiotepa was used as an example of a lipophilic compound that is rapidly and extensively absorbed into the systemic circulation.[11] Lipophilic compounds partition readily across cell membranes (hence a $C_{uro}:C_u$ ratio of 1), and are readily absorbed into the blood circulation (hence a q or blood flow-limited removal). Using a q of 95 ml/min/100 g for the bladder flow in the rat,[30] and D=0.3 × 10^-6 cm²/sec (approximated on the basis of the molecular weight of thiotepa),[31] the calculated $w_2$ (equals 0.693 (D/q)½) for thiotepa is 30 μm. For comparison, we used MMC or doxorubicin, both of which are more hydrophilic, and showed a much lower $C_{uro}:C_u$ ratio of about 1:30 and a much longer w½ of about 500 μm (experimentally determined in dogs and humans).[1,16,17] Results of the simulations indicate that, in spite of the 30-fold higher

partition across the urothelium, the more lipophilic drug showed lower concentrations in most parts of the bladder tissues (Figure 31.2). This is due to the rapid drainage of the highly lipophilic drug into the capillaries. The latter will also result in higher systemic blood concentrations and compromise the bladder targeting advantage. The ideal compound for intravesical therapy should have well-balanced lipophilic and hydrophilic properties so that it can readily partition across the urothelium, but is not rapidly absorbed into the capillaries.

## HETEROGENEITY IN CHEMOSENSITIVITY OF HUMAN BLADDER TUMORS

The response of human tumors to chemotherapeutic agents was evaluated using three-dimensional (3D) histocultures of tumors from individual patients. The major advantage of this experimental system is the maintenance of intra- and interpatient heterogeneity of drug response.[32,33] The chemosensitivity varied significantly between tumors; the drug concentrations producing 90% inhibition of DNA synthesis showed a >40-fold variation for MMC, >100-fold for doxorubicin, 40-fold for 5-fluorouridine, and 430-fold for paclitaxel.[14,34,35] In general, these effective drug concentrations are 10–100 times higher than those in monolayer cultures of human bladder tumor cells.[36-38] This significant intertumor heterogeneity in chemo-

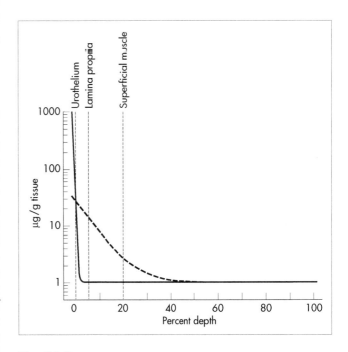

**Fig. 31.2**

Effects of physicochemical properties of a drug on its bladder tissue penetration. Computer simulations for lipophilic (solid line) and hydrophilic (broken line) compounds, using equal initial values of $C_u$ of 1000 μg/ml and $C_b$ of 1 μg/ml.

sensitivity represents a potential cause of the variable and incomplete patient response.

For MMC, the tumor sensitivity was inversely correlated with tumor malignancy, with greater activity in well-differentiated superficial tumors, and lesser activity in undifferentiated, invasive, and more rapidly proliferating tumors.[39] MMC activity is also positively correlated with the expression of its two activating enzymes: DT diaphorase (also named NQO1 or NAD(P)H:quinone oxidoreductase) and cytochrome p450 reductase.[40-49]

# OPTIMIZATION OF INTRAVESICAL CHEMOTHERAPY

## OVERVIEW

The following example illustrates our experience using a computational approach to compare the drug exposure in different parts of bladder tissues (where tumors reside) with the exposure required for drug effects, in order to predict the treatment outcome and, more importantly, to synthesize an optimal MMC treatment regimen that was predicted to nearly double its efficacy (detailed in Wientjes et al[50]).

## DRUG EXPOSURE AT TARGET TUMOR SITES

We studied the pharmacokinetics of MMC in plasma and urine of patients treated by intravesical therapy (10 patients receiving a total of 28 treatments), and the tissue pharmacokinetics in cystectomy patients and in animals (dogs and rabbits). The plasma pharmacokinetic data indicate insignificant MMC absorption into the systemic circulation. The urine and bladder tissue pharmacokinetic data were analyzed using Equations 1–3 to obtain the values of the model parameters ($V_{res}$, $k_0$ and $k_a + k_d$ for the urine pharmacokinetic model; $C_u$:$C_{uro}$ ratio, $C_u$:$C_b$ ratio, and $w^{1/2}$ for the tissue pharmacokinetic model). Note that alterations of the urine pharmacokinetic parameters will alter the $C_u$ and, therefore, the $C_{uro}$ and the CxT values in different parts of the bladder.

## DRUG EXPOSURE REQUIRED FOR ACTIVITY

Results of the MMC pharmacodynamics in 3D histocultures of patient bladder tumors indicated a >40-fold variation in tumor sensitivity. As other investigators reported higher MMC activity at acidic pH in monolayer cultures of human tumor cells,[51-54] we investigated the effect of pH on MMC activity in 3D cultures and found that the 10-fold higher activity at acidic pH compared to neutral pH was observed in monolayer cells but not in

either multilayer cultures of the same tumor cell line or histocultures of patient tumors, because of the slow equilibration between intracellular and extracellular pHs in multilayered systems (requiring at least 8 hours).[38]

## TRANSLATING IN VITRO PHARMACODYNAMICS TO IN VIVO TREATMENT EFFECT

The common denominator between in vitro and in vivo pharmacodynamics is the drug exposure under these two conditions. Equation 4 describes the relationship between drug concentration C, exposure time T, and the resulting pharmacologic effect.

$$C^n \times T = \text{effect} \qquad \text{Equation 4}$$

When n equals 1, the concentration and the exposure time are equally important in determining the effect. Concentration is more important when n is larger than 1, and time is more important when n is smaller than 1. The n value can be determined from the in vitro pharmacodynamics attained at various exposure times. To accommodate the differences in the drug concentration—time profiles under in vitro conditions (where drug concentrations remain relatively constant) and in vivo conditions (where concentrations change with time), $C^n$xT can be calculated as the time integral of $C^n$ over time (Equation 5). For MMC, the average n value was 1.24, and statistical analysis indicated that the pharmacodynamics of one-half of the 30 patient tumors were better described by an n value of 1.24, while the other half was better described by an n of 1.

$$C^n \times T = \int_0^T C^n \times dT \qquad \text{Equation 5}$$

## INTEGRATION OF PHARMACOKINETICS AND PHARMACODYNAMICS TO ESTABLISH THE PHARMACOLOGIC BASIS OF VARIABLE AND INCOMPLETE RESPONSE TO INTRAVESICAL MMC

Figure 31.3 shows the three CxT-tissue depth profiles of MMC simulated using the highest, average, and lowest $C_u$ values obtained from patients. Also shown are the drug exposures producing 90% inhibition of DNA synthesis in 30 human bladder tumors ($C^n$xT$_{90}$), placed according to the anatomical location of the tumors (e.g. Ta and T1 tumors are located on the urothelium and lamina propria, or a tissue depth of 200 and 700 μm, respectively). The probability of tumors receiving $C^n$xT$_{90}$ was 90% for Ta and 17% for T1 at the highest CxT-depth profile, 22% for Ta and 0% for T1 tumors at the average profile, and 0% for Ta and T1 tumors at the lowest profile. Note that none of the T2, T3 and T4 tumors would receive $C^n$xT$_{90}$. These data suggest that the large intra- and intersubject variability in urine/tissue pharmacokinetics and tumor chemosensitivity

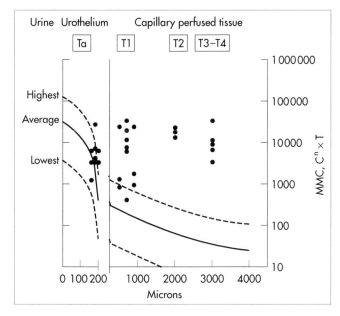

**Fig. 31.3**
Treatment efficacy simulations based on bladder wall concentrations and tumor chemosensitivity. Simulated bladder-wall tissue $C^n \times T$ versus depth profiles based on the highest, average, and lowest urine concentration profiles obtained from patients. $C^n \times T_{90}$ (●) values were calculated from the $IC_{90}$ using equation 5 and an n value of 1.24. Adapted with permission from Wientjes et al.[50]

contribute to the varying and incomplete patient response to intravesical MMC treatment.

## COMPUTER SIMULATIONS TO SELECT OPTIMAL TREATMENT CONDITIONS

We next evaluated whether increasing the drug exposure in tumors by reducing the sources of pharmacokinetic variability would produce therapeutic benefits. The goal was to identify an optimized MMC regimen that can be demonstrated, in a phase III trial with reasonable financial and patient resources, to be more efficacious than the usual community practice. The resource consideration was motivated in part by the fact that multiple previous clinical trials failed to show conclusive results on the dose-effect or treatment time-effect relationships of intravesical MMC therapy,[55–59] presumably because of the inadequate sample size (see below). We elected to use computer simulations to predict the $C^n \times T$ values in bladder tissues and, consequently, the drug effects and the clinical outcomes under various treatment conditions. This computational approach also enabled us to identify the sample size with appropriate statistical power.

In a typical intravesical treatment, the bladder is emptied by catheterization without checking for the completeness of bladder emptying, patients are not asked to refrain from fluid and caffeine intake, and the

urine pH and urine production rate are not controlled. These conditions, on average, yielded a residual urine volume of 32.4 ml, urine production rate of 1.48 ml/min, and acidic urinary pH. By controlling the catheter position and patient positioning, and by sonographically checking the residual volume, a minimal residual urine volume of 0–10 ml can be achieved. Results obtained from healthy volunteers showed that restricting fluid and caffeine intake overnight reduced the urine output to 0.63 ml/min, and administration of bicarbonate on the night before and again in the morning was sufficient to control the urine pH at about 7, which would minimize the MMC degradation. The historical intravesical MMC dose ranges from 20 to 60 mg, dissolved in 20 or 40 ml water.[2,6,55,60,61] The simulations compared the target site drug exposure at three doses, two dosing volumes, two residual urine volumes, two urine production rates, two urine pH values, and used n (pharmacodynamic parameter in Equation 4) values of 1.24; in the simulations, each parameters was altered, independently and simultaneously, to project the improvement in the target-site exposure ($C^n \times T$) for different treatment conditions (Table 31.1). As single parameters, the rank order for enhancing the $C^n \times T$ was dose > residual volume > urine production > dosing volume > urine pH > dwell time. Table 31.1 also shows the fraction of tumors exposed to the $C^n \times T_{90}$.

With the assumption that several logs of cytoreduction are required for eradicating tumor cells (i.e. 90% reduction in a regimen of weekly treatments for 6 weeks), the fraction of tumors receiving $C^n \times T_{90}$ was used to calculate the benefit offered by adjuvant MMC therapy. The results indicated marginal improvement achieved by changing individual parameters. For example, an increase of the dose from 20 to 40 mg increased the fraction of patients with Ta tumors receiving $C^n \times T_{90}$ from 22% to 56% but had no effect on patients with T1 tumors. Assuming a patient population with an equal distribution of Ta and T1 tumors, this increase in drug exposure was calculated to produce an 8% improvement in the recurrence-free rate. Interestingly, increasing the dwell time from 2 to 4 hours did not produce an improvement. This is because the drug concentration in urine at 2 hours was <10% of the initial concentration, thus resulting in a minimal increase in cumulative drug exposure. Likewise, increasing the dose from 40 mg/20 ml to 60 mg/30 ml (2 mg/ml is the maximum MMC solubility) did not show improvement because the tumor chemosensitivity was such that the 20% increase in drug exposure did not result in a greater fraction of responding tumors. Simultaneous optimization of five parameters (dose, 40 mg; dosing solution volume, 20 ml; urine-production rate constant, 0.63 ml/min; postcatheterization urine volume, 0; pH, 7) resulted in an increase in drug exposure by 5.7 (n=1) or 8.5-fold (n=1.24).

**Table 31.1** Simulations of bladder wall exposure and treatment effect*

| Variable changed | $C^nxT$ urine | $C^nxT$ at 200 μm | Improvement factor | Percent of tumors exposed to $C^nxT_{90}$ | |
|---|---|---|---|---|---|
| | | | | Ta | T1 |
| **n=1.24** | | | | | |
| Standard (Dose=20, $V_0$=20, $k_0$=1.48, $V_{res}$=32.4, pH=5, $T_{inst}$=120) | 62,179 | 674 | 1.00 | 22.2 | 0 |
| Instillation volume, from 20 to 40 ml | 24,779 | 288 | 0.77 | 55.6 | 0 |
| Dose, from 20 to 40 mg | 76,005 | 882 | 2.36 | 44.4 | 0 |
| Urine production, from 1.48 to 0.626 ml/min | 44,702 | 519 | 1.39 | 55.6 | 0 |
| Residual volume, from 32.4 to 0 ml | 62,092 | 721 | 1.93 | 22.2 | 0 |
| pH, from 5 to 7 | 32,237 | 432 | 1.16 | 22.2 | 0 |
| Instillation time, from 120 to 240 min | 32,962 | 383 | 1.02 | 22.2 | 0 |
| Optimized (Dose=40, $V_0$=20, $k_0$=0.63, $V_{res}$=0, pH=7, $T_{inst}$=120) | 274,919 | 3191 | 8.53 | 77.8 | 25.0 |
| High dose combination (Dose=60, $V_0$=30, $k_0$=0.63, $V_{res}$=0, pH=7, $T_{inst}$=120) | 332,968 | 3865 | 10.33 | 77.8 | 25.0 |
| **n=1** | | | | | |
| Standard (Dose=20, $V_0$=20, $k_0$=1.48, $V_{res}$=32.4, pH=5, $T_{inst}$=120) | 9928 | 273 | 1.00 | 22.2 | 0 |
| Optimized (Dose=40, $V_0$=20, $k_0$=0.63, $V_{res}$=0, pH=7, $T_{inst}$=120) | 56,871 | 1564 | 5.73 | 77.8 | 16.7 |

* The variables were altered and the resulting $C_u$ and $C^nxT$ were calculated using equations 1–4. Simulations were done using two n values, 1.24 and 1.

The conventional paradigm in clinical oncology is to test the effect of individual parameters. However, as shown above, doubling the dose would increase the response rate by only 8%, which would require >900 patients (>450 per arm) to detect a statistically significant difference at 80% power. Similarly, testing the effect of the remaining parameters, one at a time, would require at a minimum several thousand patients. As there are insufficient resources to support multiple trials of this magnitude, a more rational and realistic approach was to optimize the five parameters that, based on the simulation results using an n value of 1.24, would deliver $C^nxT_{90}$ to 78% and 25% of $T_a$ and T1 tumors, respectively, and would result in a 20% improvement over the standard treatment. For an n value of 1, the calculated improvement was 18%. Improvements of 18% to 20% are significant and can be detected with a modest sample size of 232 patients (116 per arm) or a total of 116 recurrences, at a 5% significance level with 80% power. These considerations led to a prospective two-arm randomized multi-institutional phase III trial.

## PHASE III TRIAL RESULTS DEMONSTRATING THERAPEUTIC BENEFITS OF THE OPTIMIZED MMC THERAPY

Fourteen academic and research centers participated in the trial. The study population consisted of patients with histologically proven transitional cell carcinoma of the bladder at high risk for recurrence due to:

- two or more episodes of histologically proven Ta, Tis, or T1 transitional cell carcinoma
- multifocal bladder tumors (defined as three or more papillary tumors present simultaneously or Tis involving at least 25% of the bladder surface area and/or in two or more biopsy sites), and/or
- primary or solitary tumors that were >5 cm in size, of grade 3, or exhibited DNA aneuploidy.

Patients with adequate bone marrow reserve, adequate renal function, and a Karnofsky performance score of 50–100 were randomized within 34 days of transurethral bladder tumor resection, by four prognostic criteria: 1) presence versus absence of Tis tumor; 2) grade 3 versus grades 1 and 2 tumors; 3) multifocal versus unifocal tumors; and 4) recurrent versus primary tumors. Patients with MMC treatments within the previous 56 weeks, prior muscle-invasive (T2–4) tumors, concurrent malignancy within the last 5 years, or pregnancy were excluded.

Patients in the optimized arm were instructed to refrain from drinking fluids for 8 hours prior to and during MMC treatment, were given oral doses of 1.3 g sodium bicarbonate the night prior to, the morning of, and 30 minutes prior to drug treatment. These patients were catheterized; their post-void residual urine volumes were measured using a bladder ultrasound instrument and reduced by repositioning the catheter and/or by changing the position of the patient, until the residual urine volume was less than 10 ml. MMC (40 mg in 20 ml sterile water) was then instilled intravesically through the Foley catheter by gravity, and retained in the bladder for 2 hours. Patients in the standard arm received a lower MMC dose (20 mg in 20 ml), were not instructed to exercise voluntary dehydration, and did not receive oral sodium bicarbonate or undergo additional postcatheterization bladder-emptying measures. MMC treatments were given weekly for 6 weeks. Primary endpoints were recurrence and time to recurrence. Patients in the two arms did not differ in demographics, disease characteristics, or history of intravesical therapy.

For hematologic toxicity, one patient in the standard arm showed a transient reduction in white blood cell count, whereas no patients in the optimized arm showed toxicity. For nonhematologic toxicity, only dysuria was statistically significantly higher in the optimized arm, and it did not result in higher frequency of treatment termination (one termination due to dysuria in each arm).

Kaplan–Meier analyses of recurrence in the intent-to-treat group and the evaluable group indicated that, in both groups, patients in the optimized arm had a statistically significantly longer time to recurrence and a higher recurrence-free fraction at all time points compared to patients in the standard arm (Figure 31.4). Improvements were found across all stratification risk groups (tumor stage, grade, focality, and recurrence, stratified log-rank test). The close alignment between the clinical outcome (18–19% improvement in

recurrence-free rate) and the simulation predictions (18–20% improvement) is noteworthy and lends support to using the effect-based, computational approach to identify/design the optimal intravesical treatment.

## ADDITIONAL INVESTIGATIONAL AND NOVEL AGENTS

### ANTHRACYCLINES

Epirubicin, a standard therapy in Europe, shows a dose-dependent efficacy between 20 and 40 mg per 40 ml, with no further improvement from 50 to 100 mg per 50 ml.[62] In a study with a 6-year follow-up, perioperative epirubicin is more effective than interferon-α in preventing recurrence.[63] Mitoxantrone shows variable activity up to the level similar to that of doxorubicin.[64-66] Pirarubicin[67-69] shows slightly better activity than saline controls. Other anthracyclines, including (2′R)-4′-O-tetrahydropyranyl-doxorubicin and amrubicin have undergone limited clinical evaluation.[70-72] Valrubicin (AD-32) provides higher bladder penetration due to its greater lipophilicity than does doxorubicin, interferes with the normal DNA breaking–resealing action of DNA topoisomerase II, and

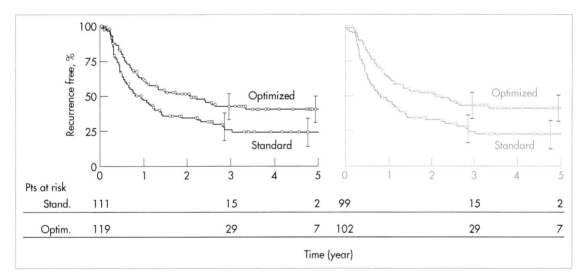

**Fig. 31.4**
Kaplan–Meier analysis of treatment outcome in (*left*) intent-to-treat and (*right*) evaluable groups. Symbols indicate censored patients, error bars show 95% confidence intervals (CI). (*Left*) In the intent-to-treat group of patients (n=230), median time to recurrence was 11.8 months in the standard arm (n=111) and 29.1 in the optimized arm (n=119). For the standard arm, the recurrence-free percentages at 1-, 3- and 5-years were 48.0 (CI: 38.4–57.7), 28.4% (CI: 18.8–38%), and 24.6% (CI: 14.9–34.3%), respectively. For the optimized arm, the recurrence-free percentages at 1-, 3- and 5-years were 61.3 (CI: 52.2–70.4), 44.5% (CI: 34.7–54.3%), and 41.5% (CI: 30.9–51.1%), respectively. (*Right*) In evaluable patients (n=201), median time to recurrence was 11.3 months in the standard arm (n=99) and 29.1 in the optimized arm (n=102). For the standard arm, the recurrence-free percentages at 1-, 3- and 5-years were 47.5 (CI: 37.6–57.4), 27.1% (CI: 17.5–36.7%), and 23.5% (CI: 14–33%), respectively. For the optimized arm, the recurrence-free percentages at 1-, 3- and 5-years were 63.3 (CI: 53.9–72.7), 44.4% (CI: 34.1–54.7%), and 42.6% (CI: 32.3–52.9%), respectively. Reproduced with permission from Au et al.[3]

causes chromosomal damage and cell cycle arrest in the G2 phase.[73] Valrubicin is approved for patients with BCG-refractory Tis tumors unsuitable for cystectomy, whereas valrubicin produces a 20% complete response rate with no evidence of disease in 8% of patients after a median follow-up of 30 months.[74] Valrubicin is not recommended in patients that can tolerate cystectomy because of the risk of progressive disease.[75]

## MITOMYCIN C-RELATED TREATMENTS

Several experimental approaches to promote MMC penetration into bladder have been evaluated. In patients with high-grade tumors after failing other treatments, combination of MMC with hyperthermia shows a 75% recurrence-free survival after 20 months of follow-up.[76,77] Application of electric current (20 mAmp for 30 minutes) enhances the urothelium penetration and systemic absorption of MMC, and improves the recurrence-free survival in high-risk patients with T1 and Tis tumors,[78] but does not ablate the marker lesions.[79] Our laboratory is evaluating the use of a chemo-sensitizer to enhance the tumor response to MMC (see below).

EO9 is an indolequinone bioreductive agent with promising preclinical activity.[80] The enzyme NQO1, important for its bioactivation, is elevated in a subset of superficial bladder tumors.[81] A phase I study showed complete disappearance of marker lesions in six of eight patients.[82]

## ANTIMETABOLITES

Gemcitabine, an active systemic agent in advanced bladder cancer, is well tolerated and shows insignificant systemic absorption when given as intravesical therapy in doses of 2 g in 50 or 100 ml saline.[83–86] 5-Fluorouracil has activity when given by long-term systemic or 6-week intravesical administration, but its activity appears to be limited to tumors with low expression of its major target enzyme, thymidylate synthase.[87,88] Oral 5-fluorouracil did not enhance the effect of perioperative intravesical doxorubicin.[89]

## ANTIMICROTUBULE AGENTS

Our MMC and doxorubicin studies suggested the following desirable properties of agents for intravesical therapy:

- higher penetration across the urothelium and longer retention in tissues
- effective against the more rapidly proliferating bladder tumors
- does not require functional p53 for apoptosis induction as 60% of bladder cancer shows high frequency of p53 mutation.[90–98]

A potential candidate is paclitaxel, which has activity against metastatic bladder cancer,[34] shows high lipophilicity and partitioning across the urothelium, tight binding to intracellular macromolecules resulting in significant drug accumulation and retention in tumor cells,[15,99] and can induce apoptosis through p53-dependent or p53-independent pathways.[100,101] An earlier phase I trial with the Food and Drug Administration (FDA)-approved paclitaxel formulation, given intravesically, did not show activity (D. Lamm, personal communication), possibly due to the sequestration of paclitaxel in Cremophor micelles.[102] Dimethyl sulfoxide (DMSO) promotes the paclitaxel release by altering the Cremophor micelle structure and promotes paclitaxel penetration into bladder tissues by disrupting the urothelium.[103] However, these beneficial effects of DMSO were compromised by the increases in urine production rate and drug permeability, and clearance by the capillaries.[104] These findings have led to the development of rapid-release, paclitaxel-loaded gelatin nanoparticles (~600 nm diameter) that release approximately 90% of the drug in 2 hours, and yield higher concentrations in the urothelium and lamina propria than the Cremophor formulation.[105] The vinca alkaloid vinorelbine showed some activity in a preliminary phase I trial.[106]

## IMMUNE STIMULATORS

Several immune stimulators (e.g. hemocyanin, bropirimine, and interferons) have shown some efficacy (see Chapter 33).

## COMBINATION THERAPY

The therapeutic value of combination chemo- or immunochemotherapy in advanced cancers is well established. There have been limited attempts to develop this modality for intravesical therapy in patients; epirubicin does not improve the response to BCG,[107] whereas a combination of the bleomycin analog peplomycin and doxorubicin shows improvement over single agents.[67]

## MOLECULAR TARGETS

Loss of tumor suppressor genes p53 and RB, over-expression of oncogenes and peptide growth factors and their ligands, and alterations in cellular adhesion molecules and tissue microenvironment all play a role in bladder tumor formation, growth, and metastasis.[108] The therapeutic targets under preclinical evaluation include: 1) epidermal growth factor receptor (EGFR), i.e. EGFR inhibitors and EGF-linked therapeutics, as superficial bladder cancer shows high EGFR expression[109,110]; and 2) p53, as its mutation is correlated with poor prognosis.[111–115] Suramin, a polysulfonated compound that broadly inhibits polypeptide growth factors, displays chemopreventive properties in a mouse superficial bladder carcinogenesis model.[116] A phase I intravesical treatment with single agent suramin showed good tolerability but limited antitumor activity.[117]

Our laboratory recently established that acidic and basic fibroblast growth factors (FGF) expressed in solid tumors are responsible for broad-spectrum resistance to anticancer drugs, and that FGF inhibitors, including monoclonal antibodies and suramin, enhance the activity of chemotherapy. The chemosensitizing effect of suramin shows an unusual dose–response relationship, occurring only at low, nontoxic doses and not at higher doses.[118–122] Results of a phase II trial in lung cancer patients indicate survival benefits of adding nontoxic doses of suramin to the standard chemotherapy (paclitaxel plus carboplatin), thus providing the clinical proof-of-concept of the suramin chemosensitization.[123,124] Separate preclinical studies have shown that nontoxic suramin treatments significantly enhanced the in vitro and/or in vivo MMC activity in xenograft and patient bladder tumors, without enhancing the host toxicity.[125] Finally, combination of chemotherapy with an FGF inhibitor is appealing as bFGF overexpression is associated with the development and chemoresistance of bladder cancer, and poor prognosis of bladder cancer patients.[126–130] Studies to identify the appropriate chemosensitizing suramin dose for intravesical therapy are ongoing in our laboratory.

## PERSPECTIVES

The therapeutic value of intravesical immuno- or chemotherapy in superficial bladder cancer is well documented. However, in spite of the theoretical advantage of being able to completely eliminate the malignant cells, these treatments have not yielded 100% recurrence-free survival. Hence, further research is needed.

For MMC, optimizing the treatment conditions to maximize the drug delivery to tumors nearly doubles the recurrence-free survival in high-risk patients to about 40%. Further improvement may be possible by enhancing MMC penetration into bladder tissues using physicochemical methods such as electromotility or hyperthermia. A second approach is patient selection. We found in the phase III MMC trial that a small subset of African–American patients performed far worse than Caucasian patients, suggesting a genetic difference in patient response.[3] A potential candidate to determine patient susceptibility is the expression of quinone reductases responsible for MMC activation, which positively correlates with MMC activity in patient bladder tumors.[131,132] Further elucidation of this mechanism may provide a pharmacogenetic approach

to preselect the patients likely to respond to intravesical MMC therapy. A third approach is to use chemosensitizers or other chemotherapeutic agents to enhance the activity of MMC. A fourth approach is to identify new agents that provide more favorable bladder penetration and retention characteristics and have high potency against bladder tumors with diverse pathobiologic properties.

An unanswered question in intravesical therapy is the optimal duration of therapy. The current approach of six weekly cycles is empirically based. Fewer treatments may be sufficient and should be evaluated. Finally, the Southwest Oncology Group Trial 8795, in which BCG was found to be superior to MMC, used an MMC protocol that was essentially identical to the standard arm in our phase III trial.[3] This consideration, together with the fact that MMC produces lower and more tolerable toxicity than BCG, suggests that it may be worthwhile to compare the optimized MMC regimen to use of BCG.

## ACKNOWLEDGEMENT

This work was supported in part by MERIT grant R37CA49816 from the National Cancer Institute, NIH, DHHS.

REFERENCES

1. Wientjes MG, Badalament RA, Wang RC, Hassan F, Au JL. Penetration of mitomycin C in human bladder. Cancer Res 1993;53:3314–3320.
2. Richie JP, Shipley WU, Yagoda A. Cancer of the bladder. In DeVita VT Jr, Hellman S, Rosenberg SA (eds): Cancer: Principles and Practice of Oncology. Philadelphia: JB Lippincott, 1989, pp 1008–1058.
3. Au JL, Badalament RA, Wientjes MG, et al. Methods to improve efficacy of intravesical mitomycin C: results of a randomized phase III trial. J Natl Cancer Inst 2001;93:597–604.
4. Paulson DF. Treatment of superficial carcinoma of the bladder. Bladder Cancer, Part B: Radiation, Local and Systemic Chemotherapy, and New Treatment Modalities. New York: Liss, 1984, pp 193–209.
5. Whitmore WF Jr. Chemotherapy for bladder cancer. J Urol 1985;134:1181–1182.
6. Herr HW. Intravesical therapy. A critical review. Urol Clin North Am 1987;14:399–404.
7. Lundholm C, Norlen BJ, Ekman P, et al. A randomized prospective study comparing long-term intravesical instillations of mitomycin C and bacillus Calmette–Guérin in patients with superficial bladder carcinoma. J Urol 1996;156:372–376.
8. Meyer JP, Persad R, Gillatt DA. Use of bacille Calmette–Guérin in superficial bladder cancer. Postgrad Med J 2002;78:449–454.
9. Lamm DL, Blumenstein BA, Crissman JD, BA et al. Maintenance bacillus Calmette–Guérin immunotherapy for recurrent TA, T1 and carcinoma in situ transitional cell carcinoma of the bladder: a randomized Southwest Oncology Group Study. J Urol 2000;163:1124–1129.
10. Traynelis CL, Lamm DL. Current status of intravesical therapy for bladder cancer. In Rous S (ed). Urology Annual. New York: Norton, 1994, pp 113–143.
11. Lunglmayr G, Czech K. Absorption studies on intraluminal thio-tepa for topical cytostatic treatment of low-stage bladder tumors. J Urol 1971;106:72–74.

12. Chai M, Wientjes MG, Badalament RA, Burgers JK, Au JL. Pharmacokinetics of intravesical doxorubicin in superficial bladder cancer patients. J Urol 1994;152:374–378.

13. Dalton JT, Wientjes MG, Badalament RA, Drago JR, Au JL. Pharmacokinetics of intravesical mitomycin C in superficial bladder cancer patients. Cancer Res 1991;51:5144–5152.

14. Song D, Wientjes MG, Gan Y, Au JL. Bladder tissue pharmacokinetics and antitumor effect of intravesical 5-fluorouridine. Clin Cancer Res 1997;3:901–909.

15. Song D, Wientjes MG, Au JL. Bladder tissue pharmacokinetics of intravesical taxol. Cancer Chemother Pharmacol 1997;40:285–292.

16. Wientjes MG, Dalton JT, Badalament RA, Drago JR, Au JL. Bladder wall penetration of intravesical mitomycin C in dogs. Cancer Res 1991;51:4347–4354.

17. Wientjes MG, Badalament RA, Au JL. Penetration of intravesical doxorubicin in human bladders. Cancer Chemother Pharmacol 1996;37:539–546.

18. Underberg WJ, Lingeman H. Aspects of the chemical stability of mitomycin and porfiromycin in acidic solution. J Pharm Sci 1983;72:549–553.

19. Beignen JH, Lingeman H, van Munster HA. Mitomycin antitumor agents: a review of their physico-chemical and analytical properties and stability. J Pharm Biomed Anal 1986;4:275–295.

20. Mellett JB, Woods LA. The comparative physiological disposition of thiotepa and tepa in the dog. Cancer Res 1960;20:524–532.

21. Colvin M. The alkylating agents. In Chabner BA (ed): Pharmacologic Principles of Cancer Treatment. Philadelphia: WB Saunders, 1982, pp 278–280.

22. Wood JH, Leonard TW. Kinetic implications of drug resorption from the bladder. Drug Metab Rev 1983;14:407–423.

23. Pauli BU, Alroy J, Weinstein RS. The ultrastructure and pathobiology of urinary bladder cancer. In Bryan GT, Cohen S (eds): The Pathology of Bladder Cancer, vol II. New York: CRC Press, 1983, pp 41–140.

24. Engelmann U, Oelsner G, Burger RA, Wagner H. Permeability of the rat bladder to cisplatinum under different conditions: comparison with mitomycin C and adriamycin. Urol Res 1983;11:39–42.

25. Engelmann U, Burger RA, Rumpelt JH, Jacobi GH. Adriamycin permeability of the rat bladder under different conditions. J Urol 1983;129:862–864.

26. Kurth KH, de Wall JG, van Oosterom HP, de Jong EAJM, Tjaden UR. Plasma levels during intravesical instillation of mitomycin C. In Liss AR (ed): EORTC Genitourinary Group Monograph 2, part B: Superficial bladder tumors. Brussels: EORTC, 1985, pp 81–93.

27. Watanabe H, Nakao M, Nakagawa S, Takada H. Size and location of tumors influencing the effect of bladder instillation therapy. Cancer Chemother Pharmacol 1987;20(Suppl):S49–S51.

28. Turnbull GJ. Ultrastructural basis of the permeability barrier in urothelium. Invest Urol 1973;11:198–204.

29. Hicks RM, Ketterer B, Warren RC. The ultrastructure and chemistry of the luminal plasma membrane of the mammalian urinary bladder: a structure with low permeability to water and ions. Philos Trans R Soc Lond B Biol Sci 1974;268:23–38.

30. Gerlowski LE, Jain RK. Physiologically based pharmacokinetic modeling: principles and applications. J Pharm Sci 1983;72:1103–1127.

31. Flessner MF, Dedrick RL, Schultz JS. A distributed model of peritoneal-plasma transport: theoretical considerations. Am J Physiol 1984;246:R597–R607.

32. Hoffman RM. Three-dimensional histoculture: origins and applications in cancer research. Cancer Cells 1991;3:86–92.

33. Weaver JR, Wientjes MG, Au JL. Regional heterogeneity and pharmacodynamics in human solid tumor histoculture. Cancer Chemother Pharmacol 1999;44:335–342.

34. Au JL, Kalns J, Gan Y, Wientjes MG. Pharmacologic effects of paclitaxel in human bladder tumors. Cancer Chemother Pharmacol 1997;41:69–74.

35. Gan Y, Wientjes MG, Badalament RA, Au JL. Pharmacodynamics of doxorubicin in human bladder tumors. Clin Cancer Res 1996;2:1275–1283.

36. Au JL, Li D, Gan Y, et al. Pharmacodynamics of immediate and delayed effects of paclitaxel: role of slow apoptosis and intracellular drug retention. Cancer Res 1998;58:2141–2148.

37. Walker MC, Parris CN, Masters JR. Differential sensitivities of human testicular and bladder tumor cell lines to chemotherapeutic drugs. J Natl Cancer Inst 1987;79:213–216.

38. Yen WC, Schmittgen T, Au JL. Different pH dependency of mitomycin C activity in monolayer and three-dimensional cultures. Pharm Res 1996;13:1887–1891.

39. Schmittgen TD, Weaver JM, Badalament RA, et al. Correlation of human bladder tumor histoculture proliferation and sensitivity to mitomycin C with tumor pathobiology. J Urol 1994;152:1632–1636.

40. Traver RD, Siegel D, Beall HD, et al. Characterization of a polymorphism in NAD(P)H: quinone oxidoreductase (DT-diaphorase). Br J Cancer 1997;75:69–75.

41. Bligh HF, Bartoszek A, Robson CN, et al. Activation of mitomycin C by NADPH:cytochrome P-450 reductase. Cancer Res 1990;50:7789–7792.

42. Hoban PR, Walton MI, Robson CN, et al. Decreased NADPH:cytochrome P-450 reductase activity and impaired drug activation in a mammalian cell line resistant to mitomycin C under aerobic but not hypoxic conditions. Cancer Res 1990;50:4692–4697.

43. Traver RD, Horikoshi T, Danenberg KD, et al. NAD(P)H:quinone oxidoreductase gene expression in human colon carcinoma cells: characterization of a mutation which modulates DT-diaphorase activity and mitomycin sensitivity. Cancer Res 1992;52:797–802.

44. Spanswick VJ, Cummings J, Smyth JF. Current issues in the enzymology of mitomycin C metabolic activation. Gen Pharmacol 1998;31:539–544.

45. Malkinson AM, Siegel D, Forrest GL, et al. Elevated DT-diaphorase activity and messenger RNA content in human non-small cell lung carcinoma: relationship to the response of lung tumor xenografts to mitomycin C. Cancer Res 1992;52:4752–4757.

46. Singh SV, Scalamogna D, Xia H, et al. Biochemical characterization of a mitomycin C-resistant human bladder cancer cell line. Int J Cancer 1996;65:852–857.

47. Mikami K, Naito M, Tomida A, Yamada M, Sirakusa T, Tsuruo T. DT-diaphorase as a critical determinant of sensitivity to mitomycin C in human colon and gastric carcinoma cell lines. Cancer Res 1996;56:2823–2826.

48. Siegel D, Beall H, Senekowitsch C, et al. Bioreductive activation of mitomycin C by DT-diaphorase. Biochemistry 1992;31:7879–7885.

49. Tomasz M, Lipman R. Reductive metabolism and alkylating activity of mitomycin C induced by rat liver microsomes. Biochemistry 1981;20:5056–5061.

50. Wientjes MG, Badalament RA, Au JL. Use of pharmacologic data and computer simulations to design an efficacy trial of intravesical mitomycin C therapy for superficial bladder cancer. Cancer Chemother Pharmacol 1993;32:255–262.

51. Atema A, Buurman KJ, Noteboom E, Smets LA. Potentiation of DNA-adduct formation and cytotoxicity of platinum-containing drugs by low pH. Int J Cancer 1993;54:166–172.

52. Pan SS, Yu F, Hipsher C. Enzymatic and pH modulation of mitomycin C-induced DNA damage in mitomycin C-resistant HCT 116 human colon cancer cells. Mol Pharmacol 1993;43:870–877.

53. Kennedy KA, McGurl JD, Leondaridis L, Alabaster O. pH dependence of mitomycin C-induced cross-linking activity in EMT6 tumor cells. Cancer Res 1985;45:3541–3547.

54. Groos E, Walker L, Masters JR. Intravesical chemotherapy. Studies on the relationship between pH and cytotoxicity. Cancer 1986;58:1199–1203.

55. Tolley DA, Parmar MK, Grigor KM, et al. The effect of intravesical mitomycin C on recurrence of newly diagnosed superficial bladder cancer: a further report with 7 years of follow up. J Urol 1996;155:1233–1238.

56. Schwaibold H, Klingenberger HJ, Huland H. Long-term results of intravesical prevention of recurrence with mitomycin C and adriamycin in patients with superficial bladder cancer. Urologe A 1994;33:479–483.

57. Giesbers AA, van Helsdingen PJ, Kramer AE. Recurrence of superficial bladder carcinoma after intravesical instillation of mitomycin-C. Comparison of exposure times. Br J Urol 1989;63:176–179.

58. van Helsdingen PJ, Rikken CH, Sleeboom HP, de Bruyn EA, Tjaden UR. Mitomycin C resorption following repeated intravesical instillations using different instillation times. Urol Int 1988;43:42–46.

59. van der Meijden AP, Debruyne FM. Treatment schedule of intravesical chemotherapy with mitomycin C in superficial bladder cancer: short-term courses or maintenance therapy. Urology 1988;31:26–29.

60. Lum BL, Torti FM. Adjuvant intravesicular pharmacotherapy for superficial bladder cancer. J Natl Cancer Inst 1991;83:682–694.

61. Huland H, Otto U. Mitomycin instillation to prevent recurrence of superficial bladder carcinoma. Results of a controlled, prospective study in 58 patients. Eur Urol 1983;9:84–86.

62. Masters JR, Popert RJ, Thompson PM, Gibson D, Coptcoat MJ, Parmar MK. Intravesical chemotherapy with epirubicin: a dose response study. J Urol 1999;161:1490–1493.

63. Rajala P, Kaasinen E, Raitanen M, Liukkonen T, Rintala E. Perioperative single dose instillation of epirubicin or interferon-alpha after transurethral resection for the prophylaxis of primary superficial bladder cancer recurrence: a prospective randomized multicenter study—FinnBladder III long-term results. J Urol 2002;168:981–985.

64. Bassi PF, Spinadin R, Carando R, et al. [Mitoxantrone chemoprophylaxis for multirecurrent multifocal superficial bladder tumours: results of a phase 2 controlled study.] Arch Ital Urol Androl 2003;75:202–204.

65. Huang JS, Chen WH, Lin CC, et al. A randomized trial comparing intravesical instillations of mitoxantrone and doxorubicin in patients with superficial bladder cancer. Chang Gung Med J 2003;26:91–97.

66. Papatsoris AG, Deliveliotis C, Giannopoulos A, Dimopoulos C. Adjuvant intravesical mitoxantrone versus recombinant interferon-alpha after transurethral resection of superficial bladder cancer: a randomized prospective study. Urol Int 2004;72:284–291.

67. Ikeda R, Chikazawa I, Kobayashi Y, et al. Prophylaxis of recurrence in superficial bladder carcinoma by intravesical chemotherapy—comparative study between instillation of combined double anticancer agents and single anticancer agent. Gan To Kagaku Ryoho 1999;26:509–514.

68. Kobayashi M, Sugaya Y, Yuzawa M, et al. [Appropriate intravesical retention time of pirarubicin concentration based on its level in tumor tissue, anti-tumor effect and side effect in intravesical instillation therapy for bladder tumor.] Gan To Kagaku Ryoho Cancer Chemother 1998;25:1771–1774.

69. Miki T, Nonomura N, Kojima Y, et al. [A randomized study on intravesical pirarubicin (THP) chemoprophylaxis of recurrence after transurethral resection of superficial bladder cancer.] Hinyokika Kiyo Acta Urol Jpn 1997;43:907–912.

70. Okamura K, Ono Y, Kinukawa T, et al. Randomized study of single early instillation of (2'R)-4'-O-tetrahydropyranyl-doxorubicin for a single superficial bladder carcinoma. Cancer 2002;94:2363–2368.

71. Tsushima T, Kobashi K, Akebi N, et al. Early phase II study of amrubicin (SM-5887) for superficial bladder cancer: a dose-finding study for intravesical chemotherapy. Gan To Kagaku Ryoho Cancer Chemother 2001;28:483–491.

72. Ohmori H, Yamato T, Asahi T. Phase I study of amrubicin hydrochloride (SM-5887) for superficial bladder cancer in intravesical chemotherapy. Gan To Kagaku Ryoho Cancer Chemother 2001;28:475–482.

73. Silber R, Liu LF, Israel M, et al. Metabolic activation of N-acylanthracyclines precedes their interaction with DNA topoisomerase II. NCI Monogr 1987;4:111–115.

74. Steinberg G, Bahnson R, Brosman S, Middleton R, Wajsman Z, Wehle M. Efficacy and safety of valrubicin for the treatment of Bacillus Calmette–Guérin refractory carcinoma in situ of the bladder. The Valrubicin Study Group. J Urol 2000;163:761–767.

75. USFDA. Valstar (Valrubicin) sterile solution for intravesical instillation: summary basis of approval equivalent. NDA 20-892. 1998. Online. Available: www.uiowa.edu/~idis/dap/valrubic.pdf.

76. Gofrit ON, Shapiro A, Pode D, et al. Combined local bladder hyperthermia and intravesical chemotherapy for the treatment of high-grade superficial bladder cancer. Urology 2004;63:466–471.

77. Colombo R, Da Pozzo LF, Lev A, et al. Local microwave hyperthermia and intravesical chemotherapy as bladder sparing treatment for select multifocal and unresectable superficial bladder tumors. J Urol 1998;159:783–787.

78. Di Stasi SM, Giannantoni A, Stephen RL, et al. Intravesical electromotive mitomycin C versus passive transport mitomycin C for high risk superficial bladder cancer: a prospective randomized study. J Urol 2003;170:777–782.

79. Brausi M, Campo B, Pizzocaro G, et al. Intravesical electromotive administration of drugs for treatment of superficial bladder cancer: a comparative Phase II study. Urology 1998;51:506–509.

80. Phillips RM, Jaffar M, Maitland DJ, et al. Pharmacological and biological evaluation of a series of substituted 1,4-naphthoquinone bioreductive drugs. Biochem Pharmacol 2004;68:2107–2116.

81. Choudry GA, Stewart PA, Double JA, et al. A novel strategy for NQO1 (NAD(P)H:quinone oxidoreductase, EC 1.6.99.2) mediated therapy of bladder cancer based on the pharmacological properties of EO9. Br J Cancer 2001;85:1137–1146.

82. Palit V, Puri R, Shah T, Flanigan GM, Loadman PM, Phillips RM. Intravesical EUquin (EO9): a new treatment for superficial bladder cancer—results of phase I study [abstract]. Proc Br Assoc Urol Surg 2004;Poster 109.

83. Palou J, Carcas A, Segarra J, et al. Phase I pharmacokinetic study of a single intravesical instillation of gemcitabine administered immediately after transurethral resection plus multiple random biopsies in patients with superficial bladder cancer. J Urol 2004;172:485–488.

84. Witjes JA, van der Heijden AG, Vriesema JLJ, Peters GJ, Laan A, Schalken JA. Intravesical gemcitabine: a phase I and pharmacokinetic study. Eur Urol 2004;45:182–186.

85. De Berardinis E, Antonini G, Peters GJ, et al. Intravesical administration of gemcitabine in superficial bladder cancer: a phase I study with pharmacodynamic evaluation. BJU Int 2004;93:491–494.

86. Laufer M, Ramalingam S, Schoenberg MP, et al. Intravesical gemcitabine therapy for superficial transitional cell carcinoma of the bladder: a phase I and pharmacokinetic study. J Clin Oncol 2003;21:697–703.

87. Kubota Y, Noguchi S, Hosaka M. UFT in bladder cancer. Oncology 1999;13:112–115.

88. Hugosson J, Bergdahl S, Carlsson G, Frosing R, Norlen L, Gustavsson B. Effects of intravesical instillation of 5-fluorouracil and interferon in patients with recurrent superficial urinary bladder carcinoma. A clinical and pharmacodynamic study. Scand J Urol Nephrol 1997;31:343–347.

89. Naito S, Iguchi A, Sagiyama K, et al. Significance of the preoperative intravesical instillation of doxorubicin and the oral administration of 5-fluorouracil in preventing recurrence after a transurethral resection of superficial bladder cancer. Kyushu University Urological Oncology Group. Int J Urol Jpn 1997;4:352–357.

90. Friedrich MG, Erbersdobler A, Schwaibold H, Conrad S, Huland E, Huland H. Detection of loss of heterozygosity in the p53 tumor-suppressor gene with PCR in the urine of patients with bladder cancer. J Urol 2000;163:1039–1042.

91. Cooke PW, James ND, Ganesan R, Burton A, Young LS, Wallace DM. Bcl-2 expression identifies patients with advanced bladder cancer treated by radiotherapy that benefit from neoadjuvant chemotherapy. BJU Int 2000;85:829–835.

92. Wu CS, Pollack A, Czerniak B, et al. Prognostic value of p53 in muscle-invasive bladder cancer treated with preoperative radiotherapy. Urology 1996;47:305–310.

93. Pfister C, Flaman JM, Dunet F, Grise P, Frebourg T. p53 mutations in bladder tumors inactivate the transactivation of the p21 and Bax genes, and have a predictive value for the clinical outcome after bacillus Calmette–Guérin therapy. J Urol 1999;162:69–73.

94. Bernardini S, Adessi GL, Billerey C, Chezy E, Carbillet JP, Bittard H. Immunohistochemical detection of p53 protein overexpression versus gene sequencing in urinary bladder carcinomas. J Urol 1999;162:1456–1501.

95. Hayakawa K, Hasegawa M, Kawashima M, et al. Comparison of effects of doxorubicin and radiation on p53-dependent apoptosis in vivo. Oncol Rep 2000;7:267–270.

96. Sato S, Kigawa J, Minagawa Y, et al. Chemosensitivity and p53-dependent apoptosis in epithelial ovarian carcinoma. Cancer 1999;86:1307–1313.

97. Lee TK, Lau TC, Ng IO. Doxorubicin-induced apoptosis and chemosensitivity in hepatoma cell lines. Cancer Chemother Pharmacol 2002;49:78–86.

98. Kawasaki T, Tomita Y, Bilim V, Takeda M, Takahashi K, Kumanishi T. Abrogation of apoptosis induced by DNA-damaging agents in human bladder-cancer cell lines with p21/WAF1/CIP1 and/or p53 gene alterations. Int J Cancer 1996;68:501–505.

99. Kuh HJ, Jang SH, Wientjes MG, Au JL. Computational model of intracellular pharmacokinetics of paclitaxel. J Pharmacol Exp Therap 2000;293:761–770.

100. Edelman MJ, Meyers FJ, Miller TR, Williams SG, Gandour-Edwards R, deVere White RW. Phase I/II study of paclitaxel, carboplatin, and methotrexate in advanced transitional cell carcinoma: a well-tolerated regimen with activity independent of p53 mutation. Urology 2000;55:521–525.

101. Lanni JS, Lowe SW, Licitra EJ, Liu JO, Jacks T. p53-independent apoptosis induced by paclitaxel through an indirect mechanism. Proc Natl Acad Sci USA 1997;94:9679–9683.

102. Nemeyer I, Wientjes MG, Au JL. Cremophor reduces paclitaxel penetration into bladder wall during intravesical treatment. Cancer Chemother Pharmacol 1999;44:241–248.

103. Schoenfeld RH, Belville WD, Jacob WH, et al. The effect of dimethyl sulfoxide on the uptake of cisplatin from the urinary bladder of the dog: a pilot study. J Am Osteopath Assoc 1983;82:570–573.

104. See WA, Xia Q. Regional chemotherapy for bladder neoplasms using continuous intravesical infusion of doxorubicin: impact of concomitant administration of dimethyl sulfoxide on drug absorption and antitumor activity. J Natl Cancer Inst 1992;84:510–515.

105. Lu Z, Yeh TK, Tsai M, Au JL, Wientjes MG. Paclitaxel-loaded gelatin nanoparticles for intravesical bladder cancer therapy. Clin Cancer Res 2004;10:7677–7684.

106. Bonfil RD, Gonzalez AD, Siguelboim D, et al. Immunohistochemical analysis of Ki-67, p21waf1/cip1 and apoptosis in marker lesions from patients with superficial bladder tumours treated with vinorelbine intravesical therapy in a preliminary phase I trial. BJU Int 2001;88:425–431.

107. Bilen CY, Ozen H, Aki FT, Aygun C, Ekici S, Kendi S. Clinical experience with BCG alone versus BCG plus epirubicin. Int J Urol Jpn 2000;7:206–209.

108. Jones P, Vogelzang N, Gomez J. Priorities of the kidney/bladder cancers progress review group, NCI. 2002. Online. Available: http://prg.nci.nih.gov/kidney/finalreport.html.

109. Bellmunt J, Hussain M, Dinney CP. Novel approaches with targeted therapies in bladder cancer. Therapy of bladder cancer by blockade of the epidermal growth factor receptor family. Crit Rev Oncol Hematol 2003;46(Suppl):S85–104.

110. Bue P, Holmberg AR, Marquez M, Westlin JE, Nilsson S, Malmstrom PU. Intravesical administration of EGF-dextran conjugates in patients with superficial bladder cancer. Eur Urol 2000;38:584–589.

111. Garcia del Muro X, Condom E, Vigues F, et al. p53 and p21 expression levels predict organ preservation and survival in invasive bladder carcinoma treated with a combined-modality approach. Cancer 2004;100:1859–1867.

112. Cordon-Cardo C. p53 and RB: simple interesting correlates or tumor markers of critical predictive nature? J Clin Oncol 2004;22:975–977.

113. Chatterjee SJ, Datar R, Youssefzadeh D, et al. Combined effects of p53, p21, and pRb expression in the progression of bladder transitional cell carcinoma. J Clin Oncol 2004;22:1007–1013.

114. Shariat SF, Tokunaga H, Zhou J, et al. p53, p21, pRB, and p16 expression predict clinical outcome in cystectomy with bladder cancer. J Clin Oncol 2004;22:1014–1024.

115. Pan CX, Koeneman KS. A novel tumor-specific gene therapy for bladder cancer. Med Hypotheses 1999;53:130–135.

116. Graham SD Jr, Napalkov P, Oladele A, et al. Intravesical suramin in the prevention of transitional cell carcinoma. Urology 1995;45:59–63.

117. Uchio EM, Linehan WM, Figg WD, Walther MM. A phase I study of intravesical suramin for the treatment of superficial transitional cell carcinoma of the bladder. J Urol 2003;169:357–360.

118. Song S, Wientjes MG, Gan Y, Au JL. Fibroblast growth factors: an epigenetic mechanism of broad spectrum resistance to anticancer drugs. Proc Natl Acad Sci USA 2000;97:8658–8663.

119. Song S, Wientjes MG, Walsh C, Au JL. Nontoxic doses of suramin enhance activity of paclitaxel against lung metastases. Cancer Res 2001;61:6145–6150.

120. Song S, Yu B, Wei Y, Wientjes MG, Au JL. Low-dose suramin enhanced paclitaxel activity in chemotherapy-naive and paclitaxel-pretreated human breast xenograft tumors. Clin Cancer Res 2004;10:6058–6065.

121. Zhang Y, Song S, Yang F, Au JL, Wientjes MG. Nontoxic doses of suramin enhance activity of doxorubicin in prostate tumors. J Pharmacol Exp Therap 2001;299:426–433.

122. Zhao L, Wientjes MG, Au JLS. Enhancement of antitumor activity of paclitaxel by suramin: unconventional dose–response relationship [abstract]. Proc Am Assoc Cancer Res 2002;43:953.

123. Villalona-Calero MA, Otterson GA, Wientjes MG, et al. Phase II evaluation of low dose suramin as a modulator of paclitaxel/carboplatin (P/C) in non-small cell lung cancer (NSCLC) patients [abstract]. Lung Cancer 2003;41(Suppl 2):149.

124. Villalona-Calero MA, Wientjes MG, Otterson GA, et al. Phase I study of low-dose suramin as a chemosensitizer in patients with advanced non-small cell lung cancer. Clin Cancer Res 2003;9:3303–3311.

125. Xin Y, Chen D, Song S-H, Lyness G, Wientjes MG, Au JL. Low-dose suramin enhances antitumor activity of mitomycin C in bladder tumors [abstract]. Proc Am Assoc Cancer Res 2004;45:461.

126. O'Brien TS, Smith K, Cranston D, Fuggle S, Bicknell R, Harris AL. Urinary basic fibroblast growth factor in patients with bladder cancer and benign prostatic hypertrophy. Br J Urol 1995;76:311–314.

127. Izawa JI, Slaton JW, Kedar D, et al. Differential expression of progression-related genes in the evolution of superficial to invasive transitional cell carcinoma of the bladder. Oncol Rep 2001;8:9–15.

128. Munro NP, Knowles MA. Fibroblast growth factors and their receptors in transitional cell carcinoma. J Urol 2003;169:675–682.

129. Allen LE, Maher PA. Expression of basic fibroblast growth factor and its receptor in an invasive bladder carcinoma cell line. J Cell Physiol 1993;155:368–375.

130. Miyake H, Hara I, Gohji K, Yoshimura K, Arakawa S, Kamidono S. Expression of basic fibroblast growth factor is associated with resistance to cisplatin in a human bladder cancer cell line. Cancer Letters 1998;123:121–126.

131. Gan Y, Mo Y, Kalns JE, et al. Expression of DT-diaphorase and cytochrome P450 reductase correlates with mitomycin C activity in human bladder tumors. Clin Cancer Res 2001;7:1313–1319.

132. Li D, Gan Y, Wientjes MG, Badalament RA, Au JL. Distribution of DT-diaphorase and reduced nicotinamide adenine dinucleotide phosphate: cytochrome p450 oxidoreductase in bladder tissues and tumors. J Urol 2001;166:2500–2505.

# Intravesical immunotherapy: BCG

## 32

*Lori A Pinke, Donald L Lamm*

## INTRODUCTION

Bacille Calmette–Guérin (BCG), a live attenuated vaccine developed against tuberculosis in 1921, is currently the most effective intravesical therapy for bladder cancer. Pearl observed that those patients with tuberculosis had significantly fewer malignancies compared with a control group. He proposed an antineoplastic effect of tuberculosis infection in 1929.[1] The use of BCG in the treatment of bladder tumors was first reported by Morales in 1976. Administration of both intradermal and intravesical Armand Frappier BCG for 6 weeks decreased the rate of tumor recurrence. As previously demonstrated in animal models, he found that limited tumor load was a crucial factor in determining the effectiveness of BCG therapy because patients with limited metastatic disease did not demonstrate remission.[2]

The first controlled trial confirming the efficacy of intravesical BCG for prophylaxis was reported by Lamm and colleagues in 1980. Thirty-seven patients were randomized to either surgical resection or resection plus intravesical and percutaneous BCG therapy. The recurrence rate after 1 year was 22% in patients receiving BCG after tumor resection, significantly lower than the 42% recurrence rate in those receiving resection alone (p=0.01).[3] Early trials also showed a role for BCG in the treatment of residual disease after surgical resection. Tumor regression was seen in 59% of patients that were incompletely resected and then received weekly doses of intravesical and intradermal BCG for 6 weeks.[4] Subsequent controlled trials comparing surgical resection alone to resection and adjuvant BCG treatment demonstrated significantly lower recurrence rates when patients received BCG. These results are summarized in Table 32.1.

These early studies established BCG as a therapeutic agent in the treatment and prevention of recurrent bladder tumors. This chapter will summarize the use of BCG in carcinoma in situ (CIS), Ta and T1 transitional cell carcinoma (TCC). Its efficacy will be compared to other standard intravesical agents. Practical issues such as dosage schedules and treatment of toxicity will be described. Finally, recent work on optimization of BCG dosing, including dose reduction and maintenance dosing, will be reviewed.

## TREATMENT INDICATIONS

Carcinoma in situ has been shown to have a high rate of progression to muscle-invasive disease, with rates ranging from 50% to 83% in long-term studies.[5-8] Intravesical immunotherapy with BCG has a major impact on this high-risk pathology with complete response rates in the range of 70% with six instillations and 84% with an additional three instillations at 3 months.[9] Brosman demonstrated a complete response

**Table 32.1** Controlled BCG trials: percent tumor recurrence

| Lead author | No. pts | No BCG (%) | BCG (%) | p Value |
|---|---|---|---|---|
| Lamm[42] | 57 | 52 | 20 | <0.001 |
| Herr[43] | 86 | 95 | 42 | <0.001 |
| Herr[44] | 49 | 100 | 35 | <0.001 |
| Yamamoto[45] | 44 | 67 | 17 | <0.05 |
| Pagano[27] | 133 | 83 | 26 | <0.001 |
| Melekos[46] | 94 | 59 | 32 | <0.02 |
| Krege[47] | 224 | 48 | 29 | <0.05 |

rate of 94% and recurrence rate of 13% using induction and an 18-month maintenance regimen with an average of 5.25 years' follow-up.[10] Patients with a complete response have a durable response as well: 65% may remain disease-free for 5 years or more.[11,12] Due to these impressive results, BCG is regarded as the best initial therapy for treatment of residual CIS and prophylaxis for recurrence and progression.

Nonmuscle-invasive TCC (Ta, T1) is another clinical situation in which recurrence and progression rates may be modified by intravesical BCG. The risk of recurrence after initial resection is 80% in patients with Ta or T1 tumors that were followed for a minimum of 20 years.[13] A subset of patients within this group are at highest risk, namely those with large, multiple, poorly differentiated tumors or concurrent CIS.

Management of T1 grade 3 tumors is particularly challenging since as much as 30% of patients may be understaged.[14] If treated with transurethral resection (TUR) alone, 50% to 80% may develop recurrences. Several nonrandomized BCG studies have shown efficacy in recurrence and progression prevention, and in disease-specific death rates. Pansadoro et al found a recurrence rate of 28% and a progression rate of 12% with a disease-specific death rate of 2% at 5 years.[15] These patients received 6 weeks of induction BCG with 3 months of maintenance. Hurle et al also demonstrated success in this patient group. Patients received induction and then monthly maintenance for 1 year. The recurrence rate was 23.5%, progression rate 13.7%, and disease-specific death rate 11.8%.[16] The management of patients with T1 grade 3 tumors is discussed in detail in Chapter 37.

## SPECIAL CIRCUMSTANCES

Prostatic urethral involvement with CIS or TCC needs to be differentiated from stromal invasion as the latter situation holds no role for BCG. Limited non-invasive urethral involvement may, however, be managed with BCG, with or without TUR. Orihuela and colleagues demonstrated that 86% of patients with mucosal involvement of the prostatic urethra had a sustained complete response in both the prostate and the bladder. They suggest that transurethral resection of the prostate (TURP) plays a crucial role by facilitating the immune response to BCG in the prostate.[17] Other authors demonstrated a local response rate of 56% to 83% in small series with limited follow-up.[18-20] BCG is a reasonable option for patients with non-invasive disease in the prostatic urethra, but care must be taken to exclude stromal involvement using staging TURP.

BCG has applications in the treatment of upper tract TCC. While the standard of care in this situation is nephroureterectomy, situations such as a solitary kidney or significant renal impairment raise the desire for preservation of the renal unit. Many different techniques

have been reported. Percutaneous resection coupled with antegrade BCG administration can be accomplished after the nephrostomy tract is well established and shows no evidence of extravasation.[21] BCG can be delivered in a retrograde manner after endoscopic resection of the ureteral orifice and placement of a ureteral stent, with subsequent intravesical BCG instillation.[22] A cystogram should be done to confirm that reflux reaches the tumor site and to determine the volume in which BCG must be delivered. (*Editor's note*: Alternatively, a single J stent can be passed suprapubically, providing convenient access to the upper tract [P. Schulam, personal communication].) A limited series of patients with solitary renal units was treated with percutaneous and ureteroscopic tumor resection and subsequent BCG; 5 of 10 were alive at 24 months with no evidence of disease.[23] Patients following this course of treatment for upper tract disease should be counseled that the price paid for preserved renal function is the risk of progressive disease.

## PATIENT SELECTION

As the previous examples demonstrate, BCG is a therapeutic option in a number of clinical scenarios. Proper patient selection serves to identify those that will benefit most from intravesical therapy. Primary low-grade Ta disease does not necessarily require additional intravesical therapy, though controlled trials and meta-analysis show that recurrence can be reduced with a single postoperative chemotherapy instillation.[24] However, if other risk factors for progression—such as multifocality, prior recurrence, large tumors, high tumor grade or lamina propria invasion—are present, immunotherapy is indicated. Stage T1 TCC carries a high recurrence rate, which may be minimized with prophylactic BCG after resection. It is well recognized that the presence of CIS poses high risk, and BCG is effective for both treatment and prophylaxis.

The success of BCG immunotherapy depends on several factors:

1. Bladder tumor burden should be minimized through transurethral resection. Murine model studies have shown improved response with cell volumes less than $10^3$ cells.
2. BCG and the remaining tumor cells must be in juxtaposition. Tumor sites away from the area of instillation may not respond.[25]
3. Success requires an immunocompetent host. Patients must be able to mount a local or systemic inflammatory response.

## DOSE OPTIMIZATION

Murine bladder tumor models have been used to evaluate immunotherapeutic agents and optimize dosing. Lamm et al reported on a series of experiments in which varying doses of BCG strains, including Tice, Pasteur, and Glaxo, were administered to mice with previously excised bladder tumors. The dose–response curve with survival as the endpoint was bell shaped. The antitumor effect peaked at a dose of $10^7$ colony-forming units, with higher doses actually decreasing the antitumor response. The presumed mechanism for this is diversion of the immune response from the tumor to BCG or impairment of the immune response due to antigenic excess.[26]

These early mouse studies set the stage for subsequent human trials to investigate the effect of dose reduction. A low dose regimen utilizing BCG Pasteur strain, 75 mg, was compared to the higher dose of 150 mg. A 6-week induction course was given, followed by a 2-year maintenance course for all responders. The time-to-failure curves showed a disease-free interval significantly higher in the low dose group compared to the high dose group (p=0.0009). Progression rates were similar. An additional benefit of low dose therapy is a reduction in side effects such as cystitis. The low dose regimen had a significantly lower (p<0.05) level of side effects compared to high dose.[27] Other researchers have confirmed the benefits of reduced doses, in doses ranging from 30 to 75 mg.[28,29]

There is an increasing body of work to suggest that maintenance therapy is another way to maximize the effectiveness of BCG. Southwest Oncology Group (SWOG) Trial 8795 randomized patients to either 50 mg Tice BCG or 20 mg mitomycin C (MMC) weekly for 6 weeks and then monthly for 1 year. The recurrence-free survival was significantly prolonged (p=0.017 proportional hazard regression) in patients receiving BCG compared to MMC.[30]

SWOG 8507 evaluated toxicity, recurrence, progression, and survival when patients with CIS or high risk TCC received either induction BCG or induction and maintenance BCG. Induction consisted of 120 mg Connaught BCG intravesically and $10^7$ colony-forming units percutaneously weekly for 6 weeks. Maintenance arm patients were treated with sets of three successive weekly intravesical and percutaneous administrations of BCG at 3 months, 6 months, and every 6 months thereafter for a total of 3 years. Median recurrence-free survival was 35.7 months in the induction group versus 76.8 months in the maintenance group (log rank, p<0.0001). The median progression-free survival was 111.5 months without maintenance, and had not been reached with over 10-years' follow-up in the maintenance arm (log rank, p=0.04). The overall 5-year survival was 78% in the induction group compared to 83% in the maintenance group, which was not statistically significant.[9]

This treatment regimen has been described as the '6 + 3' plan. The three weekly maintenance doses are crucial, because a number greater than that has a depressant effect on the immune response. During the maintenance instillations, the immune stimulation peaks at 3 weeks and may be suppressed with subsequent instillations.[31]

The suppression seen with subsequent doses may account for the lack of success seen in Palou et al's trial. This study randomized patients to a control group receiving 6-week induction alone or a maintenance group receiving an additional six instillations every 6 months (6×6) for a 2-year period. There was no significant difference in recurrence or progression compared to controls.[32]

Maintenance therapy is certainly one of the important recent topics in BCG. It seems to offer a number of advantages over traditional induction-only therapy. Immunostimulation wanes with time, and maintenance therapy serves to 'boost' the immune response. Furthermore, since TCC is a field change disease, the patient's entire urothelium remains at risk for the course of their life. Maintenance therapy maximizes the immune surveillance over the long term.

## BCG DOSING

Early BCG protocols consisted of weekly instillations of 120 mg BCG for 6 weeks. This was accompanied by an intradermal injection using the Tine or multiple puncture technique. Percutaneous injection was initiated after preliminary studies failed to demonstrate skin test conversion after only intravesical instillation. In a randomized trial, maintenance BCG had an equivalent efficacy for recurrence prevention compared to percutaneous and intravesical BCG.[33] Additional early studies for treatment of CIS showed complete response rates of 60% to 100% with intravesical BCG alone.[10,34,35]

There are currently a number of BCG strains commercially available. All of these are derived from the initial strain developed at the Pasteur Institute. Commonly used strains include Connaught, Pasteur, Tice, Armand Frappier, and Tokyo. While the individual doses for each strain may vary, their efficacy is comparable. Complete response rates in the treatment of CIS range from 60% to 79%.[12]

## EFFICACY

Intravesical chemotherapy is effective in the prevention of tumor recurrences. Comparative studies with BCG established its superiority to thiotepa, epirubicin, and doxorubicin in the prevention of recurrence (Table 32.2).

Bohle and Bock's recent meta-analysis of BCG and mitomycin demonstrated a 34% risk reduction of progression with maintenance BCG compared to mitomycin.[36] This benefit was not seen with induction-only dosing.

Recently, several large meta-analyses have demonstrated the advantages of maintenance BCG.

**Table 32.2** BCG versus chemotherapy: percent tumor recurrence

| Lead author | BCG | Chemotherapy | p Value |
|---|---|---|---|
| *Thiotepa* | | | |
| Brosman[48] | 0 | 47 | <0.01 |
| Rodrigues Netto[49] | 7 | 43 | <0.01 |
| Martinez-Pineiro[50] | 13 | 36 | <0.01 |
| *Doxorubicin* | | | |
| Lamm[11] | 53 | 78 | <0.02 |
| Martinez-Pineiro[50] | 13 | 43 | <0.01 |
| Sekine[51] | 24 | 42 | <0.05 |
| *Epirubicin* | | | |
| Van der Meijden[52] | 33 | 47 | <0.0001 |

Bohle et al compared BCG to MMC on recurrence of stages Ta and T1 TCC. BCG versus MMC had a 44% reduction in recurrence (p=0.005). This superiority was even more profound when maintenance BCG was used. There was a 57% reduction in recurrence with maintenance compared to MMC (p<0.001). Toxicity did not differ significantly between the BCG maintenance and nonmaintenance groups.[37]

A meta-analysis has also been applied to the effect of BCG and MMC on progression of TCC. There was no significant difference for the odd ratios for recurrence when BCG was compared to MMC. However, when maintenance BCG was used, there was a 34% reduction in progression compared to MMC (p=0.02).[36] Sylvester et al's meta-analysis also supports the finding that progression of TCC can be reduced with maintenance BCG. Patients receiving maintenance BCG had a 37% decrease in the odds of progression compared to controls (p=0.001).[38]

## TOXICITY

Many patients receiving BCG immunotherapy will experience some level of toxicity, either local or systemic. Preventive measures, early diagnosis, and appropriate treatment will limit adverse outcomes.

Irritative bladder symptoms such as cystitis may occur in 90% of patients.[39] Incidence of other local symptoms includes hematuria (43%), low-grade fever (29%), malaise (24%), and nausea (5%). These often occur after the third treatment as the patient's immune response peaks. Patients experiencing irritative symptoms are more likely to have them after subsequent treatments.[40] It is advisable to delay subsequent BCG treatments until symptoms resolve. If the symptoms persist for more than 48 hours or are accompanied by fever or malaise, treatment with 300 mg isoniazid daily is recommended, and consideration should be given to adding a fluoroquinolone to reduce the risk of developing isoniazid resistance. This should be continued while symptoms persist and may be reinstituted 1 day before subsequent treatments and continued for 3 days afterward.[41]

In contrast to local toxicity, systemic toxicity is far less frequent. High fever (>103°F/39.4°C) occurs in 3% of patients.[39] Because of the possibility of BCG sepsis, it is recommended that these patients be hospitalized and treated with isoniazid 300 mg and rifampin 600 mg daily. BCG is also sensitive to fluoroquinolones. These drugs, which act more quickly and also treat common gram-negative urinary infections, are most useful.

The most serious side effect of BCG therapy is sepsis. It occurs in 0.4% of patients and is commonly associated with intravascular absorption of the organism.[39] This could happen with administration following a traumatic urethral catheterization, during severe cystitis, or immediately after bladder biopsy. BCG instillation should be initiated at least 1 week after bladder tumor resection.

In a patient suspected of having BCG sepsis, attention should also be directed to the possibility of gram-negative sepsis. Treatment should cover both possibilities until final culture results are available, remembering that mycobacterial cultures are frequently negative, even in the presence of BCG infection. Initial treatment includes isoniazid 300 mg, rifampin 600 mg, and ethambutol 1200 mg daily, plus a fluoroquinolone or an aminoglycoside. If symptoms fail to respond or progress, prednisone 40 mg daily may be required to reduce the hypersensitivity response. Prednisone in this setting may be life saving and higher doses may be needed depending on the patient's symptoms. The steroid is slowly tapered when the patient improves, but may be reinstituted if symptoms recur after the taper. Patients with documented BCG sepsis should receive the triple-antibiotic treatment for 3–6 months. Additional BCG treatment is contraindicated.

Preventive measures can help to limit some of the toxicity. BCG instillation is deferred if symptoms from the previous treatment persist or if catheterization is bloody or traumatic. Log dose reduction (1/3, 1/10, 1/30, 1/100th) prevents increasing side effects. These side effects are not required to receive the benefits of maintenance BCG.

## CONCLUSION

BCG has been shown to have excellent success in the prophylaxis and treatment of CIS. Its use is expanding as high-risk groups are identified and stratified by prognostic factors. These highest risk categories are the ones that will benefit most from further refinements in BCG dosing. An already efficacious treatment can be improved as its mechanism is further elucidated and the principles of immunity followed. Maintenance therapy is the culmination of this knowledge to date.

## REFERENCES

1. Pearl R. Cancer and tuberculosis. Proc Natl Acad Sci 1929;9:97.

2. Morales A. Intracavitary bacillus Calmette–Guérin in the treatment of superficial bladder tumors. J Urol 1976;116(2):180–183.

3. Lamm DL, Thor DE, Harris SC, Reyna JA, Stogdill VD, Radwin HM. Bacillus Calmette–Guérin immunotherapy of superficial bladder cancer. J Urol 1980;124(1):38–40.

4. Morales A, Ottenhof P, Emerson L. Treatment of residual, non-infiltrating bladder cancer with bacillus Calmette–Guérin. J Urol 1981;125(5):649–651.

5. Utz DC, Hanash KA, Farrow GM. The plight of the patient with carcinoma in situ of the bladder. J Urol 1970;103(2):160–164.

6. Skinner DG, Richie JP, Cooper PH, Waisman J, Kaufman JJ. The clinical significance of carcinoma in situ of the bladder and its association with overt carcinoma. J Urol 1974;112(1):68–71.

7. Starklint H, Jensen NK, Thyro E. The extent of carcinoma in situ in urinary bladders with primary carcinomas. Acta Pathol Microbiol Scand: Section A, Pathology 1976;84(2):130–136.

8. Herr HW. Carcinoma in situ of the bladder. Semin Urol 1983;1(1):15–22.

9. Lamm DL, Blumenstein BA, Crissman JD, et al. Maintenance bacillus Calmette–Guérin immunotherapy for recurrent TA, T1 and carcinoma in situ transitional cell carcinoma of the bladder: a randomized Southwest Oncology Group Study. J Urol 2000;163(4):1124–1129.

10. Brosman SA. The use of bacillus Calmette–Guérin in the therapy of bladder carcinoma in situ. J Urol 1985;134(1):36–39.

11. Lamm DL, Blumenstein BA, Crawford ED, et al. A randomized trial of intravesical doxorubicin and immunotherapy with bacille Calmette–Guérin for transitional-cell carcinoma of the bladder. N Engl J Med 1991;325(17):1205–1209.

12. Lamm DL. BCG immunotherapy for transitional-cell carcinoma in situ of the bladder. Oncology 1995;9(10):947–952.

13. Holmang S, Hedelin H, Anderstrom C. The relationship among multiple recurrences and prognosis of patients with stages Ta and T1 TCC of the bladder followed for at least 20 years. J Urol 1995;153(6):1923–1926.

14. Pagano F, Bassi P, Galetti TP, et al. Results of contemporary radical cystectomy for invasive bladder cancer: a clinicopathologic study with an emphasis on the inadequacy of the tumor, nodes and metastases classification. J Urol 1991;145(1):45–50.

15. Pansadoro V, Emiliozzi P, Defidio L, et al. Bacillus Calmette–Guérin in the treatment of stage T1 grade 3 transitional cell carcinoma of the bladder: long-term results. J Urol 1995;154(6):2054–2058.

16. Hurle R, Losa A, Ranieri A, Graziotti P, Lembo A. Low dose Pasteur bacillus Calmette–Guérin regimen in stage T1, grade 3 bladder cancer therapy. J Urol 1996;156(5):1602–1605.

17. Orihuela E, Herr HW, Whitmore WF Jr. Conservative treatment of superficial transitional cell carcinoma of prostatic urethra with intravesical BCG. Urology 1989;34(5):231–237.

18. Bretton PR, Herr HW, Whitmore WF Jr, et al. Intravesical bacillus Calmette–Guérin therapy for in situ transitional cell carcinoma involving the prostatic urethra. J Urol 1989;141(4):853–856.

19. Schellhammer PF, Ladaga LE, Moriarty RP. Intravesical bacillus Calmette–Guérin for the treatment of superficial transitional cell carcinoma of the prostatic urethra in association with carcinoma of the bladder. J Urol 1995;153(1):53–56.

20. Palou J, Xavier B, Laguna P, Montello M, Vicente J. In situ transitional cell carcinoma involvement of prostatic urethra: bacillus Calmette–Guérin therapy without previous transurethral resection of the prostate. Urology 1996;47(4):482–484.

21. Streem SB. Percutaneous management of upper-tract transitional cell carcinoma. Urol Clin North Am 1995;22(1):221–229.

22. Bohle A, Schuller J, Knipper A, Hofstetter A. Bacillus Calmette–Guérin treatment and vesicorenal reflux. Eur Urol 1990;17(2):125–128.

23. Schoenberg MP, Van Arsdalen KN, Wein AJ. The management of transitional cell carcinoma in solitary renal units. J Urol 1991;146:700–703.

24. Sylvester R, Oosterlinck W, van der Meijden AP. A single immediate postoperative instillation of chemotherapy decreases the risk of recurrence in patients with stage TaT1 bladder cancer: a meta-analysis of published results of randomized clinical trials. J Urol 2004;171(6 Pt 1):2786–2790.

25. Lamm DL, DeHaven JI, Shriver J, Crispen R, Grau D, Sarosdy MF. A randomized prospective comparison of oral versus intravesical and percutaneous bacillus Calmette–Guérin for superficial bladder cancer. J Urol 1990;144(1):65–67.

26. Lamm DL, Reichert DF, Harris SC, Lucio RM. Immunotherapy of murine transitional cell carcinoma. J Urol 1982;128(5):1104–1108.

27. Pagano F, Bassi P, Milani C, Meneghini A, Maruzzi D, Garbeglio A. A low dose bacillus Calmette–Guérin regimen in superficial bladder cancer therapy: is it effective? J Urol 1991;146(1):32–35.

28. Lebret T, Gaudez F, Herve JM, Barre P, Lugagne PM, Botto H. Low-dose BCG instillations in the treatment of stage T1 grade 3 bladder tumours: recurrence, progression and success. Eur Urol 1998;34(1):67–72.

29. Mack D, Holtl W, Bassi P, et al. The ablative effect of quarter dose bacillus Calmette–Guérin on a papillary marker lesion of the bladder. J Urol 2001;165(2):401–403.

30. Lamm D, Blumenstein B, Crawford ED, et al. Randomized intergroup comparison of Bacillus Calmette–Guérin immunotherapy and mitomycin C chemotherapy prophylaxis in superficial transitional cell carcinoma of the bladder. Urol Oncol 1995;1:119–126.

31. de Boer EC, De Jong WH, Steerenberg PA, Aarden LA. Induction of urinary interleukin-1 (IL-1), IL-2, IL-6, and tumor necrosis factor during immunotherapy with bacillus Calmette–Guérin in superficial bladder cancer. Cancer Immunol Immunother 1992;34(5):306–312.

32. Palou J, Laguna P, Millan-Rodriguez F, Hall RR, Salvador-Bayarri J, Vicente-Rodriguez J. Control group and maintenance treatment with bacillus Calmette–Guérin for carcinoma in situ and/or high grade bladder tumors. J Urol 2001;165(5):1488–1491.

33. Lamm DL, DeHaven JI, Shriver J, Sarosdy MF. Prospective randomized comparison of intravesical with percutaneous bacillus Calmette–Guérin versus intravesical bacillus Calmette–Guérin in superficial bladder cancer. J Urol 1991;145(4):738–740.

34. deKernion JB, Huang MY, Lindner A, Smith RB, Kaufman JJ. The management of superficial bladder tumors and carcinoma in situ with intravesical bacillus Calmette–Guérin. J Urol 1985;133(4):598–601.

35. Schellhammer PF, Ladaga LE, Fillion MB. Bacillus Calmette–Guérin for superficial transitional cell carcinoma of the bladder. J Urol 1986;135(2):261–264.

36. Bohle A, Bock PR. Intravesical bacille Calmette–Guérin versus mitomycin C in superficial bladder cancer: formal meta-analysis of comparative studies on tumor progression. Urology 2004;63(4):682–687.

37. Bohle A, Jocham D, Bock PR. Intravesical bacillus Calmette–Guérin versus mitomycin C for superficial bladder cancer: a formal meta-analysis of comparative studies on recurrence and toxicity. J Urol 2003;169(1):90–95.

38. Sylvester RJ, van der MA, Lamm DL. Intravesical bacillus Calmette–Guérin reduces the risk of progression in patients with superficial bladder cancer: a meta-analysis of the published results of randomized clinical trials. J Urol 2002;168(5):1964–1970.

39. Lamm DL, van der Meijden PM, Morales A, et al. Incidence and treatment of complications of bacillus Calmette–Guérin intravesical therapy in superficial bladder cancer. J Urol 1992;147(3):596–600.

40. Berry DL, Blumenstein BA, Magyary DL, Lamm DL, Crawford ED. Local toxicity patterns associated with intravesical bacillus Calmette–Guérin: a Southwest Oncology Group Study. Int J Urol 1996;3(2):98–100.

41. Lamm DL. Complications of bacillus Calmette–Guérin immunotherapy. Urol Clin North Am 1992;19(3):565–572.

42. Lamm DL. Bacillus Calmette–Guérin immunotherapy for bladder cancer. J Urol 1985;134(1):40–47.

43. Herr HW, Pinsky CM, Whitmore WF Jr, Sogani PG, Oettgen HF, Melamed MR. Experience with intravesical bacillus Calmette–Guérin therapy of superficial bladder tumors. Urology 1985;25(2):119–123.

44. Herr HW, Pinsky CM, Whitmore WF Jr, Sogani PC, Oettgen HF, Melamed MR. Long-term effect of intravesical bacillus Calmette–Guérin on flat carcinoma in situ of the bladder. J Urol 1986;135(2):265–267.

45. Yamamoto T, Hagiwara M, Nakazono M, Yamamoto H. [Intravesical bacillus Calmette–Guérin (BCG) in the treatment of superficial bladder cancer. Prospective randomized study for prophylactic effect.] Nippon Hinyokika Gakkai Zasshi—Jpn J Urol 1990;81(7):997–1001.

46. Melekos MD, Chionis H, Pantazakos A, Fokaefs E, Paranychianakis G, Dauaher H. Intravesical bacillus Calmette–Guérin immunoprophylaxis of superficial bladder cancer: results of a controlled prospective trial with modified treatment schedule. J Urol 1993;149(4):744–740.

47. Krege S, Giani G, Meyer R, Otto T, Rubben H. A randomized multicenter trial of adjuvant therapy in superficial bladder cancer: transurethral resection only versus transurethral resection plus mitomycin C versus transurethral resection plus bacillus Calmette–Guérin. J Urol 1996;156(3):962–966.

48. Brosman SA. Experience with bacillus Calmette–Guérin in patients with superficial bladder carcinoma. J Urol 1982;128(1):27–30.

49. Rodrigues Netto Junior N, Lemos GC. A comparison of treatment methods for the prophylaxis of recurrent superficial bladder tumors. J Urol 1983;129(1):33–34.

50. Martinez-Pineiro JA, Jimenez Leon J, Martinez-Pineiro L Jr, et al. Bacillus Calmette–Guérin versus doxorubicin versus thiotepa: a randomized prospective study in 202 patients with superficial bladder cancer. J Urol 1990;143(3):502–506.

51. Sekine H, Fukui I, Yamada T, Ohwada F, Yokokawa M, Ohshima H. Intravesical mitomycin C and doxorubicin sequential therapy for carcinoma in situ of the bladder: a longer followup result. J Urol 1994;151(1):27–30.

52. van der Meijden AP, Brausi M, Zambon V, et al. Intravesical instillation of epirubicin, bacillus Calmette–Guérin and bacillus Calmette–Guérin plus isoniazid for intermediate and high risk Ta, T1 papillary carcinoma of the bladder: a European Organisation for Research and Treatment of Cancer genito-urinary group randomized phase III trial. J Urol 2001;166(2):476–489.

# Mode of action of BCG and rationale for combination immunotherapy

## 33

*Andreas Böhle, Sven Brandau*

## INTRODUCTION

Of all medical disciplines, it is exclusively in urology where immunotherapy against cancer has an established position with intravesical bacillus Calmette–Guérin (BCG) against superficial bladder carcinoma recurrences. BCG is regarded as the most successful immunotherapy to date. However, the mode of action has not yet been fully elucidated. The aim of this review is to provide a thorough overview on this complex field of research.

In 1976, Morales, Eidinger, and Bruce were the first to report on successful treatment of superficial bladder cancer with BCG.[1] Since then, BCG has become the treatment of choice for high-risk superficial bladder cancer. Intravesical BCG therapy is regarded as the most successful immunotherapy to date,[2,3] being not only superior to intravesical chemotherapy with regard to the recurrence rate of superficial bladder cancer,[4-6] but also acting beneficially on the progression rate of this tumor.[7-10] In this review we will concentrate on the immunologic mechanisms that make BCG such a powerful therapeutic agent. We describe the major findings made during the last few years when systematic analyses of patient material, detailed in vitro studies, and investigations on animal models have led to a substantially greater understanding of the mechanisms involved. BCG therapy is currently considered the most successful immunotherapy of solid tumors, and this review will provide some explanations as to why this is the case.

## GENETIC BACKGROUND

### WHAT IS BCG?

The live attenuated BCG vaccine for the prevention of disease associated with mycobacterium tuberculosis was derived from the closely related virulent tubercle bacillus *Mycobacterium bovis*[11] by Calmette and Guérin who passaged a strain of *M. bovis* 230 times in vitro between 1908 and 1921. However, because of the inability to preserve viable bacteria (such as by freezing), this live vaccine required continued passage, eventually resulting in a profusion of phenotypically different daughter strains that are collectively known as BCG. By the time lyophilized seed lots of BCG vaccines were created in the 1960s, these vaccines had been separately propagated through about 1000 additional passages (depending on the daughter strain), usually under the very conditions that effected the original attenuation.

To better understand the differences between *M. tuberculosis*, *M. bovis*, and the various BCG daughter strains, their genomic compositions were studied recently by performing comparative hybridization experiments on a DNA microarray.[12] By this method 11 regions of a virulent *M. tuberculosis* strain were found that were absent from one or more virulent strains of *M. bovis*. Five additional regions representing 38 open reading frames were present in *M. bovis*, but absent from some BCG strains. This was seen as evidence for the ongoing evolution of BCG strains since their original derivation.

In addition, contemporary BCG vaccines were compared to their progenitor strain. Because this strain was lost during World War I, the origin of current BCG vaccines could only be inferred through an evolutionary approach. Behr and coworkers[12] curated a collection of BCG daughter strains representing this global dissemination for the purpose of performing genomic comparisons. Altogether, 16 regions were found as deleted in BCG strains as compared to virulent tuberculosis. Of the 16 deletion regions, 9 are missing from BCG and all virulent *M. bovis* strains tested, 2 are missing from BCG and some of the strains of *M. bovis*, 1 is missing from all BCG strains, and 4 are missing only from certain BCG strains. Thus, BCG significantly differs from *M. bovis*, from which it was originally derived. Attenuation led to the elimination of most virulence genes which made BCG a famous vaccine against tuberculosis and a well-known immunomodulator against bladder cancer.

## THE LOCAL IMMUNE REACTION IN PATIENTS

### WHAT HAPPENS IN THE BLADDER AFTER INTRAVESICAL INSTILLATION OF BCG?

Immunotherapy with BCG results in a massive local immune response which is characterized by the induced expression of cytokines in the urine and in bladder tissue,[13] and by an influx of granulocytes as well as mononuclear cells into the bladder wall.[14,15] A large set of cytokines—including tumor necrosis factor-$\alpha$ (TNF$\alpha$), granulocyte macrophage colony-stimulating factor (GM-CSF), interferon-$\gamma$ (IFN$\gamma$), interleukin (IL) 1, IL2, IL5, IL6, IL8, IL10, IL12, and IL18—has been detected in the urine of patients treated with intravesical BCG.[16–25] Many of these cytokines are known to be involved in the initiation or maintenance of inflammatory processes. The pattern of cytokines suggests that BCG predominantly induces a T-helper type 1 (TH1) response in the bladder of patients. Nevertheless, certain TH2 cytokines (IL5 and IL10), and cytokines not specifically belonging to a TH1 or TH2 profile (e.g. IL8, GM-CSF, TNF$\alpha$), are also induced. Interestingly, in most investigations the TH2 cytokine IL4 could not be detected. Thus far, chemokines have not been intensively studied with regard to BCG therapy. Because of the significant influx of various leukocyte subpopulations after instillation of BCG, chemokines are probably also contributing to the antitumor effect of this immunotherapy. Indeed, some chemokines, such as IL8, IP10, MIP1$\alpha$, MCP1, MDC, and even eotaxin, have been detected in the urine of treated patients.[17,26,27] Finally, with regard to the cytokine response, it has to be noted that this response varies greatly between patients and that a possible correlation between cytokine expression and therapy outcome is currently under intensive investigation.[13]

In addition to these humoral mediators of inflammation, BCG-treated patients typically have characteristic granulomatous cellular infiltrates in their bladder wall. Lage et al described the presence of giant cells and epithelioid granulomas.[15] Infiltrates were surrounded by dense areas of lymphocytes and eosinophilic granulocytes. Noteworthy, instillation of BCG seems to induce a long-lasting immune response in the bladder. The bladder can be regarded as an organ that is not normally infiltrated by large numbers of immune cells. Before therapy, only low numbers of leukocytes can be detected in the suburothelial stroma of nontumor-bearing areas of the bladder. After repeated instillations of BCG, an early accumulation of granulocytes can be observed, followed by the influx of macrophages and lymphocytes.[14,28,29] Immuno-histologic analyses revealed that CD4+ cells were the predominant cell population in the granulomas of treated patients. The influx of immune cells into the bladder wall coincided with an increased expression of activation markers (HLA-DR, CD25, ICAM1) on infiltrating cells and also on the urothelium itself, which strongly expressed major histocompatibility complex (MHC) class II molecules at the end of the therapy.[14,28] It is important to note that these changes in the bladders of patients can persist for more than 1 year after the initial 6-week therapeutic induction course but commonly begin to wane after 3–6 months. This provides some of the rationale for maintenance therapy.

These investigations point to a stimulation of the local immune system in the bladder which differs significantly from nonspecific cystitis in terms of its duration and also in qualitative terms: in the case of nonspecific cystitis, or even of cystitis induced by cytostatic drugs, an early granulocytic infiltration is found and no significant influx of mononuclear cells can be observed. It is characteristic for the BCG-induced response that the early influx of granulocytes is followed by an increase of predominantly mononuclear cells (lymphocytes and macrophages). These mononuclear cells express activation markers, and cellular infiltrates can persist for at least 12 months. Through the accumulation of large numbers of immunocompetent cells, mainly in suburothelial granulomas, these infiltrates can be regarded as centers for a long-term, persisting, local immunoactivation, which is not apparent in nonspecific cystitis.

For BCG immunotherapy, as for most other therapies, the development of a so-called 'prognostic marker' which could predict therapy outcome on an individual basis is highly desirable. Based on the studies outlined above, several cytokines have been tested in this regard. Thus far, IL2 has been found to be the best candidate. Initial studies on small numbers of patients suggest that the level of urinary IL2 could have prognostic value for tumor recurrence.[22,30,31] However, the cytokine response seems to be highly variable between patients. In addition, the predictive value of urinary IL2 is still very controversial as other groups did not find a correlation of urinary cytokines and therapy outcome.[19] An interesting way of predicting the response to BCG was found by Kaempfer and coworkers[32] by analysis of the induction of IL2 and IFNγ mRNA in peripheral blood mononuclear cells during BCG treatment. Induction of IL2 mRNA was observed for patients who responded with remission, but not for those who relapsed.

## ANIMAL MODELS

In addition to the mostly descriptive studies in patients, a variety of investigations on animal models have been performed. In contrast to humans, animals can be manipulated in various ways, which makes it easier to obtain causal evidence for the involvement of a specific immune component in successful immunotherapy with BCG. The most meaningful conclusions can be drawn from animal models where the tumor is growing orthotopically in its natural immune environment (the bladder) and is treated by the intravesical route. Such a syngeneic mouse model has been developed and optimized for murine bladder cancer.[33,34]

When patients receive BCG therapy, several hundred million bacteria are instilled into the bladder. While most of these bacteria are washed out with the first postinstillation micturition, some bacteria obviously adhere to the bladder wall, although researchers are currently unable to indicate even an approximate number, mostly due to technical difficulties. Animal studies indicated that the adherence of BCG is largely mediated by a fibronectin-attachment protein on the surface of the mycobacteria and preferentially occurs at sites of electrocauterization.[35,36] Moreover, attachment of mycobacteria to the urothelium seems to be a prerequisite for effective therapy, because interruption of adherence resulted in ineffective therapy.[37]

The first conclusive evidence about the involvement of cell-mediated immunity in BCG immunotherapy came from the analysis of athymic nude mice. In contrast to efficient BCG therapy in wild-type mice, no therapeutic effect of BCG was observed in these nude mice. In addition, adoptive transfer of BCG-sensitized splenocytes syngeneic to the tumor transferred delayed-type hypersensitivity (DTH) reactivity to BCG antigens in recipient mice and restored the antitumor activity of intravesical BCG.[38] Apparently, the antitumor activity of

BCG depends on the interplay of different lymphocyte subpopulations. Depletion of either CD4+ or CD8+ cells abolished the antitumor effect of intravesical BCG therapy in mice, while DTH was only affected after depletion of CD4+ cells.[39] In a similar study, the administration of anti-asialo GM1 antibody did not significantly abrogate the antitumor activity of BCG in a model of MBT2 bladder cancer in C3H/He mice.[40] On the other hand, a recent study using an optimized murine bladder cancer model, and utilizing MB49 cells, beige mice, and anti-NK1.1 antibody, suggested that natural killer (NK) cell activity is of prime importance for the therapeutic effect of BCG. While BCG therapy was effective in wild-type mice, it was ineffective in beige mice (which are defective in some NK functions), and in mice treated with anti-NK1.1 monoclonal antibodies.[41] Based on the aforementioned studies, we conclude that T lymphocytes and most likely NK cells are required for successful BCG therapy. Nevertheless, it still has to be determined whether the respective cell populations exert their antitumor effect via direct cytotoxicity or cytokine release or both.

## WHAT IS THE FUNCTIONAL RELEVANCE OF THE INDUCTION OF MAINLY PRO-INFLAMMATORY CYTOKINES IN THE BLADDER OF TREATED INDIVIDUALS?

In a murine model, intravesical bladder tumor growth was associated with the expression of IFNγ and IL4. BCG treatment upregulated IFNγ expression and simultaneously downregulated IL4 expression, indicating the generation of a TH1-based cytokine profile.[42] In a similar model, BCG was also shown to induce TNFα.[43] The analysis of a panel of knockout (KO) mice strongly suggested an important role of the TH1/TH2 balance for effective immunotherapy with BCG. In an orthotopic bladder cancer model, therapy was effective in wild-type mice, but was completely ineffective in both IFNγ and IL12 KO mice. Interestingly, the therapeutic effect of BCG was enhanced in the absence of IL10 (IL10 KO mice).[44]

## IN VITRO MODEL INVESTIGATIONS

The in vivo studies mentioned above have been supplemented by detailed in vitro studies on isolated systems to further understand the immunostimulation with BCG and the resulting antitumor effect. These studies made clear that BCG exerts its tumor-therapeutic effect in two different ways: first, it binds to and interacts with malignant and normal urothelial cells leading, for example, to cytokine secretion by these cells and to reduced proliferation of tumor cells[45,46]; secondly, and more importantly, BCG activates directly or indirectly various immunocompetent cells which then acquire antitumor activity.

After instillation, BCG first gets into contact with the urothelial cells of the bladder. Normal and malignant urothelial cells can produce a limited array of cytokines including IL1, IL6, and TNFα in response to this mycobacterial stimulus.[47,10] In addition, short exposure to high doses of BCG, as applied during local immunotherapy, has an antiproliferative effect on certain tumor cell lines.[49]

Stimulated by the animal studies outlined above, which indicated the contribution of cell-mediated immunity to the antitumor effect of BCG, several in vitro studies have focused on the activation of mononuclear cells by BCG. It was shown that human peripheral blood mononuclear cells acquired the capacity to kill bladder tumor cells after in vitro stimulation with BCG.[46,50,51] Subsequent studies revealed that monocytes and CD4 lymphocytes serve as accessory cells in BCG-induced cell-mediated cytotoxicity.[52] This cytotoxicity is mediated by an effector cell termed BCG-activated killer cell (BAK cell) which represents a subpopulation of activated NK

cells,[41,53] and kills tumor cells via perforin without significant contribution of the FasLigand pathway.[54]

Further analyses of the activation of human peripheral blood mononuclear cells (MNCs) with BCG focused on the role of NK cells in BCG immunotherapy. NK cells are important components of the innate immune system with the potential to lyse various target cells and provide an early source of immunoregulatory cytokines.[55] NK cells recognize MHC class I molecules through so-called inhibitory NK cell receptors (iNKR) that deliver inhibitory signals and deactivate NK cell cytotoxicity. Thus, NK cells lyse targets that have lost or express insufficient amounts of MHC class I molecules, as frequently observed in tumor or virus-infected cells, including bladder tumor cells.[56] Various (mostly TH1-related) cytokines were demonstrated to augment NK cell responses. Consequently, recent mechanistic in vitro studies have uncovered the cascade of events leading to BCG-mediated NK cell activation and demonstrated a crucial role for IL12 in this context.[57]

In accordance with the patient data mentioned above, it was shown that the generation of BAK cells was dependent on the presence of TH1 cytokines such as IFNγ, IL2, and IL12[46,58] (Figure 33.1). IFNγ and IL12 are

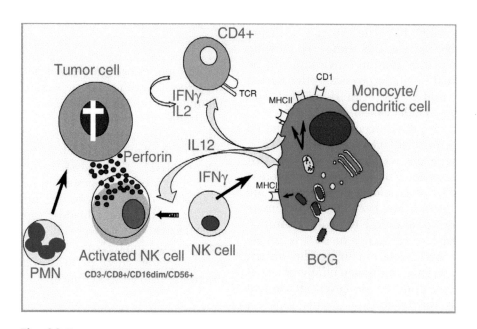

**Fig. 33.1**

The immunologic processes involved in BCG immunotherapy. During stimulation of human peripheral blood mononuclear cells with BCG, a cascade of events leads to the generation of tumor-cytotoxic natural killer (NK) cells (BAK cells). First, accessory monocytes and dendritic cells take up BCG mycobacteria and become activated. Interleukin (IL) 12 is a crucial cytokine, which is released by monocytes and dendritic cells in this process. CD4 cells also function as accessory cells by releasing cytokines. Interferon-γ (IFNγ) and IL2 are essential for BCG-induced cytotoxicity. Enhanced cytokine production then results in the activation of NK cells. A subpopulation of CD8+/CD16dim NK cells lyses tumor cells via perforin without significant contribution of the Fas/FasL pathway. The role of granulocytes (polymorphonuclear leukocytes, PMN) is under investigation. (MHC, major histocompatibility complex.)

key cytokines in directing immune responses in the TH1 direction. Indeed, as mentioned above, IFNγ and IL12 KO mice could not be successfully treated with BCG,[44] and the key role of these cytokines in BCG immunotherapy was further underscored by in vitro studies. In murine splenocyte and human peripheral blood mononuclear cell cultures, BCG induced the early production of IL12 (preceding the production of other TH1 cytokines). Inhibition of IL12 reduced BCG-induced production of IFNγ, while exogenous recombinant IL12 synergistically enhanced BCG-induced production of IFNγ.[59,60] Similarly, IFNα2b, a cytokine with various antiviral and antitumor properties, also enhanced TH1 cytokine responses and decreased IL10 (a TH2 cytokine) production in bladder cancer patients receiving BCG immunotherapy.[61] On the other hand, neutralization of IL10 enhanced IFNγ production and NK cell activation in BCG-stimulated cultures.[58,59] Taken together, these in vitro studies with immunocompetent cells of healthy donors and bladder cancer patients further substantiated the importance of the TH1/TH2 dichotomy in BCG immunotherapy.

As mentioned above, neutrophil granulocytes are the most predominant cell type in the bladder wall and urine early after instillation of BCG. At the same time, the role of this cell type in BCG immunotherapy has remained rather mysterious until now. For a long time regarded as cells contributing to undesired side effects by the release of their granule content, recent observations now suggest a possible antitumor effect of these abundant leukocytes in BCG immunotherapy.[62,63]

# MODE OF ACTION AND SHORT INTRODUCTION ON POSSIBLE IMPROVEMENTS

On the basis of all the studies mentioned in this review (and many others, which could not be cited owing to space limitations), a much clearer picture now arises with regard to the immunologic mechanism of this highly effective therapy. The initial crucial step in BCG immunotherapy seems to be the binding of mycobacteria to the urothelial lining, which is most likely dependent on the interaction of a fibronectin-attachment protein on the surface of the bacteria with fibronectin in the bladder wall. The high density of mycobacteria reduces proliferation and viability of tumor cells to a limited extent. The presence of BCG then leads to an activation of urothelial cells and antigen-presenting cells. Granulocytes and other immunocompetent mononuclear cells become attracted to the bladder wall (probably by chemokines) and a cascade of pro-inflammatory cytokines sustains the immune response. Subsequently, a largely TH1-based cytokine milieu and granuloma-like cellular foci are established in the bladder wall. This leads to eradication of residual tumor cells in several ways (Table 33.1). Within this scenario the most important effector mechanisms might be the direct antitumor activity of interferons (and perhaps other cytokines) and the cytotoxic activity of NK cells.

**Table 33.1** Components of the immune system contributing to the antitumor activity of BCG immunotherapy

| Component of immune system | Stimulation of immune cells by BCG in vitro | Animal model of immunotherapy with BCG | Analysis of material from BCG-treated patients |
|---|---|---|---|
| TH1 cytokines | Required | Detected in urine and bladder of treated mice. Proven importance in knock-out mouse models | Increased expression in urine of treated patients |
| T lymphocytes | Accessory function | Required for successful therapy | Induced in treated patients |
| NK cells | Effector function | Required for successful therapy (effector cell or IFNγ producer?) | Rare population (immunohistology is problematic) |
| Monocytic cells | Accessory function/direct killing | Unclear | Unclear |
| Granulocytes (PMN) | BCG induces PMN activation and prolongs PMN lifespan | Induced in treated mice | Induced in treated patients |
| Cellular cytotoxicity against tumor | Perforin is major killing mechanism | Unclear | Unclear (increased number of perforin-positive cells in treated patients) |
| Nitric oxide | BCG induces NOS activity in bladder cancer cells and NO production in splenocytes | NOS upregulated in a rat model of BCG immunotherapy | Nitrite locally induced in BCG patients (clinical relevance yet unclear) |

IFNγ, inteferon-γ; NK, natural killer; NO, nitric oxide; NOS, NO synthase; PMN, polymorphonuclear leukocyte(s); TH1, T-helper type 1.

## IS THERE A NEED TO IMPROVE BCG IMMUNOTHERAPY OF BLADDER CANCER AND, IF YES, HOW COULD THIS BE ACHIEVED?

Undoubtedly, immunotherapy with BCG is currently the optimal therapy for patients with superficial bladder cancer and probably the most successful immunotherapy of solid tumors.[3] On the other hand, the use of live organisms causes concern and indeed side effects and the difficulty to predict responses of patients are major drawbacks. Therefore, alternative treatment strategies using nonviable subfractions of mycobacteria have been explored. Although some reports indicate promising results with, for example cell wall extracts,[64] others show that the viability of BCG (and of an active intracellular infection?) are of prime importance for the efficacy of this immunotherapy.[65,66] Therefore, nonviable alternatives to BCG will most likely not be equally effective until adequate delivery systems have been developed and proper retention of the material in the bladder is ensured. Given the importance of cytokines for efficient BCG therapy and the direct antitumor capacity of certain cytokines,[67] current studies focus on the combination of cytokines and BCG. IFNα and IL12 seem to be the most promising candidates and have already shown some initial success in bladder cancer patients.[61,68,69] IFNα has long been recognized for its potent antiviral activity, and ongoing clinical trials are now exploring its potential in immunotherapy of cancer. Of special interest is the recent observation that either IFNα alone,[70] or a combination of BCG and IFNα,[71] might be effective in patients with superficial bladder cancer.

Although genetic manipulation of mycobacteria is somewhat difficult compared to manipulation of, for example, *Escherichia coli*, several laboratories, including our own, have succeeded in the construction of recombinant BCG strains. This now offers the opportunity to perform BCG/cytokine combination therapy by using cytokine-expressing recombinant BCG strains. Mostly it is the TH1-promoting cytokines that have been used in this context, and initial promising results have been obtained in in vitro studies and preclinical animal models.[72–74] However, during culture these cytokine-secreting BCG strains produce only low amounts of the respective recombinant protein (most strains below 1 ng/ml), and accurate in vitro studies, animal experiments, and clinical tests are needed to clarify whether patients could finally benefit from their clinical implementation.

Altogether, clinical evaluation of BCG immunotherapy of superficial bladder cancer has shown its efficacy and advantage over classical therapeutic strategies. This efficacy is based on a complex and long-lasting local immune activation as outlined in this review. The bladder as a confined compartment, in which high local concentrations of the immunotherapeutic agent and effective recruitment of immune cells can be achieved, serves as an ideal target organ for this type of immunotherapeutic approach.

## REFERENCES

1. Morales A, Eidinger D, Bruce AW. Intracavitary bacillus Calmette–Guérin in the treatment of superficial bladder tumors. J Urol 1976;116:180–183.

2. Ratliff TL, Hudson MA, Catalona WJ. Strategy for improving therapy of superficial bladder cancer. World J Urol 1991;9:95–98.

3. Chapman PB, Houghton AN. Non-antibody immunotherapy of cancer. Current Opinion in Immunology 1993;5:726–731.

4. Lamm DL, Blumenstein BA, Crawford ED, et al. A randomized trial of intravesical doxorubicin and immunotherapy with bacillus Calmette–Guérin for transitional-cell carcinoma of the bladder. N Engl J Med 1991;325:1205–1209.

5. Lamm DL, Blumenstein BA, Crawford ED, et al. Randomized intergroup comparison of bacillus Calmette–Guérin immunotherapy and mitomycin C chemotherapy prophylaxis in superficial transitional cell carcinoma of the bladder. A Southwest Oncology Group Study. Urol Oncol 1995;1:119–126.

6. Malmström P-U, Wijkström H, Lundholm C, Wester K, Busch C, Norlen BJ. 5-year follow-up of a randomized prospective study comparing mitomycin C and bacillus Calmette–Guérin in patients with superficial bladder carcinoma. J Urol 1999;161:1124–1127.

7. Herr HW, Laudone VP, Badalament RA, et al. Bacillus Calmette–Guérin therapy alters the progression of superficial bladder cancer. J Clin Oncol 1988;6(9):1450–1455.

8. Herr HW. Surgical therapy of high-risk bladder carcinoma transurethral resection (TUR): alone vs. adjuvant BCG. In Böhle A, Jocham D (eds): Optimal Therapy for Patients with High-Risk Superficial Bladder Cancer—Controversy and Consensus. Proceedings of the First Lübeck Symposium on Bladder Cancer, No. 37. Basel: Karger, 1997, pp 45–49.

9. Lamm DL, Blumenstein BA, Crissman JD, et al. Maintenance bacillus Calmette–Guérin immunotherapy for recurrent TA, T1 and carcinoma in situ transitional cell carcinoma of the bladder: a randomized Southwest Oncology Group Study. J Urol 2000;163:1124–1129.

10. Sylvester RJ, van der Meijden APM, Lamm DL. Intravesical bacillus Calmette–Guérin reduces the risk of progression in patients with superficial bladder cancer: a meta-analysis of the published results of randomized clinical trials. J Urol 2002;168:1964–1970.

11. Mahairas GG, Sabo PJ, Hickey MJ, Singh DC, Stover CK. Molecular analysis of genetic differences between Mycobacterium bovis BCG and virulent M. bovis. J Bacteriol 1996;178(5):1274–1282.

12. Behr MA, Wilson MA, Gill WP, et al. Comparative genomics of BCG vaccines by whole-genome DNA microarray. Science 1999;284:1520–1523.

13. Schamhart DHJ, de Boer EC, de Reijke TM, Kurth K-H. Urinary cytokines reflecting the immunological response in the urinary bladder to biological response modifiers: their practical use. Eur Urol 2000;37(Suppl 3):16–23.

14. Prescott S, James K, Hargreave TB, Chisholm GD, Smyth JF. Intravesical Evans strain BCG therapy: quantitative immunohistochemical analysis of the immune response within the bladder wall. J Urol 1992;147:1636–1642.

15. Lage JM, Bauer WC, Kelley DR, Ratliff TL, Catalona WJ. Histological parameters and pitfalls in the interpretation of bladder biopsies in bacillus Calmette–Guérin treatment of superficial bladder cancer. J Urol 1986;135:916–919.

16. de Boer EC, Somogyi L, de Ruiter GJW, de Reijke TM, Kurth K-H, Schamhart DH. Role of interleukin-8 in onset of the immune response in intravesical BCG therapy for superficial bladder cancer. Urol Res 1997;25:31–34.

17. Thalmann GN, Dewald B, Baggiolini M, Studer UE. Interleukin-8 expression in the urine after bacillus Calmette- Guérin therapy: a

potential prognostic factor of tumor recurrence and progression. J Urol 1997;158:1340–1344.

18. Thalmann GN, Sermier A, Rentsch C, Möhrle K, Cecchini MG, Studer UE. Urinary interleukin-8 and 18 predict the response of superficial bladder cancer to intravesical therapy with bacillus Calmette–Guérin. J Urol 2000;164:2129–2133.

19. Jackson AM, Ivshina AV, Senko O, et al. Prognosis of intravesical bacillus Calmette–Guérin therapy for superficial bladder cancer by immunological urinary measurements: statistically weighted syndromes analysis. J Urol 1998;159:1054–1063.

20. Jackson AM, Alexandroff AB, Kelly RW, et al. Changes in urinary cytokines and soluble intercellular adhesion molecule-1 (ICAM-1) in bladder cancer patients after bacillus Calmette–Guerin (BCG) immunotherapy. Clin Exp Immunol 1995;99:369–375.

21. Prescott S, James K, Hargreave TB, Chisholm GD, Smyth JF. Radio-immunoassay detection of interferon-gamma in urine after intravesical Evans BCG therapy. J Urol 1990;144:1248–1251.

22. Haaff EO, Catalona WJ, Ratliff TL. Detection of interleukin-2 in the urine of patients with superficial bladder tumors after treatment with intravesical BCG. J Urol 1986;136:970–974.

23. de Boer EC, de Jong WH, Steerenberg PA, et al. Induction of urinary interleukin-1 (IL-1), IL-2, IL-6, and tumor necrosis factor during intravesical immunotherapy with bacillus Calmette–Guérin in superficial bladder cancer. Cancer Immunol Immunother 1992;34:306–312.

24. Böhle A, Nowc C, Ulmer AJ, et al. Detection of urinary TNF, IL 1, and IL 2 after local BCG immunotherapy for bladder carcinoma. Cytokine 1990;2(3):175–181.

25. Alexandroff AB, Jackson AM, Skibinska A, James K. Production of IL-5, a classical TH2 cytokine, following bacillus Calmette–Guérin immunotherapy of bladder cancer. Int J Oncol 1996;9:179–182.

26. Poppas DP, Pavlovich CP, Folkman J, et al. Intravesical bacille Calmette–Guérin induces the antiangiogenic chemokine interferon-inducible protein 10. Urology 1998;52(2):268–275.

27. Chen X, Luo Y, Yamada H, O'Donnell MA. BCG potentiates human chemokine induction in vivo and in vitro. J Urol 2001;165(Suppl 5):114 (No. 465).

28. Böhle A, Gerdes J, Ulmer AJ, Hofstetter AG, Flad H-D. Effects of local bacillus Calmette–Guérin therapy in patients with bladder carcinoma on immunocompetent cells of the bladder wall. J Urol 1990;144:53–58.

29. de Boer EC, de Jong WH, van der Meijden APM, et al. Leukocytes in the urine after intravesical BCG treatment for superficial bladder cancer. Urol Res 1991;19:45–50.

30. Fleischmann JD, Toossi Z, Ellner JJ, Wentworth DB, Ratliff TL, Imbembo AL. Urinary interleukins in patients receiving intravesical bacillus Calmette–Guérin therapy for superficial bladder cancer. Cancer 1989;64:1447–1454.

31. de Reijke TM, de Boer EC, Kurth K-H, Schamhart DHJ. Urinary cytokines during intravesical bacillus Calmette–Guerin therapy for superficial bladder cancer: processing, stability and prognostic value. J Urol 1996;155:477–482.

32. Kaempfer R, Gerez L, Farbstein H, et al. Prediction of response to treatment in superficial bladder carcinoma through pattern of interleukin-2 gene expression. J Clin Oncol 1996;14:1778–1786.

33. Soloway M. Intravesical and systemic chemotherapy of murine bladder cancer. Cancer Res 1977;37:2918–2929.

34. Günther JH, Jurczok A, Wulf T, et al. Optimizing syngeneic orthotopic murine bladder cancer (MB49). Cancer Res 1999;59:2834–2837.

35. Ratliff TL, Palmer JO, McGarr JA, Brown EJ. Intravesical bacillus Calmette–Guérin therapy for murine bladder tumors: initiation of the response by fibronectin-mediated attachment of bacillus Calmette–Guérin. Cancer Res 1987;47:1762–1766.

36. Zhao W, Schorey JS, Bong-Mastek M, Ritchey JK, Brown EJ, Ratliff TL. Role of a bacillus Calmette–Guérin fibronectin attachment protein in BCG-induced antitumor activity. Int J Cancer 2000;86(1):83–88.

37. Kavoussi LR, Brown EJ, Ritchey JK, Ratliff TL. Fibronectin-mediated Calmette–Guérin bacillus attachment to murine bladder mucosa. Requirement of the expression of an antitumor response. J Clin Invest 1990;85:62–67.

38. Ratliff TL, Gillen DP, Catalona WJ. Requirement of a thymus-dependent immune response for BCG- mediated antitumor activity. J Urol 1987;137:155–158.

39. Ratliff TL, Ritchey JK, Yuan JJJ, Andriole GL, Catalona WJ. T-cell subsets required for intravesical BCG immunotherapy for bladder cancer. J Urol 1993;150:1018–1023.

40. Ratliff TL, Shapiro A, Catalona WJ. Inhibition of murine bladder tumor growth by bacillus Calmette–Guérin: lack of a role of natural killer cells. Clin Immunol Immunopathol 1986;41:108–115.

41. Brandau S, Riemensberger J, Jacobsen M, et al. NK cells are essential for effective BCG-immunotherapy. Int J Cancer 2001;92(5):697–702.

42. McAveney KM, Gomella LG, Lattime EC. Induction of TH1- and TH2-associated cytokine mRNA in mouse bladder following intravesical growth of the murine bladder tumor MB49 and BCG immunotherapy. Cancer Immunol Immunother 1994;39(6):401–406.

43. Shin JS, Park JH, Kim JD, Lee JM, Kim SJ. Induction of tumor necrosis factor-alpha (TNF-alpha) mRNA in bladders and spleens of mice after intravesical administration of bacillus Calmette–Guérin. Clin Exp Immunol 1995;100:26–31.

44. Riemensberger J, Böhle A, Brandau S. IFN-gamma and IL-12 but not IL-10 are required for local tumour surveillance in a syngeneic model of orthotopic bladder cancer. Clin Exp Immunol 2002;127:20–26.

45. Hawkyard SJ, Jackson AM, James K, Prescott S, Smyth JF, Chisholm GD. The inhibitory effects of interferon gamma on the growth of bladder cancer cells. J Urol 1992;147:1399–1403.

46. Thanhäuser A, Böhle A, Flad H-D, Ernst M, Mattern T, Ulmer AJ. Induction of bacillus Calmette–Guérin-activated killer cells from human peripheral blood mononuclear cells against human bladder carcinoma cell lines in vitro. Cancer Immunol Immunother 1993;37:105–111.

47. de Reijke TM, Vos PCN, Bevers RFM, de Muinck Keizer WH, Kurth R, Schamhart DHJ. Cytokine production by the human bladder carcinoma cell line T24 in the presence of bacillus Calmette–Guérin. Urol Res 1993;21:349–352.

48. Esuvaranathan K, Alexandroff AB, McIntyre M, et al. Interleukin-6 production by bladder tumors is upregulated by BCG immunotherapy. J Urol 1995;154:572–575.

49. Pryor K, Stricker P, Russell P, Golovsky D, Penny R. Antiproliferative effects of bacillus Calmette–Guerin and interferon alpha-2b on human bladder cancer cells in vitro. Cancer Immunol Immunother 1995;41(5):309–316.

50. Pryor K, Goddard J, Goldstein D, et al. Bacillus Calmette–Guerin (BCG) enhances monocyte- and lymphocyte-mediated bladder tumour cell killing. Br J Cancer 1995;71:801–807.

51. Mizutani Y, Nio Y, Fukumoto M, Yoshida O. Effects of bacillus Calmette–Guérin on cytotoxic activities of peripheral blood lymphocytes against human T24 lined and freshly isolated autologous urinary bladder transitional carcinoma cells in patients with urinary bladder cancer. Cancer 1992;69:537–545.

52. Thanhauser A, Bohle A, Schneider B, et al. The induction of bacillus Calmette–Guérin-activated killer cells requires the presence of monocytes/macrophages and T-helper type 1 cells. Cancer Immunol Immunother 1995;40:103–108.

53. Brandau S, Böhle A. Activation of natural killer cells by bacillus Calmette–Guérin. Eur Urol 2001;39:518–524.

54. Brandau S, Suttmann H, Riemensberger J, et al. Perforin-mediated lysis of tumor cells by Mycobacterium bovis bacillus Calmette–Guérin-activated killer cells. Clin Cancer Res 2000;6(9):3729–3738.

55. Cooper MA, Fehniger TA, Fuchs A, Colonna M, Caligiuri MA. NK cell and DC interactions. Trends Immunol 2004;25(1):47–52.

56. Tomita Y, Matsumoto Y, Nishiyama T, Fujiwara M. Reduction of major histocompatibility complex class I antigens on invasive and high-grade transitional cell carcinoma. J Pathol 1990;162(2):157–164.

57. Suttmann H, Jacobsen M, Reiss K, Jocham D, Bohle A, Brandau S. Mechanisms of bacillus Calmette–Guérin mediated natural killer cell activation. J Urol 2004;172(4 Pt 1):1490–1495.

58. Reiss K, Brandau S, Ulmer AJ, Flad H-D, Jocham D, Böhle A. BCG-immunotherapy of superficial bladder cancer: BCG-induced activation of MNCs is regulated by cytokines. Eur Urol 1999;36:476.

59. O'Donnell MA, Luo Y, Chen X, Szilvasi A, Hunter SE, Clinton SK. Role of IL-12 in the induction and potentiation of IFN-gamma in response to bacillus Calmette–Guérin. J Immunol 1999;163(8):4246–4252.

60. Mendez-Samperio P, Ayala-Verdin HE, Trejo-Echeverria A. Interleukin-12 regulates the production of bacille Calmette–Guérin-induced interferon-gamma from human cells in a CD40-dependent manner. Scand J Immunol 1999;50(1):61–67.

61. Luo Y, Chen X, Downs TM, DeWolf WC, O'Donnell MA. IFN-alpha 2B enhances Th1 cytokine responses in bladder cancer patients receiving Mycobacterium bovis bacillus Calmette–Guérin immunotherapy. J Immunol 1999;162(4):2399–2405.

62. Suttmann H, Lehan N, Bohle A, Brandau S. Stimulation of neutrophil granulocytes with Mycobacterium bovis bacillus Calmette–Guerin induces changes in phenotype and gene expression and inhibits spontaneous apoptosis. Infect Immun 2003;71(8):4647–4656.

63. Ludwig AT, Moore JM, Luo Y, et al. Tumor necrosis factor-related apoptosis-inducing ligand: a novel mechanism for bacillus Calmette–Guerin-induced antitumor activity. Cancer Res 2004;64(10):3386–3390.

64. Chin JL, Kadhim SA, Batislam E, et al. Mycobacterium cell wall: an alternative to intravesical bacillus Calmette–Guérin (BCG) therapy in orthotopic murine bladder cancer. J Urol 1996;156:1189–1193.

65. Kelley DR, Ratliff TL, Catalona WJ, et al. Intravesical bacillus Calmette–Guérin-therapy for superficial bladder cancer: effect of bacillus Calmette–Guérin viability on treatment results. J Urol 1985;134:48–53.

66. Shapiro A, Ratliff TL, Oakley DM, Catalona WJ. Reduction of bladder tumor growth in mice treated with intravesical bacillus Calmette–Guérin and its correlation with bacillus Calmette–Guérin viability and natural killer cell activity. Cancer Res 1983;43:1611–1615.

67. Glashan RW. A randomized controlled study of intravesical α-2b-interferon in carcinoma in situ of the bladder. J Urol 1990;144:658–661.

68. Stricker P, Pryor K, Nicholson T, et al. Bacillus Calmette–Guérin plus intravesical interferon alpha-2b in patients with superficial bladder cancer. Urology 1996;48(6):957–962.

69. Clinton SK, Canto E, O'Donnell MA. Interleukin-12. Opportunities for the treatment of bladder cancer. Urol Clin North Am 2000;27(1):147–155.

70. Papatsoris AG, Deliveliotis C, Giannopoulos A, Dimopoulos C. Adjuvant intravesical mitoxantrone versus recombinant interferon-alpha after transurethral resection of superficial bladder cancer: a randomized prospective study. Urol Int 2004;72(4):284–291.

71. O'Donnell MA, Krohn J, DeWolf WC. Salvage intravesical therapy with interferon-a2B plus low dose bacillus Calmette–Guérin is effective in patients with superficial bladder cancer in whom bacillus Calmette–Guérin alone previously failed. J Urol 2001;166:1300–1305.

72. Arnold J, de Boer EC, O'Donnell MA, Bohle A, Brandau S. Immunotherapy of experimental bladder cancer with recombinant BCG expressing interferon-gamma. J Immunother 2004;27(2):116–123.

73. O'Donnell MA, Aldovini A, Duda RB, et al. Recombinant Mycobacterium bovis BCG secreting functional interleukin-2 enhances gamma interferon production by splenocytes. Infect Immun 1994;62:2508–2514.

74. Luo Y, Chen X, Han R, O'Donnell MA. Recombinant bacille Calmette–Guérin (BCG) expressing human interferon-alpha 2B demonstrates enhanced immunogenicity. Clin Exp Immunol 2001;123(2):264–270.

# Marker tumor concept: ethical issues

34

*Laurence B McCullough*

## INTRODUCTION

The use of marker tumors raises three important issues for clinical investigators: the management of risk in the design and conduct of clinical investigation; the informed consent process, particularly the explanation of the concept of marker tumor monitoring for the effects of investigational management; and the monitoring of clinical trials by an independent panel, usually known as a Data and Safety Monitoring Board. This chapter provides a brief account of these three issues and offers practical suggestions for addressing them.

## MANAGING RISK IN DESIGN AND CONDUCT OF CLINICAL INVESTIGATION

The major sources of ethical and legal authority pertaining to research with human subjects acknowledge that clinical investigation cannot be made risk-free in all cases. It is therefore well recognized in the ethics and regulation of human subjects research that clinical investigators have an ethical and legal obligation to identify and prospectively manage risk in the design and conduct of clinical investigation. The Nuremberg Code, for example, addresses this responsibility in the design of research when it states that clinical investigation 'should be so conducted as to avoid all unnecessary physical and mental suffering and injury'.[1] This implies that investigators are responsible for the identification and reliable prediction of risk in research design.

The design of clinical investigation should minimize the risk to human subjects. One very important practical implication of this ethical and legal obligation is that, when there is a choice among alternative research designs for reliably testing a hypothesis, the least risky design should be chosen.[2] The Nuremberg Code also addresses the need to balance predicted risk against predicted benefits: 'the degree of risk taken should never exceed that determined by the humanitarian importance of the problem' that is addressed in the clinical investigation.[1] The risk–benefit ratio therefore should always be favorable, when reliable clinical ethical judgment concludes that the potential risk outweighs the benefit, research with human subjects is impermissible.

This ethical consideration also has important practical implications: 1) some forms of research, i.e. those judged too risky, are not to be undertaken; 2) research that is judged to be acceptably risky should be prospectively monitored. Should an independent monitoring process judge that results are conclusive or that unacceptable risk has occurred before the projected period of subject accrual, the trial should be stopped.

International statements on the ethics of human subjects research underscore the enduring ethical significance of these two basic ethical principles for the responsible conduct of such research. The Declaration of Helsinki requires investigators to:

- identify potential risks to subjects (principle 17)
- manage those risks 'satisfactorily' (principle 17)
- conduct research only when the risk–benefit ratio is favorable (principle 18)
- monitor research for risk occurrence and stop investigation when the risk–benefit ratio becomes unacceptable (principle 17).[3]

The International Conference on Harmonization of Technical Requirements for Registration of Pharmaceuticals for Human Use *Guidelines for Good Clinical Practice*[4] includes similar principles and acknowledges the authority of the Declaration of Helsinki, as do the *Recommendations Concerning Medical Research on Human Beings* of the Council of Europe.[5]

Current regulations for human subjects research in the United States address these ethical concerns. Risks should be minimized 'by using procedures that are consistent with sound research design and do not unnecessarily expose subjects to risk'. Risks to subjects should be 'reasonable in relation to anticipated benefits, if any, to subjects, and the importance of the knowledge that may reasonably be expected to result'.[6]

Does the risk involved in the use of marker tumors in clinical trials of treatment of superficial bladder cancer meet the ethical requirements of identifying and appropriately managing risk in human subjects research? Meijden et al identify a major scientific challenge in evaluating the efficacy of adjuvant therapy in delaying tumor recurrence: 'the unpredictable frequency and multiplicity of superficial tumor recurrence after the removal of visible tumor by endoscopic surgery'.[7] The clinical practice of leaving a single Ta, T1 bladder tumor was developed to achieve greater objectivity and reliability in measuring the effect of adjuvant therapy than could be achieved by using 'multiple tumors of indeterminate number, size and malignant characteristics'.[7] The latter approach, presumably, would result in statistically unmanageable variability in results, making it impossible to assess efficacy of adjuvant therapy reliably.

This raises a serious ethical concern. Adjuvant therapy is not benign. Responsible management of risk requires that the efficacy of this treatment should be assessed reliably, otherwise its use might result only in clinical harm to patients, which is ethically unacceptable. Moreover, clinical investigation of adjuvant therapy in the absence of a reliable method for measuring its effects on tumor recurrence could involve investigators in subjecting patients to potentially morbid clinical management that would remain of, at best, undetermined benefit and, at worst, no benefit. As a consequence, investigators could not be confident that they were not exposing subjects to risk unnecessarily, much less that the risk was offset by anticipated benefits. It follows from this ethical analysis that investigation of adjuvant therapy without a reliable measure of its efficacy would involve ethically unacceptable risk.

Meijden et al also report that the risk that the marker tumor could progress to muscle invasion is very small, about 0.9%. Using computed indices of risk of progression, they distinguish three groups: those with good, intermediate, and bad prognoses. Those with good prognoses (0% risk of progression) do not need chemotherapy, whereas those in the bad prognosis category (7% risk of progression) should receive the best chemotherapy available. Those with intermediate risk (2% risk of progression, 40–50% of all patients with Ta, T1 bladder tumors) are candidates for investigation of adjuvant therapy. For these potential subjects, it is necessary to expose them to a very small risk of tumor progression, in order to measure reliably the effect on a marker tumor of the adjuvant therapy. To minimize the risk of such research, Meijden et al propose five selection criteria[7] (Box 34.1).

Even if selection criteria are rigorously designed to minimize risk, disagreement will continue within the expert community about the merits of the use of a marker tumor to measure the effects of adjuvant therapy. Thus, the condition of equipoise would appear to be satisfied; however, in spite of available evidence about the merits of using a marker tumor (resulting, on the part of those who object, from the residual worry that leaving a marker tumor may violate the dictum of first do no harm), the expert community continues to disagree.[2,8] There is, therefore, sufficient evidence to initiate phase III trials but not sufficient evidence to judge them ethically inappropriate, because the alternative itself involves the risk of being unable to measure reliably the effects of intervention that involves nontrivial morbidity.

## THE DISCLOSURE PROCESS FOR INFORMED CONSENT FOR MARKER TUMOR STUDIES

The second major ethical issue regarding marker tumor studies concerns the information that should be provided to potential subjects during the informed consent process. All international statements on the ethics of human subjects research, from the Nuremberg Code to the latest version of the Declaration of Helsinki, make it clear that there must be an effective informed consent process and valid consent from subjects (or their surrogates) for human subjects research. The federal regulations for human subjects in research are emphatic

---

**Box 34.1** Selection criteria for a phase II marker tumor study

1. Primary or recurrent multiple Ta, T1 transitional cell carcinoma of the bladder with no palpable thickening of the bladder wall on bimanual palpation
2. Multiple tumors, but not more than seven
3. The marker tumor should be ≤1 cm in diameter
4. The histological grade of the other tumors resected at entry to the study should be either grade 1 or grade 2; patients with poorly differentiated tumors (grade 3) should be excluded
5. The presence of carcinoma in situ or muscular invasion is inappropriate for a phase II marker tumor study

After Meijden et al.[7]

in this respect. Indeed, the 'Common Rule' goes into considerable detail about the basic elements of the informed consent process and its documentation.[6]

In the case of marker tumor studies, the informed consent process should convey to potential subjects an explanation of why a marker tumor is being used, i.e.:

- to avoid subjecting patients to potentially injurious treatment without being able to reliably determine its efficacy
- that there is risk of progression to more serious forms of cancer and the predicted risk of such progression
- how the selection criteria have been chosen to minimize such risk
- how subjects will be monitored for such progression
- what will be offered to subjects whose marker tumor exhibits such progression.

Investigators should make a reasonable effort to ensure that potential subjects have developed an adequate understanding of this information and that they appreciate that the risks described could occur. It should also be made clear to potential subjects that they are free not to enroll and that they are free to withdraw at any time, with the benefits and risks of doing so being explained to them.

## MONITORING CLINICAL TRIALS

The third major ethical issue for marker tumor studies concerns their appropriate prospective monitoring, an important tool for the protection of human subjects of research. When a clinical trial involves the deliberate taking of scientifically and ethically justified risk with subjects, as is the case with marker tumor phase III trials, such clinical investigation should be monitored closely by an independent panel, usually known as a Data and Safety Monitoring Board (DSMB). The DSMB should be formally charged with reviewing and evaluating the study design and informed consent process. It should also anticipate the need to stop a trial because there is sufficient evidence either of positive results or of harmful

results of the experimental arm or because the clinical trial has no statistical probability of proving a positive result. The main advantage of the DSMB approach is that its members do not participate in the trial as investigators, reducing to a minimum their potential bias about expected results and other matters. This adds an additional level of protection to the subjects in the trial.

## CONCLUSION

Ethics is an essential component of the responsible conduct of clinical investigation. Responsible management of the ethical challenges of clinical trials is just as important as responsible management of the scientific, enrollment, and other challenges of clinical trials. Sustained attention to these ethical challenges will result in better research and increase the trust of subjects, patients, and society in general in the clinical research enterprise. This is especially the case for marker tumor studies, because they include an element of risk of tumor progression. This risk should be responsibly managed by means of a rigorous study design, appropriate informed consent process, and prospective monitoring by a DSMB.

REFERENCES

1. Nuremberg Military Tribunal. Nuremberg Code, 1947. In Reich WT (ed): Encyclopedia of Bioethics, 2nd ed. New York: Macmillan, 1995, pp 2763–2764.
2. Brody BA. The Ethics of Biomedical Research: An International Perspective. New York: Oxford University Press, 1998.
3. World Medical Association. Declaration of Helsinki. Ferney-Voltaire, France: WMA, 1996, pp 214–216.
4. International Conference on Harmonization (ICH) of Technical Requirements for Registration of Pharmaceuticals for Human Use. Guidelines on good clinical practice. Brussels: ICH, 1996, pp 219–224.
5. Council of Europe. Recommendations Concerning Medical Research on Human Beings. Strasbourg: Council of Europe, 1990, pp 241–250.
6. US Department of Health and Human Services (HHS). Regulations for the Protection of Human Subjects (45 CFR 46). Washington, DC: HHS, 1991.
7. Meijden AP, Hall RR, Kurth KH, et al. Phase II trials in Ta, T1 bladder cancer. The marker tumour concept. Brit J Urol 1996;77:634–637.
8. Freedman B. Equipoise and the ethics of clinical research. N Engl J Med 1987;317:141–145.

# The use of the marker tumor concept in Ta, T1 bladder cancer: is it justified?

## 35

*Adrian P M van der Meijden*

## INTRODUCTION

The efficacy of cancer treatment is measured by its effect on a visible lesion (primary tumor and/or metastases) and by the duration of survival. Although survival remains the most important endpoint in cancer clinical trials, this endpoint poses a problem in trials in which Ta, T1 bladder tumors are treated. The natural course of this disease is such that most tumors do not become life threatening. Many patients survive for more than 10 years and often die from other causes.[1] The most relevant clinical problem in the management of Ta, T1 bladder tumors remains the frequent and unpredictable recurrence rate, and, to a lesser degree, progression to muscle-invasive cancer.

The current standard management of superficial bladder cancer requires complete endoscopic removal of all visible tumor. Since multiple studies in Europe and the United States have shown that the general recurrence rate for all superficial disease stages is approximately 70%, adjuvant intravesical therapy provides an attractive method of potentially reducing recurrence and progression of disease; however, if complete trans-urethral resection (TUR) is performed, the urologist has no measurable marker of response to therapy by which to evaluate the impact of the adjuvant intravesical treatment.[2] In addition, a number of patients treated by TUR alone will be cured. For these patients, adjuvant therapy could be considered overtreatment.

A different situation exists for carcinoma in situ (CIS). By its multifocal nature, and the lack of visible neoplasm, it is believed that CIS cannot be eradicated by TUR. While urologists believe that TUR is ineffective for CIS, they strongly believe that TUR is the best method to eliminate Ta, T1 tumors. Although multiple clinical trials testing the benefit of adjuvant instillation therapy have been carried out, surprisingly few studies have been performed to test the adequacy and completeness of TUR. How efficient is TUR? Recent data suggest that TUR in many cases is not radical. This had led to the recommendation that a second TUR is necessary in high-risk Ta, T1 tumors.[3]

## THE MARKER TUMOR CONCEPT

The marker tumor concept was derived from phase II trials in which patients with multiple tumors, not suitable for complete TUR or not suitable for surgery, have been treated with intravesical instillation alone. In these studies, it has been observed that intravesical drugs such as thiotepa, mitomycin C, and adriamycin were able to eradicate tumor(s) in the bladder. Obviously, a direct ablative effect of the drugs on the tumor tissue is responsible for this. This observation has led to the development of the marker tumor concept. After TUR of multiple papillary tumors, one single tumor, no bigger than 1 cm, is left untouched in the bladder. This indicator lesion is the marker on which intravesical instillation therapy is tested in a phase II setting. The marker tumor concept was first described in 1981.[4] Since then, several clinical trial groups, such as the European Organisation for Research and Treatment on Cancer Genitourinary (EORTC-GU) Group, the British Medical Research Group and a Japanese clinical trial group, have studied the ablative effect of a new drug or a combination of drugs in different schedules using a marker lesion.[5–8] The currently used drugs for prophylaxis, such as mitomycin C, epirubicin, and bacillus Calmette–Guérin (BCG), provide a complete response in marker tumor studies of between 40% and 60%.

## ARGUMENTS FOR AND AGAINST

Although the concept of marker lesion has been known for over two decades, acceptance of this phase II method has not been universal—urologists believe in the efficacy of TUR! Furthermore, clinicians may find it difficult to justify leaving a visible tumor unresected in the absence of histologic confirmation of low grade and low stage. The intellectual appeal of using an existing visible lesion to test urothelial sensitivity to specific agents is high. However, if a complete response is observed in less than 40% of the patients, a given drug should not be used in a phase III trial.

Between 1903 and 1978, 13 different agents have been tested in phase III trials.[9] Of these, only a few drugs have been determined to be effective. Using a new drug directly in the prophylactic setting (phase III) is not completely harmless. The EORTC-GU Group has carried out a three-arm, phase III trial using thiotepa, doxorubicin, and cisplatin.[10] While cisplatin is very effective intravenously, 8 of 78 patients suffered from allergic shock after they were treated with cisplatin intravesically. As a consequence, the use of cisplatin intravesically has been abandoned. For many other intravesical drugs used in daily practice by urologists, the optimal dose, dwelling time, pH, etc. are still unknown, because too few phase II studies have been carried out in the past.

## HOW SAFE IS IT TO LEAVE A MARKER TUMOR?

To investigate efficacy and safety of the marker tumor concept, a careful selection of patients and trial method is necessary. The principal anxiety that a tumor may progress or metastasize has led to a limited time period in which the patient and the marker tumor are exposed to intravesical instillations. There is consensus that such a time span should not exceed 8–10 weeks. This means that the efficacy of therapy is assessed at a maximum of 10 weeks after the initial TUR. When no complete response is observed, complete TUR is carried out. The possibility of no response or even progression is therefore only relevant during these 8–10 weeks. Data from EORTC marker tumor protocols have shown that the risk of progression is very small.[2] The combined data from protocols 30864 and 30869, in which 132 patients were treated during 8 weeks with intravesical mitomycin C and epirubicin, respectively, showed T2 tumor (muscle invasive) in two cases at the first evaluation cystoscopy, 10 weeks after the start of the protocol. In EORTC protocol 30897 the sequential combination of intravesical mitomycin C and BCG was tested on a marker tumor. Of 32 eligible patients, 16 had a complete remission, 11 patients had no change, and 1 patient was not evaluable due to toxicity. Three patients had a complete disappearance of the marker but histologic confirmation was not obtained as they refused biopsy. One patient had a T2 tumor.[5]

The ablative effect of a quarter dose of BCG has been tested in 44 patients. Of these, 27 had a complete response (61%).[11] Progression to muscle invasive cancer was not observed, but CIS developed in one patient. In all four trials carried out by the EORTC-GU Group, complete response was assessed by cystoscopy, biopsy at the location where tumor was seen previously, and urine cytology. In those cases where no tumor was seen but nevertheless biopsy was taken, only 3 out of 101 biopsies revealed tumor (Ta). This observation might indicate that, when no tumor is seen and cytology is negative, a biopsy is not necessary.[12] The MRC tested BCG on a marker lesion phase II study in 94 patients, and no progression was observed.[6] Another study was carried out testing a single instillation of epirubicin on a marker tumor in 81 patients,[7] and again no progression was observed.

Evaluating the data from the six trials reported here indicates that the risk of leaving an untreated muscle-invasive tumor, or a tumor that might progress to muscle invasion during the limited time of 10–12 weeks, is 0.8% (3/383).

## WHICH PATIENTS ARE SUITABLE FOR MARKER LESION STUDIES?

Ta, T1 bladder tumors can be divided into three different prognostic categories. The EORTC, using multivariate analysis of prognostic factors, was able to estimate the risk of progression in prophylactic phase III studies during the first 3 months after TUR.[1] These risk factor assessments were confirmed by others.[13] Solitary, low-grade Ta tumors have a risk of progression during the first 3 months of TUR of 0%. Small, recurrent, low-grade-appearing tumors have been observed by others without performing a TUR.[14] In calculating the risk of leaving these low-risk tumors versus the morbidity and cost of TUR, it was found that these tumors grow slowly and that a high-grade Ta or T1 tumor develops in 6% to 7% of the patients after a mean observation time of 38 months. During the first 3 months after TUR, for intermediate-risk tumors (multiple, primary, or recurrent Ta, grade 1–2), this risk is a maximum of 2%. High-risk tumors (T1 grade 3, CIS) progress during the first 3 months in 9% of cases.

It would appear unjustified to treat patients in marker lesion studies when they belong to the low-risk group. Their excellent prognosis does not justify intensive and repetitive intravesical chemotherapy. They are optimally treated by TUR plus one immediate postoperative instillation using an intravesical chemotherapeutic drug.[15] If in high-risk patients the risk of progression is 40% to 50% in general and 7% in particular during the first 8–10 weeks, it does not seem justified to expose this category of patients to a drug or regimen with an unpredictable outcome. About one-third of all patients belong to the intermediate risk group. The risk of recurrence in this category is far more pronounced than the risk of progression. Therefore selected patients for marker tumor protocols should belong to the intermediate risk group where:

- there are primary or recurrent multiple Ta, T1 tumors
- the number of tumors is between three and seven
- the marker tumor does not exceed 1 cm
- grade 3 tumors have been excluded
- CIS has been excluded.

## CONCLUSION

The objectives of a marker tumor study are two-fold: to study the ablative or reductive activity of the investigational drug on a papillary marker lesion, and to test incidence and severity of (early) side effects.

With relatively few patients and a relatively short period of treatment (8–10 weeks) it is possible to detect whether a new drug or a combination of drugs is worth investigating further in long-term phase III trials. Expensive and inefficient long-term phase III trials may be avoided by performing marker tumor studies in patients that belong to the intermediate risk group.[16] Based on the published data, the Fourth International Bladder Consensus Conference recommended that marker tumor phase II studies should be the standard clinical practice for the evaluation of new agents.[17] Ethical considerations of such studies remain a critical issue.[18]

## REFERENCES

1. Kurth KH, Denis L, Kate ten FJW et al. Prognostic factors in superficial bladder tumors. Probl Urol 1992;6:471–483.
2. Van der Meijden APM, Hall RR, Kurth K-H, Bouffioux C, Sylvester R, and members of the EORTC Genitourinary Group. Phase II trials in Ta, T1 bladder cancer. The marker tumor concept. Br J Urol 1996;77:634–637.
3. Brausi M, Sylvester R, van der Meijden A, Kurth K-H, and members of the EORTC-SBS and QL Groups. Does the surgeon have an impact on the outcome of patients with Ta, T1, TCC. of the bladder? Results of an EORTC quality control study on TURBT. Eur Urol 2001;(S5):A466.
4. Koontz WW, Prout GR, Smith W, Frable WJ, Minnis JE. The use of intravesical thiotepa in the management of non-invasive carcinoma of the bladder. J Urol 1981;125:307–312.
5. Van der Meijden APM, Hall RR, Pavone Macaluso M, Pawinsky A, Sylvester R, Van Glabbeke M. Marker tumor response to the sequential combination of intravesical therapy with mitomycin C and BCG-RIVM in multiple superficial bladder tumors. Report from the European Organisation for Research and Treatment on Cancer-Genitourinary Group (EORTC 30897). Eur Urol 1996:29:199–203.
6. Fellows G, Parmar M, Grigor R, et al. Marker tumor response to Evans and Pasteur Bacille Calmette–Guérin in multiple recurrent pTa, PT1 bladder tumors: report from the Medical Research Council subgroup on Superficial Bladder Cancer (Urological Cancer Working Party). Br J Urol 1994;73:639–644.
7. Popert RJM, Goodall J, Coptcoat MJ. Superficial bladder cancer: the response of a marker tumor to a single intravesical instillation of epirubicin. Br J Urol 1994;74:195–196.
8. Akaza H, Hinotsu S, Aso Y, et al. BCG alone as treatment of superficial bladder cancer: can TURBT be avoided? J Urol 1995;153(2):234A.
9. Conolly JG. Chemotherapy of superficial bladder cancer. In: Conolly JG (ed): Carcinoma of the Bladder. New York: Raven, 1981, pp 165–175.
10. Bouffioux C, Denis L, Oosterlinck W, et al. Adjuvant chemotherapy of recurrent superficial transitional cell carcinoma: results of a European Organisation for Research and Treatment of Cancer randomized trial comparing intravesical instillation of thiotepa, doxorubicin and cisplatin. J Urol 1992;148:297–301.
11. Mack D, Holtl W, Bassi P, Brausi M, Ferrari P, and members of the European Organisation for Research and Treatment of Cancer Genitourinary Group. The ablative effect of quarter dose Bacillus Calmette–Guérin on a papillary marker lesion of the bladder. J Urol 2001;165:401–403.
12. Oosterlinck W, Bono AV, Mack D, Hall R, Sylvester R, de Balincourt C, Brausi M and members of the EORTC GU group. Frequency of positive biopsies after visual disappearance of superficial bladder cancer marker lesions. Eur Urol 2001;40:515–517.
13. Parmar M, Freedman L, Hargreave T, et al. Prognostic factors for recurrence and follow up policies in the treatment of superficial bladder cancer: report from the British Medical Research Council Subgroup on Superficial Bladder Cancer (Urological Cancer Working Party). J Urol 1989;142:284–288.
14. Soloway MS, Bruck DS, Kim SS. Expectant management of small recurrent non invasive papillary bladder tumors. J Urol 2003;170:438–441.
15. Sylvester RS, Oosterlinck W, van der Meijden APM. A single immediate postoperative instillation of chemotherapy decreases the risk of recurrence in patients with stage Ta, T1 bladder cancer: a meta-analysis of published results of randomized clinical trials. J. Urol 2004 171(6 Pt 1):2186–2190.
16. Van der Meijden APM. The use of the marker tumor concept in Ta, T1 bladder cancer: is it justified? Urol Oncol 2002;7:31–33.
17. Lamm DL, van der Meijden APM, Akaza H, et al. Intravesical chemo- and immunotherapy: how do we assess their effectiveness and what are their limitations and uses? Proceedings of the Fourth International Bladder Cancer Consensus Conference. Int J Urol 1995;2(S2):23–35.
18. McCullough LB. Ethical issues in the use of tumor markers in clinical investigation of the management of bladder cancer. Urol Oncol 2002;7:35–37.

# Photodynamic therapy

36

*Michael J Manyak, Unyime O Nseyo*

## INTRODUCTION

Technologic innovations have fueled improvements that have decreased length of time for surgical procedures, provided access to tissues in a less invasive manner, and augmented the armamentarium against disease processes. Despite many advances in management of malignancy, transurethral resection of superficial transitional cell carcinoma (TCC) of the bladder remains the most effective form of management for low-grade, low-stage neoplasia. However, patients with multiple, frequently recurrent, or diffuse lesions have a greater tendency for progression of their disease and are less likely to be controlled by transurethral resection alone or in combination with intravesical chemotherapy or immunotherapy.[1] Although intravesical immuno-therapy has had an impact upon recurrence and progression of superficial TCC, a subset of patients with aggressive disease are resistant to standard treatment measures and have few viable options before radical extirpative surgery.

One modality that has been evaluated for its effect on high-grade and recurrent tumors in an attempt to prevent or delay cystectomy is photodynamic therapy (PDT).[2] Tumoricidal effects of PDT are due to creation of a highly reactive oxygen species that results from activation of a photosensitizing agent contained in tissue. The agent is activated by absorbance of wavelengths of light specific for the spectrum of the agent. The relative selective retention of the photosensitizer within or around tumor cells is thought to result in more selective destruction of neoplasia while limiting damage to adjacent normal tissues. This property makes PDT attractive for use in certain malignancies where more conventional modalities prove to be less effective.

## THE HISTORY OF PHOTOSENSITIZATION

The phenomenon of photochemical sensitization was first observed and reported over a century ago by Raab who, in 1900, noted a lethal effect on paramecia exposed to light in the presence of acridine.[3] The first use of this photodynamic concept for tumor destruction occurred shortly afterwards, when Tappenier and Jesionek treated skin cancer with topically applied eosin followed by sunlight exposure.[4] Since that time, a wide range of compounds has shown photochemotoxicity. The great interest in porphyrin compounds, the most commonly used photosensitizers, can be traced to Policard's observation in 1924 of reddish fluorescence in certain human and animal tumors, which was attributed to endogenous porphyrin accumulation from hemolytic bacterial infection.[5]

Fluorescence was used again in 1942 by Auler and Banzer to determine the uptake of a bovine hemoglobin derivative called hematoporphyrin (HP) in neoplastic tissue.[6] Figge and associates extended this finding to include a variety of murine tumors as well as embryonic and traumatized tissue.[7] In 1961, Lipson and colleagues described porphyrin tumor localization after injection of a synthetic porphyrin mixture called hemato-porphyrin derivative (HPD).[8] HPD was the most commonly used photosensitizer until it was further purified to a combination of ethers and esters known as porfimer sodium (Photofrin). Nearly all human clinical trials of PDT in the last 30 years have employed porfimer sodium, but several new compounds with more desirable characteristics for clinical use may ultimately prove to be more effective photosensitizers.

## SENSITIZER DELIVERY AND RETENTION

Photodynamic therapy is a two-step process that first requires the delivery of a sensitizer to the target tissue followed by its activation with a light source. Once administered, distribution within the target tissue must be sufficient for photodestruction to occur. After intravenous administration, the sensitizer then concentrates in normal as well as neoplastic tissue. Nearly all photosensitizers studied have in common a predilection for accumulation within tissues containing significant reticuloendothelial components.[9] Normal tissues with the highest concentration of sensitizers include liver, adrenal gland, and urinary bladder, followed by pancreas, kidney, and spleen. Elevated tissue levels of the photosensitizer in liver and kidney may actually result from porphyrin metabolism and may not represent true retention. Tissues with the least concentration of sensitizer included skin, muscle, and brain, in decreasing order of concentration. Of great interest, however, are the differences noted among

sensitizers in the time to peak tissue concentration and length of retention in tissue. These differences in clearance and metabolism help explain the persistence of skin photosensitivity seen with clinical PDT using porfimer sodium that are not seen with more rapidly metabolized sensitizers.

Although sensitizer uptake is not restricted to neoplastic tissue, there is some treatment selectivity seen in animal tumor models, which may be enhanced in some human malignancies.[10] The observed treatment selectivity may be related to a sensitizer gradient between tumor and normal tissue. The ratio of tissue levels of sensitizer in skin versus tumor in animal models varies from 2:1 to 10:1, thus providing a good example of such a gradient. This phenomenon may be related either to differences in sensitizer distribution among tumor tissue compartments and subcellular components, or to differences in sensitivity between neoplastic and normal cells. However, distribution of sensitizers within tumor and the relationship to response are still not clearly understood.

Sensitizer distribution within the cell may be an important factor. Cellular uptake of porphyrins increases as the components become more lipophilic.[9] As a rule, lipophilic anionic compounds concentrate in cell membranes and subcellular components, including mitochondria, endoplasmic reticulum, and, to a lesser extent, the nucleus[11] (Figure 36.1). On the other hand,

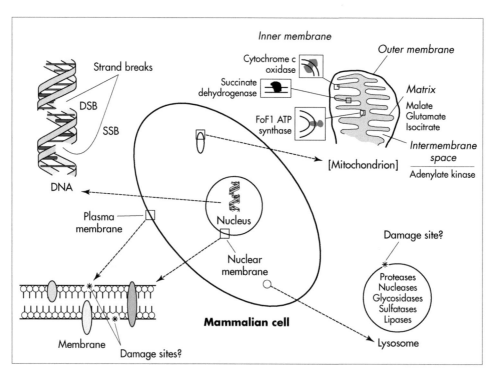

**Fig. 36.1**

Subcellular targets of photodynamic therapy in a mammalian cell. Mitchondrion insert shows three mitochondrial enzymes (FoF1 ATP synthase, cytochrome C oxidase, succinate dehydrogenase) which have been inhibited following photodynamic therapy. (DSB, double strand break; SSB, single strand break.) Reproduced with permission from J.B. Mitchell.

hydrophilic compounds tend to accumulate in lysosomes while cationic sensitizers localize in mitochondria due primarily to the differential in electrical potential across the membrane.[12] Subcellular localization may be less important, however, because cellular photodestruction occurs with all these sensitizers.

The increased concentration of HPD in traumatized or embryonic tissue suggests that the retention of porphyrin sensitizers by neoplasia may not be selective.[13,14] Although the mechanism for selective retention in tumors is unclear, it has been suggested that physiologic and anatomic characteristics of neoplasia that differ from normal tissue, coupled with photosensitizer chemical properties, are responsible for this phenomenon. This scenario contends that leakage of sensitizer occurs through the neovascular network, leading to aggregation of photosensitizer macromolecules. Clearance of these macromolecules is retarded by the dysfunctional lymphatics that accompany neoplastic growth. Once retained, the porphyrin photosensitizers can then favorably partition into hydrophobic cellular membranes. Another mechanism purported to have a role in selective sensitizer retention is the increased endocytosis in neoplastic cells mediated by low-density lipoprotein (LDL) receptors.[15] Lipophilic sensitizers such as the porphyrins tend to bind to LDL, whereas hydrophilic sensitizers favor albumin binding.[9]

Attempts to enhance sensitizer delivery, uptake, or retention have been innovative but only partially successful. Liposomes of specific lipid composition are being explored to deliver sensitizers to LDL and its receptors. A different approach has been used to stimulate biosynthesis of an endogenous sensitizer, protoporphyrin IX, by the topical administration of its precursor 5-aminolevulinic acid (5-ALA) and its esters.[16] This latter approach has been used for both fluorescent detection and treatment of TCC, and is quite attractive because of the avoidance of intravenous sensitizer administration with subsequently decreased potential for undesired side effects.[17,18]

## TIMING OF TREATMENT

The fact that there appears to be some degree of selective tumor retention of sensitizer suggests that there is an optimal time for tumor treatment after administration that would minimize damage to adjacent normal tissue. The optimal time interval between administration of porfimer sodium and clinical treatment has not been established, but most investigators wait 48–72 hours before PDT to allow clearance from nonmalignant tissues.[19] Even though the maximal tumoricidal effect is observed within a few days of intravenous porfimer

sodium administration, it takes several weeks before the amount of porfimer sodium retained within some normal tissue (as in skin) will decrease to clinically insignificant levels. Preclinical clearance kinetics and therapeutic results for other sensitizers have demonstrated a shorter optimal time interval between administration and treatment. PDT for bladder cancer using 5-ALA appears to be most effective from 2 to 4.5 hours after topical administration.[20,21]

## LIGHT DELIVERY AND TISSUE INTERACTIONS

The photosensitizer in the target tissue is excited by absorbed light of appropriate wavelength. The depth of light penetration into tissue is one variable that determines the efficacy of PDT and is a contributory factor to the generally poor results from PDT of solid tumors.[19] A threshold quantity of light energy is required to activate the photosensitizer within tissue. The depth to which this requisite light will reach depends upon both the power density of the light source applied and the tissue characteristics of the target. These optical characteristics vary with each tissue and are related in large part to the probability of a photon being absorbed per unit length of tissue, known as the absorption coefficient, and the probability of a photon being scattered per unit length of tissue, which is the scatter coefficient. The summation of these characteristics is expressed as the attenuation coefficient and provides an estimate of tissue light penetration.[22]

Light fluence in tissue decreases exponentially with the distance. Therefore, the effective penetration depth of light in tissue is inversely proportional to the effective attenuation coefficient. Evaluation of light penetration from 400 to 1100 nm through various thicknesses of several types of excised animal tissue has demonstrated a rapid rise in transmittance from 550 to 650 nm with little variance at longer wavelengths.[23] The absolute transmittance values varied for each tissue but the overall transmittance spectra remained fairly constant.

The effective attenuation coefficient is more difficult to predict in vivo because individual tissue characteristics, such as blood flow and the degree and direction in which homogeneous light distribution scatters, may affect the final light delivery. On average, the 630 nm light used for clinical PDT with porfimer sodium penetrates from 1 to 3 mm, depending on the tissue. Penetration of light from 700 to 850 nm is nearly twice that at 630 nm, making the longer visible wavelengths more attractive for photodestruction of tumors. Some of the photosensitizing agents currently under evaluation provide more efficient light absorption at wavelengths longer than 630 nm. These compounds share structural similarities with the more well-known porphyrin photosensitizers porfimer sodium and HPD: phthalocyanines, chlorins, bacteriochlorins, benzoporphyrins, purpurins, and pheophorbides have demonstrated such photosensitizing properties.

The depth of tissue destruction depends on the ability of the absorbed light to penetrate sufficiently to excite the photosensitizer, the molecular structure of which determines the wavelengths of light it absorbs. However, other biologic molecules, notably melanin and hemoglobin, can interfere with PDT, either by absorbing light intended for treatment or by producing undesirable side effects such as heat.[19] Therefore, although absorbance is greater at shorter visible light wavelengths, absorbance peaks of 630 nm or greater are usually used in PDT because of better tissue penetration (3 mm at 630 nm) and less light absorption by naturally occurring biomolecules. On the other hand, while visible light of longer wavelength is preferable for treatment of most tumors, superficial neoplastic lesions may be treated more efficiently with shorter wavelengths of visible light where deeper penetration is less critical or even undesirable.

Exposure of sensitizer-containing tissue to wavelengths that are strongly absorbed can lead to a limitation of light penetration for PDT.[9] This phenomenon can be overcome by decreasing the dose of sensitizer or by using a less efficient wavelength for exposure. However, photosensitizers also undergo photodestruction during light exposure in a process called photobleaching.[24] Photobleaching can be very useful during PDT and is felt to be the reason why normal tissue is spared photodynamic destruction. PDT requires a minimum quantity of light energy to activate the sensitizer in tissue. If photobleaching sufficient to inactivate the sensitizer occurs before the minimum light energy initiates the cytotoxic photodynamic effect, the tissue will be spared. Therefore, low levels of sensitizer in normal tissue are destroyed while the high levels of sensitizer in tumor undergo the photodynamic effect. This phenomenon suggests a drug dose dependency for efficient PDT which limits damage to adjacent normal tissue.

for a two-dimensional treatment area, and in joules/cm$^3$ for a three-dimensional volume of tissue. Earlier systems for treatment delivered 630 nm of light for porphyrin activation with an ordinary incandescent light bulb and a red filter. However, clinical PDT with these low-powered systems was limited to treatment of external lesions of rather small surface area because of the time required for treatment and the inaccessibility of internal lesions. The availability of both monochromatic light sources (lasers), with sufficient energy to initiate photodynamic activity, and optical fibers capable of delivery to previously inaccessible organs, rekindled clinical interest. The system most frequently used for PDT in the past was a tunable dye laser where the dye module could be changed to fit the absorbance spectrum of different sensitizers. Nowadays, inexpensive and reliable solid-state lasers are available as the light source of choice for PDT.

Regardless of the type of laser used, the light generated is generally transmitted along an optical fiber, permitting access to viscera otherwise inaccessible for practical PDT. Light distribution can be adapted to the target tissue configuration by modification of the optical fiber, use of multiple fibers, or with various light-scanning devices and diffusion techniques.[19,25] These types of modification allow both external and interstitial treatment of surface, intraluminal, and intracavitary lesions where contours can cause difficulty for direct light exposure to some target areas. Calculation of surface area and energy density may not be trivial in organs or body cavities with irregular contours and large treatment areas. Inaccurate determination of the treatment area may lead to delivery of excessive power, which may cause undesired thermal effects, including charring, to interfere with light absorption. Conversely, underestimation of the true treatment area could lead to treatment failure. Regardless of the method of light delivery, light doses for optimal effect in PDT range between 50 and 300 J/cm$^2$ for tumor destruction, whereas carcinoma in situ (Tis) and dysplasia may be treated with lower light doses (10–50 J/cm$^2$).[19]

## LIGHT DELIVERY SYSTEMS

Despite early observations of photodynamic effect on microorganisms, the clinical application of photosensitization did not progress until the 1970s because of a lack of sophisticated light sources. Light energy for PDT is usually measured in joules (J), with 1 J equivalent to 1 watt (W) for 1 second. The light dose for PDT is known as the energy density, and is derived by dividing the product of the power (W) and the time (seconds) by the area irradiated (cm$^2$ or cm$^3$). As a result, energy density is usually described in joules/cm$^2$

## ROLE OF OXYGEN

There is a third essential component directly involved with the porphyrin-mediated cytocidal mechanism: oxygen.[26] Photosensitized oxidation is the basis of photodynamic therapy and can result from two different types of reaction. The first step involves absorption of light energy by the photosensitizing agent to produce an excited state. The excited agent can react either with the substrate or solvent (Type I reaction) or directly with oxygen (Type II reaction)[27] (Figure 36.2). Type I reactions result in either hydrogen atom or electron

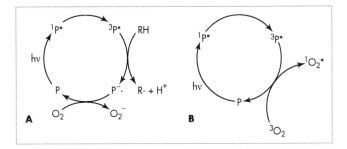

**Fig. 36.2**
A Type I, and **B**, Type II mechanisms of light energy transfer. Type II reactions with creation of singlet oxygen are predominantly involved in photodynamic therapy.

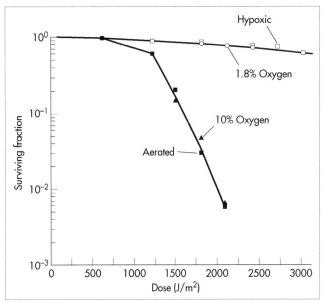

**Fig. 36.3**
Photodynamic therapy survival curves for Chinese hamster cells exposed to porfimer sodium for 2 hours followed by red light (590 nm) underaerated (closed symbols) and hypoxic (open symbols) conditions. Different symbols represent replicate experiments. Reproduced with permission from J.B. Mitchell et al.[28]

transfer, which yields radical ions that most commonly act as an oxidant. Type II reactions, however, produce singlet molecular oxygen by direct energy transfer. This latter type of reaction is felt to be the primary mechanism for the cytotoxicity of PDT. The reactive, short-lived, excited singlet oxygen state is felt to be the agent responsible for cell death and, although difficult to measure, has been directly detected in tissue and chemically trapped in situ during PDT. In vitro studies have demonstrated rapid, nearly complete cell death in an oxygenated environment during PDT but hardly any effect in an oxygen-free environment[28] (Figure 36.3). Percutaneous measurements of tumor and tissue oxygen tension show rapidly decreased levels during PDT.[29] Furthermore, vascular clamping to induce tissue hypoxia during in vivo PDT has prevented PDT side effects.[26,30] Preexisting tumor hypoxia and rapid oxygen depletion during treatment are possible reasons for treatment failures that previously have been attributed to inadequate quantities of light or photosensitizer. Although the evidence suggests that singlet oxygen is one of the major phototoxic agents at the cellular level, other photochemical products such as superoxide ion created by Type I reactions may also contribute to cell death.[31]

## CYTOTOXIC MECHANISMS OF PDT

Experimental data about mechanisms of tumor death have concerned both direct tumor effects and the impact of PDT upon tumor vasculature. Membranes are the primary cellular targets of photochemically induced singlet oxygen cellular damage, and inactivation of membrane transport systems may be one of the initial effects of PDT.[32] The most common types of membrane damage identified following porphyrin photosensitization have been DNA-protein crosslinking and lipid peroxidation.[33] The diffusion distance of singlet oxygen in cells has been estimated at 0.1 μm, which

means that damage will occur close to the site of singlet generation.[34] Due to the varied distribution of sensitizers within cells, many cellular components can be affected. Cytoplasmic organelles appear to be variably sensitive to PDT, with mitochondrial enzymes generally more sensitive to PDT than lysosomal enzymes, and nonmembrane-bound cytologic enzymes relatively insensitive. Mitochondria are the primary target of tissue containing the cationic sensitizers because of the preferential accumulation of these compounds in those structures. Photo-oxidative damage of nucleic acids and proteins may be less significant because the effect of PDT appears to be equally toxic throughout all phases of the cell cycle.

Rapid loss of cell integrity is noted regardless of the site that incurs the lethal damage. Cells begin to leak lactate dehydrogenase (LDH) almost immediately after initiation of treatment, which is followed by the release of several inflammatory and immune modulators, including eicosanoids, histamine, and eventually tumor necrosis factor.[9] When studied in vitro, cell disintegration appears to be complete within 4 hours when monitored by [51]CR-release assay. Experiments with [31]P nuclear magnetic resonance (NMR) of tumors undergoing PDT suggest a striking early drop in tumor ATP, which approached undetectable levels at 2–4 hours after PDT with a gradual return at 24–48 hours to pretreatment levels.[35]

Although initially the tumoricidal mechanisms for PDT were thought to be related to direct cytotoxic effects, other factors such as tumor vascular damage and hyperthermia appear to contribute to tumor cell death, and many investigators now believe that this mechanism is the primary cause of tumor destruction. Vascular damage may be related to reports that HPD levels are increased in tumor vascular stroma. Several reports document tumor microvasculature damage by PDT, which in some instances is noted almost immediately after initiation of treatment. These may be related to the rapid release of many vasoactive substances from cells reported from in vitro experiments. Although release of these vasoactive substances during treatment may reflect generalized inflammatory tissue response to injury, the fact that these compounds may be an important component of the PDT vascular response is supported by the greatly reduced microvascular response to PDT after prostaglandin and thromboxane $A_2$ inhibition.[36] Murine dermal photosensitivity is also decreased following administration of medications that interfere with histamine release and prostaglandin formation.[37]

Types of vascular damage include direct observation of tumor microcirculatory bleaching during PDT, microscopic arteriolar vasoconstriction and venous thrombus formation beginning during PDT, and endothelial cell necrosis in both normal and neoplastic vessels following PDT.[38-40] Vascular occlusion, however, does not usually occur until a few hours following PDT and appears irreversible.[25] This becomes important if one considers that immediate vascular occlusion would effectively cut off oxygenation to the treatment area, which may be necessary for singlet oxygen production. Peak vascular photosensitivity does not occur immediately after sensitizer injection, suggesting that time is required for the sensitizer to bind to sensitive vascular sites. The extensive in vitro cytotoxicity reported by many investigators, however, is not explained by vascular effects. Consequently, many investigators currently feel that in vivo tumor death is due to a combination of both direct cytotoxicity and disruption of tumor vasculature. In addition, apoptosis is induced by PDT, leading to a restoration of natural programmed cell death.[9]

Another potential contributor to the mechanism of PDT-induced tumor destruction is the known synergism between hyperthermia and PDT. Tumor destruction may be caused or enhanced by heat created by the intense local light doses delivered during PDT. It has also been shown in tumor models that tumor destruction is enhanced with the combination of hyperthermia and PDT, and that potentiation of these two modalities appears greatest when hyperthermia is added immediately after PDT.[41,42] This additive effect has not yet been fully explored for its potential clinical applications.

# FLUORESCENCE FOR TUMOR DETECTION

Light is used with photosensitized tissue in another fashion for diagnostic purposes. The fluorescent properties of several photosensitizing agents have intriguing potential for clinical use in detection of neoplastic as well as some benign disorders. Fluorescence is the emission of light from an excited molecule as it returns to its ground state, and it occurs at wavelengths longer than those used for excitation (Figure 36.4). Porphyrin photosensitizers produce a characteristic reddish hue in tissue when excited by absorbed light in the ultraviolet or blue–green visible light ranges. Fluorescence does indicate tumor presence but the fluorescent intensity does not necessarily predict the degree of tumor destruction, suggesting that phototoxic and fluorescent species may be separate entities following similar uptake and distribution patterns in neoplasia. It appears that the state of macromolecular aggregation may affect porphyrin tissue fluorescence.

Several early investigators independently reported fluorescence in a variety of malignant lesions.[6,7,43-45] HPD fluorescence has been used for detection of Tis and occult lung and bladder tumors. The fluorescent mapping of tumor sites prior to surgery correlated to pathologic findings in 16 patients that underwent radical cystectomy for invasive TCC or diffuse Tis.[46] Other investigators used an image intensifier to detect fluorescence of HPD at all tumor sites in eight

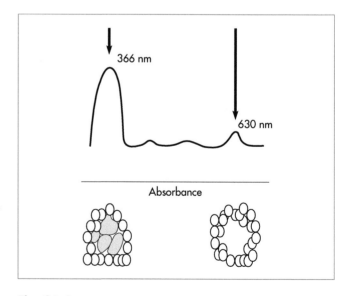

**Fig. 36.4**
Fluorescence and photodestruction during porphyrin photosensitization. Fluorescence with ultraviolet wavelength (366 nm) gives a characteristic reddish hue used in photodynamic diagnosis. Exposure of tissue to appropriate energy densities of red light at 630 nm is used for tissue destruction.

patients.[47] More recently, great promise for clinical utility of photodynamic diagnosis (PDD) with 5-ALA and its hexyl congener has been demonstrated for use in early stage bladder TCC where PDD detected between 22% and 34% of the lesions.[48-50] This subject is reviewed in detail in Chapter 17.

# PDT FOR UROLOGIC MALIGNANCY

## BLADDER TCC

The treatment of urologic malignancy was one of the earliest clinical applications for PDT following the introduction of laser technology for uniform light delivery in the 1970s. The first reported urologic use of PDT occurred in 1975 with destruction of human TCC transplants in mice with 57 $J/cm^2$.[51] The same group reported a response to PDT in a patient with bladder carcinoma the following year, and photosensitization has been used for diagnosis and treatment of bladder carcinoma since then.[52]

## UROLOGIC PDT: PRECLINICAL STUDIES

Fluorescence has been used in vitro with bladder cancer cells to study uptake, subcellular localization, and components of molecular aggregation of porphyrin photosensitizers.[53-56] The photodynamic destruction of bladder cancer cells has also been successfully accomplished in vitro, and bladder cancer cell death has been correlated with fluorescence.[53,57] Fluorescence spectroscopy has been used to study the kinetics of intravesical administration of 5-ALA in both normal and tumor-containing rat bladders.[58] Likewise, fluorescence has been used to determine the maximal tumor to normal bladder ratio of intravesical and intraperitoneal 5-ALA administration in a similar model, an important step to understanding the optimal timing of treatment.[59]

Destruction of subcutaneously transplanted and chemically induced bladder carcinomas has been successful using PDT. The first group to treat a bladder malignancy demonstrated the efficacy of PDT for bladder cancers implanted in immunosuppressed mice.[51] Others reported treatment of the Brown–Pearce carcinoma transplanted into the bladder and bladder neck of rabbits.[60] PDT is effective for destruction of transplanted, chemically induced FANFT urothelial tumors in rats using both porfimer sodium and metallopurpurins, another group of promising porphyrin sensitizers.[61,62] More recently, whole bladder PDT has been accomplished with 5-ALA using an orthotopic superficial bladder cancer rat model.[63] In another recent study by a different group, whole bladder PDT after both intravenous and intravesical porfimer sodium administration was compared to PDT after intravesical 5-ALA in the same orthotopic rat bladder tumor model.[64]

Animal studies involving PDT of normal urothelium have shown varied responses. Normal human urothelium transplanted into the mouse flank was unaffected by PDT when treated with 57 $J/cm^2$.[65] Another author using hematoporphyrin derivative (HPD) reported no damage to normal canine bladder urothelium with PDT at 200 $mW/cm^2$.[66] However, there are reports of mucosal edema with both focal light and whole bladder laser exposure without sensitizer in the normal canine bladder subjected to 30–150 $J/cm^2$. After porfimer sodium administration, superficial ulceration followed focal treatment with 180–360 $J/cm^2$, and damage through the lamina propria occurred with whole bladder exposure at 30 $J/cm^2$.[67] The same author reported treatment of a baboon which showed bladder submucosal damage after porfimer sodium administration and light exposure at 100 and 300 $J/cm^2$.[68] However, other investigators found no mucosal or submucosal damage, either in the normal canine urethra using a cylindrical fiber at 24–101 $J/cm^2$, or in the canine ureter using a cylindrical fiber at 20–39 $J/cm^2$.[69,70] One possible explanation of these varying results relates to the interval before treatment and the energy used. PDT is performed several hours after photosensitizer injection when the differential between photosensitizer retention in normal and neoplastic tissue is supposedly optimal. Survival curves for in vitro PDT cell destruction reveal a decreased effect at lower light doses, suggesting a need to accumulate a critical amount of light energy before cytotoxicity occurs. Rapid depletion of the photosensitizer may occur in tissues containing low cellular photosensitizer levels when exposed to light.[71] This phenomenon, known as photobleaching, may serve to protect normal tissues, which have lower sensitizer levels than neoplastic tissue. Therefore, experiments performed on normal tissue before photosensitizer levels have decreased would be expected to show damage. On the other hand, if sufficient time has elapsed for photosensitizer levels to decrease, PDT damage would be reduced.

## SUPERFICIAL BLADDER CARCINOMA

Transitional cell carcinoma of the bladder is responsive to PDT, with better responses generally noted for treatment of Tis.[72-74] Several early reports of PDT demonstrated some efficacy for superficial papillary lesions, but many of these studies had small numbers of patients, relatively short-term follow-up evaluation, combined complete and partial responses, or lacked data on tumor grade or size.[47,65,75-78] Energy density for treatment in these studies consisted of focal irradiation ranging from 100 to 250 J/cm$^2$. One investigator reported focal irradiation at 100 J/cm$^2$ followed by 25 J/cm$^2$ whole bladder irradiation.[65] The conclusion by several investigators that treatment is ineffective for tumors larger than 2 cm is not surprising, considering the limitations of 630 nm light penetration in tissue. One report of whole bladder PDT for prophylaxis of recurrent superficial papillary bladder carcinoma compared to observation alone suggested a significantly longer time to recurrence in the treated group but no further follow-up has been published.[79] More recent reports that include papillary lesion treatment with longer follow-up have varied response and recurrence results.[80,81] Similar findings have been noted with the use of intravesical 5-ALA for papillary tumors.[21] Most investigators would reserve PDT for patients with papillary tumors to those with multiple lesions as an adjunct to transurethral resection for residual disease.

Although the treatment of papillary lesions may be equivocal and its indications limited, it does appear that one of the most effective uses of PDT for urologic malignancy is for treatment of transitional cell Tis of the bladder. The diffuse nature of Tis requires a distribution of light evenly throughout the bladder instead of focal irradiation of tumors. Treatment for Tis has usually been performed by placement of a spherical-tipped (Figure 36.5) or cylindrical optical fiber in the approximate center of a saline-filled bladder, followed by exposure of the entire bladder epithelium simultaneously to energy densities ranging from 25 to 45 J/cm$^2$. This has occurred 48–72 hours after intravenous injection of 1.5–2.5 mg/kg of porfimer sodium, the standard sensitizer dose used in most studies of human PDT with porfimer sodium. A small preliminary study reported

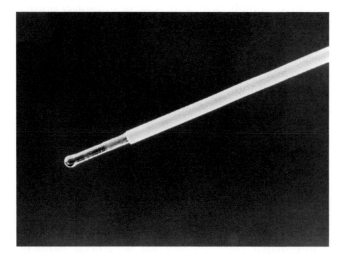

**Fig. 36.5**
Spherical tip of 600 micron optical fiber used for whole bladder photodynamic therapy. A cylindrical fiber will also give circumferential light distribution in a viscous organ.

complete response in all four patients with Tis, with recurrences in two of these patients successfully retreated by PDT.[66] A later report by this group, relating to 10 patients with Tis, 4 of them with concurrent superficially invasive papillary tumors, noted focal recurrence of Tis in 2 of the 10 patients and little or no effect on the papillary tumors.[82] Another investigator reported 11 complete responses (CR) and 3 partial responses (PR) in 16 patients with Tis, 12 of whom had PDT as their first line of treatment.[83]

There are only a few reports of PDT for bladder carcinoma with long-term follow-up. The first report evaluated 15 patients with resistant Tis 24–54 months after whole bladder PDT; 9 sustained complete response, and 2 more were rendered disease-free after retreatment with PDT.[84] Two other patients had eradication of their tumors with transurethral resection via Nd:YAG laser fulguration, and there were 2 failures of treatment. Another group later reported 58 patients with postintravesical therapy residual papillary lesions or Tis that received a single treatment of 10–60 J/cm$^2$.[80] Initial 3-month CR rates were 84% and 75% for papillary lesions and Tis, respectively, with 34 (59%) of the responders, 31 with no evidence of disease, alive with a mean follow-up of 50 months. The most recent report concerned 34 (29 Tis, 5 multiple papillary) patients with refractory disease following a single treatment using diffusion medium for light dispersal.[81] Response rates at 3 months were 44% (CR) and 12% (PR), with a mean time to recurrence of 9.8 months in the CR group. With a mean follow-up of 52 months, metastatic bladder cancer was the cause of death in only 4 of 12 patients that died, and 15 of the 22 survivors have an intact bladder, 9 with no disease and 6 with superficial disease.

The need for cystectomy following PDT has rarely been discussed and only two studies address this issue. In the report from the Bladder Photofrin Study Group, with a mean follow-up of 12 months, 14 of 36 patients (39%) required cystectomy for persistent or recurrent Tis following PDT. Although they note seven patients with bladder contracture, no cystectomies for this complication are reported.[85] In the recent study of long-term PDT outcomes, 9 of 34 patients (26%) underwent cystectomy for persistent[6] or recurrent[3] disease and 2 patients (6%) had cystectomy for bladder contracture.[81] It is important to note that all patients in both studies faced cystectomy because of intravesical treatment failure with aggressive disease; the fact that approximately only one-third of patients required cystectomy suggests that PDT is a viable option for refractive superficial disease. While it is unknown whether an earlier cystectomy would have decreased the metastatic bladder cancer death rate in the long-term study, two of the four patients that died of metastasis were not surgical candidates before invasion occurred due to concurrent morbidity.

Transitional cell carcinoma of the prostatic fossa has been mentioned as a possible target of PDT. A few anecdotal reports have suggested success with control of this fortunately rare problem, but other anecdotal reports have not been encouraging. PDT is not recommended in its current state for prostatic TCC because light penetration into the prostatic ducts is not sufficient at this time to eradicate the disease; these patients are better managed by some other form of therapy.

## SIDE EFFECTS AND COMPLICATIONS OF PDT

Enthusiasm for using PDT for refractive bladder Tis, and for widespread urologic application of PDT, is tempered by its side effects. The most common side effect of PDT with porfimer sodium is dermal photosensitivity similar to that of patients with porphyria. Patients are advised to avoid both direct and indirect sun exposure for 6–8 weeks after the intravenous injection of most porphyrin photosensitizers. The most experienced PDT investigator reports that there appears to be no relationship between phototoxic response and porfimer sodium dose in 180 patients treated for various tumors, with some type of phototoxic response experienced in 20% to 40% of patients.[86] Sunscreens are not effective unless they are opaque to visible light, from ultraviolet wavelengths to beyond 650 nm; these are not practical because of the surface area that must be covered. Attempts to alter porphyrin metabolism or inflammatory response after treatment are encouraging in animal studies but have not yet undergone clinical trials.[87] Some investigators have used indomethacin, but these anecdotal reports of decreased photosensitivity after PDT under daily oral doses await corroboration. It is encouraging that topical application of 5-ALA and its derivatives appears to bypass systemic toxicity with minor or transient skin photosensitivity.[20,21]

PDT generally does not interfere with other treatment modalities, but porfimer sodium dermal photosensitivity may be enhanced in patients previously treated with or undergoing radiation therapy, and in patients previously treated with the chemotherapeutic agent adriamycin. Patients treated with whole bladder PDT may slough tissue after treatment and frequently have irritative symptoms lasting from a few days to several weeks. There are a few reports of bladder contracture and vesicoureteral reflux following whole bladder PDT, but it is unclear whether previous radiation, intravesical BCG treatment, incorrect calculation of energy density during PDT, or overlapping treatment fields have contributed to these reports.[65,81,85] Nonetheless, severe bladder contracture with vesicoureteral reflux has occasionally led to cystectomy

following PDT.[81] Other rarely reported side effects after porphyrin sensitizer injection include nausea, vomiting, metallic taste after injection, eye photosensitivity, and liver toxicity.[2]

## SPECIAL CONSIDERATIONS FOR BLADDER PDT

Patients must be selected carefully for whole bladder PDT and attention must be paid to several details surrounding the treatment of the patient (Box 36.1). Patients should complete a staging evaluation that includes determination that the upper urinary tract and prostate do not harbor TCC (Box 36.2). Once it has been determined that PDT is appropriate for the patient, extensive patient education is initiated regarding the method of treatment and its side effects. The patient is given educational material to review, and is encouraged to raise any questions regarding treatment and after effects. An interval of 3–6 weeks before sensitizer administration allows sufficient healing to occur after bladder biopsy to avoid undue concentration of the sensitizer in inflammatory tissue.

If the patient is to receive intravenous porfimer sodium, administration occurs 48 hours before the

**Box 36.1** Exclusion criteria for whole bladder photodynamic therapy

Any tumor type other than transitional cell carcinoma

Any tumor staged T2 or greater

Metastatic bladder lesions

Transitional cell carcinoma or Tis of prostatic ducts, ureter, or urethra

Porphyria or severe liver disease

Carotenemia

Rifampicin treatment within the last 3 months

Treatment with hydroxychloroquine or related product

Inability to undergo general or regional anesthesia

Positive urine culture at time of proposed treatment

**Box 36.2** Patient evaluation for bladder photodynamic therapy

History and physical examination

Serology, blood chemistry profile

Urine culture

Metastatic evaluation: intravenous urography, retrograde pyelography, cross-sectional image studies

Cystoscopy

Urine cytology (flow cytometry optional)

Multiple bladder biopsies

Prostatic urethra biopsies (if necessary)

planned light exposure to the treatment area. However, the patient must begin to wear the appropriate sun-protective accessories (sunglasses, brimmed hat, long-sleeved shirt, long pants, socks or other foot protection, and gloves) which must continue for 6 weeks. Intravesical administration of topical photosensitizers, such as 5-ALA, may not require pretreatment photoprotection and solar precautions are only continued for 1 week post PDT. Regardless of the photosensitizer used, the patient must be protected from sunlight or intense incandescent light, including the cystoscopic xenon light source in the perioperative environment.

Once positioned, the cystoscope is anchored to avoid an important possible source of dosimetry error from optical fiber movement (Figure 36.6). The bladder is distended with saline or with diffusion medium in order to enhance light scatter. Calculation of bladder surface area is performed to determine the time of light exposure to deliver the desired energy density. Surface area has been calculated by extrapolation from an instilled volume or by transabdominal ultrasound. The optical fiber has usually been placed in the center of the bladder under direct vision or with a ureteral catheter measurement. Deviation from true center can occur with either method of placement, however, and trans-abdominal sonography may provide more accurate optical fiber placement and assist with surface area calculation[88] (Figure 36.7).

Whole bladder PDT takes about an hour to complete and patients are observed in an area protected from intense incandescent light until deemed ready for discharge or short stay admission. Patients are discharged with protective clothing and accessories, and return for an office visit at 6 weeks for assessment of skin photosensitivity. Follow-up by telephone is frequent

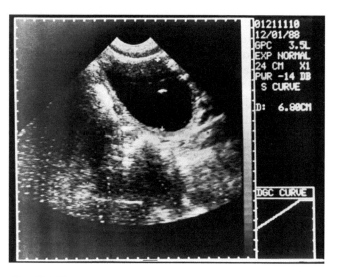

**Fig. 36.7**
Transabdominal ultrasound during whole bladder photodynamic therapy allows accurate optical fiber placement in three planes.

over the first 2 weeks or until irritative symptoms abate. Post-PDT evaluation often follows conventional recommendations with cystoscopy, cytology, and bladder biopsies at 3-month intervals.

REFERENCES

1. Heney NM, Ahmed S, Flanagan MJ, Frable W, Corder MP, Hafermann MD, Hawkins IR. Superficial bladder cancer: progression and recurrence. J Urol 1983;30:1083–1086.
2. Dougherty TJ. Photodynamic therapy (PDT) of malignant tumors. Crit Rev Oncol Hematol 1984;2:83–116.
3. Raab O. Uber die wirkung fluoreszierender staffe auf infuroriea. Z Biol 1900;19:524–546.
4. Tappenier H, Jesionek A. Therapeutische versuche mit fluoreszierenden stoffe. Muench Med Wochenschr 1903;1:2042–2044.
5. Policard A. Etudes sur les aspects offerts par des tumeur experimentales lexaminee a la lumiere de woods. C R Soc Biol 1924;91:1423–1424.
6. Auler H, Banzer G. Unter Suchungen uber die rolle der porphyrine BEI Geschwul Stkranken menschen und tieren Z Krebsforsch 1942;53:65–68.
7. Figge FHJ, Weiland GS, Manganiella LOJ. Cancer detection and therapy. Affinity of neoplastic, embryonic, and traumatized tissues for porphyrins and metalloporphyrins. Proc Soc Exp Biol Med 1948;68:640–641.
8. Lipson RL, Baldes EJ, Olsen EM. The use of a derivative of hematoporphyrin in tumor detection. J Natl Cancer Inst 1961;26:1–12.
9. Henderson BA, Dougherty TJ. How does photodynamic therapy work? Photochem Photobiol 1992;55:145–157.
10. Moan J, Sommer S. Action spectra for hematoporphyrin derivative and Photofrin II with respect to sensitization of human cells in vitro to photoinactivation. Photochem Photobiol 1984;40:631–634.
11. Moan J, Berg E, Kvam A, et al. Intracellular localization of photosensitizers. In Photosensitizing Compounds: Their Chemistry, Biology, and Clinical Use. Ciba Foundation Symposium. Chichester: Wiley, 1989, pp 95–107.
12. Oseroff AR, Ohuoha D, Ara G, et al. Intramitochondrial dyes allow selective in vitro photolysis of carcinoma cells. Proc Natl Acad Sci USA 1986;83:9729–9733.

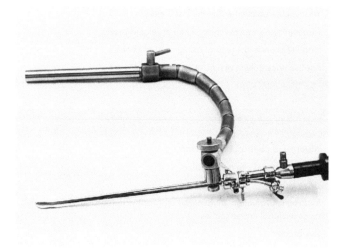

**Fig. 36.6**
Anchoring device for endoscopic photodynamic therapy. The light source must remain stable for accurate light delivery.

13. Figge FHJ, Weiland GS, Manganiella LOJ. Cancer detection and therapy. Affinity of neoplastic, embryonic, and traumatized tissues for porphyrins and metalloporphyrins. Proc Soc Exp Biol Med 1948;68:640–641.

14. Selman SH, Goldblatt PJ, Klaunig JE, et al. Localization of hematoporphyrin derivative in injured bladder mucosa. An experimental study. J Urol 1985;133:1104–1107.

15. Korbelik M, Hung J, Lam S, et al. The effects of low density lipoproteins on uptake of Photofrin II. Photochem Photobiol 1990;51:191–196.

16. Brunner H, Hausmann F, Knuechel R. New 5-aminolevulinic acid esters—efficient protoporphyrin precursors for photodetection and photodynamic therapy. Photochem Photobiol 2003;78:481–486.

17. Seidl J, Rauch J, Krieg RC, et al. Optimization of differential photodynamic effectiveness between normal and tumor urothelial cells using 5-aminolevulinic acid-induced protoporphyrin IX as sensitizer. Int J Cancer 2001;92:671–677.

18. Waidelich R, Stepp H, Baumgartner R, et al. Clinical experience with 5-aminolevulinic acid and photodynamic therapy for refractory superficial bladder cancer. J Urol 2001;165:1904–1907.

19. Manyak MJ, Russo A, Smith PD, et al. Photodynamic therapy. J Clin Oncol 1988;6:380.

20. Berger AP, Steiner H, Stenzl A, et al. Photodynamic therapy with intravesical instillation of 5-aminolevulinic acid for patients with recurrent superficial bladder cancer: a single-center study. Urology 2003;61:338–341.

21. Waidelich R, Beyer W, Knuechel R, et al. Whole bladder photodynamic therapy with 5-aminolevulinic acid using a white light source. Urology 2003;61:332–337.

22. Wilson BC, Patterson MS. The physics of photodynamic therapy. Phys Med Biol 1986;31:327.

23. Preuss LE, Bolin FP, Cain BW. A comment on spectral transmittance in mammalian skeletal muscle. Photochem Photobiol 1983;37:113.

24. Potter WR. The theory of PCT dosimetry: consequences of photodestruction of sensitizer. Photochem Photobiol 1987;46:97–101.

25. Pottier R, Truscott TG. The photochemistry of haematoporphyrin and related systems. Int J Radiat Biol 1986;50:421–452.

26. Weishaupt KR, Gomer CJ, Dougherty TJ. Identification of singlet oxygen as the cytotoxic agent in photoactivation of a murine tumor. Cancer Res 1976;36:2326–2329.

27. Foote CS. Definition of Type I and Type II photosensitized oxidation. Photochem Photobiol 1991;54:659.

28. Mitchell JB, McPherson S, DeGraff W, et al. Oxygen dependence of hematoporphyrin derivative-induced photoinactivation of Chinese hamster cells. Cancer Res 1985;45:2008–2011.

29. Tromberg BJ, Orenstein A, Kimel S, et al. In vivo tumor oxygen tension measurements for the evaluation of the efficiency of photodynamic therapy. Photochem Photobiol 1990;52:375–385.

30. Gomer CJ, Razum N. Acute skin response in albino mice following porphyrin photosensitization under oxic and anoxic conditions. Photochem Photobiol 1984;40:435–439.

31. Athar M, Elmets CA, Bickers DR, et al. A novel mechanism for the generation of super-oxide anions in hematoporphyrin derivative-mediated cutaneous photosensitization. Activation of the xanthine oxidase pathway. J Clin Invest 1989;83:1137–1143.

32. Gibson SL, Hilf R. Photosensitization of mitochondrial cytochrome c oxidase by hematoporphyrin derivative and related porphyrins in vitro and in vivo. Cancer Res 1983;43:4191–4197.

33. Moan J, Waksvik H, Christensen T. DNA single-strand breaks and sister chromatid exchanges induced by treatment with hematoporphyrin and light or by X-rays in human NHIK 3025 cells. Cancer Res 1980;40:2915–2918.

34. Moan J. On the diffusion length of singlet oxygen in cells and tissues. J Photochem Photobiol B 1990;6:343–344.

35. Hilf R, Gibson SL, Penney TL, et al. Early biochemical responses to photodynamic therapy monitored by NMR spectroscopy. Photochem Photobiol 1987;46:809–817.

36. Reed MWR, Wieman TJ, Doak KW, et al. The microvascular effects of photodynamic therapy: evidence for a possible role of cyclooxygenase products. Photochem Photobiol 1989;50:419–423.

37. Manyak MJ, Smith PD, Harrington FS, et al. Protection against dihematoporphyrin ether photosensitivity. Photochem Photobiol 1988;47:823–830.

38. Nelson JS, Liaw L-H, Berns MW. Tumor destruction in photodynamic therapy. Photochem Photobiol 1987;46:829–835.

39. Reed MWR, Wieman TJ, Doak KW, et al. The microvascular effects of photodynamic therapy. evidence for a possible role of cyclooxygenase products. Photochem Photobiol 1989;50:419–423.

40. Star WM, Marijnissen HPA, Berg-Blok A, et al. Destruction of rat mammary tumor and normal tissue microcirculation by hematoporphyrin derivative observed in vivo in sandwich observation chambers. Cancer Res 1986;46:2532–2540.

41. Waldow SM, Henderson BW, Dougherty TJ. Hyperthermic potentiation of photodynamic therapy employing Photofrin I and II: comparison of results using three animal tumor models. Lasers Surg Med 1987;7:12–22.

42. Mang TS, Dougherty TJ. Time and sequence dependent influence in in vitro photodynamic therapy (PDT) survival by hyperthermia. Photochem Photobiol 1985;42:533–540.

43. Rassmussen-Taxdal DS, Ward GE, Figge FHJ. Fluorescence of human lymphatic and cancer tissues following high doses of intravenous hematoporphyrin. Cancer 1955;8:78–81.

44. Gregorie HB Jr, Horger EO, Ward JL, et al. Hematoporphyrin-derivative fluorescence in malignant neoplasms. Ann Surg 1968;167:820–828.

45. Leonard JR, Beck WL. Hematoporphyrin fluorescence: an aid in diagnosis of malignant neoplasms. Laryngoscope 1971;81(3):365–372.

46. Benson RC Jr, Farrow GM, Kinsey JH, et al. Detection and localization of in situ carcinoma of the bladder with hematoporphyrin derivative. Mayo Clin Proc 1982;57:548–555.

47. Tsuchiya A, Obara N, Miwa M, et al. Hematoporphyrin derivative and photoradiation therapy in the diagnosis and treatment of bladder cancer. J Urol 1983;130:79–82.

48. Zaak D, Kreigmair M, Stepp H, et al. Endoscopic detection of transitional cell carcinoma with 5-aminolevulinic acid: results of 1012 fluorescence endoscopies. Urology 2001;57:690–694.

49. Zaak D, Hungerhuber E, Schneede P, et al. Role of 5-aminolevulinic acid in the detection of urothelial premalignant lesions. Cancer 2002;95:1234–1238.

50. Schmidbauer J, Witjes F, Schmeller N, et al. Improved detection of urothelial carcinoma in situ with hexaminolevulinate fluorescence cystoscopy. J Urol 2004;171:135–138.

51. Kelly JF, Snell ME, Berenbaum MC. Photodynamic destruction of human bladder carcinoma. Br J Cancer 1975;31:237–244.

52. Kelly JF, Snell ME. Hematoporphyrin derivative: a possible aid in the diagnosis and therapy of carcinoma of the bladder. J Urol 1976;115:150–151.

53. Bellnier DA, Lin C-W. Photodynamic destruction of cultured human bladder tumor cells by hematoporphyrin derivative: effects of porphyrin molecular aggregation. Photochem Photobiophys 1983;6:357–366.

54. Hisazumi H, Miyoshi N, Ueki O, et al. Cellular uptake of hematoporphyrin derivative in KK-47 bladder cancer cells. Urol Res 1984;12:143–146.

55. Shulock JR, Wade MH, Lin C-W. Subcellular localization of hematoporphyrin derivative in bladder tumor cells in culture. Photochem Photobiol 1990;51:451–457.

56. Bachor R, Scholz M, Shea CR, et al. Mechanism of photosensitization by microsphere-bound chlorin e6 in human bladder carcinoma cells. Cancer Res 1991;51:4410–4414.

57. Williams RD, Runge TC. Photodynamic therapy of human bladder cancer cells in vitro correlated with cellular fluorescence levels of Photofrin II. Photochem Photobiol 1987;46:733–737.

58. Heil P, Stocker S, Sroka R, et al. In vivo fluorescence kinetics of porphyrins following intravesical instillation of 5-aminolevulinic acid in normal and tumour-bearing rat bladders. J Photochem Photobiol 1997;38:158–163.

59. Bisson JF, Christophe M, Padilla-Ybarra JJ, et al. Determination of the maximal tumor: normal bladder ratio after i.p. or bladder

administration of 5-aminolevulinic acid in Fischer 344 rats by fluorescence spectroscopy in situ. Anticancer Drugs 2002;13:851–857.

60. Jocham D, Staehler G, Chaussy C, et al. Laserbehandlung von blasentumoren nach photosensibilisierung mit hamatoporphyrin derivat. Urologe [A] 1981;20:340–345.

61. Selman SH, Garbo GM, Keck RW, et al. Metallopurpurins and light: effect on transplantable rat bladder tumors and murine skin. Photochem Photobiol 1990;51:589–592.

62. Selman SH, Milligan AJ, Kreimer-Birnbaum M, et al. Hematoporphyrin derivative photochemotherapy of experimental bladder tumors. J Urol 1985;133:330–333.

63. Gronlund-Pakkanen S, Wahlfors J, Talja M, et al. The effect of photodynamic therapy on rat urinary bladder with orthotopic urothelial carcinoma. BJU Int 2003;92:125–130.

64. Xiao Z, Brown K, Tulip J, et al. Whole bladder photodynamic therapy for orthotopic superficial bladder cancer in rats: a study of intravenous and intravesical administration of photosensitizers. J Urol 2003;169:352–353.

65. Harty JI, Amin M, Wieman TJ, et al. Complications of whole bladder dihematoporphyrin ether photodynamic therapy. J Urol 1989;141:1341–1346.

66. Benson RC Jr, Kinsey JH, Cortese DA. Treatment of transitional cell carcinoma of the bladder with hematoporphyrin derivative phototherapy. J Urol 1983;130:1090–1095.

67. Nseyo UO, Dougherty TJ, Boyle D, et al. Experimental photodynamic treatment of canine bladder. J Urol 1985;133:311–315.

68. Nseyo UO. Photodynamic therapy. Urol Clin North Am 1992;19:591–599.

69. Manyak MJ, Matthews DM, Smith PD, et al. Photodynamic therapy: response of normal canine urethra using a cylindrical fiber. Lasers Surg Med 1988;8:301–307.

70. Manyak MJ, Matthews DM, Smith PD, et al. Response of normal canine ureter to photodynamic therapy using a cylindrical fiber. J Urol 1988;139:199–203.

71. Mang TS, Dougherty TJ, Potter WR, et al. Photobleaching of porphyrins used in photodynamic therapy and implications for therapy. Photochem Photobiol 1987;45:501–506.

72. Walther MM. The role of photodynamic therapy in the treatment of recurrent superficial bladder cancer. Urol Clin North Am 2000;27:163–170.

73. Manyak MJ. Photodynamic therapy: principles and urological applications. Semin Urol 1991;9:192–202.

74. Nseyo UO. Photodynamic therapy in the management of bladder cancer. J Clin Laser Med Surg 1996;14:271–280.

75. Hisazumi H, Misaki T, Miyoshi N. Photoradiation therapy of bladder tumors. J Urol 1983;130:685–687.

76. Misaki T, Hisazumi H, Miyoshi N. Photoradiation therapy of bladder tumors. In Doiron DR, Gomer DJ (eds): Porphyrin Localization and Treatment of Tumors. New York, Liss, 1984, pp 785–795.

77. Prout GR, Lin C-W, Benson R, et al. Photodynamic therapy with hematoporphyrin derivative in the treatment of superficial transitional cell carcinoma of the bladder. N Engl J Med 1987;317:1251–1255.

78. Tian ME. Photodynamic therapy with hematoporphyrin derivative for transitional cell carcinoma of the urinary bladder—report of 30 cases. Chung Hua Chung Liu Tsa Chih 1989;11:304–306.

79. Marcus SL, Dugan MH. Global status of clinical photodynamic therapy. Lasers Surg Med 1992;12:318–324.

80. Nseyo UO, DeHaven J, Dougherty TJ, et al. Photodynamic therapy (PDT) in the treatment of patients with resistant superficial bladder cancer: a long-term study. J Clin Laser Med Surg 1998;16:61–68.

81. Manyak MJ, Ogan K. Photodynamic therapy for refractive bladder cancer: long term outcomes of single treatment using diffusion medium. J Endourol 2003;18:633–639.

82. Benson RC Jr. Treatment of diffuse transitional cell carcinoma in situ by whole bladder hematoporphyrin derivation photodynamic therapy. J Urol 1985;134:675–678.

83. Shumaker BP, Hetzel FW. Clinical laser photodynamic therapy in the treatment of bladder carcinoma. Photochem Photobiol 1987;46:899–901.

84. Jocham D, Beer M, Baumgartner R, et al. Long-term experience with integral photodynamic therapy of Tis bladder carcinoma. Ciba Found Symp 1989;146:198–205.

85. Nseyo UO, Schumaker BJ, Klein EA, et al. Photodynamic therapy using porfimer sodium as an alternative to cystectomy in patients with refractory transitional cell carcinoma in situ of the bladder. Bladder Photofrin Study Group. J Urol 1998;160:39–44.

86. Dougherty TJ, Cooper MT, Mang TS. Cutaneous phototoxic occurrences in patients receiving Photofrin®. Lasers Surg Med 1990;10:485–488.

87. Manyak MJ, Smith PD, Harrington FS, Steinberg SM, Glatstein E, Russo A. Protection against dihematoporphyrin ether photosensitivity. Photochem Photobiol 1988;47:823–830.

88. Manyak MJ. The practical aspects of photodynamic therapy for superficial bladder cancer. Techniques Urol 1995;1:84–93.

# G3T1 bladder carcinoma

# 37

*Vito Pansadoro, Paolo Emiliozzi*

## INTRODUCTION

High-grade superficial bladder cancer infiltrating the lamina propria (G3T1) is an extremely malignant disease. Although it is superficial, it is very aggressive, with a high incidence of recurrence and progression to muscle-invasive disease. Though the optimal treatment is still controversial, a first line conservative approach is advocated today by most authors.[1]

## INCIDENCE

High-grade superficial bladder cancer accounts for 5% to 23% of all superficial transitional cell carcinomas of the bladder at first diagnosis, in several different series (Table 37.1).

## STAGING

Transurethral resection (TUR) is the most reliable procedure for clinical local staging of bladder cancer, and any treatment modality is based upon the pathology specimen obtained at TUR. However, up to 44% to 46% of patients with T1 transitional cell carcinoma of the bladder at TUR are understaged when subsequent cystectomy is performed.[15,16]

Substaging of T1 bladder cancer refers to invasion above and below the muscularis mucosae (T1A and T1B) or, alternatively, invasion above, at the level of, and below the muscularis mucosae (T1A, T1B and T1C).[17] However, a literature review showed that most series do not reveal a significant difference in terms of recurrence and progression on follow-up of substaged groups.[18]

Whether or not to maintain this subclassification remains a controversial topic. No clear prognostic value can be attributed to substaging of T1 bladder cancer (Table 37.2).

Staging may also show large discrepancies due to different interpretations of the pathologic specimen. In a pathology review of 1400 TUR specimens, only 46% of 88 G3T1 tumors were confirmed, and 10% of cases were reclassified as muscle-infiltrating tumors.[22] In yet another multicenter study, the review pathologist found that 16/54 (29%) bladder cancers initially classified as G3T1 tumors were of lower grade, while 25 bladder cancers (previously classified as lower stage) were reclassified as G3T1.[23]

**Table 37.1** Incidence of G3T1 bladder cancer in superficial bladder tumors

| Lead author (year) | Superficial cancer | G3T1 (%) |
|---|---|---|
| England (1981)[2] | 332 | 8 |
| Heney (1983)[3] | 249 | 11 |
| Smith (1986)[4] | 299 | 18 |
| Jakse (1987)[5] | 172 | 23 |
| Algaba (1987)[6] | 95 | 13 |
| Malmstrom (1987)[7] | 147 | 20 |
| Pauwels (1988)[8] | 122 | 6 |
| Abel (1988)[9] | 107 | 5 |
| Witjes (1994)[10] | 450 | 12 |
| Otto (1994)[11] | 2715 | 16 |
| Pansadoro (1995)[12] | 593 | 11 |
| Alken (1996)[13] | 631 | 12 |
| Millan-Rodriguez (2000)[14] | 1529 | 22 |

**Table 37.2** Progression for G3T1 bladder cancer according to substaging

| Lead author (year) | Follow-up (months) | Progression rate according to infiltration depth | | |
|---|---|---|---|---|
| | | Above MM (%) | At the level of MM (%) | Below MM (%) |
| Younes (1990)[19] | 56 | 25 | 25 | 89 |
| Angulo (1995)[20] | 60 | 25 | | 59 |
| Holmang (1997)[21] | 84 | 36 | | 58 |
| Kondylis (2000)[22] | 71 | 22 | | 29 |

MM, muscularis mucosae.

To reduce the risk of staging inaccuracies, interpretation of the TUR specimen should be done by an experienced pathologist with extensive experience with urothelial cancer.

## TRANSURETHRAL RESECTION

Adequate TUR is essential for the treatment of superficial bladder cancer. The technique and findings of TUR can affect proper cure and local staging of bladder cancer. When no muscle is found in the specimen after TUR for T1 bladder cancer, up to 49% of cases may be found to have muscle-infiltrating tumors at the time of the second TUR.[24] To avoid the risk of understaging and/or leaving residual tumor behind, several authors have proposed a second TUR for stage T1 bladder cancers, especially when the tumor is high grade. Infiltrating tumor is present in 4% to 28% of patients at second TUR for G3T1 bladder cancer. A literature review of second TUR for T1 bladder cancer is shown in Table 37.3.

Careful and adequate TUR must be performed, particularly when the endoscopic appearance of the tumor suggests a high-grade lesion. A second TUR after 2–6 weeks is strongly recommended for G3T1 cancers, especially when no muscle is present in the specimen: up to half of the patients may have infiltrating tumor (>T1) at second resection.

## TREATMENT

### TRANSURETHRAL RESECTION ALONE

TUR generally is the first diagnostic and therapeutic approach to bladder carcinoma. When treated with transurethral resection only, G3T1 tumors have high recurrence and progression rates. The recurrence rate is 50% to 80%, and progression to muscle invasive disease occurs in 27% to 63% of patients (Table 37.4). Up to 33% of patients with G3T1 bladder tumor treated with TUR alone will die of cancer.[41] Due to such an unacceptably high risk of recurrence and progression, TUR alone is not feasible for the treatment of G3T1 bladder cancer.

**Table 37.3** Second transurethral resection for T1 bladder cancer

| Lead author (year) | No. pts | Tumor grade | Stage at second TUR (%) | | | | |
|---|---|---|---|---|---|---|---|
| | | | T0 | Tis | Ta | T1 | T≥2 |
| Herr (1999)[24] | 58 | Any | 22 | →26← | | 24 | 28 |
| Schwaibold (2000)[25] | 60 | NA | 45 | 8 | 9 | 28 | 10 |
| Brauers (2001)[26] | 42 | 2–3 | 36 | 19 | 17 | 24 | 5 |
| Ojea Calvo (2001)[27] | 32 | Any | 41 | | →53← | | 6 |
| | 9 | 3 | 45 | | | 44 | 11 |
| Rigaud (2002)[28] | 52 | Any | 64 | 4 | 11 | 17 | 4 |
| Schips (2002)[29] | 76 | Any | 67 | | 11 | 14 | 8 |
| | 39 | 3 | 61 | | 10 | 15 | 13 |
| Grimm (2003)[30] | 34 | Any | 47 | | NA | NA | NA |
| | 7 | 3 | 14 | | | | |

NA, not applicable.

**Table 37.4** Recurrence and progression in patients with G3T1 tumor after TUR alone

| Lead author (year) | No. pts | Recurrence (%) | Progression (%) | Follow-up (months) |
|---|---|---|---|---|
| Pocock (1982)[31] | 9 | | 7 | 60 |
| Heney (1983)[3] | 33 | 79 | 48 | 36 |
| Wolf (1983)[32] | 14 | 50 | | 24 |
| RUTT (1985)[33] | 430 | | 31 | 60 |
| Jakse (1987)[5] | 31 | 80 | 33 | 60/106 |
| Algaba (1987)[6] | 12 | 67 | | 26 |
| Malmstrom (1987)[7] | 7 | | 43 | 60 |
| Kaubisch (1991)[34] | 18 | | 50 | 36 |
| Takashi (1991)[35] | 23 | | 35 | 60 |
| Mulders (1994)[36] | 48 | 75 | 27 | 48 |
| Haukaas (1999)[37] | 26 | | 38 | 108 |
| Zungri (1999)[38] | 34 | 50 | 24 | 40 |
| Paez Borda (2001)[39] | 32 | 85 | 46 | 79 |
| Kolodziej (2002)[40] | 52 | 55 | 23 | 23 |

## RADIOTHERAPY

Adjuvant radiotherapy after TUR of G3T1 bladder tumors has been proposed. However, in 1986 a study reported progression rates of 32% to 54% at 36–60 months' follow-up, with 55% disease-free survival at 5 years.[42] These results are disappointing and basically similar to those obtained with TUR alone. Based upon those results, the use of radiotherapy for superficial bladder cancer has been discouraged.[43]

More sophisticated radiotherapy has recently become available, and the outcome of radiation therapy may be improved by newer approaches. In one report, 120 patients with G3T1 or T2 bladder cancer were treated with brachytherapy.[44] Five-year disease-free survival for G3T1 was 100%. In several recent series, the results of radiotherapy for G3T1 bladder cancer seem superior to the results reported earlier (Table 37.5). However, these series are very small and the interpretation is difficult.

Until further data can confirm the encouraging results obtained with new radiotherapeutic modalities, radiation therapy should be reserved for patients with G3T1 bladder cancer refractory to intravesical immunotherapy with bacillus Calmette–Guérin (BCG), who either refuse or are unfit for surgery.[49]

## COMBINATION RADIOCHEMOTHERAPY

Rodel et al[50] treated 89 high-risk T1 cancer patients with radiotherapy alone or radiotherapy plus systemic chemotherapy with cisplatin or carboplatin and 5-fluorouracil. Six weeks after the end of treatment, 86% of the patients were free of disease at restaging TUR. At 5 years, any kind of recurrence and progression rates were 44% and 15%, respectively. At 10 years any kind of recurrence and progression rates were 64% and 40%, respectively. Overall survival was 75% at 5 years and 51% at 10 years. For G3T1 tumors (17 cases) the 5-year progression rate was 15%. Only a few centers have treated high-grade superficial bladder cancer with radiochemotherapy. Due to this limited experience, no definitive evaluation of this approach can be reasonably provided.

**Table 37.5** Progression in G3T1 tumors after radiotherapy

| | No. pts | Progression (%) | Follow-up (months) |
|---|---|---|---|
| *Older series* | | | |
| England (1981)[2] | 28 | 39 | 36 |
| Malmstrom (1987)[7] | 11 | 54 | 60 |
| Jenkins (1989)[45] | 53 | 32 | 60 |
| *Recent series* | | | |
| Mulders (1994)[36]* | 17 | 18 | 48 |
| Moonen (1994)[46] | 12 | 0 | 40 |
| Holmang (1997)[21]† | 11 | 63 | 84 |
| Bell (1999)[47] | 19 | 11 | 0 |
| Van der Steen (2002)[48] | 14 | 20 | 60 |

* Patients treated with radiotherapy between 1983 and 1988, published in 1994.

† Patients treated with radiotherapy between 1988 and 1989, published in 1997.

## INTRAVESICAL THERAPY

### BACILLUS CALMETTE–GUÉRIN

Bacillus Calmette–Guérin (BCG) immunotherapy is widely used as intravesical therapy for superficial bladder cancer. BCG reduces both recurrence and progression rates, especially in high-risk superficial tumors.[51,52] Several studies have shown that immunotherapy with BCG after TUR is superior to TUR alone for the treatment of G3T1 bladder cancer.

In a prospective study, 86 patients with high-risk superficial bladder cancer were randomized to TUR plus BCG or TUR alone.[53] At 10 years, the progression rate was 38% for patients treated with BCG and 63% for control patients. Cancer-specific survival was 75% versus 55%. Similarly, Patard and al[54] compared the results obtained in 80 patients with TUR alone or TUR plus BCG. At 61–65 months, BCG treatment was superior to TUR alone in terms of cancer-specific survival (90% versus 70%, p=0.03), recurrence rates (50% versus 90%, p<0.01), and progression rates (22% versus 47%, p=0.03).

Many authors have proposed BCG as first line treatment for primary G3T1 bladder cancer. At 22–78 months of follow up, recurrence rates are 20% to 70% and progression rates 0% to 33% (Table 37.6). In most series, the recurrence rate is 25% to 50% and progression rate 12% to 25%.

The optimal dose and schedule of BCG has not yet been established. Similar recurrence and progression rates have been reported for patients with G3T1 bladder cancers treated with full-dose and low-dose BCG regimens (see Table 37.6). In a multicenter Spanish study, Martinez-Pineiro et al[77] randomized 500 patients to either standard dose or reduced dose of BCG. At 79 months, the overall recurrence rates were 28% and 31% for standard and low-dose groups, respectively.

**Table 37.6** Results of BCG treatment for G3T1 tumors

| Lead author (year) | No. pts | Recurrence (%) | Progression (%) | Follow-up (months) |
|---|---|---|---|---|
| *Results of full-dose BCG* | | | | |
| Dal Bo (1990)[55] | 24 | 25 | 25 | 22 |
| Samodai (1991)[56] | 62 | 20 | 0 | 46 |
| Cookson (1992)[57] | 16 | 44 | 19 | 59 |
| Thanos (1994)[58] | 17 | 37 | 12 | 36 |
| Pfister (1995)[59] | 26 | 50 | 27 | 54 |
| Meng (1995)[60] | 49 | | 16 | 60 |
| Baniel (1998)[61] | 78 | 28 | 8 | 56 |
| Klan (1998)[62] | 109 | 39 | 3 | 78 |
| Gohji (1999)[63] | 25 | 40 | 4 | 63 |
| Brake (2000)[64] | 44 | 27 | 16 | 43 |
| Kondylis (2000)[22] | 49 | 65 | 24 | 71 |
| Bogdanovic (2002)[65] | 43 | 28 | 16 | 53 |
| Iori (2002)[66] | 41 | 24 | 2 | 40 |
| Kulkarni (2002)[67] | 69 | 35 | 12 | 45 |
| Patard (2002)[68]* | 50 | 50 | 22 | 61 |
| Kim (2002)[69] | 37 | 43 | 16 | 27 |
| Shahin (2003)[70] | 90 | 70 | 33 | 64 |
| Pansadoro (2003)[71] | 82 | 34 | 15 | 73 |
| Peyromaure (2004)[72] | 57 | 42 | 23 | 53 |
| *Results of low-dose BCG* | | | | |
| Mack (1995)[73] | 21 | 29 | NA | 60 |
| Vicente (1996)[74] | 95 | 40 | 11 | 46 |
| Lebret (1998)[75] | 35 | 24 | 12 | 45 |
| Hurle (1999)[76] | 51 | 25 | 18 | 85 |

\* 37% of patients treated with low dose.

NA, not applicable.

Progression rates for high-grade superficial bladder cancer were similar for both groups: 11% and 13%. Side effects were significantly lower with the reduced dose. However, there was a significantly longer disease free-survival for patients with G3T1 tumors treated with full-dose BCG. For high-risk superficial bladder cancer, time to progression was longer and the risk of death was lower with full-dose than with low-dose BCG. Based upon these data, reduced dose BCG protocols should be avoided in G3T1 bladder cancer and a standard regimen should be used, unless a reduction of toxicity is strictly required.

In another randomized study, Gruenwald et al[78] compared results in a 12-week course of BCG with those of a standard 6-week course in 70 patients with high-risk superficial carcinoma of the bladder. At a mean follow-up of 28 months, the disease-free rate was 70% for the 12-week course compared to 55% for the 6-week course. A 12-week first course of intravesical BCG may be advisable in patients with G3T1 bladder cancer.

Several papers[57,79] have shown that early recurrence of high-grade T1 bladder cancer after BCG treatment is an ominous prognostic factor: in these patients cystectomy should be performed without delay. Herr and Sogani[80] have shown that delayed cystectomy is related to a decreased survival rate.

Dinney et al[81] reported that a deferred cystectomy in patients with T1 cancer progressing to T2 stage was associated with a higher cancer-related death rate.

## MAINTENANCE

In a multicenter study, 550 patients were randomized to maintenance or no maintenance after the first course of intravesical BCG.[49] The maintenance schedule included intravesical and percutaneous BCG each week for 3 weeks at months 3, 6, 12, 18, 24, 30, and 36 after the initial treatment. Median recurrence-free survival was 36 months in the no-maintenance arm and 77 months in the maintenance arm (p<0.0001). After reviewing the literature, Lamm[82] concluded that there was an advantage of BCG over chemotherapy in improving long-term survival only if maintenance was given.

In a meta-analysis of 2410 patients comparing intravesical BCG to mitomycin, BCG was found to be superior to mitomycin in preventing tumor progression only if maintenance protocols were used.[83] In another meta-analysis of 4863 patients, BCG was compared to TUR alone or TUR and intravesical chemotherapy.[84] At 30 months, BCG reduced the progression rate from 13.8% to 9.8% (27%). The improvement was more evident for high-grade tumors.

Intravesical BCG schedules including maintenance therapy should be administered in patients with G3T1 bladder cancer.

The long-term results of BCG treatment for G3T1 bladder cancer have been evaluated. Herr followed 48

patients with G3T1 bladder cancer for 15 years. These patients had been initially randomized to TUR alone or TUR plus intravesical BCG. In this series, 81% of the patients eventually received BCG therapy.[85] Progression and cancer-related death rates were 25/48 (52%) and 15/48 (31%), respectively. Overall survival was 69%, with 24 (50%) patients with an intact bladder. Tumor progression was 35% at 1–5 years, 16% at 5–10 years, and 12% at 10–15 years. Cancer-specific deaths occurred in 25% of the patients in the first 5 years and in 10% after 5–15 years.

Long-term progression rates after BCG treatment have demonstrated that patients treated with BCG for G3T1 bladder cancer must undergo close surveillance for at least 15 years.

## INTRAVESICAL CHEMOTHERAPY

Intravesical immunotherapy with BCG seems superior to intravesical chemotherapy in reducing the recurrence rates of T1 bladder cancer. In 334 patients (303 were T1) with superficial bladder cancer treated intravesically with BCG, epirubicin or adriamycin, the risk of recurrence was significantly higher with intravesical chemotherapy than with these drugs as single agents, though the lowest recurrence rates were obtained with a combination of BCG and epirubicin.[86] In a Spanish report, 191 patients with high-risk superficial bladder cancer were treated with BCG, mitomycin or doxorubicin. At 73 months, multivariate analysis showed that BCG treatment was associated with reduced risk of disease progression.[87]

Similarly, in a Scandinavian study, Malmstrom et al[88] found that BCG, when compared with mitomycin, prolonged recurrence-free survival in high-risk superficial bladder cancer patients, but was not more effective than mitomycin in decreasing progression rates.

In two meta-analyses, BCG with a maintenance schedule was superior to mitomycin and other intravesical chemotherapeutic agents in reducing tumor recurrence and progression rates.[52,84] In yet another meta-analysis of 1901 high-risk patients with superficial bladder cancer, BCG was more effective than mitomycin in reducing recurrence rates; however, there was no advantage in terms of tumor progression.[83]

Although intravesical chemotherapy for superficial bladder cancer has not clearly demonstrated benefits in terms of progression and cancer-specific deaths, thiotepa, mitomycin, doxorubicin, and epirubicin all seem equally effective in reducing superficial bladder cancer recurrence.[89]

Several authors have reported a clinical advantage in decreasing recurrence rates with a single dose of preoperative cytotoxic intravesical chemotherapy, 30–60 minutes after completion of TUR for superficial bladder cancer.[90] However, in a study of 168 patients, with mainly G2–3T1 bladder cancers, a single dose of postoperative intravesical epirubicin did not show any advantage for patents with high-grade tumors.[91] Therefore, the role of a single dose of intravesical chemotherapy immediately following transurethral resection of bladder tumor has not been established for G3T1 cancers. Results of long-term follow-up of patients undergoing TUR and adjuvant intravesical chemotherapy for G3T1 bladder cancer are shown in Table 37.7.

Comparison between intravesical chemotherapy and BCG for the treatment of G3T1 bladder cancer is not possible. Randomized trials are not available for high-grade superficial bladder cancer. Intravesical chemotherapy may be feasible for the treatment of G3T1 bladder cancer, but it is not the primary treatment of choice.

## ALTERNATIVE AND SECOND LINE TREATMENTS

Soloway et al[89] treated 61 patients with G3T1 bladder cancer with BCG. While six patients experienced progression to muscle invasive disease, 43 patients had recurrent superficial bladder cancer (38 high-grade T1) and were retreated with TUR and a second course of BCG. At 46 months' follow-up, only nine (21%) required cystectomy (five for local progression, four for persistent high-grade T1/carcinoma in situ).

In a similar study, 34 patients with high-risk superficial bladder cancer with recurrence at 28 months (range 7–50 months) were treated with TUR and additional BCG. At 36 months, recurrence and progression (requiring cystectomy) rates were 41% and 6%, respectively.[94] In carefully selected and strictly followed patients there may be a therapeutic role for a second course of BCG treatment.

Interferon (IFN) has been used in combination with BCG. In one study, 39 patients with G3T1 bladder cancer not responding to BCG were treated with low dose BCG plus IFN$\alpha$2b.[95] At 24 months, the recurrence rate was 47%, and cystectomy was required in 10 patients (26%). Similarly, Luciani et al[96] treated 24 patients with Tis and/or T1 transitional cell carcinoma, recurrent after BCG therapy, with intravesical BCG plus IFN$\alpha$2b or valrubicin. At 28.5 months, no cancer-related deaths occurred. Fourteen patients had preserved their bladders and nine patients required cystectomy.

Combination or alternative intravesical treatments may be considered a viable, though investigational, option after BCG failure in patients at high risk for surgery.

## CYSTECTOMY

Up to 81% of patients with high-grade superficial bladder cancer refractory to BCG may progress to muscle invasion,[97] and radical cystectomy is the standard approach for patients with muscle-infiltrating bladder cancer. It is also considered to be a suitable option for the treatment of high-grade superficial bladder cancer.[98] The procedure has better acceptance than in the past due to the advent of orthotopic bladder substitutions.

Herr and Sogani[80] treated 90 patients with high-risk superficial bladder cancer with cystectomy. At 96 months, survival was 49%. Siref and Zincke treated another 32 patients with T1 (72% were high grade tumors) with cystectomy. Systemic progression occurred in 17 (53%) at 5 or more years of follow-up.[99]

Good results are obtained with cystectomy for high-grade superficial bladder cancer, with 5- and 10-year survivals of 67% to 95% and 51% to 62%, respectively (Table 37.8).

Since long-term survival after cystectomy for G3T1 bladder cancer is similar to that obtained with intravesical BCG, open surgery as first line treatment may lead to a large number of unnecessary cystectomies. However, up to 33% of patients treated with BCG may experience disease progression. Careful follow-up is needed for identification of early (3–6 months) recurrences of high-grade tumors, or progression after BCG therapy, either of which requires immediate cystectomy.

## PROGNOSTIC FACTORS

Given that a significant number of G3T1 tumors progress and require aggressive treatment, it is useful to identify patients that will not respond to intravesical immunotherapy. Clinical characteristics of the tumor and biologic markers have been studied for predictive factors.

**Table 37.7** Results of intravesical chemotherapy for G3T1 bladder cancer

| Lead author (year) | Agent | No. pts | Recurrence (%) | Progression (%) | Follow-up (months) |
|---|---|---|---|---|---|
| Bono (1994)[92] | Doxorubicin | 123 | 56 | 23 | 73 |
| Serretta (2004)[93] | Doxorubicin ± epirubicin | 137 | 51 | 9 | 24–240 |

**Table 37.8** Results for radical cystectomy in G3T1 tumors

| Lead author (year) | No. pts | 5-year survival (%) | 10-year survival (%) |
|---|---|---|---|
| Siref (1988)[99] | 32 | 67 | 57 |
| Malkowicz (1993)[100]* | 14 | 80 | |
| Amling (1994)[101]† | 91 | 76 | 62 |
| Gschwend (1998)[102] | 45 | 92 | |
| Stein (2001)[103]‡ | 208 | 74 | 51 |
| Madersbacher (2003)[104] | 77 | 76 | 58 |

* G3 in 58, G2 in 17.
† Mainly G3.
‡ 72% high grade.

## CLINICAL CHARACTERISTICS

Eighty patients with G3T1 bladder cancer were treated with intravesical BCG or chemotherapy by Solsona et al.[87] The lack of complete response to treatment at the 3-month cystoscopy (no visible tumor, negative random biopsies) was a strong predictor of invasive progression in 29 nonresponding patients. Palou et al[105] also treated 159 patients with G3T1 bladder cancer with BCG. Progression rates were 42%, 29%, and 4% according to relapse at 3 months, at 6 months, or later recurrence, respectively. In yet another report of 102 patients with high-risk superficial bladder cancer treated with BCG,[106] the risk of progression was significantly higher in patients with superficial recurrence within 6 months.

Further papers[57,79] have shown that early recurrence of high-grade T1 bladder cancer after BCG treatment is a bad prognostic factor: in these patients cystectomy should not be deferred. Sanchez-Ortiz et al[107] found a higher progression rate in patients undergoing cystectomy with a delay of more than 12 weeks.

We have reported previously on 82 patients with G3T1 bladder cancer treated with BCG.[1] At a median follow-up of 73 months, the number of lesions, history of prior superficial bladder cancer, and associated carcinoma in situ (CIS) did not significantly correlate with recurrence or progression.

In a multivariate analysis of 51 patients with G3T1 bladder tumor treated with low dose BCG, Hurle et al[76] found that only tumor size (p=0.027) and coexisting CIS (p=0.024) significantly influenced results; however, in another study in 44 patients with G3T1 cancer, Brake et al[64] found no correlation between BCG failure and CIS.

Lebret at al[108] reported that tumor size, but not the number of lesions, predicted recurrence and progression in 35 patients with G3T1 bladder cancer treated with BCG. Saint et al[106] found that tumor size and multifocality were not significantly related to BCG outcome in 102 patients with high-risk superficial bladder cancer, while previous superficial tumors and the association with CIS had a significant impact on treatment outcome.

## BIOLOGIC MARKERS

The p53 gene regulates the cell cycle and p53 mutations are found in many different tumors, including transitional cell carcinoma. The role of p53 in predicting results of BCG treatment for high-risk superficial bladder cancer has been particularly controversial. In 1998, Sarosdy[109] reviewed the literature on the subject, and established that p53 tumor suppressor gene expression did not seem to correlate with the outcome of intravesical BCG in high-grade superficial bladder cancer.

P53 overexpression by immunohistochemistry has been reported to be an independent predictive factor of recurrence for high-risk superficial bladder cancer.[106] However, since p53 immunostaining is higher in grade 3 and T1 bladder cancers, it is not clear whether the prognostic significance, if found, could be due just to the strict association with G3T1 bladder carcinoma.[110]

Llopis et al[111] studied 207 patients with T1 bladder cancer. Nearly half the patients underwent intravesical therapy with chemotherapeutic agents or BCG. In 59 patients treated with BCG, 5-year progression was 45%; p53 was significantly correlated with progression (p=0.0031).

Shariat et al[112] found that p53 did not significantly affect disease progression or survival in 43 patients with T1 bladder cancer. They found that there was a trend toward a worse prognosis for association with CIS, though it did not reach statistical value.

Grossman et al[113] evaluated 45 patients with pT1 bladder cancer retrospectively with regard to the expression of two tumor suppressor genes, p53 and RB. Patients with normal expression of both proteins (i.e. p53 negative and RB heterogeneously positive) had an excellent outcome, with no patient showing disease progression, whereas patients with abnormal expression of either or both proteins had a significant increase in progression (p=0.04 and p=0.005, respectively).

In a paper from Memorial Sloan-Kettering,[114] 19 patients with T1 bladder cancer treated with intravesical BCG were studied. p53 nuclear overexpression was related to increased progression rate before BCG therapy and in those patients with BCG refractory tumors.

Only a few investigators have studied the prognostic value of p53 in a selected population with high-grade T1 bladder cancers treated with intravesical BCG. They have not been able to confirm a correlation with treatment outcome.

Conflicting data have been reported on the prognostic value of clinical and biologic features of G3T1 bladder cancer. Although p53 may have some role in predicting the risk of progression in patients treated with TUR alone or with intravesical chemotherapy, its value in the prognosis of high-grade superficial bladder cancers treated with BCG still needs to be confirmed in large series. The association with CIS might be related to a more aggressive disease. New markers are still investigational. Future studies might clarify if additional predictive prognostic factors can help with identifying those tumors which are more likely to progress with conservative treatment. To date, no evidence of predictive value has been clearly shown for any parameter, except for early (within 3–6 months) tumor recurrence after BCG therapy, which requires aggressive therapy with cystectomy.

## CONCLUSION

G3T1 bladder cancer is an aggressive disease. When TUR alone is performed, recurrence and progression rates are extremely high. Intravesical therapy with full-dose BCG and maintenance protocols is the best conservative approach to primary G3T1 bladder cancers and should be considered as first line treatment. However, recurrence and progression have been described even up to 15–20 years after intravesical immunotherapy for G3T1 bladder cancer. These patients require strict surveillance for life. After BCG failure, second line treatments (second BCG course, intravesical chemotherapy, low-dose BCG plus IFNα2b) may be considered in carefully selected patients, or in patients that cannot or do not want to undergo surgery. Except for early recurrence after BCG, no definite prognostic factors are available to identify those patients that will experience disease progression. Patients with recurrence within 6 months should undergo cystectomy.

## REFERENCES

1. Pansadoro V, Emiliozzi P, dePaula F, Scarpone P, Pansadoro A, Sternberg CN. Long term follow-up of G3T1 transitional cell carcinoma of the bladder treated with intravesical Bacille Calmette–Guérin: 18-year experience. Urology 2002;59:227–231.
2. England HR, Paris AMI, Blandy JP. The correlation of T1 bladder tumor history with prognosis and follow-up requirements. Br J Urol 1981;53:593–597.
3. Heney NM, Ahmed S, Flannagan MJ, et al for National Bladder Cancer Collaborative Group A. Superficial bladder cancer: progression and recurrence. J Urol 1983;130:1083–1086.
4. Smith G, Elton RA, Chisholm GD, Newsam JE, Hargreave TB. Superficial bladder cancer: intravesical chemotherapy and tumor progression to muscle invasion or metastases. Br J Urol 1986;58:659–663.
5. Jakse G, Loidl W, Seeber G, Hofstadter F. Stage T1, grade 3 transitional cell carcinoma of the bladder: an unfavourable tumor? J Urol 1987;137:39–43.
6. Algaba F. Origin of high grade superficial bladder cancer. Eur Urol 1987;13:153–155.
7. Malmstrom PU, Busch C, Norlen BJ. Recurrence, progression and survival in bladder cancer. Scand J Urol Nephrol 1987;21:185–195.
8. Pauwels RPE, Schapers RFM, Smeets AWGB. Grading in superficial bladder cancer. (1) Morphological criteria. Br J Urol 1988;61:129–134.
9. Abel PD, Hall RR, Williams G. Should pT1 transitional cell cancers of the bladder be classified as superficial? Br J Urol 1988;62:235–239.
10. Witjes JA, Kiemeney LA, Schaafsma HE, Debruyne FM. The influence of review pathology on study outcome of a randomized multicentre superficial bladder cancer trial. Members of the Dutch South East Cooperative Urological Group. Br J Urol 1994;73(2):172–176.
11. Otto T, Rubben H. Management of T1 G3 bladder carcinomas. EAU Update Series 1994;2 (16):122–127.
12. Pansadoro V, Emiliozzi P, Defidio L, et al. Bacillus Calmette–Guérin in the treatment of stage T1 grade 3 transitional cell carcinoma of the bladder: long term results. J Urol 1995;154:2054–2058.
13. Alken P. Personal communication. In Sarosdy MF (ed): Management of High Grade Superficial Bladder Cancer. Role of BCG. AUA Update Ser 1998;XVII(Lesson 12):89–95.
14. Millan-Rodriguez F, Chechile-Toniolo G, Salvador-Bayarri J, Palou J, Algaba F, Vicente-Rodriguez J. Primary superficial bladder cancer risk groups according to progression, mortality and recurrence. J Urol 2000;164(3 Pt 1):680–684.
15. Dutta SC, Smith JA Jr, Shappell SB, Coffey CS, Chang SS, Cookson MS. Clinical understaging of high risk nonmuscle invasive urothelial carcinoma treated with radical cystectomy. J Urol 2001;166(2):490–493.
16. Lee SE, Jeong IG, Ku JH, Kwak C, Lee E, Jeong JS. Impact of transurethral resection of bladder tumor: analysis of cystectomy specimens to evaluate for residual tumor. Urology 2004;63(5):873–877.
17. Hasui Y, Osada Y, Kitada S, Nishi S. Significance of invasion to the muscularis mucosae on the progression of superficial bladder cancer. Urology 1994;43(6):782–786.
18. Cheng L, Weaver AL, Neumann RM, Scherer BG, Bostwick DG. Substaging of T1 bladder carcinoma based on the depth of invasion as measured by micrometer: a new proposal. Cancer 1999;86(6):1035–1043.
19. Younes M, Sussman J, True LD. The usefulness of the level of the muscularis mucosae in the staging of invasive transitional cell carcinoma of the urinary bladder. Cancer 1990;66(3):543–548.
20. Angulo JC, Lopez JI, Grignon DJ, Sanchez-Chapado M. Muscularis mucosa differentiates two populations with different prognosis in stage T1 bladder cancer. Urology 1995;45(1):47–53.
21. Holmang S, Hedelin H, Anderstrom C, Holmberg E, Johansson SL. The importance of the depth of invasion in stage T1 bladder carcinoma: a prospective cohort study. J Urol 1997;157(3):800–803.
22. Kondylis FI, Demirci S, Ladaga L, Kolm P, Schellhammer PF. Outcomes after intravesical bacillus Calmette–Guérin are not affected by substaging of high grade T1 transitional cell carcinoma. J Urol 2000;163(4):1120–1123.
23. Van Der Meijden A, Sylvester R, Collette L, Bono A, Ten Kate F. The role and impact of pathology review on stage and grade assessment of stages Ta and T1 bladder tumors: a combined analysis of 5 European Organisation for Research and Treatment of Cancer Trials. J Urol 2000;164(5):1533–1537.
24. Herr HW. The value of a second transurethral resection in evaluating patients with bladder tumors. J Urol 1999;162(1):74–76.
25. Schwaibold H, Treiber U, Kuber H, Leyh H, Hartung R. Significance of second transurethral resection for T1 bladder cancer. Eur Urol 2000;37(Suppl 2): abstract 441:111.
26. Brauers A, Buettner R, Jakse G. Second resection and prognosis of primary high risk superficial bladder cancer: is cystectomy often too early? J Urol 2001;165(3):808–810.
27. Ojea Calvo A, Nunez Lopez A, Alonso Rodrigo A, et al. Value of a second transurethral resection in the assessment and treatment of patients with bladder tumor. Actas Urol Esp 2001;25(3):182–186.
28. Rigaud J, Karam G, Braud G, Glemain P, Buzelin JM, Bouchot O. T1 bladder tumors: value of a second endoscopic resection. Prog Urol 2002;12(1):27–30.
29. Schips L, Augustin H, Zigeuner RE, et al. Is repeated transurethral resection justified in patients with newly diagnosed superficial bladder cancer? Urology 2002;59(2):220–223.
30. Grimm MO, Steinhoff C, Simon X, Spiegelhalder P, Ackermann R, Vogeli TA. Effect of routine repeat transurethral resection for superficial bladder cancer: a long-term observational study. J Urol 2003;170(2 Pt 1):433–437.

31. Pocock RD, Ponder BA, O'Sullivan JP, Ibrahim SK, Easton DF, Shearer RJ. Prognostic factors in non-infiltrating carcinoma of the bladder: a preliminary report. Br J Urol 1982;54(6):711–715.

32. Wolf H, Hojgaard K. Prognostic factors in local surgical treatment of invasive bladder cancer with special reference to the presence of urothelial dysplasia. Cancer 1983;51(9):1710–1715.

33. RUTT (Registry for Urinary Tract Tumors: Harnwegstumorregister). Jahresbericht Verh Dtsch Ges Urol 1985;37:665–669.

34. Kaubisch S, Lum BL, Reese J, Freiha F, Torti FM. Stage T1 bladder cancer: grade is the primary determinant for risk of muscle invasion. J Urol 1991;146:28–31.

35. Takashi M, Sakata T, Murase T, Hamajima N, Miyake K. Grade 3 bladder cancer with lamina propria invasion (pT1): characteristics of tumor and clinical course. Nagoya J Med Sci 1991;53(1–4):1–8.

36. Mulders PFA, Hoekstra WJ, Heybroek RPM, et al and Members of the Dutch South Eastern Bladder Cancer Group. Prognosis and treatment of T1G3 bladder tumors. A prognostic factor analysis of 121 patients. Eur J Cancer 1994;30A(7):914–917.

37. Haukaas S, Daehlin L, Maartmann-Moe H, Ulvik NM. The long-term outcome in patients with superficial transitional cell carcinoma of the bladder: a single-institutional experience. BJU Int 1999;83(9):957–963.

38. Zungri E, Martinez L, Da Silva EA, Pesqueira D, de la Fuente Buceta A, Pereiro B .T1 GIII bladder cancer. Management with transurethral resection only. Eur Urol 1999;36(5):380–384.

39. Paez Borda A, Lujan Galan M, Gomez de Vicente JM, Moreno Santurino A, Abate F, Berenguer Sanchez A. Preliminary results of the treatment of high grade (T1G3) superficial tumors of the bladder with transurethral resection. Actas Urol Esp 2001;25(3):187–192.

40. Kolodziej A, Dembowski J, Zdrojowy R, Wozniak P, Lorenz J. Treatment of high-risk superficial bladder cancer with maintenance bacille Calmette–Guérin therapy: preliminary results. BJU Int 2002;89(6):620–622.

41. Donat SM. Evaluation and follow-up strategies for superficial bladder cancer. Urol Clin North Am 2003;30(4):765–776.

42. Quilty PM, Duncan W. Treatment of superficial (T1) tumours of the bladder by radical radiotherapy. Br J Urol 1986;58:147–152.

43. Sawczuk IS, Olsson CA, deVere White R. The limited usefulness of external beam radiotherapy in the control of superficial bladder cancer. Br J Urol 1988;61(4):330–332.

44. Gonzalez Gonzalez D, Haitze van der Veen J, Ypma AF, Blank LE, Hoestra CJ, Veen RE. Brachytherapy for urinary bladder cancer. Arch Esp Urol 1999;52(6):655–661.

45. Jenkins BJ, Nauth-Misir RR, Martin JE, Fowler CG, Hope-Stone HF, Blandy JP. The fate of G3pT1 bladder cancer. Br J Urol 1989;64(6):608–610.

46. Moonen LM, Horenblas S, van der Voet JC, Nuyten MJ, Bartelink H. Bladder conservation in selected T1G3 and muscle-invasive T2–T3a bladder carcinoma using combination therapy of surgery and iridium-192 implantation. Br J Urol 1994;74(3):322–327.

47. Bell CR, Lydon A, Kernick V, Hong A, Penn C, Pocock RD, Stott MA. Contemporary results of radical radiotherapy for bladder transitional cell carcinoma in a district general hospital with cancer-centre status. BJU Int 1999;83(6):613–618.

48. Van der Steen-Banasik EM, Visser AG, Reinders JG, Heijbroek RP, Idema JG, Janssen TG, Leer JW. Saving bladders with brachytherapy: implantation technique and results. Int J Radiat Oncol Biol Phys 2002;53(3):622–629.

49. Zietman AL, Shipley WU, Heney NM, Althausen AF. The case for radiotherapy with or without chemotherapy in high-risk superficial and muscle-invading bladder cancer. Semin Urol Oncol 1997;15(3):161–168.

50. Rodel C, Dunst J, Grabenbauer GG, Kuhn R, Papadopoulos T, Schrott KM, Sauer R. Radiotherapy is an effective treatment for high-risk T1-bladder cancer. Strahlenther Onkol 2001;177(2):82–88.

51. Lamm DL, Blumenstein BA, Crissman JD, et al. Maintenance bacillus Calmette–Guérin immunotherapy for recurrent TA, T1 and carcinoma in situ transitional cell carcinoma of the bladder: a randomized Southwest Oncology Group Study. J Urol 2000;163(4):1124–1129.

52. Sylvester RJ, van der Meijden AP, Lamm DL. Intravesical bacillus Calmette–Guérin reduces the risk of progression in patients with superficial bladder cancer: a meta-analysis of the published results of randomized clinical trials. J Urol 2002;168(5):1964–1970.

53. Herr HW, Schwalb DM, Zhang ZF, et al. Intravesical bacillus Calmette–Guérin therapy prevents tumor progression and death from superficial bladder cancer: ten-year follow-up of a prospective randomized trial. J Clin Oncol 1995;113:1404–1408.

54. Patard J, Moudouni S, Saint F, et al and the Members of the Groupe Necker. Tumor progression and survival in patients with T1G3 bladder tumors: multicentric retrospective study comparing 94 patients treated during 17 years. Urology 2001;58(4):551–556.

55. Dal Bo V, Belmonte P, Veronesi A, et al. Intravesical BCG instillations in patients with carcinoma in situ and pT1G3 transitional cell carcinoma of the bladder. Eur Urol 1990;18(1):43–46.

56. Samodai L, Kiss L, Kolozsy Z, Mohacsi L. The efficacy of intravesical BCG in the treatment of patients with high risk superficial bladder cancer. Int Urol Nephrol 1991;23(6):559–567.

57. Cookson MS, Sarosdy MF. Management of stage T1 superficial bladder cancer with intravesical Bacillus Calmette–Guérin therapy. J Urol 1992;148:797–801.

58. Thanos A, Karassantes T, Davillas E, Sotiriou V, Davillas N. Bacillus Calmette–Guérin therapy for high-risk superficial bladder cancer. Scand J Urol Nephrol 1994;28(4):365–368.

59. Pfister C, Lande P, Herve JM, Barre P, Barbagelatta M, Camey M, Botto H. T1 G3 bladder tumors: the respective role of BCG and cystectomy. Prog Urol 1995;5:231–237.

60. Meng MV, Sanda MG. Comparison of intravesical BCG to radical cystectomy for high grade, T1 transitional cell carcinoma using Markov decision tree analysis. J Urol 1995;153(Suppl):466.

61. Baniel J, Grauss D, Engelstein D, Sella A. Intravesical bacillus Calmette–Guérin treatment for stage T1 grade 3 transitional cell carcinoma of the bladder. Urology 1998;52(5):785–789.

62. Klan R, Steiner U, Sauter T, et al. Zystektomie beim schlecht differenzierten T1-harnblasenkarzinom—oft zu früh? Akt Urol 1998;29:53–58.

63. Gohji K, Nomi M, Okamoto M, et al. Conservative therapy for stage T1b, grade 3 transitional cell carcinoma of the bladder. Urology 1999;53(2):308–313.

64. Brake M, Loertzer H, Horsch R, Keller K. Recurrence and progression of stage T1, grade 3 transitional cell carcinoma of the bladder following intravesical immunotherapy with Bacillus Calmette–Guérin. J Urol 2000;163:1697–1701.

65. Bogdanovic J, Marusic G, Djozic J, Sekulic V, Budakov P, Dejanovic N, Stojkov J. The management of T1G3 bladder cancer. Urol Int 2002;69(4):263–265.

66. Iori F, Di Seri M, De Nunzio C, Leonardo C, Franco G, Spalletta B, Laurenti C. Long-term maintenance bacille Calmette–Guérin therapy in high-grade superficial bladder cancer. Urology 2002;59(3):414–418.

67. Kulkarni JN, Gupta R. Recurrence and progression in stage T1G3 bladder tumour with intravesical bacille Calmette–Guérin (Danish 1331 strain). BJU Int 2002;90(6):554–557.

68. Patard JJ, Rodriguez A, Leray E, Rioux-Leclercq N, Guille F, Lobel B. Intravesical Bacillus Calmette–Guérin treatment improves patient survival in T1G3 bladder tumours. Eur Urol 2002;41(6):635–641.

69. Kim SI, Kwon SM, Kim YS, Hong SJ. Association of cyclooxygenase-2 expression with prognosis of stage T1 grade 3 bladder cancer. Urology 2002;60(5):816–821.

70. Shahin O, Thalmann GN, Rentsch C, Mazzucchelli L, Studer UE. A retrospective analysis of 153 patients treated with or without intravesical bacillus Calmette–Guérin for primary stage T1 grade 3 bladder cancer: recurrence, progression and survival. J Urol 2003;169(1):96–100.

71. Pansadoro V, Emiliozzi P, dePaula F, et al. High grade superficial (G3T1) transitional cell carcinoma of the bladder treated with intravesical Bacillus Calmette–Guérin (BCG). J Exp Clin Cancer Res 2003;22(Suppl 4):223–227.

72. Peyromaure M, Zerbib M. T1G3 transitional cell carcinoma of the bladder: recurrence, progression and survival. BJU Int 2004;93(1):60–63.

73. Mack D, Frick J. Five-year results of a phase II study with low-dose bacille Calmette–Guérin therapy in high-risk superficial bladder cancer. Urology 1995;45:958–961.

74. Vicente J, Laguna MP, Palou J. The value of conservative treatment in G3T1 bladder tumours. Eur Urol Today 1996;6:14–18.

75. Lebret T, Becette V, Barbagelatta M, et al. Correlation between p53 overexpression and response to bacillus Calmette–Guérin therapy in a high risk select population of patients with T1G3 bladder cancer. J Urol 1998;159(3):788–791.

76. Hurle R, Losa A, Ranieri A, Manzetti A, Lembo A. Intravesical bacillus Calmette–Guérin in stage T1, grade 3 bladder cancer therapy: a 7-year follow-up. Urology 1999;54(2):258–263.

77. Martinez-Pineiro JA, Flores N, Isorna S, et al for CUETO (Club Urologico Espanol de Tratamiento Oncologico). Long-term follow-up of a randomized prospective trial comparing a standard 81 mg dose of intravesical bacille Calmette–Guérin with a reduced dose of 27 mg in superficial bladder cancer. BJU Int 2002;89(7):671–680.

78. Gruenwald IE, Stein A, Rashcovitsky R, Shifroni G, Lurie A. A 12-versus 6-week course of bacillus Calmette–Guérin prophylaxis for the treatment of high risk superficial bladder cancer. J Urol 1997;157:487–491.

79. Herr HW, Klein EA, Rogatko A. Local BCG failures in superficial bladder cancer. A multivariate analysis of risk factors influencing survival. Eur Urol 1991;19(2):97–100.

80. Herr HW, Sogani PC. Does early cystectomy improve the survival of patients with high risk superficial bladder tumors? J Urol 2001;166(4):1296–1299.

81. Dinney CPN, Babkowski RC, Antelo M, et al. Relationship among cystectomy, microvessel density and prognosis in stage T1 transitional cell carcinoma of the bladder. J Urol 1998;160:1285–1290.

82. Lamm DL. Preventing progression and improving survival with BCG maintenance. Eur Urol 2000;37(Suppl 1):9–15.

83. Bohle A, Bock PR. Intravesical bacille Calmette–Guérin versus mitomycin C in superficial bladder cancer: formal meta-analysis of comparative studies on tumor progression. Urology 2004;63(4):682–686.

84. Shelley MD, Wilt TJ, Court J, Coles B, Kynaston H, Mason MD. Intravesical bacillus Calmette–Guérin is superior to mitomycin C in reducing tumour recurrence in high-risk superficial bladder cancer: a meta-analysis of randomized trials. BJU Int 2004;93(4):485–490.

85. Herr HW. Tumour progression and survival in patients with T1G3 bladder tumours: 15-year outcome. Br J Urol 1997;80(5):762–765.

86. Ali-el-Dein B, Sarhan O, Hinev A, Ibrahiem el-HI, Nabeeh A, Ghoneim MA. Superficial bladder tumours: analysis of prognostic factors and construction of a predictive index. BJU Int 2003;92(4):393–399.

87. Solsona E, Iborra I, Dumont R, Rubio-Briones J, Casanova J, Almenar S. The 3-month clinical response to intravesical therapy as a predictive factor for progression in patients with high risk superficial bladder cancer. J Urol 2000;164(3 Pt 1):685–689.

88. Malmstrom PU, Wijkstrom H, Lundholm C, Wester K, Busch C, Norlen BJ.
5-year followup of a randomized prospective study comparing mitomycin C and bacillus Calmette–Guérin in patients with superficial bladder carcinoma. Swedish–Norwegian Bladder Cancer Study Group. J Urol 1999;161(4):1124–1127.

89. Soloway MS, Sofer M, Vaidya A. Contemporary management of stage T1 transitional cell carcinoma of the bladder. J Urol 2002;167(4):1573–1583.

90. O'Donnell MA. New therapeutic strategies for non-muscle-invasive (superficial) bladder cancer. AUA Update Ser 2002;XXII(Lesson 2):9–15.

91. Ali-el-Dein B, Nabeeh A, el-Baz M, Shamaa S, Ashamallah A. Single-dose versus multiple instillations of epirubicin as prophylaxis for recurrence after transurethral resection of pTa and pT1 transitional-cell bladder tumours: a prospective, randomized controlled study. Br J Urol 1997;79(5):731–735.

92. Bono AV, Lovisolo JA, Saredi G. Transurethral resection and sequential chemo-immunoprophylaxis in primary T1G3 bladder cancer. Eur Urol 2000;37(4):478–483.

93. Serretta V, Pavone C, Ingargiola GB, Daricello G, Allegro R, Pavone-Macaluso M. TUR and adjuvant intravesical chemotherapy in T1G3 bladder tumors: recurrence, progression and survival in 137 selected patients followed up to 20 years. Eur Urol 2004;45(6):730–736.

94. Bassi P, Piazza N, Abatangelo G, et al. BCG immunotherapy of high-risk superficial bladder cancer. In Böhle A, Jocham D (eds): Optimal Therapy for Patients with High-Risk Superficial Bladder Cancer—Controversy and Consensus. Proceedings of the First Lübeck Symposium on Bladder Cancer. Basel: Karger, 1997.

95. O'Donnell MA, Krohn J, DeWolf WC. Salvage intravesical therapy with interferon-alpha 2b plus low dose bacillus Calmette–Guérin is effective in patients with superficial bladder cancer in whom bacillus Calmette–Guérin alone previously failed. J Urol 2001;166(4):1300–1304.

96. Luciani LG, Neulander E, Murphy WM, Wajsman Z. Risk of continued intravesical therapy and delayed cystectomy in BCG-refractory superficial bladder cancer: an investigational approach. Urology 2001;58(3):376–379.

97. Marth D, Studer UE, Ackermann D, Zingg EJ. Primäre Therapieversager nach intravesikalem BCG wegen Carcinoma in situ erlauben kein expektives Verhalten. Urologe [A] 1991;(Suppl. 30):A71.

98. Esrig D, Freeman JA, Stein JP, Skinner DG. Early cystectomy for clinical stage T1 transitional cell carcinoma of the bladder. Semin Urol Oncol 1997;15(3):154–160.

99. Siref LE, Zincke H. Radical cystectomy for historical and pathologic T1, N0, M0 (stage A) transitional cell cancer. Need for adjuvant systemic chemotherapy? Urology 1988;31(4):309–311.

100. Malkowicz SB, Nichols P, Lieskovsky G, Boyd SD, Huffman J, Skinner DG. The role of radical cystectomy in the management of high grade superficial bladder cancer. J Urol 1993;144:641–645.

101. Amling CL, Thrasher JB, Frazier HA, Dodge RK, Robertson JE, Paulson DF. Radical cystectomy for stages Ta, Tis and T1 transitional cell carcinoma of the bladder. J Urol 1994;151:31–36.

102. Gschwend JE, Vieweg J, Fair WR. Contemporary results of radical cystectomy for primary bladder cancer. AUA Update Ser 1998;XVIII(Lesson 13):98–103.

103. Stein JP, Lieskovsky G, Cote R, et al. Radical cystectomy in the treatment of invasive bladder cancer: long-term results in 1,054 patients. J Clin Oncol 2001;19(3):666–675.

104. Madersbacher S, Hochreiter W, Burkhard F, Thalmann GN, Danuser H, Markwalder R, Studer UE. Radical cystectomy for bladder cancer today—a homogeneous series without neoadjuvant therapy. J Clin Oncol 2003;21(4):690–696.

105. Palou J, Rosales A, Millan F, Zaragoza R, Salvador J, Vicente J. Clinical prognostic factors of recurrence and progression in TCC stage T1 G3 treated with BCG. BJU Int 2000;86(Suppl. 3):3–7.

106. Saint F, Le Frere Belda MA, Quintela R, et al. Pretreatment p53 nuclear overexpression as a prognostic marker in superficial bladder cancer treated with Bacillus Calmette–Guérin (BCG). Eur Urol 2004;45(4):475–482.

107. Sanchez-Ortiz RF, Huang WC, Mick R, Van Arsdalen KN, Wein AJ, Malkowicz SB. An interval longer than 12 weeks between the diagnosis of muscle invasion and cystectomy is associated with worse outcome in bladder carcinoma. J Urol 2003;169(1):110–115.

108. Lebret T, Becette V, Herve JM, et al. Prognostic value of MIB-1 antibody labeling index to predict response to Bacillus Calmette–Guérin therapy in a high-risk selected population of patients with stage T1 grade G3 bladder cancer. Eur Urol 2000;37(6):654–659.

109. Sarosdy MF. Management of high grade superficial bladder cancer. Role of BCG. AUA Update Ser 1998;XVII(Lesson 12):90–95.

110. Pfister C, Flaman JM, Dunet F, Grise P, Frebourg T. p53 mutations in bladder tumors inactivate the transactivation of the p21 and Bax genes, and have a predictive value for the clinical outcome after bacillus Calmette–Guérin therapy. J Urol 1999;162(1):69–73.

111. Llopis J, Alcaraz A, Ribal MJ, et al. p53 expression predicts progression and poor survival in T1 bladder tumours. Eur Urol 2000;37(6):644–653.

112. Shariat SF, Weizer AZ, Green A, et al. Prognostic value of P53 nuclear accumulation and histopathologic features in T1 transitional cell carcinoma of the urinary bladder. Urology 2000;56(5):735–740.

113. Grossman HB, Liebert M, Antelo M, Dinney CP, Hu SX, Palmer JL, Benedict WF. p53 and RB expression predict progression in T1 bladder cancer. Clin Cancer Res 1998;4(4):829–834.

114. Lacombe L, Dalbagni G, Zhang ZF, Cordon-Cardo C, Fair WR, Herr HW, Reuter VE. Overexpression of p53 protein in a high-risk population of patients with superficial bladder cancer before and after bacillus Calmette–Guérin therapy: correlation to clinical outcome. J Clin Oncol 1996;14(10):2646–2652.

# What to do when BCG fails

## 38

*Guido Dalbagni*

## INTRODUCTION

Although bacillus Calmette–Guérin (BCG) is a highly effective therapy for bladder cancer, the problem of BCG failure is significant. When the therapy fails, radical cystectomy is the gold standard. Patients are sometimes reluctant, however, to undergo major surgery for a condition that does not pose an immediate threat to their lives. Furthermore, radical cystectomy is not suitable for a subset of patients with severe comorbidities. A number of alternatives have been developed. After considering the definition of BCG failure, we will detail these therapies.

## DEFINITION OF BCG FAILURE

In evaluating salvage therapies for use after BCG failure, comparisons between therapies have been hampered by the lack of standard definitions for BCG failure and BCG-refractory transitional cell carcinoma (TCC). Some series have defined BCG failure after a single induction course of BCG[1,2]; others after two courses.[3] The latter is preferable, since it is known that patients do respond to a second cycle of BCG. Haaff et al reported the overall response in 61 patients treated with one or two courses. The 25 patients in whom the initial induction cycle failed were treated with a second course. Eight of 19 patients (42%) with carcinoma in situ (CIS) responded to the induction course, while 56% became free of tumor after additional BCG, for a cumulative response of 68% after a mean follow-up of 13.5 months. Six of 13 patients (46%) with residual tumors were rendered disease-free after one induction course, and three of seven (43%)

became free of tumor after a second treatment. The overall response was 69% with a mean follow-up of 15.2 months. Nine of 29 patients treated for prophylaxis after complete resection had a recurrence after a mean follow-up of 11.8 months. An additional induction course was given to these patients. Overall, 90% (26/29) were free of recurrence at a mean follow-up of 12.8 months.[4] Okamura et al reported the effect of repeated courses of BCG (Tokyo strain) as a prophylactic agent to prevent recurrences in patients with Ta/T1 cancer. Seventeen of 75 patients (23%) developed recurrences after a single course, and 12 received additional courses after a transurethral resection of bladder tumor (TURBT). The overall success rate was 90.7%.[5]

Bui et al reported the clinical outcome of 11 patients who received a second course after an initial complete response (CR). All patients were followed for a minimum of 5 years, and the median interval to tumor recurrence after the initial treatment was 17 months (range 9–74 months). Nine of the 11 patients achieved a CR and five were free of disease at a median follow-up of 87 months (range 64–110 months).[6] Overall, 42% to 82% of patients who did not respond to an induction course responded to a second cycle.[6–9]

These data suggest that a second course of BCG is warranted. These results also argue against defining BCG as failure to respond to a single induction course.

## TIS AFTER TWO CYCLES PORTENDS A POOR PROGNOSIS

Patients whose disease recurs after a second cycle are less likely to respond to additional BCG,[6] and are at increased risk of progression.[7] Catalona et al found that, among patients in whom two or more courses of BCG failed, the risk of developing muscle-invasive tumors or metastatic disease was 30% and 50%, respectively, while only 20% responded to additional BCG therapy.[7] Sarosdy et al reported a 28% progression and metastasis rate among patients in whom BCG and bropirimine failed and who subsequently underwent nonsurgical treatment.[3]

## PATIENTS WITH PERSISTENT TCC AFTER TWO CYCLES OF BCG DO WORSE THAN PATIENTS WITH RECURRENCE AFTER AN INITIAL RESPONSE

Harland et al reported disease progression among 10% of patients who responded to one or two courses of BCG versus 48% among those that failed to respond, with a median follow-up of 32 months.[10] The long-term outcomes of patients with Tis, treated as part of a randomized study comparing mitomycin C versus two strains of BCG, have been reported by the Dutch South East Cooperative Urological Group.[11] Of the 65% of patients who achieved a CR, 18% had progression of disease while 67% of the nonresponders had progression.[11] The cumulative response rates for the first and second 6-week courses were 56%. Ovesen et al reported a 26% progression rate among complete responders versus 77% among nonresponders with a median follow-up of 46 months.[12]

## THE DISEASE-FREE INTERVAL IS AN IMPORTANT PROGNOSTIC VARIABLE

Bretton et al reported clinical outcomes of 28 patients that received a second course of BCG. Progression occurred in 13 patients (46%), and the median duration of response to course 1 of BCG was shorter for these patients than for those with no progression. Of the 13 patients with progression, 10 (77%) had responded to course 1 for less than 21.6 months compared to only 4 of 15 (27%) without progression.[13] The conclusion of this study was that a second course of BCG was useful in patients who had a *prolonged* response to the initial treatment. Merz et al reported a high progression rate after a second course of BCG among patients whose initial response to induction BCG was followed by a recurrence within 9 months, compared to no recurrences after the second course among patients who developed recurrences after more than 12 months.[14]

These data suggest that patients with an initial CR and a late relapse are the ones most likely to benefit from a repeat course of BCG.

## PATIENTS RELAPSING WITH T1 DISEASE AFTER BCG THERAPY ARE AT HIGH RISK OF PROGRESSION

Herr and colleagues reported a progression rate of 82% among 17 patients who had stage T1 TCC at the 3-month evaluation after BCG therapy. The median time to progression was 8.5 months.[15,16] The aggressive nature of T1 TCC at the 3-month evaluation was confirmed by others.[17,18]

It seems reasonable, based on the current literature, to define BCG-refractory TCC or BCG failure as any situation associated with a high progression rate. This includes:

- persistent Tis after two consecutive BCG courses (nonresponders)
- recurrent Tis within less than 6 months of achieving a complete response after one or two courses of BCG
- recurrent Tis while on maintenance therapy
- relapse with T1 disease.

The methods of reporting the results have been inconsistent. Most studies have included all patients who received one or more courses of BCG.[19-22] Investigators have often combined patients with persistent disease (nonresponders) and patients with recurrent Tis after an initial response,[1,3] and a few studies have combined patients who were nonresponders to BCG and patients that could not complete BCG therapy because of toxicity (BCG intolerant).[3,19] Furthermore, most studies have combined all patients with papillary tumors with and without Tis. Finally, most studies have not indicated the disease-free interval after the last BCG course. These inconsistencies have led to comparisons of outcome in a very heterogeneous population.

## TREATMENT OF BCG-REFRACTORY CIS

Patients whose bladder cancer progresses after failure of intravesical therapy have been shown to fare worse than patients presenting with a de novo muscle-invasive tumor. Van der Heijden et al reported a 37% 3-year cancer-specific survival rate for the progressive group versus 65% in the de novo group.[23]

Radical cystectomy is the gold standard in patients with BCG-refractory TCC. However, those patients reluctant to undergo major surgery are usually willing to explore alternatives. Furthermore, a subset of patients with severe comorbidities are not candidates for cystectomy. Several alternative approaches have been proposed, as follows.

### INTRAVESICAL VALRUBICIN

Valrubicin is an analog of adriamycin (N-trifluoroacetyladriamycin-14-valerate [AD32]), an anthracycline with a mechanism of action different from the parent compound. Valrubicin inhibits nucleoside incorporation into DNA and RNA, leading to chromosomal damage.[24] In a phase I study of 32 patients with nonmuscle-invasive TCC, 13 patients achieved a CR with valrubicin treatment. The drug had only minor systemic side effects, and the serum levels of unmetabolized valrubicin and its two primary metabolites were very low. However, 29 patients (91%) had mild to severe irritative symptoms, which persisted for several days after each instillation.[25]

The efficacy of valrubicin was demonstrated in a phase II study of 90 patients with Tis after failure of multiple courses of intravesical therapy, including at least one course of BCG. Patients received 800 mg valrubicin weekly for 6 weeks. Nineteen patients (21%) had a CR, defined as no evidence of recurrence for at least 6 months from the initiation of therapy; 7 of these 19 had a durable response, with a median follow-up of 30 months. Forty-four patients underwent a radical cystectomy (six of whom had stage pT3 disease at cystectomy), and four patients died of bladder cancer during the 30-month follow-up. Most patients (90%) had mild to moderate local bladder symptoms, with urinary frequency in 66%, urinary urgency in 63%, and dysuria in 60%.[22]

In 1997, valrubicin was approved by the Food and Drug Administration (FDA) for the treatment of BCG-refractory Tis in patients who refuse or are unable to undergo cystectomy.

## PREAVAILABILITY: INTRAVESICAL GEMCITABINE

Gemcitabine (2',2'-difluoro-2'-deoxycytidine; Gemzar) is a novel deoxycytidine analog with a broad spectrum of antitumor activity. It was first approved in the United States for the treatment of pancreatic cancer,[26,27] but has since been found to be effective in many other tumor types. Gemcitabine has a molecular weight of 299.66, and, after intracellular activation, the active metabolite is incorporated into DNA, resulting in inhibition of further DNA synthesis. Gemcitabine may also inhibit ribonucleotide reductase and cytidine deaminase as part of its cytotoxic activity.[17] Gemcitabine is highly effective (overall response rates ranging from 22.5% to 28%) and well tolerated as both first- and second-line, single-agent therapy for the treatment of metastatic TCC.[28–30] Studies have reported a low incidence of systemic side effects. A randomized, multicenter, phase III study demonstrated that patients with unresectable or metastatic disease treated with gemcitabine plus cisplatin (GC) had survival rates similar to those of patients treated with MVAC (methotrexate, vinblastine, doxorubicin [adriamycin], and cisplatin), and GC had a better safety profile and tolerability.[31] On the basis of its excellent clinical activity, patient tolerability, and chemical characteristics, gemcitabine is a logical candidate for intravesical therapy.

Dalbagni et al reported a phase I study of intravesical gemcitabine twice a week for 3 weeks, followed by a second cycle after a week of rest, in a heavily pretreated population with BCG-refractory TCC. This study demonstrated that intravesical gemcitabine was well tolerated with minimal bladder irritation and acceptable myelosuppression. Serum levels of gemcitabine were undetectable at concentrations of 5, 10, and 15 mg/ml. However, serum gemcitabine was detected at a concentration of 20 mg/ml. Complete response as defined by a negative post-treatment cystoscopy, including a biopsy of the urothelium and negative cytology, was achieved in 7 of 18 patients (39%).[19] This was followed by a phase II study of patients with BCG-refractory TCC to determine the efficacy of gemcitabine as an intravesical agent; 28 patients completed therapy, and 16 achieved a complete response.[32]

Laufer et al reported a phase I study of weekly intravesical gemcitabine in 15 patients that had received intravesical therapy previously. Serum gemcitabine levels were undetected at concentrations of 5, 10, 15, and 20 mg/ml, while low concentrations were present in all patients receiving 40 mg/ml. However, the metabolite dFdU (2'2'-difluorodeoxyuridine) was detectable in plasma of patients receiving gemcitabine at concentrations of 15 mg/ml or higher, implying minimal absorption of gemcitabine at lower doses. The authors concluded that intravesical gemcitabine is well tolerated, with minimal toxicity. Furthermore, no evidence of recurrence at 12 weeks was noted in 9 of 13 evaluable patients.[33]

In a recent phase I study, De Berardinis and associates reported no detection of systemic gemcitabine at a concentration of 40 mg/ml. However, the inactive metabolite was detected in plasma. They were able to demonstrate activity of deoxycytidine kinase in tissue samples, an enzyme that produces 2',2'-difluoro-deoxycytidine triphosphate, the active metabolite of gemcitabine.[34]

All reports published thus far confirm the low systemic absorption of gemcitabine, the good tolerability with minimal local and systemic toxicity, and, more importantly, the efficacy of gemcitabine as an intravesical agent, even in heavily pretreated patients. This agent warrants further investigation in a large cohort of patients.

## INTRAVESICAL BCG AND INTERFERON-α

Interferons are glycoproteins that mediate host immune responses such as stimulation of phagocytes, cytokine release, enhanced natural killer cell activity, and activation of T and B lymphocytes. Intravesical interferon-α 2b (IFNα2b) has demonstrated activity in patients with nonmuscle-invasive bladder cancer.[35] Among patients with Tis enrolled in a randomized trial, two of nine that had failed earlier intravesical therapy had a CR to IFNα2b.[2]

A phase I study of low-dose BCG with different doses of IFNα2b demonstrated that this combination is well tolerated.[36] O'Donnell et al reported the efficacy of the combination in a cohort of patients who had received one or more induction courses of BCG. Of 40 patients enrolled, 63% and 53% were disease-free at 12 and 24 months, respectively.[20] The response for patients in whom a single course of BCG failed was similar to the response of those in whom multiple courses failed. There was a trend towards worse outcomes in patients with an early relapse after the induction course of BCG.[20] Punnen et al reported a durable response to low-dose BCG plus IFNα in 6 of 12 patients with nonmuscle-invasive TCC that received one or more courses of BCG.[37] Lam et al treated 32 patients with nonmuscle-invasive bladder cancer, including patients whose disease recurred after BCG. After a follow-up of 22 months, 66% were disease-free.[38]

## PHOTODYNAMIC THERAPY

Several investigators have reported the efficacy of photodynamic therapy in managing nonmuscle-invasive tumors (also reviewed in Chapter 36). This approach has also been tested in patients with BCG-refractory tumors. Nseyo et al reported the results of a multicenter trial assessing the safety and efficacy of porfimer sodium photodynamic therapy in patients in whom earlier intravesical therapy for Tis had failed. Of the 36 patients enrolled, 34 had received more than one intravesical therapy, including thiotepa, mitomycin, and doxorubicin. At 3 months, 58% achieved a complete response, but 10 of the 21 responders had a recurrence during follow-up (mean, 12 months). Fourteen patients (39%) underwent a radical cystectomy for persistent or recurrent disease, and 22% had muscle-invasive disease. Significant urinary symptoms developed, and seven patients developed bladder contractures.[39]

Photodynamic therapy after the oral administration of 5-aminolevulinic acid was performed in 24 patients with recurrent nonmuscle-invasive TCC after BCG. At a median follow-up of 36 months, 3 of 5 patients with Tis and 4 of 19 with papillary TCC were free of disease.[40]

Other alternative therapies have been investigated, including oral bropirimine, an immunostimulant which has produced remission in patients with Tis after prior intravesical therapy.[3] CR was detected in 30% of the evaluable patients that were BCG resistant. Progression to muscle-invasive or metastatic disease was documented in 6% of the patients.[3]

## CONCLUSION

- A management strategy for BCG-refractory nonmuscle-invasive cancer is suggested in Figure 38.1.
- Bropirimine is not FDA approved and is not being evaluated in clinical trials for bladder cancer.

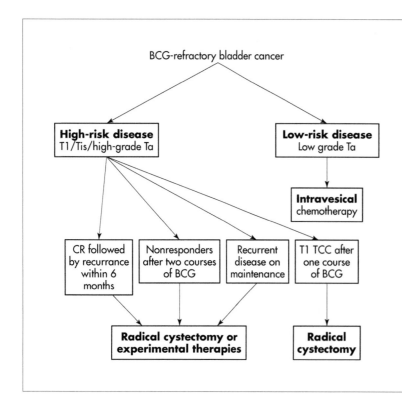

**Fig. 38.1**
Management of BCG-refractory bladder cancer. (CR, complete response; TCC, transitional cell carcinoma.)

- Valrubicin has been discontinued and is not currently available.
- Radical cystectomy still remains the standard of care for patients with BCG-refractory Tis.
- Salvage therapy for patients that refuse, or are unable to undergo, cystectomy is still under investigation.
- New promising strategies and agents warrant further investigation.

## REFERENCES

1. Klein EA, Rogatko A, Herr HW. Management of local bacillus Calmette–Guérin failures in superficial bladder cancer. J Urol 1992;147:601–605.

2. Glashan RW. A randomized controlled study of intravesical alpha-2b-interferon in carcinoma in situ of the bladder. J Urol 1990;144:658–661.

3. Sarosdy MF, Manyak MJ, Sagalowsky AI, et al. Oral bropirimine immunotherapy of bladder carcinoma in situ after prior intravesical bacille Calmette–Guérin. Urology 1998;51:226–231.

4. Haaff EO, Dresner SM, Ratliff TL, et al. Two courses of intravesical bacillus Calmette–Guérin for transitional cell carcinoma of the bladder. J Urol 1986;136:820–824.

5. Okamura T, Tozawa K, Yamada Y, et al. Clinicopathological evaluation of repeated courses of intravesical bacillus Calmette–Guérin instillation for preventing recurrence of initially resistant superficial bladder cancer [see comment]. J Urol 1996;156:967–971.

6. Bui TT, Schellhammer PF. Additional bacillus Calmette–Guérin therapy for recurrent transitional cell carcinoma after an initial complete response. Urology 1997;49:687–690; discussion 690–691.

7. Catalona WJ, Hudson MA, Gillen DP, et al. Risks and benefits of repeated courses of intravesical bacillus Calmette–Guérin therapy for superficial bladder cancer. J Urol 1987;137:220–224.

8. Kavoussi LR, Torrence RJ, Gillen DP, et al. Results of 6 weekly intravesical bacillus Calmette–Guérin instillations on the treatment of superficial bladder tumors. J Urol 1988;139:935–940.

9. Kim JC, Steinberg GD. Medical management of patients with refractory carcinoma in situ of the bladder. Drugs Aging 2001;18:335–344.

10. Harland SJ, Charig CR, Highman W, et al. Outcome in carcinoma in situ of bladder treated with intravesical bacille Calmette–Guérin. Br J Urol 1992;70:271–275.

11. van Gils-Gielen RJ, Witjes WP, Caris CT, et al. Risk factors in carcinoma in situ of the urinary bladder. Dutch South East Cooperative Urological Group. Urology 1995;45:581–586.

12. Ovesen H, Horn T, Steven K. Long-term efficacy of intravesical bacillus Calmette–Guérin for carcinoma in situ: relationship of progression to histological response and p53 nuclear accumulation. J Urol 1997;157:1655–1659.

13. Bretton PR, Herr HW, Kimmel M, et al. The response of patients with superficial bladder cancer to a second course of intravesical bacillus Calmette–Guérin. J Urol 1990;143:710–712; discussion 712–713.

14. Merz VW, Marth D, Kraft R, et al. Analysis of early failures after intravesical instillation therapy with bacille Calmette–Guérin for carcinoma in situ of the bladder. Br J Urol 1995;75:180–184.

15. Herr HW, Badalament RA, Amato DA, et al. Superficial bladder cancer treated with bacillus Calmette–Guérin: a multivariate analysis of factors affecting tumor progression. J Urol 1989;141:22–29.

16. Herr HW. Progression of stage T1 bladder tumors after intravesical bacillus Calmette–Guérin. [Erratum appears in J Urol 1991;145(4):840.] J Urol 1991;145:40–43; discussion 43–44.

17. Hurle R, Losa A, Manzetti A, et al. Intravesical bacille Calmette–Guérin in stage T1 grade 3 bladder cancer therapy: a 7-year follow-up. Urology 1999;54:258–263.

18. Solsona E, Iborra I, Dumont R, et al. The 3-month clinical response to intravesical therapy as a predictive factor for progression in patients with high risk superficial bladder cancer [see comment]. J Urol 2000;164:685–689.

19. Dalbagni G, Russo P, Sheinfeld J, et al. Phase I trial of intravesical gemcitabine in bacillus Calmette–Guérin-refractory transitional-cell carcinoma of the bladder [see comment]. J Clin Oncol 2002;20:3193–3198.

20. O'Donnell MA, Krohn J, DeWolf WC. Salvage intravesical therapy with interferon-alpha 2b plus low dose bacillus Calmette–Guérin is effective in patients with superficial bladder cancer in whom bacillus Calmette–Guérin alone previously failed. J Urol 2001;166:1300–1304; discussion 1304–1305.

21. Luciani LG, Neulander E, Murphy WM, et al. Risk of continued intravesical therapy and delayed cystectomy in BCG-refractory superficial bladder cancer: an investigational approach. Urology 2001;58:376–379.

22. Steinberg G, Bahnson R, Brosman S, et al. Efficacy and safety of valrubicin for the treatment of Bacillus Calmette–Guérin refractory carcinoma in situ of the bladder. The Valrubicin Study Group [see comment]. J Urol 2000;163:761–767.

23. van der Heijden AG, Witjes JA. Future strategies in the diagnosis, staging and treatment of bladder cancer. Curr Opin Urol 2003;13:389–395.

24. Kuznetsov DD, Alsikafi NF, O'Connor RC, et al. Intravesical valrubicin in the treatment of carcinoma in situ of the bladder. Exp Opin Pharmacother 2001;2:1009–1013.

25. Greenberg RE, Bahnson RR, Wood D, et al. Initial report on intravesical administration of N-trifluoroacetyladriamycin-14-valerate (AD 32) to patients with refractory superficial transitional cell carcinoma of the urinary bladder. Urology 1997;49:471–475.

26. Hertel LW, Boder GB, Kroin JS, et al. Evaluation of the antitumor activity of gemcitabine (2′,2′-difluoro-2′-deoxycytidine). Cancer Res 1990;50:4417–4422.

27. Burris HA 3rd, Moore MJ, Andersen J, et al. Improvements in survival and clinical benefit with gemcitabine as first-line therapy for patients with advanced pancreas cancer: a randomized trial [see comment]. J Clin Oncol 1997;15:2403–2413.

28. Moore MJ, Tannock IF, Ernst DS, et al. Gemcitabine: a promising new agent in the treatment of advanced urothelial cancer. J Clin Oncol 1997;15:3441–3445.

29. Stadler WM, Kuzel T, Roth B, et al. Phase II study of single-agent gemcitabine in previously untreated patients with metastatic urothelial cancer. J Clin Oncol 1997;15:3394–3398.

30. Lorusso V, Pollera CF, Antimi M, et al. A phase II study of gemcitabine in patients with transitional cell carcinoma of the urinary tract previously treated with platinum. Italian Co-operative Group on Bladder Cancer. Eur J Cancer 1998;34:1208–1212.

31. von der Maase H, Hansen SW, Roberts JT, et al. Gemcitabine and cisplatin versus methotrexate, vinblastine, doxorubicin, and cisplatin in advanced or metastatic bladder cancer: results of a large, randomized, multinational, multicenter, phase III study [see comment]. J Clin Oncol 2000;18:3068–3077.

32. Dalbagni G, Mazumdar M, Russo P, et al. Phase II trial of intravesical gemcitabine in BCG-refractory transitional cell carcinoma of the bladder. J Urol 2004;171:Abstract 274.

33. Laufer M, Ramalingam S, Schoenberg MP, et al. Intravesical gemcitabine therapy for superficial transitional cell carcinoma of the bladder: a phase I and pharmacokinetic study. J Clin Oncol 2003;21:697–703.

34. De Berardinis E, Antonini G, Peters GJ, et al. Intravesical administration of gemcitabine in superficial bladder cancer: a phase I study with pharmacodynamic evaluation. BJU Int 2004;93:491–494.

35. Torti FM, Shortliffe LD, Williams RD, et al. Alpha-interferon in superficial bladder cancer: a Northern California Oncology Group Study. J Clin Oncol 1988;6:476–483.

36. Stricker P, Pryor K, Nicholson T, et al. Bacillus Calmette–Guérin plus intravesical interferon alpha-2b in patients with superficial bladder cancer. Urology 1996;48:957–961; discussion 961–962.

37. Punnen SP, Chin JL, Jewett MA. Management of bacillus Calmette–Guérin (BCG) refractory superficial bladder cancer: results with intravesical BCG and interferon combination therapy. Can J Urol 2003;10:1790–1795.

38. Lam JS, Benson MC, O'Donnell MA, et al. Bacillus Calmette–Guérin plus interferon-alpha2B intravesical therapy maintains an extended treatment plan for superficial bladder cancer with minimal toxicity. Urol Oncol 2003;21:354–360.

39. Nseyo UO. Photodynamic therapy in the management of bladder cancer. J Clin Laser Med Surg 1996;14:271–280.

40. Waidelich R, Stepp H, Baumgartner R, et al. Clinical experience with 5-aminolevulinic acid and photodynamic therapy for refractory superficial bladder cancer. J Urol 2001;165:1904–1907.

# Chemoprevention of superficial bladder cancer

# 39

Anita L Sabichi, Scott M Lippman

## INTRODUCTION

Most bladder cancer patients present with superficial transitional cell carcinoma (TCC) confined to the mucosa (pTa or Tis) or the lamina propria (pT1). These patients are at approximately a 66% risk of recurrence within 5 years of resection and suffer substantial morbidity from frequent monitoring for recurrence. Several disease and treatment characteristics facilitate cancer prevention approaches in this setting. The high recurrence rate, direct methods of surveillance, and low risk of advancing stage provide an ideal setting for chemoprevention to avert recurrence. Promising preventive agents in preclinical bladder carcinogenesis models include difluoromethylornithine, isoflavanoids, and cyclooxygenase inhibitors. Ongoing clinical trials are testing the efficacy of difluoromethylornithine and the cyclooxygenase 2 inhibitor celecoxib for preventing recurrences in patients with a history of superficial bladder tumors.

The process of cancer development involves initiation, promotion, and progression to invasive disease. This multistep process provides for a generally long latency period that can potentially be exploited for intervention measures to prevent or delay progression to invasive disease. Herein lies the concept of cancer chemoprevention, which can be defined as the use of agents to prevent or delay the development of invasive cancer.

Estimates of new cancer cases in the US for 2005 placed TCC of the bladder as the fourth most common cancer in men and the eighth most common cancer in women, an overall predicted incidence of 63,210 and mortality of 13,180.[1] According to the National Cancer Institute, the prevalence of TCC in the US, with more than 499,199 cases, has surpassed the prevalence of lung cancer.[2]

As many as 70% of bladder cancer patients with TCC are classified as having superficial tumors. Superficial bladder tumors (SBTs) will progress to muscle-invasive disease in only approximately 15% of cases. Low-grade (grade 1–2) papillary tumors (pTa) have the lowest risk of progression. The 3-year rate of progression to muscle-invasive disease for Ta tumors is 4%, in contrast to up to 30% for T1 tumors. Despite a relatively low rate of progression, risk of tumor recurrence after initial diagnosis and treatment for SBTs is substantial and generally dependent upon several factors including multifocality, grade, stage, and evidence of tumor at the 3-month cystosopic examination after initial treatment. Approximately 50% of patients diagnosed with a solitary bladder tumor will experience disease recurrence within 4 years, whereas 70% of patients with multiple bladder tumors will recur within 1 year.[3–5]

Standard primary treatment for high-risk superficial TCC (e.g. T1, Tis) is transurethral resection (TUR) and adjuvant intravesical immunotherapy with bacillus Calmette–Guérin (BCG) to decrease tumor recurrence and to possibly decrease progression and improve survival. Intravesical chemotherapy and interferon are alternative therapies that can also decrease recurrence rates.[6,7] For BCG-refractory TCC, durable response rates with alternative intravesical therapies are low.[4] Despite these benefits, the long-term incidence of tumor recurrence is substantial after BCG therapy.[8] Because of this risk, long-term monitoring with regular cystoscopic evaluation, urine cytology, and/or other diagnostic biomarkers is necessary.[9,10]

Cancer chemoprevention is an exciting, relatively recent approach for improving the control of superficial TCC. Chemoprevention is designed not only to prevent cancer development but also to treat subclinical cancer.[11,12] Chemoprevention has been applied to many different tumor types, including TCC, for prevention of both primary and second tumors. With their high risk of recurrence and access to cystoscopy and urine cytology for accurate assessment of tumor development, superficial bladder cancer patients are an ideal population for cancer chemoprevention.

Discussion of cancer chemoprevention warrants review of biologic theory surrounding recurrence of TCC. Superficial TCC may recur in multiple loci throughout the bladder and/or at multiple time points. Two theories—the field defect hypothesis and the monoclonal hypothesis—have been offered to explain this frequency and multiplicity of tumor formation. According to the field defect hypothesis, various 'initiating' genetic mutations occur in carcinogen-exposed cells throughout the entire epithelial 'field', which increases susceptibility to additional genetic damage that ultimately results in cellular transformation and tumor formation. Subsequent or 'recurrent' disease after an initial TCC diagnosis is due to the development of 'second primary' tumors (SPTs) that form through successive accumulation of genetic mutations, resulting ultimately in transformation of the initiated urothelial cells. Chemical carcinogens such as the aromatic amines from cigarette smoke and aniline dyes have been implicated in this process.[13]

According to the monoclonal hypothesis, synchronous and metachronous tumors originate from propagation of a single transformed cell that spreads throughout the urothelium. Sidransky and colleagues[14] tested this theory in female patients with multiple synchronous bladder tumors and found that the tumors within the bladder of each patient had inactivation of the same X chromosome, suggesting that the tumors were monoclonal, or derived from the same progenitor cell. More recent evidence from Simon et al[15] further supports the premise that multifocal bladder tumors may be monoclonal in origin. This group analyzed the chromosomes of 32 tumors from six patients, finding identical chromosomal aberrations in all of the tumors from individual patients. Individual patients' tumor aberrations were also found in their macroscopically uninvolved adjacent urothelium, suggesting the intraepithelial spread of premalignant cells.

Takahashi et al[16] found that 80% of the patients with multifocal bladder tumors that they studied had chromosomal alterations suggestive of a monoclonal origin, and that 20% of patients had tumors arising from unique individual progenitor cells, and were not of monoclonal origin. In clinical practice, superficial bladder tumors are not characterized as recurrent or SPTs. For patient management, all TCCs appearing subsequent to the initial diagnosis are considered recurrences. Chemopreventive agents under current evaluation have shown potential effects on promotion, angiogenesis, and apoptosis, and could ultimately be shown to be effective in preventing recurrent tumors.

## CHEMOPREVENTION STRATEGIES

Chemoprevention of initial tumors is a desirable approach for individuals at a high risk of developing bladder cancer. Smoking is the most common bladder cancer risk factor, causing an estimated 48% of all bladder cancers,[17] and exposure to arylamines is the second most common risk factor.[18] These environmental carcinogens may be inactivated by acetylation, and genetic susceptibility to carcinogenesis has been associated with the loss of the N-acetyltransferase (NAT) enzyme.[9,17] Because of the sporadic nature of cancer and the long latency before its clinical appearance, very large studies are required to evaluate chemoprevention in people at the risk of, but no signs of, cancer. Initial chemoprevention studies of promising drugs have been conducted in the setting of SPT or recurrence prevention, which facilitates smaller, less costly clinical testing because event rates generally are higher than in the high-risk, noncancer setting. Patients with a history of superficial bladder cancer are an ideal population for chemoprevention. They are free of disease by conventional assessment, are followed closely, and have a high risk of developing a SPT or recurrence.

Carefully selected biomarkers may be useful as intermediate endpoints in clinical chemoprevention trials. Biomarker modulations may facilitate efficacy evaluation of the agent being studied.[10] Validated biomarkers, i.e. ones that correlate with cancer outcome, do not yet exist for this disease, but proteins such as proliferating cell nuclear antigen (PCNA) and epidermal growth factor receptor (EGFR) that are altered early in neoplasia may be relevant to cancer development.[9] Biomarkers may be relatively nonspecific and reflect cellular processes such as proliferation (e.g. PCNA, Ki67) and cell death (apoptosis). Ki67 and PCNA are nuclear antigens expressed in proliferating cells. Other biomarkers may probe the pathways that are thought to be altered by the drug being tested; for example, the retinoic acid receptor-$\beta$ may probe pathways affected by a retinoid. Other classes of biomarkers include cellular adhesion proteins (e.g. cadherins, integrins), cell cycle regulators (e.g. p53, Rb), angiogenic (e.g. VEGF) or growth factors (e.g. IGFI, EGF), and growth factor receptors (e.g. EGFR).[19] Although biomarkers can add significant value to the scientific and clinical results of chemoprevention trials, a detailed discussion of this topic is beyond the scope of this chapter and has been provided elsewhere in a recently published review of biomarkers in defining urothelial premalignant and malignant conditions.[9]

## VITAMINS

Lamm et al[20] conducted a phase III, $2 \times 2$ factorial trial involving intravesical BCG (with or without percutaneous BCG), the recommended daily allowance (RDA) of a multivitamin, and megadoses of vitamin A (40,000 IU), vitamin B6 (100 mg), vitamin C (2000 mg), vitamin E (400 IU), and zinc (90 mg) in reducing recurrence in 65 bladder cancer patients. With up to 5 years of follow-up, no significant difference in the rate of recurrence was seen in patients that did or did not receive percutaneous BCG. However, the recurrence rate in patients that received only the RDA of multivitamins was significantly higher (80%; 24/30) than in patients that also received megadoses of the vitamins A, B6, C, and E (40%; 14/35) (p=0.0011). In the megadose vitamin group, the rate of tumor recurrence was not reduced during the first 10 months of the study. This delayed effect may have occurred because of the outgrowth of residual, microscopic cancers during the initial period.

### Pyridoxine

Pyridoxine (vitamin $B_6$) has been evaluated in patients at risk for recurrent bladder cancer. The rationale supporting pyridoxine includes the concept that bladder cancer may be induced by metabolites that are produced as a result of abnormal tryptophan metabolism.[21] A Veterans Administration multicenter trial evaluated the effect of either pyridoxine or thiotepa compared with placebo in 121 bladder cancer patients.[22] Pyridoxine was significantly more effective than placebo and was equivalent to thiotepa in reducing the recurrence of bladder tumors. Another study administered pyridoxine or placebo to 291 patients with Ta or T1 bladder cancer 7–14 days following TUR.[21] No significant differences in recurrence rates or time to first recurrence occurred between the pyridoxine and placebo groups.

### Ascorbic acid

Ascorbic acid (vitamin C) is a potent reducing agent that can act as a free radical scavenger. In vivo ascorbic acid can decrease the formation of the bladder-cancer-associated carcinogenic N-nitroso compounds.[23,24] Epidemiologic studies suggest that diets containing high levels of vitamin C are associated with decreased risks of several types of cancer. For example, a cohort of 11,590 patients followed from 1981 to 1989 revealed a 0.59 relative risk of bladder cancer in patients taking vitamin C supplements (versus those who did not).[25] Another analysis revealed that bladder cancer patients had a lower vitamin C intake compared with that of a control group.[26] A reduction of nitroso-induced bladder tumor

formation in mice treated with vitamin C has also been reported.[27] However, other studies suggest there may be a vitamin C dose threshold beyond which vitamin C could promote tumorigenesis. For example, 5% dietary vitamin C in the form sodium ascorbate promoted bladder cancer in rats.[28] It has been suggested that patients with carcinogenic potential should not take high doses of vitamin C.[29]

### Alpha-tocopherol

Alpha-tocopherol (vitamin E) is another potential agent for the chemoprevention of bladder cancer with antioxidant properties and the ability to reduce the formation of nitroso compounds in animal studies.[29] An in vitro model assessing hydrogen peroxide-induced transformation of a nontumorigenic urothelial cell line demonstrated the activity of vitamin E in reducing tumor necrosis factor-$\alpha$ (TNF$\alpha$)-stimulated colony growth in soft agar.[30,31] Furthermore, the prospective Health Professionals Follow-up Study recently reported an inverse relationship between vitamin E intake and the risk of developing bladder cancer in men.[31]

## RETINOIDS

Retinoids are natural and synthetic analogs of vitamin A and were originally recognized to be important in the maintenance of cellular differentiation and epithelial integrity. This was initially demonstrated in the 1920s by Mori[32] and Wolbach and Howe[33] who noted that experimental animals developed squamous metaplasia, hyperkeratinization, and malignant transformation of multiple epithelial tissues upon severe restriction of dietary retinoids. Later work showed that a retinoid-deficient diet increased tumor formation in experimental models of bladder carcinogenesis.[34] These findings were bolstered by epidemiologic data suggesting an inverse relationship between reduced vitamin A intake and an increased incidence of bladder cancer[35] and lower serum carotenoids in patients diagnosed with bladder cancer.[36] Retinoids and retinamides were further studied and shown to be effective chemopreventive agents against bladder cancer development in numerous animal cancer models.[37–41]

Perhaps one of the most dramatic effects in the study of retinoids has been demonstrated by differentiation of acute promyelocytic leukemia (APL) cells into polymorphonuclear leukocytes by all-trans-retinoic acid (ATRA). This powerful finding led to direct clinical application of ATRA as adjunct treatment for APL patients. Initial treatment with ATRA used as a 'differentiation therapy' and followed by standard chemotherapy resulted in an improved 4-year survival compared to chemotherapy alone.[42,43]

A useful chemopreventive agent should be both effective and have minimal side effects. Vitamin A and its derivatives, such as 13-cis-retinoic acid, have been used in many chemoprevention studies but can cause side effects that significantly interfere with treatment. An early dose escalation bladder chemoprevention trial with 13-cis-retinoic acid was terminated prematurely with only 7 of 20 patients able to complete the prescribed intervention because of substantial toxicity.[44] Enrolled patients developed cheilosis, conjunctivitis, pruritus, and joint pain.

Newer synthetic retinoids, such as etretinate, and retinamides, such as N-(4-hydroxyphenyl)retinamide (fenretinide), have the ability to produce higher retinoid serum concentrations while minimizing systemic toxicity. Therapeutic retinoid effects act at a molecular and cellular level through the retinoic acid receptor heterodimers that function as transcriptional regulators. When activated, the retinoic acid transcription factor complex induces cellular differentiation and apoptosis pathways, and inhibits cellular proliferation in bladder cancer cells.[45] Less well defined are the molecular mechanisms of action of fenretinide and novel phenylretinamides. In vitro they inhibit cell growth associated with G1–G0 cell cycle arrest and induce apoptosis in bladder cancer cell lines.[45,46]

The substantial promising preclinical data on retinoids for bladder cancer chemoprevention have led to clinical trials with somewhat mixed results. Studer et al conducted a randomized prospective trial of etretinate for preventing recurrence following TUR of superficial bladder tumors.[47] Seventy-nine patients with resected Ta or T1 tumors were randomized to receive either placebo or 25 mg etretinate daily. All patients were treated for a minimum of 2 years, with median durations of 30 months for the placebo group and 33 months for the etretinate group. The mean times to the first recurrence were similar in both groups: 13.5 months (placebo) and 13.6 months (etretinate). Low-risk patients continued to be treated. The side effects, including cheilitis and mucositis, were acceptable to most patients. The time to a second recurrence was significantly longer in the etretinate group (20 months) than in the placebo group (12.7 months) (p=0.006). This delayed benefit paralleled findings in the megadose vitamin trial discussed above,[20] and suggests a benefit of prolonged treatment.

Decensi et al conducted a phase II trial of fenretinide in patients with superficial TCC and found that fenretinide improved DNA flow cytometry results.[48,49] In a more recent phase III chemoprevention trial of fenretinide,[49] Decensi and coworkers randomized 99 patients with recurrent or primary superficial bladder tumors to receive either oral fenretinide or no treatment for 2 years. Comparable tumor recurrence rates were seen in both trial arms, with 27 events in the fenretinide arm and 21 events in the control arm (p=0.36). However, reduced levels of insulin-like growth factor I (IGFI) were observed in the fenretinide group,[50] and the

investigators concluded that fenretinide may have a beneficial effect by reducing levels of IGF, high levels of which are associated with increased cancer risk. Preliminary analysis of a second randomized phase III trial of fenretinide versus placebo as adjuvant therapy in patients with superficial bladder cancer has recently been reported.[51] This study also did not show a difference in recurrence rates between the two arms.

Results from the Alpha-Tocopherol, Beta Carotene Prevention Study, a large double-blind trial evaluating the chemopreventive effects of alpha-tocopherol and beta carotene on lung and other cancers, demonstrated no significant effect of either alpha-tocopherol (relative risk [RR]=1.1, 95% CI: 0.8–1.5) or beta carotene (RR=1.0, 95% CI: 0.7–1.3) on risk of developing urothelial cancers (bladder, renal pelvis, and ureter).[52]

## DIFLUOROMETHYLORNITHINE

Difluoromethylornithine (DFMO) is an irreversible inhibitor of ornithine decarboxylase, the key enzyme that participates in polyamine biosynthesis, and which is thought to regulate growth and apoptosis in multiple cell systems. Overexpression of ornithine decarboxylase in fibroblasts enhanced soft agar colony formation and invasive behavior of these cells. Upregulation of ornithine decarboxylase by the c-myc oncogene has also been described. DFMO inhibited human bladder cancer cell growth, with a 5- to 20-fold higher concentration of DFMO required to inhibit normal human urothelial cell growth. Inhibition of polyamine synthesis by DFMO has been associated with decreased production of matrix metalloproteinases. In vivo studies revealed that DFMO reduced the incidence of papillary carcinoma induced by N-butyl-N-(4-hydroxybutyl) nitrosamine in rats.[53] Although ototoxicity has been reported at high doses, a clinical trial has demonstrated minimal ototoxicity over a 1-year period of administration,[54] making it a feasible chemopreventive agent for further investigation. A multicenter chemoprevention trial is presently underway to evaluate the efficacy of DFMO in preventing tumor recurrence in patients with superficial TCC.

## ISOFLAVONES

Increased consumption of soy products has been associated with a decreased risk of cancer for multiple tumor types including breast, prostate, and colon.[55] Isoflavones, which are found in relatively high concentration in soy products, have been associated with this phenomenon. Data from preclinical studies support the use of isoflavones as chemopreventive agents and these compounds are currently undergoing evaluation for the chemoprevention of breast and colon cancer.[56,57] Metabolites of isoflavones are excreted in the urine,[58] and soybean feeding is protective in a mouse model of bladder carcinogenesis.[59,60] The isoflavone family includes compounds such as genistein, daidzein, and biochanin-A. In a study by Su et al, these compounds inhibited the growth of J82 bladder cancer cells and induced apoptosis. Genistein induced a G2–M cell cycle arrest and a dose-dependent decrease in cdc2 kinase activity.[61]

## SELECTIVE AND NONSELECTIVE COX INHIBITORS

There has been recent interest in cyclooxygenase (COX) inhibitors as chemopreventive agents. These enzymes are responsible for the conversion of arachidonic acid to biologically active prostaglandins such as PGE2, thromboxane A2, prostacyclin, and other prostaglandins that may participate in the neoplastic process. The COX enzyme contains two adjacent active sites: one that converts arachidonic acid to prostaglandin G2 and another that is responsible for a peroxidation reaction to form prostaglandin H2. Prostaglandin H2 is then metabolized by specific enzymes in the formation of prostaglandin D2, prostaglandin E2, prostaglandin F2a, prostaglandin I2 (prostacyclin), and thromboxane A2.[62]

COX1, a 70 kD membrane protein encoded by a 22 kb gene located on chromosome 9, is constitutively expressed in many tissues and plays a role in normal physiologic processes. Only the COX1 isoform is detectable in platelets, and prostaglandins (particularly thromboxane A2 and prostacyclin) are well-known modulators of platelet function. Cytoprotective prostaglandins produced by the gastric mucosa are synthesized through COX1 and are thought to enhance mucosal blood flow. In the kidney, PGE2 produced by COX1 is essential in maintaining renal blood flow, especially during adverse physiologic conditions such as hypotension, congestive heart failure, cirrhosis, or renal insufficiency. In contrast to COX1, only low levels of COX2 have been detected in normal tissues.[62,63]

COX2 is a membrane-associated 70 kD protein. It is an inducible enzyme encoded by an 8 kb gene on chromosome 1. Increased COX2 expression occurs in response to cytokines, growth factors, and tumor promoters. Its role in tumor promotion has been of particular interest. Attempts to determine a molecular basis for the significantly lower relative risk for colon cancer in patients taking aspirin led to the discovery of high levels of COX2 expression in colorectal tumors.[62,63]

The ulcerogenic and nephrotoxic side effects of some nonsteroidal anti-inflammatory drugs (NSAIDs) such as indometacin are attributed to COX1 inhibition, whereas the anti-inflammatory action of these drugs has been attributed to COX2 inhibition. Colon carcinogenesis is inhibited by COX inhibitors in animal models. For example, inhibition of COX2 in APC delta716 knockout mice markedly suppressed tumor formation.[64] Furthermore, in patients with familial adenomatous polyposis coli (FAP), the use of NSAIDs that nonspecifically block COX isozymes significantly reduces the number and size of polyp formation.[65] A recent study has shown that a COX2-specific inhibitor also significantly reduces polyp burden in patients diagnosed with FAP.[66] The importance of COX2 as a chemopreventive target is suggested by upregulation of this enzyme in colon tumors.[67,68]

By immunostaining, most normal bladder and ureteral specimens show no staining for COX2. However, COX2 is commonly expressed in all stages of bladder cancer and has also been identified in dysplasia, which may be a malignant precursor.[69–71] These data support the association between increased expression of COX2 and bladder cancer. Increased prostaglandin synthesis may have a number of effects on bladder cancer development, including reduction of apoptosis and increased growth potential. COX2 inhibitors have been shown to inhibit growth and to promote apoptosis in multiple tumor cell types in vitro. These effects have been associated with downregulation of BCL2 in some studies.[72] Increased BCL2 expression has also been observed with COX2 upregulation, suggesting that protection from apoptosis may play a role in tumor progression.[73] Furthermore, upregulation of COX2 has been reported in association with EGF receptor activation.[74]

COX2 activity may also be counterbalanced by metabolism of prostaglandins by the enzyme prostaglandin dehydrogenase (PGDH).[75] To explore this possibility in bladder cancer, we evaluated the expression of PGDH in a series of bladder carcinoma cell lines and in normal and malignant urothelium. Diffuse expression of PGDH was consistently observed in normal bladder and ureteral urothelium. However, loss of PGDH was frequently observed in the TCC cell lines and in bladder tumors.[76] Furthermore, loss of PGDH was observed more frequently in high-grade tumors (83.3%) and in invasive tumors (75%) than in superficial, low-grade tumors (20%, p<0.025).[77]

The expression or participation of COX2 in bladder carcinogenesis has been explored in several model systems. Nimesulide, a putative COX2-specific inhibitor, has been shown to provide effective chemoprevention in a rat bladder carcinogenesis model.[78] Ibuprofen reduced the ability of a human bladder cancer cell line to invade in vitro.[79] Indometacin in the diet of mice treated with N-butyl-N-(4-hydroxybutyl) nitrosamine (BBN) significantly reduced development of tumors in the presence of the tumor promoters butylated hydroxyanisole (BHA) and sodium L-ascorbate (Na-AsA).[80] Furthermore, decreased PGE2 concentrations were found in the existing tumors in rats treated with indometacin.

A National Cancer Institute-funded multicenter chemoprevention trial testing a COX2-specific inhibitor in patients with superficial bladder cancer has recently been initiated through the University of Texas M.D. Anderson Cancer Center.[13] In this study, patients at high risk for tumor recurrence receive a 6-week course of BCG therapy. If their follow-up cystoscopy is negative for tumor recurrence, they receive an additional 3 weeks of BCG and are randomized to receive either placebo or celecoxib for a minimum of 12 months. They are then prospectively evaluated for tumor recurrence.

## CONCLUSION

Superficial bladder cancer is a common disease with a high frequency of recurrence and a comparatively low rate of progression. The high frequency of recurrence, coupled with the relative ease with which the urothelium can be surveyed with cystoscopy and urine cytology, make this disease an excellent clinical model to evaluate potential chemopreventive agents. Preclinical studies have demonstrated the effectiveness of this approach. Promising preventive agents in this setting include isoflavanoids, statins, and cyclooxygenase inhibitors. Ongoing randomized controlled trials are focusing on polyamine and COX2 inhibition as strategies for preventing disease recurrence in these patients.

## REFERENCES

1. Jemal A, Murray T, Ward E, et al. Cancer statistics, 2005. CA Cancer J Clin 2005;55(1):10–30.
2. Ries LAG, Eisner MP, Kosary CL, et al. SEER Cancer Statistics Review, 1975–2002. Bethesda, MD: National Cancer Institute, 2005.
3. Kurth KH, Bouffioux C, Sylvester R, van der Meijden AP, Oosterlinck W, Brausi M. Treatment of superficial bladder tumors: achievements and needs. The EORTC Genitourinary Group. Eur Urol 2000;37(Suppl 3):1–9.
4. Grossman HB. Superficial bladder cancer: decreasing the risk of recurrence. Oncology 1996;10(11):1617–1624; discussion 24, 27–28.
5. Bono AV. Superficial bladder cancer: state of the art. Cancer Chemother Pharmacol 1994;35(Suppl):S101–109.
6. Lamm DL, Blumenstein BA, Crissman JD, et al. Maintenance bacillus Calmette–Guérin immunotherapy for recurrent TA, T1 and carcinoma in situ transitional cell carcinoma of the bladder: a randomized Southwest Oncology Group Study. J Urol 2000;163(4):1124–1129.
7. Herr HW, Schwalb DM, Zhang ZF, et al. Intravesical bacillus Calmette–Guérin therapy prevents tumor progression and death from superficial bladder cancer: ten-year follow-up of a prospective randomized trial. J Clin Oncol 1995;13(6):1404–1408.
8. Cookson MS, Herr HW, Zhang ZF, Soloway S, Sogani PC, Fair WR. The treated natural history of high risk superficial bladder cancer: 15-year outcome. J Urol 1997;158(1):62–67.
9. Grossman HB, Schmitz-Drager B, Fradet Y, Tribukait B. Use of markers in defining urothelial premalignant and malignant conditions. Scand J Urol Nephrol Suppl 2000;205:94–104.
10. Grossman HB. Biomarkers for transitional cell carcinoma-pro. Urology 2001;57(5):847–848.
11. Lippman SM, Lee JJ, Sabichi AL. Cancer chemoprevention: progress and promise. J Natl Cancer Inst 1998;90(20):1514–1528.
12. Sporn MB, Newton DL. Chemoprevention of cancer with retinoids. Fed Proc 1979;38(11):2528–2534.
13. Sabichi AL, Lerner SP, Grossman HB, Lippman SM. Retinoids in the chemoprevention of bladder cancer. Curr Opin Oncol 1998;10(5):479–484.
14. Sidransky D, Frost P, Von Eschenbach A, Oyasu R, Preisinger AC, Vogelstein B. Clonal origin of bladder cancer. N Engl J Med 1992;326(11):737–740.
15. Simon R, Eltze E, Schafer KL, et al. Cytogenetic analysis of multifocal bladder cancer supports a monoclonal origin and intraepithelial spread of tumor cells. Cancer Res 2001;61(1):355–362.
16. Takahashi T, Habuchi T, Kakehi Y, et al. Clonal and chronological genetic analysis of multifocal cancers of the bladder and upper urinary tract. Cancer Res 1998;58(24):5835–5841.
17. Marcus PM, Hayes RB, Vineis P, et al. Cigarette smoking, N-acetyltransferase 2 acetylation status, and bladder cancer risk: a case-series meta-analysis of a gene–environment interaction. Cancer Epidemiol Biomarkers Prev 2000;9(5):461–467.
18. Castelao JE, Yuan JM, Skipper PL, et al. Gender- and smoking-related bladder cancer risk. J Natl Cancer Inst 2001;93(7):538–545.
19. Stein JP, Grossfeld GD, Ginsberg DA, et al. Prognostic markers in bladder cancer: a contemporary review of the literature. J Urol 1998;160(3 Pt 1):645–659.
20. Lamm DL, Riggs DR, Shriver JS, vanGilder PF, Rach JF, DeHaven JI. Megadose vitamins in bladder cancer: a double-blind clinical trial. J Urol 1994;151(1):21–26.
21. Newling DW, Robinson MR, Smith PH, et al. Tryptophan metabolites, pyridoxine (vitamin B6) and their influence on the recurrence rate of superficial bladder cancer. Results of a prospective, randomised phase III study performed by the EORTC GU Group. EORTC Genito-Urinary Tract Cancer Cooperative Group. Eur Urol 1995;27(2):110–116.
22. Byar D, Blackard C. Comparisons of placebo, pyridoxine, and topical thiotepa in preventing recurrence of stage I bladder cancer. Urology 1977;10(6):556–561.
23. Birt DF. Update on the effects of vitamins A, C, and E and selenium on carcinogenesis. Proc Soc Exp Biol Med 1986;183(3):311–320.
24. Mirvish SS. Role of N-nitroso compounds (NOC) and N-nitrosation in etiology of gastric, esophageal, nasopharyngeal and bladder cancer and contribution to cancer of known exposures to NOC. Cancer Lett 1995;93(1):17–48.
25. Shibata A, Paganini-Hill A, Ross RK, Henderson BE. Intake of vegetables, fruits, beta-carotene, vitamin C and vitamin supplements and cancer incidence among the elderly: a prospective study. Br J Cancer 1992;66(4):673–679.
26. Nomura AM, Kolonel LN, Hankin JH, Yoshizawa CN. Dietary factors in cancer of the lower urinary tract. Int J Cancer 1991;48(2):199–205.
27. Mokhtar NM, el-Aaser AA, el-Bolkainy MN, Ibrahim HA, el-Din NB, Moharram NZ. Effect of soybean feeding on experimental carcinogenesis—III. Carcinogenicity of nitrite and dibutylamine in mice: a histopathological study. Eur J Cancer Clin Oncol 1988;24(3):403–411.
28. Fukushima S, Imaida K, Sakata T, Okamura T, Shibata M, Ito N. Promoting effects of sodium L-ascorbate on two-stage urinary bladder carcinogenesis in rats. Cancer Res 1983;43(9):4454–4457.
29. Mirvish SS. Effects of vitamins C and E on N-nitroso compound formation, carcinogenesis, and cancer. Cancer 1986;58(8 Suppl):1842–1850.
30. Okamoto M, Oyasu R. Transformation in vitro of a nontumorigenic rat urothelial cell line by tumor necrosis factor-alpha. Lab Invest 1997;77(2):139–144.
31. Michaud DS, Spiegelman D, Clinton SK, Rimm EB, Willett WC, Giovannucci E. Prospective study of dietary supplements, macronutrients, micronutrients, and risk of bladder cancer in US men. Am J Epidemiol 2000;152(12):1145–1153.
32. Mori S. The changes in the para-ocular glands which follow the administration of diets low in fat-soluble A; with notes of the effects of the same diets on the salivary glands and the mucosa of the larynx and trachea. Johns Hopkins Hosp Bull 1922;357–360.
33. Wolbach SB, Howe PR. Tissue changes following deprivation of fat-soluble A vitamin. J Exp Med 1925;42(6):753–777.

34. Cohen SM, Wittenberg JF, Bryan GT. Effect of avitaminosis A and hypervitaminosis A on urinary bladder carcinogenicity of N-(4-(5-Nitro-2-furyl)-2-thiazolyl)formamide. Cancer Res 1976;36(7 Pt 1):2334–2339.

35. Mettlin C, Graham S. Dietary risk factors in human bladder cancer. Am J Epidemiol 1979;110(3):255–263.

36. Hicks RM. The scientific basis for regarding vitamin A and its analogues as anti-carcinogenic agents. Proc Nutr Soc 1983;42(1):83–93.

37. Sporn MB, Squire RA, Brown CC, Smith JM, Wenk ML, Springer S. 13-cis-retinoic acid: inhibition of bladder carcinogenesis in the rat. Science 1977;195(4277):487–489.

38. Moon RC, McCormick DL, Becci PJ, et al. Influence of 15 retinoic acid amides on urinary bladder carcinogenesis in the mouse. Carcinogenesis 1982;3(12):1469–1472.

39. McCormick DL, Becci PJ, Moon RC. Inhibition of mammary and urinary bladder carcinogenesis by a retinoid and a maleic anhydride-divinyl ether copolymer (MVE-2). Carcinogenesis 1982;3(12):1473–1476.

40. Croft WA, Croft MA, Paulus KP, Williams JH, Wang CY, Lower GM Jr. 13-cis-retinoic acid: effect on urinary bladder carcinogenesis by N-[4-(5-nitro-2-furyl)-2-thiazolyl]-formamide in Fischer rats. Cancer Lett 1981;12(4):355–360.

41. Becci PJ, Thompson HJ, Strum JM, Brown CC, Sporn MB, Moon RC. N-butyl-N-(4-hydroxybutyl)nitrosamine-induced urinary bladder cancer in C57BL/6 X DBA/2 F1 mice as a useful model for study of chemoprevention of cancer with retinoids. Cancer Res 1981;41(3):927–932.

42. Fenaux P, Degos L. Differentiation therapy for acute promyelocytic leukemia. N Engl J Med 1997;337(15):1076–1077.

43. Tallman MS, Andersen JW, Schiffer CA, et al. All-trans-retinoic acid in acute promyelocytic leukemia. N Engl J Med 1997;337(15):1021–1028.

44. Prout GR Jr, Barton BA. 13-cis-retinoic acid in chemoprevention of superficial bladder cancer. The National Bladder Cancer Group. J Cell Biochem Suppl 1992;16I:148–152.

45. Clifford JL, Sabichi AL, Zou C, et al. Effects of novel phenylretinamides on cell growth and apoptosis in bladder cancer. Cancer Epidemiol Biomarkers Prev 2001;10(4):391–395.

46. Waliszewski P, Waliszewska M, Gordon N, et al. Retinoid signaling in immortalized and carcinoma-derived human uroepithelial cells. Mol Cell Endocrinol 1999;148(1–2):55–65.

47. Studer UE, Jenzer S, Biedermann C, et al. Adjuvant treatment with a vitamin A analogue (etretinate) after transurethral resection of superficial bladder tumors. Final analysis of a prospective, randomized multicenter trial in Switzerland. Eur Urol 1995;28(4):284–290.

48. Decensi A, Bruno S, Costantini M, et al. Phase IIa study of fenretinide in superficial bladder cancer, using DNA flow cytometry as an intermediate end point. J Natl Cancer Inst 1994;86(2):138–140.

49. Decensi A, Torrisi R, Bruno S, et al. Randomized trial of fenretinide in superficial bladder cancer using DNA flow cytometry as an intermediate end point. Cancer Epidemiol Biomarkers Prev 2000;9(10):1071–1078.

50. Torrisi R, Mezzetti M, Johansson H, et al. Time course of fenretinide-induced modulation of circulating insulin-like growth factor (IGF)-I, IGF-II and IGFBP-3 in a bladder cancer chemoprevention trial. Int J Cancer 2000;87(4):601–605.

51. Lerner SP, Sabichi AL, Grossman HB, et al. Results of a randomized chemoprevention trial with fenretinide in non-muscle invasive bladder cancer. J Urol 2005;173:246.

52. Virtamo J, Edwards BK, Virtanen M, et al. Effects of supplemental alpha-tocopherol and beta-carotene on urinary tract cancer: incidence and mortality in a controlled trial (Finland). Cancer Causes Control 2000;11(10):933–939.

53. Uchida K, Seidenfeld J, Rademaker A, Oyasu R. Inhibitory action of alpha-difluoromethylornithine on N-butyl-N-(4-hydroxybutyl)nitrosamine-induced rat urinary bladder carcinogenesis. Cancer Res 1989;49(19):5249–5253.

54. Loprinzi CL, Messing EM, O'Fallon JR, et al. Toxicity evaluation of difluoromethylornithine: doses for chemoprevention trials. Cancer Epidemiol Biomarkers Prev 1996;5(5):371–374.

55. Messina M, Barnes S. The role of soy products in reducing risk of cancer. J Natl Cancer Inst 1991;83(8):541–546.

56. Hakkak R, Korourian S, Ronis MJ, Johnston JM, Badger TM. Soy protein isolate consumption protects against azoxymethane-induced colon tumors in male rats. Cancer Lett 2001;166(1):27–32.

57. Ingram D, Sanders K, Kolybaba M, Lopez D. Case-control study of phyto-oestrogens and breast cancer. Lancet 1997;350(9083):990–994.

58. Shelnutt SR, Cimino CO, Wiggins PA, Badger TM. Urinary pharmacokinetics of the glucuronide and sulfate conjugates of genistein and daidzein. Cancer Epidemiol Biomarkers Prev 2000;9(4):413–419.

59. Zhou JR, Mukherjee P, Gugger ET, Tanaka T, Blackburn GL, Clinton SK. Inhibition of murine bladder tumorigenesis by soy isoflavones via alterations in the cell cycle, apoptosis, and angiogenesis. Cancer Res 1998;58(22):5231–5238.

60. Hursting SD, Perkins SN, Phang JM, Barrett JC. Diet and cancer prevention studies in p53-deficient mice. J Nutr 2001;131(11 Suppl):3092S–3094S.

61. Su SJ, Yeh TM, Lei HY, Chow NH. The potential of soybean foods as a chemoprevention approach for human urinary tract cancer. Clin Cancer Res 2000;6(1):230–236.

62. Dubois RN, Abramson SB, Crofford L, et al. Cyclooxygenase in biology and disease. FASEB J 1998;12(12):1063–1073.

63. Taketo MM. Cyclooxygenase-2 inhibitors in tumorigenesis (part I). J Natl Cancer Inst 1998;90(20):1529–1536.

64. Oshima M, Dinchuk JE, Kargman SL, et al. Suppression of intestinal polyposis in Apc delta 716 knockout mice by inhibition of cyclooxygenase 2 (COX-2). Cell 1996;87(5):803–809.

65. Giardiello FM, Offerhaus GJ, DuBois RN. The role of nonsteroidal anti-inflammatory drugs in colorectal cancer prevention. Eur J Cancer 1995;31A(7–8):1071–1076.

66. Steinbach G, Lynch PM, Phillips RK, et al. The effect of celecoxib, a cyclooxygenase-2 inhibitor, in familial adenomatous polyposis. N Engl J Med 2000;342(26):1946–1952.

67. Kargman SL, O'Neill GP, Vickers PJ, Evans JF, Mancini JA, Jothy S. Expression of prostaglandin G/H synthase-1 and -2 protein in human colon cancer. Cancer Res 1995;55(12):2556–2559.

68. Sano H, Kawahito Y, Wilder RL, et al. Expression of cyclooxygenase-1 and -2 in human colorectal cancer. Cancer Res 1995;55(17):3785–3789.

69. Komhoff M, Guan Y, Shappell HW, et al. Enhanced expression of cyclooxygenase-2 in high grade human transitional cell bladder carcinomas. Am J Pathol 2000;157(1):29–35.

70. Mohammed SI, Knapp DW, Bostwick DG, et al. Expression of cyclooxygenase-2 (COX-2) in human invasive transitional cell carcinoma (TCC) of the urinary bladder. Cancer Res 1999;59(22):5647–5650.

71. Shirahama T. Cyclooxygenase-2 expression is up-regulated in transitional cell carcinoma and its preneoplastic lesions in the human urinary bladder. Clin Cancer Res 2000;6(6):2424–2430.

72. Liu XH, Yao S, Kirschenbaum A, Levine AC. NS398, a selective cyclooxygenase-2 inhibitor, induces apoptosis and down-regulates bcl-2 expression in LNCaP cells. Cancer Res 1998;58(19):4245–4249.

73. Tsujii M, DuBois RN. Alterations in cellular adhesion and apoptosis in epithelial cells overexpressing prostaglandin endoperoxide synthase 2. Cell 1995;83(3):493–501.

74. Coffey RJ, Hawkey CJ, Damstrup L, et al. Epidermal growth factor receptor activation induces nuclear targeting of cyclooxygenase-2, basolateral release of prostaglandins, and mitogenesis in polarizing colon cancer cells. Proc Natl Acad Sci USA 1997;94(2):657–662.

75. Tong M, Tai HH. Induction of NAD(+)-linked 15-hydroxyprostaglandin dehydrogenase expression by androgens in human prostate cancer cells. Biochem Biophys Res Commun 2000;276(1):77–81.

76. Liebert M, Chen IL, Gebhardt D, et al. Loss of expression of prostaglandin dehydrogenase in human bladder cancers. Proc Am Assoc Cancer Res 1998; p 118.

77. Gee JR, Montoya RG, Khaled HM, Sabichi AL, Grossman HB. Cytokeratin 20, AN43, PGDH, and COX-2 expression in transitional and squamous cell carcinoma of the bladder. Urol Oncol 2003;21(4):266–270.

78. Okajima E, Denda A, Ozono S, et al. Chemopreventive effects of nimesulide, a selective cyclooxygenase-2 inhibitor, on the development of rat urinary bladder carcinomas initiated by N-butyl-N-(4-hydroxybutyl)nitrosamine. Cancer Res 1998;58(14):3028–3031.

79. Cook GP, Hampton JA. Effects of ibuprofen on the in vitro invasiveness of a human transitional cell carcinoma. Anticancer Res 1997;17(1A):365–368.

80. Shibata MA, Hasegawa R, Shirai T, Takesada Y, Fukushima S. Chemoprevention by indomethacin of tumor promotion in a rat urinary bladder carcinogenesis model. Int J Cancer 1993;55(6):1011–1017.

# Surrogate endpoint biomarkers

40

*Robert W Veltri*

## INTRODUCTION

The etiology and pathogenesis of bladder cancer is characterized by a complex matrix of host-determined (genetic and behavioral) and epigenetic or environmentally determined factors, which interact to generate cytologic and histologic alterations in the normal urothelium manifested as atypia, dysplasia, and/or anaplasia.[1-7] The incubation (latent) period for development of bladder cancer has been estimated to be about 20–25 years with a range of 5–50 years.[2-8] Chemical carcinogens such as benzidine-based dyes as well as 4,4'-methylenedianaline (MDA) and 4,4'-methylenebis (2-chloroanaline) (MBOCA) derived from occupational sources[8-12] are potent inducers of bladder cancer. Also, the by-products of pyrolysis from tobacco (aromatic hydrocarbons including β-naphthylamine and nitrosamines) are established bladder carcinogens.[9,13] Numerous other suspected carcinogens and cofactors (promoters) have been implicated in the cause of bladder cancer. Some of these include therapeutic drugs, chronic inflammation, bladder outlet obstruction, stones, coffee, saccharine, cyclamates, urinary tract infections, infestation with *Schistosoma haematobium*, etc.[1-3,9-14]

## BACKGROUND

It is generally accepted that bladder cancer develops along two biologic pathways, presenting about two-thirds of the time as a nonmuscle-invasive papillary type of disease growing out into the lumen of the bladder; following treatment, recurrence occurs in 60% to 70% of patients.[15,16] The second pathway develops as carcinoma in situ (CIS), and has a high propensity to invade and progress.[15,16] The molecular evolution of these two pathologic disease states when they become progressive has common elements of genomic instability which are demonstrable by microsatellite analysis or chromosome comparative hybridization (CGH).[15-19] However, the CIS pathway also has clear evidence of significant mutations in p53, deletion of the retinoblastoma (Rb) gene, and often losses of chromosome 9.[15-19] The genomic destabilization demonstrable by microsatellite analysis and CGH alone are insufficient to explain the mechanism of tumor progression. Progression requires other alterations at the level of oncogenes (amplifications), tumor suppressor genes (mutations and deletions), and methylation of promoter regulatory elements of genes important to cell growth, adhesion, death, motility, and invasion that are also required to drive tumor progression.[15-21] In the final analysis, understanding the biology and molecular evolution of bladder cancer provides opportunities for the improved early detection and treatment of patients with nonmuscle-invasive, locally advanced, and aggressive metastatic disease regardless of the histopathologic type—transitional cell carcinoma (TCC) or squamous cell carcinoma (SCC)—and racial origin. However, there is one critical additional feature of bladder cancer that produces a significant clinical dilemma for long-term management of the bladder cancer patient and that is tumor clonality.[22]

Tumor clonality has a significant impact on selection and implementation of surrogate endpoint biomarkers (SEBs); however, our current understanding of this phenomenon remains highly contentious with evidence supporting both monoclonality as well as oligoclonality.[21-29] The basis for this controversy depends, in part, on several variables including the biology of the type and amount of tumor being assessed (TCC versus SCC); the stage, grade, and location of the tumor; the method of sample collection and preservation; and the molecular analysis technology used. A recent in-depth analysis of the literature covering clonality, genetic, epigenetic, and tumor microenvironment of the transformed urothelium generated two theories to help explain this controversy[22]:

- a 'clonogenic theory' for multifocal and recurrent tumors suggesting they originate from a single clone
- a 'field change' resulting from multiple hits of molecular targets throughout the bladder and occasionally upper urinary tract generating multiple transformation events that evolve into mature tumors at different times.

Extreme examples that clearly demonstrate this divergence of scientific opinion of bladder cancer molecular heterogeneity range from one study involving global epigenetic (DNA methylation) mapping to assess multifocal low-grade tumors yielding evidence of oligoclonality,[29] to evaluation of complex multi-compartment muscle-invasive, high-grade bladder carcinoma demonstrating monoclonality based upon microsatellite analysis.[30,31] Therefore, once bladder cancer is diagnosed, and the pathologic as well as the molecular staging criteria already place the tumor at risk for progression, it might be best to treat it as an oligoclonal disease and perform additional testing to verify the presence or absence of a 'field effect' using organ-mapping biopsies to evaluate multiple molecular targets.[22] Certainly, in the future, one could envision highly engineered customized urine proteomic profiles and/or cDNA microarrays or biomarker panels, based upon comprehensive molecular pathology bladder cancer databases, to make such an assessment a part of routine clinical work-up of the bladder cancer patient. The urologist and patient should benefit from an earlier total characterization of the patient's bladder tumor pathologic and molecular grade and stage. This would allow for a more informed treatment plan that could include a profile of surrogate biomarkers as well as true clinical endpoints for characterizing each patient's risk for toxicity associated with the therapeutic regimen selected as well as a likelihood of a marked partial or complete clinical response. This approach should eventually lead to customized therapy guided by accurate pathologic (tumor and field areas) and newer molecular grading and staging criteria, resulting in the identification of clear specific molecular defects to target in patients with cancer of the upper and/or lower urinary tracts.[22,32,33]

In the area of biomarkers for bladder cancer detection there exists extensive literature, which is covered under the subject of cell- and soluble urine-based biologic markers (biomarkers) and urine proteomics in order to improve detection of primary and recurrent bladder cancer.[21,32-35] These topics are thoroughly addressed in Chapters 10, 12, 13, and 20 of this treatise on bladder cancer. The validation of any new detection biomarker will vary considerably, because this must always be decided based upon current accepted practice guidelines that include cytopathology and cystoscopy with biopsy interpretation. However, these fundamental pathologic and clinical practices vary considerably with regard to sensitivity and specificity.[35-37] Add to these variables the assay technical complexity, as well as clinical accuracy and reproducibility of the assay as has been demonstrated in numerous clinical trials, and the results in routine clinical practice often do not reproduce those achieved in controlled clinical trials.[34-39]

For biomarkers that finally do make it to the clinic following regulatory approval, several fail to become accepted into routine clinical practice, perhaps due to flaws in the original clinical trial designs that may have included methods of specimen acquisition and preservation, central versus multiple test site processing of clinical samples, variations in interpreting the cytology, and biopsy. An example of one such test that has proved to work well in conjunction with routine cytology to detect bladder cancer is the fluorescent in situ hybridization (FISH) test that employs four molecular targets to detect bladder cancer.[36-40] The final step in this process of acceptance into clinical practice concerns the cost–benefit analysis as it relates to a biomarker replacing cystoscopy; although the final decision is not yet in, there is evidence mounting that this first step may be feasible.[39,41]

# DEFINITIONS

Most of the above cited critical clinical biomarker validation issues carry over into this review because ultimately it will be the patient's response to an intervention, as well as the urologist's acceptance of the technology into routine clinical practice, that will become the basis for concluding efficacy of 'surrogate endpoint biomarkers' (SEBs). The following is an attempt to survey the field of SEBs as it applies to bladder cancer and to apply definitions established by the Biomarkers Definitions Working Group,[42] which include the following:

1. *Biologic marker* (biomarker): 'A characteristic that is objectively measured and evaluated as an indicator of biologic or pathogenic processes, or pharmacologic responses to a therapeutic intervention.' Biomarkers have been used for diagnosis, staging, prognosis, and for monitoring response to an intervention.

2. *Clinical endpoint biomarker* (CEB): 'A characteristic or variable that reflects how a patient feels, functions, or survives.' The authors further state that such endpoints are the most credible and distinct measurements or analyses of disease characteristics observed in a study or clinical trial involving a therapeutic intervention.[42]

3. *Surrogate endpoint biomarker* (SEB): As it relates to the use of a surrogate biomarker for evaluation of a treatment, in 1989 Prentice developed a formal and statistical definition of a surrogate as 'a response variable for which a test of the null hypothesis of the relationship to the treatment groups under comparison is also a valid test of the corresponding null hypothesis based upon the true endpoint'.[43] Prentice also provided a set of objective statistical criteria that could be applied if the endpoint is binary. Subsequently, Freedman supplemented these criteria using the 'proportion explained', which is the proportion of treatment effect mediated by the SEB.[44] Finally, Buyse and Molenberghs[45] replaced the 'proportion explained' with two quantities:

 • the relative effect linking the treatment response to both the surrogate (S) and true (T) endpoints
 • the individual level association between the surrogate (S) and true (T) endpoints, after accounting for treatment response ('adjusted association').

For the purposes of this review, the definition used is simply stated as: 'A biomarker that is intended to substitute for a clinical or "true" endpoint.'[42]

Therefore, the definition applied here includes treatment assessment as defined above and potentially other applications as they apply to an SEB, i.e. it is expected to predict clinical benefit (or harm) or lack of benefit (or harm), based upon established epidemiologic, therapeutic, pathophysiologic, or other scientific evidence (Box 40.1).[42] Importantly, as mentioned above, SEBs represents a subset of bio-

markers that prove clinically useful primarily in determining, for example, the value of a therapeutic or chemopreventive agent. Occasionally, an SEB may be applied in natural history of disease or epidemiologic studies. An effective SEB that has been applied in a clinical trial ultimately should become a part of clinical practice in the management of the disease being studied.

The position of the Food and Drug Administration (FDA) on the use of a SEB is one of cautious optimism. They will accept the use of a SEB based upon the above definitions, provided that the clinical trial using a SEB will continue beyond approval until a clinical or 'true' benefit outcome is determined and the use of the SEB has been validated.[46] Any clinical trial designed with the use of a SEB will include in the design sufficient follow-up to eventually prove the clinical (true endpoint) benefit predicted by the SEB and that such studies will be carried out with due diligence. The reason the FDA is so cautious relates to the limitations that exist to the application of surrogate endpoints in place of true clinical endpoints; for example, the sample size for the application of a SEB in a clinical trial may be lower than what would be required for a true clinical endpoint. However, the true clinical endpoint may be more demanding, especially in randomized phase III clinical trials for new treatments as opposed to phase II clinical trials, which are preliminary studies of efficacy.[47,48] In the case of bladder cancer clinical trials, if the patient cohort has advanced disease or is at high risk for progression, the clinical or 'true' endpoint is likely to be achievable within a reasonable time frame (1–5 years) and hence both the SEB and the clinical endpoint can be validated.

## PROPOSED SEB EVALUATION AND VALIDATION

### PHASE I: IDENTIFY

Identification of strong SEB candidates should be based upon highly specific molecular targets, substantiated by multiple, well-designed published studies and targeted to clinically achievable and useful outcomes (epidemiologic; assessment of treatment intervention; predicts toxicity, pathologic status, and clinical benefit, etc.) with nominal sample sizes that include controls. In addition, the assay format and patient cohort demographics need to be comparable so as to allow data pooling.

### PHASE II: REASSESS

Phase II involves reassessment of SEB candidates employing well-characterized approved and HIPAA (Health Insurance Portability and Accountability Act)

---

**Box 40.1** Surrogate biomarker objectives

1. Therapy
 • Select patients
 • Evaluate toxicity
 • Select effective drug dose
 • Predict clinical response
 • Predict nonclinical response (e.g. quality of life)

2. Epidemiology
 • Predict occupational risk
 • Predict smoking risk
 • Predict susceptibility (genetic) risk

3. Prognosis
 • Extent of cancer (pathologic stage)
 • Type (transitional cell carcinoma, squamous cell carcinoma, or mixed)
 • Grade
 • Molecular grade and staging

compliant larger sample sets that target the surrogate and true clinical outcome of interest. Notable for this phase of development is the requirement for a single assay format (immunoassay or molecular based) that is standardized, accurate, and reproducible. Under these conditions, in the case of bladder cancer, because the incidence is lower, these studies, in order to be successful, usually require multi-institutional participation to achieve the sample size criterion required for statistical validity. These studies should be prospective if the 'true' clinical endpoint occurs within a reasonable time frame (e.g. 1–3 years), with high grade or stage T1 with CIS or T2–4 disease, and retrospective if the clinical outcome takes much longer and the biomarker can be reliably assessed in archived material; for example, in the case of low-grade Ta superficial disease, where recurrence may be a shorter-term clinical endpoint, but in the case of progression it might take several years and one may be assessing a chemopreventive agent.

## PHASE III: VALIDATE

In this phase the candidate SEB is validated with new prospective multi-institutional IRB (Institutional Review Board) approved and HIPAA compliant patient cohorts. These studies should be designed and carried out prospectively, and include both the surrogate and clinical endpoints; they must also include appropriate control populations. At this point the assay protocol is fully validated as a standard operating procedure (SOP) with appropriate laboratory quality systems documentation in place.[49] The ultimate objective is to ensure that every aspect of test design, development, production, installation, clinical laboratory certifications, and servicing related to the laboratory procedure are thoroughly documented, implemented, and maintained. These studies will also provide a basis for regulatory approval of the SEB in a service pathology laboratory environment, hospital or doctor's office, dependent on the level of assay complexity.

## PHASE IV: ESTABLISH

In this phase the SEB is established as a clinical guideline to manage patients. In order to apply the new technology for patient care, the test will need to have been formatted and delivered commercially, and this will require appropriate regulatory approval for purposes of reimbursement authorization by Medicare or third party payers. The regulatory approval process will vary considerably depending on the type of assay, and its level of complexity, as well as the laboratory testing environment where the test will be provided. If the test is to be manufactured for commercial distribution, and is to be delivered from an automated instrument platform, then FDA approval is required.

Notably at this time, the FDA is structured to approve the safety and effectiveness of a medical device to meet specific claims (monitoring, screening, prognosis, etc.) of new cancer biomarker assays, either under a 510(k) notification (based upon an existing or predicate or equivalent device; examples include the BTA or NMP22 urine test) or a premarket approval (PMA). However, in the case of a new cancer biomarker for prognosis, it is likely to be classified as a class III medical device unless it was introduced or delivered for interstate commerce or commercial distribution before May 28, 1976, therefore requiring a PMA process, which can be quite complex, time consuming, and costly. Any reclassification of a class III medical device to class I or II requires a stringent review of the new device to determine if it has sufficient regulatory controls to provide reasonable assurance of its safety and effectiveness for its intended use. On January 21, 2004, the FDA cleared for reclassification a new breast cancer test manufactured by Veridex LLC (a Johnson & Johnson company) from a class III to a class II device. This decision was based upon solid evidence for good manufacturing practices and performance data to verify claims.[50,51] The new device is referred to as CellSearch™ Epithelial Cell Kit/CellSpotter™ Analyzer, and the FDA now defines this generic type of device as 21 CFR 866.6020—immunomagnetic circulating cancer cell selection and enumeration system—which consists of biologic probes, fluorochromes, and other reagents; preservation and preparation devices; and semi-automated analytical instruments to select and count circulating cancer cells in a prepared sample of whole blood. This device is intended for adjunctive use in monitoring or predicting breast cancer disease progression, response to therapy, and for the detection of recurrent disease. Interestingly, there are at least two recent manuscripts describing detection of peripheral blood circulating bladder cancer cells in patients with advanced disease: one uses MUC7 as the biomarker and reverse transcriptase-polymerase chain reaction (RT-PCR) for detection,[52] the other uses the CD45 biomarker and immunomagnetic technology to detect such cells.[53]

## SEBS IN THE MANAGEMENT OF BLADDER CANCER

With the above background, definitions, and suggested schema for development of SEBs for specific applications in the management of bladder cancer, do we actually have any bladder cancer biomarkers that can meet these criteria for any use defined in Box 40.1. After review of several publications, as well as review of select bladder cancer clinical trials, the following likely SEB candidates have been chosen for consideration: Figure

40.1 demonstrates the sourcing process for SEB selection; Figure 40.2 illustrates a possible therapeutic intervention model adapted from the Biomarkers Definitions Working Group.[42] The basis for a decision to choose an intervention for curing bladder cancer other than cystectomy requires that the alternative be equally efficacious and be based upon accurate staging and grading of the disease.[54,55] The current review would suggest adding an additional quality assurance layer to accurately stage and grade the cancer at the molecular level.[16–33]

A number of recent reviews list some potential prognostic biomarkers that predict recurrence and/or progression in bladder cancer that can be categorized as oncogenes (i.e. cH-ras, c-myc, Her2/neu) or tumor suppressor genes based upon loss of heterozygosity and CGH technology that are located on chromosomes 9, 13, and 17 and include several clinically important genes (p16$^{INK4A}$, RB, p53, p21$^{WAF/Cip1}$, p27$^{Kip1}$, cyclins D and E).[56–58] In addition, next generation technology has utilized molecular profiling with cDNA microarrays to analyze mRNA from bladder cell lines and tissue to identify new candidate biomarkers as well as substantiate biomarkers identified by the other methods described above.[59–62] Finally, several investigators have also used this global approach using cDNA microarrays as well as global assessment of epigenetic and gene-specific methylation patterns to characterize bladder cancer recurrence and progression.[29,63–66]

The results of these surveys have generated several specific candidate biomarkers and molecular profiles that target recurrence, progression, and new potential

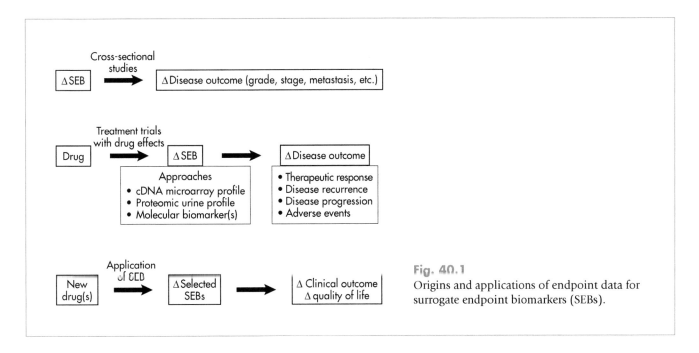

**Fig. 40.1**
Origins and applications of endpoint data for surrogate endpoint biomarkers (SEBs).

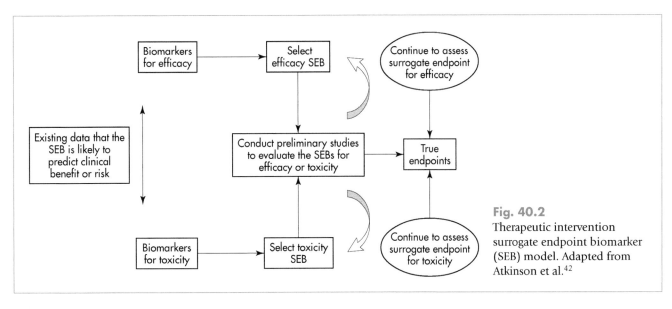

**Fig. 40.2**
Therapeutic intervention surrogate endpoint biomarker (SEB) model. Adapted from Atkinson et al.[42]

therapeutic targets that involve biologic characteristics of invasion and metastasis, including oncogenes, tumor suppressor genes, promoter methylation patterns, programmed cell death, angiogenesis, etc. It should also be borne in mind that bladder cancer is not one disease, but rather it may take two separate pathways to disease progression with markedly different time requirements for evolution. This dual pathway of bladder cancer pathogenesis is illustrated in a review by Marta Sanchez-Carbayo (Figure 40.3).[60] Even this model, however, lacks the integration of possible roles of promoter gene-specific methylation,[66] stroma field effects,[22,67] and other chromosome deletions[55,68] that have been demonstrated in bladder carcinoma. With this overview as a backdrop, it is possible to review a few very specific likely SEB candidates for bladder cancer using the four phase development criteria outlined above and the schema presented in Figure 40.2.

## MUTATION IN FIBROBLAST GROWTH RECEPTOR FACTOR 3 (FGFR3)

Point mutations of the FGFR3 gene are well documented in achondroplasia and thanatophoric dysplasia, and were observed in sporadic cancers including bladder cancer.[69] Mutations in bladder cancer

have proven to be strong correlates to a good prognosis.[70,71] Recently, point mutations in the FGFR3 gene have been reported to occur in 88% of the well-differentiated transitional cell carcinoma (Ta) grade 1 tumors that had a most favorable prognosis, whereas only 16% of grade 3 tumors having a poor prognosis demonstrated such mutations.[72] The assay format is a DNA, PCR-based procedure that has been shown to be accurate and highly reproducible. Therefore, the FGFR3 gene is a candidate SEB that may be useful for molecular grading and staging of superficial Ta papillary tumors, and potentially useful for stratification of patients for chemoprevention trials and certain therapeutic trials for patients lacking such mutations. It can therefore be concluded that this candidate SEB is ready for phase III according to the above scheme.

## CYTOGENETICALLY DETERMINED LOSS OF CHROMOSOME 9

This chromosomal aberration is the first and most common genetic loss identified in bladder cancer.[56,57] Chromosome 9 monosomy has proved accurate in predicting recurrence.[74] Stadler et al[74] subsequently confirmed that chromosome 9 losses (9p21) occurred early in bladder oncogenesis and before p53 alterations

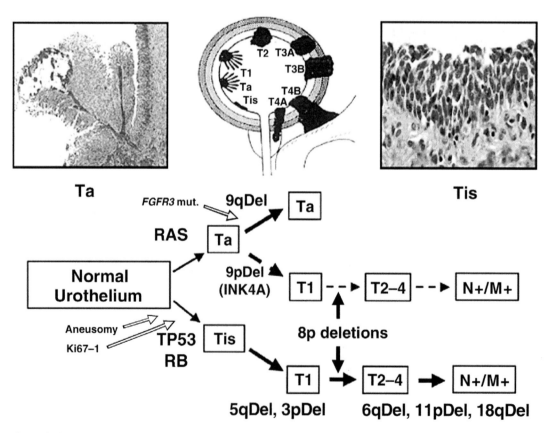

**Fig. 40.3**
Two major progression pathway molecular models for bladder cancer. Modified from Sanchez-Carbayo.[60]

or development of aneusomy or genomic destabilization, making it a useful early marker to identify patients at high risk for disease progression.[73,74] This has been repeatedly illustrated in several models such as the one shown in Figure 40.3 for the molecular pathway to progression of bladder cancer. The author therefore proposes that a second phase III candidate SEB for molecular staging of bladder cancer should be chromosome 9 assessment by FISH analysis for microsatellite markers on chromosome 9p21. The proper reagents and methodology for assaying these aberrances is readily available, and the assay can be reproducibly performed using FISH.[73–75] In fact, the 9p21 marker is also one of the FISH probes included in the commercially available four-marker bladder detection Vysis assay.[40]

## CELL CYCLE REGULATORY PATHWAY (P53, P21, PRB/P16)

The importance of one or more members of this group of prognostic indicators has provided reproducible results for molecular staging and prognosis and recently for the prediction of clinical outcome.[56,76–78] A limitation of this approach has been the application of immuno-histochemistry technology utilizing a variety of specific antibodies with different requirements for meeting performance specifications. However, most of these problems have been resolved and investigators have moved toward use of similar reagents and methods.[78,79] Recent follow-up investigations by at least one group have generated strong support for p53, p21, and other members of the cell cycle regulatory repertoire being predictive of clinical outcome.[80] In fact, a National Cancer Institute (NCI) sponsored multicenter clinical trial has been established, which is to enroll 760 patients from over 30 hospitals around the world. The trial is termed 'MVAC in Organ-Confined Bladder Cancer Based on p53 Status'. The protocol can be found on the NCI website http://www.nci.nih.gov/clinicaltrials/ or at http://www.hopkinskimmelcancercenter.org/clinicaltrials/index.cfm?action=3&protocolnumber=J9849/. The other genes being assessed in the cystectomy specimens include RB, p21, and p16. Patients are registered for the trial within 9 weeks of their cystectomy. The tumor is then analyzed for p53; abnormal p53 cases go to randomization for MVAC or routine follow-up, with normal p53 cases also going to routine follow-up. Clearly, p53 and possibly p21 can be considered prognostic molecular staging SEBs that meet the phase III criteria outlined above.

At present there is no phase IV SEB for bladder cancer as defined above. However, there are some upcoming candidate phase II biomarkers that should provide new SEB applications for development as outlined in Box 40.1 and categorized below:

- *Epidemiology*: use of biomarkers for genotoxicity[81–83]
- *Prognosis*: aberrant methylation, either global or gene-specific[66,84,85]; high throughput cDNA microarray patterns[60–64]; image-based nuclear morphometric analysis[86–90]
- *Therapy*: applications for targeted gene, immuno- and radiotherapy.[91–95]

## CONCLUSION

Numerous other molecular- and immunoassay-based technologies are omitted from this review; however, most of these biomarkers are being evaluated for detection and diagnosis, not as SEBs as surrogates for clinical outcomes. The future of the SEB field will require close attention to a system for selection, technology validation, and a well-conceived clinical trial design to implement the SEB in a manner that will eventually lead to making its application a 'clinical practice guideline'.

Whenever this entire process is initiated, or moving from phase II to phases III–IV, it will be extremely critical to work in close association with the FDA to preplan SEB forecasted regulatory claims that are being anticipated. These discussions will require significant cross-talk that will involve clear and concise discussions about the technologies, as well as the biomarkers intended for use, and all limitations relating to the manufacture, distribution, sale, and reimbursement-related issues surrounding the use of the instrumentation and reagents as well as test result interpretation. All the groups involved in discovery, development, and release to market of new SEBs—academic leaders, diagnostic companies, large pharmacologic and government agencies—will need to participate in the discussions with the FDA in order to ensure success. The final layer to this process will be to strive for the application of ISO9000-rated processes that will put in place the necessary documentation for adherence to 'quality systems'[49] practices in the manufacture of instrumentation, reagents, kits, etc. as well as the delivery of these tests and results to the end users (hospitals, service clinical pathology laboratories, and doctors' offices) on behalf of the final recipients of the reported results for implementation, the doctor and the patient.

### REFERENCES

1. Greenlee RT, Hill-Harmon MB, Murray T, Thun M. Cancer statistics. CA Cancer J Clin 2001;51:15–36.
2. Smart CR. Bladder cancer survival statistics. J Occup Med 1990;32:927–928.
3. el-Mawla NG, el-Bolkainy MN, Khaled HM. Bladder cancer in Africa: update. Semin Oncol 2001;12:174–178.
4. Prout GR, Wesley MN, Greenberg RS, et al. Bladder cancer: race differences in extent of disease at diagnosis. Cancer 2000;89:349–358.

5. Michaud DS, Clinton SK, Rimm EB, Willet WC, Giovannucci E. Risk of bladder cancer by geographic region in a U.S. cohort of male health professionals. Epidemiology 2001;6:719–726.

6. Mostofi FK, Davis CJ, Sesterhenn IA. Current understanding of pathology of bladder cancer and attendant problems. J Occup Med 1990;32:793–796.

7. Feldman AR, Kessler L, Myers MH, Naughton MD. The prevalence of cancer: estimates based on the Connecticut tumor registry. N Engl J Med 1986;315:1394–1397.

8. Hoover R, Cole P. Temporal aspects of bladder carcinogenesis. N Engl J Med 1973;288:1040–1045.

9. Kogevinas M, Trichopoulos D. Urinary bladder cancer. In Adami HO, Hunter D, Trichopoulos V (eds): Textbook of Cancer Epidemiology. New York: Oxford University Press, 2002, pp 446–466.

10. Ward E, Carpenter A, Markowitz S, et al. Excess number of bladder cancers in workers exposed to ortho-toluidine and aniline. J Natl Cancer Inst 1991;83:501–506.

11. Marsh GM, Leviton LC, Talbott EO, et al. Drake chemical workers' health registry study: 1. Notification and medical surveillance of a group of workers at high risk of developing bladder cancer. Am J Ind Med 1991;19:291–301.

12. Schulte PA, Ringen K, Hemstreet GO, Ward E. Occupational cancer of the urinary tract. J Occup Med 1987;2:85–107.

13. Morrison AS, Buring JE, Veerhoek WG, et al. An international study of smoking and bladder cancer. J Urol 1984;131:650–654.

14. Mostafa MH, Shewata SA, O'Connor PJ. Relationship between schistosomiasis and bladder cancer. Clin Microbiol Rev 1999;12:97–111.

15. Jones PA, Droller MJ. Pathways of development and progression in bladder cancer: new correlations between clinical and molecular mechanisms. Semin Urol 1993;11(4):177–192.

16. Spruck CH, Ohneseit PF, Gonzalez-Zulueta M, et al. Two molecular pathways to transitional cell carcinoma of the bladder. Cancer Res 1994;54:784–788.

17. van Tilborg Angel AG, de Vries A, de Bont M, Groenfeld LE, van der Kwast TH, Zwarthoff EC. Molecular evolution of multiple recurrent cancers of the bladder. Hum Mol Genet 2000;9:2973–2980.

18. Brandau S, Bohle A. Bladder cancer I. Molecular and genetic basis of carcinogenesis. Eur Urol 2001;39:491–497.

19. Knowles MA. What we could do now: molecular pathology of bladder cancer. J Clin Pathol 2001;54:215–221.

20. Brandau S, Bohle A. Bladder cancer I. Molecular and genetic basis of carcinogenesis. Eur Urol 2001;39:491–497.

21. Kausch I, Bohle A. Bladder cancer II. Molecular aspects and diagnosis. Eur Urol 2001;39:498–506.

22. Duggan BJ, Gray SB, McKnight JJ, Watson CJ, Johnston SR, Williamson KE. Oligoclonality in bladder cancer: the implication for molecular therapies. J Urol 2004;171:419–425.

23. Paiss T, Wöhr G, Hautmann RH, Mattfeldt T, Müller M, Haeussler J, Vogel W. Some tumors of the bladder are polyclonal in origin. J Urol 2002;167:718–723.

24. Hafner C, Knuechel R, Zanardo L, et al. Evidence for oligoclonality and tumor spread by intraluminal seeding in multifocal urothelial carcinomas of the upper and lower urinary tract. Oncogene 2001;20:4909–4915.

25. Louhelainen J, Wukström H, Hemminki K. Allelic losses demonstrate monoclonality of multifocal bladder tumors. Int J Cancer 2000;87:522–527.

26. Kang C-H, Yu T-J, Hsieh H-H, et al. The development of bladder tumors and contralateral upper urinary tract tumors after primary transitional cell carcinoma of the upper tract. Cancer 2003;98:1620–1626.

27. Vriesema JLJ, Aben KKH, Witjes JA, Kiemeney LALM, Schalken JA. Superficial and metachronous invasive bladder carcinomas are clonally related. Int J Cancer 2001;93:699–702.

28. Takahashi T, Habuchi T, Kakehi Y, Okuno H, Terachi T, Kato T, Ogawa O. Molecular diagnosis of metastatic origin in a patient with metachronous multiple cancers of the renal pelvis and bladder. Urology 2000;56:331–333.

29. Markl ID, Cheng J, Liang G, Shibata D, Laird PW, Jones PA. Global and gene-specific epigenetic patterns in human bladder cancer genomes are relatively stable in vivo and in vitro over time. Cancer Res 2001;61:5875–5884.

30. Hartmann A, Rosner RU, Schlake G, Dietmaier W, Zaak D, Hofstaedter F, Knuechel R. Clonality and genetic divergence in multifocal low-grade superficial urothelial carcinoma as determined by chromosome 9 and p53 deletion analysis. Lab Invest 2000;80:709–718.

31. Diaz-Cano SJ, Blanes A, Matilla A, Wolfe HJ. Molecular evolution and intratumor heterogeneity by topographic compartments in muscle invasive transitional cell carcinoma of the urinary bladder. Lab Invest 2000;80:278–289.

32. Saint F, Salomon L, Quintela R, Cicco A, Hoznek A, Abbou CC, Chopin DK. Do prognostic parameters of remission versus relapse after Bacille Calmette-Guérin (BCG) immunotherapy exist? Analysis of a quarter century of literature. Eur Urol 2003;43:351–361.

33. Sidransky D. Emerging molecular markers of cancer. Nat Rev 2002;2:210–219.

34. Mariani AJ, Mariani MC, Macchioni C, Stams UL, Hariharan A, Moriera A. The significance of adult hematuria: 1,000 hematuria evaluations including a risk–benefit and cost-effectiveness analysis. J Urol 1989;141:350–355.

35. Bastacky S, Ibrahim S, Wilczynski SP, et al. The accuracy of urinary cytology in daily practice. Cancer 1999;87:118–128.

36. Witjes JA. Bladder carcinoma in situ in 2003: state of the art. Eur Urol 2004;45:142–146.

37. Dey P. Urinary markers in bladder carcinoma [review]. Clin Chim Acta 2004;340:57–65.

38. Friedrich MG, Hellstrom A, Toma MI, Hammerer P, Huland H. Are false-positive urine markers for the detection of bladder carcinoma really wrong or do they predict tumor recurrence? Eur Urol 2003;43:146–151.

39. Simon MA, Lokeshwar VB, Soloway MS. Current bladder cancer tests: unnecessary or beneficial? Crit Rev Oncol/Hematol 2003;47:91–107.

40. Veeramachaneni R, Nordberg ML, Shi R, Herrera GA, Turbat-Herrera EA. Evaluation of fluorescence in situ hybridization as an ancillary tool to urine cytology in diagnosing urothelial carcinoma. Diag Cytopathol 2003;28:301–307.

41. Lotan Y, Roehrborn CG. Cost-effectiveness of a modified care protocol substituting bladder tumor markers for cystoscopy for the follow-up of patients with transitional cell carcinoma of the bladder: a decision analytical approach. J Urol 2002;167:75–79.

42. Atkinson AJ, Magnuson WG, Colburn WA, et al. Biomarkers and surrogate endpoints: preferred definitions and conceptual framework. Commentary. Clin Pharmacol Ther 2001;69:89–95.

43. Prentice RL. Surrogate markers endpoints in clinical trials: definition and operational criteria. Stat Med 1989;8:431–440.

44. Freedman LS, Graubard BI, Schatzkin A. Statistical validation of intermediate endpoints for chronic diseases. Stat Med 1992;11:167–178.

45. Buyse M, Molenberghs G. Approximate inference in generalized linear mixed models. J Am Stat Assoc 1993;88:9–25.

46. Food and Drug Modernization Act 1997. Title 21 Code of Federal Regulations, Part 314, Subpart H, Section 314.500. Washington, DC: Food and Drug Administration, 1997.

47. DeMets DL. Statistical issues in interpreting clinical trials. J Intern Med 2004;255:529–537.

48. Schatzkin A, Gail M. The promise and peril of surrogate end points in cancer research. Nat Rev 2002;2:1–9.

49. Berte LM, Nevalainen DE. Quality Systems for the Laboratory. Chicago: American Society of Clinical Pathologists, 2000.

50. Tibbe AG, de Grooth BG, Greve J, Dolan GJ, Terstappen LW. Imaging technique implemented in CellTracks system. Cytometry 2002;47(4):248–255.

51. Hayes DF, Walker TM, Singh B, et al. Monitoring expression of HER-2 on circulating epithelial cells in patients with advanced breast cancer. Int J Oncol 2002;21:1111–1117.

52. Kinjo M, Okegawa T, Horie S, Nutahara K, Higashihara E. Detection of circulating MUC7-positive cells by reverse transcription-polymerase

chain reaction in bladder cancer patients. Int J Urol 2004;11(1):38–43.

53. Meye A, Bilkenroth U, Schmidt U, et al. Isolation and enrichment of urologic tumor cells in blood samples by a semi-automated CD45 depletion autoMACS protocol. Int J Oncol 2002;21(3):521–530.

54. Stein JP, Skinner DG. Results with radical cystectomy for treating bladder cancer: a 'reference standard' for high-grade, invasive bladder cancer. BJU Int 2003;92:12–17.

55. Stein JP. Indications for early cystectomy. Urology 2003;62:591–595.

56. Kausch I, Böhle A. Molecular aspects of bladder cancer: III. prognostic markers of bladder cancer. Eur Urol 2002;41:15–29.

57. Quek ML, Quinn DI, Daneshmand S, Stein JP. Molecular prognostication in bladder cancer—a current perspective. Eur J Cancer 2003;39:1501–1510.

58. Stein JP, GrossFeld GD, Ginsberg DA, et al. A contemporary review of the literature. J Urol 1998;160:645–659.

59. Duggan BJ, McKnight JJ, Williamson KE, et al. The need to embrace molecular profiling of tumor cells in prostate and bladder cancer. Clin Cancer Res 2003;9:1240–1247.

60. Sanchez-Carbayo M. Use of high-throughput DNA microarrays to identify biomarkers for bladder cancer. Clin Chemistry 2003;49:23–31.

61. Dyrskjot L, Thykjaer T, Kruhoffer M, et al. Identifying distinct classes of bladder carcinoma using microarrays. Nat Genet 2003;33:90–97.

62. Sanchez-Carbayo M, Cordon-Cardo C. Applications of array technology: identification of molecular targets in bladder cancer. Br J Cancer 2003;89:2172–2177.

63. van Tilborg AAG, de Vries A, de Bont M, et al. Molecular evolution of multiple recurrent cancers of the bladder. Hum Mol Genet 2003;9:2973–2980.

64. Sanchez-Carbayo M, Socci ND, Charytonowicz E, et al. Molecular profiling of bladder cancer using cDNA microarrays: defining histogenesis and biological phenotype. Cancer Res 2002;62:6973–6980.

65. Sanchez-Carbayo M, Socci ND, Lozano JJ, et al. Gene discovery in bladder cancer progression using cDNA microarrays. Am J Pathol 2003;163:505–516.

66. Muruyama R, Toyooka S, Toyooka KO, et al. Aberrant promoter methylation profile of bladder cancer and is relationship to clinicopathological features. Cancer Res 2001;61:8659–8663.

67. Paterson RF, Ulbright TM, MacLennan GT, et al. Molecular genetic alterations in the laser-capture-microdissected stroma adjacent to bladder carcinoma. Cancer 2003;98:1830–1836.

68. Knowles MA. What we could do now: molecular pathology of bladder cancer. J Clin Pathol 2001;54:215–221.

69. Sibley K, Stern P, Knowles MA. Frequency of fibroblast growth factor receptor 3 mutations in sporadic tumours. Oncogene 2001;20:4416–4468.

70. Billerey C, Chopin D, Aubriot-Lorton MH, et al. Frequent FGFR3 mutations in papillary non-invasive bladder (pTa) tumors. Am J Pathol 2001;158:1955–1959.

71. van Rhijn BW, Lurkin I, Radvanyi F, Kirkels WJ, van der Kwast TH, Zwarthoff EC. The fibroblast growth factor receptor 3 (FGFR3) mutation is a strong indicator of superficial bladder cancer with low recurrence rate. Cancer Res 2001;61(4):1265–1268.

72. Bas WG, van Rhijn AN, van der Kwast TH, et al. Molecular grading of urothelial cell carcinoma with fibroblast growth factor receptor 3 and MIB-1 is superior to pathologic grade for the prediction of clinical outcome. J Clin Oncol 2003;21:1912–1921.

73. Jung I, Reeder JE, Cox C, et al. Chromosome 9 monosomy by fluorescence in situ hybridization of bladder irrigation specimens is predictive of tumor recurrence. J Urol 1999;162:1900–1903.

74. Stadler WM, Steinberg G, Yang X, et al. Alterations of the 9p21 and 9q33 chromosomal bands in clinical bladder cancer specimens by fluorescence in situ hybridization. Clin Cancer Res 2001;7:1676–1682.

75. Cheng L, Bostwick DG, Li G, Zhang S, Vortmeyer AO, Zhuang Z. Conserved genetic findings in metastatic bladder cancer: a possible utility of allelic loss of chromosomes 9p21 and 17p13 in diagnosis. Arch Pathol Lab Med 2001;125:1197–1199.

76. Stein JP, GrossFeld GD, Ginsberg DA, et al. A contemporary review of the literature. J Urol 1998;160:645–659.

77. Chatterjee SJ, Datar R, Youssefzadeh D, et al. Combined effects of p53, p21, and pRb expression in the progression of bladder transitional cell carcinoma. J Clin Oncol 2004;22(6):1007–1013.

78. Tokunaga H, Shariat SF, Green AE, Brown RM, Zhou J-H, Benedict WF, Lerner SP. Correlation of immunohistochemical molecular staging of bladder biopsies and radical cystectomy specimens. Int J Radiol 2001;51:16–22.

79. Cordon-Cardo C. p53 and RB: simple interesting correlates or Tumor markers of critical predictive nature? [Editorial] J Clin Oncol 2004;22:975–977.

80. Shariat SF, Tokunaga H, Zhou JH, Kim JH, Ayala GE, Benedict WF, Lerner SP. P53, p21, pRB, and p16 expression predict clinical outcome in cystectomy with bladder cancer. J Clin Oncol 2004;22:1014–1024.

81. Taylor JA, Umbach DM, Stephens E, et al. The role of N-acetylation polymorphisms in smoking-associated bladder cancer: evidence of a gene–gene exposure three way interaction. Cancer Res 1998;58:3603–3610.

82. Hein DW, Doll MA, Fretland AJ, et al. Molecular genetics and epidemiology of the NAT1 and NAT2 acetylation polymorphisms. Cancer Epidemiol Biomarkers Prev 2000;9:29–42.

83. Thier R, Bruning T, Roos PH, Rihs HP, Golka K, Ko Y, Bolt HM. Markers of genetic susceptibility in human environmental hygiene and toxicology: the role of selected CYP, NAT, and GST genes. Int J Environ Health 2003;206:149–171.

84. Markl IDC, Cheng J, Liang G, Shibata D, Laird PW, Jones PA. Global and gene-specific epigenetic patterns in human bladder cancer genomes are relatively stable in vivo and in vitro over time. Cancer Res 2001;61:5875–5884.

85. Lee M-G, Kim H-Y, Byun D-S, et al. Frequent epigenetic inactivation of RASSF1A in human bladder cancer. Cancer Res 2001;61:6688–6692.

86. Shankey TV, Jin J-K, Dougherty S, Gandhi K, Pyle J. An overview of clinical applications for multi-parameter flow and image cytometry of urologic malignancies. Cancer Mol Biol 1994;1:19–25.

87. Palcic B. Nuclear texture: can it be used as a surrogate endpoint biomarker? J Cell Biochem 1994;19(Suppl):40–46.

88. Richman A, Mayne S, Jekel J, Albertsen P. Image analysis combined with visual cytology in the early detection of recurrent bladder carcinoma. Cancer 1998;82(9):1738–1748.

89. Slaton JW, Dinney CPN, Veltri RW, Miller MC, Liebert M, O'Dowd GJ, Grossman HB. DNA ploidy enhances the cytological prediction of recurrent transitional cell carcinoma of the bladder. J Urol 1997;158:806–811.

90. Veltri RW, Partin AW, Miller, MC. Quantitative nuclear grade (QNG): a new image analysis-based biomarker of clinically relevant nuclear structure alterations. J Cell Biochem 2000;35(Suppl):151–157.

91. Altieri DC. Validating survivin as a cancer therapeutic target. Nat Rev 2003;3:48–54.

92. Sjostrom J, Blomqvist C, Heikkila P, et al. Predictive value of p53, mdm-2, p21, and mib-1 for chemotherapy response in advanced breast cancer. Clin Cancer Res 2000;6:3103–3110.

93. Rotterud R, Berner A, Holm R, Skovlund E, Fossa SD. p53, p21 and mdm-2 expression vs. response to radiotherapy in transitional cell carcinoma of the bladder. BJU Int 2001;88:202–208.

94. Decensi A, Torrisi R, Bruno S, et al. Randomized trial of fenretinide in superficial bladder cancer using DNA flow cytometry as an intermediate end point. Cancer Epidemiol Biomarkers Prev 2000;9:1071–1078.

95. Saint F, Salomon L, Quintela R, Cicco A, Hoznek A, Abbou CC, Chopin DK. Do prognostic parameters of remission versus relapse after Bacille Calmette–Guérin (BCG) immunotherapy exist? Analysis of a quarter century of literature. Eur Urol 2003;43:351–361.

# T2–4

# Follow-up strategies in superficial bladder cancer

## 41

*Juan Palou, José Segarra*

## INTRODUCTION

Bladder cancer healthcare costs are the highest among adults who have solid tumors since superficial transitional cell cancer is a life-long disease that may recur and progress. Even though transurethral resection of bladder tumor (TURBT), endovesical chemotherapy, and immunotherapy decrease the recurrence and progression rate, the persistent possibility of developing new tumors obliges the urologist to perform life-long follow-up.[1] The general recommendation for cystoscopic surveillance every 3 months for the first year, every 6 months for the second year, and then yearly for all patients with superficial bladder cancer[2] is no longer acceptable, since superficial bladder cancer is a heterogeneous disease with a variable propensity for recurrence and progression.[3]

It is possible to establish general guidelines, however, in order to choose the most appropriate surveillance schedule based on a patient's particular tumor characteristics. A recent study[4] from the United Kingdom and Ireland demonstrated a complete lack of consensus regarding long-term surveillance recommendations. There is a genuine need to establish follow-up schedules based on our contemporary understanding of bladder cancer biology.

## NATURAL HISTORY OF SUPERFICIAL BLADDER CANCER

### TRANSURETHRAL RESECTION OF THE PRIMARY BLADDER TUMOR

The most important first investigation is the diagnostic cystoscopy and TURBT. It should be conducted or supervised by experienced urologists,[5] since this first maneuver will influence the finding of persistence of disease or early recurrence at 3 months. The aims are to identify tumor(s), to remove them completely, and biopsy any suspicious areas of the bladder that may harbor occult malignancy. Care must be taken in performing this evaluation and resection since the incidence of residual tumor after primary TURBT is known to be quite high. Klän et al[6] found residual tumor in 43% of their patients at the time of restaging (second) TURBT and Herr[7] found this in an even higher percentage of patients (76%).

It is important to consider the differences in recurrence or persistence at 3 months in different centers. Investigators working with the European Organisation for Research and Treatment of Cancer (EORTC) have reported recurrence rates of 21% to 43.8% in patients with solitary tumors (1975–1978). Interestingly, this rate of recurrence declined in studies performed a decade later to 3% to 5.3% (1987–1989). In patients with multiple tumors, recurrence rates were initially found to be 50% to 61.5% but this fell to between 14.4% and 24.6% in more contemporary trials.[8] Brausi et al have presented results which corroborate the different recurrence and progression rates of solitary and multifocal tumors.[9] These authors suggested that the quality of the transurethral resection (TUR) performed by the individual surgeons may be responsible for their results.

In 1991, Kolozsy provided data supporting the need for a proper first resection.[10] In our experience with 936 patients with nonmuscle-invasive bladder cancer (Ta or T1) that underwent a thorough and complete primary TURBT, the recurrence rate was 10% and the progression rate was 1% at 3–4 months.[11] In 114 patients with T1G3 tumors, with or without carcinoma in situ (CIS) and treated with bacillus Calmette–Guérin (BCG), the recurrence and progression rates at 3 months were 9.6% and 3.5%, respectively. With such a low incidence of recurrence and progression rate at 3 months, there was no clear indication for a second early TURBT. We suggest a second resection in patients with no muscle identified in the specimen, incomplete resection or, in doubtful cases, coming from other centers.[12,13]

## RECURRENCE

Prognostic factors for recurrence are multiplicity, recurrence at 3 months, size of the tumor, and anaplasia.[13,14] Based on these prognostic factors, the following risk groups have been developed related to recurrence and progression[1]:

- Low-risk tumors including single, Ta, G1, <3 cm diameter
- High-risk tumors including T1G3, multifocal or highly recurrent, CIS
- Intermediate-risk tumors which include all other tumors, Ta-1, G1–2, multifocal, >3 cm diameter.

Fitzpatrick et al advocated that a patient with a negative cystoscopy at 3 months had a 79% chance of being free of disease for 10 years; conversely, 90% of patients with tumor at first cystoscopy had recurrence.[15] Parmar et al considered multiplicity and recurrence at 3 months as the main prognostic factors for recurrence.[16] These two parameters provided the most predictive information related to recurrence, which is independent of the stage:

- Good risk (60% of the cases) included those patients with a solitary tumor at presentation and no new occurrence at first cystoscopy. The recurrence rate for these patients was 20% 1 year following TURBT.
- Medium risk (30% of the cases) included those patients that have either multiple tumors at diagnosis, and are tumor-free at first cystoscopy, or have a solitary tumor with a new occurrence at first cystoscopy. These patients have a recurrence risk of 40% at 1 year and 60% at 2 years.
- Poor risk (10% of the cases) included those patients having multiple tumors at presentation and a new occurrence at first cystoscopy. This group has a recurrence rate of 50% at 6 months and 90% by 1–2 years.

The pattern of recurrence of these risk groups will determine the follow-up schedule.[17–20] Holmäng et al proposed discontinuing cystoscopy follow-up 5–10 years after the last recurrence in patients with a solitary, low-grade tumor.[17] These data also indicated that patients with more than 10 recurrences will have recurrences until death or cystectomy. Recurrence more than 4 years after the resection of the primary lesion was also an ominous sign. In patients with multiple and highly recurrent tumors, shorter intervals of follow-up should be considered during the first years.[20]

## PROGRESSION

The Medical Research Council (MRC) classification is useful in order to understand the risk of recurrence, but is not useful from the point of view of progression. Hall et al[19] previously considered the particularly poor prognosis of T1G3 tumors based on a 29% progression rate, and suggested that these tumors be considered as a unique group.

In long-term follow-up studies, progression in grade and stage up to 37% occurs in patients with TaG1 lesions using a definition of progression as upgrading to G2 or T1 tumors[20]; however, only 3.3% progressed to muscle-invasive disease. Heney et al reported a progression rate of 30% in patients with T1 tumors and 4% in Ta tumors.[21]

It is important to consider that, even though some low-grade superficial bladder cancers may progress to muscle-invasive disease, the majority of patients will experience a superficial recurrence with an increase of grade and stage before they become invasive. Morris et al reported that patients that were tumor-free for more than 2 years did not develop invasive bladder cancer.[22]

The higher risk of recurrence and progression in high-grade tumors and CIS obliges more frequent follow-up and for the lifetime of the patient.[17,23] In our group,[13] with a multivariate analysis of 1529 patients with primary superficial bladder carcinoma with multiple random biopsies, a clear difference was established related to progression:

- Low-risk patients, including solitary Ta–T1G1 without CIS, had a risk of recurrence of 37% and progression of 0%.
- Medium-risk patients, including multiple T1G1, TaG2, solitary T1G2 without CIS, had a risk of recurrence of 45% and progression of 1.8%.
- High-risk patients, including multiple T1G2, Ta–T1G3, primary CIS or any tumor associated with CIS, had a risk of recurrence of 54% and progression of 15%.

Comparing low- and medium-risk groups to high-risk groups, the high-risk group must be followed more frequently and life-long.

## METHODS OF PATIENT FOLLOW-UP

Methods of follow-up in superficial bladder cancer must consider effectiveness, sensitivity, specificity, cost, and discomfort to the patients. Urologists need to work out the best combination in order to offer the optimum approach without jeopardizing the future well-being of the patient.

## CYSTOSCOPY

The development of flexible cystoscopy has reduced the fear of frequent outpatient cystoscopy in patients with nonmuscle-invasive bladder cancer. Up to 33% will have urinary symptoms (such as stranguria and frequency) after flexible cystoscopy.[24] Cystoscopy offers the possibility of a complete evaluation of the bladder including dome and anterior wall with ease, so that a complete examination of the bladder can be done with safety. Hall et al recommend only rigid cystoscopy under general anesthesia for patients from the poor risk group, because of the high probability of tumor recurrence and the greater need for resection.[19]

Cystoscopy may correctly predict stage and grade in the follow-up of patients with recurrent papillary bladder tumors identified on outpatient flexible cystoscopy.[25] This may also lead to the possibility of treating them safely with outpatient fulguration. With primary tumors there may not be such a good correlation between macroscopic appearance and pathology, so TUR is mandatory.[26]

At 3 months, cystoscopy should be performed in all patients. There are multiple potential causes of persistent bladder tumor at the first follow-up cystoscopy, including incomplete resection of the primary tumor, implantation at traumatized sites in the bladder, rapid growth of epithelial malignancy, and tumor present but not noticed at the first endoscopy.[9,14,27]

It is not unusual to find erythematous lesions after BCG at 3 months (65%) and 6 months (20%) that may suggest the diagnosis of recurrence.[28] In the absence of a positive cytology, no biopsy should be undertaken in order to reduce the risk that patients would be overbiopsied and treated.[29] At the first follow-up cystoscopy, CIS is normally found only in patients with a prior history of CIS. In these patients the presence of any abnormality with cytology or cystoscopy should prompt a biopsy.[29,30] In the follow-up of patients with a previous history of TCC, a biopsy should be done for any red patches after more than 6 months following completion of intravesical BCG, if there is no maintenance treatment, in order to rule out CIS.

It is not uncommon to notice a pseudotumor-like inflammatory reaction, which can be misinterpreted. In a series of 114 patients with T1G3 tumors treated with BCG, of 14 macroscopic tumor lesions at 3 months, 36% were granulomatous reactions.[28] When there is a papillary lesion, the possibility of a positive biopsy is higher (86.4%).[29]

## ECHOGRAPHY

It would be advantageous to find an effective, non-invasive alternative to cystoscopy. Echography has been used by different centers but the advantages and risks have not yet been established. Transabdominal echography examination is an easy and non-invasive method that, with a full bladder, can provide information about any endoluminal alteration of the bladder wall. Size and location of the tumor are the main variables in the diagnostic possibilities of ultrasonography. Malone et al detected only 38% of tumors less than 5 mm in diameter.[31] Boccon-Gibod et al could detect tumors as small as 2.5 mm, but missed lesions that developed in the dome.[32] Bladder wall trabeculation, prostate protrusion into the bladder, clots, calcifications, and persistence of sutures all may lead to a false diagnosis of a bladder tumor. Obesity may also make the detection of a tumor difficult.

Transabdominal ultrasonography has been used for the detection of recurrent bladder tumors with a sensitivity that ranges from 50% to 82%.[33,34] Provided that certain precautions are taken, this technique can decrease the frequency of cystoscopy.[35] A small, prospective randomized study of 97 patients demonstrated the usefulness of examining patients with transabdominal ultrasound, without any differences with regard to recurrence, progression, and tumor-related death between the two groups.[36]

## CYTOLOGY

Cytology is considered standard in the follow-up because of its high specificity (97–100%). The sensitivity varies, and ranges from 25% in low-grade tumors to 90% to 95% in high-grade tumors.[37] The main objective of cytology is to detect high-grade recurrence. A negative cytology does not exclude the presence of a papillary lesion in the bladder. A positive cytology in the absence of macroscopic tumor may help in the diagnosis of flat lesions of the bladder and alert the urologist to look for the presence of extravesical TCC disease.

## TUMOR MARKERS

The ideal test for bladder cancer detection should be highly sensitive and specific, cost-effective, and non-invasive, and produce results instantaneously (point of care). To date, no tumor marker test for the detection of bladder cancer fulfils these criteria. Recently, Vriesema et al reported that most patients preferred cystoscopy to urinary marker testing when bladder tumor marker sensitivity was lower than 90%, suggesting that patients want to be sure that they have no tumor.[38]

A variety of methods are used, including abnormal blood group antigen expression and the detection of tumor antigens, growth factors, protein fragments, and chromosomal abnormalities. Although the utility of urine tumor markers is extensively analyzed in Chapter 20, it is important to briefly note that several markers have been developed as potential tests to detect the presence of TCC in the urinary tract. Globally, a sensitivity of 50% to 90% and a specificity of 60% to 90% have been demonstrated.[37] Since there is a higher sensitivity of these markers than cytology in low-grade tumors, a tumor marker test would probably be a good option for this group of patients.

Future studies will need to demonstrate the feasibility of using only markers in low-risk disease instead of cytology, but, for now, use of both is recommended. A protocol that would decrease the number of invasive procedures and cost has merit if it does not compromise patient care.[39] Future results of the usefulness of echography, combined with point-of-care urine biomarker tests, may open a window for non-invasive follow-up of patients with low- and medium-risk tumors.

## PROPOSAL OF FOLLOW-UP

The classic recommendation for cystoscopic surveillance has been every 3 months for the first year, every 6 months for the second year, and yearly thereafter. Even though this schedule may be correct globally, it is no longer acceptable since we can reliably identify risk groups of tumors that have a different pattern of recurrence and progression. Different recommendations have been proposed including cystoscopy and cytology at different intervals, according to risk stratification of patients (Boxes 41.1–41.4).

The clear difference in recurrence rates, according to the criteria of the MRC,[16,19] determined by counting the

**Box 41.1** Recommendations of the European Association of Urology[1]

First cystoscopy at 3 months in all cases; a second resection at the site of the transurethral resection is advised at 4–6 weeks in high-grade lesions, though not yet established

Low risk tumors: cystoscopy at 3 months, 12 months and then yearly for 5 years

High risk tumors: cystoscopy every 3 months for the first 2 years, every 4 months in the third year, every 6 months thereafter for up to 5 years and then yearly life-long

Intermediate risk group: lies in between low and high risk, and follow-up up to 10 years

With any disease recurrence, the cystoscopy schedule restarts from the beginning

Tumor markers and echography not yet established

**Box 41.2** Recommendations of the National Comprehensive Cancer Network[56]

First cystoscopy at 3 months in all cases

Cystoscopy and cytology every 3 months for 1 year

After the first year, every 3–6 months until the fifth year, then annually

**Box 41.3** Recommendations of the British Medical Research Council Subgroup on superficial bladder cancer[19]

First cystoscopy at 3 months in all cases

Good risk: flexible cystoscopy at 12 months and annually thereafter

Medium risk: flexible cystoscopy every 3 months for the first year; if free of disease, annual flexible cystoscopy thereafter

Poor risk (10% of the cases): rigid cystoscopy every 3 months for the first year

**Box 41.4** Recommendations of the Comité de Cancérologie de l'Association Française d'Urologie[57]

First cystoscopy at 3 months in all cases

Low risk: cystoscopy at 6 and 12 months and annually thereafter until the fifth year, and then annual echography until 10 years

Medium risk: cystoscopy and cytology at 6 and 12 months, then annually until 15 years

High risk: cystoscopy and cytology every 3 months for the first year, every 6 months for the second year, and then annually for 15 years

number of tumors at initial presentation and the status of the bladder at the first follow-up cystoscopy, is an easy way to classify patients and to recommend an appropriate follow-up strategy. A risk-adapted follow-up schedule and utilization of cystoscopy and biomarkers should result in significant cost savings.[39] The possibility of incomplete resection, missing a tumor in another location, implantation of cells or rapid growth of TCC in multifocal disease leads to an early cystoscopy at 3 months as an accepted standard common to all patients, regardless of risk group. In a multivariate analysis, only findings at first cystoscopy, presence of papillary urothelial neoplasms of low malignant potential versus grades 1–3, but not tumor stage and the number of tumors, had prognostic significance for recurrence.[40] Only first cystoscopy findings and grade had prognostic significance for time to stage progression.[40] In patients with papillary urothelial neoplasm of low malignant potential (LMP), or low-grade carcinoma with a negative first cystoscopy, an alternative follow-up strategy could use repeat echography at 12 months and periodic voided urine markers, which have a higher sensitivity compared to cytology for low-grade disease, and there is a negligible risk of progression.

The medium and poor risk groups (excluding high-grade tumors and CIS) according to the MRC correlate to intermediate tumors of the European Association of

Urology (EAU) or medium risk as suggested by Fundació Puigvert.[41] This group of patients may be classified together as having multiple or recurrent low-grade tumors, and should be followed-up with cystoscopy and cytology. Future studies will need to demonstrate whether it is appropriate to follow this group combining echography/cystoscopy and tumor markers and/or cytology.

Regarding the duration of follow-up, it appears advisable to stop follow-up in patients with a single TaG1 tumor in the absence of recurrence over 5 years. In all other cases, annual follow-up is advisable for up to 10 years, with life-long surveillance.[42] In patients with multiple and recurrent tumors, recurrences continue to appear for up to 10–12 years.[22,40,42] Patients with recurrences during the first 4 years after TUR may continue to have life-long recurrences.[40]

High-grade tumors and the presence of CIS are associated with a high risk for progression, and, consequently, closer follow-up is advised in order to detect high-grade recurrences or progression as soon as possible.[41,43] The grade or association with CIS determines the risk group, irrespective of multiplicity of tumors or early recurrence. A solitary T1G3 tumor should never be included as good risk.[44] For recurrent tumors, the follow-up should be according to the risk group of the new tumor. A follow-up proposal that takes account of these issues is outlined in Box 41.5.

---

**Box 41.5** Follow-up proposal

1. Solitary low grade tumor
   - Flexible cystoscopy and tumor marker at 3 months
   - Echography and tumor marker at 12 months
   - Echography and tumor marker annually for 5 years
2. Multiple low-grade or recurrent tumor
   - Flexible cystoscopy and cytology at 3 months
   - Flexible cystoscopy and cytology every 3 months for 1 year
   - Flexible cystoscopy and cytology every 6 months for 5 years and then annually up to 10 years
   - Consider echography and tumor markers
3. Carcinoma in situ and/or high-grade nonmuscle invasive bladder cancer
   - Flexible cystoscopy and cytology at 3 months
   - Flexible cystoscopy and cytology every 3 months for 2 years
   - Flexible cystoscopy and cytology every 4 months at the third year
   - Flexible cystoscopy and cytology every 6 months

---

## PROSTATIC URETHRA FOLLOW-UP

TCC of the prostate may occur in 8% to 48% of patients.[45–50] Prostatic urethral involvement tends to be more common in patients with CIS of the bladder,[45,47] as well as those with tumor multifocality and involvement of the bladder neck.[48,50–52]

In the series of Herr and Donat,[51] with a minimum follow-up of 15 years, of the 72% of patients with superficial bladder cancer with associated CIS and treated with BCG, 39% had relapsed in the prostate at a median follow-up of 28 months. Non-invasive disease occurred in 62%, while 38% had stromal invasion.

Solsona et al[53] strongly recommended frequent directed biopsies of the prostatic urethra during initial and repeated cystoscopic examinations; however, details of frequency and technique were not provided. For patients with positive cytology at follow-up, in the absence of macroscopic bladder carcinoma, it is mandatory to evaluate the bladder and the prostatic urethra with multiple biopsies.[53]

With a positive cytology during the first 6 months of follow-up after conservative management of a superficial bladder carcinoma, bladder recurrence is most likely to be the cause.[54] If positive cytology appears in longer-term follow-up, and no tumor is detected in the bladder or prostatic urethra, the upper urinary tract should always be evaluated.[55]

### REFERENCES

1. Oosterlinck W, Lobel B, Jakse G, Malmström PU, Stöckle M, Sternberg C. Guidelines on bladder cancer. Eur Urol 2002;41:105–112.
2. Tolley DA, Hargreave TB, Smith PH, et al. Effect of intravesical mitomycin C on recurrence of newly diagnosed superficial bladder cancer: interim report from the Medical Research Council Subgroup on Superficial Bladder Cancer (Urological Cancer Working Party). BMJ 1998;296:1759–1761.
3. Donat SM. Evaluation and follow-up strategies for superficial bladder cancer. Urol Clin North Am 2003;30:765–776.
4. Wazait HD, Al-Bhueissi SZ, Patel HR, Nathan MS, Miller RA. Long-term surveillance of bladder tumors: current practice in the United Kingdom and Ireland. Eur Urol 2003;43:485–488.
5. Abel PD. Follow-up of patients with superficial transitional cell carcinoma of the bladder. In Pagano F, Fair WR (eds): Superficial Bladder Cancer. Oxford: Ed Isis, 1997.
6. Klän R, Loy V, Huland H. Residual tumors discovered in routine recurrent transurethral resection in patients with stage T1 transitional cell carcinoma of the bladder. J Urol 1991;146:316–318.
7. Herr HW. The value of a second transurethral resection in evaluating patients with bladder tumors. J Urol 1999;162:74–76.
8. Kurth KH, Bouffioux C, Sylvester R, van der Meijden AP, Oosterlink W, Brausi M. Treatment of superficial bladder tumors: achievements and needs. The EORTC Genitourinary Group. Eur Urol 2000;37(Suppl 3):1–9.
9. Brausi M, Collette L, Kurth K, et al. Variability in the recurrence rate at first follow-up cystoscopy after TUR in stage Ta T1 transitional cell carcinoma of the bladder: a combined analysis of seven EORTC studies. Eur Urol 2002;41:523–531.
10. Kolozsy Z. Histopathological 'self control' in transurethral resection of bladder tumors. Br J Urol 1991;67:162–164.
11. Millán F, Palou J, Chéchile G, Montlleó M, Huguet J, Salvador J. The value of a second transurethral resection in evaluating patients with bladder tumors. J Urol 2001;162:1258.
12. Herr HW, Donat SM, Dalbagni G. Correlation of cystoscopy with histology of recurrent papillary tumors of the bladder. J Urol 2002;168:978–980.
13. Millán Rodriguez F, Chéchile Toniolo G, Salvador Bayarri J, Palou Redorta J, Vicente Rodríguez J. Multivariate analysis of the prognostic factors of primary superficial bladder cancer. J Urol 2000;163:73–78.
14. Kurth KH, Denis L, Bouffioux CH, Sylvester R, Debruyne FM, Pavone Macaluso M, Oosterlink W. Factors affecting recurrence and progression in superficial bladder cancer tumors. Eur J Cancer 1995;31A(11):1840–1846.

15. Fitzpatrick JM, West AB, Butler MR, Lane V, O'Flynn JD. Superficial bladder tumors (stage pTa, grades 1 and 2): the importance of recurrence pattern following initial resection. J Urol 1986;135:920–922.

16. Parmar MKB, Freedman LS, Hargreave TB, et al. Prognostic factors for recurrence and follow-up policies in the treatment of superficial bladder cancer. J Urol 1989;142:284–288.

17. Holmäng S, Hedelin H, Anderström C, Johansson SL. The relationship among multiple recurrences, progression and prognosis of patients with stages Ta and T1 transitional cell cancer of the bladder followed for at least 20 years. J Urol 1995;153:1823–1827.

18. Prescott S, Tolley DA. Cystoscopy in bladder cancer. BMJ 1994;308:718

19. Hall RR, Parmar MKB, Richards AB, Smith PH. Proposal for changes in cystoscopy follow up of patients with bladder cancer and adjuvant intravesical chemotherapy. BMJ 1994;308:257–260.

20. Leblanc B, Duclos AJ, Benard F, et al. Long-term follow-up of initial Ta grade 1 transitional cell carcinoma of the bladder. J Urol 1999;162:1946–1950.

21. Heney NM, Ahmed S, Flanagan MJ, et al. Superficial bladder cancer: progression and recurrence. J Urol 1983;130:1083–1086.

22. Morris SB, Gordon EM, Shearer RJ, et al. Superficial bladder cancer: for how long should a tumor-free patient have check cystoscopies? Br J Urol 1995;75:193–196.

23. Cookson MS, Herr HW, Zhang ZF, Soloway S, Sogani PC, Raif WR. The treated natural history of high risk superficial bladder cancer: 15 year outcome. J Urol 1997;158:62–67.

24. Denholm SW, Conn IG, Newsam JE, Chisholm GD. Morbidity following cystoscopy: comparison of flexible and rigid techniques. Br J Urol 1990;66:152–154.

25. Herr HW, Donat M, Dalbagni G. Correlation of cystoscopy with histology of recurrent papillary tumors of the bladder. J Urol 2002;168:978–980.

26. De León Morales E, Arango Toro O, Lorente Garín JA, Cortadellas Angel R, Bielsa Gali O, Gelabert Mas A. La impresión cistoscópica frente al diagnóstico histológico en los tumores vesicales. ¿Coinciden? Actas Urol Esp 2003;27(1):18–21.

27. Brausi M, Collette L, Kurth K, et al. Variability in the recurrence rate at first follow-up cystoscopy after TUR in stage Ta T1 transitional cell carcinoma of the bladder: a combined analysis of seven EORTC studies. Eur Urol 2002;41:523–531.

28. Pieras Ayala E, Palou J, Rodríguez-Villamil L, Millán Rodríguez F, Bayarri JS, Vicente Rodríguez J. Seguimiento cistoscópico de los tumores vesicales G3T1 iniciales tratados con BCG. Arch Esp De Urol 2001;54:211–217.

29. Dalbagni G, Rechtschaffen T, Herr HW. Is transurethral biopsy of the bladder necessary after 3 months to evaluate response to bacillus Calmette–Guérin therapy? J Urol 1999;162:708–709.

30. Skemp NM, Fernandez ET. Routine bladder biopsy alters Bacille Calmette–Guérin treatment: is it necessary? Urology 2002;59:224–226.

31. Malone PR, Weston-Underwood J, Aron PM, et al. The use of transabdominal ultrasound in the detection of early bladder tumors. Br J Urol 1986;58:520–522.

32. Boccon-Gibod L, Le Portz B, Godefroy D, Steg A. Suprapubic ultrasonography in the follow-up of superficial bladder tumors. Eur Urol 1985;11:317–319.

33. Davies AH, Cranston D, Meagher T, Fellows GJ. Detection of recurrent bladder tumors by transrectal and abdominal ultrasound compared with cystoscopy. J Urol 1989;64:409–411.

34. Granados EA, de la Torre P, Palou J. La ecografía y la cistoscopia: dos medios diagnósticos en el tumor vesical (1ª parte). Actas Urol Esp 1990;15:538–542.

35. Vallancien G, Veillon B, Cartón M, Brisset JM. Can transabdominal ultrasonography of the bladder replace cystoscopy in the followup of superficial bladder tumors? J Urol 1986;136:32–34.

36. Olsen LH, Genster HG. Prolonging follow-up intervals for non-invasive bladder tumors: a randomized controlled trial. Scand J Urol Nephrol Suppl 1995;172:33–36.

37. Malkowicz SB. Management of superficial bladder cancer. In Walsh PC, Retik AB, Vaughan ED, Wein AJ, et al (eds): Campbell's Urology, 8th ed. Philadelphia: Saunders, 2002.

38. Vriesema JLJ, Poucki MH, Kiemeney LALM, Witjes JA. Patient opinion of urinary tests versus flexible urethrocystoscopy in follow-up examination for superficial bladder cancer: a utility analysis. Urology 2000;56:793–797.

39. Lotan Y, Roehrborn CG. Cost-effectiveness of a modified care protocol substituting bladder tumor markers for cystoscopy for the followup of patients with transitional cell carcinoma of the bladder: a decision analytical approach. J Urol 2002;167:75–79.

40. Holmäng S, Johansson SL. Stage TA-T1 bladder cancer: the relationship between findings at first followup cystoscopy and subsequent recurrence and progression. J Urol 2002;167:1634–1637.

41. Millán F, Chéchile G, Salvador J, et al. Multivariate analysis of the prognostic factors of primary superficial bladder cancer. J Urol 2000;163:73–78.

42. Thompson RA Jr, Campbell EW Jr, Kramer HC, Jacobs S, Naslund MJ. Late invasive recurrence despite long-term surveillance for superficial bladder cancer. J Urol 1993;149:1010–1011.

43. Vicente Rodríguez J, Salvador Bayarri J, Chéchile Toniolo G, Millán Rodríguez F, Palou Redorta J. Tumores vesicales superficiales iniciales: nuestra experiencia. Nuestro criterio. Actas Urol Esp 2000;24:522–529.

44. Prescott SW, Tolley DA. Cystoscopy in bladder cancer. BMJ 1994;308:718.

45. Orihuela E, Herr WH, Whitmore WF. Conservative treatment of superficial transitional cell carcinoma of the prostatic urethra with intravesical BCG. Urology 1989;34:231–237.

46. Hillyard RW, Ladaga L, Schellhammer PF. Superficial transitional cell carcinoma of the bladder associated with mucosal involvement of the prostatic urethra: results of treatment with intravesical bacillus Calmette–Guérin. J Urol 1988;139:290–293.

47. Bretton PR, Herr HW, Whitmore WF, et al. Intravesical bacillus Calmette–Guérin therapy for in situ transitional cell carcinoma involving the prostatic urethra. J Urol 1989;141:853–856.

48. Nixon RG, Chang SS, Lafleur BJ, Smith JA, Cookson MS. Carcinoma in situ and tumor multifocality predict the risk of prostatic urethral involvement at radical cystectomy in men with transitional cell carcinoma of the bladder. J Urol 2002;167(2 Pt 1):502–505.

49. Revelo MP, Cookson MS, Chang SS, Shook MF, Smith JA Jr, Shappell SB. Incidence and location of prostate and urothelial carcinoma in prostates from cystoprostatectomies: implications for apical sparing surgery. J Urol 2004;171(2 Pt 1):646–651.

50. Wood DP, Montie JE, Pontes JE, VanderBrug Medendorp S, Levin HSJ. Transitional cell carcinoma of the prostate in cystoprostatectomy specimens removed for bladder cancer. J Urol 1989;141:346–349.

51. Herr HW, Donat SM. Prostatic tumor relapse in patients with superficial bladder tumors: 15-year outcome. J Urol 1999;161:1854–1857.

52. Pieras AE, Palou J, Rodríguez-Villamil L, Millán Rodríguez F, Salvador Bayarri J, Vicente Rodruiguez J. Cytoscopic follow-up of initial G3T1 bladder tumors treated with BCG. Arch Esp de Urol 2001;54:211–217.

53. Solsona E, Iborra I, Ricós JV, Monrós JL, Dumont R, Casanova J, Calabuig C. Recurrence of superficial bladder tumors in prostatic urethra. Eur Urol 1991;19:89–92.

54. Schwalb DM, Herr HW, Fair WR. The management of clinically unconfirmed positive urine cytology. J Urol 1993;150:1751–1756.

55. Schwalb DM, Herr HW, Sogani PC, et al. Positive urine cytology following a complete response to intravesical bacillus Calmette–Guérin therapy: pattern of recurrence. J Urol 1994;152(2 Pt 1):382–387.

56. National Comprehensive Cancer Network. Practice guidelines in oncology: bladder cancer: including upper tract tumors and transitional cell carcinoma of the prostate, version 1.2002. Oncology 1998;12(7A):225–271.

57. Gattegno B, Chopin D. Surveillance of superficial bladder tumors. Progrès en Urologie 2001;11:1151–1157.

# The natural history of invasive bladder cancer

42

*George R Prout Jr*

## INTRODUCTION

The natural history of any cancer, unless it is on the skin and not treated, is truly not known. Biopsy and many other factors may alter the developmental course of the neoplasm, so this chapter might be better entitled the 'treated history' of human bladder cancer.

It follows, then, that to understand what we do know, we must begin with observations of the behavior of malignancies in treated states and to record characteristics of a given set of histologically similar lesions. We must recognize that, until the Second World War was over, the concept of bladder cancer was in an astonishingly confused state because there was a mountain of data that mixed noninvasive tumors, the majority, with invasive tumors. Thus, the concept that physicians could cure most of these cancers was firmly in place—and rightly so. But this chapter deals with tumor types, nodal involvement, modes of transmission, and other variables that are intimately involved with bladder cancer. While it is not the intent to deal with these items alone, it is they that record the history of invasive bladder cancer, and thus are the footprints we must follow.

## TUMOR TYPES

There were some who recognized the problem of invasive versus noninvasive tumors, but it required an outspoken few to cause others to recognize the problem. Jewett and Marshall were among those who spoke, and they and their trainees began to create a network that isolated and defined the problem;[1-3] this, of course,

required pathologists with both an interest and a commitment.[4]

## CARCINOMA IN SITU

It is not possible to attack the whole world of invasive bladder cancer without starting at the beginning, and that is with carcinoma in situ (CIS), which is where most invasive carcinoma has its beginning. The neoplasm(s) are high grade; some lack the necessary mechanisms to invade and so they push the 'normal' mucosa aside. Upon reaching the prostatic urethra, as many do, the cells plunge down the ejaculatory ducts and invade the prostatic substance. CIS was first described by Melicow,[5] Masina,[6] and Melicow and Hollowell.[7] It was initially found in bladders with invasive carcinomas and probably viewed as a curiosity. Since it was found in circumstances in which the damage was already done, it was not immediately seized and studied.

Two types of CIS have been described: the primary form (rare, uncommon) and the secondary (associated with other urothelial tumors).[8,9] Time and/or some subtle changes in neoplastic expression are not so uncommon.[10] This type of CIS is often encountered when field change is present and the neoplastic processes are visible, largely microscopically. We set out to enumerate these changes by studying the courses of 129 patients with low-grade, low-stage (Ta, T1) bladder cancer.[11] We found that in 15% of the patients with grade 1 and half of the 55 patients with grade 2 disease, the cancer progressed to muscle invasion. There was sufficient mucosa around the base of 75 of these tumors to search for abnormalities and CIS was found in 12.

These patients had 38 recurrences (3.1 tumors in 2.9 years per patient from the onset of symptoms to diagnosis), and 10 of them developed invasive disease.

Other opinions concerning CIS hold that the disease may be present for years before progressing and that when CIS alone is present, invasion is not common.[12,13] Others have reported contrasting experiences.[14,15] This is a serious disorder and, even if successfully treated initially, frequently returns.

With the advent of BCG it was clear that not only CIS but also other resistant, superficial carcinomas could be managed. These experiences tended to somewhat diminish the intensity with which CIS was pursued, but the problems did not vanish. Both CIS and superficial, high-grade cancer continued to create problems, and still do.[16-19]

## GRADE 1 BLADDER CANCER

There is an obvious separation between low- and high-grade bladder cancer. Surprisingly, all low-grade cancer is not associated with low-grade recurrences, although this is generally true. In a search for grade 1 bladder cancer followed for up to 10 years, we reviewed the collected data from the National Bladder Cancer Group and found detailed data on 178 patients that fit this category.[20] Of these patients, 122 had single tumors, 75% of which were less than 2 cm in size. Patients with multiple tumors were at a significant risk for recurrence, and 90% had recurrence. There were five patients whose recurrences were T1: one of these had CIS before the T1 tumor. Three patients developed muscle invasion and one of these had a cystectomy with cure. One patient refused treatment and died in uremia. There were no hallmarks to indicate change, although nearly all of the downgraded tumors were approximately 2 years from their first tumor event. A major question raised by this series is why, after many recurrences, they stopped recurring?

## BLOOD VESSEL INVASION

There are a few reports dealing with blood vessel invasion alone. One of these is by Bell et al, who used a special stain to identify elastic tissue in the walls of the vessels (Verhoeff–van Gieson stain).[21] They found blood vessel invasion (V+) in 42% of the 74 specimens they studied: the deeper the lesion, the greater the involvement. Progressing from stage A to stage C (Jewett–Strong–Marshall), the blood vessel involvement increased from 12% to 75%. Squamous cell carcinoma involved vessels more commonly than did transitional cell carcinoma; the 5-year survival was 32% for the former and 48% for the latter.

Because of difficulty in distinguishing between lymphatics, small venules, and capillaries, convention has placed these together in reporting involvement. Jewett and Strong, Jewett and Ebersole, and Soto et al described considerable heterogeneity in invasive carcinoma.[1,3,22] Solid, flat tumors invade in a tentacular fashion while tumors with a papillary surface extend on a broad front and do so less deeply. Soto et al made another observation of importance: tumors with a papillary surface had vascular involvement in about 25% of the specimens while solid tumors had blood vessel involvement in 66% of specimens.

In an analysis of data from the Surgical Adjuvant Bladder Study, Slack and Prout analyzed the results of a study of 214 patients with muscle-invasive bladder cancer, some of whom were treated with preoperative radiotherapy and some not, and, postoperatively, some with 5-fluorouracil and some not.[23] (The last part of the protocol was abandoned because of negative effect.) The results of the study clearly indicated that radiosensitive tumors were more frequently without papillary, lymphatic involvement (L–), and P0 (no residual tumor) in the final surgical specimen (85% 5-year survival); patients at the other extreme (solid, lymphatic invasion [L+], radiotherapy) had a 5-year survival of 20%. Missing data compromised these results.

In treating a select group of patients (medical inoperability, technically unresectable disease, advanced age, or patient self-selection), Shipley et al used full-dose radiotherapy.[24] These patients were clinical stages T2 and T3, and those with a papillary surface had a 5-year survival rate of 63%. None of those with solid morphology survived 5 years. In the same vein, Heney et al examined the slides of 86 patients with muscle invasion and found that those with solid configuration fared much more poorly than those with papillary surfaces (27% versus 50% at 5 years).[25] Of the 86 patients, 24 were N+. The presence of V+ conferred a much greater likelihood of N+ (38%) than when V– was present (6/38). Small vessel and nodal involvement resulted in a 5-year survival of 21%, while those without invasion of this type had a 42% 5-year survival. V+ in the N– group conferred a 30% 5-year survival, and when there was no small vessel involvement observed, a 52% 5-year survival was experienced. Clinical staging provided a 5-year survival of 77% for T2 patients, 33% for T3 patients, and 14% for T4 patients.

Support for these findings comes from Batata et al who analyzed the Memorial Sloan-Kettering Cancer Center experience.[26] They found that size of tumor was associated with survival. Tumors larger than 4 cm were associated with a 5-year survival of 6%. Patients with smaller tumors had a 5-year survival of 48%. Batata et al also found that patients with invasive tumors whose surface was papillary had a 51% 5-year survival versus patients with solid tumors whose 5-year survival was 33%. Further, they reported that V+ in the operative specimen produced a 14% 5-year survival; if V–, the 5-year survival was 41%.

## NODAL INVOLVEMENT

In the past, involved lymph nodes were a dire sign.[27,28] About 30% of the surgical failures were found to have no pelvic nodal metastases but instead had pulmonary, bony, and/or hepatic metastases.[29] The reasons for these skips are not clear. Curiously, reports dealing with pelvic lymphadenectomy, rarely, if ever, comment on this. Does this event contribute to the deaths reported in patients with negative adenectomies? Quite likely.

Skinner was one of the first to report on a significant number of survivors with positive pelvic nodes after cystectomy (36% 5-year survival).[30] This experience was greatly enlarged upon by Lerner et al who related an experience with 132 patients with positive nodes.[31] Worthy of emphasis is the fact that 11% of the failures in this group were in the pelvis, speaking for the benefit of the node dissection performed. Droller, in a commentary on the paper, raised issues with some of the authors' conclusions, engaging in a debate that still continues.[32] One matter does, however, seem clear: patients with certain positive node characteristics can be cured by the appropriate node dissection.

Recently, Vieweg et al reviewed the Memorial Sloan-Kettering experience regarding cystectomy when positive nodes were found.[33] They did so to identify tumor characteristics, i.e. vascular, lymphatic invasion, papillary surface, or solid. The tumors had a solid morphology of 95.8%, and 95.4% had lymphatic or vascular invasion. Because the review was retrospective, the extent of the nodal involvement (microscopic or gross) could not be determined. Cancer was confined to the bladder in 23% of the patients and nonconfined in 77%. The 5-year survival for N1 patients was 44.2% and for N2 was 26.6%. No N3 patient survived 5 years. The authors point out that routine pathologic procedures involving step-sectioning of lymph nodes may account for missed tumor deposits in more than 30% of specimens examined.[34]

Lymph node involvement has been central in evaluating all forms of therapy. Among the several reports of lymph nodes and their impact on survival, that of Smith and Whitmore relates to the percentage of involvement by site.[35] From a series of dissections they found that 16% had paravesical nodes involved, obturator nodes 74%, external iliac nodes 65%, and presacral nodes 25%. (Our literature is replete with 'obturator node involvement' yet a search through the anatomical literature reveals, at most, reference to one 'obturator node', or none. These nodes are most likely part of the external iliac chain on the posterior wall of the artery.)

Leissner et al have done a magnificent job of defining numbers and sites of nodes related to the bladder.[36] This cooperative group has named 12 anatomical regions and three levels of dissection to which all tissues of a cystectomy and node removal are assigned. During the procedure, each surgeon removed tissue that was identified and placed in the specific area from which it was removed. There were, on average, 43.1 lymph nodes removed from a sample of 290 patients, of whom 81 had metastases.

## CONCLUSION

This piece of history is not all-inclusive. Many clinicians, oncologists, and pathologists have made important contributions to the subject at hand. There simply isn't room for the product of all those good people.

REFERENCES

1. Jewett HJ, Strong GH. Infiltrating carcinoma of the bladder: relationship of depth of penetration of the bladder wall to the incidence of local extension and metastases. J Urol 1946;55:366–372.
2. Marshall VF. Symposium on bladder cancer: current clinical problems regarding bladder tumors. Cancer 1956;9:543–550.
3. Jewett HJ, Eversole SL. Characteristics of modes of local invasion. J Urol 1960;83:383–389.
4. Jewett HJ, King LR, Shelley WM. A study of 365 infiltrating bladder cancers: relationship of certain pathologic characteristics to prognosis after extirpation. J Urol 1964;92:668–678.
5. Melicow MM. Histological study of vesical urothelium intervening between gross neoplasms in total cystectomies. J Urol 1952;68:261–279.
6. Masina F. Mucosal changes in relation to bladder tumors. Br J Urol 1952;24:344–351.
7. Melicow MM, Hollowell JW. Intra-urothelial cancer: carcinoma in situ, Bowen's disease of the urinary system. Discussion of 30 cases. J Urol 1952;68:763–772.
8. Melamed MR, Voutsa NG, Grabstald H. Natural history and clinical behaviour of in situ carcinoma of the human urinary bladder. Cancer 1964;17:1533–1545.
9. Farrow GM, Utz DC, Rife CC. Morphological and clinical observation of patients with early bladder cancer treated with total cystectomy. Cancer Res 1976;36:2495–2501.
10. Hiatt HH, Watson JD, Winston JA (eds). Origins of Human Cancer. Cold Spring Harbor Conference on Cell Proliferation, vol 4, Parts A, B, C. New York: Cold Spring Harbor Laboratory, 1977.
11. Prout GR Jr, Barton BA, Griffin PP, Friedell GH. Treated history of noninvasive grade 1 transitional cell carcinoma. J Urol 1992;148:1413–1419.
12. Farrow GM, Utz DC. Observations on the microinvasive transitional cell carcinoma of the bladder. Clin Oncol 1982;1:609–615.
13. Orozco RE, Martin AA, Murphy WM. Carcinoma in situ of the urinary bladder: clues to host involvement in human carcinogenesis. Cancer 1994;74:115–122.
14. Hudson MA, Herr HW. Carcinoma in situ of the urinary bladder. J Urol 1995;153:564–572.
15. Prout GR Jr, Griffin PP, Daly JJ, Heney NM. Carcinoma in situ of the urinary bladder with and without associated vesical neoplasms. Cancer 1983;52:524–532.
16. Herr HW. Tumor progression and survival in patients with T1G3 bladder tumors. Br J Urol 1997;80:762–765.

17. Cookson MS, Herr HW, Shang ZF, et al. The treated natural history of high risk superficial bladder cancer: 15 year outcome. J Urol 1997;158:62–67.

18. Prout GR Jr, Griffin PP, Daly JJ. The outcome of the conservative management of carcinoma in situ of the urinary bladder. J Urol 1987;188:766–770.

19. Cookson MS, Sarosdy ML. Management of stage 1 superficial bladder cancer with intravesical BCG. J Urol 1992;148:797–801.

20. Prout GR Jr, Barton BA, Griffin PP, Friedell GH. The treated history of non-invasive grade 1 transitional cell carcinoma. J Urol 1992;148:1413–1419.

21. Bell JT, Burney SW, Friedell GH. Blood vessel invasion in human bladder cancer. J Urol 1971;105:675–678.

22. Soto EA, Friedell GH, Tiltman AJ. Bladder carcinoma as seen in giant sections. Cancer 1977;39:447–455.

23. Slack NH, Prout GR Jr. The heterogeneity of invasive bladder carcinoma and different responses to treatment. J Urol 1980;123:644–652.

24. Shipley WU, Rose MA, Perrone TL, et al. Full-dose irradiation for patients with invasive bladder carcinoma: clinical and histological factors prognostic of improved survival. J Urol 1985;134:679–683.

25. Heney NM, Proppe K, Prout GR Jr, Griffin PP, Shipley WU. Invasive bladder cancer: tumor configuration, lymphatic invasion and survival. J Urol 1983;130:895–897.

26. Batata MA, Chu FCH, Hilaris BS, et al. Factors of prognostic and therapeutic significance in patients with bladder cancer. Int J Radiat Oncol Biol Phys 1981;7:757–761.

27. Van der Werf-Messing B. Carcinoma vesicae treated at the Rotterdam Radiotherapy Institute between 1950 and 1974. Rotterdam: Erasmus University Press, 1975.

28. Marshall VF. The relation of the preoperative estimate to the pathologic demonstration of the extent of vesical neoplasms. J Urol 1952;68:714–723.

29. Babaian RJ, Johnson DE, Llamas L, et al. Metastases from transitional cell carcinoma of the urinary bladder. Urology 1980;16:142–144.

30. Skinner DG. Management of invasive bladder cancer: a meticulous node dissection can make a difference. J Urol 1982;128:34–36.

31. Lerner SP, Skinner DG, Lieskovsky G, et al. The rationale for en bloc pelvic lymph node dissection for bladder cancer patients with nodal metastases: long-term results. J Urol 1993;149:758–764; discussion 764–765.

32. Droller MJ. Editorial comments. J Urol 1993;149:764.

33. Vieweg J, Gschwend JE, Herr HW, Fair WR. Pelvic lymph node dissection can be curative in patients with node positive bladder cancer. J Urol 1999;161:449–454.

34. Wilkinson EJ, Hause L. Probability of lymph node sectioning. Cancer 1974;33:1269–1274.

35. Smith JA, Whitmore WF. Regional lymph node metastases from bladder cancer. J Urol 1981;126:591–593.

36. Leissner J, Ghoneim MA, Abol-Enein JW, et al. Extended radical lymphadenectomy in patients with urothelial bladder cancer: results of a prospective multicenter study. J Urol 2004;171:139–144.

# Selection and perioperative management of patients undergoing radical cystectomy and urinary reconstruction

# 43

*Melissa R Kaufman, Joseph A Smith Jr*

## INTRODUCTION

Radical cystectomy is a formidable surgical procedure. Moreover, many patients with invasive bladder cancer have significant comorbidity considering the median age at diagnosis and the strong association with a history of cigarette smoking. Optimal patient preparation and perioperative management are therefore essential in decreasing both the morbidity and mortality from this operation. This chapter defines some of the selection criteria, the preoperative evaluation, and the perioperative management of patients undergoing radical cystectomy.

## WHO ARE CANDIDATES

Radical cystectomy is the treatment of choice for muscle invasive or recurrent high-grade transitional cell carcinoma of the bladder.[1] The median survival for patients not cured by surgery is limited.[2] Patients with unresectable local disease may have significant morbidity from bleeding, pelvic pain, or voiding symptoms. Combined, these factors create strong incentives to proceed with cystectomy in patients with disease not controllable by transurethral methods. Historically, a significant number of patients were excluded from cystectomy because of advanced age and/or significant comorbidity.[3] Improvements in surgical technique and postoperative management have expanded the patient population considered eligible for surgery.[4]

There are few data which allow calculation of how many patients are excluded from radical cystectomy by being declared medically unfit for surgery. Undoubtedly, this categorization is appropriate for a distinct minority for whom alternative treatment methods must be considered.[5] However, the overwhelming majority of patients in whom cystectomy is indicated on the basis of tumor status should be considered candidates for surgery despite the attendant risks.[6]

## AGE

In most reported series, the typical patient undergoing cystectomy is in the sixth or seventh decade of life.[7] There are a number of reports, however, detailing the morbidity and mortality of the operation in octogenarians or even nonagenarians.[8] Chronologic age is only one consideration and must be correlated with comorbidity. Most series have shown that elderly patients tolerate cystectomy with morbidity not substantially different from that of younger patients.[9-12]

The choice of urinary diversion may be influenced in part by age. Parekh et al were unable to show any significant increase in morbidity for patients undergoing continent orthotopic neobladder reconstruction over that of patients undergoing ileal conduit cutaneous diversion.[13] Nonetheless, continent reconstruction is a more lengthy procedure, and it seems logical that morbidity may be somewhat increased, especially in the elderly. Further, the quality-of-life advantages afforded by continent reconstruction may be of less importance in older patients.[14] In properly motivated and informed patients, orthotopic neobladder can be offered even to those over 80 years of age. In general, however, most elderly patients are better served by an ileal conduit.

## COMORBIDITY

With any operation, including radical cystectomy, the risk of postoperative complications correlates with preexisting comorbid medical conditions. The American Society of Anesthesiologists (ASA) scoring system separates anesthetic risk by comorbid factors and has been shown to stratify anesthetic risk accurately (Box 43.1).[15]

The correlation of transitional cell carcinoma of the bladder with a history of smoking compounds the problem.[16,17] Other comorbid related conditions that occur commonly in populations of patients undergoing radical cystectomy include coronary artery disease, a risk or history of cerebrovascular accident (CVA), and peripheral vascular disease. Chronic obstructive pulmonary disease is frequently observed in patients being considered for radical cystectomy.

Nevertheless, many patients with significant comorbidity tolerate cystectomy well with proper attention to perioperative management as discussed below. Even in elderly ASA Class 3 or 4 patients, cystectomy can be performed with acceptable morbidity and limited mortality.[6,18] Overall, very few patients should be considered unfit for cystectomy strictly because of age or comorbidity.

## PREOPERATIVE EVALUATION AND MANAGEMENT

One of the keys to limiting postoperative morbidity is proper evaluation of presurgical medical conditions (Table 43.1). Although elimination or complete correction of many comorbid conditions is not feasible, appropriate control and evaluation can help minimize or prevent postoperative complications.[19] Studies have shown that an undue delay between the diagnosis of invasive bladder cancer and radical cystectomy can adversely affect both pathologic findings and survival.[20,21] In general, time periods of greater than 90 days between diagnosis and surgery are associated with a worse prognosis. However, an expeditious and thorough evaluation of the patient's general medical condition should not be compromised.

## CORONARY ARTERY DISEASE

Although an electrocardiogram is obtained routinely before anesthesia, a cardiac stress test should also be considered, even in asymptomatic patients.[22] Sometimes a correctable ischemia or arrhythmia is uncovered. Identifiable ischemia on a stress test should be evaluated with coronary angiography. When

---

**Box 43.1** American Society of Anesthesiologists physical class classification

*Class 1:* No organic, physiological, biochemical, or psychiatric disturbance

*Class 2:* Mild to moderate systemic disturbance that may or may not be related to the reason for surgery, such as anemia, morbid obesity, diabetes mellitus, chronic bronchitis, or essential hypertension

*Class 3:* Severe systemic disturbance, which may or may not be related to the reason for surgery, such as poorly controlled hypertension, diabetes mellitus with vascular complications, chronic obstructive pulmonary disease that limits activity, or history of myocardial infarction

*Class 4:* Severe systemic disturbance that is life threatening with or without surgery, such as congestive heart failure, persistent angina, or advanced hepatic dysfunction

*Class 5:* Moribund patient who has little chance of surviving, but undergoes surgery as a last resort

---

**Table 43.1** Common cystectomy comorbidities and evaluation/treatment strategies

| Comorbidity | Preoperative evaluation | Postoperative evaluation |
|---|---|---|
| Coronary artery disease | Electrocardiogram | Routine monitoring of vital signs |
| | Exercise or pharmacologic stress testing | Careful fluid management |
| | Cardiology consultation | Restart cardiac medications |
| Cerebrovascular disease | Carotid duplex analysis | Neurologic examinations |
| Chronic obstructive pulmonary disease | Cessation of smoking | Bronchodilators |
| | Chest x-ray | Aggressive pulmonary toilet |
| | Pulmonary consultation as indicated | Incentive spirometry |
| | | Respiratory therapy as indicated |
| Diabetes mellitus | Blood glucose, HgA1c testing | Blood glucose testing |
| | Ensure proper management with oral agents | Sliding scale insulin |
| Nutritional status | Rare indication for total parenteral nutrition | Oral feeding as rapidly as feasible |
| | | High-calorie supplements |
| | | Total parenteral nutrition for prolonged ileus |

appropriate, percutaneous coronary artery stents should be placed.[23] Occasionally, findings requiring coronary artery bypass grafts are discovered. Although this surgery would obviously delay cystectomy beyond the preferred time period, and introduce a risk of tumor progression, correction of significant coronary artery occlusive disease preoperatively may be indicated to decrease the risk of perioperative myocardial infarction and death.

Preoperative correction or control of cardiac arrhythmias is essential. In general, cardiology consultation would be appropriate. An attempt to determine the etiology of new onset or previously undiagnosed atrial fibrillation or other arrhythmias should be undertaken. The ventricular response should be controlled and premature contractions suppressed to ensure optimal cardiac output.

## CEREBROVASCULAR DISEASE

Carotid artery evaluation should be considered, especially in patients with a history of coronary artery occlusive disease or peripheral vascular disease. Auscultation of the neck could reveal a carotid bruit. Doppler ultrasound is an easy and noninvasive method for evaluation of the carotid artery. Significant stenosis may require preoperative consultation with a vascular surgeon or neurosurgeon.[24] Transient hypotension which could occur during surgery might precipitate a devastating CVA in the face of significant carotid artery occlusion.

## CHRONIC OBSTRUCTIVE PULMONARY DISEASE

Although the underlying lung damage from chronic obstructive pulmonary disease (COPD), especially when cigarette induced, is not reversible, preoperative measures to optimize lung function can be important. Even short-term cessation of smoking can improve recovery.[25] Bronchodilators and pulmonary toilet can be important preoperative adjuncts to aggressive postoperative pulmonary care. Although clinical recognition of lung disease is often sufficient to identify patients at risk for postoperative pulmonary complications, spirometry may be useful if there is uncertainty concerning the presence or extent of lung impairment.[26] Baseline arterial blood gases have not been proven to enhance risk assessment or postoperative management.

## DIABETES

Type 2 diabetes is an extremely common and increasingly frequent problem. Further, many patients with type 2 diabetes have poor long-term blood glucose control reflected by elevated hemoglobin-A1c (HgA1c) levels.

Elevated blood glucose and HgA1c have been correlated to increased mortality in critically ill surgical patients.[27,28] Prior to cystectomy, HgA1c levels should be obtained and optimal diabetic control attained. Diet, exercise, and weight loss often allow effective management of many individuals with type 2 diabetes. If oral agents and other measures are unsuccessful, insulin administration may be necessary to correct hyperglycemia.

## NUTRITIONAL STATUS

Some patients with bladder cancer have experienced significant weight loss or poor nutrition, perhaps as a consequence of a locally advanced tumor. The National Veterans Affairs Surgical Risk Study demonstrated that preoperative hypoalbuminemia, reflecting malnutrition, correlates with significantly increased morbidity and mortality.[29] Currently, preoperative intravenous nutrition is rarely indicated or necessary. However, use of high caloric supplements may be helpful in some situations to optimize nutritional status without unduly delaying surgery. Historically, total parenteral nutrition has been used in select patients to reverse a catabolic status, and to facilitate wound healing and recovery after cystectomy.[30] Early and aggressive use of postoperative parenteral nutrition should be considered, especially in patients with poor preoperative nutritional status.

## AZOTEMIA

Invasive bladder cancer may occlude the ureteral orifice and cause hydronephrosis. In the face of a normal contralateral kidney, renal function may not be compromised with unilateral obstruction. In this setting, relief of the obstruction is not necessary prior to cystectomy. With bilateral obstruction, or with impaired function of the contralateral kidney and unilateral obstruction, azotemia may be present. Significant azotemia should be corrected prior to surgery.[31] Cystoscopic placement of ureteral stents is usually difficult when obstruction results from invasive bladder cancer because the tumor obscures the trigone and ureteral orifice. A percutaneous nephrostomy tube may be required. Depending upon the degree and duration of obstruction, postobstructive diuresis may occur after placement of a nephrostomy tube.

# PREOPERATIVE PREPARATION

## PREPARATION FOR BLOOD TRANSFUSION

Radical cystectomy is an operation with the potential for significant intraoperative blood loss.[32-34] In addition, anemia is a common preoperative finding, either because of chronic disease or because of hematuria. Profound anemia should be corrected preoperatively with blood transfusions. Indeed, even in patients with a normal serum hematocrit preoperatively, possible need for blood transfusion should be anticipated. Although bleeding is not usually massive and sudden with cystectomy, the median intraoperative blood loss is such that a substantial number of patients require a blood transfusion.[33] A type and screen may be sufficient, depending upon how long it takes to obtain fully cross-matched blood in a given hospital. For most patients, however, blood should be typed and cross-matched preoperatively so that it can be administered in a timely fashion if required.

## BOWEL PREPARATION

Thoughts about both the value and method of bowel preparation have evolved in recent years.[35] Undoubtedly, though, minimizing contamination of the operative field is desirable and is facilitated by a mechanical bowel preparation. With an ileal conduit, minimal contamination should occur with division of the bowel and anastomosis of the ureters. Isolation and cleansing of a small bowel segment used for construction of a continent reservoir can also minimize contamination. An effective mechanical bowel preparation becomes more important when the colon is used for urinary tract reconstruction. Regardless of the method used for reconstruction, there is a low but definite risk of rectal injury with cystectomy. A decision to perform primary closure of a recognized rectal injury is facilitated by minimizing fecal spillage.

Various methods are used for mechanical cleansing of the bowel.[35] Most commonly, an oral polyethylene glycol electrolyte solution (GoLYTELY) is administered. However, this requires consumption of a large amount of fluid, and can cause vomiting or abdominal cramping and pain. In particular, many elderly patients tolerate this poorly and may be unable to complete the bowel preparation. Dehydration from the induced diarrhea can also be problematic. Oral sodium phosphate solutions have been shown to have an equivalent mechanical cleansing effect and require consumption of less fluid.[36]

Antibiotic bowel preparation may also be important. The classic Nichols preparation consists of 1 g each of oral neomycin and erythromycin base at 1300, 1400, and 2300 hours the day prior to surgery.[37] The addition of intravenous antibiotics, preferably a third generation cephalosporin, used at maximum dosage and administered at the ideal time before, during, and for 24 hours after surgery, is the preferred regimen to decrease wound infection rates for bowel surgery.[38]

## PREOPERATIVE MEDICATIONS

In general, instructions about withholding preoperative medications are delivered to the patient by the anesthesiologist. However, it is important for the surgeon to be aware of medicines that should be withheld and the time required for washout.[39,40] Warfarin should be discontinued 5 days prior to surgery. Depending upon the reason for which long-term warfarin is being used, a window wherein low molecular weight heparin is used to bridge the time of discontinuation until readministration of warfarin may be important. In particular, patients with mechanical heart valves should be maintained with such a window. Aspirin and nonsteroidal anti-inflammatory drugs should be withheld at least 7 days prior to surgery because of their antiplatelet effect. Clopidogrel and ticlopidine, inhibitors of platelet aggregation, should be stopped 7 days preoperatively. Metformin, a commonly used oral medication for glycemic control in patients with type 2 diabetes, should be withheld for at least 1 day prior to surgery.

Antihypertensives usually are continued until the day prior to surgery. Depending on blood pressure control and the medications themselves, the anesthesiologist may allow oral intake of some antihypertensives on the morning of surgery with a small sip of water. Otherwise, patients generally are kept with nothing by mouth for at least 8 hours prior to the surgery to avoid aspiration. Although currently not frequently used, psychotropic monoamine oxidase inhibitors must be discontinued 2 weeks preoperatively.

## INTRAOPERATIVE PATIENT MONITORING

Intraoperative monitoring is the responsibility of the anesthesiologist but requires input from the surgeon. The two should communicate about the anticipated length of surgery, the method of urinary reconstruction, and the potential for significant blood loss depending upon tumor size and stage. At a minimum, a large-bore peripheral intravenous cannula should be available for administration of blood products. Insertion of a central line is not routinely required. However, in patients with significant cardiovascular comorbidity, the presence of a central line could allow rapid insertion of a pulmonary artery catheter. An automatic, inflatable arm cuff is usually sufficient for monitoring blood pressure. A radial artery catheter, however, allows continuous blood pressure monitoring as well as evaluation of serial arterial blood gasses when oxygenation is an issue. This may be particularly applicable in patients with chronic obstructive pulmonary disease or cardiovascular comorbidity.

# POSTOPERATIVE CARE

## LOCATION

Each surgeon must make a decision about the appropriate hospital area for early postoperative recovery depending upon circumstances within the hospital. Not all hospitals provide equivalent care in different units. Fewer than 5% of our patients undergoing cystectomy require transfer to the intensive care unit postoperatively.[41] In some circumstances, we utilize an intermediate care unit when continuous cardiac monitoring is desirable, especially in patients with a history of arrhythmia or intraoperative rhythm disturbances. Most often, though, patients are transferred from the recovery room to the urology ward, where there are nurses experienced in the postoperative care of patients undergoing cystectomy.

We utilize an incision that does not extend above the level of the umbilicus for cystectomy, even with urinary reconstruction. In these circumstances, even in patients with significant COPD, extubation in the operating room or recovery room is feasible. Sometimes, however, there is delayed return of a good respiratory effort. In this situation, overnight intubation and ventilatory support are important. Efforts to wean the patient from the ventilator as soon as possible should be undertaken and usually are feasible on the first postoperative day.

## PAIN MANAGEMENT

Pain is one of the most frequently expressed concerns for patients undergoing surgical procedures. Beyond the physical discomfort and mental anguish associated with pain, poor analgesic control after cystectomy can increase the rate of complications. Mobility may be limited in a patient with poor pain control, increasing the risk of postoperative pneumonia or thromboembolic complications. Inappropriate use of narcotics can occasionally lead to respiratory depression and frequently contributes to ileus. Further, mental status changes with narcotic administration can lead to confusion or even combativeness and dislodgement of drains or tubes.[25]

Fortunately, the lower midline abdominal incision used for cystectomy does not frequently cause significant pain after surgery. The pain associated with a surgical incision depends not only on the length but also on the location. Upper abdominal incisions interfere more with respiratory efforts. Further, separation of muscles along the natural plane of the linea alba avoids the need for actual incision of muscular tissue. Other than pain from the surgical incision itself, bowel distension from ileus is the most common cause of postoperative pain. A vicious cycle can ensue with administration of narcotics for pain relief which, in turn, exacerbates or prolongs ileus.

Occluded stents may also be a source of postoperative pain, usually flank pain. The pain can be severe and colicky. Irrigation of stents to maintain patency should be performed in patients complaining of flank pain. Occasionally, radiographic imaging to ensure proper stent placement can be helpful.

For all of these reasons, postoperative pain management is an important aspect of care for patients undergoing cystectomy. Epidural catheters can be an effective method for analgesia after surgery. However, there are also potential problems with epidural catheters. First, insertion and maintenance of the catheter itself require additional steps. Rather than facilitating mobility, the presence of an epidural catheter may limit ambulation. In our experience, the use of an epidural catheter has not decreased the severity or duration of postoperative ileus. The catheter may become dislodged and provide ineffective pain control.

Patient-controlled analgesia allows more effective pain control and may also result in less overall narcotic usage than periodic administration of parenteral narcotics. A basal rate of analgesic administration (usually morphine sulfate) is maintained, and the patient makes a decision about when an additional bolus is required. Patients should be encouraged to use bolus administration as necessary but to limit narcotic use as much as possible.

Ketorolac, a nonsteroidal anti-inflammatory drug, is an effective analgesic and may have particular applicability in a postoperative setting. We routinely administer ketorolac 30 mg in the postanesthesia care unit and continue a dose of 15 mg every 6 hours for 24 hours postoperatively. Most often, this provides excellent analgesia and limited narcotics are required as supplements. Because of a risk of renal dysfunction with prolonged administration, ketorolac generally should be discontinued 24–48 hours postoperatively and its use withheld altogether in patients with azotemia.[42] In addition, there is some risk of gastrointestinal toxicity or hemorrhagic complications.[43]

## DEEP VENOUS THROMBOSIS PROPHYLAXIS

In most surgical series, thromboembolic complications are the leading cause of mortality and a significant source of morbidity in patients undergoing radical cystectomy.[8] Multiple factors contribute to the risk of thromboembolic problems including comorbidity, the underlying malignancy, and the generally prolonged duration of surgery. Although many guidelines recommend routine anticoagulant prophylaxis for patients undergoing cystectomy, most clinicians are concerned about the risk of hemorrhagic complications.

Although intraoperative bleeding may not be directly affected, postoperative bleeding, pelvic hematoma, and hematuria may all occur in patients on anticoagulant prophylaxis.

Numerous studies have shown that, in order to obtain the maximal effect, any form of prophylaxis used must be administered preoperatively.[44] Low-dose warfarin, mini-dose heparin, and low molecular weight heparin probably have nearly equal efficacy in preventing thromboembolic complications. Further, all have been shown to be superior to no prophylactic anticoagulants in terms of decreasing both deep venous thrombosis (DVT) and pulmonary embolus (PE). Prolonged lymphatic drainage may occur more frequently in patients on anticoagulants, leading to lymphocele formation.[45] However, with intraperitoneal procedures such as radical cystectomy and pelvic lymph node dissection, the entire peritoneum is open and there is less likelihood of loculation of lymphatic fluid.

Other measures are also important. It is generally agreed that early ambulation is important and should be encouraged. Pneumatic calf compression devices have not been proven to be of benefit for radical cystectomy but are commonly used and recommended on the basis of their value with other surgical procedures.[46,47]

In a patient with a suspected DVT, Doppler ultrasonography should be performed. While the accuracy is more limited for calf thrombosis, the test has greater than 95% sensitivity and specificity for proximal venous thrombosis, the most common source of pulmonary embolus.[48] If a Doppler study confirms the presence of DVT, anticoagulant therapy should be administered with unfractionated heparin.[49] The goal of therapy is a partial thromboplastin time 2–2.5 times the control value. Oral warfarin should be initiated immediately as a delay of 5–7 days may occur before therapeutic levels are achieved. Continuation of anticoagulant therapy is usually recommended for a minimum of 3 months after a postoperative thromboembolic event.

If DVT or PE is diagnosed within the first 48 hours after surgery, consideration should be given to placement of an inferior vena cava filter, although there may be a reluctance to administer full dose anticoagulation in the early postoperative period. Even with a filter in place, however, anticoagulant therapy should be initiated once the patient gets beyond the immediate postoperative state.

A clinical suspicion of pulmonary embolus requires prompt diagnosis and treatment. Ventilation perfusion scans frequently are indeterminate in the postoperative period because of atelectasis and/or pneumonia. The diagnosis can be confirmed by pulmonary arteriography or helical computed tomography (CT) scan. Thrombolytic therapy is playing an increasing role in treatment of an acute PE, especially in a patient with clinically significant respiratory compromise.

## GASTROINTESTINAL MANAGEMENT

Historically, patients undergoing major abdominal surgery, especially procedures with a bowel anastomosis, were maintained on nasogastric suction until bowel function returned. In some centers, gastrostomy tube placement has been used to avoid the discomfort of prolonged nasogastric suction. Increasingly, nasogastric tubes are being omitted after abdominal surgery. Nasogastric tubes remove the naturally produced gastric juices as well as air from endogenous production and swallowing. Thus, they may help prevent postoperative distension or vomiting. Nonetheless, most patients do not require nasogastric suction after cystectomy, and placement of a gastrostomy tube seems needlessly invasive.

There is some additional information suggesting that early enteral feeding can help prevent some of the immunosuppression which occurs after surgery and may help promote peristalsis. We performed a randomized prospective study which showed no difference between patients receiving oral intake on the second postoperative day and those kept without food until bowel sounds and bowel function returned (unpublished data). There was an identical rate of abdominal distension in around 10% of patients in both groups requiring insertion of a nasogastric tube.

The pathway we use maintains the patient nil by mouth for at least 24 hours after surgery but nasogastric tubes are not used routinely.[50,51] By the second or third postoperative day, a full liquid diet may be initiated and advanced as tolerated. The stepwise progression from clear liquids to full liquids to a regular diet is not necessarily maintained. In fact, we usually avoid a clear liquid diet alone as many patients prefer full liquids and there is no evidence that a clear liquid diet is tolerated better. Bisacodyl suppositories are used beginning on the second or third postoperative day. This helps promote emptying of the colon and rectum. However, small bowel ileus is likely unaffected.

In a patient with abdominal distension beyond the fourth or fifth postoperative day, a diagnosis of partial small bowel obstruction must be considered. Anastomotic stricture or edema, internal hernia, or obstruction from fibrous tissue can all cause either partial or complete small bowel obstruction after cystectomy. A radiographic flat plate film of the abdomen can be helpful. While distended small bowel typically is visualized in either circumstance, gas in the colon or rectum is more suggestive of ileus. Clinical findings are also important. Bowel sounds are usually diminished or absent when distension is from ileus, whereas they may be hyperactive and with intermittent rushes when small bowel obstruction is present.

Unless there is evidence of an acute intraperitoneal process, the initial management in a patient with ileus versus partial small bowel obstruction is nasogastric suction. Prolonged ileus is the most common cause of delayed hospital discharge and usually resolves spontaneously.[51] Histamine receptor antagonists or proton pump inhibitors may help prevent some of the gastric discomfort. If an apparent ileus fails to resolve after a period of nasogastric suction, an abdominal CT scan should be considered. Sometimes an intra-peritoneal fluid collection such as urinoma or abscess, especially in a patient with fever, can be the source of a prolonged ileus. Administration of oral contrast with small bowel follow-through occasionally is helpful. A water-soluble contrast agent should be used. Ready passage of the contrast, especially into a dilated colon, is consistent with ileus. Parenteral nutrition should be considered in patients with prolonged ileus, and surgical exploration should be deferred unless there are signs of acute obstruction. The overwhelming majority of patients eventually have resolution of the ileus and do not require exploration. Sometimes, however, partial small bowel obstruction can mimic ileus, and surgical exploration is required if there is no resolution of the small bowel distention.

## MANAGEMENT OF DRAINAGE TUBES

The number and type of drainage tubes used after cystectomy is very much dependent upon the philosophy of the individual surgeon. In general, however, a closed suction drain should be placed in the pelvis. The drain evacuates lymphatic fluid, blood, and any urine which may extravasate from either the ureteral anastomosis or the suture line of the reservoir or conduit. Since the drain is intraperitoneal, some output can be expected under the best of circumstances. In general, we remove the drain when the overall output is less than 100 cc in 24 hours. If drainage is excessive or prolonged, it can be submitted for chemistry studies. A creatinine level exceeding the serum level indicates the presence of urine in the drainage. Also, indigo carmine given intravenously will stain the drainage blue if there is urine present. Most often, watchful waiting is appropriate even in the face of a urine leak as spontaneous healing can be expected. If the urine leakage is readily evacuated by the drain, the patient may tolerate this well and even begin oral feeding. If there are indwelling stents, their patency should be confirmed. If no stents are present, or if the drainage persists, an intravenous pyelogram may help detect the source of the urine leakage and allow placement of a nephrostomy tube and internal stent if appropriate.

Ureteral stents frequently are placed across the ureterointestinal anastomosis. Depending upon the method of reconstruction, these may exit through the ileal conduit stoma, through a separate skin stab wound, or alongside a urethral Foley catheter. In any event, their patency should be maintained by periodic irrigation. There is no strong evidence that stents prevent or even reduce the risk of ureterointestinal anastomotic stricture, but they can avoid temporary obstruction from edema and divert the urine to external drainage while anastomotic healing occurs.[52] The duration for which stents are left indwelling is also a matter of individual surgeon philosophy. However, we typically will remove the stents prior to patient discharge.

Some surgeons place a drainage catheter within an ileal conduit to promote urine drainage while the suture or staple line along the base of the conduit heals. This tube may be redundant if there are indwelling ureteral stents. Further, because it can interfere with secure maintenance of a stomal appliance, removal prior to discharge is usually advised.

With a continent cutaneous reservoir, pouch drainage usually occurs via a Malecot catheter which exits either above or below the abdominal stoma. Since most continent cutaneous reservoirs are constructed from right colon, a large amount of mucus is produced and periodic tube irrigation is indicated to maintain patency. These tubes typically are left indwelling for up to several weeks until the patient is facile with intermittent catheterization.

With an orthotopic reservoir, a urethral Foley catheter is placed. Simultaneous placement of a Malecot tube in the suprapubic region is used by some surgeons as a security measure. We have found this unnecessary, and a 20 Fr. urethral Foley catheter alone has provided adequate drainage. The anastomotic integrity usually is sufficient so that a catheter could be replaced if there were premature autodeflation of the catheter balloon. The patient is discharged with the catheter in place with the intent that it be removed approximately 3 weeks later.

## STOMAL THERAPY

Although many patients are motivated to avoid an abdominal stoma, an ileal conduit can provide good quality of life and be a relatively trouble-free method for urinary diversion. However, proper placement and maintenance of the stoma are essential. The stomal site should be selected preoperatively. Usually, the stoma is placed in either the right lower or the right upper quadrant of the abdomen depending upon the patient's body habitus, abdominal creases, or scars from prior surgical incisions. Use of mesh for closure of a ventral or inguinal hernia can also affect placement.

A trained stomal therapist should be available to mark the patient preoperatively. The patient is examined in a sitting, standing, and lying position. The belt line is determined. The stomal therapist may mark both a primary and a secondary site to allow the surgeon some flexibility as intraoperative findings such as adhesions or short mesentery length can dictate placement of the stoma in a specific location.

The patient and the patient's family should be engaged in changing the stomal appliance as soon as possible after surgery. Many patients have a natural aversion to a stoma initially but quickly become comfortable with it and adept at changing the appliance. Selection of proper wafer size and determination of whether use of an abdominal belt is indicated are important considerations.

**Table 43.2** Radical cystectomy—ileal conduit pathway: pre- and early postoperative care

| | Preoperative preparation | Day of surgery/postoperatively | Postoperative days 1–2 |
|---|---|---|---|
| Goals | Informed consent process<br>Preop testing/labs completed within 30 days of surgery<br>Patient and family verbalize understanding of preop teaching | Tolerates procedure without complication<br>Recovers uneventfully from anesthesia<br>Drains and stents patent and functioning<br>Pain controlled, temperature <101°F | Tolerates ambulation with assistance<br>Drains and stents patent and functioning<br>Pain controlled, temperature <101°F<br>Urine output >30 cc/hr |
| Care reminder | Vital signs<br>Height and weight | Vital signs and temperature q.q.h.<br>Assess stoma/peristomal skin q.q.h.<br>Check pouch/dressing q.q.h.<br>Strict intake and output | Vital signs and temperature q.q.h.<br>Assess stoma/peristomal skin q.q.h.<br>Check pouch q.q.h., dressing off POD 2<br>Strict intake and output |
| Treatment | History and physical<br>Consent signed | Incentive spirometer q.h.<br>SCD on 7 hr, off 1 hr<br>TED hose, knee high<br>TCDB q.h.<br>Jackson-Pratt drain empty and record q8h | Incentive spirometer q.h.<br>SCD on 7 hr, off 1 hr<br>TED hose, knee high<br>TCDB q.h.<br>Jackson-Pratt drain empty and record q8h |
| Activity | Ad lib | Bedrest | Out of bed to chair POD 1, then ambulate<br>Ambulate in hallway t.i.d. POD 1 |
| Diet | Clear liquid diet day prior to surgery<br>NPO after midnight | NPO | NPO |
| Tests | Complete blood count<br>Chest x-ray (posteroanterior and lateral) if indicated<br>Basic metabolic panel if indicated<br>Type and crossmatch 2 units packed red blood cells | Potassium 0500 POD 1<br>Hematocrit 0500 POD 1 and POD 2 | |
| Medication | Bowel preparation day prior to surgery<br>GoLYTELY, neomycin, flagyl | D5 ½ NS + 20 mEq KCl @ 150 cc/hr<br>Cefotetan 1 g IV on call to OR then 1 g IV q12h × 2 doses<br>Ketorolac 30 mg IV in PACU then 15 mg IV q6h × 36 hr<br>Analgesic IV/PCA<br>Famotidine 20 mg IV q12h<br>Individualized patient medications | D5 ½ NS + 20 mEq KCl @ 150 cc/hr<br>Cefotetan 1 g IV on call to OR then 1 g IV q12h × 2 doses<br>Ketorolac 30 mg IV in PACU then 15 mg IV q6h × 36 hr<br>Analgesic IV/PCA<br>Famotidine 20 mg IV q12h<br>Individualized patient medications |
| Consults | Enterostomal RN to mark stoma<br>Anesthesia preop evaluation clinic<br>RN practitioner consult<br>CM consult | Enterostomal RN teaching<br>Social work consult | Enterostomal RN teaching |
| Teaching | Orientation to medical center when/where to arrive for surgery, parking, family waiting/visitation<br>MD instructions on procedure anticipated risks/benefits<br>Preop processes concerning cystectomy/ileal conduit | Postop routines to anticipate, IS, TCDB<br>Use of PCA | Patient to receive written educational materials<br>'About Your Urostomy' booklet |
| Discharge planning | Initiate discharge planning, assess home/family support<br>Anticipated length of stay<br>Notify CM for special needs<br>Coordinate with primary care provider, development disability services, prn<br>Autologous blood donation prn | Home health care referral | |

CM, case manager; IS, incentive spirometer; IV, intravenous; NPO, nil per os; PACU, postanesthesia care unit; PCA, patient-controlled analgesia; PO, per os (orally); POD, postoperative day; PRN, according to circumstances, RN, registered nurse; SCD, sequential compression devices; TED, thromboembolic disease; TCDB, turn/cough/deep breathe.

## DISCHARGE PLANNING

A patient should be afebrile, ambulatory without assistance, and tolerating an oral diet before discharge is considered. Even under these circumstances, strong family support and good education are essential. Although a patient may be able to maintain self-hygiene, assistance in food preparation and cleanup as well as aspects of daily living are necessary for a period of time. Sometimes family members are either unavailable or unable to provide the necessary care.

**Table 43.3** Radical cystectomy—ileal conduit pathway: ongoing postoperative care and follow-up

| | Postoperative days 3–4 | Postoperative days 5–7 | Postoperative follow-up |
|---|---|---|---|
| Goals | Pain controlled, temperature <101°F<br>Wafer/pouch intact without leakage<br>Drain output decreasing to 100 cc/day<br>Ambulates with assistance<br>Return of bowel function with flatus/bowel movement | Pain controlled, temperature <101°F<br>Wafer/pouch intact without leakage<br>Patient/family demonstrate urostomy care and verbalize understanding of procedure of pouch/wafer change<br>Ambulates with assistance<br>Return of bowel function, tolerates diet<br>Patient/family understand discharge instructions and home care | Pain controlled<br>Wound healing adequate<br>Tolerates baseline activity |
| Care reminder | Vital signs and temperature q.q.h.<br>Assess stoma/peristomal skin q.q.h.<br>Check pouch q.q.h.<br>Strict intake and output | Vital signs and temperature q.q.h.<br>Assess stoma/peristomal skin q.q.h.<br>Check pouch q.q.h.<br>Strict intake and output | Vital signs and temperature |
| Treatment | Incentive spirometer q.h.<br>SCD on 7 hr, off 1 hr<br>TED hose, knee high<br>TCDB q.h.<br>Jackson-Pratt drain empty and record q8h | Incentive spirometer q.h.<br>SCD on 7 hr, off 1 hr<br>TED hose, knee high<br>TCDB q.h.<br>D/C drains on day of discharge | |
| Activity | Ambulate in hallway t.i.d. | | Ad lib |
| Diet | NPO | Full liquid diet advance to regular diet as tolerated | Regular |
| Tests | Hematocrit 0500 POD 4<br>BMP 0500 POD 4 | | |
| Medication | D5 ½ NS + 20 mEq KCl/L @ 150 cc/hr<br>Analgesic IV/PCA<br>Famotidine 20 mg IV q12h<br>Individualized patient medications | Decrease and D/C IV fluids when taking PO<br>Analgesic PO<br>D/C famotidine when taking PO<br>Trimethoprim-sulfamethoxazole (Bactrim DS) PO b.i.d. × 17 days, alternatively nitrofurantoin (Macrodantin) 100 mg PO q.h.s. × 17 days<br>Individualized patient medications | |
| Consults | – | – | |
| Teaching | | Discharge self-care and activity:<br>    May shower<br>    Walking and stairs okay<br>    No lifting over 5 lbs<br>    No driving<br>    Keep wound clean and dry<br>Discharge medications:<br>    Milk of Magnesia for constipation<br>    Percocet for pain<br>    Bactrim or Macrodantin × 17 days<br>Reportable signs and symptoms:<br>    How and when to contact surgeon<br>    Call for temperature >101°F, wound erythema, increased tenderness, nausea, and emesis<br>Pouch/wafer change | |
| Discharge planning | | Discharge prescriptions written and received<br>Follow-up appointment scheduled and confirmed 2–4 weeks, depending on surgeon preference<br>Home health care arrangements completed prior to discharge | |

D/C, discontinue. See Table 43.2 for explanation of other acronyms.

Visiting nurses can allow a patient to return to a home environment even when some assistance is required. In other situations, an intermediate care facility can provide a bridge between inpatient hospitalization and a return home. The key to all of these measures is proper preparation and education of both the patient and immediate family members or care providers.

## CLINICAL PATHWAYS

All aspects of perioperative care are facilitated by use of a clinical pathway.[53] The pathway document outlines the minimal care necessary for the ideal patient (Tables 43.2 and 43.3). Further, the pathway allows the patient to anticipate various aspects of care and to participate in recovery. Especially with an operation as complex as cystectomy, deviations from a pathway or use of additional procedures or testing is common. Thus, it is incumbent upon the clinician to provide careful oversight and involvement rather than simply allowing the pathway to serve as a default guide.

## CONCLUSION

The morbidity and mortality from radical cystectomy have diminished significantly over the last few decades. Some of this is a consequence of improved surgical technique and better understanding of the anatomy. To a great extent, though, the improvements can be attributed to advances in perioperative care. Sometimes this means eliminating or withholding unnecessary procedures or treatments, especially those which are invasive in themselves. In other circumstances, it requires active intervention. In all situations, familiarity with available knowledge and experience is essential in providing optimal results.

### REFERENCES

1. Stein JP, Lieskovsky G, Cote R, et al. Radical cystectomy in the treatment of invasive bladder cancer: long-term results in 1,054 patients. J Clin Oncol 2001;19:666–675.
2. Quek ML, Stein JP, Clark PE, et al. Natural history of surgically treated bladder carcinoma with extravesical tumor extension. Cancer 2003;98:955–961.
3. Montie JE, Wood DP Jr. The risk of radical cystectomy. Br J Urol 1989;63:483–486.
4. Thrasher JB, Crawford ED. Current management of invasive and metastatic transitional cell carcinoma of the bladder. J Urol 1993;149:957–972.
5. Shipley WU, Kaufman DS, Zehr E, et al. Selective bladder preservation by combined modality protocol treatment: long-term outcomes of 190 patients with invasive bladder cancer. Urology 2002;60:62–68.
6. Farnham SB, Cookson MS, Alberts G, et al. Benefit of radical cystectomy in the elderly patient with significant co-morbidities. Urol Oncol 2004;22:178–181.
7. Lynch CF, Cohen MB. Urinary system. Cancer 1995;75:316–329.
8. Hendry WF. Morbidity and mortality of radical cystectomy (1971–78 and 1978–85). J R Soc Med 1986;79:395–400.
9. Chang SS, Alberts G, Cookson MS, et al. Radical cystectomy is safe in elderly patients at high risk. J Urol 2001;166:938–941.
10. Peyromaure M, Guerin F, Debre B, et al. Surgical management of infiltrating bladder cancer in elderly patients. Eur Urol 2004;45:147–154.
11. Game X, Soulie M, Seguin P, et al. Radical cystectomy in patients older than 75 years: assessment of morbidity and mortality. Eur Urol 2001;39:525–529.
12. Soulie M, Straub M, Game X, et al. A multicenter study of the morbidity of radical cystectomy in select elderly patients with bladder cancer. J Urol 2002;167:1325–1328.
13. Parekh DJ, Gilbert WB, Koch MO, et al. Continent urinary reconstruction versus ileal conduit: a contemporary single-institution comparison of perioperative morbidity and mortality. Urology 2000;55:852–855.
14. Dutta SC, Chang SC, Coffey CS, et al. Health related quality of life assessment after radical cystectomy: comparison of ileal conduit with continent orthotopic neobladder. J Urol 2002;168:164–167.
15. American Society of Anesthesiologists. New classification of physical status. Anesthesiology 1963;24:111.
16. Morrison AS. Advances in the etiology of urothelial cancer. Urol Clin North Am 1984;11:557–566.
17. Burch JD, Rohan TE, Howe GR, et al. Risk of bladder cancer by source and type of tobacco exposure: a case-control study. Int J Cancer 1989;44:622–628.
18. Parekh DJ, Clark T, O'Connor J, et al. Orthotopic neobladder following radical cystectomy in patients with high perioperative risk and co-morbid medical conditions. J Urol 2002;168:2454–2456.
19. Miller DC, Taub DA, Dunn RL, et al. The impact of co-morbid disease on cancer control and survival following radical cystectomy. J Urol 2003;169:105–109.
20. Chang SS, Hassan JM, Cookson MS, et al. Delaying radical cystectomy for muscle invasive bladder cancer results in worse pathological stage. J Urol 2003;170:1085–1087.
21. Sanchez-Ortiz RF, Huang WC, Mick R, et al. An interval longer than 12 weeks between the diagnosis of muscle invasion and cystectomy is associated with worse outcome in bladder carcinoma. J Urol 2003;169:110–115; discussion 115.
22. Eagle KA, Berger PB, Calkins H, et al. ACC/AHA guideline update for perioperative cardiovascular evaluation for noncardiac surgery—executive summary: a report of the American College of Cardiology/American Heart Association Task Force on Practice Guidelines (Committee to Update the 1996 Guidelines on Perioperative Cardiovascular Evaluation for Noncardiac Surgery). Online. Available: www.acc.org/clinical/guidelines/perio/update/periupdate_index.htm.
23. Park KW. Preoperative cardiac evaluation. Anesthesiol Clin North America 2004;22:199–208.
24. Beneficial effect of carotid endarterectomy in symptomatic patients with high-grade carotid stenosis. North American Symptomatic Carotid Endarterectomy Trial Collaborators. N Engl J Med 1991;325:445–453.
25. Richardson JD, Cocanour CS, Kern JA, et al. Perioperative risk assessment in elderly and high-risk patients. J Am Coll Surg 2004;199:133–146.
26. Rock P, Passannante A. Preoperative assessment: pulmonary. Anesthesiol Clin North America 2004;22:77–91.
27. Connery LE, Coursin DB. Assessment and therapy of selected endocrine disorders. Anesthesiol Clin North America 2004;22:93–123.
28. Coursin DB, Connery LE, Ketzler JT. Perioperative diabetic and hyperglycemic management issues. Crit Care Med 2004;32:S116–125.
29. Gibbs J, Cull W, Henderson W, et al. Preoperative serum albumin level as a predictor of operative mortality and morbidity: results from the National VA Surgical Risk Study. Arch Surg 1999;134:36–42.
30. Askanazi J, Hensle TW, Starker PM, et al. Effect of immediate postoperative nutritional support on length of hospitalization. Ann Surg 1986;203:236–239.

31. Krishnan M. Preoperative care of patients with kidney disease. Am Fam Physician 2002;66:1471–1476.

32. Ahlering TE, Henderson JB, Skinner DG. Controlled hypotensive anesthesia to reduce blood loss in radical cystectomy for bladder cancer. J Urol 1983;129:953–954.

33. Chang SS, Smith JA Jr, Wells N, et al. Estimated blood loss and transfusion requirements of radical cystectomy. J Urol 2001;166:2151–2154.

34. Park KI, Kojima O, Tomoyoshi T. Intra-operative autotransfusion in radical cystectomy. Br J Urol 1997;79:717–721.

35. Ferguson KH, McNeil JJ, Morey AF. Mechanical and antibiotic bowel preparation for urinary diversion surgery. J Urol 2002;167:2352–2356.

36. Oliveira L, Wexner SD, Daniel N, et al. Mechanical bowel preparation for elective colorectal surgery. A prospective, randomized, surgeon-blinded trial comparing sodium phosphate and polyethylene glycol-based oral lavage solutions. Dis Colon Rectum 1997;40:585–591.

37. Nichols RL, Broido P, Condon RE, Gorbach SL, Nyhus LM. Effect of preoperative neomycin–erythromycin intestinal preparation on the incidence of infectious complications following colon surgery. Ann Surg 1973;178:453–459.

38. Mangram AJ, Horan TC, Pearson ML et al. Guideline for prevention of surgical site infection, 1999. Centers for Disease Control and Prevention (CDC) Hospital Infection Control Practices Advisory Committee. Am J Infect Control 1999;27:97–134.

39. Mercado DL, Petty BG. Perioperative medication management. Med Clin North Am 2003;87:41–57.

40. Pass SE, Simpson RW. Discontinuation and reinstitution of medications during the perioperative period. Am J Health Syst Pharm 2004;61:899–914.

41. Chang SS, Cookson MS, Hassan JM, et al. Routine postoperative intensive care monitoring is not necessary after radical cystectomy. J Urol 2002;167:1321–1324.

42. Haragsim L, Dalal R, Bagga H, et al. Ketorolac-induced acute renal failure and hyperkalemia: report of three cases. Am J Kidney Dis 1994;24:578–580.

43. Strom BL, Berlin JA, Kinman JL, et al. Parenteral ketorolac and risk of gastrointestinal and operative site bleeding. A postmarketing surveillance study. JAMA 1996;275:376–382.

44. Heit JA. Perioperative management of the chronically anticoagulated patient. J Thromb Thrombolysis 2001;12:81–87.

45. Koch MO Jr, Smith JA. Low molecular weight heparin and radical prostatectomy: a prospective analysis of safety and side effects. Prostate Cancer Prostatic Dis 1997;1:101–104.

46. Cisek LJ, Walsh PC. Thromboembolic complications following radical retropubic prostatectomy. Influence of external sequential pneumatic compression devices. Urology 1993;42:406–408.

47. Chandhoke PS, Gooding GA, Narayan P. Prospective randomized trial of warfarin and intermittent pneumatic leg compression as prophylaxis for postoperative deep venous thrombosis in major urological surgery. J Urol 1992;147:1056–1059.

48. Ramzi DW, Leeper KV. DVT and pulmonary embolism: Part I. Diagnosis. Am Fam Physician 2004;69:2829–2836.

49. Ramzi DW, Leeper KV. DVT and pulmonary embolism: Part II. Treatment and prevention. Am Fam Physician 2004;69:2841–2848.

50. Baumgartner RG, Wells N, Chang SS, et al. Causes of increased length of stay following radical cystectomy. Urol Nurs 2002;22:319–323.

51. Chang SS, Baumgartner RG, Wells N, et al. Causes of increased hospital stay after radical cystectomy in a clinical pathway setting. J Urol 2002;167:208–211.

52. Regan JB, Barrett, DM. Stented versus nonstented ureteroileal anastomoses: is there a difference with regard to leak and stricture? J Urol 1985;134:1101–1103.

53. Chang SS, Cookson MS, Baumgartner RG, et al. Analysis of early complications after radical cystectomy: results of a collaborative care pathway. J Urol 2002;167:2012–2016.

# Radical cystectomy—technique and outcomes

44

*John P Stein, Donald G Skinner*

## INTRODUCTION

In the United States, bladder cancer is the fourth most common cancer in men and the eighth most common in women, with transitional cell carcinoma (TCC) comprising nearly 90% of all primary bladder tumors.[1] Although the majority of patients present with superficial bladder tumors, 20% to 40% of patients will either present with or ultimately develop muscle-invasive disease. Invasive bladder cancer is a lethal malignancy. If left untreated, over 85% of patients die of the disease within 2 years of the diagnosis.[2] Furthermore, in a certain percent of patients with high-grade bladder tumors without involvement of the lamina propria disease will recur/progress and/or fail intravesical management. Such patients may be best treated with an earlier cystectomy when survival outcomes are optimal.[3]

The rationale for an aggressive treatment approach employing radical cystectomy for high-grade, invasive bladder cancer is based on several important observations:

1. The best long-term survival rates, coupled with the lowest local recurrences, are seen following definitive surgery removing the primary bladder tumor and regional lymph nodes.[4,5]
2. The morbidity and mortality of radical cystectomy has significantly improved over the past several decades.
3. TCC tends to be a tumor that is resistant to radiation therapy, even at high doses.
4. Chemotherapy alone, or in combination with bladder-sparing protocols, has not demonstrated long-term local control and survival rates equivalent to those with cystectomy.[6]

5. Radical cystectomy provides accurate pathologic staging of the primary bladder tumor (p stage) and regional lymph nodes, thus selectively determining the need for adjuvant therapy based on precise pathologic evaluation.

For the aforementioned reasons, radical cystectomy has become a standard and arguably is the best definitive form of therapy for high-grade, invasive bladder cancer today.

The evolution and improvement in lower urinary tract reconstruction, particularly orthotopic diversion, has been a major component in enhancing the quality of life of patients requiring cystectomy. Currently, most men and women can safely undergo orthotopic lower urinary tract reconstruction to the native, intact urethra following cystectomy.[7] Orthotopic reconstruction most closely resembles the original bladder in both location and function, provides a continent means to store urine, and allows volitional voiding via the urethra. The orthotopic neobladder eliminates the need for a cutaneous stoma, urostomy appliance, and the need for intermittent catheterization in most cases. These efforts have improved the quality of life of patients who must undergo bladder removal, and have also stimulated patients and physicians to consider radical cystectomy for high-grade, invasive bladder cancer at an earlier, more curable stage.[8]

At the University of Southern California (USC) a dedicated effort has been made to improve continually upon the surgical technique of radical cystectomy and to provide an acceptable form of urinary diversion, without compromise of a sound cancer operation.[9–11] Certain technical issues regarding radical cystectomy and an appropriate extended bilateral pelvic iliac lymphadenectomy are critical in order to minimize local recurrence and positive surgical margins, and to maximize cancer-specific survival. Attention to surgical detail is important in optimizing the successful clinical outcomes of orthotopic diversion, maintaining the rhabdosphincter mechanism and urinary continence in these patients.[11]

Herein, the detailed surgical approach and technical aspects of radical cystectomy in men and women are described. This surgical approach also includes a description of an extended lymphadenectomy. We believe this is an important component in radical cystectomy and the clinical outcomes of patients with high-grade, invasive bladder cancer. A growing body of evidence exists to suggest that a more extended lymphadenectomy may be beneficial in both lymph node-positive and lymph node-negative patients with bladder cancer.[12-16] Although the exact limits of the lymphadenectomy for patients with bladder cancer undergoing cystectomy are currently debated, we advocate a lymph node dissection with the boundaries to include initiation at the level of the inferior mesenteric artery (superior limits of dissection), extending laterally over the inferior vena cava/aorta to the genitofemoral nerve (lateral limits of dissection), and distally to the lymph node of Cloquet medially (on Cooper's ligament) and the circumflex iliac vein laterally. This dissection should also include bilaterally all obturator, hypogastric, and presciatic lymph nodes, as well as the presacral lymph nodes.

## INDICATIONS FOR CYSTECTOMY

Invasive bladder cancer includes a spectrum of tumors ranging from infiltration of the superficial lamina propria (T1), to extension into (T2), and through (T3) the muscularis propria. Traditionally, tumor invasion of the smooth muscle bladder muscularis propria has been an absolute indication for radical cystectomy. In addition, there is sufficient evidence to suggest that certain high-grade tumors invading the lamina propria (T1) are at increased risk for muscularis propria invasion and/or tumor progression,[3,17-22] and may be best treated with an early radical cystectomy. Furthermore, superficial bladder tumors with lymphovascular invasion,[19,23] those with prostatic urethral involvement,[24] or those associated with carcinoma in situ (CIS),[25,26] in conjunction with a poor response to repeated transurethral resection and intravesical therapy,[22] may also be at high risk and could benefit from an early and aggressive therapeutic scheme such as radical cystectomy.

## PREOPERATIVE EVALUATION

Complete clinical staging for bladder cancer should evaluate the retroperitoneum and pelvis along with common metastatic sites, including the lungs, liver, and bones. A chest x-ray, liver function tests, and serum alkaline phosphatase should be obtained routinely. Patients with an elevated serum alkaline phosphatase and/or complaints of bone pain should undergo a bone scan. A computed tomography (CT) scan of the chest is obtained when pulmonary metastases are suspected by history, or because of an abnormal chest x-ray. A CT scan of the abdomen and pelvis is routinely performed to evaluate the pelvis and retroperitoneum for any significant lymphadenopathy or local contiguous spread. This radiographic evaluation should also be performed in patients with suspected metastases, elevated liver functions tests, or a bladder tumor associated with hydronephrosis, or in patients with an extensive primary bladder tumor that is either clinically nonmobile or fixed; the results of these studies may have an impact upon the decision for neoadjuvant therapy. However, CT scan of the primary bladder is neither sufficiently sensitive nor specific to evaluate the degree of bladder wall tumor invasion or to determine accurately the pelvic lymph node involvement with tumor.[27,28]

## EN BLOC RADICAL CYSTECTOMY AND PELVIC–ILIAC LYMPHADENECTOMY: SURGICAL TECHNIQUE

### PREOPERATIVE PREPARATION

Patients undergoing radical cystectomy are admitted on the morning of the day before surgery. All patients receive a mechanical and antibacterial bowel preparation the day before surgery. Intravenous hydration must be considered in these patients to prevent dehydration upon arrival at the operating room. In addition, all patients should be evaluated and counseled by the enterostomal therapy nurse prior to surgery. A clear liquid diet may be consumed until midnight, after which time the patient takes nothing per mouth. A standard modified Nichols bowel preparation[29] is initiated the morning of admission: 120 ml castor oil laxative (Neoloid) by mouth at 09:00; 1 g neomycin by mouth at 10:00, 11:00, 12:00, 13:00, 16:00, 20:00, and 24:00; and 1 g erythromycin base by mouth at 12:00, 16:00, 20:00, and 24:00. This regimen is generally well tolerated, obviates the need for enemas, and maintains nutritional and hydrational support. Intravenous crystalloid fluid hydration is begun in the evening before surgery in those patients admitted to the hospital on the day before surgery, and maintained to ensure an adequate circulating intravascular volume as the patient enters the operating room. This may be particularly important in the elderly, frail patient with associated comorbidities.

Patients over 50 years of age at our institution routinely undergo prophylactic digitalization prior to cystectomy unless a specific contraindication exists. Patients younger than 50 years of age are not routinely digitalized. Digoxin is given orally: 0.5 mg at 12:00, 0.25 mg at 16:00, and 0.125 mg at 20:00. Our experience with preoperative digitalization in patients undergoing cystectomy has been positive and there is evidence suggesting that preoperative digitalization may reduce the risk of perioperative dysrhythmias and congestive heart failure in the elderly patient undergoing an extensive operative procedure.[30,31] Attention to fluid management is important in these elderly patients, particularly on postoperative days three and four when mobilization of third-space fluid is highest, subsequently necessitating liberal use of diuretics. In addition, intravenous broad-spectrum antibiotics are administered en route to the operating room, providing adequate tissue and circulating levels at the time of incision.

Preoperative evaluation and counseling by the enterostomal therapy nurse is a critical component to the successful care of all patients undergoing cystectomy and urinary diversion. Patients determined to be appropriate candidates for orthotopic reconstruction are instructed how to catheterize per urethra should it be necessary postoperatively. All patients are site marked for a cutaneous stoma, instructed in the care of a cutaneous diversion (continent or incontinent form), and instructed in proper catheterization techniques should medical, technical or oncologic factors preclude orthotopic reconstruction. The ideal cutaneous stoma site is determined only after the patient is examined in the supine, sitting, and standing position. Proper stoma site selection is important to patient acceptance, and to the technical success of lower urinary tract reconstruction should a cutaneous form of diversion be necessary. Incontinent stoma sites are best located higher on the abdominal wall, while stoma sites for continent diversions can be positioned lower on the abdomen (hidden below the belt line) since they do not require an external collecting device. The use of the umbilicus as the site for catheterization may be employed with excellent functional and cosmetic results.

## PATIENT POSITIONING

The patient is placed in the hyperextended supine position with the superior iliac crest located at the fulcrum of the operating table (Figure 44.1). The legs are slightly abducted so that the heels are positioned near the corners of the foot of the table. In the female patient considering orthotopic diversion, the modified frog-leg or lithotomy position is employed, allowing access to the vagina. Care should be taken to ensure that all pressure points are well padded. Reverse Trendelenburg

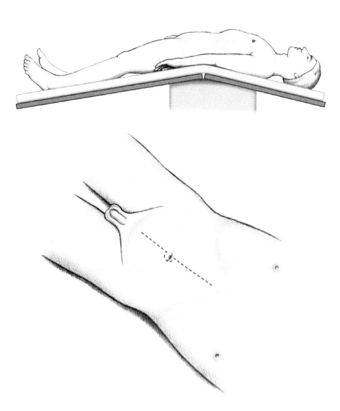

**Fig. 44.1**
Proper patient positioning for cystectomy in the male patient. Note that the iliac crest is located at the break of the table.

position levels the abdomen parallel with the floor and helps to keep the small bowel contents in the epigastrium. A nasogastric tube is placed, and the patient is prepped from nipples to mid-thighs. In the female patient the vagina is also fully prepped. After the patient is draped, a 20 Fr. Foley catheter is placed in the bladder and left to gravity drainage. A right-handed surgeon stands on the patient's left-hand side of the operating table.

## INCISION

A vertical midline incision is made extending from the pubic symphysis to the cephalad aspect of the epigastrium. The incision should be carried lateral to the umbilicus on the contralateral side of the marked cutaneous stoma site. When the umbilicus is considered as the site for a catheterizable stoma, the incision should be directed 2–3 cm lateral to the umbilicus at this location. The anterior rectus fascia is incised, the rectus muscles retracted laterally, and the posterior rectus sheath and peritoneum entered in the superior aspect of the incision. As the peritoneum and posterior fascia are incised inferiorly to the level of the umbilicus, the urachal remnant (median umbilical ligament) is identified, circumscribed, and removed en bloc with the cystectomy specimen (Figure 44.2). This maneuver prevents early entry into a high-riding bladder, and

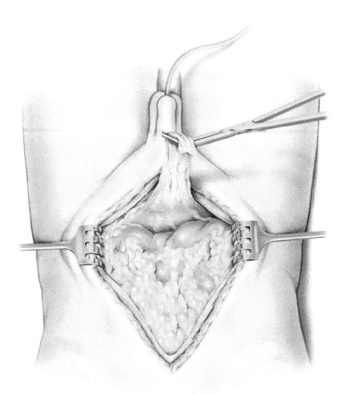

**Fig. 44.2**
Wide excision of the urachal remnant and medial umbilical ligaments en bloc with the cystectomy specimen.

ensures complete removal of all bladder remnant tissue. Care is taken to remain medial and avoid injury to the inferior epigastric vessels (lateral umbilical ligaments), which course posterior to the rectus muscles. If the patient has previously had a cystotomy or segmental cystectomy, the cystotomy tract and cutaneous incision should be circumscribed full-thickness and excised en bloc with the bladder specimen. The medial insertion of the rectus muscles attached to the pubic symphysis can be slightly incised, maximizing pelvic exposure throughout the operation.

## ABDOMINAL EXPLORATION

A careful, systematic intra-abdominal exploration is performed to determine the extent of disease, and to evaluate for any hepatic metastases or gross retroperitoneal lymphadenopathy. The abdominal viscera are palpated to detect any concomitant unrelated disease. If no contraindication exists at this time, all adhesions should be incised and freed.

## BOWEL MOBILIZATION

The bowel is mobilized beginning with the ascending colon. A large right-angle Richardson retractor elevates the right abdominal wall. The cecum and ascending colon are reflected medially to allow incision of the

lateral peritoneal reflection along the avascular/white line of Toldt. The mesentery to the small bowel is then mobilized off its retroperitoneal attachments cephalad (toward the ligament of Treitz) until the retroperitoneal portion of the duodenum is exposed. This mobilization facilitates a tension-free urethroenteric anastomosis if orthotopic diversion is performed. Combined sharp and blunt dissection facilitate mobilization of this mesentery along a characteristic avascular fibroareolar plane. Conceptually, the mobilized mesentery forms an inverted right triangle: the base formed by the third and fourth portions of the duodenum, the right edge represented by the white line of Toldt along the ascending colon, the left edge represented by the medial portion of the sigmoid and descending colonic mesentery, and the apex represented by the ileocecal region (Figure 44.3). This mobilization is critical in setting up the operative field, and facilitates proper packing of the intra-abdominal contents into the epigastrium.

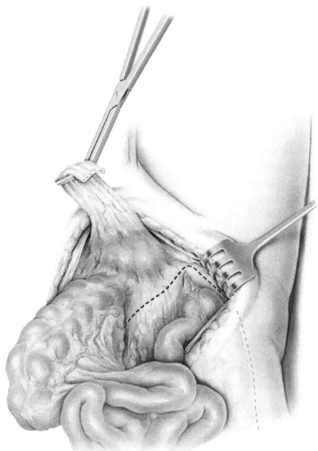

**Fig. 44.3**
View of the pelvis from overhead after the ascending colon and peritoneal attachments of the small bowel mesentery have been mobilized up to the level of the duodenum. This mobilization allows the bowel to be properly packed in the epigastrium and exposes the area of the aortic bifurcation which is the starting point of the lymph node dissection.

The left colon and sigmoid mesentery are then mobilized to the region of the lower pole of the left kidney by incising the peritoneum lateral to the colon along the avascular/white line of Toldt. The sigmoid mesentery is then elevated off the sacrum, iliac vessels, and distal aorta in a cephalad direction up to the origin of the inferior mesenteric artery (IMA) (Figure 44.4). This maneuver provides a wide mesenteric window through which the left ureter will pass (without angulation or tension) for the ureteroenteric anastomosis at the terminal portions of the operation. This sigmoid mobilization helps identify the IMA and facilitates retraction of the sigmoid mesentery, particularly when the superior limits of the lymph node dissection are performed. Care should be taken to dissect along the base of the mesentery and to avoid injury to the inferior mesenteric artery and blood supply to the sigmoid colon.

After mobilization of the bowel, a self-retaining retractor is placed. The right colon and small intestine are carefully packed into the epigastrium with three moist lap pads, followed by a moistened towel rolled to the width of the abdomen. The descending and sigmoid colon are not packed and remain as free as possible, providing the necessary mobility required for the ureteral and pelvic lymph node dissection.

Successful packing of the intestinal contents is an art and prevents their annoying spillage into the operative field. Packing begins by sweeping the right colon and small bowel under the surgeon's left hand along the right sidewall gutter. A moist open lap pad is then swept with the right hand along the palm of the left hand, under the viscera along the retroperitoneum and sidewall gutter. In similar fashion, the left sidewall gutter is packed, ensuring not to incorporate the descending or sigmoid colon. The central portion of the small bowel is packed with a third lap pad. A moist rolled towel is then positioned horizontally below the lap pads, but cephalad to the bifurcation of the aorta.

Occasionally, prior to placement of the first moist lap pad, a mobile greater omental apron can be used to facilitate packing of the intestinal viscera in a fashion similar to that with lap pad. After the bowel has been packed, a wide Deaver retractor is placed with gentle traction on the previously placed packing to provide cephalad exposure.

## URETERAL DISSECTION

The ureters are most easily identified in the retroperitoneum just cephalad to the common iliac vessels. They are carefully dissected into the deep pelvis (several centimeters beyond the iliac vessels) and divided between two large hemoclips. A section of the proximal cut ureteral segment (distal to the proximal hemoclip) is sent for frozen section analysis to ensure the absence of carcinoma in situ or overt tumor. The ureter is then slightly mobilized in a cephalad direction and tucked under the rolled towel to prevent inadvertent injury. Frequently, an arterial branch from the common iliac artery or the aorta needs to be divided to provide adequate ureteral mobilization. In addition, the rich vascular supply emanating laterally from the gonadal vessels should remain intact and undisturbed. These attachments are an important blood supply to the ureter, which ensure an adequate vascular supply for the ureteroenteric anastomosis at the time of diversion. This is particularly important in irradiated patients. Leaving the proximal hemoclip on the divided ureter during the exenteration allows for hydrostatic ureteral dilation and facilitates the ureteroenteric anastomosis. In women, the infundibulopelvic ligaments are ligated and divided at the level of the common iliac vessels.

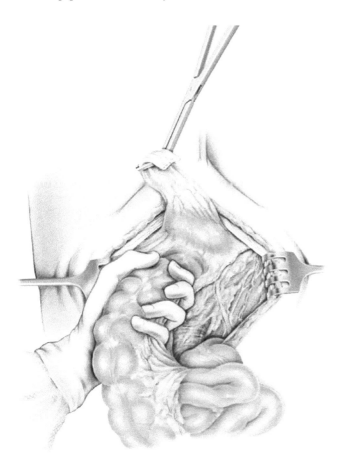

**Fig. 44.4**
View of the pelvis from overhead, after the ascending colon and small bowel have been packed in the epigastrium. Note that the sigmoid mesentery is mobilized off the sacral promontory and distal aorta up to the origin of the inferior mesenteric artery.

## PELVIC LYMPHADENECTOMY

A meticulous pelvic lymph node dissection is routinely performed with radical cystectomy. The extent of the lymphadenectomy may vary depending on the patient and surgeon preference. An accumulating body of evidence suggests that a more extended lymphadenectomy may be beneficial in patients undergoing cystectomy for high-grade, invasive bladder cancer.[12-16] When performing a salvage procedure following definitive radiation treatment (greater than 5000 cGy), a more limited pelvic lymphadenectomy may be performed or even abandoned if there appears to be a significant risk of iliac vessel and obturator nerve injury.[32]

For a combined common and pelvic iliac lymphadenectomy, the lymph node dissection is initiated at the IMA (superior limits of dissection), and extends laterally over the inferior vena cava to the genitofemoral nerve, representing the lateral limits of dissection. Distally, the lymph node dissection extends to the lymph node of Cloquet medially (on Cooper's ligament) and the circumflex iliac vein laterally.

The cephalad portion (at the level of the IMA) of the lymphatics is ligated with hemoclips to prevent lymphatic leak, while the caudal (specimen) side is ligated only when a blood vessel is encountered. Frequently, small anterior tributary veins originate from the vena cava just above the bifurcation. These should be clipped and divided. In men, the spermatic vessels are retracted laterally and spared. In women the infundibulopelvic ligament, along with the corresponding ovarian vessels, has been ligated previously and divided at the pelvic brim as described earlier.

All fibroareolar and lymphatic tissues are dissected caudally off the aorta, vena cava, and common iliac vessels over the sacral promontory into the deep pelvis. The initial dissection along the common iliac vessels is performed over the arteries, skeletonizing them. As the common iliac veins are dissected medially, care is taken to control small arterial and venous branches coursing along the anterior surface of the sacrum. Electrocautery is helpful at this location and allows the adherent fibroareolar tissue to be swept off the sacral promontory down into the deep pelvis with the use of a small gauze sponge. Significant bleeding from these presacral vessels can occur if not properly controlled. Hemoclips are discouraged in this location as they can be easily dislodged from the anterior surface of the sacrum, and troublesome bleeding can occur.

Once the proximal portion of the lymph node dissection is completed, a finger is passed from the proximal aspect of dissection under the pelvic peritoneum (anterior to the iliac vessels), distally toward the femoral canal. The opposite hand can be used to strip the peritoneum from the undersurface of the transversalis fascia and connects with the proximal dissection from above. This maneuver elevates the peritoneum and defines the lateral limit of peritoneum to be incised and removed with the specimen. The peritoneum is divided medial to the spermatic vessels in

men, and lateral to the infundibulopelvic ligament in women. The only structure encountered is the vas deferens in the male or round ligament in the female; these structures are clipped and divided.

A large right-angled rake retractor (e.g. Israel) is used to elevate the lower abdominal wall, including the spermatic cord or remnant of the round ligament, to provide distal exposure in the area of the femoral canal. Tension on the retractor is directed vertically toward the ceiling, and care is taken to avoid injury to the inferior epigastric vessels. This approach provides excellent exposure to the distal external iliac vessels. The distal limits of the dissection are then identified: the circumflex iliac vein crossing anterior to the external iliac artery distally, the genitofemoral nerve laterally, and Cooper's ligament medially. The lymphatics draining the ipsilateral leg, particularly medial to the external iliac vein, are carefully clipped and divided to prevent lymphatic leakage. This includes the lymph node of Cloquet (also known as Rosenmuller), which represents the distal limit of the lymphatic dissection at this location. The distal external iliac artery and vein are then circumferentially dissected and skeletonized, with care being taken to ligate an accessory obturator vein

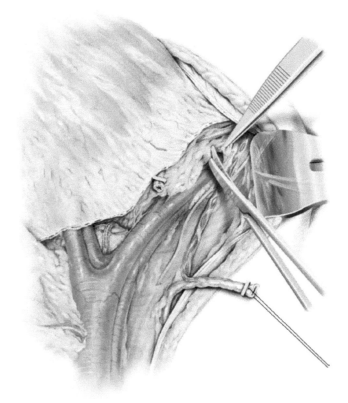

**Fig. 44.5**
Skeletonizing the external iliac artery and vein. Note that the vessels are dissected completely free up to the level of the origin of the hypogastric artery. This allows for the vessels to be carefully retracted medially and the psoas fascia incised to allow passage of a gauze sponge.

(present in 40% of patients) originating from the inferomedial aspect of the external iliac vein.

Following completion of the distal limits of dissection, the proximal and distal dissections are joined. The proximal external iliac artery and vein are skeletonized circumferentially to the origin of the hypogastric artery (Figure 44.5). Care should be taken to clip and divide a commonly encountered vessel arising from the lateral aspect of the proximal external iliac vessels coursing to the psoas muscle. The external iliac vessels (artery and vein) are then retracted medially, and the fascia overlying the psoas muscle is incised medial to the genitofemoral nerve. On the left side, branches of the genitofemoral nerve often pursue a more medial course and may be intimately related to the iliac vessels, in which case they are excised.

At this point, the lymphatic tissues surrounding the iliac vessels are composed of a medial and a lateral component attached only at the base within the obturator fossa. The lateral lymphatic compartment (freed medially from the vessels and laterally from the psoas) is bluntly swept into the obturator fossa by retracting the iliac vessels medially, and passing a small gauze sponge lateral to the vessels along the psoas and pelvic sidewall (Figure 44.6). This sponge should be passed anterior and distal to the hypogastric vein and

directed caudally into the obturator fossa. The external iliac vessels are then elevated and retracted laterally, and the gauze sponge carefully withdrawn from the obturator fossa with gentle traction using the left hand (Figure 44.7). This maneuver effectively sweeps all lymphatic tissue into the obturator fossa, and facilitates identification of the obturator nerve deep to the external iliac vein. The obturator nerve is best identified proximally, and carefully dissected free from all lymphatics. The obturator nerve is then retracted laterally along with the iliac vessels (Figure 44.8). At this point, the obturator artery and vein should be carefully entrapped between the index finger (medial to the obturator nerve) laterally and the middle finger medially with the left hand. This isolates the obturator vessels exiting the obturator canal along the pelvic floor. These vessels are then carefully clipped and divided, making certain to stay medial to the obturator nerve. The obturator lymph node packet is then swept medially toward the sidewall of the bladder, and small tributary vessels and lymphatics from the pelvic sidewall and ligated. The nodal packet will be removed en bloc with the cystectomy specimen.

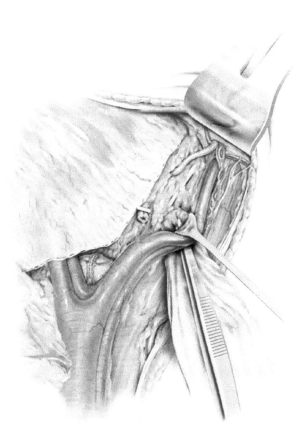

**Fig. 44.6**
Passing a small gauze sponge lateral to the external iliac vessels and medial to the psoas muscle.

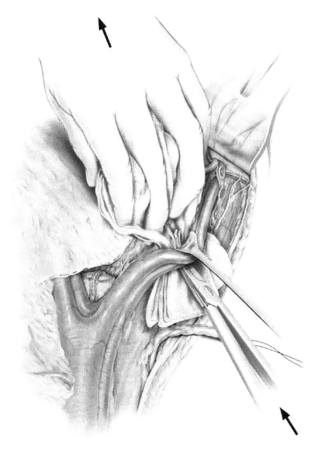

**Fig. 44.7**
Withdrawing the gauze sponge with the left hand. This aids in dissecting and clearing the obturator fossa, sweeping all fibroareolar and lymphatic tissue toward the bladder.

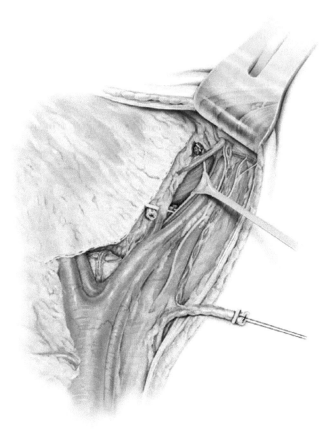

**Fig. 44.8**
Obturator fossa cleaned. This allows proper identification of the obturator nerve passing deep to the external iliac vein.

## LIGATION OF THE LATERAL VASCULAR PEDICLE TO THE BLADDER

Following dissection of the obturator fossa and division of the obturator vessels, the lateral vascular pedicle to the bladder is isolated and divided. Developing this plane isolates the lateral vascular pedicle to the bladder; a critical maneuver in performing a safe cystectomy with proper vascular control. Isolation of the lateral vascular pedicle is performed with the left hand. The bladder is retracted toward the pelvis, placing traction and isolating the anterior branches of the hypogastric artery. The left index finger is passed medial to the hypogastric artery, posterior to the anterior visceral branches, and lateral to the previously transected ureter. The index finger is directed caudally toward the endopelvic fascia, parallel to the sweep of the sacrum. This maneuver defines the two major vascular pedicles to the anterior pelvic organs: the lateral pedicle anterior to the index finger, composed of the visceral branches of the anterior hypogastric vessel, and the posterior pedicle posterior to the index finger, composed of the visceral branches between the bladder and rectum.

With the lateral pedicle entrapped between the left index and middle fingers, firm traction is applied vertically and caudally. This facilitates identification and

isolation of individual branches off the anterior portion of the hypogastric artery (Figure 44.9). The posterior division of the hypogastric artery, including the superior gluteal, iliolumbar, and lateral sacral arteries, is preserved in order to avoid gluteal claudication. Distal to this posterior division, the hypogastric artery may be ligated for vascular control, but should not be divided since the lateral pedicle is easier to dissect if left in continuity. The largest and most consistent anterior branch to the bladder, the superior vesical artery, is usually isolated and individually ligated and divided easily. The remaining anterior branches of the lateral pedicle are then isolated and divided between hemoclips down to the endopelvic fascia, or as far as is technically possible. With blunt dissection the index finger of the left hand helps identify this lateral pedicle, and protects the rectum as it is pushed medially. Right-angle hemoclip appliers are ideally suited for proper

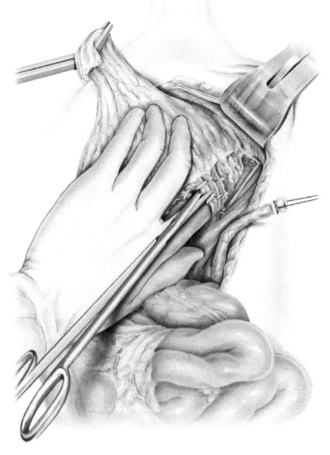

**Fig. 44.9**
Isolation of the lateral vascular pedicle. The left hand is used to define the right lateral pedicle, extending from the bladder to the hypogastric artery. This plane is developed by the index finger (medial) and the middle finger (lateral), exposing the anterior branches of the hypogastric artery. This vascular pedicle is clipped and divided down to the endopelvic fascia. Traction with the left hand defines the pedicle, allows direct visualization, and protects the rectum from injury.

placement of the clips. Hemoclips are positioned as far apart as possible to ensure that 0.5–1 cm of tissue projects beyond each clip when the pedicle is divided. This prevents the hemoclips from being dislodged and thus causing unnecessary bleeding. Occasionally, in patients with an abundance of pelvic fat, the lateral pedicle may be thick and require division into two manageable pedicles. The inferior vesicle vein serves as an excellent landmark because the endopelvic fascia is just distal to this structure. Incision of the endopelvic fascia just lateral to the prostate may help to identify the distal limit of the lateral pedicle.

## LIGATION OF THE POSTERIOR PEDICLE TO THE BLADDER

Following division of the lateral pedicles, the bladder specimen is retracted anteriorly, exposing the cul-de-sac (pouch of Douglas). The surgeon elevates the bladder with a small gauze sponge under the left hand, while the assistant retracts the peritoneum of the rectosigmoid colon in a cephalad direction. This provides excellent exposure to the recess of the cul-de-sac and places the peritoneal reflection on traction, facilitating the proper division. The peritoneum lateral to the rectum is incised and extended anteriorly and medially across the cul-de-sac to join the incision on the contralateral side (Figure 44.10).

An understanding of the fascial layers is critical for the appropriate dissection of this plane. The anterior and posterior peritoneal reflections converge in the cul-de-sac to form Denonvillier's fascia, which extends caudally to the urogenital diaphragm (Figure 44.11, arrow). This important anatomic boundary in the male separates the prostate and seminal vesicles anterior to the rectum posterior. The plane between the prostate and seminal vesicles and the anterior sheath of Denonvillier's fascia will not develop easily. However, the plane between the rectum and the posterior sheath of Denonvillier's (fascia) so called Denonvillier's space should develop easily with blunt and sharp dissection. Therefore, the peritoneal incision in the cul-de-sac must be made slightly on the rectal side rather than the bladder side. This allows proper and safe entry and development of Denonvillier's space between the anterior rectal wall and the posterior sheath of Denonvillier's fascia (Figure 44.12). With a posterior sweeping motion of the fingers, the rectum can be carefully swept off of Denonvillier's fascia (with the seminal vesicles, prostate, and bladder anteriorly in men), and off of the posterior vaginal wall in women. This sweeping motion, when extended laterally, helps to thin and develop the posterior pedicles, which appear like a collar emanating from the lateral aspect of the rectum. Care should be taken when developing this posterior plane more caudally because the anterior rectal fibers reflect anteriorly, are often adherent to the specimen, and can offer resistance to blunt dissection. In

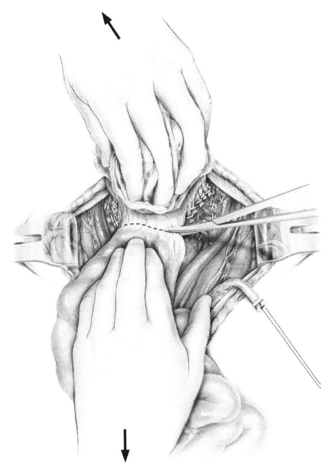

**Fig. 44.10**
The peritoneum lateral to the rectum is incised down into the cul-de-sac, and carried anteriorly over the rectum to join the opposite side. Note that the incision should be made precisely so the proper plane behind Denonvillier's fascia can be developed safely.

this region, just cephalad (proximal) to the urogenital diaphragm, sharp dissection may be required to dissect the anterior rectal fibers off the apex of the prostate in order to prevent rectal injury at this location.

Several situations may impede the proper development of this posterior plane. Most commonly, when the incision in the cul-de-sac is made too far anteriorly, proper entry into Denonvillier's space is prevented. Improper entry can occur between the two layers of Denonvillier's fascia, or even anterior to this, making the posterior dissection difficult and increasing the risk of rectal injury. Furthermore, posterior tumor infiltration or previous high-dose pelvic irradiation can obliterate this plane, making the posterior dissection difficult. To prevent injury to the rectum in these situations, sharp dissection should be performed under direct vision. In order to prevent a rectal injury it is important to avoid blunt dissection with the finger in areas where normal tissue planes have been obliterated by previous surgery or radiation. Sharp dissection under

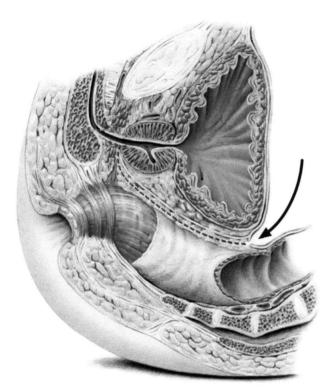

**Fig. 44.11**
The formation of Denonvillier's fascia. Note that it is derived from a fusion of the anterior and posterior peritoneal reflections. Denonvillier's space lies behind the fascia. To successfully enter this space and facilitate mobilization of the anterior rectal wall off Denonvillier's fascia, the incision in the cul-de-sac is made close to the peritoneal fusion on the anterior rectal wall side, and not on the bladder side.

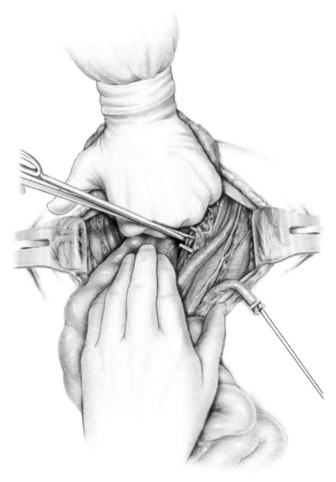

**Fig. 44.12**
After the peritoneum of the cul-de-sac has been incised, the anterior rectal wall can be swept off the posterior surface of the Denonvillier's fascia. This effectively defines the posterior pedicle that extends from the bladder to the lateral aspect of the rectum on either side.

direct vision will dramatically reduce the potential for rectal injury. If a rectotomy occurs, a two- or three-layer closure is recommended. A diverting proximal colostomy is not routinely required unless gross contamination occurs, or if the patient has received previous pelvic radiation therapy. If orthotopic diversion or vaginal reconstruction is planned, an omental interposition is recommended in order to help prevent fistulization.

Once the posterior pedicles have been defined, they are clipped and divided to the endopelvic fascia in the male patient. The endopelvic fascia is then incised adjacent to the prostate, medial to the levator ani muscles (if not done previously), to facilitate the apical dissection. In the female patient, the posterior pedicles, including the cardinal ligaments, are divided 4–5 cm beyond the cervix. With cephalad pressure on a previously placed vaginal sponge stick, the apex of the vagina can be identified, and incised posteriorly just distal to the cervix. The vagina is then circumscribed anteriorly with the cervix attached to the cystectomy specimen. If concern exists regarding an adequate surgical margin at the posterior or base of the bladder, then the anterior vaginal wall should be removed en bloc with the bladder specimen; vaginal reconstruction

will be required if sexual function is desired. It is our preference to spare the anterior vaginal wall if orthotopic diversion is planned. This eliminates the need for vaginal reconstruction, helps to maintain the complex musculofascial support system, and helps to prevent injury to the pudendal innervation to the rhabdosphincter and proximal urethra, both important components to the continence mechanism in women. The anterior vaginal wall is then sharply dissected off the posterior bladder down to the region of the bladder neck (vesicourethral junction), which is identified by palpating the Foley catheter balloon. At this point, the specimen remains attached only at the apex in men and vesicourethral junction in women.

## ANTERIOR APICAL DISSECTION IN THE MALE PATIENT

Only after the cystectomy specimen is completely freed and mobile posteriorly is attention directed anteriorly to the pelvic floor and urethra. All fibroareolar connections between the anterior bladder wall, prostate, and undersurface of the pubic symphysis are divided. The endopelvic fascia is incised adjacent to the prostate, and the levator muscles are carefully swept off the lateral and apical portions of the prostate. The superficial dorsal vein is identified, ligated, and divided. With tension placed posteriorly on the prostate, the puboprostatic ligaments are identified, and only slightly divided just beneath the pubis, lateral to the dorsal venous complex that courses between these ligaments. Extensive dissection in this region along the pelvic floor should be carefully avoided. The puboprostatic ligaments need to be incised only enough to allow for a proper apical dissection of the prostate. The apex of the prostate and the membranous urethra now become palpable.

Several methods can be used to control the dorsal venous plexus. One may carefully pass an angled clamp beneath the dorsal venous complex, anterior to the urethra (Figure 44.13). The venous complex can then be ligated with a 2-0 absorbable suture and divided close to the apex of the prostate. If any bleeding occurs from the

transected venous complex, it can be oversewn with an absorbable (2-0 polyglycolic acid) suture. In a slightly different fashion, the dorsal venous complex may be gathered at the apex of the prostate with a long Allis clamp (Figure 44.14). This may help better define the plane between the dorsal venous complex and the anterior urethra. A figure-of-eight 2-0 absorbable suture can then be carefully placed under direct vision anterior to the urethra (distal to the apex of the prostate) around the gathered venous complex. This suture is best placed with the surgeon facing the head of the table and holding the needle driver perpendicular to the patient. The suture is then tagged with a hemostat. This maneuver avoids the passage of any instruments between the dorsal venous complex and rhabdo-sphincter, which could potentially injure these structures and compromise the continence mechanism. After the complex has been ligated, it can be sharply divided with excellent exposure to the anterior surface of

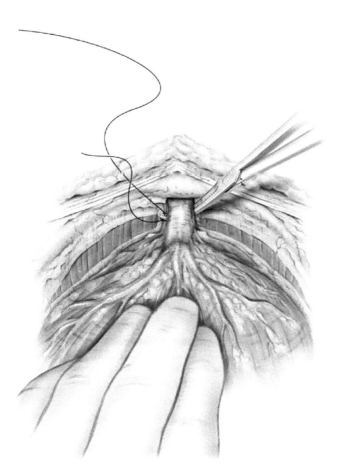

**Fig. 44.13**
Control of the dorsal venous complex. A right-angled clamp can be passed posterior to the venous complex and anterior to the urethra. An absorbable suture can be passed to ligate the complex distal to the apex of the prostate.

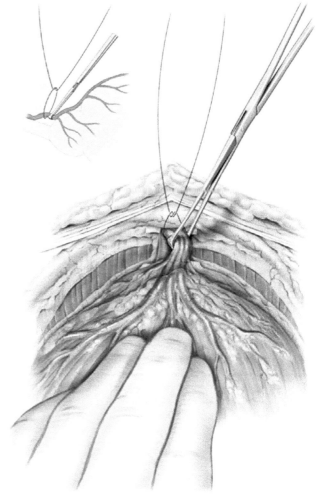

**Fig. 44.14**
The dorsal venous complex is gathered with an Allis clamp distal to the apex of the prostate. This maneuver defines the plane between the dorsal venous complex and urethra.

the urethra. Once the venous complex has been severed, the suture can be used to further secure the complex. The suture is then used to suspend the venous complex anteriorly to the periosteum to help reestablish anterior fixation of the dorsal venous complex and puboprostatic ligaments and thus possibly enhance continence recovery (Figure 44.15). The anterior urethra is now exposed.

Regardless of the aforementioned technique to control the dorsal venous complex, the urethra is then incised 270° just beyond the apex of the prostate. Six 2-0 polyglycolic acid sutures are placed in the anterior urethra, carefully incorporating only the mucosa and submucosa of the striated urethral sphincter muscle anteriorly. Next, two posterior urethral sutures are placed incorporating the rectourethralis muscle or the caudal extent of Denonvillier's fascia. The posterior

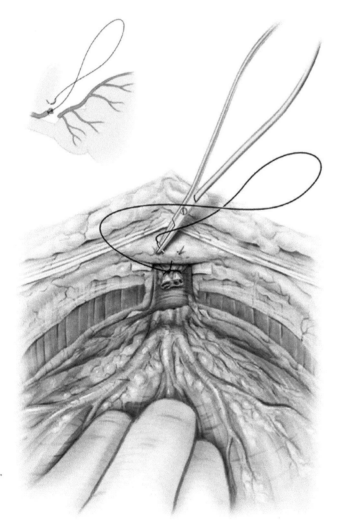

**Fig. 44.15**
An absorbable suture is carefully passed in a figure-of-eight fashion anterior to the urethra around the gathered dorsal venous complex to control the vascular structure. The dorsal venous complex is completely divided. The previously placed suture is then used to further secure the venous complex. The complex is then fixed anteriorly to the periosteum.

urethra can then be divided and the specimen removed after dividing the Foley catheter between clamps in order to avoid spillage of bladder contents.

Alternatively, the dorsal venous complex can simply be sharply transected prior to securing vascular control of the dorsal venous complex. Cephalad traction on the prostate elongates the proximal and membranous urethra and allows the urethra to be skeletonized laterally by dividing the so-called 'lateral pillars', extensions of the rhabdosphincter. Again, a section comprising the anterior two-thirds of the urethra is divided, exposing the urethral catheter. The urethral sutures are then placed. Six 2-0 polyglycolic acid sutures are placed, equally spaced, into the urethral mucosa and lumen anteriorly. The rhabdosphincter, the edge of which acts as a hood overlying the dorsal venous complex, is included in these sutures if the dorsal venous complex was sharply incised. This maneuver compresses the dorsal vein complex against the urethra for hemostatic purposes. The urethral catheter is then drawn through the urethrotomy, clamped on the bladder side, and divided. Cephalad traction on the bladder side with the clamped catheter occludes the bladder neck, prevents tumor spill from the bladder, and provides exposure to the posterior urethra. Two additional sutures are placed in the posterior urethra, again incorporating the rectourethralis muscle or distal Denonvillier's fascia. The posterior urethra is then divided and the specimen removed. Bleeding from the dorsal vein is usually minimal at this point. If additional hemostasis is required, one or two anterior urethral sutures can be tied to stop the bleeding. Regardless of the technique, frozen section analysis of the distal urethral margin of the cystectomy specimen is then performed in order to exclude tumor involvement.

If a cutaneous form of urinary diversion is planned, urethral preparation is slightly modified. Once the dorsal venous complex is secured and divided, the anterior urethra is identified. The urethra is mobilized from above as far distally as possible into the pelvic diaphragm. With cephalad traction, the urethra is stretched above the urogenital diaphragm, a curved clamp is placed as distal on the urethra as feasible and divided distal to the clamp. Care must be taken to avoid rectal injury with this clamp. This is prevented by placing gentle posterior traction with the left hand or index finger on the rectum and ensuring the clamp is passed anterior. The specimen is then removed. Mobilization of the urethra as distally as possible facilitates secondary urethrectomy should it be necessary. The levator musculature can then be reapproximated along the pelvic floor to facilitate hemostasis.

## ANTERIOR DISSECTION IN THE FEMALE

The wide female pelvis allows for better anterior exposure in a woman, particularly at the vesicourethral junction. However, urologists may be less familiar with pelvic surgery in women than in men. In addition, paravaginal vascular control may be troublesome in women, and the venous plexus anterior to the urethra is less well defined in women. When orthotopic diversion is considered in female patients undergoing cystectomy, several technical issues critical to the procedure must be addressed in order to maintain the continence mechanism in these women.

When the posterior pedicles are developed in women, the posterior vagina is incised at the apex just distal to the cervix (Figure 44.16). This incision is carried anteriorly along the lateral and anterior vaginal walls forming a circumferential incision. The anterior lateral vaginal wall is then grasped with curved Kocher clamps. This provides countertraction and facilitates dissection between the anterior vaginal wall and the bladder specimen. Careful dissection of the proper plane will prevent entry into the posterior bladder and also reduce

the amount of bleeding in this vascular area (Figure 44.17). Development of this posterior plane and vascular pedicle is best performed sharply and carried just distal to the vesicourethral junction. Palpation of the Foley catheter balloon assists in identifying this region. This dissection effectively maintains a functional vagina.

In the case of a deeply invasive posterior bladder tumor in a woman, with concern of an adequate surgical margin, the anterior vaginal wall should be removed en bloc with the cystectomy specimen. After dividing the posterior vaginal apex, the lateral vaginal wall subsequently serves as the posterior pedicle and is divided distally. This leaves the anterior vaginal wall attached to the posterior bladder specimen. The Foley catheter balloon again facilitates identification of the vesicourethral junction. The surgical plane between the vesicourethral junction and the anterior vaginal wall is then developed distally at this location. A 1 cm length of

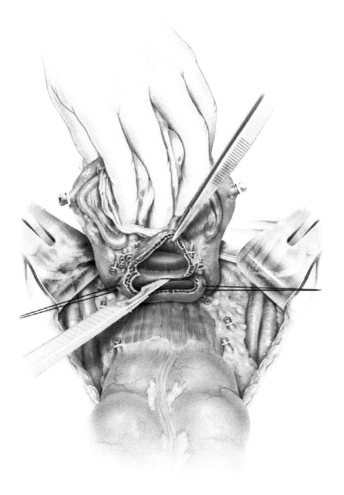

**Fig. 44.16**
In women, the vagina is incised distal to the cervix. Note that cephalad traction on the posterior aspect of the vagina facilitates the incision of the anterior vaginal wall. Slight dissection of the posterior vaginal wall off the rectum provides mobility to the vaginal cuff.

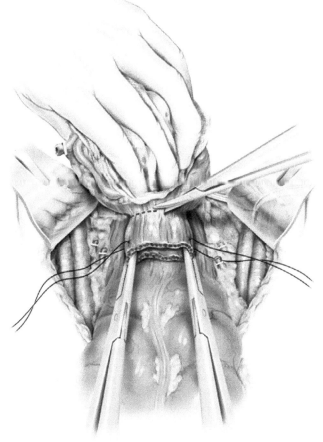

**Fig. 44.17**
Dissection of the anterior vaginal wall off of the bladder. Note caudal traction of the cystectomy specimen with countertraction applied to the vagina in a cephalad direction. Dissection continues only slightly distal to the level of the vesicourethral junction. This can be identified by palpation of the Foley balloon in the bladder (not shown).

proximal urethra is mobilized while the remaining distal urethra is left intact with the anterior vaginal wall. Vaginal reconstruction by a clam shell (horizontal) or side-to-side (vertical) technique is required. Other means of vaginal reconstruction may include a rectus myocutaneous flap, detubularized cylinder of ileum, a peritoneal flap, or an omental flap.

It is emphasized that no dissection should be performed anterior to the urethra along the pelvic floor. The endopelvic fascia should remain undisturbed and not opened in women considering orthotopic diversion. This prevents injury to the rhabdosphincter region and corresponding innervation, which is critical in maintaining the continence mechanism. Anatomic studies have demonstrated that the innervation of this rhabdosphincter region in women arises from branches off the pudendal nerve that course along the pelvic floor posterior to the levator muscles.[33,34] Any dissection performed anteriorly may injure these nerves and compromise the continence status.

When the posterior dissection is completed (with care to dissect just distal to the vesicourethral junction), a Satinsky vascular clamp is placed across the bladder neck. The Satinsky vascular clamp placed across the catheter at the bladder neck prevents any tumor spill from the bladder. With gentle traction the proximal urethra is completely divided anteriorly, distal to the bladder neck and clamp. The urethra is situated more anteriorly in women than in men, and the urethral sutures can be placed easily after the specimen is completely removed (Figure 44.18). Ten to 12 sutures are placed. Frozen section analysis is performed on the distal urethral margin of the cystectomy specimen in order to exclude tumor. Once hemostasis is obtained, the vaginal cuff may be closed in two layers with absorbable sutures. The vaginal cuff is then anchored via a colposacralpexy using a strut of Marlex mesh to the sacral promontory. This fixates the vagina without angulation or undue tension. Note that at the terminal portions of the surgical procedure, a well-vascularized omental pedicle graft is placed between the reconstructed vagina and neobladder, and secured to the levator ani muscles to separate the suture lines and prevent fistulization (Figure 44.19).

If a cutaneous diversion is planned in the female patient, the posterior pedicles are developed as previously mentioned. Attention is then directed anteriorly, and the pubourethral ligaments are divided. A curved clamp is placed across the urethra, and the anterior vaginal wall is opened distally and incised circumferentially around the urethral meatus. The vaginal cuff is closed as previously described and suspended. Alternatively, a perineal approach may be used for this dissection with complete removal of the entire urethra.

Following removal of the cystectomy specimen, the pelvis is irrigated with warm sterile water. The presacral

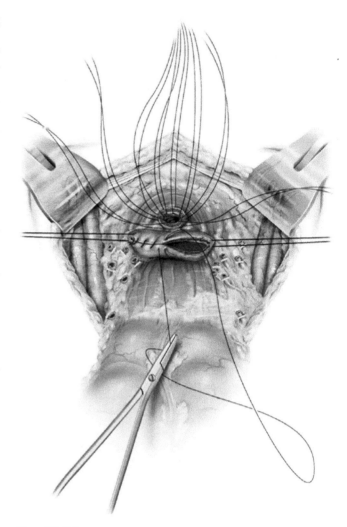

**Fig. 44.18**
View of the female pelvis from above with the partially opened vaginal cuff and the urethral sutures placed.

nodal tissue previously swept off the common iliac vessels and sacral promontory into the deep pelvis is collected and sent separately for pathologic evaluation. Nodal tissue in the presciatic notch bilaterally, anterior to the sciatic nerve, is also sent for histologic analysis. Hemostasis is obtained and the pelvis is packed with a lap pad while attention is directed to the urinary diversion.

The use of various tubes and drains postoperatively is important. The pelvis is drained with a 1-inch Penrose drain for urine or lymph leak for 3 weeks, and a large suction hemovac drain for the evacuation of blood for 24 hours. A gastrostomy tube with an 18 Fr. Foley catheter is placed routinely, utilizing a modified Stamm technique that incorporates a small portion of omentum (near the greater curvature of the stomach) interposed between the stomach and the abdominal wall.[35] This provides a simple means of draining the stomach and prevents the need for an uncomfortable nasogastric tube while the postoperative ileus resolves.

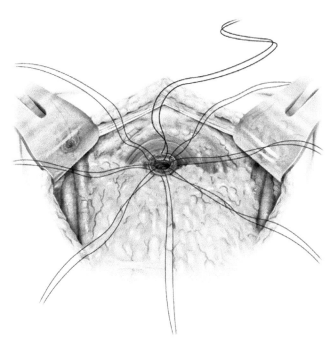

**Fig. 44.19**
View of the female pelvis. Note a vascularized omental pedicle graft is situated anteriorly covering the reconstructed vagina/vaginal cuff. The urethra and sutures will be placed into the neobladder (not shown). The omental graft is secured to the pelvic floor to prevent fistulization between the neobladder and vaginal cuff.

## POSTOPERATIVE CARE

A meticulous, team-oriented approach to the care of these generally elderly patients undergoing radical cystectomy helps reduce perioperative morbidity and mortality. Patients are best monitored in the surgical intensive care unit (ICU) for at least 24 hours or until stable. Careful attention to fluid management is imperative as third-space fluid loss in these patients can be tremendous and deceiving. Patients with compromised cardiac or pulmonary function may require invasive cardiac monitoring with a pulmonary artery catheter placed prior to surgery to precisely ascertain the cardiac response to fluid shifts. A combination of crystalloid and colloid fluid replacement is given on the night of surgery, and converted to crystalloid on postoperative day 1. Prophylaxis against stress ulcer is initiated with a histamine receptor ($H_2$) blocker. Intravenous broad-spectrum antibiotics are continued in all patients and subsequently converted to oral antibiotics as the diet progresses. Pulmonary toilet is encouraged with incentive spirometry, deep breathing, and coughing.

Prophylaxis against deep vein thrombosis is important in patients undergoing extensive pelvic operations for malignancies. The anticoagulation is initiated in the recovery room with 10 mg of sodium warfarin via a nasogastric or the gastrostomy tube. The daily dose is adjusted to maintain a prothrombin time in the range of 18–22 seconds. If the prothrombin time exceeds 22–25 seconds, 2.5 mg of vitamin K is administered intramuscularly to prevent possible bleeding. Pain control by a patient-controlled analgesic (PCA) system provides comfort and enhances deep breathing and early ambulation. If digoxin was given preoperatively, it is continued until discharge. The gastrostomy tube is generally removed on postoperative day 7, or later if bowel function is delayed. The catheter and drain management is specific to the form of urinary diversion. Some patients may develop a prolonged ileus or some other complication that delays the quick return of oral intake. In such circumstances, total parenteral nutrition (TPN) is wisely instituted earlier rather than later, so that the patient will not become farther behind nutritionally.

## DISCUSSION

Understanding that invasive bladder cancer can be a lethal disease, we have adopted an early and aggressive surgical approach.[3,4] This includes a radical cystectomy with a meticulous and extended bilateral pelvic iliac lymph node dissection. We firmly believe radical cystectomy provides the best local pelvic control of the disease. In addition, radical cystectomy provides accurate evaluation of the primary bladder tumor (p stage), along with the regional lymph nodes. This pathologic evaluation allows the application of adjuvant treatment strategies based on clear histopathologic determination, not clinical staging, which has been associated with significant errors in 30% to 50% of patients.[3,27,28,36,37] This, coupled with the evolution and application of orthotopic lower urinary tract reconstruction in both men and women, has provided patients with a more acceptable means to store and eliminate urine.[7]

Generally, most invasive TCCs are high-grade tumors. These bladder tumors originate in the bladder mucosa, and progressively invade the lamina propria and, sequentially, the muscularis propria, perivesical fat, and contiguous pelvic structures, with an increasing incidence of lymph node involvement with disease progression (Table 44.1).[4,16,38,39] In over 2200 patients undergoing radical cystectomy from four large contemporary cystectomy series, the cumulative incidence of node-positive bladder cancer at the time of surgery was 25%. Radical cystectomy with an appropriate lymphadenectomy effectively removes the primary bladder tumor and the regional lymph nodes that may contain metastases in a significant number of patients undergoing the procedure. In the USC series of 1054 patients undergoing radical cystectomy for TCC, the incidence of lymph node metastases correlated with the primary bladder tumor stage.[4] Patients with

**Table 44.1** Incidence of lymph node metastasis following radical cystectomy in contemporary series: correlation to primary bladder tumor

| Lead author | Period | No. pts | No (%) lymph node metastases | Bladder tumor stage* No. (%) | | | | |
|---|---|---|---|---|---|---|---|---|
| | | | | P0, Pis, Pa, P1 | P2A | P2B | P3 | P4 |
| Poulsen[16] | 1990–1997 | 191 | 50 (26%) | 2 (3%) | 4 (18%) | 7 (25%) | 33 (51%) | 4 (44%) |
| Vieweg†[38] | 1980–1990 | 686 | 193 (28%) | 10 (10%) | 12 (9%) | 22 (23%) | 97 (43%) | 52 (41%) |
| Leissner‡[39] | 1999–2002 | 290 | 81 (28%) | 1 (2%) | 5 (13%) | 12 (22%) | 53 (44%) | 10 (50%) |
| Stein[4] | 1971–1997 | 1054 | 246 (24%) | 19 (5%) | 21 (18%) | 35 (27%) | 113 (45%) | 58 (43%) |
| Totals | | 2221 | 570 (25%) | | | | | |

\* TNM staging system: 1997 AJCC.[50]
† 6 patients with carcinoma in situ of prostatic ducts with lymph node positive disease classified as Pis.
‡ Multicenter trial.

nonmuscle-invasive tumors demonstrated a 5% incidence of node-positive disease, compared with 18% in patients with superficial muscle-invasive bladder tumors (P2A), 27% with deep muscle-invasive bladder tumors (P2B), and approximately 45% of patients with extravesical tumor extension of the primary bladder tumor (P3 and P4) (Table 44.1).

## MORBIDITY AND MORTALITY OF RADICAL CYSTECTOMY AND LYMPHADENECTOMY

The early clinical results and outcomes with regard to the morbidity and mortality of radical cystectomy were disappointing. Lack of universal acceptance of this procedure was attributed to the considerable complication rate and the need for improvements in urinary diversion. Prior to 1970, the perioperative complication rate of radical cystectomy was approximately 35%, with a mortality rate of nearly 20%. However, with contemporary medical, surgical, and anesthetic techniques, along with better patient selection, the mortality and morbidity from radical cystectomy have dramatically decreased. We reported a

3% mortality rate in the USC series (Table 44.2),[4] which is similar to that in other contemporary series of radical cystectomy.[5,16,36–39] Importantly, we found that the administration of preoperative therapy (radiation and/or chemotherapy), and the form of urinary diversion performed (continent or incontinent) did not appear to increase the mortality rate of patients undergoing radical cystectomy.[4]

The early complication rate following radical cystectomy often associated with significant comorbidities should not be underestimated in this elderly group of patients. The median age of patients undergoing cystectomy in our series was 66 years (range 22–93 years). In this series of 1054 patients, 28% developed an early complication within the first 3 months of surgery (Table 44.2).[4] These early complications included all those related to the cystectomy, perioperative care, and urinary diversion. The administration of preoperative therapy (radiation and/or chemotherapy) and the form of urinary diversion did not significantly alter the early complication rate in these cystectomy patients. Most early complications following radical cystectomy are unrelated to the urinary diversion (85% diversion

**Table 44.2** Perioperative mortality and early complication rate following cystectomy at USC

| | | No. pts | Perioperative mortality* | Early complication† |
|---|---|---|---|---|
| Form of urinary diversion | Conduit‡ | 278 (26%) | 8 (3%) | 83 (30%) |
| | Continent§ | 776 (74%) | 19 (2%) | 209 (27%) |
| Preoperative adjuvant therapy | None | 884 (84%) | 26 (3%) | 247 (28%) |
| | Radiation only | 108 (10%) | 1 (1%) | 30 (30%) |
| | Chemotherapy only | 49 (5%) | 0 | 12 (25%) |
| | Radiation and chemotherapy | 13 (1%) | 0 | 3 (23%) |
| Totals | | 1054 | 27 (3%) | 292 (28%) |

\* Any death within 30 days of surgery or prior to discharge.
† Any complications within the first 3 months postoperative.
‡ Including ileal and colon conduits.
§ Including continent cutaneous, orthotopic, and rectal reservoirs.

unrelated), and can be managed conservatively without the need for reoperation in approximately 90% of patients.[40] In our experience, the most common early, diversion-unrelated complication is dehydration, while the most common early, diversion-related complication following radical cystectomy is urinary leakage.

Although we have found that preoperative treatment with chemotherapy and/or radiation therapy does not increase the perioperative morbidity or mortality, neoadjuvant treatment strategies have not been routinely employed in our patients prior to radical cystectomy for invasive bladder cancer. Preoperative radiation therapy is considered only in those patients with a history of a previous partial cystectomy or those that have experienced extravesical tumor spill at the time of endoscopic management of the primary bladder tumor.[41] Furthermore, although there has been a recent interest in the application of neoadjuvant chemotherapy in patients with muscle-invasive bladder cancer,[42] the routine administration of this is clearly a debatable issue.[43] We have been, and continue to be, strong advocates of postoperative adjuvant chemotherapy when given to high-risk patients, on the basis of accurate pathologic evaluation of the primary bladder tumor and regional lymph nodes.[4,44]

We have also evaluated the clinical outcomes of radical cystectomy in elderly patients (80 years of age or more) requiring therapy for bladder cancer.[45] We found that in appropriately selected individuals the perioperative morbidity and mortality of elderly patients is similar to that of younger patients undergoing the same operation. Our data are similar to those in other reports.[46,47] Collectively, this suggests that an aggressive surgical approach is a viable treatment strategy for properly selected elderly individuals who are in generally good health and require definitive management for bladder cancer. It is clear that physiologic age may be more important than chronologic age when determining who is an appropriate candidate for radical cystectomy. Proper patient selection, and strict attention to perioperative details, along with a dedicated and meticulous surgical approach, are all critical components to minimize the morbidity and mortality of surgery, and to ensure the best clinical outcomes in patients following radical cystectomy (see also Chapter 43 for additional discussion of patient preparation and perioperative management).

## PATHOLOGIC STAGE AND SUBGROUPS

The pathologic stage of the primary bladder tumor and the presence of lymph node metastases are perhaps the most important survival determinants in patients undergoing cystectomy for bladder cancer (Table 44.3).[4] These pathologic determinants may also be categorized into certain pathologic subgroups that provide risk stratification. It is this pathologic evaluation and subgroup stratification that most precisely directs the need for adjuvant therapy in the appropriately selected individual. The pathologic subgroups are defined as organ-confined, lymph node-negative tumors (P0, Pa, Pis, P1, P2A, P2B), nonorgan-confined (extravesical) lymph node-negative tumors (P3, P4), and lymph node-positive disease (N+). The recurrence-free and overall survival for the entire 1054 patients in the USC series at 5 years was 68% and 66%, and 60% and 43%, respectively, at 10 years (Table 44.3, Figure 44.20). In this cohort, most deaths occurring within the first 3 years after radical cystectomy are attributed to bladder cancer recurrences. However, with continued follow-up (after 3 years), most deaths in this elderly group of patients are primarily related to other comorbid diseases, unrelated to bladder cancer.

## ORGAN-CONFINED, LYMPH NODE-NEGATIVE TUMORS

In the USC series, 56% of patients demonstrated pathologically organ-confined, lymph node-negative bladder tumors.[4] The survival results in this pathologic subgroup of patients are excellent (Table 44.3, Figure 44.21). The recurrence-free survival in this subgroup of organ-confined, lymph node-negative bladder tumors was 85% at 5 years and 82% at 10 years. Importantly, we found no significant survival differences among superficially noninvasive (Pis, Pa), lamina propria invasive (P1), and muscle-invasive (P2A, P2B) tumors— as long as the tumor was confined to the bladder and there was no evidence of lymph node tumor involvement. Similar outcomes for patients with pathologic superficial bladder tumors following cystectomy have been previously reported.[5,37] These data support the notion that the ideal outcome for patients with high-grade, invasive bladder cancer occurs when the primary bladder tumor is confined to the bladder, without evidence of extravesical extension or lymph node metastases. Significant delays in treatment of patients with invasive bladder cancer obviously should be avoided. There is evidence to suggest that prolonged delays may lead to more advanced pathologic stages and decreased survival in patients with muscle-invasive bladder cancer.[48] Furthermore, it should be emphasized that care should be taken in delaying a more definitive therapy in patients with high-risk superficial bladder tumors, or those tumors that are superficial but have not responded appropriately to conservative forms of therapy.[3]

## EXTRAVESICAL, LYMPH NODE-NEGATIVE TUMORS

Nonorgan-confined (extravesical) lymph node-negative tumors were found in approximately 20% of our

**Table 44.3**  Recurrence-free and overall survival after radical cystectomy

| Pathologic stage* | No. pts | Probability of surviving and remaining recurrence-free (P ± SE) | | | |
| --- | --- | --- | --- | --- | --- |
| | | Recurrence-free | | Overall survival | |
| | | 5 years | 10 years | 5 years | 10 years |
| P0, Pa, Pis | | | | | |
| N– | 208 | 0.89 ± 0.02 | 0.85 ± 0.03 | 0.85 ± 0.03 | 0.67 ± 0.04 |
| N+ | 5 | 0.60 ± 0.22 | 0.60 ± 0.22 | 0.40 ± 0.22 | 0.40 ± 0.22 |
| All pts P0, Pa, Pis | 213 | 0.88 ± 0.02 | 0.85 ± 0.03 | 0.84 ± 0.03 | 0.67 ± 0.04 |
| P1 | | | | | |
| N– | 194 | 0.83 ± 0.03 | 0.78 ± 0.04 | 0.76 ± 0.03 | 0.52 ± 0.04 |
| N+ | 14 | 0.43 ± 0.13 | 0.43 ± 0.13 | 0.50 ± 0.13 | 0.42 ± 0.13 |
| All pts P1 | 208 | 0.80 ± 0.03 | 0.75 ± 0.04 | 0.74 ± 0.03 | 0.51 ± 0.04 |
| P2A | | | | | |
| N– | 94 | 0.89 ± 0.03 | 0.87 ± 0.04 | 0.77 ± 0.04 | 0.57 ± 0.06 |
| N+ | 21 | 0.50 ± 0.11 | 0.50 ± 0.11 | 0.52 ± 0.11 | 0.52 ± 0.11 |
| All pts P2A | 115 | 0.81 ± 0.04 | 0.80 ± 0.04 | 0.72 ± 0.04 | 0.56 ± 0.05 |
| P2B | | | | | |
| N– | 98 | 0.78 ± 0.05 | 0.76 ± 0.05 | 0.64 ± 0.05 | 0.44 ± 0.06 |
| N+ | 35 | 0.41 ± 0.09 | 0.37 ± 0.09 | 0.40 ± 0.08 | 0.26 ± 0.08 |
| All pts P2B | 133 | 0.68 ± 0.04 | 0.65 ± 0.05 | 0.58 ± 0.04 | 0.39 ± 0.05 |
| P3 | | | | | |
| N– | 135 | 0.62 ± 0.05 | 0.61 ± 0.05 | 0.49 ± 0.04 | 0.29 ± 0.05 |
| N+ | 113 | 0.29 ± 0.05 | 0.29 ± 0.05 | 0.24 ± 0.04 | 0.12 ± 0.04 |
| All pts P3 | 248 | 0.47 ± 0.04 | 0.46 ± 0.04 | 0.38 ± 0.03 | 0.22 ± 0.03 |
| P4 | | | | | |
| N– | 79 | 0.50 ± 0.06 | 0.45 ± 0.07 | 0.44 ± 0.06 | 0.23 ± 0.06 |
| N+ | 58 | 0.33 ± 0.07 | 0.33 ± 0.07 | 0.26 ± 0.06 | 0.20 ± 0.05 |
| All pts P4 | 137 | 0.44 ± 0.05 | 0.41 ± 0.05 | 0.33 ± 0.04 | 0.22 ± 0.04 |
| Organ-confined† | | | | | |
| N– | 594 | 0.85 ± 0.02 | 0.82 ± 0.02 | 0.78 ± 0.02 | 0.56 ± 0.0 |
| N+ | 75 | 0.46 ± 0.06 | 0.44 ± 0.06 | 0.45 ± 0.06 | 0.37 ± 0.06 |
| All pts | 669 | 0.80 ± 0.02 | 0.77 ± 0.02 | 0.74 ± 0.02 | 0.54 ± 0.02 |
| Extravesical‡ | | | | | |
| N– | 214 | 0.58 ± 0.04 | 0.55 ± 0.04 | 0.47 ± 0.04 | 0.27 ± 0.04 |
| N+ | 171 | 0.30 ± 0.04 | 0.30 ± 0.04 | 0.25 ± 0.04 | 0.17 ± 0.03 |
| All pts | 385 | 0.46 ± 0.03 | 0.44 ± 0.03 | 0.37 ± 0.03 | 0.22 ± 0.03 |
| LN– pts | 808 | 0.78 ± 0.02 | 0.75 ± 0.02 | 0.69 ± 0.02 | 0.49 ± 0.02 |
| LN+ pts | 246 | 0.35 ± 0.03 | 0.34 ± 0.03 | 0.31 ± 0.03 | 0.23 ± 0.03 |
| Total group | 1054 | 0.68 ± 0.02 | 0.66 ± 0.02 | 0.60 ± 0.02 | 0.43 ± 0.02 |

LN–, without lymph node involvement (node-negative); LN+, with lymph node involvement (node-positive); pts, patients.
* 1997 TNM staging system.[50]
† Organ confined, including P0, Pa, Pis, P1, P2, and P2B bladder tumors.
‡ Extravesical, including P3 and P4 bladder tumors.

patients undergoing cystectomy (Table 44.3, Figure 44.21).[4] In this pathologic subgroup, no obvious survival differences between extravesical P3 and P4 tumors were observed. The recurrence-free survival in this pathologic subgroup of extravesical, nonorgan-confined, lymph node-negative tumors was 58% at 5 years, and 55% at 10 years. Clearly, patients with these locally advanced tumors have higher recurrence rates and lower survival rates than the subgroup of patients with organ-confined tumor and lymph node-negative

tumors.[49] Consequently, adjuvant treatment strategies may be considered for the latter.

In 1997, the TNM (tumor, node, metastases) staging system for bladder cancer was modified by the American Joint Committee on Cancer (AJCC) and the UICC.[50] The revised TNM classification stratifies extravesical tumor involvement (previously defined as pT3B) into microscopic (pT3A) and gross (pT3B) extravesical tumor extension. In order to determine the clinical significance of this new pathologic subgrouping, we evaluated the

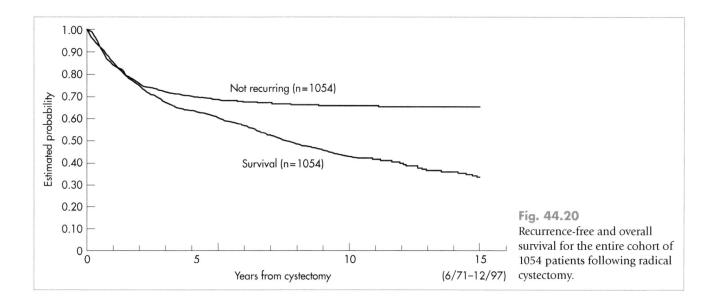

**Fig. 44.20**
Recurrence-free and overall survival for the entire cohort of 1054 patients following radical cystectomy.

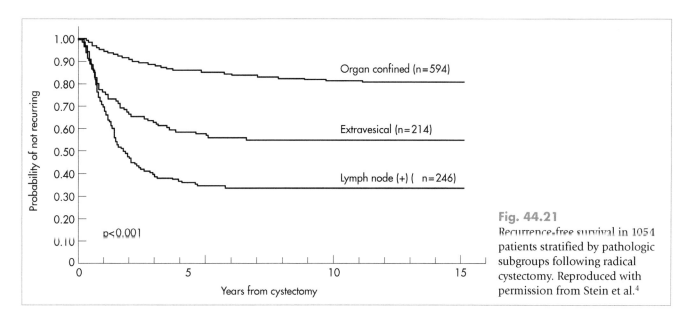

**Fig. 44.21**
Recurrence-free survival in 1054 patients stratified by pathologic subgroups following radical cystectomy. Reproduced with permission from Stein et al.[4]

clinical outcomes following radical cystectomy in our group of patients with pathologic pT3 disease stratified by microscopic and gross extravesical tumor involvement.[49] We found no significant difference in the recurrence-free and overall survival in patients when evaluating for pT3A and pT3B extravesical tumor extension. The incidence of lymph node involvement was not different between the groups (approximately 45%). However, as one would expect, the presence of lymph node involvement was associated with a higher risk of recurrence and worse overall survival. Because no differences were observed between the clinical outcomes for patients with pT3A and pT3B disease, we believe they should be treated similarly. Furthermore, the fact that future staging systems may classify these tumors collectively may also facilitate comparisons with historical cystectomy series.

## LYMPH NODE-POSITIVE DISEASE

Despite our aggressive treatment philosophy and approach to bladder cancer, 24% of our patients demonstrated lymph node-positive disease at the time of cystectomy (Table 44.1, Figure 44.21).[4] This underscores the virulent and metastatic capabilities of high-grade, invasive bladder cancer. Although patients with lymph node tumor involvement are a high-risk group of patients, nearly one-third of these patients in our series are alive at 5 years, and 23% at 10 years. It is possible that the surgical approach (with an extended pelvic–iliac lymph node dissection) may provide some advantage with long-term survival in selected individuals with lymph node-positive disease. The impact of adjuvant therapy in this group of patients, although difficult to assess and subject to selection bias, may also play a role in the outcomes of patients with lymph node-positive disease.[4] In fact, in a separate analysis of lymph node-positive patients, we found that the administration of adjuvant chemotherapy was a significant and independent predictor for recurrence and overall survival.[13]

The prognosis in patients with lymph node-positive disease can be stratified by the number of lymph nodes involved (tumor burden), and by the p stage of the primary bladder tumor.[4] In our cystectomy series, patients with fewer than five positive lymph nodes had better survival rates than patients with five or more lymph nodes involved. A significant difference was also observed when patients were stratified by their primary bladder stage. Patients with lymph node-positive disease and organ-confined bladder tumors had a significantly better recurrence-free survival than those with nonorgan-confined, lymph node-positive tumors. Similar results with lymph node-positive tumors following cystectomy have been reported previously.[5,38]

We believe that the number of lymph nodes involved with tumor and the extent of the lymph node dissection are both important variables for patients undergoing cystectomy for bladder cancer. We recently reexamined our 246 patients with lymph node tumor involvement following radical cystectomy,[13] to evaluate other prognostic factors in this high-risk group of patients. This reevaluation subsequently stimulated the concept of 'lymph node density'—an important prognostic factor that better stratifies lymph node-positive patients following radical cystectomy. Lymph node density (defined as the total number of positive lymph nodes divided by the total number of lymph nodes removed) accounts for the extent of the lymph node dissection (number of lymph nodes removed) and the tumor burden (number of positive lymph nodes) following radical cystectomy for patients with lymph node-positive disease. Lymph node density incorporates these concepts simultaneously.

If lymph tumor burden and the extent of the lymphadenectomy are important variables in patients with lymph node-positive disease, it is only logical that lymph node density is also important. In fact, we found lymph node density to be a significant and independent prognostic variable in patients with lymph node metastases and that it may best stratify this high-risk group of patients (Figure 44.22).[13] It is possible that future staging systems, and the application of adjuvant therapies in clinical trials, should consider applying these concepts to better stratify this high-risk group of patients after radical cystectomy. Regardless, patients with any lymph node involvement remain at high risk for disease recurrence and should be considered for adjuvant treatment strategies.

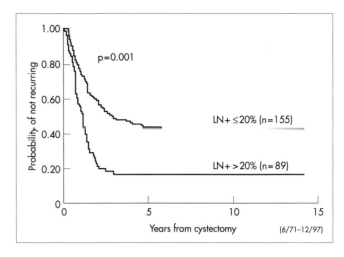

**Fig. 44.22**
Recurrence-free survival in 244 patients with lymph node positive disease stratified by lymph node density (20% or less and greater than 20%). (Reproduced with permission from Stein et al.[13])

## RECURRENCE FOLLOWING CYSTECTOMY

Recurrence following radical cystectomy for bladder cancer is not unusual and correlates directly to the pathologic stage and subgroup. In our report of 1054 patients with long-term follow-up (median 10 years), recurrences were classified as local (pelvic), distant, and urethral. Local recurrences, by definition, are those tumor recurrences that occur within the soft tissue field of exenteration. Distant recurrences are defined as those that occur outside the pelvis, while urethral tumors are classified as a new primary tumor that occurs in the retained urethra. Overall, 30% of the 1054 patients in the USC series experienced a local or distant tumor recurrence. The median time to any recurrence was 12 months, with 86% of all patients developing their recurrence within the first 3 years postoperatively. Of the 311 patients in our series that developed a recurrence, 75% of all recurrences were distant (median time to distant recurrence, 12 months), and 25% of all recurrences were only local (median time to local recurrence, 18 months).

### PELVIC (LOCAL) RECURRENCE

Radical cystectomy clearly provides the best local (pelvic) control of the disease. Of the 311 patients in our series that developed a recurrence, the median time to distant recurrence was 12 months while the median time to local recurrence was 18 months.[4] The use of a high-dose, short course of preoperative radiation therapy does not reduce the risk of pelvic recurrence.[41] Nearly all patients suffering a pelvic recurrence following cystectomy will die of their disease despite additional and even aggressive therapeutic efforts.

## METASTATIC (DISTANT) RECURRENCE

Recurrences following radical cystectomy are most commonly found at distant sites. Distant recurrences can also be stratified by pathologic subgroups. In our series, patients with organ-confined, lymph node-negative tumors demonstrated a 13% recurrence rate, which increased to 32% for those with extravesical lymph node-negative tumors, and 52% for patients with lymph node-positive tumors.[4] Patients at high risk for tumor recurrence clearly should be considered for adjuvant chemotherapy protocols.

## URETHRAL RECURRENCE

It is generally believed that urethral tumors, in patients with a history of bladder cancer following radical cystectomy, represent a second manifestation of the multicentric defect of the primary transitional cell mucosa that led to the original bladder tumor. The term 'urethral recurrence' may therefore be somewhat misleading, suggesting a failure of definitive treatment of the bladder cancer as the etiology of the urethral lesion. Rather, most urethral tumors probably represent simply another occurrence of the TCC in the remaining urothelium. As radical cystectomy has emerged as the most effective therapy for invasive bladder cancer, and as orthotopic diversion to the native intact urethra has increasingly been performed, the fate of the retained urethra has become an increasingly important oncologic issue.

The advent of orthotopic lower urinary tract reconstruction has arguably improved the quality of life in patients following radical cystectomy for bladder cancer. Approximately 90% of all patients undergoing cystectomy for TCC of the bladder at our institution receive an orthotopic neobladder substitute. From an oncologic perspective, only those patients found to have a positive margin at the proximal urethra (distal to the apex of the prostate in men and just distal to the bladder neck in women) on intraoperative frozen section are absolutely excluded from orthotopic reconstruction. This enthusiasm to preserve the native urethra following radical cystectomy and allow for orthotopic reconstruction has rightfully increased concerns for the potential for urethral recurrence in these patients.

Prior to the orthotopic era in women, urethral tumor recurrence was not considered an important oncologic issue, as the entire urethra was routinely removed at the time of cystectomy. With a better understanding of female pelvic anatomy and the innervation of the rhabdosphincter and continence mechanism in women,[33] along with the identification of various pathologic risk factors for urethral tumor involvement

in these patients, orthotopic diversion has now become a commonly performed form of urinary diversion in women following cystectomy.[51] We have demonstrated that tumor involving the bladder neck is the most important risk factor for urethral tumor involvement in women.[52,53] Although bladder neck involvement is a significant risk factor for urethral tumors, not all women with tumor involving the bladder neck will have urethral tumors. Approximately 50% of women with tumor at the bladder neck will have a urethra free of tumor. In this situation, the patient may potentially be considered an appropriate candidate for orthotopic diversion. Furthermore, we have shown that intraoperative frozen-section analysis of the distal surgical margin provides an accurate and reliable means to evaluate the proximal urethra, and currently is the primary pathologic factor that determines appropriate candidacy for orthotopic diversion.[53] With this selection process, we have not, to date, had a female urethral recurrence.[51]

A growing number of male patients with the urethra reconstructed following cystectomy exist today, and longer follow-up will expose them to a greater risk for a urethral recurrence. The historical incidence of second primary tumors in the retained urethra following cystectomy for bladder cancer ranges from 6% to 10%.[54] Specific clinical and pathologic risk factors may include multifocal tumors, carcinoma in situ, tumor involvement of the prostate (particularly invasion of the prostatic stroma), and the form of urinary diversion performed (orthotopic or cutaneous).[54-60]

We recently evaluated our clinical experience regarding the incidence and associated risk factors for urethral tumors in a large group of male patients undergoing radical cystectomy and urinary diversion for TCC of the bladder with long-term follow-up.[61] We analyzed the clinical and pathologic results of 768 consecutive male patients undergoing radical cystectomy with the intent to cure for high-grade, invasive bladder cancer (median follow-up 13 years); 397 men (52%) underwent an orthotopic urinary diversion (median follow-up 10 years) and 371 men (48%) underwent a cutaneous urinary diversion (median follow-up 19 years). Overall, a total of 45 patients (7%) developed a urethral recurrence, with an overall median time to occurrence of 2 years (range 0.2–13.6 years): 16 men (5%) with an orthotopic, and 29 men (9%) with a cutaneous form of urinary diversion.

In this cohort of male patients, multiple risk factors were analyzed with regard to second primary tumors of the urethra.[61] In a multivariable analysis, two important variables were identified that significantly increased the risk of a urethral tumor recurrence following cystectomy, including any prostate tumor involvement and the form of urinary diversion. The estimated 5-year probability of a urethral recurrence was 5% without any prostate involvement, and increased to 12% and 18% with superficial (prostatic urethra and ducts) and invasive (stroma) prostate involvement, respectively. Furthermore, patients undergoing an orthotopic diversion demonstrated a significantly lower risk of urethral recurrence than those undergoing a cutaneous form of urinary diversion.

The overall management of the urethra in male patients treated for high-grade invasive bladder cancer is an important issue. This concern has become even more critical from an oncologic perspective since the advent of orthotopic diversion. The indications and timing of a prophylactic urethrectomy in those undergoing cystectomy and a cutaneous diversion are debatable. This may include urethrectomy at the time of cystectomy, based on preoperative clinical parameters or the intraoperative frozen-section analysis of the urethral margin, or a delayed urethrectomy based on final pathologic evaluation of the cystectomy specimen.

Our long-term findings provide some insight regarding the issue of management of the retained urethra in both men and women following cystectomy for bladder cancer. We believe that intraoperative frozen-section analysis of the proximal urethra by an experienced pathologist is a reliable and accurate means to determine candidacy for orthotopic diversion in all patients. It has been our practice to construct an orthotopic neobladder in men and women whose intraoperative frozen section of the proximal urethra is without tumor. Our data suggest that this approach does not appear to increase the risk of a urethral recurrence in these patients.[53,54,61] Male patients with known prostatic tumor involvement should not necessarily be excluded from receiving an orthotopic substitute if the intraoperative biopsy is normal. Similarly, female patients with bladder neck involvement should not necessarily be excluded from having an orthotopic neobladder if the intraoperative biopsy is normal. All patients should be carefully counseled regarding the careful follow-up, the long-term risks of a urethral recurrence, and the possible need for urethrectomy following cystectomy for TCC of the bladder.

## IMPORTANCE OF SURGICAL TECHNIQUE

The dedication of the surgeon and technical commitment to a properly performed cystectomy and adequate lymphadenectomy are important to the success and clinical outcomes in patients with high-grade bladder cancer. The importance of surgical technique is well illustrated in the role this may have played in a recently reported randomized multi-institutional cooperative group trial.[42] In this prospective study, 270 patients underwent cystectomy with half of the patients receiving neoadjuvant chemotherapy. In a separate analysis of this trial, various surgical factors were subsequently analyzed.[43] Of these 270 patients, 24 had no lymph node dissection, 98 had a limited dissection of the obturator lymph nodes only, and 146 patients had a so-called standard (not extended) pelvic lymph node dissection. The 5-year survival rates for these groups were 33%, 46%, and 60%, respectively. The median number of lymph nodes removed for the entire cohort was 10. As expected, the survival rate for patients with <10 lymph nodes removed was significantly lower than in patients with >10 lymph nodes removed (44% versus 61%, respectively). In a multivariate analysis, the extent of the lymph node dissection, number of lymph nodes removed, and the number of cases performed by the individual surgeon were the most significant factors influencing survival in patients undergoing cystectomy for bladder cancer.[43] It is emphasized that, although this well-publicized study was not intended to analyze the surgical approach and/or technical differences in the treatment of bladder cancer, it was the surgical factors and not neoadjuvant chemotherapy that were most critical as predictors in the outcomes of these patients.[40]

Although the current standard for high-grade, invasive bladder cancer remains radical cystectomy, a current trend in urologic oncology has been to minimize the surgical approach, attempting organ preservation without compromising the cancer outcomes. So-called sexual-function-preserving cystectomy has recently been advocated for some patients with bladder cancer to improve clinical outcomes including continence, potency, and fertility. This surgical (modified cystectomy) approach generally includes sparing the prostate, vasa deferentia, and seminal vesicles while resecting the prostatic adenoma (in some cases) and reconstructing the lower urinary tract to the prostate. In appropriately selected young men who require cystectomy, and for whom potency and fertility remain relevant issues, this may be an important technique that will preserve erectile function, improve voiding, and maintain the ability to reproduce. In fact, our group at USC was one of the first to describe and promote a modified, prostate-sparing cystectomy in carefully selected male patients, with nonurothelial malignancies or nonmalignant bladder diseases, that necessitated cystectomy but not necessarily prostatectomy.[62] We continue to emphasize that this modified technique can be performed in certain appropriately selected young men requiring cystectomy but must not let it compromise the control of cancer.

Recently, various prostate-sparing techniques have been reported in patients with TCC of the bladder undergoing radical cystectomy.[63-67] The rationale for this technique includes improvement in urinary continence results (compared with continence following orthotopic diversion to the urethra), enhancement in erectile preservation and function, and maintenance of fertility in younger patients. Several important oncologic issues must be considered, including the risks of adenocarcinoma of the prostate in nearly 40% of men and TCC involving the prostate in patients undergoing cystectomy for bladder cancer. In addition, it could be argued that the functional and clinical results with orthotopic reconstruction are indeed very good and, in the properly selected patient, nerve-sparing techniques can also be performed to preserve erectile function. Until we better define the long-term oncologic risks associated with prostate-sparing techniques, all patients considering these procedures should provide proper informed consent and be advised that radical cystectomy remains the standard therapy for high-grade, invasive bladder cancer.

## CONCLUSION

Unlike other therapies, radical cystectomy pathologically stages the primary bladder tumor and regional lymph nodes. This histologic evaluation provides important prognostic information and identifies high-risk patients who may benefit from adjuvant therapy. Our data suggest that patients with extravesical tumor extension, or with lymph node-positive disease, appear to be at increased risk for recurrence and may be considered for adjuvant chemotherapy strategies.[4] Additionally, the recent application of molecular markers, based on pathologic staging and analysis, may also serve to identify patients at risk for tumor recurrence who may benefit from adjuvant forms of therapy.[68]

The clinical results and outcomes following radical cystectomy demonstrate good survival, with excellent local recurrence rates for high-grade, invasive bladder cancer. These results provide sound data, and a standard to which other forms of therapy for invasive bladder cancer can be compared. Furthermore, improvements in orthotopic urinary diversion have improved the quality of life in patients following cystectomy. Continence rates following orthotopic diversion are good and provide patients with a more natural voiding pattern per urethra. Contraindications to orthotopic urinary diversion are the presence of tumor within the urethra or extending to the urethral margin as determined by frozen-section analysis of the distal surgical margin at the time of cystectomy, compromised renal function (creatinine >2.5 ng/ml), or the presence of inflammatory bowel disease. Even in patients with locally advanced disease, orthotopic diversion can be employed without concern over subsequent tumor-related reservoir complications.

The question whether patients have a better quality of life following cystectomy or following bladder-sparing protocols, which require significant and prolonged treatment to the bladder with the potential for tumor recurrence, has not been elucidated. Currently, orthotopic diversion should be considered the diversion of choice in all cystectomy patients, and the urologist should have a specific reason why an orthotopic diversion is *not* performed. Patient factors such as frail general health, motivation, or comorbidity, and the cancer factor of a positive urethral margin, may disqualify some patients. Nevertheless, the option of lower urinary tract reconstruction to the intact urethra has been shown to decrease physician reluctance and increase patient acceptance to undergo earlier cystectomy when the disease may be at a more curable stage.[8]

In conclusion, a properly performed radical cystectomy with an appropriate lymphadenectomy provides the best survival rates, with the lowest reported local recurrence rates for high-grade, invasive bladder cancer. The surgical technique is critical to optimize the best clinical and technical outcomes in patients undergoing this procedure. Advances in lower urinary tract reconstruction provide a reasonable alternative for patients undergoing cystectomy, and have improved the quality of life of those patients requiring removal of their bladders.

REFERENCES

1. Jemal A, Thomas A, Murray T, Thun M. Cancer statistics 2002. CA Cancer J Clin 2002;52:23–47.
2. Prout G, Marshall VF. The prognosis with untreated bladder tumors. Cancer 1956;9:551–558.
3. Stein JP. Indications for early cystectomy. Urology 2003;62:591–595.
4. Stein JP, Lieskovsky G, Cote R, et al. Radical cystectomy in the treatment of invasive bladder cancer: long-term results in 1054 patients. J Clin Oncol 2001;19:666–675.
5. Ghoneim MA, El-Mekresh MM, El-Baz MA, El-Attar IA, Ashamallah A. Radical cystectomy for carcinoma of the bladder: critical evaluation of the results in 1,026 cases. J Urol 1997;158:393–399.
6. Montie JE. Against bladder sparing: surgery. J Urol 1999;162:452–455.
7. Stein JP, Skinner DG. Orthotopic bladder replacement. In Walsh PC, Retik AB, Vaughan ED, Wein AJ (eds): Campbell's Urology, 8th ed. Philadelphia: WB Saunders, 2002, pp 3835–3864.
8. Hautmann RE, Paiss T. Does the option of the ileal neobladder stimulate patient and physician decision toward earlier cystectomy? J Urol 1998;159:1845–1850.
9. Stein JP, Skinner DG. Radical cystectomy in the female. Atlas Urol Clin North Am 1997;5(20):37–64.
10. Stein JP, Skinner DG, Montie JE. Radical cystectomy and pelvic lymphadenectomy in the treatment of infiltrative bladder cancer. In Droller MJ (ed): Bladder Cancer: Current Diagnosis and Treatment. Totowa, NJ: Humana Press, 2001, pp 267–307.
11. Stein JP, Quek MD, Skinner DG. Contemporary surgical techniques for continent urinary diversion: continence and potency preservation. Atlas Urol Clin North Am 2001;9:147–173.
12. Stein JP. The role of lymphadenectomy in bladder cancer. Am J Urol Rev 2003;1:146–148.
13. Stein JP, Cai J, Groshen S, Skinner DG. Risk factors for patients with pelvic lymph node metastases following radical cystectomy with en bloc cystectomy: the concept of lymph node density. J Urol 2003;170:35–41.
14. Herr HW, Bochner BH, Dalbagni G, Donat SM, Reuter VE, Bajorin DF. Impact of the number of lymph nodes retrieved on outcome in

patients with muscle invasive bladder cancer. J Urol 2002;167:1295–1298.

15. Leissner J, Hohenfellner R, Thuroff JW, Wolf HK. Lymphadenectomy in patients with transitional cell carcinoma of the urinary bladder; significance for staging and prognosis. Br J Urol Int 2000;85:817–823.

16. Poulsen AL, Horn T, Steven K. Radical cystectomy; extending limits of pelvic lymph node dissection improves survival for patients with bladder cancer confined to the bladder wall. J Urol 1998;160:2015–2019.

17. Freeman JA, Esrig D, Stein JP, et al. Radical cystectomy for high risk patients with superficial bladder cancer in the era of orthotopic urinary reconstruction. Cancer 1995;76:833–839.

18. Anderstrom C, Johansson S, Nilsson S. The significance of lamina propria invasion on the prognosis of patients with bladder tumors. J Urol 1980;124:23–26.

19. Heney NM, Ahmed S, Flanagan MJ, Frable W, Corder MP, Hafermann MD, Hawkins IR. Superficial bladder cancer: progression and recurrence. J Urol 1983;130:1083–1086.

20. Dalesio O, Schulman CC, Sylvester R, et al. Prognostic factors in superficial bladder tumors. A study of the European Organization for Research on Treatment of Cancer: Genitourinary Tract Cancer Cooperative Group. J Urol 1983;129:730–733.

21. Herr HW, Jakse G, Sheinfeld J. The T1 bladder tumor. Semin Urol 1990;8:254–261.

22. Fitzpatrick JM. The natural history of superficial bladder cancer. Semin Urol 1993;11:127–136.

23. Malkowicz SB, Nichols P, Lieskovsky G, Boyd SD, Huffman J, Skinner DG. The role of radical cystectomy in the management of high grade superficial bladder cancer (PA, P1, PIS and P2). J Urol 1990;144:641–645.

24. Schellhammer PF, Bean MA, Whitmore WF Jr. Prostatic involvement by transitional cell carcinoma: pathogenesis, patterns, and prognosis. J Urol 1977;118:399–403.

25. Prout GR Jr, Griffin PP, Daly JJ, Henery NM. Carcinoma in situ of the urinary bladder with and without associated vesical neoplasms. Cancer 1983;52:524–532.

26. Utz DC, Farrow DM. Management of carcinoma in situ of the bladder: a case for surgical management. Urol Clin North Am 1980;7:533–540.

27. Voges GE, Tauschke E, Stockle M, Alken P, Hohenfellner R. Computerized tomography: an unreliable method for accurate staging of bladder tumors in patients who are candidates for radical cystectomy. J Urol 1989;142:972–974.

28. Pagano F, Bassi P, Galetti TP, Meneghini A, Milani C, Artibani W, Garbeglio A. Results of contemporary radical cystectomy for invasive bladder cancer: a clinicopathologic study with an emphasis on the inadequacy of the tumor, nodes and metastases classification. J Urol 1991;145:45–50.

29. Nichols RL, Broido P, Condon RE, Gorbach SL, Nyhus LM. Effect of preoperative neomycin–erythromycin intestinal preparation on the incidence of infectious complications following colon surgery. Ann Surg 1973;178:453–462.

30. Pinaud MLJ, Blanloeil YAG, Souron RJ. Preoperative prophylactic digitalization of patients with coronary artery disease—a randomized echocardiographic and hemodynamic study. Anesth Analg 1983;62:685–689.

31. Burman SO. The prophylactic use of digitalis before thoracotomy. Ann Thorac Surg 1972;14:359–368.

32. Crawford ED, Skinner DG. Salvage cystectomy after radiation failure. J Urol 1980;123:32–34.

33. Colleselli K, Stenzl A, Eder R, Strasser H, Poisel S, Bartsch G. The female urethral sphincter: a morphologic and topographical study. J Urol 1998;160:49–50.

34. Grossfeld GD, Stein JP, Bennett CJ, Ginsberg DA, Boyd SD, Lieskovsky G, Skinner DG. Lower urinary tract reconstruction in the female using the Kock ileal reservoir with bilateral ureteroileal urethrostomy: update of continence results and fluorodynamic findings. Urology 1996;48:383–388.

35. Buscarini M, Stein JP, Lawrence MA, Skinner DG. Tube gastrostomy following radical cystectomy and urinary diversion: surgical technique and experience in 709 patients. Urology 2000;56:150–152.

36. Frazier HA, Robertson JE, Dodge RK, and Paulson DF. The value of pathologic factors in predicting cancer-specific survival among patients treated with radical cystectomy for transitional cell carcinoma of the bladder and prostate. Cancer 1993;71:3993–4001.

37. Amling CL, Thrasher JB, Frazier HA, Dodge RK, Robertson JE, Paulson DF. Radical cystectomy for stages Ta, Tis and T1 transitional cell carcinoma of the bladder. J Urol 1994;151:31–35.

38. Viewig J, Gschwend JE, Herr HW, Fair WR. The impact of primary stage on survival in patients with lymph node positive bladder cancer J Urol 1999,161.72–76.

39. Leissner J, Ghoneim MA, Abol-Enein H, et al. Extended radical lymphadenectomy in patients with urothelial bladder cancer: results of a prospective multicenter study. J Urol 2004;171:139–144.

40. Stein JP, Dunn MD, Quek ML, Miranda G, Skinner DG. The orthotopic T-pouch ileal neobladder: experience with 209 patients. J Urol 2004;172:584–587.

41. Skinner DG, Lieskovsky G. Contemporary cystectomy with pelvic node dissection compared to preoperative radiation therapy plus cystectomy in management of invasive bladder cancer. J Urol 1984;131:1069–1072.

42. Grossman HB, Natale RB, Tangen CM, et al. Neoadjuvant chemotherapy plus cystectomy compared with cystectomy alone for locally advanced bladder cancer. N Engl J Med 2003;349:859–866.

43. Herr HW. Surgical factors in bladder cancer: more (nodes) + more (pathology) = less (mortality). BJU Int 2003;92:187–188.

44. Skinner DG, Daniels JA, Russell CA, et al. The role of adjuvant chemotherapy following cystectomy for invasive bladder cancer: a prospective comparative trial. J Urol 1991;145:459–467.

45. Figueroa AJ, Stein JP, Dickinson M, et al. Radical cystectomy for elderly patients with bladder carcinoma. An updated experience with 404 patients. Cancer 1998;83:141–147.

46. Koch MO, Smith JA Jr. Influence of patient age and co-morbidity on outcome of a collaborative care pathway after radical prostatectomy and cystoprostatectomy. J Urol 1996;155:1681–1684.

47. Chang SS, Alberts G, Cookson MS, Smith JA Jr. Radical cystectomy is safe in elderly patients at high risk. J Urol 2001;166:938–941.

48. Sanchez-Ortiz RF, Huang WC, Mick R, Van Arsdalen KN, Wein AJ, Malkowicz SB. An interval longer than 12 weeks between the diagnosis of muscle invasion and cystectomy is associated with worse outcome in bladder carcinoma. J Urol 2003;169:110–115.

49. Quek ML, Stein JP, Clark PE, et al. Microscopic and gross extravesical extension in pathologic staging of bladder cancer. J Urol 2004;171:640–645.

50. AJCC Cancer Staging Manual, 5th ed. Philadelphia: Lippincott-Raven, 1997, pp 241–243.

51. Stein JP, Ginsberg DA, Skinner DG. Indications and technique of the orthotopic neobladder in women. Urol Clin North Am 2002;29:725–734.

52. Stein JP, Cote RJ, Freeman JA, et al. Indications for lower urinary tract reconstruction in women after cystectomy for bladder cancer: a pathological review of female cystectomy specimens. J Urol 1995;154:1329–1333.

53. Stein JP, Esrig D, Freeman JA, et al. Prospective pathologic analysis of female cystectomy specimens: risk factors for orthotopic diversion in women. Urology 1998;51:951–955.

54. Freeman JA, Esrig D, Stein JP, Skinner DG. Management of the patient with bladder cancer. Urethral recurrence. Urol Clin North Am 1994;21:645–651.

55. Freeman JA, Tarter TA, Esrig D, et al. Urethral recurrence in patients with orthotopic ileal neobladders. J Urol 1996;156:1615–1619.

56. Stenzl A, Bartsch G, Rogatsch H. The remnant urothelium after reconstructive bladder surgery. Eur Urol 2002;41:124–131.

57. Levinson AK, Johnson DE, Wishnow KI. Indications for urethrectomy in an era of continent urinary diversion. J Urol 1990;144:73–75.

58. Hardeman SW, Soloway MS. Urethral recurrence following radical cystectomy. J Urol 1990;144:666–669.

59. Stockle M, Gokcebay E, Riedmiller H, Hohenfellner R. Urethral tumor recurrences after radical cystoprostatectomy: the case for primary cystoprostatourethrectomy? J Urol 1990;143:41–42; discussion 43.

60. Tobisu K, Tanaka Y, Mizutani T, Kakizoe T. Transitional cell carcinoma of the urethra in men following cystectomy for bladder cancer:

multivariate analysis for risk factors. J Urol 1991;146:1551–1553; discussion 1553–1554.

61. Stein JP, Clark, P, Miranda G, Cai J, Groshen S, Skinner DG. Urethral tumor recurrence following cystectomy and urinary diversion: clinical and pathologic characteristics in 768 male patients. J Urol 2005;173(4):1163–1168.

62. Spitz A, Stein JP, Lieskovsky G, Skinner DG. Orthotopic urinary diversion with preservation of erectile and ejaculatory function in men requiring radical cystectomy for nonurothelial malignancy: a new technique. J Urol 1999;161:1761–1764.

63. Vallancien G, El Fettouh HA, Cathelineau X, Baumert H, Fromont G, Guillonneau B. Cystectomy with prostate sparing for bladder cancer in 100 patients: 10-year experience. J Urol 2002;168:2413–2417.

64. Ghanem AN. Experience with 'capsule sparing' cystoprostadenectomy for orthotopic bladder replacement: overcoming the problems of impotence, incontinence and difficult urethral anastomosis. BJU Int 2002;90:617–620.

65. Horenblas S, Meinhardt W, Ijzerman W, Moonen LFN. Sexuality preserving cystectomy and neobladder; initial results. J Urol 2001;166:837–840.

66. Colombo R, Bertini R, Salonia A, et al. Nerve and seminal sparing radical cystectomy with orthotopic urinary diversion for selected patients with superficial bladder cancer: an innovative surgical approach. J Urol 2001;165:51–55.

67. Colombo R, Bertini R, Salonia A, et al. Overall clinical outcomes after nerve and seminal sparing radical cystectomy for the treatment of organ confined bladder cancer. J Urol 2004;171:1819–1822.

68. Stein JP, Grossfeld GD, Ginsberg DA, et al. Prognostic markers in bladder cancer: a contemporary review of the literature. J Urol 1999;160:645–659.

# Cystectomy in the female

45

*Aristotelis G Anastasiadis, Susan Feyerabend, Markus A Kuczyk,
Arnulf Stenzl*

## INTRODUCTION

The Czech surgeon Pawlik reported the first cystectomy in a female more than a century ago.[1] He described an implantation of the ureters into the vagina with a good postoperative result regarding continence as well as a survival of 16 years. Other physicians could not achieve similar results and therefore this technique of urinary diversion was subsequently abandoned. Until recently, women undergoing cystectomy for bladder cancer received urinary diversion either into the intact rectosigmoid or into the abdominal skin.[2-6] Despite increasing popularity for orthotopic neobladders after cystectomy in men with bladder cancer during the last decade, a similar approach for female patients was thought not to be appropriate because of the need for a concomitant total urethrectomy.[7]

However, results of a combined series from two institutions have indicated that selected women with transitional cell cancer (TCC) undergoing radical cystectomy can safely be spared a portion of their urethra.[8,9] The remaining urethral segment would be sufficient for a continence mechanism when anastomosed to a low-pressure intestinal reservoir. Important aspects which have to be taken into consideration in female patients with TCC prior to cystectomy and urinary diversion are discussed in this chapter. These aspects include anatomical considerations, patient selection, and surgical techniques, as well as oncologic and functional outcome.

## INCIDENCE OF URETHRAL TUMORS IN BLADDER CANCER OF THE FEMALE—IS URETHRA-SPARING CYSTECTOMY ONCOLOGICALLY SAFE?

An important question when considering urethra-sparing cystectomy in female patients is whether there is a risk of compromising oncologic outcome. In order to use the urethra for bladder reconstruction, about 80% of the urethra should be preserved.[10] Within the urethra, the level of transition between transitional and squamous epithelium varies considerably. With increasing age, the transition zone moves cranially and can even cover the whole urethra, bladder neck, and part of the trigone, probably due to the influence of estrogen.[11,12] Since the bladder neck and a small portion of the proximal urethra are resected during surgery, only a very short segment, in some patients even none, of the remnant urethra will be covered by transitional cell epithelium, whereas the major part of the urethral mucosa will consist of either regular or metaplastic squamous epithelium. Therefore, often only squamous metaplasia is found at the level of urethral dissection. To the authors' knowledge, no data describe a TCC recurrence on squamous epithelium after removal of the entire urothelium of the bladder during cystectomy.

Several studies have tried to address the risk of urethral tumors in the remnant female urethra after cystectomy. In retrospective analyses, Stein et al[13] and Coloby et al[14] step-sectioned urethrocystectomy specimens of female bladder cancer patients and found urethral tumor involvement in 7 of 65 (10.7%) and 3 of 47 (6.4%) patients, respectively. A strong correlation with cancer at the bladder neck and/or the trigone was found in both studies, and a subtotal urethrectomy was suggested. On the other hand, De Paepe et al[15] found carcinoma in situ or papillary tumors in the urethra in 8 of 22 (36%) patients and suggested that a urethrectomy should be performed in all women undergoing radical cystectomy for TCC of the bladder. It should be borne in mind, however, that there were only 22 patients included in this report and that no details about the localization of either primary tumor in the bladder or secondary tumors in the urethra were provided.

Ashworth[16] and Stenzl et al[17] also evaluated the incidence of secondary urethral tumors of more than 600 patients treated for bladder cancer. In these series, the incidence of secondary urethral tumors was 1.4% and 2%, respectively. Interestingly, women showed a lower incidence of urethral involvement than male patients from the same institution.[18]

## ANATOMY OF THE FEMALE URETHRA

The sphincter system of the female urethra consists of smooth muscle layers, which are controlled by autonomic nerves, and striated muscle layers innervated by somatic nerves. The autonomic nerve branches for the smooth muscle portion of the urethral sphincter originate from the pelvic plexus.[19,20] The innervation of the voluntary sphincter system is controversial: although most authors suggest that branches of the pudendal nerve provide the nerve supply to this sphincter,[21,22] others have suggested that the autonomic nervous system is responsible for its innervation.[23]

Women treated with distal partial urethrectomy, for example for complicated diverticula or tumors, remain continent unless a major portion of the middle third of the urethra is resected.[24] It is, therefore, generally accepted that the bladder neck, together with an adequate proximal urethral segment, is sufficient for urinary continence in women. Fetal and adult cadaver studies have demonstrated that the entire rhabdo-sphincter, which is innervated by the pudendal nerve caudally, is located in the caudal half of the urethra and merges approximately halfway with the mid-layer of the proximal smooth musculature.[25] Smooth muscle fibers of the outer and inner layer, innervated by the autonomic nervous system, however, are present throughout the whole length of the urethra.

Nerve fibers originating from the pelvic plexus located dorsolaterally from the rectum have been traced on their route to the bladder neck and urethra to run dorsal to the distal ureter, underneath the lateral vesical pedicle and along the lateral walls of the vagina.[26] An anterior exenteration with complete resection of the vagina with the caudal margin below the bladder neck would therefore result in the dissection of the majority, if not all, of the autonomic nerves to the female urethra. As a consequence, a careful dissection of the lateral vaginal walls, bladder neck, and proximal urethra would leave the majority of plexus fibers to the urethra intact, thus preserving the sphincter mechanism.[77–79]

The suspensory fascial reinforcements of the remnant urethra will not be compromised if a nerve-sparing cystectomy is performed, since care is taken to stay as close as possible to the urethra proximally and to avoid any dissection caudal to the level of the urethral division.

Another important aspect is the lymphatic drainage of the remnant urethra after cystectomy. Bladder tumors which are close to, but not adjacent to, the bladder neck and show grossly enlarged lymph nodes preoperatively may cause reverse lymphatic tumor cell drainage to the external inguinal lymph nodes. This could increase the risk of periurethral tumor cell nests in the remnant urethra. One should therefore consider the status of the pelvic and inguinal nodes in addition to the location of the primary tumor in selecting female patients for orthotopic reconstruction. If preoperatively performed biopsies of these areas are positive for cancer, this is a relative contraindication for orthotopic urinary diversion.

## PATIENT SELECTION CRITERIA

Female candidates for creation of an orthotopic neobladder to the urethra should be selected according to tumor extension, urethral competence, performance status, and motivation (Box 45.1).[10] Preoperatively, bimanual and endoscopic tumor evaluation, a computed tomography (CT) scan of the abdomen and thorax, and a bone scan, as well as biopsies of the bladder neck, should be performed. Urethral competence should be assessed by the patient's history, endoscopy, radiography, and intraluminal urethra pressure profile (UPP).

Patients with an orthotopic neobladder need strength and motivation for continence training and should be able to adhere to simple rules, for example, a certain micturition pattern in the early postoperative period. An acceptable performance status and motivation are therefore necessary. This includes the understanding and handling of specific problems, such as possible urinary retention or increased post void residuals that may require intermittent catheterization, or nocturnal and diurnal incontinence.

## SURGICAL TECHNIQUE

The technique of anterior exenteration and concomitant lymphadenectomy has been described elsewhere in the

1. Tumor extension
   - Tumor/carcinoma in situ at bladder neck
   - Urethral tumor
   - Any positive surgical margin on frozen section
   - ≥N2
   - Any tumor involvement of inguinal nodes
   - M+

2. Urethral competence
   - History of stress incontinence ≥Grade II due to sphincteric incompetence
   - Marked urethral hypermobility
   - $P_{rest}$ <30 cm $H_2O$ in the intraluminal urethra pressure profile (UPP)
   - Full dose radiation to the urethra

3. Performance status and motivation
   - Any reduced performance status, e.g. Karnofsky index ≤90%
   - No motivation to undergo intensive continence training if necessary
   - No motivation to wear pads if necessary
   - No motivation or dexterity for clean intermittent catheterization if necessary

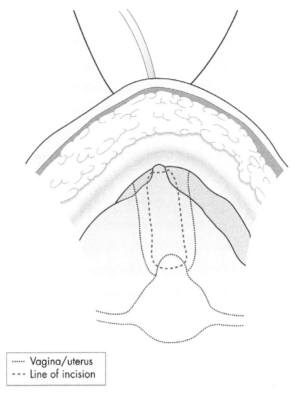

····· Vagina/uterus
--- Line of incision

**Fig. 45.1**
Incision line during nerve-sparing cystectomy in order to preserve autonomic nerve fibers to the remnant urethra. Adapted from Stenzl A, Draxl H, Posch B, Colleselli K, Falk M, Bartsch G. The risk of urethral tumors in female bladder cancer: can the urethra be used for orthotopic reconstruction of the lower urinary tract? J Urol 1995;153:950–955.

literature. Therefore, in the present chapter we will describe only those variations which are relevant for female patients undergoing an orthotopic reconstruction of the lower urinary tract. All our patients receive an ileal low-pressure reservoir with an antireflux protection for the upper urinary tract and direct anastomosis of the pouch to the remnant urethra. To facilitate intraoperative catheterization of the pouch after dividing the Foley catheter during cystectomy, the patient can be placed in a low lithotomy position. In most cases, however, we place the patient in a simple supine position to avoid possible complications related to positioning.

During pelvic lymphadenectomy care is taken to minimize dissection in the region of the upper hypogastric nerve crossing the common iliac artery. Special attention is then directed towards dissection and resection of the inner genitalia. After mobilization of the ovaries, tubes and uterus, only the vaginal fundus and the anterior vaginal wall down to the level of the subsequent urethral dissection are resected (Figure 45.1). The dorsal half of the vaginal fundus is incised circumferentially around the cervical insertion or scar from a previous hysterectomy. The line of incision is continued ventrally and caudally to include an approximately 2 cm wide segment of the ventral wall of the vagina. The bladder neck and proximal urethra are then carefully 'peeled' out of the surrounding connective tissue and fascia. Care is taken to incise the endopelvic fascia medially, where it leaves the bladder surface. The dissection of the proximal urethra is performed by incising the fascia longitudinally in the midline and staying as close to the urethral wall as possible in order

to avoid damage to the nerve fibers coursing to the remnant urethra (Figure 45.2). The proximal urethra with its Foley catheter is clamped with a strong Overholt clamp and dissected approximately 0.5–1 cm distal to the bladder neck (Figure 45.3). The specimen is then removed and a transverse frozen section of the urethra is sent for intraoperative pathologic evaluation.

Squamous metaplasia was present in all our specimens, but no tumor or dysplasia was diagnosed at the level of urethral dissection. In obese patients, a ureteral catheter placed in an antegrade fashion may be an additional help in guiding the final pouch catheter transurethrally prior to closure of the urethroileal anastomosis. The vaginal defect is closed transversely with a running 0 polyglycolic acid (PGA) suture (Figure 45.4). If necessary, continence training devices may be introduced into the resulting small vaginal pouch. If the patient is sexually active, the vaginal defect might also be closed with a small-detubularized ileal patch.

Any low-pressure reservoir can be anastomosed to the remnant urethra with preferably six 2-0 synthetic absorbable sutures. We have observed that caudal migration of the pouch into the pelvis may result in

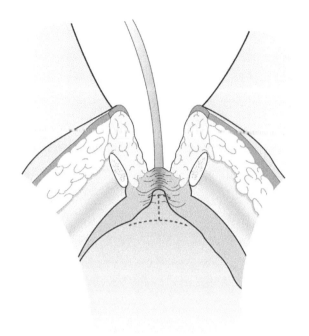

**Fig. 45.2**
Adult anatomic specimen of the bladder neck and urethra with part of the pubic bone removed. When following the dashed line of incision (- - -) during dissection and staying close to the urethra and bladder neck respectively, neither the majority of the autonomic nerves to the remnant urethra nor the urethral suspensory system will be damaged. Adapted from Stenzl A, Draxl H, Posch B, Colleselli K, Falk M, Bartsch G. The risk of urethral tumors in female bladder cancer: can the urethra be used for orthotopic reconstruction of the lower urinary tract? J Urol 1995;153:950–955.

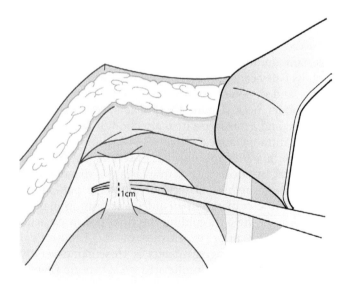

**Fig. 45.3**
The urethra is clamped and dissected approximately 0.5–1 cm caudal of the bladder neck. Adapted from Stenzl A, Draxl H, Posch B, Colleselli K, Falk M, Bartsch G. The risk of urethral tumors in female bladder cancer: can the urethra be used for orthotopic reconstruction of the lower urinary tract? J Urol 1995;153:950–955.

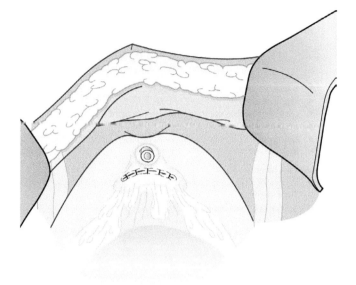

**Fig. 45.4**
After removal of the specimen, the vagina is closed transversely. Any low-pressure reservoir can now be anastomosed to the remnant urethra. A J-shaped omentum flap or additional attachment sutures of the pouch to the pelvic wall are advocated to improve postoperative micturition results. Adapted from Stenzl A, Draxl H, Posch B, Colleselli K, Falk M, Bartsch G. The risk of urethral tumors in female bladder cancer: can the urethra be used for orthotopic reconstruction of the lower urinary tract? J Urol 1995;153:950–955.

intestinal folds that may cause intermittent obstructive valves at the ileourethral anastomosis. Instead of anastomosing the spout-like residual opening, which is connected to the urethra in the hemi-Kock or T-pouch, we therefore now employ a technique used in other pouches, in which a circular ileal opening close to the mesentery at the lowest part of the pouch is anastomosed to the urethra.[30]

At the end of the procedure, a J-shaped omentum flap is brought down and around the bottom of the pouch.[17] Alternatively, portions of the ileal pouch adjacent to this anastomosis can be sutured to the anterior and lateral pelvic walls as well as the remnant vaginal stump to avoid both the formation of obstructive folds over the urethral anastomosis and the formation of a 'pouchocele' due to a postoperative descensus of the reservoir. Initial attempts to perform a 'neobladder neck suspension' to improve early continence were not successful because of urinary retention. Suspension of the vaginal vault with remnant portions of the round ligaments or fascial strips to prevent kinking of the pouch and subsequent retention have been suggested recently, but long-term results are not yet available.

Both ureteroileal anastomoses are stented with 7 Fr. single J-shaped ureteral catheters, which are brought out either transurethrally along the urethral catheter or through the lower abdominal wall. Pelvic drains are removed on the fifth postoperative day, ureteral catheters after approximately 8–10 days, and the 20 Fr. urethral catheter after 14 days, if a previous pouchogram shows no extravasation.

# RESULTS

## ONCOLOGIC RESULTS

In a multicenter study, the combined data of 102 women aged 28–79 (mean 59) years who underwent a urethra-sparing cystectomy and orthotopic urinary diversion were reviewed.[31] Surgery was performed for bladder cancer (n=96), cervical cancer (n=2), vaginal cancer (n=1), cancer of the fallopian tube (n=1), uterine sarcoma (n=1), or rectal cancer (n=1). The histology of the 96 bladder cancers was TCC in 81, adenocarcinoma in 8, squamous cell cancer in 5, small cell carcinoma in 1, and unclassified in 1 patient. The mean follow-up time was 26 months. At completion of the study, 88/102 patients were alive and 83/102 patients were alive and disease free.

The bladder neck was free of tumor in all patients. The bladder neck and up to 1 cm of the proximal urethra were removed with the specimen. An ileal orthotopic neobladder was performed if staging biopsies of the bladder neck and intraoperative frozen section of the urethral margin revealed no tumor. No perioperative deaths were reported, and early and late complications requiring secondary interventions occurred in 5% and 12% of patients, respectively. With 88 of 102 patients alive and 83 of 102 patients disease free, a disease-specific survival of 74% and a disease-free survival of 63% could be estimated at 5 years. The remnant urethra was monitored via voided cytology and endoscopically. Three pelvic recurrences occurred in patients with gynecologic tumors and one in a patient with adenocarcinoma of the bladder, but none of them in the area of the urethra or its supplying autonomic nerves.

The incidence of concomitant secondary malignant involvement of gynecologic organs in female cystectomy specimens has been evaluated in a recent study.[32] Overall gynecologic organ involvement was documented in 16 of 609 patients (2.6%). Although the majority of these women were diagnosed with squamous cell bladder carcinoma, which may not be representative for many geographic areas, first evidence is provided that the risk of secondary malignant involvement of genital organs in female cystectomy specimens is low. Therefore, the routine removal of involved gynecologic organs during radical cystectomy in women may be an issue of discussion in the future.

## FUNCTIONAL OUTCOME

### VOIDING PATTERN

A routine postoperative urodynamic evaluation of the pouch and remaining urethra is not necessary, but was performed in 15 patients.[10] The voiding pattern, including volumes at each micturition, was evaluated by a detailed questionnaire. To obtain the maximum pouch volume, the average of three maximum volumes was calculated and was used as a value up to which the pouch was filled during urodynamic testing. The calculated bladder capacity in these women ranged from 400 to 750 (mean 560) cc. Post void residuals ranged from 0 to 150 cc.

The intraluminal pouch pressures at rest were below 30 cm $H_2O$ in all patients except one, who showed intermittent peak pressures of up to 38 cm $H_2O$ after 6 months. Maximum intraluminal urethral pressures in the UPP ranged from 30 to 35 (mean 32) cm $H_2O$, which was virtually unchanged, from preoperative values with an average of 33.4 (range 28–42) cm $H_2O$.

### DIURNAL AND NOCTURNAL CONTINENCE

For the evaluation of diurnal and nocturnal continence we used definitions from the literature.[7] In patients followed for more than 6 months postoperatively, daytime and nocturnal continence could be achieved in 85.5% and 79%, respectively. Interestingly, only 25% of preoperatively irradiated patients for gynecologic malignancies have regained diurnal continence, whereas all other patients have Grade I–II stress incontinence. We therefore consider a full course of preoperative radiation a relative contraindication for this surgical procedure. Urodynamic results from patients included in the multicenter study mentioned above are also available.[31] Daytime and nocturnal continence rates with maximally one pad for safety were 82% and 72%, respectively. Twelve patients (12%) were unable to empty their bladders completely and needed some form of catheterization.

Urinary retention or unacceptably large post void residuals in patients with an ileal valve obstructing the neobladder outlet partially or completely could be treated successfully. This entity, first described in 1997,[10] can be observed endoscopically when positioning the cystoscope just below the bladder neck and draining the pouch. This problem can be resolved completely by incising these valves carefully.

### SEXUAL FUNCTION

Another important aspect of nerve-preserving surgery is that of sexual function. Similar to male erectile physiology, nitric oxide (NO) plays a major role in vasodilation in clitoral tissues.[33] Autonomic nerves are responsible not only for NO-mediated changes in the clitoris, but also for vasoactive intestinal polypeptide (VIP) mediated vasodilation and secretion of the vaginal mucosa. The latter plays a major role during the phase of sexual arousal. Neurotransmitters, in turn, are able to modulate the sensitivity of sensory nerve fibers to central or peripheral stimuli.[34] Similar to erectile dysfunction in men, female sexual dysfunction (FSD) can be a sequela of pelvic surgery with a major impact on quality of life, relationships, and psychosocial function.

Although sexual function may play only a minor role for many cancer patients, for a subset of patients it represents an important aspect of quality of life. Unfortunately, data on sexual function of cancer patients remain scant in the literature. In addition, FSD in cancer patients is extremely difficult to evaluate because of its complexity due to somatic and psychological aspects, which are often intertwined.[35] More studies are needed in this field to further optimize surgical techniques and to improve patients' quality of life.

## CONCLUSION

Recent larger series confirm our initial results, showing that sparing the urethra after cystectomy will not compromise oncologic outcome and can be used satisfactorily for orthotopic reconstruction of the lower urinary tract in female patients. Diurnal and nocturnal continence rates of 87.5% and 79%, respectively, and clean intermittent catheterization in 10% after 6 months are comparable to results in larger male series and justify the use of orthotopic neobladders as a procedure of choice in selected females.

We now know that urinary continence of any bladder substitution can be maintained despite removal of the bladder neck and the adjacent proximal urethra. In our anatomic studies as well as those of others, no prominent sphincteric structure was present in either the female bladder neck or the cranial urethra. The bulk of the striated intrinsic sphincter ('rhabdosphincter') is located in the mid to caudal third of the urethra and will not be removed with proximal urethrectomy, as described above. Its innervation via the pudendal nerve will not be compromised during the surgical procedure.

Controversy still exists as to whether dissecting autonomic nerves to the urethra when performing a subtotal colpectomy and resection of the bladder neck including a wide margin of surrounding tissue will compromise long-term results. As yet, we do not know if these autonomic nerves are needed for satisfactory function of the urethral smooth muscles, nor can we determine to what extent these nerves can be spared at

each individual surgery. Based on available anatomic and functional studies, however, it is suggested that most of the autonomic innervation of the remnant urethra should stay intact postoperatively to preserve both muscular resistance and continence despite removal of a safe segment of the proximal urethra for oncologic reasons.[19,36]

Over the years, it was possible to further improve postoperative functional results by:

1. leaving the posterior and lateral vaginal walls intact when performing a nerve-sparing anterior exenteration—this can be achieved by carefully dissecting out the bladder neck and the proximal urethra;
2. removing 0.5–1 cm of the cranial urethra en bloc with the cystectomy specimen and obtaining a frozen section of the whole urethral circumference;
3. using previous experience with low-pressure reservoirs in male patients;
4. preventing complications related to a downward migration of the pouch by using either a J-shaped omentum flap or stay sutures between the pouch wall and the surrounding pelvic structures.[37,38]

## REFERENCES

1. Pawlik K. Extirpace mechyre mocoveho, Lekaru Ceskych 1890;29:705–706.
2. Bricker E. Bladder substitution after pelvic evisceration. Surg Clin North Am 1950;30:1511–1521.
3. Clarke B, Leadbetter W. Ureterosigmoidostomy: collective review of results in 2,897 reported cases. J Urol 1955;73:999–1008.
4. Fisch MWR, Müller SC, Hohenfellner R. The sigma-rectum pouch (Mainz pouch II). Scand J Urol Nephrol (Suppl) 1992;142:187–188.
5. Ghoneim M. The modified rectal bladder: a bladder substitute controlled by the anal sphincter. Scand J Urol Nephrol 1992;142:89–91.
6. Gilchrist R, Merricks J, Hamlin H. Construction of a substitute bladder and urethra. Surg Gynecol Obstet 1950;90:752–760.
7. Skinner DG, Boyd SD, Lieskovski G, Bennett C, Hopwood B. Lower urinary tract reconstruction following cystectomy: experience and results in 126 patients using the Kock ileal reservoir with bilateral ureteroileal urethrostomy. J Urol 1991;146:756–760.
8. Cancrini A, de Carli P, Fattahi H, Pompeo V, Cantiani R, von Heland M. Orthotopic ileal neobladder in female patients after radical cystectomy: 2-year experience. J Urol 1994;153:956–958.
9. Stein J, Stenzl A, Esrig D, et al. Lower urinary tract reconstruction following cystectomy in women using the Kock ileal reservoir with bilateral utereroileal urethrostomy: initial clinical experience. J Urol 1994;152:1404–1408.
10. Stenzl A, Colleselli K, Bartsch G. Update of urethra-sparing approaches in cystectomy in women. World J Urol 1997;15:134–138.
11. Packham D. The epithelial lining of the female trigone and urethra. Br J Urol 1971;43:201–208.
12. Wiener D, Koss L, Salaby B, Freed S. The prevalence and significance of Brunn's nests, cystitis cystica, and squamous metaplasia in normal bladders. J Urol 1979;122:317–323.
13. Stein J, Cote R, Freeman J, et al. Indications for lower urinary tract reconstruction in women following cystectomy for bladder cancer: a pathologic review of female cystectomy specimens. J Urol 1995;154:1329–1333.
14. Coloby P, Kakizoe T, Tobisu KI. Urethral involvement in female bladder cancer patients: mapping of 47 consecutive cysto-urethrectomy specimens. J Urol 1994;152:1438–1442.

15. De Paepe M, Andre R, Mahadevia P. Urethral involvement in female patients with bladder cancer. A study of 22 cystectomy specimens. Cancer 1990;65:1237–1242.

16. Ashworth A. Papillomatosis of the urethra. Br J Urol 1956;28:3–11.

17. Stenzl A, Colleselli K, Poisel S, Feichtinger H, Bartsch G. The use of neobladders in women undergoing cystectomy for transitional cell cancer. World J Urol 1996;14:15–21.

18. Erckert M, Stenzl A, Falk M, Bartsch G. The incidence of urethral tumor involvement in male bladder cancer patients. World J Urol 1996;14:3–8.

19. Baader B, Baader SL, Herrmann M, Stenzl A. Anatomical bases of the autonomic innervation of the female pelvis. Urologe A 2004;43:133–149.

20. Wein A, Levin R, Barrett D. Voiding function: relevant anatomy, physiology, and pharmacology. In Gillenwater J, Grayhack J, Howards S, Duckett J (eds): Adult and Pediatric Urology, 2nd ed. Chicago: Year Book, 1991, pp 933–999.

21. Gosling JA, Dixon JS, Critchley HO, Thompson SA. A comparative study of the human external sphincter and periurethral levator ani muscles. Br J Urol 1981;53:35–41.

22. Tanagho EA, Meyers FH, Smith DR. Urethral resistance: its components and implications. II. Striated muscle component. Invest Urol 1969;7:195–205.

23. Donker P, Droes J, Van Ulden B. Anatomy of the musculature and innervation of the bladder and the urethra. In Williams D, Chisholm G (eds): Scientific Foundations of Urology, vol II. London: Heinemann, 1976, p 32.

24. Neuwirth H, Stenzl A, de Kernion J. Urethral cancer. In Haskell C (ed): Cancer Treatment. Philadelphia: Saunders, 1990, pp 762–764.

25. Strasser H, Ninkovic M, Hess M, Bartsch G, Stenzl A. Anatomic and functional studies of the male and female urethral sphincter. World J Urol 2000;18:324–329.

26. Colleselli K, Stenzl A, Eder R, Strasser H, Poisel S, Bartsch G. The female urethral sphincter: a morphological and topographical study. J Urol 1998;160:49–54.

27. De Petriconi R, Kleinschmidt K, Flohr P, Paiss T, Hautmann R. Ileal neobladder with anastomosis to the female urethra. Urologe A 1996;35:284–290.

28. Mills RD, Studer UE. Female orthotopic bladder substitution: a good operation in the right circumstances. J Urol 2000;163:1501–1504.

29. Stenzl A, Draxl H, Posch B, Colleselli K, Falk M, Bartsch G. The risk of urethral tumors in female bladder cancer: can the urethra be used for orthotopic reconstruction of the lower urinary tract? J Urol 1995;153:950–955.

30. Studer U, Ackermann D, Casanova G, Zingg E. Three years experience with an ileal low pressure bladder substitute. Br J Urol 1989;63:43–52.

31. Stenzl A, Jarolim L, Coloby P, et al. Urethra-sparing cystectomy and orthotopic urinary diversion in women with malignant pelvic tumors. Cancer 2001;92:1864–1871.

32. Ali-El-Dein B, Abdel-Latif M, Mosbah A, Eraky I, Shaaban AA, Taha NM, Ghoneim MA. Secondary malignant involvement of gynecologic organs in radical cystectomy specimens in women: is it mandatory to remove these organs routinely? J Urol 2004;172:885–887.

33. Burnett AL, Calvin DC, Silver RI, Peppas DS, Docimo SG. Immunohistochemical description of nitric oxide synthase isoforms in the human clitoris. J Urol 1997;158:75–78.

34. McKenna KE. The neurophysiology of female sexual dysfunction. World J Urol 2002;20:93–100.

35. Anastasiadis AG, Davis AR, Sawczuk IS, et al. Quality of life aspects in kidney cancer patients: data from a national registry. Supp Care Cancer 2003;11:700–706.

36. Stenzl A, Anastasiadis AG, Corvin S, Feil G, Strasser H, Kuczyk M. Advantages of nerve sparing pelvic surgery—results of experimental and clinical studies. Urologe A 2004;43:141–149.

37. Stenzl A, Höltl L. Orthotopic bladder reconstruction in women—what we have learned over the last decade? Crit Rev Oncol Hematol 2003;47:147–154.

38. Stenzl A. Current concepts for urinary diversion in women. EAU Update Series 2003;1:91–99.

# Nerve-sparing radical cystectomy

46

*Marc S Chuang, Gary D Steinberg, Mark P Schoenberg*

## INTRODUCTION

Bladder cancer is the second most common genitourinary malignancy, with transitional cell carcinoma (TCC) comprising nearly 90% of all primary bladder cancers. Although the majority of patients present with superficial bladder tumors, 20% to 40% either present with or develop invasive disease.[1]

The first cystectomy was performed in the late 1800s.[2] However, early techniques were associated with high rates of morbidity and mortality. Young and Davis[3] indicated that high mortality rates and poor success rates made cystectomy unjustifiable. In 1939, Hinman[4] reported a mortality rate of 34.5% in a series of 250 cystectomies. More recently, improvements in surgical anesthetic techniques as well as perioperative care have reduced the mortality rate of radical cystectomy to 1% to 3%.[1,5,6]

During the 1960s and 1970s, various regimes of preoperative radiation were used in an attempt to improve survival after cystectomy; however, these failed to demonstrate any additional benefit.[7] In the largest series to date, Stein et al[1] evaluated their long-term experience with 1054 patients diagnosed with invasive bladder cancer. They were able to demonstrate excellent long-term, recurrence-free survival in patients with organ-confined, lymph-node-negative disease. Patients with lymph node involvement or extravesical extension had a significantly higher probability of recurrence. Patients could also be stratified by the extent of lymph node involvement. The overall recurrence rate was 30%. These data and data from similar studies support aggressive surgical management of invasive bladder carcinoma.[8,9] Thus, radical cystectomy is currently considered the gold standard for muscle invasive disease.[10]

With improved survival following radical cystectomy, increased emphasis was placed on quality of life issues. In 1982, Walsh and Donker demonstrated that impotence following radical prostatectomy arises from injury to the pelvic nerve plexus that provides autonomic innervation to the corpora cavernosa.[11] The technique for radical prostatectomy and cystoprostatectomy was therefore modified to avoid injury to these cavernous nerves and preserve potency. In 1985, Lepor and associates reported a detailed three-dimensional model of the course of the cavernous nerves in the region of the prostate based on microscopic step-sections taken from a human cadaver.[12] In 1987, Schlegel and Walsh demonstrated the exact relationship of the cavernous nerves to the seminal vesicles and bladder (Figure 46.1).[13] This study demonstrated that the pelvic plexus is located retroperitoneally on the lateral wall of the rectum, 5–11 cm from the anal verge with its midpoint related to the tip of the seminal vesicle. The cavernous branches travel in a direct route from the pelvic plexus toward the posterolateral base of the prostate. Because the bulk of the pelvic plexus and its important branches are located lateral and posterior to the seminal vesicles, these vesicles can be used as an intraoperative landmark to avoid injury to the pelvic plexus when ligating the posterior pedicle of the bladder. Using this technique in 25 patients, the authors reported an 83% potency rate among patients undergoing cystectomy without urethrectomy.

Pritchett et al[14] questioned the cancer control of the nerve-sparing technique when they were able to demonstrate lymph nodes in the tissue left behind during the preservation of the neurovascular bundle. As

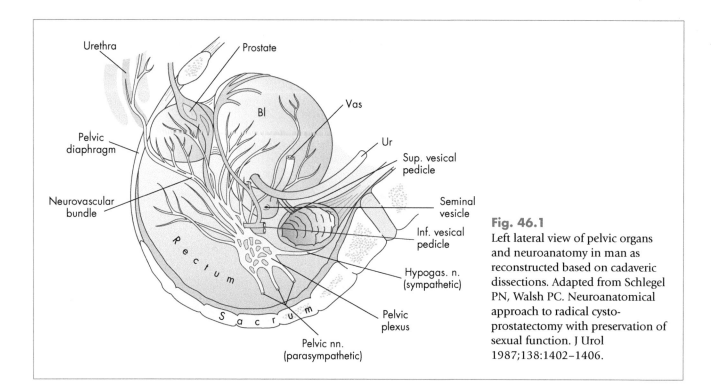

Urethra

Prostate

Pelvic
diaphragm

BI

Vas

Ur

Sup. vesical
pedicle

Neurovascular
bundle

Seminal
vesicle

Inf. vesical
pedicle

Rectum

Hypogas. n.
(sympathetic)

Sacrum

Pelvic
plexus

Pelvic nn.
(parasympathetic)

**Fig. 46.1**
Left lateral view of pelvic organs
and neuroanatomy in man as
reconstructed based on cadaveric
dissections. Adapted from Schlegel
PN, Walsh PC. Neuroanatomical
approach to radical cystoprostatectomy with preservation of
sexual function. J Urol
1987;138:1402–1406.

these lymph nodes were thought to potentially represent the first site of metastasis, the authors cautioned against using this technique. Brendler et al[15] reviewed their results using the nerve-sparing technique in 76 men, and demonstrated a 5-year actuarial local recurrence rate of 7.5%; 64% of patients that underwent cysto-prostatectomy alone were potent at follow-up. Therefore it was concluded that the nerve-sparing technique did not compromise cancer control, and had the added benefit of preserving potency in most men. Schoenberg et al[16] reviewed the long-term follow-up in the same cohort of patients. They demonstrated a disease-specific 10-year survival rate for all stages of bladder cancer of 69%, and a 10-year survival rate free of local recurrence of 94%. The overall potency rate was 42%. Recovery of sexual function following nerve-sparing cystectomy correlated with patient age: 62% in men aged 40–49 years old, 47% in men 50–59 years old, 43% in men 60–69 years old, and 20% in men 70–79 years old. Marshall et al[17] were able to demonstrate a 71% potency rate in patients that underwent total ileocolic neobladder reconstruction following nerve-sparing cystectomy for transitional cell carcinoma.

Despite the encouraging potency results reported by some investigators, sexuality after urinary diversion remains a significant patient concern. After cystectomy there is an overall decrease in sexual desire, interaction with one's partner, and sexual activities. Hart et al[18] found that concerns with sexual function were one of the most common complaints following radical cystectomy and urinary diversion. Moderate to severe sexual dissatisfaction was noted in 47% of patients

compared to 16% prior to surgery. However, men with severe postoperative erectile dysfunction demonstrated a statistically significant improvement in sexual function and satisfaction following penile prosthesis implantation. Henningsohn and colleagues[19] reported that 94% of men had some degree of erectile dysfunction following radical cystectomy compared to 48% in age-matched controls. Importantly, in this cohort of patients no attempt was made at nerve sparing.

In properly selected patients, nerve-sparing cystectomy can be performed safely. It offers long-term survival and recurrence rates similar to the standard radical cystectomy, and can preserve potency in the majority of patients. Nevertheless, patients should be counseled preoperatively regarding the possibility of permanent sexual dysfunction.

## PREOPERATIVE PREPARATION

Prior to surgery, patients meet with an enterostomal therapist to learn about urinary diversion and to become familiar with various stomal appliances. Most patients are understandably anxious about having a stoma, and discussion with a trained enterostomal therapist preoperatively and perhaps meeting with other ostomy patients greatly reduces psychological stress before surgery. An optimal stomal site is selected by examining the patient in various positions (sitting, reclining, and standing). This ensures that placement will be away from any sites that might affect proper seating of the urinary appliance, such as bony prominences, skin creases, scars, and clothing. The proper site is marked indelibly so that during preoperative skin preparation the marking will not wash away. This is helpful even in patients in whom urinary tract reconstruction without a stoma is planned because operative findings may make a stoma necessary. However, the majority of patients today should have a continent urinary diversion.

The day prior to surgery patients are started on a low residue diet and instructed to drink 3–4 liters of Go-Lytely. One gram of a second-generation cephalosporin is given intravenously on call to the operating room and every 8 hours for the next 24 hours. Thromboembolism-deterrent (TED) hose compression stockings are placed prior to induction of anesthesia, and subcutaneous heparin is administered for deep vein thrombosis prophylaxis.

# SURGICAL TECHNIQUE

## POSITION

Patients are positioned supine with the umbilicus positioned over the break of the table. The table is tilted into slight Trendelenburg position.

## INCISION AND EXPOSURE

A 22 Fr. catheter with a 30 cc balloon is passed into the bladder and the balloon is inflated with 40–50 cc of saline.

A midline abdominal incision is made from the symphysis pubis to just below the umbilicus. The anterior rectus fascia is incised, and the rectus muscles parted bluntly in the midline, exposing the transversalis fascia, which is incised from the symphysis pubis up to the semilunar line of Douglas. It is important to incise the transversalis fascia before developing the space of Retzius to avoid injuring the inferior epigastric vessels.

The space of Retzius is then developed and the peritoneum is mobilized on either side of the bladder by blunt finger dissection. Careful cranial mobilization of the peritoneum along the pelvic sidewall exposes the iliac vessels and vas deferens. The vas deferens is used as a tractor on each side to complete the mobilization of the peritoneum above the bifurcation of the common iliac vessels and to develop a pocket in the retro-peritoneum over the psoas muscle just medial to the spermatic vessels. The vas deferens is divided, the ureter is identified, and a vessel loop is placed around the ureter. This is performed bilaterally, typically by opening the peritoneum and dividing the urachus as well as the lateral peritoneal 'wings' of the bladder. The peritoneal

incision is then extended downward obliquely on each side towards the internal inguinal ring. This dissection is facilitated by having first mobilized the peritoneum from the pelvis on each side as previously described, enabling the surgeon to place one hand in the pelvis behind the mobilized peritoneum to provide traction and exposure while the peritoneal incision is extended from above. Care should be taken not to incise the peritoneum too close to the bladder; by incising the peritoneum directly against the surgeon's hand, inadvertent injury to the bladder is avoided. A self-retaining retractor is positioned in the abdomen and the intestines are packed out of the pelvis.

## PELVIC LYMPHADENECTOMY

Pelvic lymphadenectomy is performed, removing all fibroareolar tissue along the external iliac vessels and obturator fossa bilaterally. The limits of this dissection are:

- lateral—genitofemoral nerve;
- medial—bladder;
- cephalad—bifurcation of common iliac artery;
- caudad—circumflex iliac vein.

The lymph node dissection is begun by opening the fibroareolar tissue sheath surrounding the external iliac artery from the femoral canal up to and above the common iliac bifurcation. After all nodal tissue is circumferentially swept off the external iliac artery, the sheath overlying the external iliac vein is incised. This dissection is often aided by the use of a large vein retractor to elevate the external iliac artery and vein. In dissecting the distal portion of the external iliac vein, care should be taken not to injure the accessory obturator vein which exists in about 25% of patients; it courses from the distal external iliac vein into the obturator canal. The lymphatic channels at the distal extent of the dissection are secured with large hemoclips, particularly those draining into the node of Cloquet, and then divided.

The lateral extent of dissection is performed by blunt finger dissection along the psoas muscle, carefully lifting the nodal package medially off the genitofemoral nerve, thus allowing the package to drop behind the iliac vessels. Lifting the package medially allows the fibroareolar tissue to be bluntly freed off the pelvic sidewall into the obturator fossa. Frequently, small perforator vessels can be coagulated and divided to prevent subsequent inadvertent tearing and bleeding.

The proximal portion of the lymph node dissection is completed by gently lifting the package with caudal traction and teasing out the lymphatic channels which are fulgurated and divided. Great care must be utilized at the proximal extent of the dissection to prevent accidental transection of the obturator nerve. The nodal package is fractured off of the obturator nerve and attachments to the bladder. Typically the entire nodal package can be removed in toto.

Bleeding is usually minimal during this dissection, and small vessels are usually easily controlled with fulguration. Occasionally, the hypogastric vein may be injured as the lymph node package is being removed, and bleeding can be quite profuse and difficult to control. In this situation, it is best to simply place a small sponge over the vein and leave it for 10–15 minutes. The bleeding will almost always tamponade spontaneously, and attempts at suture ligation or fulguration are more likely to worsen bleeding than control it.

## OPENING AND PACKING OF THE ABDOMEN

Once the peritoneal incisions have been carried to the level of the hypogastric arteries, they are extended cephalad about 10 cm along the colic gutters bilaterally. Attachments of the sigmoid colon to the peritoneum are dissected sharply to facilitate mobilization of the colon.

One of the most critical steps in radical cystoprostatectomy is proper packing of the intestines out of the operative field. This must be done precisely and requires practice. Three moistened Mikulicz pads and a rolled moist towel are used to pack the small bowel and right colon into the epigastrium. An opened moist lap pad is packed cephalad into each colic gutter and a third lap pad is used to pack the central small bowel. A rolled moist towel is then placed horizontally over the lower edge of the Mikulicz pads with the open edges placed cephalad into each pericolic gutter.

## TRANSECTION OF URETERS AND DIVISION OF PROXIMAL VESICAL PEDICLES

Once pelvic lymphadenectomy is completed, the ureters are identified bilaterally as they cross the external iliac arteries. The ureters are encircled with vessel loops and dissected distally under mild traction. If a continent urinary reconstruction which requires greater ureteral length is planned, it may be necessary to dissect the ureters, particularly the left, almost to the level of the bladder.

Precise identification, ligation, and division of the vascular pedicles to the bladder are facilitated by understanding that the pedicles to the bladder cross anterolateral to the ureter. Dissecting over the ureters prior to ureteral transection allows the individual vesical vascular pedicles to be identified and ligated close to the hypogastric vessels. This avoids mass ligation of the pedicles that frequently results in avulsion and considerable bleeding. The ureters should be traced almost to the ureterovesical junction before transection, allowing division of the obliterated umbilical, superior, and middle vesical pedicles.

After the vascular pedicles have been divided and the ureters mobilized distally, the ureters are dissected proximally for an appropriate distance to allow subsequent anastomosis to the intestinal reservoir. On the left side, it may be necessary to carry this dissection almost to the lower pole of the kidney, particularly in obese patients. However, additional mobilization risks devascularization of the ureter. Once the ureters have been mobilized both caudad and cephalad, a right-angled clamp is placed distally on each ureter, and they are divided. Frozen sections are obtained of the distal margins to ensure there is no dysplasia or carcinoma. If there is, the ureters must be sectioned higher until normal margins are obtained. The distal ureteral stumps are ligated with a 2-0 silk suture.

## MOBILIZATION OF THE BLADDER FROM THE RECTUM

The peritoneum overlying the dome of the bladder is incised transversely about 2 cm above the rectum. It is important to incise the peritoneum since this will allow the plane between the bladder and rectum to be developed properly; however, care should be taken not to incise too deeply as this may cause inadvertent injury to the bladder. Once the peritoneum has been incised, a plane behind the bladder is developed, initially by sharp dissection; the dissection is then continued bluntly. The surgeon places one hand behind the bladder palm up and sweeps the fingers backward to dissect the rectum from the bladder. Usually this plane develops quite easily unless the patient has had previous radiotherapy or surgery. It is important to continue the sharp dissection until the seminal vesicles have been exposed. The seminal vesicles can be visualized by elevating the posterior wall of the bladder with a Deaver retractor (Figure 46.2).

Once the seminal vesicles have been identified, the remaining vascular pedicles to the bladder are ligated and divided immediately lateral to the seminal vesicle on each side. Visualization of the seminal vesicles allows these pedicles to be transected anterior to the neurovascular bundle but posterior to the bladder. However, in cases where there is induration or the possibility of extravesical disease, one must widely excise the lateral tissue and neurovascular bundle.

In dividing the vascular pedicles to the bladder, there may be significant venous bleeding that is difficult to control with suture ligation. In such cases, it may be helpful to open the endopelvic fascia bilaterally, transect the puboprostatic ligaments, and ligate the deep dorsal vein of the penis.

## DIVISION OF PUBOPROSTATIC LIGAMENTS AND CONTROL OF DORSAL VEIN

The dissection from above is continued until the pedicles adjacent to the seminal vesicles have been ligated and divided. At this point, the inferior vesical

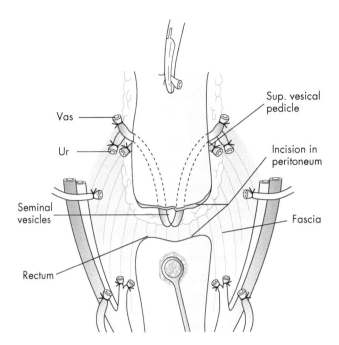

**Fig. 46.2**
Peritoneal reflection in rectovesical cul-de-sac has been incised and bladder is elevated from rectum. Tips of seminal vesicles are seen. Adapted from Schlegel PN, Walsh PC. Neuro-anatomical approach to radical cystoprostatectomy with preservation of sexual function. J Urol 1987;138:1402–1406.

pedicles are the only remaining vessels to the bladder as in a nerve-sparing radical prostatectomy. However, in some patients, visualization of the seminal vesicles may be difficult and in those cases the dissection should cease and begin anteriorly.

The catheter balloon is positioned under the malleable blade and drawn cephalad to expose the prostate, taking care not to tear the bladder. The fat overlying the prostate is dissected away using a forceps. This dissection should start on the anterolateral surface of the prostate, avoiding dissecting in the midline which may injure the superficial branch of the deep dorsal vein of the penis. It is important, however, to remove as much fat as possible in order to properly expose the puboprostatic ligaments.

The endopelvic fascia is then wiped with a moist sponge stick on each side lateral to the prostate. This exposes the fascia, and frequently a small ovale in the fascia will be seen just lateral to the deep dorsal vein of the penis. Using this opening, the endopelvic fascia is incised sharply about 1 cm lateral to the prostate. Care should be taken to incise only the fascia and to incise lateral to the prostate to avoid injuring the lateral branches of the dorsal vein complex. The incision is begun sharply and then extended both anteriorly and posteriorly using the index finger. A sponge stick is then used to displace the prostate posteriorly.

If the entire fat lateral to the dorsal vein has been dissected away and the endopelvic fascia has been

opened completely, the puboprostatic ligaments will be visualized easily. These ligaments are avascular, but the dorsal vein runs immediately between them, and frequently in continuity. Therefore, before transecting these ligaments, it is important to develop the plane both laterally and medially to the ligaments using sharp dissection. This must be done carefully but completely in order to avoid injuring the dorsal vein when the ligaments are transected. The ligaments should be transected close to the prostate before attempting to ligate the dorsal vein complex.

The dorsal vein is suture ligated distally and proximally. The dorsal vein is transected sharply. Additional bleeders may be suture ligated with a circle-tapered UR needle, using a sponge stick to displace the prostate posteriorly. The dorsal vein must be controlled completely in order to visualize and preserve the neurovascular bundles for potency.

## MOBILIZATION OF THE PROSTATE

The final phase of nerve-sparing cystoprostatectomy is dissection of the prostate and ligation and division of the inferior vesical pedicles. Dissection of the prostate is done as in a nerve-sparing radical prostatectomy. Following division of the dorsal vein, the urethra is dissected just distal to the prostate. Care should be taken not to injure the neurovascular bundles which lie immediately lateral to the urethra at this point. An umbilical tape then is passed around the urethra and gentle traction is exerted cephalad. Using a Kitner dissector, the urethra is dissected from the urogenital diaphragm, removing only urethral mucosa and smooth muscle, leaving the striated muscle of the urogenital diaphragm behind. This dissection continues until the membranous urethra has been liberated completely from the urogenital diaphragm. Even in patients in whom nerve sparing is not a consideration, pelvic dissection of the membranous urethra greatly facilitates the perineal dissection if a urethrectomy is subsequently required. The anterior urethra is then gently pulled out of the urogenital diaphragm and transected distal to the urogenital diaphragm. The catheter is transected, the posterior wall of the urethra divided, and the catheter drawn cephalad into the wound.

In patients in whom an orthotopic continent diversion is planned, the urethra must be handled similar to a nerve-sparing radical prostatectomy. In brief, the anterior wall of the urethra is transected just distal to the prostate until the Foley catheter comes into view. A right-angled clamp pulls the catheter into the pelvis and the catheter is transected. With use of a right-angled clamp, the space between the rectum, striated urethral sphincter, rectourethralis muscle, and posterior wall of the urethra is developed. The neurovascular bundles are posterolateral at this point. The tissue on top of the clamp is then transected sharply to free the prostate from the rectum. This is a critical step in all nerve-sparing radical pelvic operations, and must be done carefully and precisely to avoid injuring the underlying neurovascular bundles which lie immediately posterolateral to the rectourethralis. Elevating the rectourethralis muscle before incising it allows preservation of the underlying neurovascular bundles and avoids injuring the rectum.

The lateral pelvic fascia on each side of the prostate is then incised; this allows the neurovascular bundles to drop posteriorly. The small vascular branches to the apex of the prostate are then gently mobilized with a fine right-angled clamp, secured proximally with small metal clips, and divided. Following division of the apical vascular branches, the neurovascular bundles fall laterally, allowing the larger lateral pedicles to be ligated and divided (Figure 46.3). When the prostate has been mobilized cranially to the level of the seminal vesicles, Denonvilliers' fascia overlying the seminal vesicles is incised transversely. Once the seminal vesicles have been exposed from below, a plane of communication between the cranial and caudal dissection is formed, allowing the remaining vascular pedicles to the prostate and bladder to be divided immediately lateral to the seminal vesicles. The bladder, prostate, and seminal vesicles are removed en bloc, and the intact neurovascular bundles can be visualized in the pelvis. Urinary tract reconstruction is then performed.

## WIDE EXCISION OF THE NEUROVASCULAR BUNDLE

The primary goal of radical cystoprostatectomy must be eradication of cancer. Whenever the tumor encroaches upon the posterior pedicle, the neurovascular bundle should be widely excised to ensure adequate surgical margins. The anatomic radical cystoprostatectomy allows mobilization of the neurovascular bundles off the rectum, permitting wider surgical margins that incorporate all perivesical tissues lateral to the hypogastric vessels. Thus, improved surgical margins can be achieved while still preserving potency in the majority of patients, even when only a single neurovascular bundle is preserved.

## POSTOPERATIVE CARE

TED hose compression stockings remain on for at least 48 hours and subcutaneous heparin is administered until the patient is ready for discharge. Ambulation is begun the day following surgery. Intravenous antibiotics are administered for 24 hours postoperatively; usually, a second-generation cephalosporin is given. Ureteral stents are left in place for 7–10 days to allow healing of the ureterointestinal anastomoses. Drains are left in the pelvis until the ureteral stents have been removed. Patients are usually discharged between the sixth and eighth postoperative day.

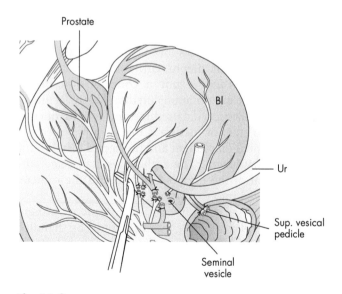

**Fig 46.3**
Schematic illustration of division of left posterior pedicle along lateral edge of left seminal vesicle. Note that cavernous nerves are preserved posteriorly. Adapted from Schlegel PN, Walsh PC. Neuroanatomical approach to radical cystoprostatectomy with preservation of sexual function. J Urol 1987;138:1402–1406.

### REFERENCES

1.  Stein JP, Lieskovsky G, Cote R, et al. Radical cystectomy in the treatment of invasive bladder cancer: long-term results in 1,054 patients. J Clin Oncol 2001;19(3):666–675.

2.  Jimenez VK, Marshall FF. Surgery of bladder cancer. In Walsh PC et al (eds): Campbell's Urology, 8th ed. Philadelphia: WB Saunders, 2002, pp 2819–2844.

3.  Young HH, Davis DM. Young's Practice of Urology, vol 12. Philadelphia: WB Saunders, 1926.

4.  Hinman F. The technique and late results of ureterointestinal implantation and cystectomy for cancer of the bladder. Int Soc Urol Rep 1939;7:464–524.

5.  Bracken RB, McDonald MW, Johnson DE. Complications of single stage radical cystectomy and ileal conduit. Urology 1981;27:141–146.

6.  Hendry WF. Morbidity and mortality of radical cystectomy (1971–1978 and 1978–1985). J Roy Soc Med 1981;79:395–400.

7.  Skinner DG, Lieskovsky G (eds). Management of invasive and high grade bladder cancer. In Diagnosis and Management of Genitourinary Cancer. Philadelphia: WB Saunders, 1988, pp 295–312.

8.  Quek ML, Stein JP, Clark PE, et al. Natural history of surgically treated bladder carcinoma with extravesical tumor extension. Cancer 2003;98(5):955–961.

9.  Skinner DG, Stein JP, Lieskovsky G, et al. 25-year experience in the management of invasive bladder cancer by radical cystectomy. Eur Urol 1998;33(Suppl 4):25–26.

10. Stein JP, Ginsberg DA, Skinner DG. Indications and technique of the orthotopic neobladder in women. Urol Clin North Am 2002;29:725–734.

11. Walsh PC, Donker PJ. Impotence following radical prostatectomy: insight into etiology and prevention. J Urol 1982;128:492.

12. Lepor H, Gregerman M, Crosby R, Mostofi FK, Walsh PC. Precise localization of the autonomic nerves from the pelvic plexus to the corpora cavernosa: a detailed anatomical study of the adult male pelvis. J Urol 1985;133:207–212.

13. Schlegel PN, Walsh PC. Neuroanatomical approach to radical cystoprostatectomy with preservation of sexual function. J Urol 1987;138:1402–1406.

14. Pritchett TR, Schiff WM, Klatt E, Lieskovsky G, Skinner DG. The potency-sparing radical cystectomy: does it compromise the completeness of the cancer resection? J Urol 1988;140: 1400–1403.

15. Brendler CB, Steinberg GD, Marshall FF, Mostwin JL, Walsh PC. Local recurrence and survival following nerve-sparing radical cystoprostatectomy. J Urol 1990;144:1137–1141.

16. Schoenberg MP, Walsh PC, Breazeale DR, Marshall FF, Mostwin JL, Brendler CB. Local recurrence and survival following nerve sparing radical cystoprostatectomy for bladder cancer: 10-year followup. J Urol 1996;155:490–494.

17. Marshall FF, Mostwin JL, Radebaugh LC, Walsh PC, Brendler CB. Ileocolic neobladder post-cystectomy: continence and potency. J Urol 1991;145:502–504.

18. Hart S, Skinner EC, Meyerowitz BE, Boyd S, Lieskovsky G, Skinner DG. Quality of life after radical cystectomy for bladder cancer in patients with an ileal conduit, or cutaneous or urethral Koch pouch. J Urol 1999;162:77–81.

19. Henningsohn L, Steven K, Kallestrup EB, Steineck G. Distressful symptoms and well-being after radical cystectomy and orthotopic bladder substitution compared with a matched control population. J Urol 2002;168:168–175.

# Laparoscopic radical cystectomy and urinary diversion

# 47

*Inderbir S Gill, Ingolf Tuerk*

## INTRODUCTION

Ongoing technical and technologic developments have refined various laparoscopic procedures such that they have become viable alternatives to their conventional open surgical counterparts. With the worldwide acceptance of laparoscopic techniques, initially in the management of upper urinary tract pathology, and more recently for laparoscopic radical prostatectomy, a natural progression has been made to applying these techniques to bladder surgery. In the United States in 2004, bladder cancer was diagnosed in 44,640 men and 15,600 women, leading to 8780 and 3930 deaths, respectively.[1] Radical cystectomy is currently the accepted standard of treatment for patients with localized muscle invasive bladder cancer. Since the initial report of laparoscopic radical cystectomy (LRC) with bilateral pelvic lymphadenectomy/ileal conduit urinary diversion performed entirely intracorporeally by Gill and colleagues[2] in 2000, more than 225 cases from over 20 institutions worldwide have been reported[3] (Table 47.1).[2,4-20] In this chapter, we review the current worldwide experience with LRC and urinary diversion, focusing on historical background, laboratory experience, surgical technique, current controversies and future directions.

## HISTORICAL BACKGROUND

In early 1992, Parra et al described the initial report of laparoscopic simple cystectomy in a female patient suffering from pyocystis of a retained bladder.[21] This patient had previously undergone open surgical supravesical diversion for management of neurogenic bladder; accordingly, urinary diversion was not performed as part of the laparoscopic procedure. In 1995, Sanchez et al described the first report of laparoscopic-assisted radical cystectomy with an ileal conduit formed extracorporeally in a 64-year-old woman with invasive bladder cancer.[22] Puppo et al reported the first small series of laparoscopic-assisted transvaginal radical cystectomies in five females, wherein the ileal conduit was created via a mini-laparotomy incision after completion of the LRC.[23] In another publication, the same group reported cutaneous ureterostomies in nine patients with advanced pelvic cancer.[24]

While these early studies established the technical feasibility of LRC, it was not until 2000 that LRC and ileal conduit were performed completely intracorporeally in the initial two clinical cases after successful pilot studies in animals had been performed at the Cleveland Clinic.[2] To date, the ileal conduit, the orthotopic ileal neobladder (Studer), and the sigmoid–rectum pouch (Mainz II) have all been created purely laparoscopically with exclusively intracorporeal suturing techniques.[4,8]

## EXPERIMENTAL LAPAROSCOPIC URINARY DIVERSION IN ANIMAL MODELS

Experimental studies of urinary diversion have formed the basis for the subsequent clinical experience. Anderson et al investigated the feasibility of laparoscopic-assisted Mainz II (sigmoid–rectum) pouch in nine mini pigs.[25] The cystectomy and dissection of ureter and large bowel were performed laparoscopically, and the Mainz II pouch was created extracorporeally by

**Table 47.1** World experience with laparoscopic radical cystectomy (LC) and urinary diversion

| Technique | Lead author | Institution/location | No. pts | Comment on abstract/manuscript or technique |
|---|---|---|---|---|
| Purely laparoscopic | Gill IS[2,4-7] | Cleveland, USA | 30 | Purely laparoscopic reconstruction of the urinary diversion |
|  | Tuerk, I[8,9] | Massachusetts, USA and Berlin, Germany | 15 | Mainz II continent sigmoid–rectum pouch |
| Laparoscopic assisted | Van Velthoven R[5] | Brussels, Belgium | 22 | Extracorporeal reconstruction, variety of diversions |
|  | Basillote JB[10] | Irvine, USA | 13 | Comparison between LC and open radical cystectomy, extracorporeal reconstruction |
|  | Hemal AK[11] | New Delhi, India | 11 | Emphasis on complications of the initial experience with LC, extracorporeal ileal conduit |
|  | Simonato A[12] | Milan, Italy | 10 | Detailed steps of LC with illustrations. A variety of diversions including intracorporeal and extracorporeal reconstruction |
|  | Denewer A[13] | Mnsoura, Egypt | 10 | Salvage cystectomy after radical radiotherapy. A modified ureterosigmoidostomy diversion through a mini-laparotomy (8 cm) |
|  | Abdel-Hakim AM[14] | Cairo, Egypt | 9 | Extracorporeal reconstruction of ileal neobladder |
|  | Castillo O[5] | Santiago, Chile | 7 | Extracorporeal reconstruction, Studer neobladder |
|  | Paz A[5] | Ashkelon, Israel | 7 | Comparison between LC and open radical cystectomy, extracorporeal reconstruction |
|  | Popken G[5] | Berlin, Germany | 7 | Extra/intracorporeal reconstruction with a variety of diversions |
|  | Puppo P[7] | Pietra Ligure, Italy | 5 | First transvaginal and laparoscopic approach for bladder cancer. Ileal conduit was accomplished through a mini-laparotomy at the stoma site |
|  | Xiao LC[5] | Guangzhou, China | 5 | Extracorporeal reconstruction, Indiana pouch |
|  | Huan SK[5] | Chi Mei, Taiwan | 4 | Extracorporeal reconstruction, Indiana pouch |
|  | Sung GT[5] | Pusan, Korea | 4 | Extracorporeal ileal conduit |
|  | Guazzoni G[15] | Milan, Italy | 3 | Nerve sparing LC with extracorporeal W-shaped neobladder |
|  | Pedraza R[5] | New York, USA | 2 | Patients underwent LC with total ureterectomy and creation of pyelocutaneous ileal conduit intracorporeally |
| Hand assisted | McGinnis DE[16] | Bryn Mawr, USA | 7 | Hand-assisted LC with extracorporeal ileal conduit |
|  | Fan EW[5] | Chi Mei, Taiwan | 6 | Hand-assisted laparoscopic bilateral nephroureterectomy with radical cystectomy (end stage renal disease) |
|  | Peterson AC[17] | Tacoma, USA | 1 | First reported case of hand-assisted LC with extracorporeal ileal conduit |
| Robotic assisted | Menon M[18] | Detroit, USA | 14 | Nerve-sparing robotic-assisted LC |
|  | Balaji KC[19] | Omaha, USA | 3 | LC with robotic assistance for intracorporeal suturing of the ureter–ileal conduit anastomosis (two patients with interstitial cystitis) |
|  | Beecken WD[20] | Frankfurt, Germany | 1 | First reported case of robotic-assisted LC with intracorporeal orthotopic neobladder |
| Other | Goharderakhshan R[7] | Harbor City, USA | 25 | Series focusing on complications associated with LC. Reconstructive technique not detailed |
|  | Vallancien G[7] | Paris, France | 20 | Prostate-sparing cystectomy. Reconstructive technique not detailed |

Adapted from Moinzadeh & Gill.[3]

open techniques. Forty-four percent of animals developed stones across metallic staple lines used to create the Mainz II pouch.

The major technical difficulty encountered in performing a laparoscopic urinary diversion remains the performance of intracorporeal reconstruction. Reconstructive techniques have been performed by three different approaches: performing the entire procedure intracorporeally, performing extracorporeal suturing and returning the diversion into the abdomen for intracorporeal completion, or performing urinary diversion through a mini-laparotomy. Investigators at the Cleveland Clinic were the first to demonstrate the feasibility of creating urinary diversion following cystectomy with ileal loop (in 10 surviving pigs) and orthotopic ileal neobladder (Studer) (in 12 surviving pigs) using completely intracorporeal laparoscopic techniques.[26,27] These laparoscopic procedures duplicated principles of open surgery and demonstrated that reconstruction of bowel could be performed with purely intracorporeal freehand suturing techniques without complications such as ileoureteral or ileourethral anastomotic strictures or leakage.

## INDICATIONS AND CONTRAINDICATIONS

Proper patient choice/identification is crucial during the early learning experience for any emerging technique. Currently, we offer LRC to patients with organ-confined, non-bulky bladder malignancy as determined by preoperative radiographic and clinical findings. We have no experience with LRC in the presence of prior radiotherapy and neoadjuvant chemotherapy, or morbidly obese patients. These factors currently constitute relative contraindications because of the potential increase in technical challenge. In relatively obese patients, difficulty may be expected in delivering a loop of ileum through an obese abdominal wall to the skin level. Prior abdominal surgery per se is no longer considered as an absolute contraindication to laparoscopic surgery. Attention must be paid to avoid intra-abdominal injury upon insertion of the initial access port at the beginning of the procedure.

## SURGICAL TECHNIQUES

### LAPAROSCOPIC RADICAL CYSTECTOMY

Surgical technical steps of LRC aim to mirror established open surgical techniques. Typically a five- or six-port transperitoneal technique is employed similar to that for a standard laparoscopic prostatectomy. The retrovesical dissection is performed initially. In the male, a transverse periotomy is created in the rectovesical cul-de-sac, and the vas deferens is divided bilaterally. Dissection is performed towards Denonvilliers' fascia, which is incised horizontally to provide visualization of the yellowish prerectal fat, signifying proper entry into the plane between the rectum posteriorly and the prostate and bladder anteriorly. Unlike the procedure in a laparoscopic radical prostatectomy, the seminal vesicles and vas deferens are not mobilized individually but maintained en bloc with the bladder specimen. The lateral and posterior vascular pedicles of the bladder and prostate are developed with blunt dissection and controlled bilaterally with sequential firings of the endoscopic GIA stapler. Both ureters are clipped and divided close to the bladder, and the distal ureteral margin is sent for frozen section evaluation. The proximal cut end of each ureter is temporarily clip-occluded to facilitate hydrostatic distension.

An inverted V-shaped peritoneotomy is created, starting lateral to the right medial umbilical ligament, proceeding up towards the umbilicus where the urachus is incised, and extending lateral to the left medial umbilical ligament. In this manner, the urachus is divided high, near the umbilicus. The anterior surface of the bladder is mobilized with the entire perivesical fat being maintained with the bladder specimen. The endopelvic fascia is incised bilaterally and the dorsal vein secured with a stitch, similar to that used in a laparoscopic radical prostatectomy. In the male patient the puboprostatic ligaments and the prostatourethral junction are divided sharply, maintaining an adequate stump of sphincter-active urethra. The few remaining prostate attachments are divided, and the specimen immediately entrapped in an Endocatch-II bag. Frozen section biopsy of the cut end of the urethral stump is confirmed to be negative for cancer.

In the female, a sponge stick in the vagina or Koh colpotomiser system allows the vaginal apex to be identified and incised. After complete dissection of the bladder and surrounding structures (uterus/fallopian tube/ovary), the specimen is placed in an impervious, plastic-enclosed bag and retrieved through either the vagina, the rectum, or a midline 5 cm incision. Frozen section of distal ureteral margin and the cut end of the urethral stump are confirmed to be negative for malignancy.

### EXTENDED PELVIC LYMPH NODE DISSECTION (PLND)

Given the absence of pelvic lymphadenopathy on preoperative computed tomography, which is further corroborated by intraoperative laparoscopic inspection, cystectomy is performed initially, followed by PLND. Right lymphadenectomy is carried out first. The patient is tilted 30° up on the right side in the 30° Trendelenburg head-down position. The lateral border of dissection is developed along the genitofemoral nerve by dividing the fibroareolar tissue and exposing the iliopsoas muscle. The lymphatic tissue packet is completely lifted en bloc off of the surface of the iliopsoas muscle and swept medially. Tissue anterior to the external iliac artery and vein is then individually split longitudinally using J-hook electrocautery, skeletonizing the two vessels circumferentially. It should be noted that the external iliac vein typically appears as a flat ribbon at standard (15 mmHg) pneumo-peritoneum pressures. To facilitate identification of the external iliac vein in case of doubt, pneumoperitoneum pressures can be decreased to 5 mmHg to allow redistension of the vein.[6]

Cephalad dissection along the proximal common iliac artery is facilitated by the fact that the transected ureter has already been mobilized away during the cystectomy procedure. The circumferentially mobilized common iliac is retracted with a vessel loop to completely retrieve fatty tissue in the area distal to the aortic bifurcation. The hypogastric artery is mobilized with care taken not to injure the internal iliac vein. The released packet is rolled medially, posterior to the mobilized external iliac artery and vein, and delivered into the pelvis. Dissection along the medial aspect of the packet identifies the obturator nerve. Distally the lymphatics caudal to the node of Cloquet are clipped and transected. To guard against local seeding, care must be taken to avoid cutting into any enlarged lymph node(s). The entire specimen is immediately placed in an Endocatch bag without the specimen touching adjacent tissues. Lymphadenectomy is performed on the left side in similar fashion with the patient tilted 30° up on that side. Bilateral lymphadenectomy specimens are entrapped separately, extracted intact, and submitted separately for analysis.

## LAPAROSCOPIC-ASSISTED ILEAL CONDUIT URINARY DIVERSION

Informed consent is obtained with a discussion of risks including, but not limited to, adjacent organ and bowel injury, and open conversion. Full mechanical bowel preparation with 4 liters of polyethylene glycol is performed, oral antibiotics are administered, and the patient is admitted on the morning of surgery. Preoperative antibiotic prophylaxis with a second-generation cephalosporin and lower extremity compressive devices are routine. Once general anesthesia is induced, a nasogastric tube is inserted, the abdomen and genitalia are properly draped, and a 16 Fr. Foley catheter is placed from the sterile field.

Pneumoperitoneum is obtained and a five-port transperitoneal technique is employed: a primary 10 mm trocar at the umbilicus, two 10 mm trocars at each lateral pararectal line 10 cm above the pubic symphysis, and two 5 mm trocars 2–3 cm medial and superior to the anterior–superior iliac spines.

Both ureters are dissected proximally, clipped, and transected close to the ureterovesical junction. The cut ends are sent for frozen section analysis. Two 4-0 vicryl holding sutures are placed at the distal ends of the ureters for subsequent identification and atraumatic manipulation. The vascular pedicles of the bladder and prostate are controlled with serial applications of an articulating endoscopic GIA laparoscopic stapler. The urethra is sectioned at the prostate apex, completing the bladder excision. The bladder is placed into a laparoscopic retrieval bag, which in female patients can be retrieved through an opening in the anterior vaginal wall. In males, the specimen bag is retrieved at the end of the operation by extending one of the port sites.

The ureters are dissected for a distance sufficient to reach the proximal end of the loop. Care is taken to preserve periureteral tissue and thus the ureteral vascular supply. Blunt dissection is used to develop a tunnel posterior to the sigmoid mesocolon and anterior to the sacrum. The left ureter is passed under the sigmoid colon using the previously placed holding suture. Ureteral length is once again confirmed to assure that both ureters reach the proximal portion of the ileal segment in order to avoid undue tension on the anastomoses. A previously marked stoma site away from desired trocar sites should not compromise optimal port placement. When the stoma site is separate from all trocars, a 4.5 cm infraumbilical incision is made. The specimen is retrieved. The color-coded ureteral holding sutures are exteriorized. A 15 cm segment of ileum is selected with care to spare 15–20 cm proximal to the ileocecal junction. The segment of bowel is delivered through the incision and isolated with a GIA stapler. The mesentery is appropriately divided with care to preserve the major mesenteric vasculature. The isolated segment is dropped posteriorly.

Applications of a GIA 55 mm stapler are used to create a side-to-side, functional, end-to-end ileoileal anastomosis along the antimesenteric border of the small bowel. The open end of the anastomosis is then closed using a Ta 55 mm stapler. The end staple line is imbricated with interrupted, absorbable suture. The window through the mesentery is then closed with interrupted absorbable suture to prevent internal hernia formation.

Gentle traction on the ureteral holding sutures pulls the distal ureters into the operative field. The ureters are gently spatulated for approximately 1 cm. Bilateral ureteral 6 Fr. single J stents are passed into the renal pelvis. The ureters are sequentially implanted into the proximal end of the ileal segment in a standard Bricker fashion. The proximal end of the ileal conduit is replaced into the abdominal cavity. The ureteral stents are exteriorized through the ileal segment.

The rectus fascia is partially closed, leaving space through which the conduit passes. The ileal segment is secured to the fascia using interrupted 2-0 polyglactin sutures. The stoma is matured in the standard open fashion. In the obese patient, ureteroileal anastomoses performed through an incision may require excessive proximal ureteral mobilization. In these cases, the stoma is matured first, and the ureteroileal anastomoses are performed completely intracorporeally.

Postoperative management is as with the comparable open procedure. Patients receive prophylaxis for deep venous thrombosis, and ambulation is begun on the first postoperative day. The nasogastric tube is removed once bowel function returns, and the diet is advanced accordingly. The drain is removed once output diminishes. The stents are removed between postoperative days 10 and 12 as outpatient procedure.

## PURE LAPAROSCOPIC ILEAL CONDUIT URINARY DIVERSION

A 15 cm segment of ileum is selected while sparing the distal 15–20 cm of ileum. The efferent limb should reach the abdominal wall at the previously marked stoma site without undue tension or mesenteric kinking. The segment of bowel is isolated with an endoscopic GIA stapler by transecting proximally and distally. The mesentery is divided below these areas with care to preserve the major mesenteric vasculature. Endoscopic staplers, the harmonic scalpel, or serial application of laparoscopic clips can be used to transect the mesentery with complete hemostasis. The isolated segment is dropped posteriorly.

The stapled edges of the distal and proximal ileum are removed sharply. Applications of an endoscopic GIA stapler are used to create a side-to-side, functional, end-to-end anastomosis along the antimesenteric border of the small bowel. The open end of the anastomosis is then closed using an endoscopic Ta stapler. The end staple line is imbricated intracorporeally with interrupted, absorbable suture. The window through the mesentery is then closed with interrupted absorbable suture to prevent internal hernia formation.

The previously marked stoma site is matured in the standard everting fashion. The ileal segment is secured to the fascia using interrupted 2-0 polyglactin sutures. A previously marked stoma site away from desired trocar sites should not compromise optimal port placement.

Creating the stoma first greatly facilitates intracorporeal suturing of the ureteroileal anastomosis by providing a point of fixation for the ileal segment. Gentle traction on the ureteral holding sutures pulls the distal ureters to the proximal end of the ileal segment. The ureters are spatulated for approximately 1 cm. Six French single J stents are grasped by a laparoscopic right-angle clamp and inserted though the stoma into the conduit lumen. The right angle clamp tents the ileal loop at the desired ileotomy site. A laparoscopic electrosurgical J-hook is used to create the ileostomy, and the stent is delivered into the abdominal cavity. The ureters are sequentially implanted in a standard Bricker fashion. The apices are fixed to the bowel using three interrupted 4-0 poliglecaprone sutures. The remainder of the ureteral implantation is performed using a running 4-0 poliglecaprone suture. The stent is passed into the renal pelvis on each side when 80% of the anastomosis is complete.

The ureters and ileal diversion are inspected for any undue tension. The abdominal cavity is irrigated with sterile antibiotic solution. Once meticulous hemostasis is assured, a flat Jackson-Pratt drain is placed through a lateral 5 mm trocar site into the pelvis. The port sites are closed in the usual fashion with fascial closure for all sites ≥10 mm under direct vision with 0 polyglactin.

Postoperative management is as with the comparable open procedure. Patients receive prophylaxis for deep venous thrombosis and ambulation is begun on the first postoperative day. The nasogastric tube is removed once bowel function returns, and the diet is advanced accordingly. The drain is removed once output diminishes. The stents are removed between postoperative days 10 and 12.

## PURE LAPAROSCOPIC ORTHOTOPIC ILEAL NEOBLADDER

Preoperative preparation and LRC are performed as previously described. The left ureter is transposed to the right side posterior to the sigmoid colon.

A 65 cm segment of ileum is selected with care to spare the distal 15–20 cm proximal to the ileocecal junction (Figure 47.1A). The mid-portion of the segment should reach the urethral stump without undue tension or mesenteric kinking. The ileum, with its mesenteric pedicle, is isolated with an endoscopic GIA stapler. Endoscopic staplers, the harmonic scalpel, or serial application of laparoscopic clips can be used to transect the mesentery with complete hemostasis. The isolated segment is dropped posteriorly. An endoscopic GIA stapler is used to create a side-to-side, functional, ileoileal anastomosis along the antimesenteric border. The open end of the anastomosis is closed using an endoscopic Ta stapler. The end staple line is imbricated intracorporeally with interrupted, absorbable suture.

The staple lines are removed and the bowel lumen is cleansed using a suction-irrigation device. Care is taken to preserve the proximal 10 cm as an afferent Studer limb for the ureteral anastomosis. The remaining 55 cm is incised along its antimesenteric side using monopolar electrocautery, endoshears, and/or harmonic scalpel. The posterior plate of the neobladder is created by suturing the medial edges of the detubularized bowel in a running fashion with 2-0 polyglactin such that the bowel forms a J-shaped configuration (Figure 47.1B).

The anterior plate of the neobladder is partially closed using another running 2-0 polyglactin suture. Before completion of the anterior wall, both ileoureteral stents are delivered into the Studer limb and retrieved into the peritoneal cavity through two separate ileotomy incisions at the proposed site of ureteroileal anastomoses. The anterior enterotomy is left open at its inferior-most portion in order to create the urethroneovesical anastomosis.

The most dependent portion of the ileal plate is delivered to the urethral stump. The anastomosis is started at the 6 o'clock position with two running 2-0 poliglecaprone sutures in a parachute fashion and extended to the 12 o'clock position on either side. The sutures are then tied to each other. Once the anastomosis is complete, a 22 Fr. Foley catheter is placed (Figure 47.2).

A                                          B

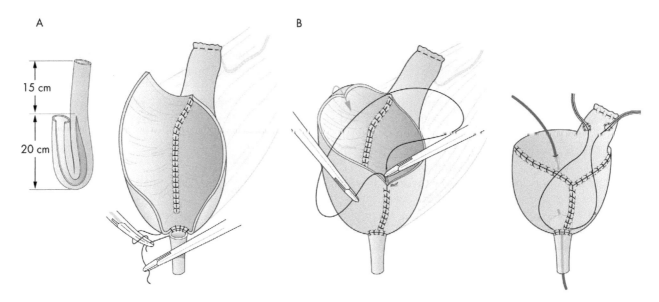

**Fig. 47.1**
**A** Completed posterior neobladder plate and suturing of urethroneovesical anastomosis. **B** Anterior suture line and completed neobladder with drains. (Adapted with permission from The Cleveland Clinic Foundation.)

The ureters are spatulated for approximately 1 cm. Bilateral ureteral 6 Fr. single J stents are passed into the renal pelvis. The stents are exteriorized through the wall of the neobladder and then through one of the lateral 5 mm port sites. The ureters are sequentially implanted into the proximal portion of the ileal segment in a standard Bricker fashion.

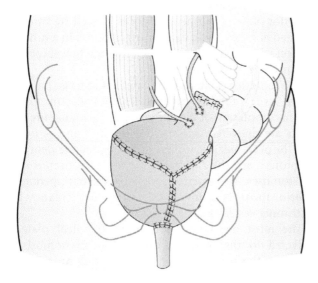

**Fig. 47.2**
Completed neobladder in the pelvis. (Adapted with permission from The Cleveland Clinic Foundation.)

The ureters and ileal neobladder are inspected in situ for any undue tension. A flat Jackson-Pratt drain is placed through a lateral 5 mm trocar site into the small pelvis. The port sites are closed in the usual fashion with fascial closure for all sites ≥10 mm under direct vision with 0 polyglactin.

Postoperative management is as with the comparable open procedure. Patients receive prophylaxis for deep venous thrombosis, and ambulation is begun on the first postoperative day. The nasogastric tube is removed once bowel function returns, and the diet is advanced accordingly. The drain is removed once output diminishes. The stents are removed between postoperative days 10 and 12. The Foley catheter is removed one day following stent removal after absence of leak is confirmed on cystogram.

## CLINICAL STUDIES OF LAPAROSCOPIC RADICAL CYSTECTOMY AND URINARY DIVERSION

Notable advantages of LRC appear to be decreased blood loss, less postoperative pain, and earlier return to activity. The decreased blood loss (approximately 300–400 cc) is likely due to clear visualization and delicate hemostatic handling of the bladder pedicles with linear stapling devices, in addition to the tamponade effects afforded by the $CO_2$ pneumoperitoneum pressure. Although total operative times in the initially published series were 7–11 hours,[2,4,8] in more recent series the operative times have been reduced to 4.3–8.3 hours.[12]

It is likely that, with further experience, operative times will continue to decrease as, in the authors' experience, the LRC part of the procedure now comprises approximately 2 hours. More recently, a retrospective study of 13 laparoscopically assisted radical cystectomies with ileal neobladder compared with the 11 procedures employing the open approach revealed no statistically significant difference in operative time.[10] It should be noted, however, that in this study, radical cystectomy was performed laparoscopically and the reconstructive portion (ileal orthotopic neobladder) was performed through a 15 cm low Pfannenstiel incision.

Although the initial clinical publications focused on laparoscopic surgical techniques, recent reports have described the use of robotic assistance,[19,20,28] as well as hand assistance.[5,16,17] The perceived advantage of these various assisted laparoscopic techniques (open, robotic, or hand) compared to pure laparoscopic technique is their decreased learning curve for surgeons when transitioning from open to laparoscopic pelvic urologic surgery.[18,29] Surgical robotic systems provide multiangled movement with endo-wrist instruments and three-dimensional stereoscopic visualization. Recently, Balaji et al reported on the feasibility of robot-assisted totally intracorporeal laparoscopic ileal conduit in three patients, although each case took more than 10 hours.[19] The benefits of robotic applications in large series of patients remain unknown.

Seminal and prostate-sparing cystectomy may represent an alternative in young patients in whom preservation of both sexual potency and urinary continence are important.[15] However, from an oncologic point of view, long-term outcomes are the key to confirming whether this surgery can be proposed as a valid option for treatment of young, fully potent, and socially active patients with organ-confined bladder malignancy.

# ONCOLOGIC OUTCOMES

A major area of laparoscopic approach for bladder malignancy remains to prove its acceptability for long-term, disease-free survival. So far, most of the publications of LRC reported the institutions' initial experience focusing on technique and perioperative results. Recently Hrouda et al reviewed a total of nine articles on LRC with available follow-up.[30] Among the total of 102 patients described in these nine articles, there were no instances of positive margins or inadvertent incisions in the bladder. However, the small number of patients and the short duration of follow-up (maximum of 2 years) do not permit any conclusions about oncologic outcome (Table 47.2).[6,8,10-14,18,23]

Although reports of oncologic outcomes of LRC are limited, Gupta et al reported 2-year follow-up of five patients having undergone LRC with ileal loop creation with good outcomes.[31] More recently, authors from the same institution added both follow-up and complications data in their initial report of experiences with 11 patients undergoing LRC.[11] One patient had surgical margins positive for tumor and received cisplatin-based chemotherapy; he had no recurrence in their follow-up period. At a mean of 18.4 months follow-up, all patients had normal renal function and preserved upper tracts with no evidence of metastasis and no local recurrence.

Recent emphasis on extended pelvic lymphadenectomy for transitional cell carcinoma of the bladder deserves discussion. Finelli et al reported their analysis of 22 cases of laparoscopic pelvic lymphadenectomy for bladder cancer.[6] The initial 11 patients that underwent a limited dissection were compared with the subsequent 11 consecutive patients that had an extended lymphadenectomy. Bilateral extended lymphadenectomy

**Table 47.2** Oncologic outcomes

| Lead author (year) | No. pts | Technique (reconstruction) | Margins | Lymphadenectomy (n node, range) | Mean (range) months at stated follow-up | No. pts overall survival |
|---|---|---|---|---|---|---|
| Puppo (1995)[23] | 5 | Lap (extra) | Not stated | Limited (not stated) | 10.8 (6–18) | 5 |
| Denewer (1999)[13] | 10 | Lap (extra) | Not stated | Limited (not stated) | Not stated | 9 |
| Tuerk (2001)[8] | 5 | Lap (purely intra) | 5/5 negative | Limited (not stated) | Not stated | 5 |
| Abdel-Hakim (2002)[14] | 9 | Lap (extra) | 9/9 negative | Limited (n=2–4) | Not stated | 9 |
| Simonato (2003)[12] | 10 | Lap (extra) | 10/10 negative | Limited (not stated) | 12.3 (5–18) | 10 |
| Menon (2002)[18] | 17 | Robot (extra) | 17/17 negative | Limited (n=4–27) | Not stated (2–11) | 17 |
| Hemal (2004)[11] | 11 | Lap (extra) | 10/11 negative | Limited (not stated) | 18.4 (1–48) | 10 |
| Basillote (2004)[10] | 13 | Lap (extra) | 12/13 negative | Limited (not stated) | Not stated | 13 |
| Gill (2004)[6] | 22 | Lap (purely intra) | 21/22 negative | 11/22 Extended (n=21, 6–30) | 11 (2–43) | 18 |

Adapted from Hrouda et al.[30]
Extra, extracorporeal; intra, Intracorporeal; Lap, laparoscopic; Robot, robotic-assisted.

required approximately 1.5 hours compared to the 30–45 minutes required for the limited template. With a limited lymphadenectomy, the median and mean number of lymph nodes retrieved were 3 and 6 (range 1–15) versus 21 and 18 (range 6–30) for the extended template (p=0.001). The median nodal yield of the extended laparoscopic lymphadenectomy was in keeping with series of open surgical procedures recommending that at least 10–15 lymph nodes be removed.[32] No patient developed port-site or local recurrence over the short follow-up of 11 months (range 2–43 months).

## FUNCTIONAL OUTCOMES AND COMPLICATIONS

LRC is a complex procedure and requires advanced laparoscopic expertise. While increasing numbers of publications regarding LRC have demonstrated the technical feasibility of the surgery, a critical appraisal of the attendant complications is essential (Table 47.3).[6,7,10–13,18] Sharp et al[7] reported the outcomes in the Cleveland Clinic of the initial 21 cases of LRC, all with intracorporeally created urinary diversion. Six major (29%) and nine minor (45%) complications were reported. The major complications, all of which required reoperation, were small bowel obstruction (three), and one each of ureteroileal anastomotic leak, urethrovaginal fistula, and bowel perforation with delayed death. Minor complications were related mainly to prolonged ileus.

In the initial experiences since 1999 of 11 patients that underwent LRC and an open-hand sewn ileal conduit, Hemal et al reported one case with positive margin and five others (45%) with procedure-specific complications.[11] There were three intraoperative complications including injury to the external iliac vein in one patient and a small rectal tear in two, all repaired by laparoscopic free-hand suturing. Other laparoscopic-related complications were subcutaneous emphysema in one patient and hypercarbia, necessitating conversion to open surgery in another. The authors concluded that LRC is associated with complications similar to those

**Table 47.3** Complications in the papers with complication descriptions (n=10 or more)

| Lead author (year) | No. pts | No. of complications | Description of complications (→treatment and event) |
|---|---|---|---|
| Basillote (2004)[10] | 13 | 8<br>4 major (31%) | 1 ureteral obstruction (→percutaneous nephrostomy)<br>1 bladder neck contracture (→reoperation)<br>1 epididymal abscess (→orchidectomy)<br>1 wound dehiscence (→reoperation)<br>1 obturator nerve paresis (→physical therapy)<br>1 pyelonephritis (→intravenous antibiotics)<br>1 pouchitis (→intravenous antibiotics)<br>1 positive margin at prostate apex (prostate cancer) |
| Simonato (2003)[12] | 10 | 5 | 2 metabolic acidosis (→sodium bicarbonate administration)<br>1 Grade 3 bilateral hydronephrosis<br>1 Grade 2 bilateral hydronephrosis<br>1 Grade 2 monolateral hydronephrosis |
| Denewer (1999)[13] | 10 | 6 | 1 external iliac artery clipped (→vascular resection anastomosis from open part), leading to 1 postoperative deep venous thrombus (→thrombolytics)<br>1 reactionary hemorrhage (→re-exploration) (→delayed death)<br>1 urine leak (→conservative drainage)<br>1 pelvic collection (→ultrasound-guided drainage)<br>1 pyelonephritis (→parenteral antibiotics) in diabetes patient |
| Menon (2002)[18] | 17 | 15 | 13 bilharziasis with periureteric, perivesicular and perivesical scarring<br>1 bleeding (→re-exploration)<br>1 for a malfunction of lens (→open conversion) |
| Hemal (2004)[11] | 11 | 6<br>3 major (27%) | 2 small rectal tear (→laparoscopic suturing)<br>1 external iliac vein injury (→laparoscopic suturing)<br>1 subcutaneous emphysema (→resolved over 4 days)<br>1 hypercarbia (→open) (→delayed death, 4 weeks after surgery)<br>1 positive margin (→cisplatin-based chemotherapy) |
| Gill (2004),[6] (2004)[7] | 22 | 16<br>6 major (27%) | 6 prolonged ileus (→conservative management)<br>3 bowel obstruction (→open conversion)<br>2 deep venous thrombosis (→thrombolytics)<br>1 urethrovaginal fistula (→open conversion)<br>1 bowel perforation (→open conversion) (→delayed death)<br>1 ureteroileal leak (→open conversion)<br>1 postoperative bleed (→laparoscopic suturing)<br>1 deep pelvic vein injury (→laparoscopic suturing) |

**Table 47.4** Operative outcomes

| Lead author (year) | No. pts | Technique (reconstruction) | Urinary diversion | Mean (range) operative duration (h) | Blood loss (ml) (transfusion) | Ileus (days) | Length of stay (days) | Time to oral intake (days) | Time to return to work (days) | Follow-up months (range) | Functional outcomes |
|---|---|---|---|---|---|---|---|---|---|---|---|
| Puppo (1995)[23] | 5 | Transvaginal and lap-assisted (extra) | Ileal conduit, 4 Cutaneous, 1 | 7.2 (6–9) | (3 trans used 2–6 units) | 2.6 (2–4) | 10.6 (7–18) | 2–4 | Not stated | 11 (6–16) | 4/5 discharged with no postop. complications 1 discharged after 18 days due to obesity and diabetic problems |
| Denewer (1999)[13] | 10 | Lap-assisted (extra) | Sigmoid pouch, 10 (extra) | 3.6 (3.3–4.1) | (mean 2.2 units, range 2–3) | Not stated | 10–13 | Not stated | Not stated | Not stated | All continent 1 ureterosigmoid urine leak 1 pyelonephritis |
| Tuerk (2001)[8] | 5 | Purely intracorporeal laparoscopic | Sigmoid–rectum pouch, 5 (purely intra) | 7.4 (6.9–7.9) | 245 (150–300) | Not stated | 10 (in all 5) | Liquid 3 | Not stated | Not stated | All 5 continent and no obstruction of upper urinary tract in urogram on 10th postop. day |
| Abdel-Hakim (2002)[14] | 9 | Lap-assisted (extra) | Orthotopic, 9 (extra) | 8.3 (6.5–12) | 150–500 | Not stated | Not stated | 3 | Not stated | Not stated | No complications in pouchgram on 10th postop. day |
| Simonato (2003)[12] | 10 | Lap-assisted (extra) | Orthotopic, 6 Sigmoid, 2 Cutaneous, 2 (extra) | Orthotopic, 7.1 Sigmoid, 5.8 Cutaneous, 4.7 | 310 (220–440) | 3.3 (1–5) | Orthotopic, 8.1 Sigmoid, 8 Cutaneous, 5 | 3–6 | Not stated | 12.3 (5–18) | 2 bilateral hydronephrosis and metabolic acidosis 1 monolateral hydronephrosis |
| Menon (2002)[18] | 17 | Robotic-assisted (extra) | Orthotopic, 14 Ileal conduit, 3 (extra) | Orthotopic, 5.1 Ileal conduit, 4.3 | <150 | Not stated | Not stated | Not stated | Not stated | Not stated | 13 bilharziasis with periureteric, perivesicular and perivesical scarring |
| Hemal (2004)[11] | 11 | Lap-assisted (extra) | Ileal conduit, 11 (extra) | 6.1 (4.3–8) | 530 (300–900) | Not stated | 10.5 | Not stated | 26 | 18.4 (1–48) | All had normal renal function and preserved upper urinary tracts |
| Basillote (2004)[10] | 13 | Lap-assisted (extra) | Orthotopic, 13 (extra) | 8.0 (±77 min) | 1000 ± 414 | Not stated | 5.1 ± 1.2 | Liquid 2.8 Solid 4.1 | 11.0 ± 1.9 | Not stated | 1 ureteral obstruction 1 bladder neck contracture 1 obturator nerve paresis |
| Gill (2004),[6] (2003)[7] | 22 | Purely intracorporeal laparoscopic | Ileal conduit, 14 Orthotopic, 6 (intra) Indiana, 2 (extra) | 8.6 | 490 | 6 prolonged ileus 3 bowel obstruction | Not stated | 8 | Not stated | 11 (2–43) | 1 ureteroileal leak 1 urethrovaginal fistula |

Adapted from Hrouda et al.[30]
Extra, extracorporeal; Intra, intracorporeal; Lap, laparoscopic.

seen with other laparoscopic and open surgical procedures, especially during the initial period.

A recent retrospective study comparing 11 men that underwent open approach with 13 men that underwent laparoscopically assisted radical cystectomy with ileal neobladder suggested that the laparoscopic approach provided a significant decrease in postoperative pain (parenteral morphine equivalent use: open, 144 versus laparoscopy, 61, P=0.042) and quicker recovery (start of oral liquids: open, 5 versus laparoscopy, 2.8, P=0.004; start of oral solids: open, 6.1 versus laparoscopy, 4.1, P=0.002; hospital stay: open, 8.4 days versus laparoscopy, 5.1 days, P=0.0004; resumption of light work: open, 19 versus laparoscopy, 11, P=0.0001) without a significant increase in operative time and with similar complication rate.[10] The authors concluded that LRC contributes to decreased postoperative pain and quicker recovery with complication rates similar to those of the open approach (Table 47.4).[6–8,10–14,18,23]

At the time of writing, the authors have performed more than 50 laparoscopic radical cystectomies at their respective institutions. LRC is now a well-established technique, typically performed in less than 2 hours with a blood loss of 50–100 cc. Because we have noted neither significant reduction of morbidity nor earlier return of bowel function associated with the entire urinary diversion procedure performed completely intracorporeally, we now perform the urinary diversion part of the procedure through a mini-laparotomy incision. Double-teaming this with a surgeon who performs an open procedure has resulted in time savings of up to 2 hours, with increased confidence in the bowel and ureteral reconstructive parts of the operation. We have noted a considerable reduction in bowel-related complications more recently in contrast to our earlier, completely intracorporeal experience. While requirement for blood transfusion continues to be minimal, hospital stay continues to range from 3 to 6 days, depending on the time it takes for bowel function gradually to return, the rate-limiting part of the procedure. Unquestionably, LRC with urinary diversion is an advanced undertaking, and is best reserved for teams with considerable experience in laparoscopic and open pelvic surgery. To date, more than 241 laparoscopic radical cystectomies have been performed at more than 15 centers worldwide.

## FUTURE DIRECTIONS

LRC is being performed in an increasing number of centers that have significant experience with other laparoscopic urologic surgery, particularly prostatectomy. However, the most challenging aspect is the laparoscopic reconstructive part of the procedure. Most laparoscopic surgeons should exercise caution with completely intracorporeal urinary diversion until more experience is gained.

Although there is considerable difference of opinion and clinical practice regarding urinary diversion as well as bladder substitution, currently orthotopic ileal neobladders represent the most physiological bladder substitute after radical cystectomy for malignancy and have been used in both men and women. However, there are considerable disadvantages of using intestinal segments in urinary tract reconstruction including metabolic changes, mucus production, and tumor formation. These disadvantages may be exaggerated in patients with compromised renal function. Consequently, the search for the perfect urinary bladder substitute continues. In the future, novel bladder substitutes such as tissue engineering[33] and ureteral augmentation[34] or the use of absorbable endoscopic staples may decrease the technical difficulty associated with laparoscopic reconstruction.

## CONCLUSION

As growing experience is reported from the major medical centers throughout the world, minimally invasive surgery for bladder malignancy and urinary diversion is gaining acceptance as an alternative to open surgical procedures. Refinements in instrumentation and techniques can only provide additional improvements. Careful prospective evaluations of oncologic and functional outcomes are awaited in order to define LRC as a viable alternative to standard open radical cystectomy.

## REFERENCES

1. Jemal A, Tiwari RC, Murray T, et al. Cancer statistics, 2004. CA Cancer J Clin 2004;54:8–29.
2. Gill IS, Fergany A, Klein EA, et al. Laparoscopic radical cystoprostatectomy with ileal conduit performed completely intracorporeally: the initial two cases. Urology 2000;56:26–29.
3. Moinzadeh A, Gill IS. Review of laparoscopic radical cystectomy. Cancer 2005; in press.
4. Gill IS, Kaouk JH, Meraney AM, et al. Laparoscopic radical cystectomy and continent orthotopic ileal neobladder performed completely intracorporeally: the initial experience. J Urol 2002;168:13–18.
5. Abstracts: 21st World Congress on Endourology and SWL, September 21–24. J Endourol 2003;17(Suppl):A80.
6. Finelli A, Gill IS, Desai MM, Moinzadeh A, Magi-Galluzzi C, Kaouk JH. Laparoscopic extended pelvic lymphadenectomy for bladder cancer: Technique and initial outcomes. J Urol 2004;172:1809–1812.
7. Abstracts: American Urological Association Annual Meeting, April 26–May 1, 2003, Chicago, IL. 2003, 169(Suppl).
8. Tuerk I, Deger S, Winkelmann B, Schonberger B, Loening SA. Laparoscopic radical cystectomy with continent urinary diversion (rectal sigmoid pouch) performed completely intracorporeally: the initial 5 cases. J Urol 2001;165:1863–1866.
9. Abstracts: NE-AUA 72th Annual Meeting September 11–14, 2003, Quebec, Canada. 2003, Abstract 42.
10. Basillote JB, Abdelshehid C, Ahlering TE, Shanberg AM. Laparoscopic assisted radical cystectomy with ileal neobladder: a comparison with the open approach. J Urol 2004;172:489–493.

11. Hemal AK, Kumar R, Seth A, Gupta NP. Complications of laparoscopic radical cystectomy during the initial experience. Int J Urol 2004;11:483–488.

12. Simonato A, Gregori A, Lissiani A, Bozzola A, Galli S, Gaboardi F. Laparoscopic radical cystoprostatectomy: a technique illustrated step by step. Eur Urol 2003;44:132–138.

13. Denewer A, Kotb S, Hussein O, El-Maadawy M. Laparoscopic assisted cystectomy and lymphadenectomy for bladder cancer: initial experience. World J Surg 1999;23:608–611.

14. Abdel-Hakim AM, Bassiouny F, Abdel Azim MS, et al. Laparoscopic radical cystectomy with orthotopic neobladder. J Endourol 2002;16:377–381.

15. Guazzoni G, Cestari A, Colombo R, et al. Laparoscopic nerve- and seminal-sparing cystectomy with orthotopic ileal neobladder: the first three cases. Eur Urol 2003;44:567–572.

16. McGinnis DE, Hubosky SG, Bergmann LS. Hand-assisted laparoscopic cystoprostatectomy and urinary diversion. J Endourol 2004;18:383–386.

17. Peterson AC, Lance RS, Ahuja S. Laparoscopic hand assisted radical cystectomy with ileal conduit urinary diversion. J Urol 2002;168:2103–2105.

18. Menon M, Shrivastava A, Tewari A, et al. Laparoscopic and robot assisted radical prostatectomy: establishment of a structured program and preliminary analysis of outcomes. J Urol 2002;168:945–949.

19. Balaji KC, Yohannes P, McBride CL, Oleynikov D, Hemstreet GP 3rd. Feasibility of robot-assisted totally intracorporeal laparoscopic ileal conduit urinary diversion: initial results of a single institutional pilot study. Urology 2004;63:51–55.

20. Beecken WD, Wolfram M, Engl T, et al. Robotic-assisted laparoscopic radical cystectomy and intra-abdominal formation of an orthotopic ileal neobladder. Eur Urol 2003;44:337–339.

21. Parra RO, Andrus CH, Jones JP, Boullier JA. Laparoscopic cystectomy: initial report on a new treatment for the retained bladder. J Urol 1992;148:1140–1144.

22. Sanchez de Badajoz E, Gallego Perales JL, Reche Rosado A, Gutierrez de la Cruz JM, Jimenez Garrido A. Laparoscopic cystectomy and ileal conduit: case report. J Endourol 1995;9:59–62.

23. Puppo P, Perachino M, Ricciotti G, Bozzo W, Gallucci M, Carmignani G. Laparoscopically assisted transvaginal radical cystectomy. Eur Urol 1995;27:80–84.

24. Puppo P, Ricciotti G, Bozzo W, Pezzica C, Geddo D, Perachino M. Videoendoscopic cutaneous ureterostomy for palliative urinary diversion in advanced pelvic cancer. Eur Urol 1995;28:328–333.

25. Anderson KR, Fadden PT, Kerbl K, McDougall EM, Clayman RV. Laparoscopic assisted continent urinary diversion in the pig. J Urol 1995;154:1934–1938.

26. Fergany AF, Gill IS, Kaouk JH, Meraney AM, Hafez KS, Sung GT. Laparoscopic intracorporeally constructed ileal conduit after porcine cystoprostatectomy. J Urol 2001;166:285–288.

27. Kaouk JH, Gill IS, Desai MM, et al. Laparoscopic orthotopic ileal neobladder. J Endourol 2001;15:131–142.

28. Menon M, Hemal AK, Tewari A, et al. Nerve-sparing robot-assisted radical cystoprostatectomy and urinary diversion. BJU Int 2003;92:232–236.

29. Binder J, Jones J, Bentas W, et al. [Robot-assisted laparoscopy in urology. Radical prostatectomy and reconstructive retroperitoneal interventions]. Urologe A 2002;41:144–149.

30. Hrouda D, Adeyoju AA, Gill IS. Laparoscopic radical cystectomy and urinary diversion: fad or future? BJU Int 2004;94:501–505.

31. Gupta NP, Gill IS, Fergany A, Nabi G. Laparoscopic radical cystectomy with intracorporeal ileal conduit diversion: five cases with a 2-year follow-up. BJU Int 2002;90:391–396.

32. Stein JP, Cai J, Groshen S, Skinner DG. Risk factors for patients with pelvic lymph node metastases following radical cystectomy with en bloc pelvic lymphadenectomy: concept of lymph node density. J Urol 2003;170:35–41.

33. Atala A. Tissue engineering for the replacement of organ function in the genitourinary system. Am J Transplant 2004;4(Suppl 6):58–73.

34. Desai MM, Gill IS, Goel M, et al. Ureteral tissue balloon expansion for laparoscopic bladder augmentation: survival study. J Endourol 2003;17:283–293.

# Role of extended pelvic lymphadenectomy

48

*Bernard H Bochner, Seth P Lerner*

## HISTORICAL PERSPECTIVE AND RATIONALE FOR RADICAL CYSTECTOMY AND LYMPHADENECTOMY

Anatomic studies define the external and internal iliac and the obturator as the primary lymphatic drainage sites of the bladder and the common iliac sites as the secondary. In addition, there are lymphatics which drain the trigone and the posterior wall directly to the presacral lymph node.[1] Following the identification of the primary and secondary lymphatic drainage basins of the bladder within the pelvis, it remained to be determined whether a therapeutic advantage could be gained through their excision at the time of cystectomy. Experience with a similar radical surgical approach for cervical cancer, in which a therapeutic pelvic lymphadenectomy was combined with a total exenterative procedure, demonstrated not only that it could safely be executed but that it also potentially improved outcome.[2]

Early experience with radical cystectomy and regional lymphadenectomy for patients with nodal metastases suggested that, despite a more aggressive surgical approach, most node-positive patients experienced an exceedingly poor long-term outcome. Lymph node metastases thus appear to be surrogate markers for systemic disease. In 1956, Whitmore and Marshall published their experience of 100 consecutive bladder cancer patients undergoing radical cystectomy and a regional pelvic lymphadenectomy.[3] In 32 patients with node-positive disease, only 22% were reported alive at 1 year. Three patients (9%) survived 2 years and only 1 (3%) was alive at 3 years, the majority developing metastatic disease. While these data represented an overall improvement in outcome in node-positive patients, the poor survival in patients with regionally advanced disease led many to question whether radical cystectomy was indicated in the presence of positive regional nodes.

## PATIENTS WITH PELVIC NODE METASTASES ARE CURABLE

Supported by reports of success with the Wertheim technique for cervical cancer, which included removal of the external and internal iliac as well as the common iliac lymph nodes, along with a total hysterectomy, Leadbetter and Cooper proposed inclusion of a thorough pelvic lymph node dissection that included the hypogastric, external iliac, presacral, and common iliac lymphatics at cystectomy.[4] Subsequently, Skinner championed the benefits of a thorough lymph node dissection at the time of cystectomy and presented compelling evidence supporting its therapeutic benefits.[5] Contemporary experience with patients whose bladder cancer has involved the regional pelvic lymph nodes establishes a significantly more favorable outcome following radical cystectomy and pelvic lymphadenectomy than described in earlier reports.

Current reports note that approximately 25–33% of all patients with invasive bladder cancer involving the regional lymph nodes will be rendered disease free following radical cystectomy and a thorough pelvic lymph node dissection (Table 48.1).[6-9] Stein and colleagues reported their updated series of 1054 bladder cancer patients including 246 patients with pathologic

**Table 48.1** Outcome following radical cystectomy and pelvic lymphadenectomy for patients with node metastases

| Author | No. pts | Median survival (months) | 5-yr survival (%) | 10-year survival (%) |
|---|---|---|---|---|
| Mills et al[6] | 83 | 20 | 29 | NS |
| Stein et al[7] | 246 | ~24 | 31 | 23 |
| Vieweg et al[8] | 193 | ~21 | 25 | 20.8 |
| Ghoneim et al[9] | 188 | 11 | 23.4 | NS |
| BCRC | 211 | 24 | 33 | 19 |

BCRC, Bladder Cancer Research Consortium (Baylor College of Medicine, UT Southwestern Johns Hopkins); NS, not significant.

evidence of regional lymph node involvement. At 5 and 10 years, 35% and 34% of all lymph node-positive bladder cancer patients, respectively, were found to be free of disease following radical cystectomy and an extended pelvic lymphadenectomy, which included all nodes from the aortic bifurcation distally to the inguinal ligament.[7] The Memorial Sloan-Kettering experience with 193 contemporary node-positive bladder cancer patients that received radical cystectomy and a more limited pelvic lymph node dissection (PLND)—proximal limit at the bifurcation of the common iliac vessels—reported a 31% disease-specific survival and 25% overall survival at 5 years.[8] Ghoneim et al found 188 (18%) node-positive patients among 1026 patients with bladder cancer treated with radical cystectomy and pelvic lymphadenectomy that included the nodes at the distal common iliac vessels. Squamous cell carcinoma accounted for 59% of these patients and 85% were associated with bilharziasis.[9] The 5-year survival was 23.4% in the node-positive patients. Mills et al reported a 29% overall survival in 83 node-positive patients that underwent cystectomy and pelvic lymphadenectomy that included nodes from the bifurcation of the common iliac distally.[6] Other groups have similarly documented that, overall, approximately 25–33% of all patients with regional metastatic bladder cancer can be expected to survive 5 years following radical cystectomy and PLND. These data are confounded to some extent by the fact that many of the patients were treated with perioperative systemic chemotherapy. Pelvic lymphadenectomy is essential to identify patients with node metastases and to accurately stage the cancer, but the true contribution of the node dissection per se to overall survival in patients treated with chemotherapy is difficult to ascertain in these retrospective series.

## MORBIDITY

Several studies have compared the morbidity of a pelvic lymphadenectomy that generally includes the external iliac, hypogastric, and obturator lymph nodes to an extended node dissection initiated at the aortic bifurcation or the inferior mesenteric artery (IMA), including the common iliac nodes and often the presacral nodes. Poulsen et al reported a similar incidence of lymphoceles of 1.5% versus 1.6%, respectively.[10] In a study comparing two institutions' experience with radical cystectomy and a limited versus extended node dissection, the median operative time was 53 minutes longer in the extended dissection group. There was no difference in 30-day surgical morbidity, with the exception of a higher incidence of pneumonia in the limited dissection group.[11] Leissner et al described detailed lymph node mapping in a multicenter trial involving six centers.[12] Most surgeons felt that a dissection that began at the origin of the IMA added 60 minutes to a cystectomy and node dissection that was initiated distal to the common iliac arteries. They also noted that the extended dissection allowed performance of the cystectomy more rapidly without affecting the blood loss.

## PATHOLOGIC STAGE OF THE PRIMARY TUMOR AND NUMBER OF POSITIVE NODES IMPACTS SURVIVAL

### INCIDENCE

The incidence of nodal metastasis increases with more advanced pathologic tumor stage (Table 48.2).[13] Patients with nodal metastasis but otherwise organ-confined bladder primary tumors have a better prognosis than node-positive patients with non-organ-confined tumors. The number of positive nodes also impacts survival independent of the primary tumor stage. In the original series of 132 patients with node metastases reported from the University of Southern California, the 5-year survival probability of patients with organ-confined cancer was 50% compared to 18% for patients with non-organ-confined cancer (Table 48.2).[14] Stein et al corroborated these findings in a recent update including 246 node-positive patients (Figure 48.1).[7] Vieweg et al reported outcomes from the

**Table 48.2** Impact of pathologic tumor stage on incidence and survival in node-positive disease after radical cystectomy

| | Overall incidence positive nodes 20–25% in contemporary radical cystectomy series[13] | | | |
|---|---|---|---|---|
| | **P0–P1** | **P2** | **P3** | **P4** |
| 8 series | 0–6 | 6–30 | 27–59 | 43–59 |

| | Survival probability impacted by pathologic T stage (p<0.001)[14] | | | |
|---|---|---|---|---|
| **Path. stage** | **No. pts** | **2 years** | **5 years** | **10 years** |
| P0–P2 | 43 | 74 | 50 | 37 |
| P3, P4 | 89 | 45 | 18 | 12 |

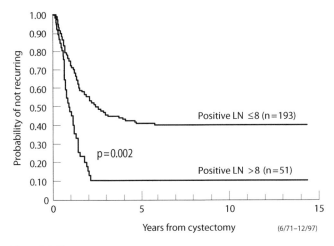

**Fig. 48.1**
Recurrence-free survival in 244 patients with lymph node (LN) positive disease stratified by total number of lymph nodes involved with tumor (8 or fewer versus more than 8). (Reprinted from Stein et al[16] with permission from Elsevier.)

Memorial Sloan-Kettering Cancer Center series with a 51% 5-year overall survival in 44 P0–P3a, LN+ patients compared to a 17% 5-year survival in 149 patients with P3b–P4, N+ disease.[15]

## VOLUME OF DISEASE

A similar stratification of outcome can be observed when considering the volume of disease at the level of the regional lymph nodes. If the number of positive nodes or size of the involved node(s) is considered as a measure of the extent of tumor involvement of the regional nodes, patients with fewer involved nodes or smaller tumor-bearing nodes have been found to have an improved outcome. Vieweg et al reported the 5-year disease-specific survival of 193 node-positive patients that underwent cystectomy based on TNM node staging (1987 system) as 44%, 27%, and 0% for N1, N2, and N3 patients, respectively.[15] The median survival for these three groups was 3.1, 1.9, and 0.9 years, respectively (p=0.0006). Lerner et al noted that patients with fewer

than six involved lymph nodes exhibited a significantly improved 5-year survival compared to patients with more than six positive nodes.[14] An update of this series found that eight or fewer nodes involved was an optimized cut-off in that patients with eight or fewer involved nodes (n=193) demonstrated a 41% 5-year recurrence-free survival and 37% overall 5-year survival compared to 10% and 4%, respectively, in patients with more than eight involved nodes (n=51), p<0.001 (see Figure 48.1).[16] Other series have confirmed similar differences in outcome, as noted in a study by Mills et al, in which patients with fewer than five involved lymph nodes did significantly better than those with more involved nodes (5-year survival of approximately 50% versus 10%).[6]

## NUMBER OF NODES REMOVED

The number of nodes removed is also important in node-negative patients. Herr demonstrated that disease-specific survival was favorably impacted in node-negative patients with an increasing number of nodes removed (Figure 48.2).[17] The presumed explanation for this is that low node counts may lead to decreased sensitivity for detecting node metastases and these patients may in fact be understaged. Higher node counts more accurately identify patients that are true node negative.

## LOCATION OF NODES

The location of nodal disease may also have an impact. There are lymph nodes embedded in the perivesical tissue and these are frequently identified in radical cystectomy specimens. Bella and colleagues identified perivesical lymph nodes in 32 of 198 patients treated with radical cystectomy.[18] Metastatic disease in these nodes was identified in 14 of these patients and in 10 of 14 this was the only site of node metastases. These patients had a worse outcome compared to similar staged patients and perivesical node metastasis was an independent predictor of overall and disease-specific survival.

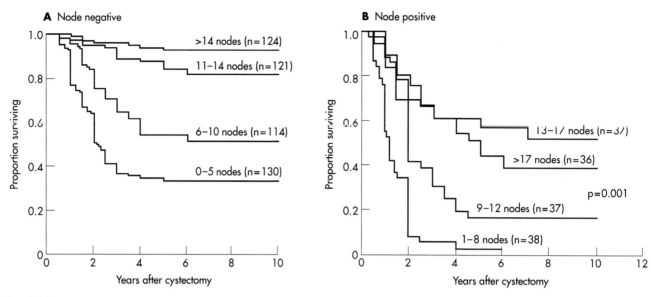

**Fig. 48.2**

Data from Memorial Sloan Kettering Cancer Center indicating that the number of nodes removed impact survival in both node-negative and node-positive patients. **A** Disease-specific survival for node-negative patients by node-examined quartiles. **B** Disease-specific survival for node-positive patients by node-examined quartiles. (Reprinted from Herr et al[17] with permission from Elsevier.)

## SIZE OF NODES

Additional measurements of the burden of disease, such as the size of the involved nodes or the presence of extracapsular lymph node extension by tumor within the regional lymph nodes, may also prove to be prognostically important. Mills et al reported that patients with involved nodes greater than 0.5 cm or the presence of extracapsular extension within the involved nodes demonstrated a lower survival.[6] Multivariate analysis of the relative importance of the number of positive nodes, size of involved nodes or the presence of extracapsular lymph node perforation demonstrated that only the presence of extracapsular perforation remained independently predictive of outcome, with a hazard ratio of 2.61 (1.69–3.54).[6]

## THE NUMBER OF POSITIVE NODES IN CONTEXT OF NUMBER OF NODES REMOVED

While the number of lymph nodes involved with metastatic disease contains important prognostic information, simultaneous consideration of the extent of the lymphadenectomy performed appears to further enhance the prognostic significance. For example, consider two patients, both with four positive lymph nodes identified after cystectomy. The first patient had a total of 10 lymph nodes evaluated pathologically while the second patient had 40 lymph nodes analyzed.

Should both patients be considered similarly staged? Would both patients have a similar anticipated outcome?

Data from both the University of Southern California and the Memorial Sloan-Kettering Cancer Center suggest that evaluation of the number of involved nodes in the context of the total number of lymph nodes removed provides a more accurate means to identify higher risk node-positive patients (Figure 48.3).[16,19] Using

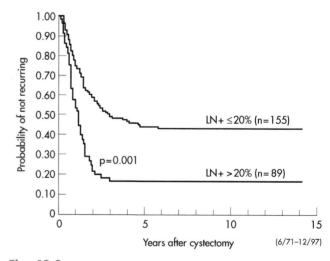

**Fig. 48.3**

Recurrence-free survival in 244 patients with lymph node positive (LN+) disease stratified by lymph node density (20% or less versus more than 20%). Data from the University of Southern California. (Reprinted from Vieweg et al[15] with permission from Elsevier.)

information obtained from the ratio of positive lymph nodes to the total number of lymph nodes evaluated (density of positive lymph nodes), both institutions have independently demonstrated an improved stratification of node-positive patients into differing risk groups. Using 20% as a cut-off for the percentage of involved lymph nodes, a 44% versus 17% 5-year recurrence-free survival probability was observed for patients with less than or more than 20% of their total nodes involved with disease, respectively.[16] An even greater difference in outcome was reported using a ratio-based analysis in a series of 162 node-positive patients that had undergone cystectomy and lymphadenectomy.[19] The 5-year disease-specific survival of patients with <20% of total nodes involved was approximately 65% compared to 5% for patients with >20% of evaluated lymph nodes involved with tumor. The ratio of positive nodes to total nodes removed and the number of nodes removed provided independent prognostic information, whereas pathologic stage was not significant in the multivariate analysis.[19] Furthermore, these variables were also associated with local pelvic recurrence.

## EXTENT OF LYMPHADENECTOMY

### IMPORTANCE

Given the importance of staging information provided by the lymphadenectomy, the question of the extent of the dissection required for adequate staging or therapeutic value remains to be clarified. An established set of necessary anatomic boundaries and extent (or number of lymph nodes) of the lymph node dissection that would provide optimal staging and therapeutic efficacy for bladder cancer is presently not available. The lack of prospectively validated studies has led to ongoing controversy regarding the necessary extent of dissection.

Wishnow et al attempted to determine the rate of involvement of the pelvic lymph nodes within the common iliac chain or more distally in the obturator, hypogastric, and external iliac nodes in bladder cancer patients undergoing radical cystectomy.[20] In a series of 130 patients with grossly negative lymph nodes at the time of cystectomy, 88% of whom had common iliac nodes resected, 18 (14%) patients were identified with microscopically involved nodes. Of these 18 patients, 17 had one or two positive nodes. None of the 17 patients had common iliac or lateral external iliac lymph nodes involved. Based on these findings, the authors recommended confining the proximal limit of the lymph node dissection to the bifurcation of the common iliac vessels for patients with no evidence of grossly positive lymph nodes.

More recently, at the Memorial Sloan-Kettering Cancer Center, a series of 144 bladder cancer patients undergoing radical cystectomy were prospectively evaluated to determine the site of regional lymph node involvement.[21] Eighteen patients (14%) were found to have microscopically involved regional lymph nodes including four with disease involving the common iliac nodes. In this series all but one patient with common iliac nodes had simultaneous involvement of a more distal lymph node region (hypogastric, obturator, or external iliac), suggesting that excision of the common iliac nodes would benefit a subset of microscopically node-positive patients.

Additional information on the distribution of positive pelvic nodes is provided by a multicenter, prospective trial in which all patients underwent an extended PLND (proximal limits of dissection at or above the bifurcation of the aorta).[12] Of the 290 patients evaluated in this series, 81 (27.9%) demonstrated evidence of tumor involvement in 599 pelvic nodes. Involved nodes above the bifurcation of the common iliac vessels comprised 35% of all positive nodes. A total of 20 patients (6.9%) demonstrated involvement of the common iliac nodes without evidence of disease within the more distal nodal regions (obturator, hypogastric, or external iliac). While exact information on the nature of the nodes (gross or microscopically enlarged) was not available, in the 29 patients with only a single lymph node metastasis, 10% were located above the bifurcation of the common iliac vessels, providing further strong support for the need to extend the dissection to minimally include the common iliac chain. Indeed, if the obturator lymph nodal regions were the only sites excised, 74% of all positive nodes would have been inadequately eradicated.

Vazina and colleagues reported a retrospective node mapping study of 43 node-positive patients treated by a single surgeon with radical cystectomy and extended pelvic lymphadenectomy.[22] Positive nodes above the common iliac bifurcation were identified in 30% and 50% of patients with pT3 or pT4 disease, respectively. All but one patient with positive nodes at or above the common iliac bifurcation had positive nodes at more distal sites. This study also noted node metastases in the presacral region in 5% of patients. Importantly, 3 of 10 patients with pT2 tumors and positive nodes distal to the common iliac bifurcation had presacral node metastases. These data support inclusion of the presacral nodes as part of the standard node dissection template.

### OUTCOME

The data describing the relationship between the extent of the node dissection and outcome are provided by single-institution, retrospective reviews. Poulsen et al reported a comparative analysis of two consecutive series of bladder cancer patients undergoing either a limited (proximal limit at the bifurcation of the common iliac vessels) or extended (including the nodes up to the level of the bifurcation of the aorta) lymphadenectomy performed at the time of radical cystectomy.[10] Previously untreated bladder cancer patients were included in the study in which 126 underwent an extended lymphadenectomy (between 1993 and 1997) and 68 received a limited lymph node dissection (between 1990 and 1993). The two groups were well matched demographically, with a slightly higher percentage of extravesical tumors in the extended lymphadenectomy group. As anticipated, the extended node dissection yielded a greater number of lymph nodes than the more limited excision (25 versus 14, p<0.001). Both groups had a similar proportion of node-positive patients, 27% in the extended and 24% in the limited lymph node groups. Despite the increased number of more advanced tumors in the extended dissection group, a similar 5-year recurrence-free survival, risk of local recurrence, and risk of distant metastasis were observed. In the subgroup of patients with organ-confined primary tumors, however, patients that underwent an extended dissection benefited with an improved 5-year recurrence (85% versus 64%, p<0.02).

Leissner and colleagues presented their analysis of 302 patients that received an extended lymph node dissection at the time of radical cystectomy for bladder cancer. They noted that patients with a greater number of lymph nodes identified in their pathology report had an improved disease-free and overall survival as well as improved local tumor control.[23] At 5 years, 51% of patients with ≤15 lymph nodes removed were alive and disease free compared to 65% for those with ≥16 lymph nodes evaluated. The improvement in local control was also significant, with pelvic recurrences identified in 27% compared to 17% of patients with ≤15 and ≥16 lymph nodes evaluated, respectively (p<0.01). Herr et al confirmed a similar improved outcome in 322 patients, in which those that underwent a more extensive node dissection, as represented by a greater number of lymph nodes identified in the pathology report, exhibited an improved overall survival.[24] All patients underwent cystectomy without preoperative radiation, or neoadjuvant or adjuvant chemotherapy. Of the 258 patients with negative nodes, the median number of nodes evaluated was 8, and for the 64 node-positive patients the median number of nodes was 11. The 5-year overall survival for node negative patients was 82% versus 41% for those patients with 9 or more nodes removed versus 8 or fewer nodes removed. For patients with node positive disease, approximately 44% versus 20% of patients with 11 or more versus fewer than 11 nodes removed, respectively. While these data provide additional evidence of the importance of a complete node dissection, the number of nodes removed in both

node-negative and node-positive patients is lower than that reported by other institutions.

A recent analysis of 101 node-positive patients from Studer's group in Berne, Switzerland, emphasizes the importance of extranodal extension as an independent determinant of progression-free survival in patients with N1 or N2 disease.[25] In their series, the proximal limit of dissection was the common iliac artery at the level of the crossing of the ureter, and the median number of nodes removed was 21 (range 10–43). While number of nodes removed stratified as <5 or ≥5, node density of 20% and pathologic tumor stage were associated with outcome by univariate analysis, only extranodal extension was an independent predictor of progression by multivariate analysis. These data suggest that the number of lymph nodes reported may function mainly as a surrogate measure of the extent of dissection performed. If this is true then one would expect that if all patients received a similar PLND, outcomes would not be significantly affected by the number of lymph nodes reported by the pathologist. Variation in lymph node reporting and individual lymph node content, as well as other less well characterized variables, may all affect the number of lymph nodes reported despite similar anatomic dissections.

Additional supportive data obtained from a national cohort of patients are provided by a multivariate analysis of Surveillance, Epidemiology and End Results (SEER) registry data on 1923 radical cystectomy patients. This retrospective study found that the number of lymph nodes examined was positively associated with an improved survival, particularly in patients with higher stage disease. Patients with at least four lymph nodes evaluated demonstrated an improved outcome; however, patients with 10–14 nodes reported exhibited the greatest improvement in overall survival.[26]

A sobering statistic from this trial is that 40% of the patients had no nodes or fewer than four nodes removed with the cystectomy specimen, suggesting that a large number of patients may be undertreated surgically. This is an issue which should be addressed at each opportunity through continuing medical education programs, and the concept of the important contributions of pelvic lymphadenectomy should be incorporated into residency training programs as well.

## IS LATERALITY IMPORTANT?

The ability to limit the dissection to the ipsilateral side of the pelvis in patients with tumors located on one side of the bladder has also been proposed. Wishnow et al suggested that when there was clear laterality of the primary bladder tumor, lymph node metastases were confined to the ipsilateral side.[20] Contemporary data, however, clearly show that, despite a clear laterality of the primary bladder tumor, contralateral nodal involvement will frequently be identified. Leissner et al found that of 32 node positive patients with primary tumors located specifically to one side of the bladder, the risk of contralateral lymph node involvement was only slightly less than that found for the ipsilateral nodes.[12] Sentinel node studies have also confirmed that the initial node region involved with disease may be located in the contralateral side of the primary tumor.[27]

## SURGICAL STANDARD FOR BLADDER CANCER AND CURRENT PRACTICE

The establishment of the minimum number of lymph nodes needed for adequate staging, prognosis or improved outcome would provide a surgical standard that could be widely applied. Such standards have been established for the surgical management of colorectal, breast, and gastric cancers.[28-30] No such standard has been established to date for lymphadenectomy for bladder cancer. Major difficulties in establishing such a standard include the wide variation in reported node yields following either limited or extended dissections and the lack of prospective studies validating any such 'standard'. The variable extent of surgical dissection and differing techniques used for pathologic review contribute to the differences in reported median node number. Other variables include individual anatomic variation in the number of nodes present,[31] surgeon, patient age, and pretreatment. Our data indicate a range of 2–80 with a median of 26 nodes removed.[21] While increasing data confirm that surgeon experience is related to outcome following major surgical procedures,[32] Leissner et al demonstrated that node yield following radical cystectomy was not related to surgical experience.[23] In this series, some surgeons with the highest surgical volume reported the lowest node yields. In fact, in a single surgeon series from Baylor College of Medicine, the range of lymph nodes identified ranged from 2 to 80, despite consistent application of pelvic lymphadenectomy in 176 consecutive patients.[22] Recent data from Memorial Sloan-Kettering Cancer Center evaluating the factors associated with node yield variability in a series of 144 consecutive radical cystectomies demonstrated that only the extent of the dissection was associated with overall node yield within a group of four experienced surgeons.[21] Patient age, neoadjuvant systemic chemotherapy, the time from transurethral resection or prior use of bacillus Calmette–Guérin (BCG) did not exhibit a statistical association with node count. In contrast, others have found that increasing patient age is associated with lower node yields after an extended dissection.[12]

The way in which the nodes are submitted to pathology also affects the number of nodes reported. By sending separate nodal packets from the different anatomic node regions as opposed to an en bloc submission with the main specimen, Bochner et al reported a 3.5-fold increase in the number of reported nodes for a standard dissection and a 1.6-fold increase in node yield for an extended dissection.[33]

## CONCLUSION

Anatomic and clinical experience with invasive bladder cancer has established the natural pathways of disease progression. Decades of experience with radical surgery for the management of muscle invasive bladder cancer clearly emphasizes the role that surgical quality may play in patient outcome. Future advances in establishing surgical standards for the treatment of bladder cancer will require well-controlled prospective trials that directly compare varying extents of surgery to their ability to provide local and distant disease control, as well as disease-specific survival. This will set the stage for clear benchmarks that can then be broadly applied to clinical practice. Technologic innovation in radiologic imaging will facilitate prospective identification of patients harboring occult pelvic lymph node metastases that will not only improve the accuracy of pretreatment staging but also facilitate appropriate surgical planning.

REFERENCES

1. H.R. In Anatomy of the Human Lymphatic System. Ann Arbor, MI: Edwards Brothers, 1938, p 214.
2. Brunschwig A. Extended surgery in advanced cancer. Ann Surg 1951;133(4):574–576.
3. Whitmore WF Jr, Marshall VF. Radical surgery for carcinoma of the urinary bladder: one hundred consecutive cases four years later. Cancer 1956;9(3):596–608.
4. Leadbetter WF, Cooper JF. Regional gland dissection for carcinoma of the bladder; a technique for one-stage cystectomy, gland dissection, and bilateral uretero-enterostomy. J Urol 1950;63(2):242–260.
5. Skinner DG. Management of invasive bladder cancer: a meticulous pelvic node dissection can make a difference. J Urol 1982;128(1):34–36.
6. Mills RD, Turner WH, Fleischmann A, et al. Pelvic lymph node metastases from bladder cancer: outcome in 83 patients after radical cystectomy and pelvic lymphadenectomy. J Urol 2001;166(1):19–23.
7. Stein JP, Lieskovsky G, Cote R, et al. Radical cystectomy in the treatment of invasive bladder cancer: long-term results in 1,054 patients. J Clin Oncol 2001;19(3):666–675.
8. Vieweg J, Gschwend JE, Herr HW, et al. Pelvic lymph node dissection can be curative in patients with node positive bladder cancer. J Urol 1999;161(2):449–454.
9. Ghoneim MA, el-Mekresh MM, el-Baz MA, el-Attar IA, Ashamallah A. Radical cystectomy for carcinoma of the bladder: critical evaluation of the results in 1,026 cases. J Urol 1997;158(2):393–399.
10. Poulsen AL, Horn T, Steven K. Radical cystectomy: extending the limits of pelvic lymph node dissection improves survival for patients with bladder cancer confined to the bladder wall. J Urol 1998;160(6 Pt 1):2015–2019; discussion 2020.
11. Brossner C, Pycha A, Toth A, et al. Does extended lymphadenectomy increase the morbidity of radical cystectomy? BJU Int 2004;93(1):64–66.

12. Leissner J, Ghoneim MA, Abol-Enein H, et al. Extended radical lymphadenectomy in patients with urothelial bladder cancer: results of a prospective multicenter study. J Urol 2004;171(1):139–144.

13. Lerner S, Skinner D. Radical cystectomy for bladder cancer. In Vogelzang NJ, Scardino PT, Shipley WU, Coffey DS (eds): Comprehensive Textbook of Genitourinary Oncology, 2nd ed. Philadelphia: Lippincott Williams & Wilkins, 2000, pp 425–447.

14. Lerner SP, Skinner DG, Lieskovsky G, et al. The rationale for en bloc pelvic lymph node dissection for bladder cancer patients with nodal metastases: long-term results. J Urol 1993;149(4):758–764, discussion 764–765.

15. Vieweg J, Gschwend JE, Herr HW, et al. The impact of primary stage on survival in patients with lymph node positive bladder cancer. J Urol 1999;161(1):72–76.

16. Stein JP, Lieskovsky G, Cote R, et al. Risk factors for patients with pelvic lymph node metastases following radical cystectomy with en bloc pelvic lymphadenectomy: concept of lymph node density. J Urol 2003;170(1):35–41.

17. Herr HW. Extent of surgery and pathology evaluation has an impact on bladder cancer outcomes after radical cystectomy. Urology 2003;61(1):105–108.

18. Bella AJ, Stitt LW, Chin JL, Izawa JI. The prognostic significance of metastatic perivesical lymph nodes identified in radical cystectomy specimens for transitional cell carcinoma of the bladder. J Urol 2003;170(6 Pt 1):2253–2257.

19. Herr HW. Superiority of ratio based lymph node staging for bladder cancer. J Urol 2003;169(3):943–945.

20. Wishnow KI, Johnson DE, Ro JY, et al. Incidence, extent and location of unsuspected pelvic lymph node metastasis in patients undergoing radical cystectomy for bladder cancer. J Urol 1987;137(3):408–410.

21. Bochner BH, Cho D, Herr HW, et al. Prospectively packaged lymph node dissections with radical cystectomy: evaluation of node count variability and node mapping. J Urol 2004;172(4 Pt 1):1286–1290.

22. Vazina A, Dugi D, Shariat SF, et al. Stage specific lymph node metastasis mapping in radical cystectomy specimens. J Urol 2004;171(5):1830–1834.

23. Leissner J, Hohenfellner R, Thuroff JW, et al. Lymphadenectomy in patients with transitional cell carcinoma of the urinary bladder; significance for staging and prognosis. BJU Int 2000;85(7):817–823.

24. Herr HW, Bochner BH, Dalbagni G, et al. Impact of the number of lymph nodes retrieved on outcome in patients with muscle invasive bladder cancer. J Urol 2002;167(3):1295–1298.

25. Fleischmann A, Thalmann GN, Markwalder R, Studer UE. Extracapsular extension of pelvic lymph node metastases from urothelial carcinoma of the bladder is an independent prognostic factor. J Clin Oncol 2005;23(10):2358–2365.

26. Konety BR, Joslyn SA, O'Donnell MA. Extent of pelvic lymphadenectomy and its impact on outcome in patients diagnosed with bladder cancer: analysis of data from the surveillance, epidemiology and end results program data base. J Urol 2003;169(3):946–950.

27. Sherif A, De La Torre M, Malmstrom PU, Thorn M. Lymphatic mapping and detection of sentinel nodes in patients with bladder cancer. J Urol 2001;166(3):812–815.

28. Siewert JR, Fink U, Sendler A, et al. Relevant prognostic factors in gastric cancer: ten-year results of the German Gastric Cancer Study. Ann Surg 1998;228(4):449–461.

29. Mathiesen O, Carl J, Bonderup O, Panduro J. Axillary sampling and the risk of erroneous staging of breast cancer. An analysis of 960 consecutive patients. Acta Oncol 1990;29(6):721–725.

30. Caplin S, Cerottini JP, Bosman FT. For patients with Dukes' B (TNM Stage II) colorectal carcinoma, examination of six or fewer lymph nodes is related to poor prognosis. Cancer 1998;83(4):666–672.

31. Weingartner K, Ramaswamy A, Bittinger A, et al. Anatomical basis for pelvic lymphadenectomy in prostate cancer: results of an autopsy study and implications for the clinic. J Urol 1996;156(6):1969–1971.

32. Birkmeyer JD, Stukel TA, Siewers AE, et al. Surgeon volume and operative mortality in the United States. N Engl J Med 2003;349(22):2117–2127.

33. Bochner BH, Herr HW, Reuter VE. Impact of separate versus en bloc pelvic lymph node dissection on the number of lymph nodes retrieved in cystectomy specimens. J Urol 2001;166(6):2295–2296.

# Role of sentinel node detection

49

*Per-Uno Malmström, Amir Sherif*

## INTRODUCTION

The original concept of a sentinel node was first described by Gould et al in discussing a cancer of the parotid gland[1] and it was clinically implemented by Cabanas in treating penile carcinoma.[2] It was proposed that the lymphatic drainage from a primary tumor goes to one particular regional lymph node—called the sentinel node—and then continues to other nodes. The tumor status of the sentinel node was believed to reflect the status of the regional lymphatic field. For more than 10 years the concept evolved and, based on dynamic investigations of lymphatic drainage in each patient, it was clearly shown that the site of the sentinel node was specific for each individual. It is now established that more than one sentinel node may exist in the same individual.[3] Use of lymphatic mapping and sentinel node biopsy to identify patients with lymph node metastasis is well established in those with malignant melanoma[4] and intensively studied in those with breast cancer.[5-7] The method has also been applied in patients with gastrointestinal cancer.[8]

Two types of marker are used to identify the sentinel node: dye and radioactive tracer. These markers are usually injected near the tumor or intratumorally (breast cancer), transported in the lymph capillaries, and accumulate through phagocytosis by macrophages in the sentinel node. In the pioneering works regarding melanoma and breast cancer, blue dyes, either patent blue or lymphazurine blue, were the only markers of the sentinel node. Alex et al used radioactive tracer and identified the sentinel node perioperatively with a hand-held gamma-detection tube.[9] Currently, preoperative lymphoscintigraphy is often part of the method for locating the sentinel node in malignant melanoma and breast cancer, and finding the draining regional lymph node basin in some cases, such as in midline melanoma. During surgery the sentinel node is identified with a hand-held gamma-detection tube to measure high radioactivity compared with the background radioactivity in the operative field. It is also recognized with dye and by visualizing blue-colored lymph vessels leading into a blue-colored gland.

We applied the latter technique in patients with invasive bladder cancer that were candidates for cystectomy with pelvic lymph node dissection.[10] We examined whether sentinel nodes could be identified in these patients, evaluated the aforementioned different techniques of detection, and investigated whether the histologic status of the identified sentinel node reflected that of the routinely excised lymphatic field.

The detection rate of sentinel nodes was 85%. In 8 of 13 cases, sentinel node(s) were preoperatively detected with lymphoscintigraphy. Using perioperative dye marker in combination with perioperative injection of radioactive tracer, Albures identified 11 sentinel nodes, 7 of which corresponded to previously identified sentinel nodes determined by lymphoscintigraphy. In our study we chose Albures for its large mean particle size (250–500 nm) and consequently slow kinetics. This contrasts with Nanocoll (25–50 nm) used by most investigators in the fields of breast cancer and malignant melanoma detection. Utilizing this quality we expected to find that the radioactive tracer would remain for a longer period in the lymphatic system and would also be detectable perioperatively the day after primary injection. Nanocoll is expected to have a quicker velocity due to the lower molecular weight, and thus to serve better for isolated perioperative injections without 1 day's preoperative lymphoscintigraphy.

In three cases in which the dye failed, the Geiger meter found two previously scintigraphically detected sentinel nodes, while one of the cases was detected solely with the Geiger meter. In two patients all three methods failed. In four patients lymphatic node metastases were detected on final histopathology. Each patient had one metastasis, and the metastatic deposits were restricted to detected sentinel nodes. Only one of these proved to be an obturator node. The main drawbacks of this study were the small number of patients and the limited lymph node dissection, confined only to the obturator fossa and to any positive findings by scintigraphy. A new study in collaboration with another center has recently started with the goal to include 150–200 patients and to perform an extended lymph node dissection in order to cover the entire pelvic lymphatic drainage of the bladder. The surgical aim is to include all lymphatic tissue from the obturator fossa bilaterally, the iliac regions up to the aortic bifurcation and any positive findings detected elsewhere in the surgical field. A preliminary evaluation of that trial reported that the sentinel nodes were detected in 81% (29/36) of investigated patients.[11] Almost half of these nodes were located outside the obturator fossa. Nineteen patients had lymph node metastases, detected with the sentinel node technique in 16. In three patients, sentinel nodes were considered false negatives: two patients had macroscopic lymph node metastases found at surgery and in one patient there was a positive node located on the vesical wall. Sentinel node biopsy might thus in the future become an attractive alternative to an extended lymphadenectomy, especially in the context of laparoscopic[12] or robot-assisted cystectomy.

## TECHNICAL CONSIDERATIONS

We used a 3.7 Fr. Williams cystoscopy needle, directing it with the help of an Albarran bridge. On the basis of previous experience from tracer injection in other solid tumors with successful identification of sentinel nodes, we injected in four different positions surrounding the tumor or tumor base (Figure 49.1). We had also, a priori, decided not to inject the tumor itself, but rather near to it, in visibly nontumorous tissue. Subsequently, research on vascular endothelial growth factor C (VEGF-C) distribution and local tumor-specific lymph-angiogenesis has supported this approach from a biological point of view (see below).

The depth of the injections may also pose a technical challenge. We had initially decided to attempt injecting in the detrusor muscle per se, thus trying to avoid shallow sub- or intraurothelial injection sites. We had postulated that the maximum lymphatic drainage should be found in the muscular layer and not in the urothelial layer. It is also important to avoid an

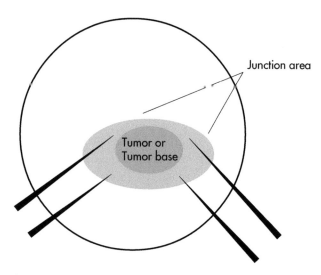

**Urinary bladder**

**Fig. 49.1**
Injection technique, where the four injections of tracer are placed near the tumor in the peritumoral junction area.

excessively deep penetration of the needle, causing a perforation of the bladder wall and, theoretically, an extravesical deposition of the tracer, creating a false positive detection on lymphoscintigraphy (Figure 49.2).

## FALSE NEGATIVE DETECTION

Several investigators have discussed the possible mechanisms of false negative detection, i.e. failure to

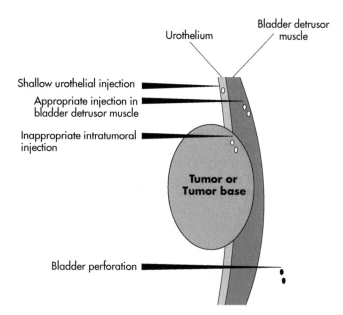

**Fig. 49.2**
Injection into the bladder detrusor muscle, where care is taken to avoid shallow injection, deep penetration with bladder perforation, and intratumoral injection.

detect nodes that actually are sentinel nodes and may even contain metastatic deposits.[3,7] The most plausible reason for a false negative result is illustrated in Figure 49.3. It is postulated that a node that is completely infested by metastatic cells might be incapable of receiving [99m]Tc-Albures and/or blue dye marker. Thus, there is actually no microanatomic possibility for uptake, and the tracers continue to the next sentinel node. The prerequisite for this scenario is that the undetected node is metastatic. For an undetected nonmetastatic node, no explanatory model has been formulated. The reasons might be mainly macrotechnical as shown in Figure 49.2, illustrating inadequate injections that are too shallow, too deep, or intratumoral.

## MOLECULAR PROFILING

In order to study the biology behind the first steps of dissemination of cancer cells, sentinel lymph node metastases were compared to corresponding primary tumors.[13] The latter were microdissected and separate specimens from the central portion and invasive front were sampled. Eight of the 13 patients from the first study were selected: four patients with and four without nodal metastases. Their molecular profiles were analyzed for p53 genomic structure, and immuno-histochemical expression of p53, pRB, Ki 67, and E-cadherin. Furthermore, microvessel density and apoptosis were assessed. The genotypes were identical in the central part and invasive front. The first metastases in sentinel nodes had a similar molecular profile, but in half of the patients, signs of clonal evolution were detected. Biomarker expression in most patients showed only small and insignificant variations between tumor compartments and the sentinel node. The findings are summarized in Figure 49.4.

Thus the data indicated that invasive urinary bladder carcinomas were monoclonal proliferations with mainly homogenous biomarker profiles. The implications of these findings might be the natural selection of clones that are more apt to metastasize. However, we were unable to determine whether clonal evolution takes place prior to dissemination, or if a selective survival mechanism materializes at the new site of expansion, i.e. in the sentinel node.

## CT-ENHANCED LYMPHOSCINTIGRAPHY

The problems of planar lymphoscintigraphy have mainly been localizing the detected node(s) in their exact anatomic position. A new technique has recently evolved, in which the picture of planar lympho-scintigraphy is fused with a computed tomography (CT) scan performed during the same imaging session (Figure

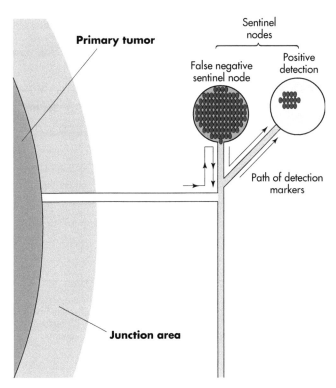

**Fig. 49.3**
A hypothetical model depicting the possible reason for nondetection of a sentinel node, i.e. false negative node. A sentinel node that is full of metastatic deposits cannot receive any tracer, and the latter is redirected to another more accepting sentinel node.

49.5).[14-17] We have explored the utility of this method in invasive bladder cancer, and the preliminary results have shown two main findings. Primarily, we can now identify the exact anatomic localization of the sentinel node(s). The second achievement in this pilot study, which included six patients, was the significantly higher detection rate of sentinel nodes. A total of 20 sentinel nodes were detected in five of six patients with the CT-enhancement, while planar pictures visualized only two sentinel nodes in two of six patients. Two patients had lymph node metastases, and the other four were node negative. The combined methods visualized five of six metastatic sentinel nodes, while planar lympho-scintigraphy detected only one of six nodal metastases. No patient was understaged on the basis of the final histopathologic stage (TNM classification).[18]

## THE SENTINEL NODE CONCEPT

### LYMPHANGIOGENESIS

The concept of lymphangiogenesis is rapidly evolving in different fields of cancer research. In short, the capacity of the tumor to communicate through tumor-specific

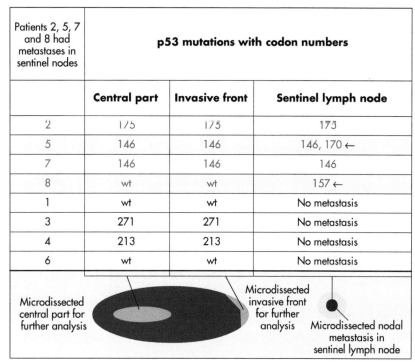

| Patients 2, 5, 7 and 8 had metastases in sentinel nodes | p53 mutations with codon numbers | | |
|---|---|---|---|
| | **Central part** | **Invasive front** | **Sentinel lymph node** |
| 2 | 175 | 175 | 175 |
| 5 | 146 | 146 | 146, 170 ← |
| 7 | 146 | 146 | 146 |
| 8 | wt | wt | 157 ← |
| 1 | wt | wt | No metastasis |
| 3 | 271 | 271 | No metastasis |
| 4 | 213 | 213 | No metastasis |
| 6 | wt | wt | No metastasis |

Microdissected central part for further analysis

Microdissected invasive front for further analysis

Microdissected nodal metastasis in sentinel lymph node

**Fig. 49.4**
Study on molecular profiling in bladder tumors with metastatic sentinel nodes versus unmetastasized. P53 mutations are considered important markers of clonality. In patients 5 and 8, a clonal evolution in the genomic expression of p53 was found in the metastatic sentinel node deposit.

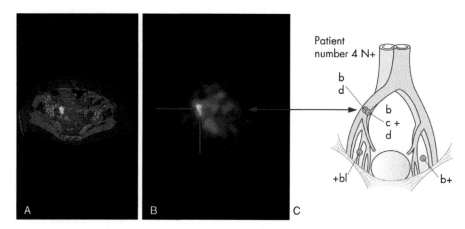

Patient number 4 N+

**Fig. 49.5**
**A** Fused picture of CT scan and planar lymphoscintigraphy. **B** Enlarged picture of two sentinel nodes over the right common iliac region. **C** Total yield in the same patient schematically illustrated. Of the four sentinel nodes detected, three were ultimately found to be metastatic (N+). None of the nodes was detected by planar lymphoscintigraphy (a); all four nodes were detected by SPECT-technique (b); the metastatic sentinel node over the right common iliac artery was also detected intraoperatively by both gamma-meter detection (c) and visual detection of blue dye tracer (d).

lymphatic vessels that connect to the physiologic lymphatic drainage of the organ itself may be one possible explanation of lymphatic spread. Investigators have identified VEGF-C as the main substance promoting the tumor-specific formation of lymph vessels.[19,20] VEGF-C acts as a ligand on the endothelial receptor VEGFR-3,[21] promoting new vessel formation.

The data suggest that it is mainly preexisting lymphatic endothelium from the peritumoral area that is activated, and not bone-marrow-recruited endothelial progenitor cells.[22] The relationship between elevated levels of VEGF-C and the occurrence of nodal metastasis has been shown to have significance in a number of solid tumors such as breast cancer[23] and gastric cancer.[24] Interestingly, investigators from Boston have recently verified that the maximum VEGF-C expression, and consequently the maximum formation of lymphatic vessels, takes place in the peripheral zone of the tumor, and not in the center or the core of the primary tumor.[25] Thus the junction area between the alien tumor and the hosting organ forms a zone of communication and transportation. This opens up new research opportunities for sentinel node detection. It can be postulated that high levels of VEGF-C induce lymphatic vessel formation, and once functional connections are established to the physiologically normal system, draining nodes can be detected as the specific sentinel node(s), with or without established metastases present at the moment of detection and surgery.

The initial report describing VEGF-C upregulation as a marker of risk for nodal metastases in invasive bladder cancer has shown similar results.[26] Analysis of induction of angiogenesis in other solid tumors[27] and in bladder cancer[28] has pointed to local hypoxia as one key event. Whether this is also the case for lymphangiogenesis has not yet been investigated. Thus, in the near future, it will be of interest to investigate the concept of VEGF-C expression in conjunction with sentinel node detection. A hypothetical model is illustrated in Figures 49.6 and 49.7.

## CHEMOATTRACTION

The regulation of leukocyte trafficking and homing to specific organs and targets in need of leukocyte presence is coordinated utilizing chemokines. They interact with G-protein-coupled receptors, and the net result is a directed flow of leukocytes to their specific targets. Müller et al investigated the possibility of a similar

system of chemoattraction in metastatic breast cancer cells.[29] A quantitative analysis of all known chemokine receptors in human breast cancer lines was performed. The investigators isolated mRNA and utilized flow cytometry analysis to determine receptor expression while in vivo expression was confirmed by immunohistochemistry. Chemotaxis and chemoinvasion assays were undertaken, and, finally, antibodies that were directed against the specific receptors were used to inhibit formation of metastasis in vivo. The chemokine receptors CXCR4 and CXCR7 were found to be highly expressed in human breast cancer cells and metastases. Their respective ligands CXCL12 and CCL21 demonstrated significant peak levels in target organs.

The same concept has subsequently been applied to other solid tumors with similar results.[30-34] The first abstract describing this concept in urothelial bladder cancer was presented in 2004,[35] when Retz et al reported that urothelial bladder cancer utilizes the chemokine receptor CXCR4 with its corresponding chemokine ligand CXCL12.

Blending the concepts of chemoattraction and sentinel nodes would facilitate analysis of the specific chemoattractive mechanisms found in sentinel nodes, with or without metastases at the time of detection and surgery. A similar investigation of control, or negative, nodes, i.e. nonsentinel nodes, might further add to the knowledge in this specific field. In Figure 49.8 a hypothetical model illustrates all three concepts of sentinel node, VEGF-C-induced tumor-specific lymph vessels, and the chemoattractive forces postulated to be involved. The force involved is the attraction of an

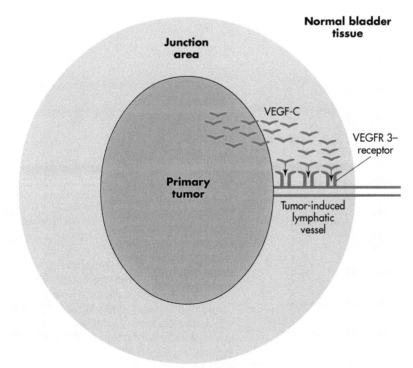

**Fig. 49.6**
A model for tumor-induced lymphangiogenesis in which the ligand VEGF-C couples to the endothelial VEGFR-3 receptor and enhances the formation of the tumor-specific lymphatic network.

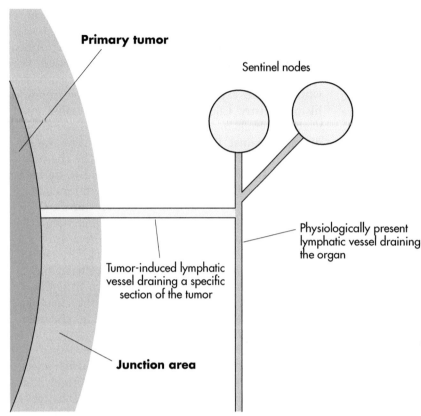

**Fig. 49.7**
Tumor-induced lymphatic vessels connect to the physiologically present lymphatic vessels draining the organ; thus the corresponding node(s) are now defined as the tumor-draining nodes, i.e. the sentinel node(s).

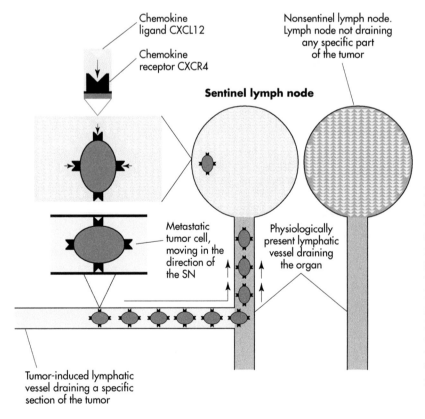

**Fig. 49.8**
Homing mechanisms for dissemination of tumor cells to target organs, e.g. lymph nodes. Lymph nodes, sentinel or nonsentinel, contain an abundance of the chemokine CXCL12. The metastatic cells containing the chemokine receptor CXCR4 on their surface are attracted to a gradient of higher concentrations of the ligand. The net result is the increasing influx of metastatic cells into the target organ. The prerequisite for this is the microanatomic connection between tumor-induced lymphatic vessels and the local physiologic system. Nodes unconnected would primarily not receive metastatic cells, while so-called sentinel nodes (SN) would.

abundance of chemokine ligand CXCL12 found in the target organ. The metastatic cell expresses the corresponding chemokine receptor CXCR4 on its surface, and disseminated metastatic cells follow a gradient of CXCL12. This is only possible once there is a microanatomic connection between the peripheral active zone of the tumor and the host, i.e. once there is a VEGF-C-induced connection to the physiologically draining node and the sentinel node(s).

Thus the chemoattraction cannot take place between as yet unconnected lymph nodes despite their abundance of CXCL12. Hypothetically it can be assumed that tumors and/or metastatic cells, being incapable of expressing CXCR4 on their surface, may not have the capacity to be attracted, and thus, even though the actual tumor might have a large volume, it will remain localized and undisseminated. Conversely, such a model could also explain why more aggressive but still low-volume tumors might have an overexpression of CXCR4 and thus metastasize more readily and earlier in the natural history of the specific patient.

## CONCLUSION

Sentinel node detection in node staging of malignant urologic tumors is a new diagnostic approach still being explored at the experimental level. The advantages over conventional roentgenologic procedures could be in the method's reproducibility both pre- and perioperatively, thus making possible the dynamic assessment of the lymphatic field in each patient. New techniques of visualization might be of importance for more detailed and exact detection of sentinel nodes with or without metastatic deposits. The clinical implications for improved accuracy of nodal staging relate to the clinician's concepts of radical surgery, extent of surgery, choice of urinary diversion, and the need for adjuvant oncologic therapy.

Sentinel node detection per se may also provide a gateway for further investigation of the actual mechanisms pertaining to lymphatic dissemination. It can be postulated that nodes, both sentinel and nonsentinel, harvested in a prospective manner, plus well-prepared scientific questions, might provide the ideal model for studying the molecular biology of metastatic capacity, lymphangiogenesis, homing of metastatic cells, immunologic response to tumor assault, and other vital key events leading to established spread of the primary tumor.

REFERENCES

1. Gould EA, Winship T, Philbin PH, Kerr HH. Observations on a 'sentinel node' in cancer of the parotid. Cancer 1960;13:77–78.

2. Cabanas RM. An approach for the treatment of penile carcinoma. Cancer 1977;39(2):456–466.

3. Nieweg OE, Tanis PJ, Kroon BB. The definition of a sentinel node. Ann Surg Oncol 2001;8(6):538–541.

4. Morton DL, Wen DR, Wong JH, et al. Technical details of intraoperative lymphatic mapping for early stage melanoma. Arch Surg 1992;127(4):392–399.

5. Giuliano AE, Kirgan DM, Guenther JM, Morton DL. Lymphatic mapping and sentinel lymphadenectomy for breast cancer. Ann Surg 1994;220:391–398.

6. Giuliano AE. Current status of sentinel lymphadenectomy in breast cancer. Ann Surg Oncol 2001;8(Suppl 9):52S–55S.

7. Keshtgar MRS, Ell PJ. Clinical role of sentinel-lymph-node biopsy in breast cancer. Lancet Oncol 2002;3(2):105–110.

8. Thörn M. Lymphatic mapping and sentinel node biopsy: is the method applicable to patients with colorectal and gastric cancer? Eur J Surg 2000;166:755.

9. Alex JC, Weaver DL, Fairbank JT, Rankin BS, Krag DN. Gamma-probe-guided lymph node localization in malignant melanoma. Surg Oncol 1993;2(5):303–308.

10. Sherif A, De La Torre M, Malmström PU, Thorn M. Lymphatic mapping and detection of sentinel nodes in patients with bladder cancer. J Urol 2001;166(3):812–815.

11. Liedberg F, Chebil G, Davidsson T, Malmström P-U, Sherif A, Månsson W. Is the sentinel concept applicable in bladder cancer? Scand J Urol Nephrol 2003;37(Suppl 214):24. (The Congress of the Scandinavian Association of Urology, Bergen, Norway, June 10–13, 2003.)

12. Kamprath S, Possover M, Schneider A. Laparoscopic sentinel lymph node detection in patients with cervical cancer. Am J Obstet Gynecol 2000;182(6):1648.

13. Malmström P-U, Ren Z-P, Sherif A, De La Torre M, Wester K, Thörn M. Early metastatic progression of bladder carcinoma: molecular profile of primary tumor and sentinel lymph node. J Urol 2002;168:2240–2244.

14. Kretschmer L, Altenvoerde G, Meller J, Zutt M, Funke M, Neumann C, Becker W. Dynamic lymphoscintigraphy and image fusion of SPECT and pelvic CT-scans allow mapping of aberrant pelvic sentinel lymph nodes in malignant melanoma. Eur J Cancer 2003;39(2):175–183.

15. Even-Sapir E, Lerman H, Lievshitz G, et al. Lymphoscintigraphy for sentinel node mapping using a hybrid SPECT/CT system. J Nucl Med 2003;44(9):1413–1420.

16. Lerch H, Jigalin A, Gasthaus K, Kunze K, Mainusch O, Lehmann P. Three-dimensional localization of sentinel lymph nodes using combined emission and transmission SPECT data. Clin Nucl Med 2003;28(1):1–4.

17. Wurm TM, Eichhorn K, Corvin S, Anastidis AG, Bares R, Stenzl A. Anatomic-functional image fusion allows intraoperative sentinel node detection in prostate cancer patients. Abstract 854, AUA-San Francisco 2004. J Urol 2004;171(4)Suppl 226.

18. Sherif A, Garske U, De La Torre M, Malmström P-U, Thörn M. CT-enhanced lymphoscintigraphy in detecting sentinel lymph nodes of invasive bladder cancer. Abstract 315, AUA-San Francisco 2004. J Urol 2004;171(4)Suppl 83.

19. Kukk E, Lymboussaki A, Taira S, Kaipainen A, Jeltsch M, Joukov V, Alitalo K. VEGF-C receptor binding and pattern of expression with VEGFR-3 suggests a role in lymphatic vascular development. Development 1996;122(12):3829–3837.

20. Saharinen P, Tammela T, Karkkainen MJ, Alitalo K. Lymphatic vasculature: development, molecular regulation and role in tumor metastasis and inflammation. Trends Immunol 2004;25(7):387–395.

21. Yulong H. Suppression of tumor lymphangiogenesis and lymph node metastasis by blocking vascular endothelial growth factor receptor 3 signaling. J Natl Cancer Inst 2002;94:819–825.

22. He Y, Rajantie I, Ilmonen M, et al. Preexisting lymphatic endothelium but not endothelial progenitor cells are essential for tumor lymphangiogenesis and lymphatic metastasis. Cancer Res 2004;64(11):3737–3740.

23. Skobe M, Hawighorst T, Jackson DG, et al. Induction of tumor lymphangiogenesis by VEGF-C promotes breast cancer metastasis. Nat Med 2001;7(2):192–198.

24. Yonemura Y, Endo Y, Fujita H, et al. Role of vascular endothelial growth factor C expression in the development of lymph node metastasis in gastric cancer. Clin Cancer Res 1999;5:1823–1829.

25. Padera TP, Kadambi A, di Tomaso E, et al. Lymphatic metastasis in the absence of functional intratumor lymphatics. Science 2002;296(5574):1883–1886.

26. Takihana Y, Tsuchida T, Kamiyama M, et al. A real-time quantitative analysis for vascular endothelial growth factor (VEGF) C may be correlated with lymph node metastasis in urinary bladder cancer Abstract 732, AUA-San Francisco 2004. J Urol 2004;171(4)Suppl 194.

27. Laderoute KR, Alarcon RM, Brody MD, et al. Opposing effects of hypoxia on expression of the angiogenic inhibitor thrombospondin 1 and the angiogenic inducer vascular endothelial growth factor. Clin Cancer Res 2000;6(7):2941–2950.

28. Reiher FK, Ivanovich M, Huang H, Smith ND, Bouck NP, Campbell SC. The role of hypoxia and p53 in the regulation of angiogenesis in bladder cancer. J Urol 2001;165(6 Pt 1):2075–2081.

29. Müller A, Homey B, Soto H, et al. Involvement of chemokine receptors in breast cancer metastasis. Nature 2001;410(6824):50–56.

30. Wiley HE, Gonzalez EB, Maki W, Wu MT, Hwang ST. Expression of CC chemokine receptor-7 and regional lymph node metastasis of B16 murine melanoma. J Natl Cancer Inst 2001;93(21):1638–1643.

31. Mashino K, Sadanaga N, Yamaguchi H, et al. Expression of chemokine receptor CCR7 is associated with lymph node metastasis of gastric carcinoma. Cancer Res 2002;62(10):2937–2941.

32. Schrader AJ, Lechner O, Templin M, et al. CXCR4/CXCL12 expression and signalling in kidney cancer. Br J Cancer 2002;86(8):1250–1256.

33. Scotton CJ, Wilson JL, Scott K, et al. Multiple actions of the chemokine CXCL12 on epithelial tumor cells in human ovarian cancer. Cancer Res 2002;62(20):5930–5938.

34. Hwang JH, Hwang JH, Chung HK, et al. CXC chemokine receptor 4 expression and function in human anaplastic thyroid cancer cells. J Clin Endocrinol Metab 2003;88(1):408–416.

35. Retz M, Sidhu SS, Dolganov GM, Lehmann J, Carrol PR, Basbaum C. Chemokine receptor CXCR4 mediates migration and invasion of bladder cancer cells. Abstract 723, AUA-San Francisco 2004. J Urol 2004;171(4)Suppl 192.

# Management of the urethra in the cystectomy patient

50

*Hendrik van Poppel*

## INTRODUCTION

Over the past 10 years, the indications for urethrectomy at the time of cystectomy have undergone substantial modification. While years ago a prophylactic urethrectomy was performed in many patients with cutaneous diversions, it has become clear that only patients with invasion from transitional cell carcinoma (TCC) at the level of the prostatic urethra or bladder neck have a substantial risk of developing subsequent urethral recurrence. Since the introduction of bladder replacement procedures, the indications for prophylactic urethrectomy have become more and more restricted. The pre- or intraoperative assessment of the prostatic urethra in males and of the bladder neck in females is the most important issue determining appropriate management of the urethra in patients with bladder cancer.

### HISTORICAL PERSPECTIVE

Historically, there have been many reasons to advocate a prophylactic urethrectomy at the time of cystectomy for bladder cancer. Bladder replacement has now become a well-accepted procedure after cystectomy in both males and females and nowadays prophylactic urethrectomy is mandatory only in very unusual circumstances.[1]

The overall recurrence rate in the remnant urethra after cystectomy is about 10%.[2] Urethral recurrence may happen early or late after cystectomy and frequently is associated with advanced disease with distant metastases not found earlier because follow-up of the remnant urethra was not well established. At the time of symptomatic recurrence many patients have already developed metastatic disease. When a delayed urethrectomy has to be performed for urethral recurrence, the procedure is technically much more difficult, especially at the level of the urethral stump because of postoperative fibrotic changes.

The philosophy regarding prophylactic urethrectomy has changed dramatically, however, since the introduction of bladder replacement procedures using the native urethra. This has substantially reduced the patients' and urologists' reluctance to perform a cystectomy. The risk for urethral recurrence must, however, be weighed against the gain in quality of life, and recommendations for follow-up of the remnant urethra need to be established. Any patient that is a good candidate for cystectomy is a potential candidate for a bladder substitute connected to the urethra provided that the risk of recurrence, and subsequent tumor progression, is minimal.[3]

## ETIOLOGY AND RISK FACTORS FOR URETHRAL INVASION AND RECURRENCE

The origin of TCC in the prostate is not clearly understood. The tumor might extend in continuity from the bladder, starting at the bladder neck and the proximal prostatic urethra, growing along the urothelium into the prostatic ducts and the prostatic stroma. In this situation a urethral recurrence is nothing more than tumor persistence after cystoprostatectomy. Alternatively, TCC of the prostate can arise from implantation of cells shed from the primary tumor or de novo from urothelium affected by the same carcinogenic process that induced tumor growth in the bladder.[4]

Retrospective analyses of large cystectomy series have identified specific pathologic characteristics of primary bladder tumors that can help to predict a higher risk for urethral recurrence. These include high tumor stage and grade, multifocal recurrent tumors, upper tract involvement, carcinoma in situ (CIS), trigonal or bladder neck invasion, and involvement of the prostatic urethra, particularly invasion of the stroma of the prostate.[5-9] When all these situations would indicate prophylactic urethrectomy, the majority of bladder cancer patients would be in need of a cutaneous diversion because of the necessity to perform a prophylactic urethrectomy.[4]

The importance of prostatic urethral involvement was first recognized half a century ago when, in a cystectomy series, 71% of the urethral recurrences occurred in patients that had TCC in the prostatic urethra.[10] This association was later confirmed by other investigators that recognized different stages of prostatic urethral involvement.[5] There was a clear distinction between the presence of TCC limited to the urethral mucosa (TpU), invasion in the prostatic ducts (TpD), and invasion to the prostatic stroma (TpS) with, respectively, 0%, 25%, and 64% of urethral recurrence after cystectomy. Other groups have reported analogous figures of, respectively, 0%, 10%, and 30%.[11] These studies indicate that the invasion of the prostatic stroma is the single best prognostic indicator for development of urethral recurrence.

The association between the presence of CIS in the bladder and urethral recurrence is widely recognized. However, it has been shown in whole-mount step-sections that CIS of the bladder is not correlated with TCC of the prostatic urethra.[12] Conversely, CIS of the bladder neck and the trigone is clearly correlated with TCC of the prostate but not directly correlated with urethral recurrences.[12] Therefore, CIS at the bladder neck is a risk factor for TCC of the prostatic urethra and the latter is a risk factor for urethral recurrence.[9] The presence of CIS in the bladder or even at the bladder neck is not per se an absolute contraindication for urethral preservation.[6]

## INVESTIGATION OF THE PROSTATIC URETHRA BEFORE AND DURING SURGERY

A rigorous pre- and intraoperative assessment of the prostatic urethra is mandatory since the invasion into the prostatic urethra is the most relevant prognosticator of urethral recurrence. For this purpose prostatic urethra cold-cup biopsies or transurethral resection biopsies were proposed.[13] In a prospective study of the prostatic involvement prior to cystectomy, a transurethral resection biopsy of the prostate accurately identified 9 out of 10 patients with prostatic involvement.[13] Core needle biopsies or needle aspirations were much less accurate. Consequently, 5 and 7 o'clock paracollicular biopsies have been advocated to identify involvement with TCC.[14,15] Recently, however, the value of this approach has been challenged. In a series of 371 consecutive patients that underwent cystectomy with negative preoperative paracollicular biopsies, urethral recurrence was diagnosed in 13 (3.5%) after a median time of 1 year.[16,17] The follow-up in these reports is, however, too short to definitively discourage the practice of transurethral resection (TUR) biopsying of the prostatic urethra.

At a time when even more bladder substitution procedures are performed, significantly more authors have chosen not to perform preoperative paramontanal biopsies and rather to rely on intraoperative frozen section analysis of the urethral resection margin at the prostatic apex.[6,18-22] This means that intraoperative assessment proved to be reliable for selection of patients that can have an orthotopic reconstruction, without subjecting the patients to unnecessary preoperative biopsies.[22] It is important, therefore, that all patients be counseled preoperatively about continent and incontinent diversion should intraoperative findings show that orthotopic bladder replacement is not feasible. The advantage of the preoperative assessment of the prostatic urethra with TUR biopsies is that patients can be counseled efficiently before surgery about what type of diversion probably will be performed.

## FOLLOW-UP OF THE RETAINED URETHRA AFTER CYSTOPROSTATECTOMY

### URETHRAL RECURRENCE

One could presume that the introduction of the orthotopic neobladder and the increased frequency of conservation of the urethra would be associated with an increased recurrence rate in the retained urethra. The largest published series evaluating the recurrence rate of urethral TCC in patients with a cutaneous diversion and an intact defunctionalized urethra and in patients that had a neobladder and a functional urethra[6] reported an overall probability of urethral recurrence for all 436 male patients of 7.8% at 5 years. For patients with an ileal neobladder, this figure was 2.9% and in those with a cutaneous diversion, 11.1%. The 5-year urethral recurrence rate was significantly higher in patients with prostatic involvement, but was only 5% in patients with a neobladder as compared with 24% in those with a

Bricker diversion. The recently presented update of results in an even larger sample of 768 patients,[22] confirmed a urethral tumor recurrence rate of approximately 7% and clearly showed that patients undergoing orthotopic diversion and those without any prostate involvement with TCC had a significantly lower incidence of urethral recurrence. These results clearly indicate that a functional orthotopic neobladder may decrease the risk of developing recurrent TCC in the retained urethra.

The explanation of this finding remains incompletely elucidated. It is well known that primary malignancies are rare in the small bowel and even less common in the ileum,[23] and a number of intrinsic physiologic, biochemical, genetic, and immunologic characteristics of the ileum have been suggested.[6] On the other hand, the decreased risk of recurrent TCC in a urethra connected to an ileal neobladder might have nothing to do with its juxtaposition to ileum and exposure to ileal secretory products. The simple continued exposure to urine may be a responsible factor or there might be an unknown systemic cancer protective effect of the orthotopic reservoir.[4] Conversely, there may be a systemic effect of the non-orthotopic reservoir, which increases the risk of urethral recurrence in the defunctionalized urethra.[6]

These data have changed the management of the remnant urethra, the only absolute contraindications for bladder replacement being the presence of overt TCC in the anterior urethra and a positive frozen section of the urethral margin during cystectomy.[6,20–22]

Although reliable pre- or intraoperative tools are available to recognize patients at risk for urethral recurrence, there is always a (small) risk of tumor growth in the remnant urethra. This urethral recurrence should be detected while still curable by secondary urethrectomy or even by more conservative (endoscopic) treatment modalities. Follow-up of the retained urethra is mandatory, especially in those with cutaneous diversions, given their higher propensity to malignant change.[4]

Unfortunately, urethral recurrence can remain asymptomatic for a long time, and in many patients symptoms occur at the time of evolution to a metastatic stage. Clinically, carcinoma of the urethra is manifested as a bloody urethral discharge, penile or perineal pain, or a mass in the urethra or perineum. This is not the clinical picture that the urologist wants to face, but this type of recurrence has been reported to occur up to 20 years after cystectomy.[13] Once overt carcinoma becomes clinically manifest, the prognosis is indeed poor and nearly all patients will die within 5 years.[13,23] This poor outcome is related to the fact that the lamina propria is the only barrier between the urethral mucosa and the cavernous corpora.[14] If there were no reliable tests to detect urethral recurrence earlier, one would have to advocate prophylactic urethrectomy in many cases. This emphasizes the importance of careful routine follow-up with urethral cytology and/or urethroscopy.

## URETHRAL WASH CYTOLOGY

Urethral wash cytology has been proposed for routine screening of patients with retained urethras.[24] Practically, a 14 Fr. catheter is introduced to the proximal blind end of the urethra. Normal saline (10–15 ml) is used to wash the urethra while the patient actively contracts the external urethral sphincter and pelvic floor. The efflux is collected in an equal volume of a fixative and the specimen is then processed for cytologic examination.[4] In a review of urethral wash cytology performed every 6 months, lifelong, all recurrences were diagnosed while still confined to the urethra.[14] No patient developed a symptomatic urethral recurrence. No patient had false positive results or clinically obvious tumor in the absence of positive cytology. Therefore, urethral wash cytology of the remnant urethra, performed twice a year, was claimed to have a 100% sensitivity and specificity to detect urethral recurrence at a stage that was curable.[25] One might decrease the number of unnecessary urethral washings by selecting only those patients with CIS in the surgical specimen or in the precystectomy biopsies and thus reduce the frequency to a once yearly washing cytology. However, this approach has not been shown to be sufficiently safe until now, and every bladder cancer patient has a chance, though small in many of them, of developing a urethral recurrence.

The value of regular urethral cytology washings has recently been challenged. When the outcome was compared between patients that had routine urethral wash cytology and those that were not followed by urethral wash cytology but presented with bleeding or urethral discharge, there was no significant survival difference[26] or any statistically significant effect on disease progression.[27] Despite these data, this author does not discourage the continued use of urethral wash cytology since it is simple, well tolerated, and minimally invasive. In addition, symptoms such as urethral discharge may be overlooked by patients and, therefore, until prospective, preferably multi-institutional, evaluations are performed, the author continues to advocate close surveillance with routine urethral washing.[26] Monitoring the residual urethra with urethral washing cytology can spare patients a urethrectomy by allowing conservative endoscopic treatment and help to prevent the development of invasive carcinomas in this organ.[27,28]

In addition to urethral wash cytology, many urologists are performing routine urethroscopy. It has been proposed that urethrocystoscopies be performed twice a year for 3 years and then once yearly.[21]

## TECHNIQUE OF SIMULTANEOUS URETHRECTOMY

When a patient cannot undergo a bladder substitution, the immediate urethrectomy can be performed en bloc with the cystoprostatectomy or after intraoperative decision making. While a delayed urethrectomy for urethral recurrence would most likely need to be performed through a perineal incision, a simultaneous urethrectomy could be done by a perineal or a prepubic approach.

### PERINEAL APPROACH

A urethrectomy performed through a perineal incision will add an hour to an already long and demanding operation.[14] A two-team approach by a perineal surgeon and an abdominal surgeon can somewhat shorten the procedure. The perineal urethrectomy will, however, also add to the morbidity and mortality. Indeed, an increased incidence of deep venous thrombosis was reported in patients undergoing a simultaneous perineal urethrectomy.[18] This outcome is probably related to the perineal pain and discomfort that is responsible for delayed mobilization of the patient after perineal urethrectomy.

### PREPUBIC APPROACH

The prepubic approach for simultaneous urethrectomy can avoid these problems. The technique was first described in 1989 by Van Poppel et al[29] and then further refined and detailed (Figures 50.1–50.8).[30,31] It was shown to be a safe technique without major

complications. There is no need to place the patient in a lithotomy position, saving time and decreasing postoperative thromboembolic complications. The disadvantage of the classic perineal approach, hindering early postoperative mobilization, is thus avoided. The few complications are mainly due to hemorrhage and can be avoided by intraoperative hemostasis and adequate postoperative management.[37]

An interesting modification of the technique using urethral stripping was presented more recently.[33] It is clear that the entire urethra comprising the fossa navicularis and the urethral meatus needs to be excised since carcinoma can recur even at this distant level.[13]

## MANAGEMENT OF URETHRAL RECURRENCE IN PATIENTS WITH A NEOBLADDER

Patients followed with routine urethral wash cytology that were noted to have positive cytology findings and subsequently underwent therapeutic urethrectomy fared well.[14,25] Several reports have dealt with the therapeutic possibilities ranging from endoscopic treatments to formal urethrectomy and construction of an alternative continent/incontinent cutaneous or rectosigmoid diversion.[34,35] The median time to urethral recurrence is 24 months, and all diagnostic means should therefore be applied regularly during that time in order to detect superficial recurrences before any invasion has occurred that would necessitate urethrectomy.

The endoscopic approaches proposed for urethral recurrence are TUR,[20,34,36,37] instillation therapy with 5-fluorouracil,[2] and even bacillus Calmette–Guérin

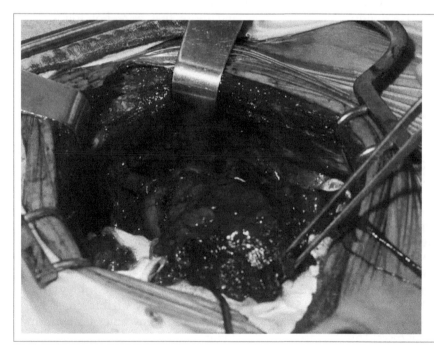

**Fig. 50.1**
Dissection of the membranous urethra through the pelvic floor. Reproduced from Van Poppel & Baert.[31]

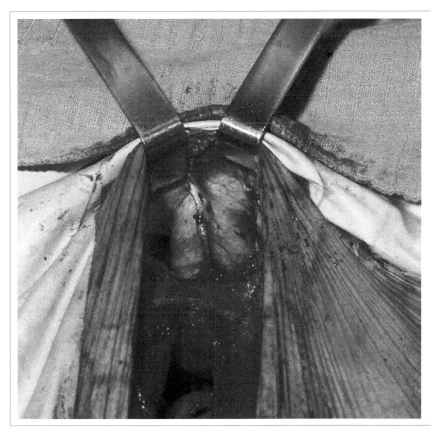

**Fig. 50.2**
Prepubic exposure of the penile shaft.
Reproduced from Van Poppel & Baert.[31]

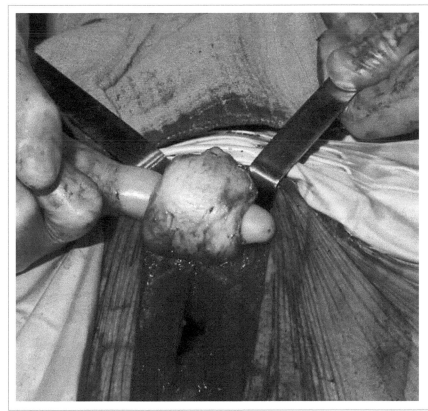

**Fig. 50.3**
Inversion of the penis dissected upon Buck's
fascia. Reproduced from Van Poppel &
Baert.[31]

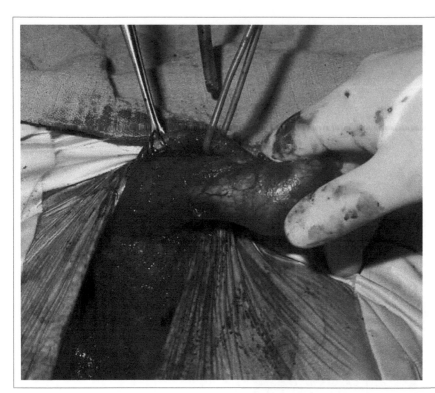

**Fig. 50.4**
Separation of the corpus spongiosum from
the corpora cavernosa. Reproduced from
Van Poppel & Baert.[31]

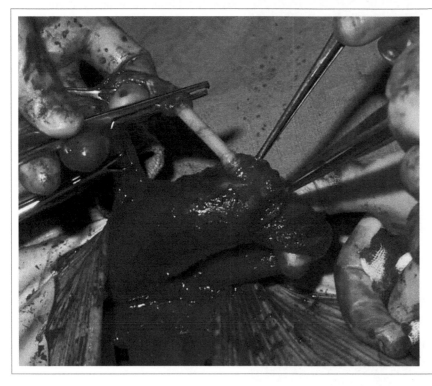

**Fig. 50.5**
Transection of the glandular urethra.
Reproduced from Van Poppel & Baert.[31]

(BCG), which was indeed shown to be effective in urethral CIS.[34,38]

In the case of urethrectomy, pathologic evaluation has revealed a varied histology. About one-third of the specimens showed no evidence of disease (pT0) on pathologic examination. The authors explain this phenomenon by the occurrence of denudation of the urethral epithelium during urethral washing. It might be that vigorous saline irrigation during cytology specimen acquisition effectively washes away the neoplastic urothelium, particularly in cases of focal carcinoma in situ. Denudation of the mucosa during the operative procedure due to urethral manipulation is another possible explanation.[26]

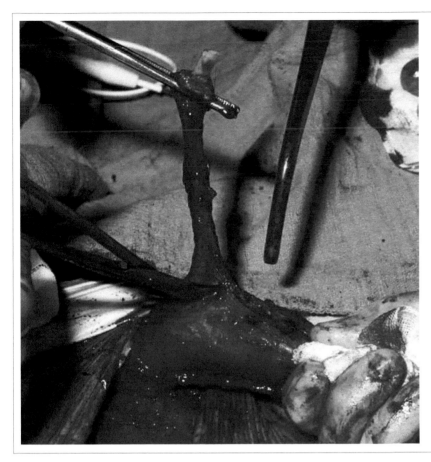

**Fig. 50.6**
Dissection of the urethra towards the
bladder. Reproduced from Van Poppel &
Baert.[31]

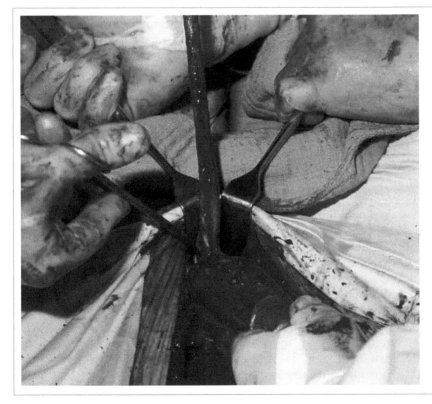

**Fig. 50.7**
Blunt dissection of the bulbous urethra.
Reproduced from Van Poppel & Baert.[31]

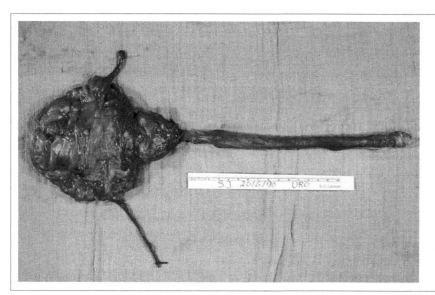

**Fig. 50.8**
In continuity removed cystoprostato-
urethrectomy specimen. Reproduced from
Van Poppel & Baert.[31]

## GUIDELINES FOR THE FEMALE URETHRA

Orthotopic bladder reconstruction has been much less widely applied in women, mainly because of more frequent voiding dysfunction in the female as well as a perceived increased risk for local recurrence. In the classic cystectomy with cutaneous diversion in women, urethrectomy is performed routinely. The female urethra, however, can also be preserved when invasive bladder cancer does not involve the trigone. It has been shown that the female continence mechanism may adequately function after cystectomy.[39-42] The key point is the preservation of the distal two-thirds of the urethra, and limiting the dissection above the endopelvic fascia in order to preserve the innervation of the sphincter by the pudendal nerve.

Urethral tumors occur only in female patients with TCC at the level of the bladder neck.[39] While some authors have recommended intraoperative frozen section at the urethral margin as the best method for determining patients' suitability for orthotopic reconstruction,[40] others have stated that a preoperative assessment is preferable because the quality of permanent imbedded sections is superior and because small tumor clusters and mucosal atypia can be missed by frozen section.[42]

Preservation of the female urethra is possible when the primary tumor does not involve the bladder neck. Before considering a bladder substitution in female patients, assessment of the sphincteric function is absolutely mandatory. When there is any doubt about continence before surgery, video-urodynamic studies are necessary. The successful functional outcome is not comparable with that in men because of the more frequent problems of incontinence and—even more common—hypercontinence. It is imperative that the radical nature of cancer surgery remains uncompromised.

Because follow-up of the remnant urethra in the female cannot be achieved with urethral wash cytology, and the value of sampling with a urethral swab has not been extensively studied, the physician must rely mainly on the voided urine specimen and on urethroscopy.

## CONCLUSION

The indications for total urethrectomy at the time of cystectomy have undergone substantial modification. Historically, urethrectomy was performed in patients with multifocal tumors, diffuse CIS, and prostatic urethral involvement. Recent studies have shown that prostatic stromal invasion and diffuse CIS of the prostatic urethra are the primary risk factors. Routine preoperative prostatic urethral biopsies prior to cystectomy are not always performed but frozen section analysis of the urethral margin can be relied upon when deciding whether to proceed with neobladder construction. Suggested algorithms are described in Figures 50.9–50.11 to guide overall management and gender-specific management of the urethra.

In patients that are not candidates for a neobladder and have known prostatic stromal involvement by tumor, an en bloc urethrectomy is performed, preferably through a prepubic approach. In women, a classic radical cystectomy includes removal of the urethra and the anterior vaginal wall. In patients that are candidates for neobladders, a cystoscopy and preoperative bladder neck biopsies can be performed or, as in men, intraoperative frozen sections of the bladder neck are proposed to select those that could undergo bladder substitution. In women that are not candidates for neobladder, the urethra is routinely resected. When the urethra is not resected, early diagnosis of urethral recurrence remains important and urethral wash cytology and urethroscopy can help to detect

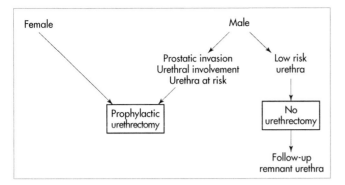

**Fig. 50.9**
Management of the urethra in the cystectomy patient, candidate for cutaneous diversion.

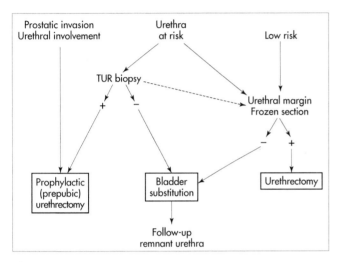

**Fig. 50.10**
Management of the urethra in the male cystectomy patient, candidate for orthotopic bladder substitution. (TUR, transurethral resection.)

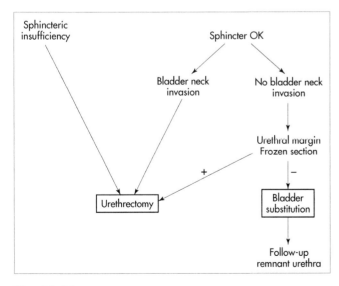

**Fig. 50.11**
Management of the urethra in the female cystectomy patient, candidate for orthotopic bladder substitution.

recurrences at a stage when conservative measures can still provide a cure and avoid the need for a delayed urethrectomy.

## REFERENCES

1. Carrion R, Seigne J. Surgical management of bladder carcinoma. Cancer Control 2002;9:284–292.
2. Freeman JA, Ersig D, Stein JP, Skinner DG. Management of the patient with bladder cancer. Urethral recurrence. Urol Clin North Am 1994;21:645–651.
3. Hautman RE, de Petriconi R, Gottfried H-W, Kleinschmidt K, Mattes R, Pais T. The ileal neobladder: complications and functional results in 363 patients after 11 years follow-up. J Urol 1999;161:422–428.
4. Van Poppel H, Sorgeloose T. Radical cystectomy with or without urethrectomy? Crit Rev Oncol/Hematol 2003;47:141–145.
5. Hardeman SW, Soloway MS. Urethral recurrence following radical cystectomy. J Urol 1990;144:666–669.
6. Freeman JA, Tarter TA, Ersig D, et al. Urethral recurrence in patients with orthotopic ileal neobladders. J Urol 1996;156:1615–1619.
7. Tobisu KI, Tanaca Y, Mizutani T, Mizutane T, Kakizoe T. Transitional cell carcinoma of the urethra in men following cystectomy for bladder cancer: multivariate analysis for risk factors. J Urol 1991;146:1551–1554.
8. Bell CR, Gujral S, Collins CM, Sibley GN, Persad RA. Review. The fate of the urethra after definitive treatment of invasive transitional cell carcinoma of the urinary bladder. BJU Int 1999;83:607–612.
9. Nixon RG, Chang SS, Lafleur BJ, Smith JA Jr, Cookson MS. Carcinoma in situ and tumor multifocality predict the risk of prostatic urethral involvement at radical cystectomy in men with transitional cell carcinoma of the bladder. J Urol 2002;167:502–505.
10. Ashworth A. Papillomatosis of the urethra. Br J Urol 1956;28:3.
11. Levinson AK, Johnson DE, Wishnow KI. Indications for urethrectomy in era of continent urinary diversion. J Urol 1990;144:73–75.
12. Wood DP, Montie JE, Pontes JE, Vanderberg Medendorp S, Levin HS. Transitional cell carcinoma of the prostate in cystoprostatectomy specimens removed for bladder cancer. J Urol 1989;141:346–349.
13. Schelhammer PE, Withmore FW. Transitional cell carcinoma of the urethra in men having cystectomy for bladder cancer. J Urol 1976;115:56–60.
14. Hickey DP, Soloway MS, Murphy WM. Selective urethrectomy following cystoprostatectomy for bladder cancer. J Urol 1986;136:828–830.
15. Wood DP, Montie JE, Pontes E, Levin HS. Identification of transitional cell carcinoma of the prostate in bladder cancer patients: a prospective study. J Urol 1989;141:83–85.
16. Donat SM, Wei DC, McGuire MS, Herr HW. The efficacy of transurethral biopsy for predicting the long-term clinical impact of prostatic invasive bladder cancer. J Urol 2001;165:1580.
17. Varol C, Burkhard F, Thalmann G, Studer UE. Urethral recurrence following cystectomy for bladder cancer: prevention and detection in patients with orthotopic bladder substitutes. J Urol 2003;169(Suppl):103; Abstr. 399.
18. Studer UE, Zingg EJ. Ileal orthotopic bladder substitutes. What have we learned from 12 years' experience with 200 patients? Urol Clin North Am 1997;24:781–793.
19. Elmajian AD. Indications for urethrectomy. Semin Urol Oncol 2001;19:37–44.
20. Iselin CE, Cary CN, Webster GD, Vieweg J, Paulson DF. Does prostate transitional cell carcinoma preclude orthotopic bladder reconstruction after radical cystoprostatectomy for bladder cancer? J Urol 1997;158:2123–2126.
21. Lebret T, Hervé J-M, Barré P, et al. Urethral recurrence of transitional cell carcinoma of the bladder. Predictive value of preoperative latero-montanal biopsies and urethral frozen sections during prostatocystectomy. Eur Urol 1998;33:170–174.
22. Stein JP, Clark PE, Cai J, Groshen S, Miranda G, Skinner DG. Urethral tumor recurrence following cystectomy and urinary diversion: clinical and pathological characteristics in 768 patients. J Urol 2004;171(Suppl):80; Abstr. 306.

23. Taggart DP, Imrie WC. A new pattern in histologic predominance and distribution of malignant disease of the small intestine. Surg Gynec Obstet 1987;165:515–518.

24. Wolinska WH, Melamed MR, Schellhammer PF, Whitmore WF Jr. Urethral cytology following cystectomy for bladder carcinoma. Am J Surg Pathol 1977;1:225.

25. Tongaonkar HB, Dalal AV, Kulkarni JN, Kamat MR. Urethral recurrences following radical cystectomy for invasive transitional cell carcinoma of the bladder. Br J Urol 1993;72:910.

26. Lin DW, Herr H, Dalbagni G. Value of urethral wash cytology in the retained male urethra after radical cystoprostatectomy. J Urol 2003;169:961–963.

27. Knapik JA, Murphy WM. Urethral wash cytopathology for monitoring patients after cystoprostatectomy with urinary diversion. Cancer 2003;99:352–356.

28. Couts AG, Grigor MK, Fowler JW. Urethral dysplasia and bladder cancer in cystectomy specimens. Br J Urol 1985;57:535–541.

29. Van Poppel H, Strobbe E, Baert L. Prepubic urethrectomy. J Urol 1989; 1536–1537.

30. Van Poppel H, Baert L. Prepubic urethrectomy. In Hohenfellner R, Novick A, Fichtner J (eds): Innovations in Urologic Surgery. Oxford: Isis Medical Media, 1997, pp 295–302.

31. Van Poppel H, Baert L. Prophylactic urethrectomy: When and how? In Petrovich Z, Baert L, Brady LW (eds): Carcinoma of the Bladder: Innovations in Management. Berlin: Springer-Verlag, 1998, pp 143–153.

32. Van Poppel H, Baert L. Innovative technique for urethrectomy. Prepubic technique and results in 41 patients. Progr Clin Biol Res 1991;370:147–150.

33. Hiebl R, Langen PH, Haben B, Polsky MS, Steffens J. Prepubic urethrectomy with urethral stripping. J Urol 1999;162:127–128.

34. Huguet J, Palou J, Serrallach M, Solé Balcells FJ, Salvador J, Villavicencio H. Management of urethral recurrence in patients with Studer ileal neobladder. Eur Urol 2003;43:495–498.

35. Bartoletti R, Natali A, Gacci M, Rizzo M, Selli C. Urethral carcinoma recurrence in ileal orthotopic neobladder: urethrectomy and conversion in a continent pouch with abdominal stoma. J Urol Int 1999;62:213–216.

36. Miller MI, Benson MC. Management of urethral recurrence after radical cystectomy and neobladder creation by urethroscopic resection and fulguration. J Urol 1996;156:1760.

37. Studer U, Danuser H, Hochreiter W. Summary of 10 years' experience with ileal low-pressure bladder substitute combined with an afferent tubular isoperistaltic segment. World J Urol 1996;14(1):29–39.

38. Witjes IA, Debruyne FM, Van Der Meijden AP. Treatment of carcinoma in situ of the urethra with intraurethra instillations of Bacillus Calmette–Guérin: case report and review of the literature. Eur Urol 1991;20:170–172.

39. Coloby PJ, Kakizoe T, Tobisu K, et al. Urethral involvement in female bladder cancer patients: mapping of 47 consecutive cysto-urethrectomy specimens. J Urol 1994;152:1438–1442.

40. Stein JP, Cote RJ, Freeman JA, et al. Indications for lower urinary tract reconstruction in women after cystectomy for bladder cancer: a pathological review of female cystectomy specimens. J Urol 1995;154:1329–1333.

41. Stenzl A, Draxl H, Posch B, et al. The risk of urethral tumors in female bladder cancer: can the urethra be used for orthotopic reconstruction of the lower urinary tract? J Urol 1995;153:950–955.

42. Mills RD, Studer UE. Female orthotopic bladder substitution: a good operation in the right circumstances. J Urol 2000;163:1501–1504.

# Primary bladder sparing therapy

# Role of radical cystectomy in patients with unresectable and/or locoregionally metastatic bladder cancer

## 51

S Machele Donat

## INTRODUCTION

Approximately 19% of patients with bladder cancer will present with locally advanced disease, 3% with distant metastases, and about 25% with unsuspected positive regional nodes discovered at the time of cystectomy.[1-9] Although radical cystectomy with pelvic lymph-adenectomy cures the majority of patients with invasive tumors confined to the bladder (stage pT1–2), and about half of those with microscopic extravesical tumor spread (stage pT3a), it cures only a minority of those with low-volume pelvic nodal (N1) or locally advanced disease (stage pT3b–4), and rarely cures those with extensive node-positive (N2–3) or metastatic (M+) bladder cancer.[2-9] The 5-year survival of non-organ-confined bladder cancer following cystectomy alone is reported in the vicinity of 43% for node-negative patients and 23% in node-positive patients, even in series in which an extended pelvic nodal dissection is standard practice (Table 51.1).[3-9] These findings indicate that the most important cause of surgical failure is the presence of occult metastasis outside the field of surgery, and, therefore, surgery alone in the treatment of locally advanced unresectable bladder cancer, gross regional nodal disease, and/or limited metastatic disease is destined to failure.[2-9,10]

Similarly, combination chemotherapy (methotrexate, vinblastine, adriamycin (doxorubicin), and cisplatin: MVAC) used alone will result in a major response in 39% to 72% of patients and a complete response in 20% to 36% of patients; however, the response is rarely durable, with the median survival approximately 1 year and only 4% to 9% of patients surviving more than 5 years.[11,12] These findings indicate that the use of either surgery or chemotherapy alone in advanced disease is unlikely to be curative. Therefore, both local tumor control and eradication of systemic disease are important treatment issues in terms of improved long-

**Table 51.1** Survival rates following radical cystectomy alone for locally advanced (extravesical tumor) and regionally node-positive (gross) bladder cancer

| Series (year) | Overall % node-positive patients | Stage pT3b–4, N0 % 5-year survival | Stage pT3b–4, N2–3 % 5-year survival |
|---|---|---|---|
| Stein (2001)[3] | 23 | 47 | 24 |
| Dalbagni (2001)[4] | 36 | 26 | 13 |
| Mills (2001)[6] | 18 | – | 29 |
| Herr (2001)[5] | 23 | – | 24 |
| Frank (2002)[8] | 22 | – | 15 |
| Maderbacher (2003)[7] | 24 | 56 | 26 |
| Herr (2003)[9] | 23 | 42 | 28 |
| **Totals** | **24** | **43** | **23** |

term survival and as a secondary goal in palliation of symptoms when cure is not possible.

Improvements in tumor response rates to combination chemotherapy, such as MVAC and more recent, less toxic cisplatin-based regimens, have given rise to the concept of multimodality therapy using surgery as an adjunct to chemotherapy to remove any previously unresectable and/or residual disease in an effort to improve survival.[11-13] The term 'postchemotherapy surgery' is often used interchangeably with the term 'salvage cystectomy' to describe radical cystectomy in patients that have failed a bladder-sparing approach or to describe a planned radical cystectomy following neoadjuvant chemotherapy in patients with surgically resectable muscle-invasive bladder cancer. For the purposes of this chapter, we will specifically discuss the concept of using surgery as an adjunct to combination chemotherapy in the treatment of patients that present with unresectable non-organ-confined or locally advanced bladder cancer, grossly positive regional nodal disease, and/or limited surgically resectable metastatic disease.

## CLINICAL BACKGROUND

Radical cystectomy cures less than half of patients with measurable extravesical tumor spread, secondary to high-volume pelvic disease, positive lymph nodes in 40% or more, and preexisting distant metastases, increasing the risk for tumor relapse and surgical failure.[2-10] However, contemporary cystectomy series have reported higher survival among patients with resectable pelvic masses and negative lymph nodes, with 5-year survival rates in the range of 43% compared with 23% in those with grossly positive nodes (see Table 51.1).[3-9] Collectively, the data from these series suggest that few patients with bulky pelvic tumors and positive lymph nodes are cured with surgery alone and argue for combining multiagent chemotherapy with radical cystectomy.

The use of systemic chemotherapy has been explored in both the neoadjuvant (preoperative) and adjuvant (postoperative) settings, with recent studies showing that neoadjuvant chemotherapy improves the survival of patients that are potentially curable by cystectomy.[14-16] A cooperative group-randomized study (SWOG 8710, Intergroup-0080) in patients with muscle-invasive bladder cancer found a clinically significant improvement (p=0.04) in survival with a median survival time 2.6 years longer among patients that received neoadjuvant chemotherapy than in those that received cystectomy alone.[14] The 5-year survival rate was 57% in the chemotherapy-plus-cystectomy group versus 43% in the cystectomy-alone group (p=0.06). A significantly higher proportion of deaths from bladder cancer occurred in the cystectomy-alone group than in the group receiving combination therapy (p=0.002),

translating into a 14% reduction in absolute mortality and a 5% improvement in 5-year survival rate for the group receiving combination therapy. Furthermore, the survival benefit in the neoadjuvant MVAC group was strongly related to a significant improvement in tumor downstaging, with 38% having no evidence of cancer at cystectomy, compared with 15% of the patients in the cystectomy-alone group (p<0.001).

Of great interest for the treatment of locally advanced cancer patients was the observation that patients with locally advanced extravesical disease (stage T3 or T4) derived significant benefit (p=0.04) from neoadjuvant MVAC chemotherapy with a median survival time of 65 months in the MVAC-plus-cystectomy group compared with 24 months in the cystectomy-alone group. This translated into a 10% reduction in mortality in the combination-therapy group compared with the cystectomy-alone group in those with advanced disease (T3 or T4). For patients with clinical T2 tumors, the 5-year survival was improved by only 5%, whereas patients with stage T3B–4 tumors had a 20% improvement in 5-year survival (Figure 51.1).

Millikan et al also addressed combined chemotherapy and surgery in patients heavily weighted to have pathologic extravesical tumor extension and nodal involvement (94/140 or 67%), randomizing them to receive either two courses of neoadjuvant MVAC followed by cystectomy plus three additional cycles of chemotherapy, or, alternatively, to have initial cystectomy followed by five cycles of adjuvant chemotherapy.[17] Although there was no difference in outcome between the two groups, by intent-to-treat, 81 patients (58%) remained disease free, with a median follow-up of 6.8 years. Of particular relevance was the finding of a nearly 40% cure rate among patients with pathologically proven lymph node metastasis, better than any reported outcome with surgery alone in a similar cohort (see Table 51.1).[2-9] In addition, all patients in this study with pathologically extravesical extension also had nodal involvement, supporting an improved cure fraction among patients with locally advanced bladder cancer by a combination of multiagent chemotherapy and surgery. Collectively, these promising combination-therapy experiences suggest that therapeutic chemotherapy may improve survival after radical cystectomy, even for more advanced bladder cancer, and provide an impetus to explore further combined modality approaches in treatment of advanced bladder cancer.

## RATIONALE FOR POSTCHEMOTHERAPY SURGERY

Postchemotherapy surgery as an adjuvant treatment in locally advanced (≥pT3A) or limited metastatic (N+,

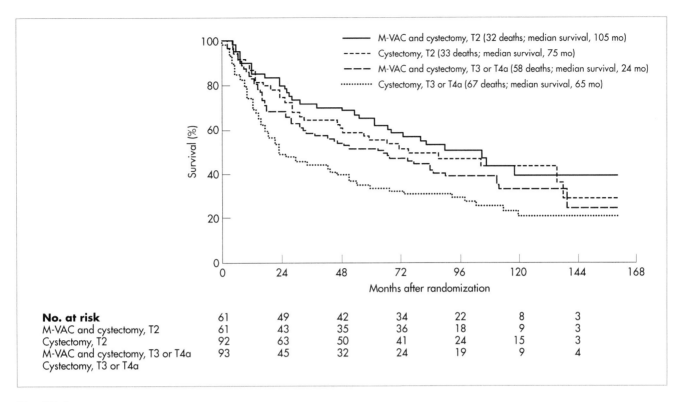

**Fig. 51.1**
Survival analysis for neoadjuvant chemotherapy plus cystectomy versus cystectomy alone in locally advanced bladder cancer.
Reproduced with permission from Grossman et al.[14] Copyright © 2003 Massachusetts Medical Society. All rights reserved.

M+) bladder cancer has become a viable treatment option in select patients with the advent of more effective combination chemotherapy. The concept of combined modality therapy utilizing combination chemotherapy and radical surgery has evolved following several critical clinical observations over the past two decades.

- Available chemotherapy has limited curative potential in patients with locally advanced or metastatic urothelial tumors.[11,12,18]
- The majority of patients with nodal metastases tend to have recurrence at the initial sites of clinical disease following chemotherapy.[18]
- Extended lymph node dissection appears to contribute to long-term survival in a small subset of patients.[2-9]
- Incidence of both local recurrence and distant relapse following surgery increases with pathologic stage despite extended surgical dissection.[2-9,19]
- Improved modern combination chemotherapy can render disease surgically resectable in patients that initially might not have been surgical candidates.[20]

The challenge remains in the proper selection of patients that may benefit from postchemotherapy surgery, the optimal combination and dosing of systemic therapy, the optimal sequence for surgery and

systemic therapy, and the extent of surgery to be performed.[11,13,21] There are compelling arguments for both neoadjuvant and adjuvant chemotherapy (Table 51.2). On one hand, upfront cystectomy may palliate symptoms such as clot retention, urinary incontinence, and ureteral obstruction, all of which would complicate the delivery of adequate and timely chemotherapy. On the other hand, perioperative complications may delay the timing of needed chemotherapy. Of note, in The University of Texas M.D. Anderson Cancer Center series reporting on cystectomy with adjuvant MVAC versus cystectomy with both pre- and postoperative MVAC, investigators found no difference in perioperative morbidity; however, patients were more likely to be able to receive at least two cycles of chemotherapy if given before surgery rather than after, even though there was no difference in the eventual outcome between the two groups.[17] The Memorial series evaluating post-chemotherapy surgery in patients with unresectable or regionally metastatic disease also noted no increase in operative mortality or surgical morbidity although the surgery was more technically challenging.[22]

The role of surgery in patients with locally advanced bladder cancer and/or regionally metastatic disease in whom the timing of adjuvant chemotherapy may be critical is controversial and evolving. Inaccuracy in clinical staging remains a significant problem, with staging errors reported in the 35% to 65% range (Table 51.3).[17,23] Although computed tomography (CT) is routinely used for preoperative staging, it is relatively limited in its ability to distinguish extravesical spread of tumor and fails to detect positive lymph nodes in over half of cases.[24,25] These inaccuracies are accentuated in the postchemotherapy setting, where it can often be difficult to discern fibrosis/necrosis from viable tumor. This is especially important, particularly in light of the observations by Dimopoulos et al, who noted a higher incidence of relapse at earlier sites of disease in patients that had clinically responded to chemotherapy.[18]

## BLADDER-SPARING PROCEDURES IN LOCALLY ADVANCED BLADDER CANCER

Although radical cystectomy usually is advised after chemotherapy for invasive bladder cancers,[26] selected patients may be treated by partial cystectomy if they achieve a major reduction in tumor size and a complete endoscopic response to neoadjuvant chemotherapy. Herr and Scher reported a small series of 26 patients that underwent a partial cystectomy after MVAC, of which 17 (65%) survived beyond 5 years, including 14 (54%) with an intact functioning bladder.[27] The group with the best prognosis was patients found to have no tumor (pT0) in their surgical specimens, with a 5-year survival rate of 87% (14/16) compared with 30% (3/10) among patients with residual invasive cancer. Overall, 12 patients (46%) developed bladder recurrences, of which 5 (18%) were invasive and 7 (26%) were superficial. The experience indicates that neoadjuvant chemotherapy may permit bladder sparing in highly selected patients that have significant downsizing of their tumors located in sites favorable to partial cystectomy; however, they remain at risk for the development of new tumors in the bladder, the majority of which may be treated successfully by local therapy or salvage cystectomy.

## POSTCHEMOTHERAPY SURGERY FOR UNRESECTABLE AND NODE-POSITIVE BLADDER CANCER

After the MVAC regimen became established in 1983 as effective chemotherapy against metastatic bladder cancer,[28] it became reasonable to consider chemotherapy and surgery for patients with locally advanced but inoperable disease. Donat et al reported their initial experience with 41 consecutive patients that had stage pT4b,N2–3,M0 unresectable or extensive node-positive bladder cancer treated with MVAC followed by an attempt at postchemotherapy radical cystectomy.[20] Of the 41 patients, 34% achieved a complete clinical response, and 29 (71%) were deemed surgical candidates and underwent surgical exploration, with cystectomy being accomplished in 24. Cystectomy was

**Table 51.2** Advantages of neoadjuvant chemotherapy versus adjuvant chemotherapy

| Neoadjuvant therapy | Adjuvant therapy |
|---|---|
| Measurable disease to assess response | Chemotherapy is limited to those that will benefit (based on pathologic staging) |
| Downstaging of the tumor allows better surgery | Local symptoms may be relieved, allowing easier delivery of chemotherapy |
| Surgical complications may delay needed therapy | No delay in definitive local therapy |
| Allows identification of candidates for bladder-sparing procedures | Avoids any increase in surgical morbidity secondary to chemotherapy side effects |
| Improves survival | May improve survival |

**Table 51.3** The inaccuracy of clinical staging*

| Clinical T stage | Pathologic stage† | | | | | | |
|---|---|---|---|---|---|---|---|
| | No. pts | P0/Pa/Pis | P1 | P2 | P3A | P3B | Node-positive disease |
| T1 | 113 | 17 | 73 (65%) | 16 | 2 | 5 (4%) | 10 (9%) |
| T2 | 181 | 22 | 23 | 65 (36%) | 34 | 37 (20%) | 33 (18%) |
| T3a | 104 | 5 | 8 | 6 | 48 (46%) | 37 (36%) | 29 (28%) |
| T3b | 56 | 3 | 1 | 6 | 13 | 33 (59%) | 32 (57%) |
| **Totals** | **454** | | | | | | **104 (22%)** |

* Clinical stage matched pathologic stage in 48%.
† Reflects stages of the cystectomy specimen only.
Adapted from Herr.[23]

not performed in 17 patients that had not responded to chemotherapy or refused the treatment. After a minimum follow-up of 4 years (range 4–7 years), nine patients (22%) survived and remained free of disease, including seven with a pathologic complete response in the bladder (complete response to chemotherapy) and two after resection of residual viable bladder cancer (complete response to MVAC plus surgery). There was an overall survival advantage for those that underwent chemotherapy with postchemotherapy surgery (p=0.009), with the authors concluding that chemotherapy allowed for potentially curative surgery to be performed as a combined modality strategy in patients whose disease was initially unresectable.

An update of the Memorial experience from 1984 to 1999 examining patients with unresectable and regionally metastatic bladder cancer treated with cisplatin-based chemotherapy regimens again showed patients responding to chemotherapy had a longer survival.[22] Of 207 patients, 92 (44%) responded sufficiently to undergo postchemotherapy surgery with the intent of removing all residual disease. Of these, 80 (39%) underwent surgery, and 12 refused surgery. Tumor progression while on chemotherapy or poor performance status accounted for the 115 patients that did not undergo cystectomy. Of the 80 patients that underwent surgery, 34 (42%) survived 9 months to 5 years, including 20 of 46 (41%) with complete resection of residual viable disease. Of 60 patients that received MVAC and had mature follow-up of 5 years or more, 10 of 34 (29%) survived after resection of persistent tumor. Postchemotherapy surgery did not benefit patients that failed to achieve a major clinical response to chemotherapy, and only one of 12 patients (8%) that refused surgery survived longer than 5 years.

The M.D. Anderson Cancer Center reported similar findings in a group of 11 patients that underwent postchemotherapy retroperitoneal lymph node dissection for nonvisceral metastasis restricted to the retroperitoneal nodes, 7 concurrently with cystectomy and 4 at the time of relapse in the retroperitoneum.[29] Although all 11 patients showed major clinical responses to chemotherapy, 9 had residual viable tumor in the retroperitoneal nodes. The 4-year disease-specific and recurrence-free survival rates were 36% and 27%, respectively. Of the 7 patients with a complete clinical response, only 1 had a true pathologic complete response, again emphasizing the inaccuracy of clinical staging in the postchemotherapy setting.

These two series demonstrate that postchemotherapy surgical resection of metastatic bladder cancer can be curative in selected patients. Further, the inaccuracy of clinical methods for assessing a complete response to chemotherapy alone and the high relapse rate at initial sites of disease suggest that surgical resection of prechemotherapy sites of local–regional disease may improve relapse-free survival.

## POSTCHEMOTHERAPY SURGERY FOR METASTATIC BLADDER CANCER

Although the role of surgical excision of viable residual cancer following chemotherapy to achieve complete response is well defined in other genitourinary tumors such as testis cancer, it is not yet established in urothelial cancer. However, in the original MVAC series,[28] 13 patients that underwent complete postchemotherapy resection of viable metastatic tumor achieved a median survival of 25 months, and several survived 5 years, indicating a possible benefit in selected patients. Following this initial experience, Dodd et al evaluated 203 patients with unresectable primary tumors and metastatic transitional cell carcinoma that received therapeutic MVAC chemotherapy.[30] Fifty responding patients underwent postchemotherapy surgery for suspected or known residual disease. In 17 patients, no viable tumor was found at surgery, pathologically confirming a complete response to chemotherapy, and in 30 patients residual viable bladder cancer was completely resected, and the patient had a complete response to chemotherapy plus surgery. Figure 51.2 shows that, of those 30 patients obtaining a complete response by the combination of surgery and chemotherapy, 7 (33%) remained alive at 5 years. Similarly, of 41% discovered at surgery to have a complete pathologic response to chemotherapy alone, those patients with unresectable primary tumors and metastases restricted to lymph node sites were most likely to survive 5 years. Of 7 patients that underwent postchemotherapy resection of visceral metastasis, 3 survived after thoracotomy to resect residual lung disease.

The most recent collective experience from the Memorial Sloan-Kettering Cancer Center includes a total of 276 patients, 89 (32%) of whom achieved major responses after cisplatin-based chemotherapy in nodal or distant metastatic sites and subsequently underwent postchemotherapy surgery.[13] Thirty of the 89 patients (34%) survived 5 years after postchemotherapy surgery, and 27 (30%) patients had no viable tumor in the resected specimen, confirming a complete response to chemotherapy. In 54 patients, residual, viable cancer was completely resected, resulting in a complete response utilizing chemotherapy plus surgery. Eighteen of these 54 patients (33%) remain alive at 5 years, a result similar to the results observed for patients that attained a complete response to chemotherapy alone (44%). Of the 14 responding patients that refused surgery, only 1 (7%) survived for 3 years. Table 51.4 summarizes survival outcome reported in the three Memorial series of patients after postchemotherapy resection of residual viable local or metastatic bladder cancer.[13,28,30] About a third of patients that undergo resection survive up to 5 years, and many have resection of both pelvic and distant metastatic sites of disease.

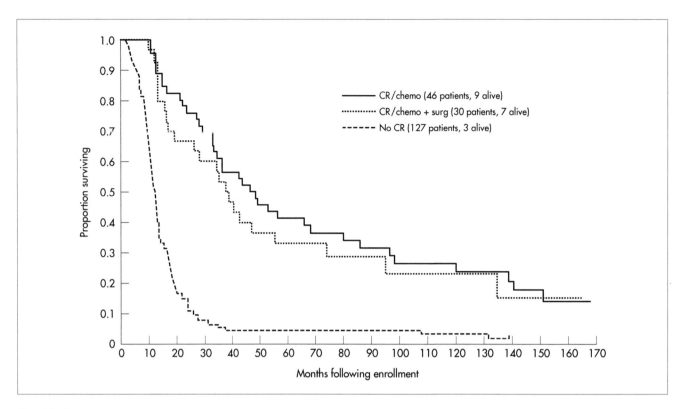

**Fig. 51.2**
Outcomes of postchemotherapy surgery after treatment with MVAC in patients with unresectable or metastatic transitional cell carcinoma. From Dodd PM, McCaffrey JA, Herr HW, et al. Outcome of post-chemotherapy surgery after treatment with MVAC in patients with unresectable or metastatic transitional cell carcinoma. Journal of Clinical Oncology 1999;17:2546–2552. Reprinted with permission from the American Society of Oncology.

**Table 51.4** Postchemotherapy surgery for unresectable primary and node-positive bladder cancer: MSKCC experience 1984–1999

| Pathologic findings at surgery | No. pts clinically resectable postchemotherapy | % Complete clinical response to chemotherapy | % Alive (3–5 years) |
| --- | --- | --- | --- |
| Residual cancer | 54 | 7 (13%) | 18 (33%) |
| No residual cancer | 27 | 14 (52%) | 12 (44%) |
| Unresectable disease | 8 | 0 (0%) | 0 (0%) |
| Refused surgery | 14 | 10 (71%) | 1 (7%) |
| **Overall** | **103/276 (37%)** | **CR 30%, PR 57%, NR 13%** | **31/103 (30%)** |

CR, complete response; NR, no response; PR, partial response.
Adapted from Herr et al.[13]

A recent M.D. Anderson Cancer Center experience specifically focused on 31 patients with metastatic bladder cancer that underwent metastasectomy performed with intent of rendering them free of disease.[31] All gross disease was completely resected in 30 patients (97%), including lung metastases in 24 cases (77%), distant lymph node metastases in 4 (13%), brain metastases in 2 (7%) and subcutaneous metastases in 1 (3%). The majority of patients (22 or 71%) underwent resection in the postchemotherapy setting; 4 (13%) received chemotherapy adjuvantly, and 5 (16%) underwent surgical resection alone. The results in this highly selected cohort, with 33% alive at 5 years after metastasectomy, again suggest that resection of metastatic disease is feasible and may contribute to long-term disease control, especially when integrated with chemotherapy in patients that would otherwise succumb to disease. These experiences suggest that optimal candidates for surgery include patients whose post-chemotherapy sites of disease are restricted to the bladder or pelvis, lymph nodes, or solitary visceral metastases and who have a major response to chemotherapy.

On the other hand, surgical resection of metastatic deposits unresponsive to chemotherapy is rarely reported or practiced, except to achieve palliation in selected cases. Otto et al reported their experience with resection of metastatic bladder cancer in 70 patients that failed to respond to MVAC chemotherapy.[32] Resected sites of disease included lymph nodes, peritoneum, skin, bone, lung, and liver. Seventy-six percent of the patients had multiple sites of disease, while 24% had a solitary site of disease. The median survival time was 7 months, with 30% and 19% surviving 1 and 2 years, respectively. Although the surgery did not appear to prolong survival, 42 of the 51 patients (83%) appeared to benefit from surgery in terms of tumor-related symptoms and improved performance scores. The WHO performance score changed from 3.3 to 2.1 (p=0.005). The authors reported no major adverse effects of surgery in such patients, although symptomatic patients felt worse after surgery.

## SELECTION OF PATIENTS FOR POSTCHEMOTHERAPY SURGERY

Selection of patients that should undergo and are most likely to benefit from postchemotherapy surgery is evolving, but several generalizations can be made on the basis of previous experience.

1. A major clinical response (complete or partial) to chemotherapy portends the best chance for long-term survival with postchemotherapy surgery, based on the fact that there were no patients surviving 5 years in any of the reported series among patients that achieved less than a major response to chemotherapy despite postchemotherapy surgery.
2. Visceral metastasis, especially liver and bone, portends a poor outcome despite complete surgical resection of visible disease. This is in contrast to patients with locally advanced primary, pelvic soft tissue, and regional or distant nodal disease.
3. Limited nodal (one or two positive nodes) or a solitary (rather than multiple) visceral/lung lesion is most likely to benefit from surgical resection.
4. Long-term survival is greatest when disease is restricted to the bladder, pelvis, and regional nodes following chemotherapy. The majority of patients having residual tumor after chemotherapy in both distant sites and the bladder experience a rapid recurrence and death.
5. A complete clinical response to chemotherapy as measured by radiographic shrinkage of tumor, negative urine cytology, and negative transurethral or needle biopsy does not obviate the need for postchemotherapy surgical resection considering reports of less than 7% survival in this setting and a very high relapse rate at prior sites of disease, both locally and distantly. Unlike neoadjuvant chemotherapy given to patients with operable

tumors confined to the bladder, TUR biopsies and CT images to evaluate advanced bladder cancer generally confirm absence of tumor progression, but not pathologic tumor response, rendering them of little use in selecting patients for postchemotherapy surgery.[24,25,29,33]

## CONCLUSION

Platinum-based chemotherapy is the primary treatment for metastatic bladder cancer;[34] however, used alone it is rarely curative, with tumor relapse in the bladder, pelvic soft tissue, and lymph nodes a common finding even after a complete clinical response to chemotherapy.[11,12,18] Current postchemotherapy clinical staging methods are imprecise, with minimal correlation between a clinical complete response to chemotherapy and the final pathologic specimen, limiting its usefulness in determining which patients may defer surgery.[13,20,22,29,30] The best correlation for survival after postchemotherapy surgery is the achievement of a major or complete clinical response to chemotherapy.[5,11,13,20,22] Current data show that many patients with advanced bladder cancer have residual viable cancer even after achieving a major response to chemotherapy. However, with complete resection of known or suspected sites of residual disease, up to 33% of these patients will survive up to 5 years. Furthermore, the need for postchemotherapy surgery in the setting of a complete clinical response is supported by the finding that over 90% of those that refused surgery died of recurrent metastatic bladder cancer.[13] Although a complete pathologic response promises the best prognosis, with 5-year survival of up to 58%, as many as 41% of patients achieve a complete response and 5-year survival with the combination of chemotherapy and surgery.[22] Conversely, patients that do not achieve a major response to chemotherapy, or that experience progression of disease while on chemotherapy, do not appear to benefit from postchemotherapy surgery with few, if any, surviving 5 years even with surgery,[13,17,20,22,30] although there may be a palliative benefit in selected patients.[32]

More effective chemotherapy regimens have made postchemotherapy surgery a viable option for selected patients with locally advanced or metastatic bladder cancer and suggest that a multidisciplinary approach to the treatment of these patients should be considered. Although the surgery is technically challenging, it may be done safely in experienced hands and provides improved survival in some and palliation in many more.

REFERENCES

1. Jemal A, Tiwari RC, Murray T, et al. Cancer statistics 2004. CA Cancer J Clin 2004;54(1):8–29.

2. Vieweg J, Gschwend JE, Herr HW. Pelvic lymph node dissection can be curative in patients with node-positive bladder cancer. J Urol 1999;161:449–454.

3. Stein JP, Lieskovsky G, Skinner DG. Radical cystectomy in the treatment of invasive bladder cancer: long-term results in 1,054 patients. J Clin Oncol 2001;19:666–675.

4. Dalbagni G, Genega E, Herr HW, et al. Cystectomy for bladder cancer: a contemporary series. J Urol 2001;165:1111–1116.

5. Herr HW, Donat SM. Outcome of patients with grossly node positive bladder cancer after pelvic lymph node dissection and radical cystectomy. 2001;J Urol 165:62–64.

6. Mills RD, Turner WH, Fleishmann A, et al. Pelvic node metastases from bladder cancer: outcome in 83 patients after radical cystectomy and pelvic lymphadenectomy. J Urol 2001;166:19–23.

7. Maderbacher S, Hochreiter W, Studer UE. Radical cystectomy for bladder cancer today—homogeneous series without neoadjuvant therapy. J Clin Oncol 2003;21:690–696.

8. Frank I, Cheville JC, Zincke H. Transitional cell carcinoma of the urinary bladder with regional lymph node involvement treated by cystectomy. Cancer 2003;97(10):2425–2431.

9. Herr HW. Superiority of ratio based lymph node staging for bladder cancer. J Urol 2003;169:943–945.

10. Quek ML, Stein JP, Clark PE, et al. Natural history of surgically treated bladder carcinoma with extravesical tumor extension. Cancer 2003;98(5):955–961.

11. Bajorin DF, Dodd PM, Mazumdar M, et al. Long-term survival in metastatic transitional cell carcinoma and prognostic factors predicting outcome of therapy. J Clin Oncol 1999;17:3173–3181.

12. Saxman SB, Propert KJ, Einhorn LH, et al. Long-term followup of a phase III intergroup study of cisplatin alone or in combination with VAC in patients with metastatic urothelial carcinoma. J Clin Oncol 1997;15:2564–2569.

13. Herr HW, Donat SM, Bajorin DF. Bladder cancer, the limits of surgical excision. When/how much? Urol Oncol 2001;6:221–224.

14. Grossman HB, Natale RB, Tangen CM, et al. Neoadjuvant chemotherapy plus cystectomy compared with cystectomy alone for locally advanced bladder cancer. N Engl J Med 2003;349:859–866.

15. Advanced Bladder Cancer (ABC) Meta-analysis Collaboration. Neoadjuvant chemotherapy in invasive bladder cancer: a systematic review and meta-analysis. Lancet 2003;361:1927–1934.

16. Winquist E, Kirchner TS, Segal R, et al. Neoadjuvant chemotherapy for transitional cell carcinoma of the bladder: a systematic review and meta-analysis. J Urol 2004;171:561–569.

17. Millikan RE, Dinney CPN, Swanson D, et al. Integrated therapy for locally advanced bladder cancer: a final report of a randomized trial of cystectomy plus adjuvant MVAC versus cystectomy with both preoperative and postoperative MVAC. J Clin Oncol 2001;19:4005–4013.

18. Dimopoulos MA, Finn L, Logothetis CJ. Pattern of failure and survival of patients with metastatic urothelial tumors relapsing after cis-platinum chemotherapy. J Urol 1994;151:598.

19. Stein JP, Skinner DG. Results with radical cystectomy for treating bladder cancer: a 'reference standard' for high-grade, invasive bladder cancer. BJU Int 2003;92:12–17.

20. Donat SM, Herr HW, Bajorin DF. MVAC chemotherapy and cystectomy for unresectable bladder cancer. J Urol 1996;156:368–371.

21. Millikan R, Siefker-Radtke A, Grossman HB. Neoadjuvant chemotherapy for bladder cancer. Urol Oncol: Semin Orig Investig 2003;21:464–467.

22. Herr HW, Donat SM, Bajorin DF. Post-chemotherapy surgery in patients with unresectable or regionally metastatic bladder cancer. J Urol 2001;165:811–814.

23. Herr HW. Uncertainty and outcome of invasive bladder tumors. Urol Oncol 1996;2:92–95.

24. See WA, Fuller JR. Staging of advanced bladder cancer: current concepts and pitfalls. Urol Clin North Am 1992;19:663–683.

25. Herr HW, Hilton SH. Routine CT scan in cystectomy patients: does it change management? Urology 1996;47(3):324–325.

26. Schultz PK, Herr HW, Zhang Z-F, et al. Neoadjuvant chemotherapy for invasive bladder cancer: prognostic factors for survival of patients treated with MVAC with 5-year follow-up. J Clin Oncol 1994;12:1394–1401.

27. Herr HW, Scher HI. Neoadjuvant chemotherapy and partial cystectomy for invasive bladder cancer. J Clin Oncol 1994;12:975–980.

28. Sternberg CN, Yagoda A, Scher HI, et al. Preliminary results of MVAC for transitional cell carcinoma of the urothelium. J Urol 1985;133:403–407.

29. Sweeney P, Millikan R, Donat SM, et al. Is there a therapeutic role for post-chemotherapy retroperitoneal lymph node dissection in metastatic transitional cell carcinoma of the bladder? J Urol 2003;169:2113–2117.

30. Dodd PM, McCaffrey JA, Herr HW, et al. Outcome of post-chemotherapy surgery after treatment with MVAC in patients with unresectable or metastatic transitional cell carcinoma. J Clin Oncol 1999;17:2546–2552.

31. Siefker-Radtke AO, Walsh GL, Pisters LL, et al. Is there a role for surgery in the management of metastatic urothelial cancer? The M.D. Anderson experience. J Urol 2004;171:145–148.

32. Otto T, Krege S, Suhr J, et al. Impact of surgical resection of bladder cancer metastases refractory to systemic therapy on performance score: a Phase II trial. Urology 2001;57:55–59.

33. Schultz PK, Herr HW, Zhang Z-F, et al. Neoadjuvant chemotherapy for invasive bladder cancer: prognostic factors for survival of patients treated with MVAC with 5-year follow-up. J Clin Oncol 1994;12:1394–1401.

34. Raghavan D. Progress in the chemotherapy of metastatic cancer of the urinary tract. Cancer 2002;97:2050–2055.

# Radical TURBT

52

*Eduardo Solsona*

## INTRODUCTION

Radical cystectomy is the gold standard of therapy for patients with muscle-invasive bladder cancer. Although the quality of life of patients treated with radical cystectomy has improved substantially with the use of orthotopic, continent urinary diversions and preservation of sexual potency in selected cases, morbidity is high and there is no doubt that patients with their own bladders, even after undergoing one or more transurethral resections of the bladder (TURBs), have less morbidity and a better quality of life than patients treated with cystectomy. For this reason, bladder preservation programs have been developed for patients with muscle-invasive bladder cancer.[1-3] TURB is a fundamental procedure for the diagnosis and staging of bladder cancer. However, TURB alone is controversial as a therapeutic approach to invasive bladder cancer due to the different patterns of tumor spread (frontal, tentacular) and the presence of microfoci, both surrounding and at a distance from the primary tumor. This makes it difficult to achieve complete tumor resection. Nevertheless, retrospective studies of TURB alone have demonstrated the feasibility of this approach in patients with low invasive disease. In selected series, 5-year survival rates ranging from 31% to 53% have been reported.[4,5]

## RATIONALE

In large series, the incidence of attaining P0 at cystectomy is approximately 12%.[6-9] The lack of residual cancer suggests that in some instances patients may be overtreated by cystectomy and that the tumor was completely controlled with TURB during the diagnostic work-up.

Cystectomy has little or no survival impact on patients with distant micrometastases, which are the main cause of failure. Consequently, many of these patients initially could have potentially been treated successfully with TURB alone. The incidence of P0, therefore, constitutes the main rationale for the use of radical TURB in selected patients with invasive bladder cancer. However, the absence of residual tumor in the cystectomy specimen does not necessarily mean that patients are cured with cystectomy, as the 5-year cause-specific survival rate in some series is around 80%.[8,10-13]

On the other hand, in univariate and multivariate analyses, a complete TURB is a good prognostic factor in patients included in bladder preservation programs with radiochemotherapy,[14,15] as well as in patients treated with cystectomy after preoperative radiotherapy[16] or with radical radiotherapy.[17] The prognostic value also suggests a potential therapeutic effect of complete TURB in patients with invasive bladder cancer.

## RETROSPECTIVE STUDIES

In a retrospective study from Western Sweden, Holmäng et al[18] reported that cystectomy was superior to TURB and to radiotherapy in patients with clinical stages T2–3 bladder carcinoma when 5-year tumor-related mortality was evaluated, with rates of 56.6%, 75%, and 81.8%, respectively. In this study, patients unfit for cystectomy were treated with TURB or radiotherapy. Consequently, the survival rates with these approaches are not totally comparable. In another retrospective study of 114 patients with invasive bladder cancer, TURB resulted in a better 5-year overall survival rate than did cystectomy or radiotherapy or preoperative radiotherapy plus cystectomy.[19] However, combination therapy was slightly superior for patients with stage B2 (cT2b) disease. Both studies were retrospective and some important selection bias may have occurred.

A review of retrospective studies of patients with invasive bladder cancer initially treated with TURB revealed the results shown in Table 52.1.[4,5,19-23] Although some patients were salvaged with cystectomy after an invasive recurrence, 5-year survival rates ranged from 31% to 58.8%. This was particularly remarkable in patients with clinical stage B1 (cT2a) disease. However, this survival rate is inferior to that of patients treated with cystectomy—56% to 68% and 59% to 81% in P2a and P2b respectively.[6,9,24] Although cystectomy is superior to TURB in terms of survival, these results also demonstrated that a group of patients with invasive bladder cancer could be cured with TURB as monotherapy. The problem is how to identify clinically those patients in whom TURB can provide local control of the tumor. For this reason, it is important to analyze the prospective studies.

**Table 52.1** Survival in retrospective studies of patients treated with TURB alone

| Lead author (reference) | No. pts | 5-Year cancer-specific survival (%) | | |
| --- | --- | --- | --- | --- |
| | | General | B1 (cT2a) | B2 (cT2b) |
| Flocks[21] | 126 | 47 | 54 | 43 |
| Milner[5] | 190 | 53 | 57 | 23 |
| Barnes[20] | 114 | 40 | | |
| O'Flynn[23] | 123 | 52 | 59 | 20 |
| Barnes[4] | 75 | 31 | | |
| Henry[19] | 43 | 52 | 63 | 38 |
| Kondas[22] | 27 | 48.8 | 54.6 | 20 |
| Total | 698 | 45.8 | 58.8 | 31 |

## PROSPECTIVE STUDIES

Only two prospective studies dealing with TURB as a therapeutic approach in patients with invasive bladder cancer have been published. The basic aim of both series was to achieve a complete resection of invasive bladder tumor limited to the muscularis propria, T2a–b (2002 TNM classification). However, since the unreliability of the clinical staging assessment with respect to pathologic staging precludes its use as an inclusion criterion, Herr used the absence of invasive tumor on a repeat TURB performed 2–3 weeks after a complete TURB of the primary tumor as an inclusion criterion.[25]

Solsona et al systematically performed a fractionated TURB in large papillary tumors or small mixed or sessile tumors, including, first, resection of the exophytic part of the tumor, then removal of the endophytic part. Once the endophytic part was completely removed macroscopically, five or more biopsies were taken from the healthy appearing muscularis propria of the tumor bed; cold-cup biopsies of the perivesical fat were then performed, if this structure had been reached during the TURB.[76,77] If all of these biopsies were negative, TURB was then considered radical and patients were included in a surveillance program. Although the inclusion criteria used by Herr[25] and Solsona et al[26,27] were not completely identical, initial results were comparable, with a progression rate of 33.3% and 27.7%, a cause-specific survival of 82.2% and 80.5%, and a bladder preservation rate of 67% and 75.2%, respectively (Table 52.2). More importantly, with a minimum follow-up of more than 10 years, the results continued to be comparable with slight modifications with respect to the initial evaluation (Table 52.3). Patients in both series were carefully selected, which is an important consideration that limits comparison of these results to survival of contemporary patients treated with radical cystectomy. Herr compared the survival of patients in his series with patients that fulfilled the same inclusion criteria but refused TURB and patients that preferred radical cystectomy.[28] The 10-year disease-specific survival was 76% in 99 patients that received TURB as definitive therapy (57% with bladder

**Table 52.2** Prospective studies of patients treated with TURB alone

| Series (year) | Herr 1987[25] | Solsona et al 1998[27] |
| --- | --- | --- |
| No. patients | 45 | 133 |
| No recurrence (%) | 9 (20) | 61 (45.8) |
| Recurrence: cT1A (%) | 21 (46.6) | 35 (26.2) |
| Progression (%) | 15 (33.3) | 37 (27.7) |
| cT≥2M0 | 13 (28.8) | 30 (22.4) |
| cT0M1 | 2 (4.4) | 7 (5.3) |
| Cancer-specific survival (%) | 37 (82.2) | 107 (80.5) |
| Bladder preservation (%) | 30 (67) | 100 (75.2) |
| Median follow-up | 5.1 (3–7 years) | 83 (11–183 months) |

**Table 52.3** 10-year outcome in prospective studies of TURB alone

| Series (year) | Herr (2001)[28] | Solsona (2004)* |
| --- | --- | --- |
| No. patients | 99 | 133 |
| Progression: T≥2- (%) | 34 (34) | 40 (30) |
| Cancer-specific survival (%) | 75 (76) | 106 (79.7) |
| Bladder preservation (%) | 57 (57) | 96 (72.1) |
| Cystectomy (%) | 34 (34) | 11 (8.9) |

\* Unpublished data, presented at the XXth Congress of the European Association of Urology 2005.

preserved) compared with 71% in 52 patients that had immediate cystectomy (p=0.3).

In Herr's series, of the 99 patients treated with TURB, 82% of 73 that had T0 on restaging TURB survived versus 57% of the 26 patients that had residual T1 tumor on restaging TURB (p=0.003).[28] Survival rates in patients that were P0 at cystectomy did not differ significantly between prospective studies of TURB (Table 52.4).

Of 133 patients in Solsona et al's series, 92 were followed for more than 15 years; 79 of these patients have died, 21 of tumor and 58 from intercurrent diseases.[27] The cause-specific survival was 77.2%, the progression rate was 31.5%, and the bladder preservation rate was 70.6% (Table 52.5). These figures strongly confirm the feasibility of TURB as monotherapy in a carefully selected group of patients with invasive bladder cancer. Although progression and recurrence occurred after 10 years, the negative impact on cause-specific survival was minimal.

**Table 52.4** Survival comparisons between patients with P0 at cystectomy and TURB alone (prospective studies)

| Author (reference) | No. pts | 5-year cancer-specific survival (%) |
|---|---|---|
| Radical cystectomy | | |
| Mathur[11] | 3 | 2 (67) |
| Brendler[10] | 13 | 12 (92.3) |
| Pagano[8] | 25 | 17 (67) |
| Thrasher[13] | 66 | 50 (75) |
| Stein[9] | 39 | 36 (92) |
| Total | 146 | 117 (8.1) |
| Radical TURB | | 10-year cancer-specific survival (%) |
| Herr[28] | 99 | 75 (76) |
| Solsona[27] | 133 | 106 (79.7) |
| Total | 232 | 181 (78.1) |

**Table 52.5** Prospective studies: 15-years' outcome

| No. patients | 92 |
|---|---|
| Overall survival (%) | 13 (14.1) |
| Cancer-specific survival (%) | 71 (77.2) |
| Patients lost for follow-up (%) | 9 (9.7) |
| Recurrence: T1A (%) | 29 (31.5) |
| Progression: T≥2- (%) | 29 (31.5) |
| Bladder preservation (%) | 65 (70.6) |
| Patients alive with bladder (%) | 12 (13) |

## JUSTIFICATION OF THE RESULTS IN THE PROSPECTIVE STUDIES

These excellent results may have occurred for several reasons. The Spanish approach to bladder preservation in patients with invasive bladder cancer clearly relies heavily on patient selection. As previously mentioned, patients with negative biopsies of the muscularis propria after a macroscopically complete TURB were included in a surveillance program. However, patients with positive biopsies of the muscularis propria of the tumor bed were usually treated with radical cystectomy. Since 1989, these patients have been offered cystectomy or three courses of cisplatin-based systemic chemotherapy in order to preserve the bladder. Of these patients, 64 chose cystectomy and 61 chose TURB plus systemic chemotherapy. A significantly higher survival rate was achieved in patients treated with radical TURB alone as compared to patients treated with more aggressive procedures—TURB plus systemic chemotherapy or cystectomy (Figure 52.1). This clearly reflects patient selection. These patients met the same inclusion criteria used in both studies. The presence or absence of residual

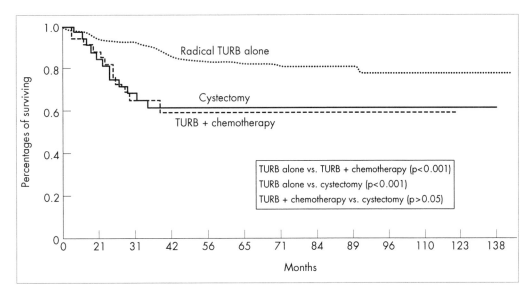

**Fig. 52.1**
Survival comparison between the three series of the bladder preservation programs.

cancer on the biopsies of the muscularis propria of the tumor bed was the single most important variable in decision making regarding treatment selection. Univariate and multivariate analyses were performed in order to determine how this and other variables affected survival outcomes (Table 52.6). On univariate analysis, morphology, biopsies of the tumor bed, and treatment selection were all statistically significant factors. However, on multivariate analysis, biopsy of the tumor bed was the only independent prognostic variable. Thus, biopsy of the muscularis propria of the tumor bed which is macroscopically free of tumor is an important prognostic factor that differentiates between two groups: one with a good prognosis (negative biopsies of muscularis propria) and the other with a poor prognosis (positive biopsies of muscularis propria). This is despite the use of the most radical therapies in the latter group, including systemic chemotherapy.

The key to good results achieved by radical TURB alone in prospective studies is close follow-up and patient selection. The most important factor is biopsy of the tumor bed which, when negative, selects a group of patients with a good prognosis, and confirms the radicality of the endoscopic tumor resection. The prognostic value of radical TURB was also corroborated in a recent review by Dunst et al[15] in bladder preservation programs using multimodal approaches.

## CONCERNS

Radical TURB in a very select group of patients with invasive bladder cancer can be a feasible alternative to cystectomy. All bladder preservation programs should provide long-term follow-up because patients remain at risk of disease progression throughout their lives. In series from Herr[28] and Solsona et al,[27] progression and recurrence developed after 5 and 10 years. With long-term follow-up many patients may die of causes that are not tumor related, and relapse percentages can be misleading. When at-risk patients were evaluated sequentially, the incidence rates of nonmuscle-invasive recurrence and progression were similar, with the highest proportion of events occurring during the first 3 years. Afterwards, the frequency dramatically decreased, but continued to occur up to 15 years. Patients developed distant metastases without local bladder tumor recurrence during the first 3 years. Thereafter, progression was due to invasive local recurrence (Table 52.7). This means that progression occurred primarily during the first 3 years, representing 67% of patients that progressed. Thereafter, the percentage was 17.5% in 3–5 years, 12.5% in 5–10 years, 2.5% in 10–15 years, and none after 15 years. According to these data, a strict follow-up schedule is proposed, including endoscopic evaluation every 3 months during the first 3 years due to the risk of recurrence during this period. Subsequent follow-up every 6 months is recommended up to the fifth year and then annually up to the tenth year. On the first endoscopic evaluations at 3 months, as well as in the second evaluation at 6 months, a new TURB of the scar tissue where the tumor was initially located is strongly recommended, along with routine urinary cytology, random biopsies, and bimanual examination in order to identify residual tumors. When these initial follow-up evaluations are negative, cystoscopy and

**Table 52.6** Prognostic factors for cancer-specific survival including 133 patients with negative biopsies of tumor bed treated with radical TURB alone and 125 patients with positive biopsies of the tumor bed, 61 treated with TURB plus chemotherapy and 64 with radical cystectomy

| Univariate analysis Variables incuded | Percentages | p value |
|---|---|---|
| Recurrent tumor (yes vs. no) | 26.3 vs. 24.1 | 0.6903 |
| Biopsies of tumor bed (positive vs. negative) | 33.6 vs. 20.3 | 0.0004 |
| Age (continuous) | 25.4 vs. 27.2 | 0.9716 |
| Grade (2 vs. 3) | 20 vs. 28.9 | 0.097 |
| Tumor morphology (papillary vs. sessile) | 21.2 vs. 29.5 | 0.0452 |
| Number of tumors (unique vs. multiple) | 25.1 vs. 34.3 | 0.4284 |
| Sex (women vs. men) | 43.1 vs. 25 | 0.1381 |
| Tumor size (≥3 cm vs. >3 cm) | 26.6 vs. 26.1 | 0.7421 |
| Bladder Tis associated (yes vs. no) | 31.9 vs. 25.6 | 0.3955 |
| Treatment: TURB alone vs. TURB + chemotherapy vs. Radical cystectomy | 20.3 vs. 36 31.2 | 0.0007 0.0015 |
| **Multivariate analysis Variables** | **p value** | **Exp (B)** |
| Biopsies of muscularis propria (tumor bed) | 0.0007 | 2.6423 |

**Table 52.7** Final outcome: sequential assessment

| | Minimum months of follow-up | | | | | | |
|---|---|---|---|---|---|---|---|
| | Initial (%) | ≥12 (%) | ≥24 (%) | ≥36 (%) | ≥60 (%) | ≥120 (%) | ≥180 (%) |
| Pts at risk | 130 | 132 | 128 | 118 | 98 | 50 | 17 |
| Progression | 40 (30) | 25 (18.9) | 22 (17.2) | 12 (10.1) | 6 (6.1) | 2 (4) | 0 |
| T≥2,M0 | 33 (24.8) | 19 (14.4) | 19 (14.8) | 12 (10.1) | 6 (6.1) | 2 (4) | 0 |
| T0,M1 | 7 (5.2) | 6 (4.5) | 3 (2.3) | 0 | 0 | 0 | 0 |
| Recurrence: T1A | 40 (30) | 26 (19.7) | 18 (12.7) | 15 (12.7) | 8 (8.1) | 8 (6) | 0 |

cytology can be performed in the outpatient clinic and biopsies performed if needed in response to abnormal results. In order to evaluate locoregional progression, CT scans and chest x-rays should be performed every 6 months for 3 years.

The greatest concern associated with this approach is the progression rate: 34% in Herr's series[28] and 32% in Solsona et al's series.[27] It is important to clarify that some patients were understaged (invasive recurrence at the 3-month evaluation) and other patients developed true progression (after a disease-free interval).

Attempting to address both problems, Solsona et al carried out univariate and multivariate analyses including clinical–pathologic variables (Table 52.8).[22] Regarding true progression, the presence of carcinoma in situ (CIS) was the only significant variable in the multivariate analysis. However, this variable was clinically irrelevant since the biologic behavior of CIS in these patients was similar to that in patients with nonmuscle-invasive bladder tumors associated with CIS. In consequence, the initial presence of CIS is not an exclusion criterion for patients with muscle-invasive bladder tumors included in a bladder preservation program of radical TURB, but these patients do need intravesical bacillus Calmette–Guérin (BCG) as adjuvant therapy. The recurrence rate of nonmuscle-

invasive bladder cancer was not very high in Solsona et al's and Herr's series and did not affect prognosis.[27,28] Therefore, intravesical therapy should be used only in patients with bladder-associated CIS and for patients that develop nonmuscle-invasive recurrences.

With respect to understaging, no single variable was statistically significant, but a relationship between tumor size and morphology was noted. Stratifying variables, such as tumor size of more than 3 cm and solid morphology had a close relationship to understaging, reaching statistical significance (p=0.0236). When the primary tumor had a papillary morphology, size had no prognostic value (p=0.647) following radical transurethral resection of bladder tumor (TURBT).[27] However, given the relationship with understaging, one must be very cautious about using radical TURB alone for patients with solid tumors of more than 3 cm.

In a separate analysis, p53 overexpression was tested in a pilot study of 60 patients in Solsona et al's series.[27] Among these patients, 10/18 (55.5%) with p53 overexpression and 16/42 (38%) with negative p53 developed progression. This difference was not statistically significant. Recently, Herr[28] observed a significantly superior local progression-free rate of 68% and survival of 82% in patients with no residual tumor

**Table 52.8** Predictive factors for progression differentiating between understaging (progression at 3-months' evaluation in the scar) and true progression (after a progression-free interval): univariate analysis

| Univariate analysis Variables | True progression percentages (p value) | Understanding percentages (p value) |
|---|---|---|
| Tumor size (≤3 cm vs. >3 cm) | 23.1 vs. 24.5 (0.813) | 1.9 vs. 8.5 (0.057) |
| Age (≤65 vs. >65 years) | 25 vs. 20.7 (0.791) | 7.5 vs. 3.7 (0.652) |
| Grade (2 vs. 3) | 20.3 vs. 26 (0.445) | 1.5 vs. 10.1 (0.117) |
| Tumor morphology (papillary vs. sessile) | 22.1 vs. 25 (0.517) | 3.9 vs. 9.6 (0.135) |
| No. tumors (unique vs. multiples) | 22.8 vs. 26.3 (0.968) | 6.1 vs. 5.5 (0.532) |
| Primary vs. recurrent tumors | 23.1 vs. 25 (0.698) | 6.8 vs. 0 (0.250) |
| Sex (women vs. men) | 13.9 vs. 18.7 (0.686) | 12.5 vs. 5.1 (0.072) |
| Bladder Tis (yes vs. no) | 17 vs. 42.4 (0.013) | 6.9 vs. 3.1 (0.346) |
| **Multivariate analysis: True progression** Variable | **p value** | **Exp (B)** |
| Bladder Tis | 0.026 | 2.27 |

(T0) upon repeat TURB versus 28% and 57%, respectively, in those with nonmuscle-invasive residual tumors (T1A). In summary, patients with invasive bladder cancer that are the best candidates for TURB as monotherapy are those patients with negative biopsies of the muscularis propria of the tumor bed or no residual tumor at repeat TURB after a macroscopically initial complete resection, regardless of size if the primary tumor is papillary, and less than 3 cm if the primary tumor is sessile.

Another concern is that some tumors might have been overstaged pathologically because of confusion between muscularis mucosae and muscularis propria. The histologic structures of muscularis mucosae and propria are different: smooth muscle fibers are associated with blood vessels in muscularis mucosae and thick muscle fibers in muscularis propria. However, in fragmented biopsies it is difficult to determine whether the smooth muscle present represents muscularis mucosae or muscularis propria. The necessary presence of muscularis propria with no tumor invasion in the third sample from the fractionated TURB as an inclusion criterion is crucial in the differentiation between both muscular structures. Pathologists can compare the histologic structure of the muscle fibers from the third sample clearly as muscularis propria and the second sample which should include muscle fibers infiltrated by tumor.

## COMMENTS

The importance of these prospective studies is that they have been able to identify a group of patients with muscle-invasive bladder tumors whose survival rates are approximately equivalent to those of patients with P0 in cystectomy specimens. This select group of patients represents 21% and 19%, respectively, of patients with invasive bladder tumors treated at the Memorial Sloan-Kettering Cancer Center and the Instituto Valenciano de Oncología.

Whether radiochemotherapy associated with radical TURB might improve the outcome of radical TURB is not entirely clear. One of the most important aims of radiochemotherapy in combination with TURB is to eliminate residual tumor after TURB. The incidence of negative biopsies indicating persistent muscle-invasive cancer at the initial 3-month follow-up in Solsona et al's series was 6.7%.[26] Therefore, only a modest number of patients may have benefited from additional radiation and chemotherapy, while all of these patients would have suffered the toxicity and long-term side effects of these radiochemotherapy programs. In fact, radio-chemotherapy programs have never been prospectively compared to radical TURB alone or to cystectomy.

In a recent meta-analysis the survival benefit of neoadjuvant chemotherapy programs was small but significant, i.e. 5%.[29]

The role of pelvic lymphadenectomy in this group of patients is also controversial. The incidence of lymph node metastases in patients with P2 ranges from 9.9% to 20%,[29,30-33] 12.6% in P2A tumors,[33] and from 0% to 5% in P0 tumors.[30,31] Because our patients are potentially those with P0 in the cystectomy specimen, the incidence of micrometastases in lymph nodes should be very low. This incidence could be included in the 5.2% of patients that develop distant metastases with no bladder-invasive recurrence and those with synchronous bladder tumors. Taking into account the low incidence of occult positive lymph nodes and that the 5-year survival rate ranges from 14% to 40% in cases of positive lymph nodes in patients treated with cystectomy and lymphadenectomy, in this selected group of invasive bladder cancer patients the potential survival benefit should be minimal, adding unnecessary morbidity in most of the patients.

## CONCLUSION

The key to success of radical TURB is careful patient selection according to very strict inclusion criteria based upon fractionated TURB performed in patients suspected of having invasive bladder tumors including those with large papillary tumors, tumors with thick papillae, or sessile tumors less than 3 cm, or using a second TURB after a complete initial TURB as selection criteria. A second TURB with no tumor in chips, or with negative biopsies on muscular layer and perivesical fat of tumor bed, supports the use of radical TURB as initial monotherapy.

Regardless of these very careful patient selections, with long-term follow-up the progression rate is high. Consequently, a strict follow-up schedule is mandatory, particularly during the first 3 years. At the first endoscopic evaluation, a TURB of the scar tissue where the initial tumor was located is essential in order to preclude understaging. This approach achieves similar cause-specific survival for patients with P0 on cystectomy specimen.

In summary, a small and select group of patients with invasive bladder cancer, identified by a second TURB with no tumor in chips or with negative biopsies of the muscular layer and perivesical fat of the tumor bed, can be treated with TURB as an initial monotherapy.

## REFERENCES

1. Kachnic LA, Kaufmann DS, Griffin FE, et al. Bladder preservation by combined modality therapy for invasive bladder cancer. J Clin Oncol 1997;15:1022–1029.

2. Rödel C, Grabenbauer GG, Kühn R, et al. Combined-modality treatment and selective organ preservation in invasive bladder cancer: long-term results. J Clin Oncol 2002;20:3061–3071.

3. Sternberg CN, Pansadoro V, Calabro F, et al. Can patient selection for bladder preservation be based on response to chemotherapy? Cancer 2003;97:1644–1652.

4. Barnes RW, Dick AL, Hadley HL, Johnston OL. Survival following transurethral resection of bladder carcinoma. Cancer Res 1977;37:2895–2897.

5. Milner WA. The role of conservative surgery in the treatment of bladder tumours. Br J Urol 1954;26:375.

6. Dalbagni G, Genega E, Hashibe M, et al. Cystectomy for bladder cancer: a contemporary series. J Urol 2001;165:1111–1116.

7. Frazier HA, Robertson JE, Dodge RK, Paulson DF. The value of pathological factors in predicting cancer-specific survival among patients treated with radical cystectomy for transitional cell carcinoma of the bladder and prostate. Cancer 1993;71:3993–4001.

8. Pagano F, Bassi P, Galetti TP, et al. Results of contemporary radical cystectomy for invasive bladder cancer: a clinicopathological study with an emphasis on the inadequacy of the tumor, nodes, and metastasis classification. J Urol 1991;145:45–50.

9. Stein JP, Lieskovsky G, Cote R, et al. Radical cystectomy in the treatment of invasive bladder cancer: long-term results in 1054 patients. J Clin Oncol 2001;19:666–675.

10. Brendler C, Steinberg GD, Marshall FF, Mostwin JL, Walsh PC. Local recurrence and survival following nerve-sparing radical cystoprostatectomy. J Urol 1990;144:1137–1140.

11. Mathur VK, Krahn HP, Ramsey EW. Total cystectomy for bladder cancer. J Urol 1981;125:784–786.

12. Stein JP, Freeman JA, Boyd SD, et al. Radical cystectomy in the treatment of invasive bladder cancer: long-term results in a large group of patients. J Urol 1998;159:213.

13. Thrasher JB, Frazier HA, Robertson JE, Paulson DF. Does stage pT0 cystectomy specimen confer a survival advantage in patients with minimally invasive bladder cancer? J Urol 1994;152:393–396.

14. Fung CY, Shipley WU, Young RH, et al. Prognostic factors in invasive bladder carcinoma in a prospective trial of preoperative adjuvant chemotherapy and radiotherapy. J Clin Oncol 1991;9:1533–1542.

15. Dunst J, Rodel C, Zietman A, Schrott KM, Sauer R, Shipley WU. Bladder preservation in muscle-invasive bladder cancer by conservative surgery and radiochemotherapy. Semin Surg Oncol 2001;20:24–32.

16. Fossa SD, Waehre H, Aass N, Jacobsen AB, Olsen DR, Ous S. Bladder cancer definitive radiation therapy of muscle-invasive bladder cancer. A retrospective analysis of 317 patients. Cancer 1993;72:3036–3043.

17. Gospodarowicz MK, Hawkins NV, Rawlings GA, et al. Radical radiotherapy for muscle invasive transitional cell carcinoma of the bladder: failure analysis. J Urol 1989;142:1488–1453.

18. Holmäng S, Hedelin H, Anderstrom C, Johansson SL. Long-term followup of all patients with muscle invasive (stages T2, T3 and T4) bladder carcinoma in a geographical region. J Urol 1997;158:389–392.

19. Henry K, Miller J, Mori M, Loening S, Fallon B. Comparison of transurethral resection to radical therapies for stage B bladder tumors. J Urol 1988;140:964–967.

20. Barnes RW, Bergman RT, Hadley HL, Love D. Control of bladder tumors by endoscopic surgery. J Urol 1967;97:864.

21. Flocks RH. Treatment of patients with carcinoma of the bladder. JAMA 1951;145:295–301.

22. Kondas J, Vaczi L, Scecso L, Konder G. Transurethral resection for muscle-invasive bladder cancer. Int Urol Nephrol 1993;25:557–567.

23. O'Flynn JD, Smith JD, Hanson JS. Transurethral resection for the assessment and treatment of vesical neoplasms. A review of 800 consecutive cases. Eur Urol 1975;1:38.

24. Marderbacher S, Hochreiter W, Bukhard F, Thalmenn GN, Danuse H, Studer U. Radical cystectomy for bladder cancer today—a homogeneous series without neo-adjuvant therapy. J Clin Oncol 2003;21:690–696.

25. Herr HW. Conservative treatment of muscle-infiltrating bladder cancer prospective experience. J Urol 1987;138:1162–1163.

26. Solsona E, Iborra I, Ricós JV, Monrós JL, Dumont R. Feasibility of transurethral resection for muscle-infiltrating carcinoma of the bladder: prospective study. J Urol 1992;147:1513.

27. Solsona E, Iborra I, Ricós JV, Monrós JL, Casanova J, Calabuig C. Feasibility of transurethral resection for muscle infiltrating carcinoma of the bladder: long-term followup of a prospective study. J Urol 1998;159:95–98; discussion 98–99.

28. Herr HW. Transurethral resection of muscle-invasive bladder cancer: 10-year outcome. J Clin Oncol 2001;19:89–93.

29. (No authors) Neoadjuvant chemotherapy in invasive bladder cancer: a systematic review and meta-analysis. Lancet 2003;361:1927–1934.

30. Lerner SP, Skinner DG, Lieskovsky G, et al. The rationale for en bloc pelvic lymph node dissection for bladder cancer patients with nodal metastases: long-term results. J Urol 1993;149:758–764; discussion 764–765.

31. Poulsen AL, Horn T, Steven K. Radical cystectomy extending the limits of pelvic lymph node dissection improves survival for patients with bladder confined to the bladder wall. J Urol 1998;160:2015–2020.

32. Vieweg J, Gschwend JE, Herr HW, Fair WR. Pelvic lymph node dissection can be curative in patients with node positive bladder cancer. J Urol 1999;161:449–454.

33. Leissner J, Hohenfellner R, Thuroff JW, Wolf HK. Lymphadenectomy in patients with transitional cell carcinoma of the urinary bladder; significance for staging and prognosis. BJU Int 2000;85:817–823.

# Partial cystectomy 53

*Yair Lotan, David A Swanson, Arthur I Sagalowsky*

## INTRODUCTION

Bladder cancer is the fourth most common cancer in men (6%) and the tenth most common cancer in women (2%), accounting in men for 3% of cancer deaths in the year 2004 in the US.[1] On average, 15% to 30% of all patients with bladder cancer are diagnosed with muscle-invasive tumors and radical cystectomy represents the gold standard therapy.[2] In an effort to reduce the morbidity of radical cystectomy, attempts have been made to utilize bladder-preserving therapy such as aggressive transurethral resection (TUR) followed by combined chemotherapy/radiotherapy or partial cystectomy. The advantage of partial cystectomy over TUR is that it allows for complete pathologic staging of the tumor and pelvic lymph nodes with preservation of normal bladder and sexual function. The popularity of this procedure peaked in the 1950s and 1960s, but reports in the 1970s emphasized the problems, particularly high recurrence rates. Unfortunately, partial cystectomy virtually disappeared thereafter, despite the fact that good results are possible, even with T2 and T3 tumors. Many of the recurrences were due, not to incomplete removal of tumor, but to the appearance of new tumors, suggesting that patient selection is critically important to the potential for success of partial cystectomy.[3-7]

Although partial cystectomy can be performed when adequate transurethral biopsy cannot be confidently performed because of location or other considerations, and it may be appropriate as palliative therapy in highly selected patients instead of radical cystectomy, our discussion in this chapter will focus on its potential to provide definitive therapy for transitional carcinoma of the bladder.

## INDICATIONS

As stated, the most important factor in performing a successful partial cystectomy is proper patient selection. Bladder cancer is an aggressive disease that places the entire urothelium at risk. Once it metastasizes, treatment options such as radical cystectomy, radiotherapy, and systemic chemotherapy do not significantly change the overall survival rates.[8,9] Accordingly, the best opportunity to cure patients of their disease is offering the appropriate treatment at the start of therapy. In fact, a review of the literature concluded that only 5.8% to 18.9% of patients with muscle-invasive bladder cancer were suited for partial cystectomy, and that would be considered too permissive by many.[10] Another study evaluating initial management of all stages of bladder cancer in Canada found that only 3.5% of cases underwent partial cystectomy or open excision as their initial treatment.[11] At The University of Texas M.D. Anderson Cancer Center, 842 radical cystectomies were performed between January 1982 and January 1993. In that same period, 36 patients (4.1% of all patients requiring extirpative surgery) underwent partial cystectomy as a planned procedure, selected with intent to cure, because radical cystectomy was deemed unnecessary to remove all tumor.

In well-selected patients, partial cystectomy offers outcomes equivalent to those of radical cystectomy. Early recurrences are due to incomplete tumor excision, either because of unrecognized tumor or inadequate surgical margins. Conceptually, radical cystectomy is simply a partial cystectomy with the widest possible margins! New tumors in the remnant bladder, obviously an argument for removing the entire bladder, can be minimized by selecting patients with a solitary tumor and no antecedent history of prior transitional carcinoma of the bladder. Candidates for partial cystectomy should have a solitary lesion in the mobile portion of the bladder (particularly the dome and posterior wall) where it is possible to resect the tumor with a margin of at least 2 cm. As such, larger lesions increase the difficulty of complete resection with negative margins and there is a practical limit to the size of lesion that will allow for a partial cystectomy. While the need for ureteral reimplantation can increase the difficulty of the procedure, it is not an absolute contraindication.[12] Although there is no intrinsic reason for not permitting ureteral reimplantation, it is a strong relative contraindication because it provides an added check that the tumor is located in an appropriate position to ensure success. The surgeon will not be tempted to offer it to patients whose tumor is on the bladder base (where the results have been historically poorer), and will not be tempted to 'cheat' and take <2 cm margin of normal mucosa around the tumor to avoid reimplanting the ureter. Evaluation should be performed either cystoscopically or with random bladder biopsies to confirm that all other areas in the bladder have normal mucosa. Furthermore, patients should have a good bladder capacity with a normally functioning bladder.

Those patients with urachal adenocarcinomas, or tumors in bladder diverticula, represent special categories of patients that may specifically benefit from partial cystectomy. Some previous reports also recommended partial cystectomy for tumors that are inaccessible to TUR or large enough to make TUR technically difficult.[12] However, as stated earlier, if partial cystectomy is being offered to such patients, they should fulfill the other criteria of first tumor, solitary tumor, and tumor located where it is possible to achieve a 2 cm margin. Sternberg et al recommended using response to chemotherapy as the basis for selecting patients for partial cystectomy.[13] Only those patients that attained a complete or partial response to combination chemotherapy (methotrexate, vinblastine, adriamycin (doxorubicin), and cisplatin: MVAC) with solitary lesions in favorable anatomic locations were eligible for partial cystectomy but the results were reasonably good. Similarly, Herr and Scher recommended somewhat expanding the indications for performing partial cystectomy in patients that responded well to neoadjuvant chemotherapy.[14]

The main contraindications to partial cystectomy include the presence of carcinoma in situ (CIS) and multifocal disease, as well as a history of prior tumors. The risk of developing recurrence increases with the presence of multicentric disease (p<0.03) and when neoplasm is found at the margin of resection (p<0.05).[3,15]

## CANCER IN BLADDER DIVERTICULUM

Because of the absence of a muscular layer, resection of cancer in a bladder diverticulum is difficult and carries a high risk of perforation. These cancers are also prone to early metastases.[16–18] Partial cystectomy offers a good treatment option for patients with isolated tumors in a diverticulum or those difficult to resect. It is important that they fulfill the other criteria for a partial cystectomy including a solitary lesion with negative random biopsies, no prior history of bladder tumors, and the ability to achieve a 2 cm negative margin. Furthermore, partial cystectomy is not ideal for large high-grade or invasive tumor, as the most important predictor of outcome is the stage of the tumor.[19] In order to improve outcomes, Garzotto et al recommended combining partial cystectomy with chemotherapy or radiation therapy.[20] Unfortunately, there are no randomized trials comparing combination therapies with partial cystectomy due to the infrequent nature of cancers in bladder diverticula.

## NON-TRANSITIONAL CELL CARCINOMA

Partial cystectomy has been utilized successfully for management of nontransitional cell carcinoma of the bladder. A multitude of case reports describe the use of partial cystectomy for benign lesions such as leiomyoma,[21] inflammatory pseudotumor,[22] neurofibroma,[23] pheochromocytoma,[24] and paragangliomas.[25] While partial cystectomy has been used for treatment of bladder sarcomas, recurrences have been reported, and these tumors should be widely excised.[26,27]

Partial cystectomy can also be necessary[27] in cases with non-urologic malignancies such as locally advanced colorectal carcinoma. If clear margins are achievable then those patients can have good local control without sacrificing survival.[28,29]

## ADENOCARCINOMA AND URACHAL TUMORS

Adenocarcinomas of the bladder are rare and often aggressive cancers. They can be primary or urachal in origin.[30] In one of the largest series of adenocarcinoma of the bladder (n=185), el-Mekresh and colleagues found an overall 5-year disease-free survival of 55%.[31] Only three factors had a significant impact on survival: the tumor pathologic stage, grade of the tumor, and lymph node involvement. They recommended radical cystectomy over partial cystectomy in managing these tumors. While partial cystectomy was appropriate for some patients, Xiaoxu et al also found poor 3-year survival rates (33%) after partial cystectomy for primary adenocarcinoma of the bladder.[32]

There is generally less controversy about performing partial cystectomy for urachal tumors, in large part because they commonly appear in a location where the procedure is technically possible. In evaluating the surgical management of urachal tumors at the Mayo Clinic, Henly et al found that these cancers comprised only 0.22% of bladder cancers diagnosed at their institution over a 35-year period.[33] They found no difference in 5-year survival of patients with partial and those with radical cystectomy (43% and 50%, respectively). They attributed the low survival to the aggressiveness of the disease. Herr recommended performing an extended partial cystectomy, including complete excision of the umbilicus, overlying peritoneum, and posterior rectus fascia lateral to the medial obliterated umbilical ligaments.[34] He found that 10 of 12 patients were free of disease at 1–13 years with no recurrences in bladder or pelvis. Santucci and coauthors also found that 88% of patients (n=16) with well-differentiated colonic-type adenocarcinomas of the urachus were cured by partial cystectomy.[35]

## PREOPERATIVE CONSIDERATIONS

The main objective of preoperative evaluation is proper staging of the bladder tumor. Cystoscopy with random bladder biopsy can help exclude patients with multifocal disease or CIS. Bimanual examination under anesthesia allows for evaluation of the extent of tumor involvement and bladder mobility. When there is a concern regarding bladder function, an evaluation of bladder capacity is in order. Preoperative testing should include a computed tomography (CT) scan and chest radiograph to look for evidence of metastatic disease. The overall health of the patient should also be assessed in determining appropriateness of surgical intervention.

## SURGICAL TECHNIQUE

The surgical technique has been well described elsewhere.[10,36,37] The main objectives include:

1. bilateral pelvic lymphadenectomy
2. full mobilization of the bladder with ligation of the superior vesical artery on the affected side or the vas deferens, if necessary
3. identification of the tumor either cystoscopically or through a small vertical cystotomy in order to avoid cutting across tumor
4. excision of the tumor with a clear 2 cm margin of normal bladder

5. watertight closure of the bladder and pelvic drain. A Foley catheter is preferred over a suprapubic tube due to the risk of spilling tumor cells into the pelvis or along the suprapubic tube tract.

One of us (DAS) believes strongly that the procedure should be done extraperitoneally.

After mobilizing the anterior and lateral aspects of the bladder, the surgeon should peel the parietal peritoneum from the bladder with blunt and sharp dissection, leaving the peritoneum attached only over the area adjacent to the tumor (Fig. 53.1). Next, the peritoneum is cut so that a patch is left adherent to the bladder overlying the tumor. The peritoneal defect is closed, and the peritoneum and contents are packed out of the way, converting the remainder of the operation to an extravesical one before the cystotomy is performed.

Of concern during partial cystectomy is recurrence of disease in the wound or pelvis secondary to spillage of tumor cells during surgery. Recurrence rates range from 0% to 40% and can lead to significant morbidity and mortality (Table 53.1). While most authors recommend only carefully packing the pelvis to prevent tumor spill from the bladder, that approach protects the pelvis better than the wound, and several other techniques have been advocated. In one approach, the area of tumor is identified endoscopically, and clamps (e.g. Pean or Satinsky) are used to isolate the area of bladder that is to be excised. The tumor is removed and the cut edge is oversewn without opening the bladder.[38] During this maneuver, one surgeon identifies the tumor cystoscopically while the other places clamps that

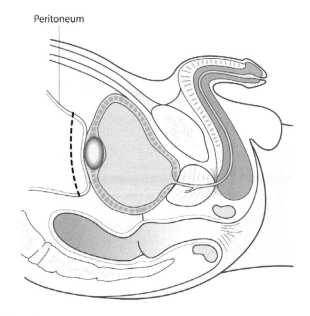

Peritoneum

**Fig. 53.1**
The appearance after dissecting the peritoneum off the bladder except for that portion overlying the tumor. The peritoneum is then opened (dashed line), a peritoneal patch left attached to the bladder over the tumor, and the peritoneal defect closed.

**Table 53.1** Partial cystectomy series with operative mortality and recurrence rates

| Authors | Years of accrual | No. pts | Operative mortality (%) | Overall recurrence (%) | Wound recurrence (%) | Bladder recurrence (%) |
|---|---|---|---|---|---|---|
| Dandekar et al[42] | 1984–1993 | 32 | 3.1 | 43.8 | 0 | 43.8% (n=14/32); Bladder (n=12/32); Superficial (n=5); Invasive (n=7); Distant (n=2) |
| Kaneti[15] | 25 years | 62 | 1.6 | 38.0 | NA | 41 patients received postoperative XRT, only 1 needed cystectomy |
| Lindahl et al[12] | 1958–1978 | 55 | 7.3 | 58.0 | NA | NA |
| Schoborg et al[44] | 1955–1975 | 45 | 4.4 | 70.0 | NA | NA |
| Faysal & Freiha[7] | 1962–1977 | 117 | 0.0 | 78.0 | 3.4 | 54 patients received XRT; 14 patients had cystectomy and 9 had salvage cystectomy |
| Merrell et al[47] | 1958–1973 | 54 | NA | 29.0 | NA | 10 had XRT and 2 had cystectomy |
| Brannan et al[48] | 1950–1974 | 49 | 2.0 | NA | 0 | 12 patients received XRT with 5 receiving salvage cystectomy |
| Cummings et al[4] | 1945–1971 | 101 | 0.0 | 49.0 | NA | NA |
| Novick & Stewart[3] | 1960–1972 | 50 | 0.0 | 50 (n=25) | NA | 15 patients had pelvic recurrence or metastases |
| Evans & Texter[49] | 25 years | 47 | 0.0 | NA | NA | 10 patients with repeat partial cystectomy and 8 patients requiring cystectomy |
| Utz et al[5] | 1945–1965 | 153 | 3.0 | NA | 2 | 50 |
| Resnick & O'Conor[6] | 1955–1965 | 102 | NA | 75.6 | 7.8 | Overall (75.6%); resection margin recurrence (29.4%) |
| Long et al[50] | 1940–1971 | 27 | 20.0 | NA | 40 | NA |
| Magri[43] | 1952–1959 | 104 | 9.6 | 32.7 | 11.5 | 21.2 |

NA, not applicable; XRT, radiotherapy.

exclude the tumor with a 2 cm margin. Two sets of clamps are used with one closing the normal bladder and the other closing the tumor side. This prevents spillage of cancer cells as the tumor is excised. Other recommendations include the instillation of intravesical chemotherapy such as mitomycin C into the bladder prior to beginning the procedure to reduce the number of viable cancer cells.[38] While the evidence for benefit of such an approach is sparse, mitomycin C has been shown to prevent bladder tumor cell implantation and reduce recurrence of superficial bladder cancers.[39–41] One caveat, however, is that it is important to irrigate the bladder carefully before opening it to prevent systemic absorption of the intravesical agent.

Urinary leakage from the bladder closure is not infrequent and can usually be managed conservatively.[36,42] Other complications include wound infection, which rarely can lead to sepsis. Cases of bladder wall necrosis leading to vesicocutaneous fistulas and peritonitis have also been reported, but not recently.[12] When the ureter has been reimplanted, ureteric fistulae and ureteral anastomotic strictures have occurred.[15]

Decreased bladder capacity can cause problems with bladder function. Cummings et al found that 18% (19/101) of their patients experienced compromised bladder function with significant irritative symptoms, with five patients requiring palliative diversion.[4]

## POSTOPERATIVE COMPLICATIONS

Complications after partial cystectomy can be divided into those that occur perioperatively (<30 days) and those that appear long term (>30 days). Operative mortality is less than 5% in most large series but has been reported as high as 20% (see Table 53.1). These series are not contemporary, however, and there is no reason to believe the mortality should be any higher than for radical cystectomy, and is probably lower.

## FOLLOW-UP AND OUTCOMES

The use of perioperative radiation therapy as an adjuvant to partial cystectomy has been shown to improve survival in some series[43] but to have no benefit in others.[5,6] It should be emphasized, however, that most of the papers discussing preoperative radiation therapy were written in an era when this approach was common, if not standard, for patients undergoing extirpative surgery for bladder cancer—including radical cystectomy. One difficulty in assessing benefits of adjuvant radiation therapy is the significant selection bias in treating those patients more likely to have recurrence[4,5,44] as well as treating patients only after they show evidence of local recurrence.[6] The important fact to remember is that it is possible to perform partial cystectomy safely after preoperative doses up to 5000 cGy, and possibly higher, as long as the bladder volume is sufficient. Even after 5000 cGy, the bladder will usually expand with time to approach normal volumes, although this is less likely after higher preoperative doses.

Patients with bladder cancer undergoing partial cystectomy require close monitoring. Overall recurrence rates have been reported from 29% to 78% (see Table 53.1). Most recurrences are new tumors and occur in the bladder secondary to the multifocal nature of bladder cancer. Consequently, cystoscopy and cytology should

be continued at 3-month intervals for at least 2 years, and then at appropriate intervals thereafter on a schedule similar to that for tumors managed endoscopically.[36] Unfortunately, patients may experience distant metastases, especially with high-grade and high-stage tumors, and regular CT scans of the abdomen and pelvis, plus chest x-rays, are recommended.

Survival for patients with bladder cancer who undergo partial cystectomy depends on the grade and stage of the tumor (Table 53.2). Overall, 5-year survival ranging from 40% to 80% has been reported in various series and depends on the stage distribution of bladder cancer in the study cohort. Patients with low-grade and low-stage tumors have the best overall survival.[12] It should be emphasized, however, that even T2 and T3 tumors can be controlled with partial cystectomy if all tumor is excised. For adverse prognostic features such as extensive

**Table 53.2** Partial cystectomy series with 5- and 10-year survival rates

| Authors | No. pts | 5-year survival (overall (%) | A | B1 | B2 | C | D | 10-year survival |
|---|---|---|---|---|---|---|---|---|
| Dandekar et al[42] | 32 | 80.1 | | T2=100% (n=5) | T3a=88.5% (n=18) | T3b=45.7% (n=9) | | NA |
| Kaneti[15] | 62 | 50.0 | 0–A=68% (n=15/23) | B=40% (n=8/20) | | 33% (n=26) | 0% (n=0/3) | 22 |
| Lindahl et al[12] | 55 | 47.1 | | | | | | 35.4 |
| Schoborg et al[44] | 45 | NA | 0–A=69% (n=9/13) | 29% (n=2/7) | 50% (n=3/6) | 12% (n=2/17) | 100% (n=1/1) | 0–A=37% (n=3/8); B1=0% (n=0/5); B2=20% (n=1/5); C=0% (n=0/15); D=0% (n=0/1) |
| Faysal & Freiha[7] | 117 | 40.0 | 58% (n=7/12) | 29% (n=4/14) | 32% (n=8/25) | 7% (n=1/15) | 0% (n=0/2) | NA |
| Merrell et al[47] | 54 | 48.0 | | 67% (n=21) | 37% (n=16) | 25% (n=8) | 0% (n=5) | Overall=30%; B1=33% (n=18); B2=25% (n=12); C=0% (n=2); D=0% (n=3) |
| Brannan et al[48] | 49 | 57.7 | 68.8% (n=11/16) | 54.5% (n=6/11) | 62.5% (n=5/8) | 33% (n=3/9) | | Overall=32.4%; A=45.5% (n=5/11); B1=44.4% (n=4/9); B2=20% (n=1/5); C=11% (n=1/9) |
| Cummings et al[4] | 101 | 60 | 79% (n=23/29) | 80% (n=17/21) | 45% (n=10/22) | 6% (n=1/17) | | NA |
| Novick & Stewart[3] | 50 | NA | 67% (n=10/15) | B=53% (n=8/15) | | 17% (n=1/6) | 25% (n=1/4) | A=67% (n=4/6); B=44% (n=4/9); C=0% (n=0/3); D=0% (n=0/4) |
| Evans & Texter[49] | 47 | 46.7 | 68% (n=17/26) | 42% (n=3/7) | 14% (n=1/7) | 0% (n=0/7) | | NA |
| Utz et al[5] | 153 | 43.3 | 68% (n=17/26) | 47% (n=18/38) | 40% (n=14/35) | 29% (n=11/38) | 0% (n=0/19) | NA |
| Resnick & O'Conor[6] | 102 | 41.9 | 70.7% (n=17/24) | 76.9% (n=10/13) | 18.3% (n=3/16) | 13% (n=2/7) | 20% (n=1/5) | NA |
| Long et al[50] | 27 | NA | 75% (n=6) | 48% (n=7) | 23% (n=5) | 11% (n=11) | | NA |
| Magri[43] | 104 | 41.8 | Ta=80% (8/10) | T2=38.4% (10/26) | | T3=26.3% (5/19) | | NA |

NA, not applicable.

invasion of the perivesical fat or nodal metastases, adjuvant chemotherapy is appropriate, as it would be if the patient had undergone a radical cystectomy.

The experience at the M.D. Anderson Cancer Center illustrates the potential efficacy of partial cystectomy for muscle-invasive tumors. From January 1982 through July 1996, 24 patients with muscle-invasive tumors (transitional cell carcinoma 23, squamous cell carcinoma 1) underwent partial cystectomy as definitive therapy with intent to cure. There were 13 patients with T2, four with T3a, and seven with T3b tumors. With a median follow-up of 36 months (range 6–165), of 17 patients with no bladder recurrences, four died of intercurrent disease, and two of metastatic bladder cancer. Eleven patients were alive, although, in truth, three patients were at risk for recurrence for <12 months. Seven patients had recurrent tumors in their bladder remnants:

- two were treated with TUR-BT ± Bacillus Calmette–Guérin (BCG) and remain clinically free of disease (NED)
- two were NED after delayed radical cystectomy
- one received MVAC adjuvant chemotherapy for N1 disease with good response
- two patients, however, died of metastatic disease after late recurrence.

Patient P.L.M. received five courses of adjuvant MVAC after partial cystectomy for pT3b tumor with vascular invasion. He had a grade 2 Ta solitary recurrence 33 months after partial cystectomy, and a grade 3 T1 recurrence 8 months after that. Evaluation soon afterwards revealed metastases to lungs, bones, adrenal gland, and retroperitoneal lymph nodes, and he died 43 months after his original surgery.

Patient J.E.H. underwent partial cystectomy for T3b tumor, followed by five courses of CISCA (cisplatin, cyclophosphamide (Cytoxan), adriamycin). He did well until 89 months later at which time he had a grade 3 T1 recurrence, which was treated with TUR-BT and BCG. Fifty months later, his cytology became positive, and he was found to have transitional cell carcinoma in the prostatic ducts and stroma, with positive pelvic lymph nodes found on CT scan. He underwent salvage chemotherapy and became clinically NED; TUR biopsy of the prostate revealed only a single focus of transitional cell carcinoma in the prostatic ducts. However, salvage surgery was delayed for medical reasons and he developed bony metastases 156 months after his partial cystectomy. He died of disease shortly thereafter.

## CONCLUSION

Considering the relatively poor survival outcomes for patients with partial cystectomy historically, it can be concluded that patient selection is critical in determining the best treatment course for patients with invasive bladder cancer. Bladder preservation with partial cystectomy and combined therapy, either neoadjuvant or adjuvant chemotherapy, or possibly combined trimodality surgery–chemotherapy–radiation therapy, may improve survival outcomes in selected patients.[13,14,45,46] It is apparent that some patients, even with T2 or T3 tumors if solitary and without prior history of bladder cancer, can be treated successfully with partial cystectomy with or without adjuvant therapy, but they are still at risk of developing recurrent bladder cancer. Although many of the recurrences will be superficial and potentially manageable endoscopically, some will be invasive and some patients may develop metastatic disease. It is *critically* important that all patients treated for T2 or T3 disease with partial cystectomy be followed with regular cystoscopies and urinary cytologies for their *lifetimes*. If invasive disease occurs, delayed radical cystectomy is the most conservative approach. Nonetheless, with the appropriate caveats, partial cystectomy can be effective therapy for 3% to 4% of patients that need extirpative surgery for bladder cancer, and many patients are very grateful for the opportunity to preserve normal bladder and sexual function.

## REFERENCES

1. Jemal A, Tiwari RC, Murray T, et al. Cancer statistics, 2004. CA Cancer J Clin 2004;54:8–29.
2. Lerner SP, Skinner E, Skinner DG. Radical cystectomy in regionally advanced bladder cancer. Urol Clin North Am 1992;19:713–723.
3. Novick AC, Stewart BH. Partial cystectomy in the treatment of primary and secondary carcinoma of the bladder. J Urol 1976;116:570–574.
4. Cummings KB, Mason JT, Correa RJ Jr, Gibbons RP. Segmental resection in the management of bladder carcinoma. J Urol 1978;119:56–58.
5. Utz DC, Schmitz SE, Fugelso PD, Farrow GM. Proceedings: a clinicopathologic evaluation of partial cystectomy for carcinoma of the urinary bladder. Cancer 1973;32:1075–1077.
6. Resnick MI, O'Conor VJ Jr. Segmental resection for carcinoma of the bladder: review of 102 patients. J Urol 1973;109:1007–1010.
7. Faysal MH, Freiha FS. Evaluation of partial cystectomy for carcinoma of bladder. Urology 1979;14:352–356.
8. Borden LS Jr, Clark PE, Hall MC. Bladder cancer. Curr Opin Oncol 2003;15:227–233.
9. Pashos CL, Botteman MF, Laskin BL, Redaelli A. Bladder cancer: epidemiology, diagnosis, and management. Cancer Pract 2002;10:311–322.
10. Sweeney P, Kursh ED, Resnick MI. Partial cystectomy. Urol Clin North Am 1992;19:701–711.
11. Hayter CR, Paszat LF, Groome PA, Schulze K, Mackillop WJ. The management and outcome of bladder carcinoma in Ontario, 1982–1994. Cancer 2000;89:142–151.
12. Lindahl F, Jorgensen D, Egvad K. Partial cystectomy for transitional cell carcinoma of the bladder. Scand J Urol Nephrol 1984;18:125–129.
13. Sternberg CN, Pansadoro V, Calabro F, et al. Can patient selection for bladder preservation be based on response to chemotherapy? Cancer 2003;97:1644–1652.
14. Herr HW, Scher HI. Neoadjuvant chemotherapy and partial cystectomy for invasive bladder cancer. J Clin Oncol 1994;12:975–980.

15. Kaneti J. Partial cystectomy in the management of bladder carcinoma. Eur Urol 1986;12:249–252.

16. Das S, Amar A D. Vesical diverticulum associated with bladder carcinoma: therapeutic implications. J Urol 1986;136:1013–1014.

17. Yu CC, Huang JK, Lee YH, Chen KK, Chen MT, Chang LS. Intradiverticular tumors of the bladder: surgical implications—an eleven-year review. Eur Urol 1993;24:190–196.

18. Melekos MD, Asbach HW, Barbalias GA. Vesical diverticula: etiology, diagnosis, tumorigenesis, and treatment. Analysis of 74 cases. Urology 1987;30:453–457.

19. Golijanin D, Yossepowitch O, Beck SD, Sogani P, Dalbagni G. Carcinoma in a bladder diverticulum: presentation and treatment outcome. J Urol 2003;170:1761–1764.

20. Garzotto MG, Tewari A, Wajsman Z. Multimodal therapy for neoplasms arising from a vesical diverticulum. J Surg Oncol 1996;62:46.

21. Sakellariou P, Protopapas A, Kyritsis N, Voulgaris Z, Papaspirou E, Diakomanolis E. Intramural leiomyoma of the bladder. Eur Radiol 2000;10:906–908.

22. Poon KS, Moreira O, Jones EC, Treissman S, Gleave ME. Inflammatory pseudotumor of the urinary bladder: a report of five cases and review of the literature. Can J Urol 2001;8:1409–1415.

23. Cheng L, Scheithauer BW, Leibovich BC, et al. Neurofibroma of the urinary bladder. Cancer 1999;86:505–513.

24. Kozlowski PM, Mihm F, Winfield HN. Laparoscopic management of bladder pheochromocytoma. Urology 2001;57:365.

25. Cheng L, Leibovich BC, Cheville JC, et al. Paraganglioma of the urinary bladder: can biologic potential be predicted? Cancer 2000;88:844–852.

26. Iczkowski KA, Shanks JH, Gadaleanu V, et al. Inflammatory pseudotumor and sarcoma of urinary bladder: differential diagnosis and outcome in thirty-eight spindle cell neoplasms. Mod Pathol 2001;14:1043–1051.

27. Martin SA, Sears DL, Sebo TJ, Lohse CM, Cheville JC. Smooth muscle neoplasms of the urinary bladder: a clinicopathologic comparison of leiomyoma and leiomyosarcoma. Am J Surg Pathol 2002;26:292–300.

28. Balbay MD, Slaton JW, Trane N, Skibber J, Dinney CP. Rationale for bladder-sparing surgery in patients with locally advanced colorectal carcinoma. Cancer 1999;86:2212–2216.

29. Weinstein RP, Grob BM, Pachter EM, Soloway S, Fair WR. Partial cystectomy during radical surgery for nonurological malignancy. J Urol 2001;166:79–81.

30. Burnett AL, Epstein JI, Marshall FF. Adenocarcinoma of urinary bladder: classification and management. Urology 1991;37:315–321.

31. el-Mekresh MM, el-Baz MA, Abol-Enein H, Ghoneim MA. Primary adenocarcinoma of the urinary bladder: a report of 185 cases. Br J Urol 1998;82:206–216.

32. Xiaoxu L, Jianhong L, Jinfeng W, Klotz LH. Bladder adenocarcinoma: 31 reported cases. Can J Urol 2001;8(5):1380–1383.

33. Henly DR, Farrow GM, Zincke H. Urachal cancer: role of conservative surgery. Urology 1993;42:635–639.

34. Herr HW. Urachal carcinoma: the case for extended partial cystectomy. J Urol 1994;151:365–366.

35. Santucci RA, True LD, Lange PH. Is partial cystectomy the treatment of choice for mucinous adenocarcinoma of the urachus? Urology 1997;49:536–540.

36. Jiminez VK, Marshall FF. Surgery of bladder cancer. In Walsh PC, Retik AB, Stamey TA, Vaughan (eds): Campbell's Urology. Philadelphia: Saunders, 2002, p 2841.

37. Boileau MA. Segmental or partial cystectomy. In Johnson DE, Boileau MA (eds): Genitourinary Tumors: Fundamental Principles and Surgical Techniques. New York: Grune & Stratton, 1982, p 457.

38. Haddad FS. Partial cystectomy for bladder cancer. A new technique. Urology 1991;38:458–459.

39. Pode D, Horowitz AT, Vlodavsky I, Shapiro A, Biran S. Prevention of human bladder tumor cell implantation in an in vitro assay. J Urol 1987;137:777–781.

40. Zincke H, Benson RC Jr, Hilton JF, Taylor WF. Intravesical thiotepa and mitomycin C treatment immediately after transurethral resection and later for superficial (stages Ta and Tis) bladder cancer: a prospective, randomized, stratified study with crossover design. J Urol 1985;134:1110–1114.

41. Solsona E, Iborra I, Ricos JV, Monros JL, Casanova J, Dumont R. Effectiveness of a single immediate mitomycin C instillation in patients with low risk superficial bladder cancer: short and long-term followup. J Urol 1999;161:1120–1123.

42. Dandekar NP, Tongaonkar HB, Dalal AV, Kulkarni JN, Kamat MR. Partial cystectomy for invasive bladder cancer. J Surg Oncol 1995;60:24–29.

43. Magri J. Partial cystectomy: a review of 104 cases. Br J Urol 1962;34:74–87.

44. Schoborg TW, Sapolsky JL, Lewis CW Jr. Carcinoma of the bladder treated by segmental resection. J Urol 1979;122:473–475.

45. Angulo JC, Sanchez-Chapado M, Lopez JI, Flores N. Primary cisplatin, methotrexate and vinblastine aiming at bladder preservation in invasive bladder cancer: multivariate analysis on prognostic factors. J Urol 1996;155:1897–1902.

46. Sternberg CN, Arena MG, Calabresi F, et al. Neoadjuvant M-VAC (methotrexate, vinblastine, doxorubicin, and cisplatin) for infiltrating transitional cell carcinoma of the bladder. Cancer 1993;72:1975–1982.

47. Merrell RW, Brown HE, Rose JF. Bladder carcinoma treated by partial cystectomy: a review of 54 cases. J Urol 1979;122:471–472.

48. Brannan W, Ochsner MG, Fuselier HA Jr, Landry GR. Partial cystectomy in the treatment of transitional cell carcinoma of the bladder. J Urol 1978;119:213–215.

49. Evans RA, Texter JH Jr. Partial cystectomy in the treatment of bladder cancer. J Urol 1975;114:391–393.

50. Long RT, Grummon RA, Spratt JS Jr, Perez-Mesa C. Carcinoma of the urinary bladder. Comparison with radical, simple, and partial cystectomy and intravesical formalin. Cancer 1972;29:98–105.

# Optimal radiotherapy for bladder cancer

54

*Michael F Milosevic, Robert Bristow, Mary K Gospodarowicz*

## INTRODUCTION

There is extensive experience using radiation, either alone or in combination with surgery or chemotherapy to treat muscle-invasive bladder cancer. The goal of radiation treatment is to eradicate the tumor while preserving the structure and function of the bladder and other surrounding normal tissues. The utility of radiation in treating cancer arises because of differences in the radiation response of tumors and normal tissues. In general, tumor cells are less able than normal cells to repair DNA damage produced by radiation. DNA and other intracellular damage from radiation induce downstream molecular events leading to cell death. Differences in the molecular and cellular radiation responses of malignant and normal tissues result in a favorable therapeutic ratio. The tumoricidal effects of carefully planned and delivered radiation treatment should outweigh the potential for serious toxicity to normal surrounding tissues. Advances in high-precision, image-guided radiotherapy, coupled with an improved understanding of bladder cancer radiobiology and specific targeting of molecular pathways that contribute to radiation resistance, have the potential to dramatically improve tumor control in bladder cancer patients while maintaining normal bladder function.

This chapter will review the current literature concerning the use of radiation to treat muscle-invasive bladder cancer, including patient selection, treatment planning and delivery, and the results of radiation alone or in combination with neoadjuvant or concurrent chemotherapy. Much of the evidence for radiotherapy is based on large series of unselected patients treated at single institutions over many years. Many of these patients received radiotherapy instead of cystectomy because of advanced age, concurrent medical problems, or extensive disease at the time of diagnosis. Most were treated before the introduction of modern, high-precision, image-guided radiation planning and delivery techniques. Therefore, the current literature reflects the worst possible results of radiotherapy rather than the optimal outcomes that might be achieved in patients that are carefully selected using clinical, radiographic, and novel molecular markers of response, and treated with biologically targeted, high-precision techniques. This chapter will emphasize possible approaches to improving the outcome of patients with bladder cancer through the integrated application of emerging radiobiologic and technologic concepts. In particular, the radiobiology of bladder cancer will be discussed with a focus on molecular markers of radiation response that might be used in the future to select optimal patients for radiotherapy or stratify patients in clinical studies. These biomarkers of tumor response are also potential targets for novel molecular-based agents that can be used in combination with radiation to improve the therapeutic outcome.

## PATIENT SELECTION FOR RADIOTHERAPY

Radiotherapy for muscle-invasive bladder cancer, administered with the aim of permanently controlling the tumor and preserving normal bladder function, is most appropriate in situations in which the prior probability of achieving this goal is high. Numerous factors may influence the success of radiotherapy in patients with bladder cancer, and they can be broadly classified as those relating to the characteristics of the tumor, the bladder, and the patient. Table 54.1[6–9,22] summarizes the results of multivariate analyses of local control and survival in several large contemporary series.

In general, there is limited evidence to support the use of radiotherapy to treat superficial bladder cancer. Given the effectiveness and convenience of other management strategies, radiation should be reserved for circumstances in which these other options have either been exhausted or are otherwise inappropriate for patient-specific reasons.

## TUMOR FACTORS FOR LOCAL CONTROL

Sustained local control of muscle-invasive bladder cancer treated with radiotherapy is strongly influenced by the bulk of local disease at the time of treatment, and the propensity for new tumors to develop in the bladder after treatment. Advanced T category, large tumor size, the presence of an extravesical mass, and hydronephrosis have all been associated with either incomplete response to radiation or local disease recurrence.[1–10] Overall, approximately 50% of patients treated with external beam radiotherapy have complete regression of disease: 50% to 70% of those with T2 or T3a disease and 40% to 50% with T3 or T4a tumors.[1,2,4,5,11–13] Sustained local control can be

expected in 30% to 50% and 20% to 30% of patients with T2 and T3 disease, respectively.[2,6,14] A gross complete transurethral resection of the bladder tumor before radiotherapy has been associated with improved local control,[7,15] although this has not been observed consistently.[4,13,16]

Treatment of bladder cancer with radiotherapy is associated with long-term risk of new tumor development in the preserved bladder. For example, Gospodarowicz et al[6] reported a continuous decline in local relapse-free rate and cause-specific cystectomy-free survival to beyond 10 years in 355 patients treated with radiotherapy alone. Patients at greatest risk of new tumor development are those with multifocal superficial disease at the time of initial diagnosis.[6–9,17] Extensive carcinoma in situ (CIS), when present in association with muscle-invasive bladder cancer, is a particularly strong adverse prognostic factor for sustained local control with radiotherapy.[1,18,19] Wolf et al[19] reported the development of new bladder cancers after radiotherapy in 58% of patients with dysplasia or CIS at initial presentation, but in none of the patients without concomitant CIS. Zietman et al[20] described the Massachusetts General Hospital experience with superficial disease recurrence in 121 patients who presented initially with muscle-invasive cancer and were treated with a combination of surgery, radiation, and chemotherapy. Superficial disease recurrence was seen at 57 sites in 32 patients (26%), at a median interval of 2.1

**Table 54.1** Prognostic factors by multivariate analysis for local control and survival following treatment with radiotherapy, with or without chemotherapy

| Lead author (year) | No. pts | Local control | Survival |
|---|---|---|---|
| Gospodarowicz (1991)[6]* | 355 | T stage | Grade<br>T stage<br>Tumor bulk<br>Hydronephrosis |
| Fossa (1993)[22] | 308 | | Age<br>Year of treatment†<br>T category<br>Serum creatinine |
| Mameghan (1995)[8] | 342 | Multifocal disease<br>Hydronephrosis<br>T stage | |
| Moonen (1998)[9] | 379 | Multifocal disease<br>Radiation dose | Age<br>T category |
| Rodel (2002)[7] | 415 | Multifocal disease | Age<br>Extent of TURBT<br>T category<br>Lymphatic invasion<br>Treatment‡ |

\* Cause-specific survival.
† 1980–1985 versus 1986–1990.
‡ Radiotherapy alone, versus radiotherapy + carboplatin, versus radiotherapy + cisplatin, versus radiotherapy + 5-fluorouracil/cisplatin; p=0.06.
TURBT, transurethral resection of bladder tumor prior to radiotherapy.

years from the completion of initial treatment. CIS associated with the original muscle-invasive tumor was a strong predictor of subsequent superficial recurrence. Conservative treatment with transurethral resection and intravesical therapy was undertaken in 27 patients, 10 of whom eventually required cystectomy because of further superficial recurrence or progression to invasive cancer. There was no difference in survival among patients who remained permanently free of disease following initial treatment and those who developed a superficial recurrence. These results indicate that, while CIS is associated with reduced long-term disease control in the bladder, it is not an absolute contraindication to the use of radiotherapy in patients with muscle-invasive disease, and should be considered in the context of other tumor- and patient-related factors when treatment options are evaluated.

## TUMOR FACTORS FOR SURVIVAL

The prognostic factors for survival are similar to those for local control, and generally reflect primary tumor bulk. Patients with T2 tumors have an expected survival of 30% to 50%, and those with T3 disease a survival of 15% to 35%.[1-6,9,11-14,21-25] In addition, advanced age at diagnosis, high histologic grade, and gross residual disease at the completion of transurethral resection of the bladder prior to radiotherapy have all been associated with reduced survival.[1,6,7,9,22]

Several surgical series have demonstrated pelvic lymph node metastases at diagnosis in 10% to 50% of patients with muscle-invasive bladder cancer depending on primary tumor extent.[26-29] Nodal metastases imply a high risk of occult distant metastases, a high risk of recurrence outside of the pelvis following local treatment alone, and significantly lower survival relative to node-negative patients. Nevertheless, the impact of nodal metastases on the outcome of bladder cancer patients treated with radiotherapy has not been extensively studied. This in part reflects the difficulty of reliably identifying subclinical nodal disease in the absence of surgical dissection. Very few of the modern radiotherapy series have described the prognostic impact of nodal status at diagnosis. Rodel et al[7] showed that lymph node involvement was predictive of inferior local control by univariate analysis, but not by multivariate analysis. However, patients with positive nodes were more likely to develop distant metastases independent of other tumor-, patient-, and treatment-related factors. The potential for radiotherapy, with or without concurrent chemotherapy to control bulky nodal disease, is limited by normal tissue toxicity and the relatively modest doses that can be delivered safely.[30] In addition, these patients are at particularly high risk of having occult distant metastases. Patients in this situation desiring bladder conservation should be managed by multimodality strategies that incorporate initial chemotherapy followed by consolidative pelvic radiotherapy for complete responders.

## PATIENT FACTORS

Radiotherapy is generally tolerated well in elderly patients[31] and in those with concurrent medical problems, and this has contributed to an imbalance in the underlying likelihood of long-term survival between patients who undergo cystectomy and those treated with radiotherapy. However, the benefit of definitive radiotherapy with bladder conservation is likely to be limited in situations in which pretreatment bladder function is compromised and in patients at high risk of developing intolerable acute or long-term treatment complications. Those with severe irritable bladder symptoms due to factors such as longstanding outflow obstruction, chronic infection, multiple prior transurethral resections, or prior intravesical chemotherapy may have permanent impairment of bladder function after radiotherapy that diminishes the benefit of organ preservation. Anatomic and technical factors that limit the accuracy and reproducibility of radiation delivery, and increase the likelihood of missing the target—such as atonic bladders and large bladder diverticula—may contribute to a higher risk of local tumor recurrence and treatment complications. New image-guided radiation delivery systems may help to overcome these challenges.

Overall, the ideal candidate for definitive radiotherapy with bladder preservation has a small, solitary tumor less than 5 cm in size with no associated CIS, no evidence of lymph node or distant metastases, and a normal (or normally functioning) bladder. The patient must be highly motivated to preserve the bladder, committed to frequent invasive follow-up examinations, and willing to accept the uncertainty that accompanies life-long bladder surveillance and the possibility of requiring treatment of new, superficial, invasive, or metastatic disease.

## RADIOTHERAPY TREATMENT PLANNING AND DELIVERY

The goal of radiotherapy is to eradicate all gross and microscopic tumor in the bladder and often also in the pelvic lymph nodes, while minimizing patient toxicity. Therefore, the success of radiotherapy depends not only on the selection of appropriate patients, but also on knowledge of tumor patterns of spread, accurate localization of the primary tumor and lymph node metastases, selection of appropriate treatment volumes to encompass all tumor and exclude as much normal tissue as possible, and careful tracking of tumor movement. The bladder is not a fixed structure but rather varies in size and position as a function of urine volume and rectal contents. Compensation for frequent variations in bladder positioning and tumor movement during a fractionated course of treatment is an important component of the radiotherapy treatment plan.

## RADIOTHERAPY FOR THE PRIMARY BLADDER TUMOR

Radiotherapy for bladder cancer implies the need for accurate and reproducible delivery of multiple radiation fractions to the gross tumor and regions of subclinical disease extension. Microscopic infiltrative tumor is likely to be present in the lamina propria, muscularis propria, and lymphovascular spaces adjacent to the primary tumor, although the degree of extension beyond gross disease has not been studied and is likely to be highly variable. Disease may also extend into paravesical tissues. The location and extent of gross tumor determined from diagnostic and staging tests—including cystoscopy, pelvic computed tomography (CT), and pelvic magnetic resonance imaging (MRI)—should be integrated with results of CT imaging of the patient in the treatment position to develop a three-dimensional radiotherapy plan. CT-based treatment planning has been shown to be more accurate than conventional planning techniques that rely on cystogram alone.[32–35] However, there probably is significant interobserver variability in the definition of gross tumor using CT, particularly in the region of the trigone and bladder neck.[36,37] This may be improved in the future with the use of planning MRI and registration of the CT and MR images. MRI provides greater soft tissue resolution than CT, and valuable information about the extent of local disease. Figure 54.1 shows

axial, sagittal and coronal images of a tumor extensively involving the dome and posterior wall of the bladder and causing ureteric obstruction and hydronephrosis.

The clinical target volume (CTV) for treatment of the primary bladder tumor is often considered to be the entire bladder. However, lateralized solitary tumors that can be accurately localized are probably safely treated with a reduced CTV that encompasses the gross tumor and a surrounding margin to account for microscopic disease extension. Cowan et al[38] reported the results of a three-arm phase III study in which patients with bladder cancer were randomized to either whole-bladder treatment, or escalated dose partial-bladder treatment with two different dose regimens. The median irradiated pelvic volume was 61% lower in the partial-volume arms of the study than in the whole-bladder arm. While statistically significant, there were no differences in complete response, sustained local control, long-term survival, or toxicity; the trial was closed early due to slow accrual and only 72 patients of a planned 123 reached the clinical endpoint of failure of local control.

Variability in the position of the bladder tumor from day to day during a course of fractionated radiotherapy theoretically may be minimized by asking patients to completely empty their bladders immediately prior to imaging for treatment planning, and prior to receiving each radiation fraction. However, the efficacy of this maneuver has not been rigorously evaluated, and there still may be significant changes in bladder volume depending on factors such as the interval between voiding and treatment delivery, the state of hydration of the patient, and the use of diuretic medications or beverages. Movement may also be influenced by extrinsic pressure, such as might arise from differences in rectal filling,[39] and by the characteristics of the tumor, including size and degree of extravesical extension. Turner et al[39] demonstrated interfraction bladder wall movement of at least 1.5 cm in 18 of 30 patients, with

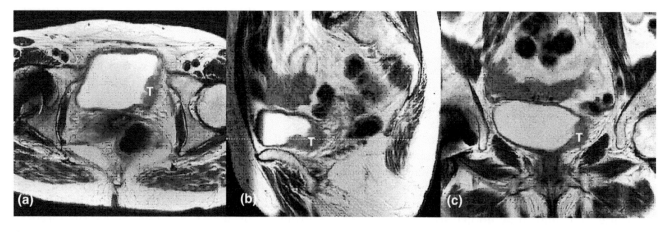

**Fig. 54.1**
(a) Axial, (b) sagittal, and (c) coronal $T_2$-weighted MR images of a muscle-invasive bladder tumor (T) involving the left posterolateral wall. MR provides high-resolution images of bladder cancer that can be used to accurately determine radiation treatment volumes.

the greatest movement being seen in those with large initial bladder volumes. Bladder movement resulted in inadequate coverage of the CTV in 10 patients. An isotropic planning target volume (PTV) of 2 cm around the CTV was recommended to account for random internal movement.[39] Muren et al[40] studied 20 patients with bladder cancer using weekly CT scans. In 89% of the repeat scans during treatment, the bladder wall extended beyond the bladder contour as outlined using the original planning CT. The greatest displacements during treatment occurred along the superior, left, anterior, and posterior aspects of the bladder and measured up to 3.6 cm. Anisotropic margins (CTV–PTV) of 1.1–2.3 cm were necessary to encompass all bladder displacements simultaneously except in the most extreme cases. Similarly, Meijer et al[37] advocated anisotropic margins (CTV–PTV) of 2.3 cm superiorly and 1 cm inferiorly (behind the symphysis) and laterally.

The choice of radiation treatment margin around the gross bladder tumor is likely to influence not only local control, but also toxicity. In a recent analysis, conformal three- or four-field treatment plans for 15 patients were developed using either isotropic margins of 1 cm around the bladder wall CTV, or wider anisotropic margins of 1.2 cm laterally and 2 cm elsewhere. The wider margins were associated with a 1.5- to 2.4-fold increase in the volume of small bowel and rectum receiving greater than 50% of the prescribed dose. The fractional rectal volume receiving greater than 75% of the prescribed dose was 3.6- to 5-fold higher. The higher doses to critical normal structures correlated with model predictions of higher complication rates.[41] In the future, image-guided radiotherapy that allows day-to-day optimization of the treatment volumes should further reduce the possibility of accidentally underdosing mobile tumors while at the same time minimizing the dose to critical adjacent normal tissues. Figure 54.2 is an axial image through the bladder acquired using cone-beam CT[42] that is integrated with the radiation treatment unit. Anatomic imaging prior to each daily fraction and correction of errors would greatly improve the accuracy of bladder cancer radiotherapy.

## RADIOTHERAPY FOR PELVIC LYMPH NODE METASTASES

Pelvic lymph node metastases occur in 10% to 50% of patients with muscle-invasive bladder cancer.

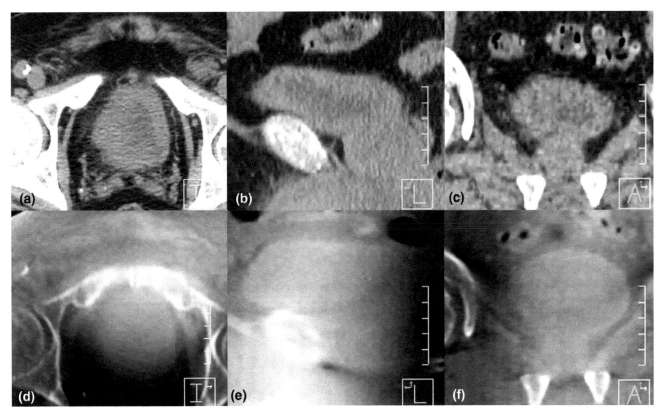

**Fig. 54.2**
(a) Axial and reconstructed (b) sagittal and (c) coronal planning CT images in a patient with bladder cancer. (d) Axial, (e) sagittal, and (f) coronal cone-beam CT images in the same patient acquired during treatment. The cone-beam CT imager is incorporated into the radiation treatment unit. Daily imaging prior to radiation and correction for patient positioning errors and internal organ movement have the potential to greatly improve the accuracy of bladder cancer radiotherapy.

Radiotherapy treatment volumes historically have encompassed pelvic lymph nodes, whether or not there is radiographic evidence of gross nodal metastases. However, the benefit of nodal irradiation in bladder cancer has not been extensively studied. Several surgical series have suggested long-term survival of 15% to 30% in patients with nodal metastases who undergo thorough lymph node dissection at the time of cystectomy.[27,28,43–49] By extrapolation, there may also be a benefit of aggressive nodal treatment in patients who are managed primarily with radiotherapy. Pelvic lymph node radiation typically is delivered using a four-field technique, which encompasses a large volume of small bowel and rectum. Therefore, the dose of radiation that can be prescribed safely is limited by the radiation tolerance of these critical normal tissues, and is probably inadequate to control gross or, in some cases, even 'bulky' subclinical nodal disease that is near the threshold of radiographic detection. Intensity modulated radiotherapy (IMRT), which allows the radiation dose to be 'sculpted' in three dimensions to a predefined lymph node volume while excluding surrounding normal tissue, may facilitate higher lymph node doses.[30] Figure 54.3 shows an optimized radiation treatment plan in which the whole bladder and pelvic lymph nodes are treated with IMRT to facilitate dose escalation with relative sparing of the surrounding normal tissues.

## CONVENTIONAL RADIATION FRACTIONATION

Using current radiation techniques, the dose that can be delivered safely to pelvic lymph nodes is limited by the radiation tolerance of the surrounding normal tissues, and is typically 40–50 Gy in 1.8–2.0 Gy daily fractions. The future implementation of precision IMRT techniques may allow escalation of the lymph node dose, with the expectation of improved nodal control.[30]

Radiation doses of 50–70 Gy in 1.8–2.5 Gy fractions over 4–7 weeks are commonly used to treat the primary bladder tumor. The clinical dose–response relationship for bladder cancer is poorly defined, and it remains unclear to what extent differences in total dose in this range influence local tumor control and patient survival. In practice, the prescribed dose is usually determined by the radiation tolerance of the surrounding normal tissues on the assumption that a higher bladder cancer dose will always be desirable and produce improved local control. Therefore, phase III randomized studies comparing different conventionally fractionated dosage schedules have never been undertaken. At least four case series have suggested improved local tumor control with doses greater than 55–60 Gy,[2,13,17,50] although others have found no evidence to support such a relationship.[3,10] The dose–response relationship in these and

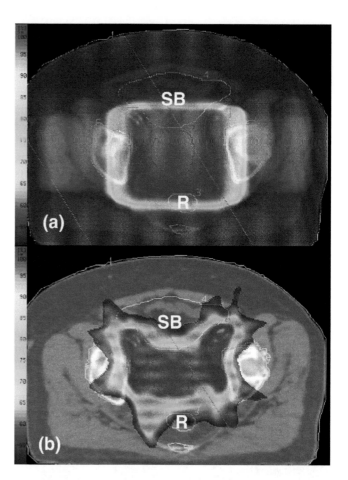

**Fig. 54.3**
Radiation treatment plans for bladder cancer (including the pelvic lymph nodes) using (a) a standard four-field approach, and (b) intensity-modulated radiotherapy (IMRT). The IMRT plan results in relative dose sparing of the small bowel (SB) and rectum (R).

other retrospective studies may have been obscured to some extent by differences among the dose strata in the distribution of other important tumor-, patient-, and treatment-related factors.

## SIDE EFFECTS OF RADIOTHERAPY

Conventionally fractionated radiotherapy to total doses of less than 70 Gy is typically well tolerated by patients with bladder cancer. Most experience acute gastro-intestinal and lower urinary tract side effects during treatment that usually are easily controlled with dietary modification and medications. Late complications primarily affect the bowel and normal bladder, and typically arise from 1 to 4 years after treatment is completed. Approximately 75% of late complications are present by 3 years.[5,14] Late bladder side effects, which include urinary frequency, dysuria, and hematuria, have been reported in 7% to 15% of patients,[2,5,6,14,51] and in some circumstances necessitate cystectomy. Severe gastrointestinal toxicity is seen in 6% to 17% of patients.[5,6,14] Doses above 70 Gy are likely to be associated with an unacceptably high rate of serious complications if delivered using standard radiation techniques,[3] but may be feasible in the future with image-guided intensity-modulated radiotherapy.

## FOLLOW-UP AFTER RADIOTHERAPY

Patients with muscle-invasive bladder cancer are at risk of developing progressive tumor both in the bladder and at metastatic sites after completing radiation treatment. This underscores the importance of life-long bladder surveillance and prompt treatment of bladder recurrences.[20] Several studies have demonstrated that new superficial disease in the bladder following radiotherapy, including new CIS, can often be managed effectively with transurethral resection and intravesical bacillus Calmette–Guérin (BCG).[20,52,53] However, persistent or new muscle-invasive cancer usually implies the need for salvage cystectomy. Most modern radiotherapy series have reported salvage cystectomy rates of only 20% to 30% of patients.[2,6,7,22,51,54,55] Many patients referred for radiotherapy have bulky unresectable tumors and a high risk of occult micrometastases, or concurrent medical problems, making them unsuitable for initial surgery. For the same reasons, these patients often are not considered for salvage cystectomy in the event of radiation failure. However, cystectomy frequently is the only remaining option for patients with recurrent localized muscle-invasive bladder cancer. In general, all patients with residual or recurrent bladder cancer following radiotherapy should be evaluated for cystectomy.

The rate of bladder cancer regression following radiotherapy influences both the optimal timing of cystoscopy to evaluate response and the optimal timing of salvage cystectomy. Several reports have identified disease status at the completion of radiotherapy (with or without concurrent chemotherapy) as an important prognostic factor for overall patient outcome.[6,7] In most radiotherapy series, response has been evaluated 1–3 months after completion of treatment.[6,7] However, the Massachusetts General Hospital has adopted a policy of earlier evaluation.[56] After initial thorough transurethral resection, patients receive induction radiotherapy to a dose of approximately 40 Gy with concurrent cisplatin chemotherapy. Cystoscopy is performed 2–4 weeks later to assess disease regression. Patients that have had complete regression receive consolidative radiotherapy, while those with residual bladder cancer proceed to immediate cystectomy. The advantage is early cystectomy after only a modest dose of radiotherapy, which should maximize the curative potential of cystectomy and minimize toxicity. However, early response assessment before completion of full-course radical radiotherapy theoretically may decrease the likelihood of bladder preservation if slow responders, who would have achieved complete regression of disease given sufficient time, are evaluated prematurely. Although there has not been a randomized comparison of early versus delayed response assessment and cystectomy, the results from several series suggest comparable results with respect to local control, patient survival, the proportion of patients undergoing cystectomy, and treatment complications.[6,7,9,56] At the Princess Margaret Hospital, it is our practice to assess response no later than 6 weeks after completing radiotherapy.

## PATIENT OUTCOME FOLLOWING RADIOTHERAPY FOR BLADDER CANCER

There is substantial evidence that radiotherapy is effective treatment for bladder cancer. However, many patients with muscle-invasive disease have bulky tumors at presentation and are at high risk of harboring occult lymph node or distant metastases. Radiotherapy and chemotherapy are therefore frequently used in combination with the aim of enhancing local tumor control, reducing metastasis development, and improving patient survival.

### RADIOTHERAPY ALONE

Table 54.2[2–6,9,11–14,21–25,32] summarizes the published experience with external beam radiotherapy alone as treatment for bladder cancer. Most are retrospective descriptions of the experience at a single institution over several decades, and often do not consider changes with time in patient assessment, imaging, stage classification, radiotherapy technique, and supportive treatment. Management strategies vary from institution to institution, including the criteria for salvage cystectomy, making detailed comparisons of results problematic. Nevertheless, there are consistent patterns among the studies with respect to both short- and long-term response to radiation. Together, they provide strong evidence that a substantial proportion of patients, particularly those with small tumors at presentation, are cured with radiotherapy and maintain normal bladder function.

Radical external beam radiotherapy produces complete regression of muscle-invasive bladder cancer in approximately 70% of patients,[1,2,4,5,11–13] and 30% to 50% have sustained local control (complete tumor regression without subsequent recurrence in the bladder).[2,6,14] Nevertheless, distant metastases develop in more than 50% of patients,[1] and long-term overall survival is in the range of only 25% to 30%.[1,3,5,9,22]

**Table 54.2** External beam radiotherapy alone for muscle-invasive bladder cancer

| Lead author (year) | No. Pts | 5-year survival by T category (%) | | | |
| | | T2 | T3 (T3a/T3b) | T4 | Overall |
| --- | --- | --- | --- | --- | --- |
| Goffinet (1975)[23] | 384 | 35–42 | 20 | | |
| Yu (1985)[24] | 356 | 42 | (35/23) | | |
| Goodman (1981)[25] | 470 | | | | 38 |
| Duncan (1986)[5] | 963 | 40 | 26 | 12 | 30 |
| Blandy (1988)[11] | 614 | 27 | 38 | 9 | |
| Jenkins (1988)[12]* | 182 | 46 | 35 | | 40 |
| Gospodarowicz (1991)[6]* | 355 | 50 | (38/28) | | 46 |
| Johnson (1991)[14]* | 319 | 31 | 16 | 6 | 28 |
| Davidson (1990)[21]* | 709 | 49 | 28 | 2 | 25 |
| Greven (1990)[2] | 116 | 59 | 10 | 0 | |
| Smaaland (1991)[13] | 146 | 26 | 10† | | |
| Fossa (1993)[22] | 308 | 38‡ | 14§ | | 24 |
| Vale (1993)[4] | 60 | 38 | 12 | | |
| Pollack (1994)[3] | 135 | 42 | 20 | 0 | 26 |
| Moonen (1998)[9] | 379 | 25 | 17 | | 22 |
| Borgaonkar (2002)[32]* | 163 | 48 | 26 | | 45 |

\* Cause-specific survival.
† T3/T4.
‡ T2/T3a.
§ T3b/T4.

Salvage cystectomy for progressive or recurrent disease after radiotherapy, which is an important part of the integrated management plan, has historically been undertaken in less than 30% of patients.[1,2,22,54] This, at least in part, reflects the poor general health, age, and prognosis of patients treated with radiation, who often have concomitant medical contraindications to surgery. Overall, approximately 80% of patients that survive long-term following external beam radiotherapy have intact, well-functioning bladders.[7]

## RADIOTHERAPY AND CONCURRENT CHEMOTHERAPY

Rodel et al[7] recently updated their large accumulated experience in 415 patients with T1–4 bladder cancer. More than 50% of patients had T3 or T4 disease. All were treated with transurethral resection followed by pelvic radiotherapy. Chemotherapy with cisplatin, carboplatin, and/or 5-fluorouracil (5-FU) was used concurrently with radiation in 289 patients. Complete tumor regression occurred in 72% of patients, as assessed by cystoscopy and biopsy 6 weeks after completing treatment. Among patients that achieved a complete response, 50% remained free of any relapse in the bladder at 10 years, and 64% had no recurrence of muscle-invasive disease. Overall, 20% of patients underwent salvage cystectomy. Distant metastases

developed in 35% of patients. The 10-year cause-specific survival was 42%.

In other studies, the Massachusetts General Hospital has pursued an aggressive program of bladder conservation with conservative surgery, radiation, and chemotherapy in selected patients since 1986. Patients initially underwent a thorough transurethral resection, followed by induction treatment with radiotherapy to 40 Gy, and concurrent cisplatin chemotherapy. Those with complete regression of disease proceeded to consolidative radiotherapy (a further 24–25 Gy with chemotherapy), while those with residual disease underwent cystectomy. Among 190 patients, 82% completed treatment according to protocol. Sixty percent of patients treated with chemoradiation alone remained free of bladder cancer long term. Superficial disease recurred in the bladder in 24 patients, and in the majority of cases was managed conservatively with further resection and intravesical chemotherapy. A muscle-invasive recurrence developed in 16%. The 10-year cause-specific survival rates were 60% overall, and 45% with an intact bladder. Bladder function was normal by urodynamic assessment in 75% of these patients.[56,57]

The only phase III trial of radiotherapy and concurrent chemotherapy was conducted by the National Cancer Institute of Canada[58] and is summarized in Table 54.3 along with other neoadjuvant and concurrent chemoradiation studies.[59–63] Patients

**Table 54.3** Randomized studies of combination radiation and chemotherapy

| Lead author (year) | No. pts | Stage | Experimental arm | Control arm | 3–5 year survival* |
|---|---|---|---|---|---|
| Shearer (1988)[59] | 423 | T3 | ± Neo and Adj MTX | RT alone 64 Gy or preRT 44 Gy + cyst | 39% vs. 37%, NS |
| Wallace (1991)[60] | 255 | T2–4 | ± Neo Cis | RT alone | NS |
| Coppin (1996)[58]† | 99 | T2–4 | ± Con Cis ×3 with induction RT | Induction RT 40 Gy RT boost 20 Gy or Cyst | 47% vs. 33%, NS |
| Shipley (1998)[61] (RTOG 89-03) | 123 | T2–4 | ± Neo CMV ×2 after TURBT | TURBT RT 39.6 Gy + Con Cis RT boost 25.2 Gy + Cis if CR Cyst if no CR | 48% vs. 49%, NS |
| Ghersi (1999)[63] | 976 | T2–4 | ± Neo CMV ×3 | RT or Cyst | 55% vs. 50%, NS |
| Senglov (2002)[62] | 153 | T2–4 | ± Neo Cis and MTX ×3 | RT or Cyst | 29% vs. 29%, NS |

\* Experimental versus control arm.
† Improved pelvic control.
Adj, adjuvant; Cis, cisplatin; CMV, cisplatin, methotrexate, vinblastine; Con, concurrent; CR, complete response; Cyst, cystectomy; MTX, methotrexate; Neo, neoadjuvant; NS, not significant; preRT, planned preoperative RT; RT, radiotherapy; TURBT, transurethral resection of bladder tumor.

with T2–4b urothelial carcinoma of the bladder received local regional therapy alone (full-dose radiotherapy or preoperative radiotherapy and cystectomy), with or without concurrent cisplatin. There was no difference in overall survival or distant relapse-free survival. However, patients that received concurrent chemotherapy had a significantly lower rate of pelvic recurrence than those treated with radiation alone. There was no difference in the risk of serious side effects.

## NEOADJUVANT CHEMOTHERAPY AND RADIOTHERAPY

Initial phase II studies of neoadjuvant chemotherapy suggested improved local control and prolonged survival.[64–66] However, phase III studies have, in general, failed to confirm these results. The largest phase III neoadjuvant study comprised 976 patients with T2–4 bladder cancer randomized to receive three cycles of chemotherapy with cisplatin, methotrexate and vinblastine (CMV) followed by cystectomy or radiotherapy, versus the same treatment without chemotherapy.[63] A total of 485 patients underwent cystectomy; 415 were treated with radiotherapy and 76 received preoperative radiation followed by cystectomy. There was no difference in overall survival between the chemotherapy and no-chemotherapy arms (55% versus 50%, respectively). Locoregional control was not affected by chemotherapy, although there was a suggestion that the development of metastasis was delayed.

Although the results of individual phase III randomized studies of neoadjuvant chemotherapy have been disappointing, a recent meta-analysis that combined individual data from 2688 patients in 10 studies has shown a survival advantage with combination platinum-based chemotherapy.[67] There

was a 13% relative reduction in the risk of death and an improvement in survival at 5 years from 45% to 50%. Local disease-free survival and metastasis-free survival were also improved (relative risk reductions of 13% and 18%, respectively).

## HIGH PRECISION RADIATION TREATMENT FOR BLADDER CANCER

The potential of radiotherapy to eradicate bladder cancer has been limited over the years by technologic factors that prevented the accurate and reproducible delivery of sufficient radiation dose to the primary tumor and pelvic lymph nodes while at the same time sparing important adjacent normal tissues and minimizing toxicity. Little appreciation of the potential for the bladder and tumor to move between and during radiation fractions, coupled with inadequate treatment planning and delivery, has probably contributed to inadvertent underdosing of tumor and an excess number of local treatment failures. In addition, the radiation dose that can be delivered safely to pelvic lymph nodes is limited because of normal tissue tolerance to between 45 and 50 Gy, which is insufficient for reliable control of gross nodal disease or even 'bulky' subclinical metastases that are just below the threshold of radiographic detection. Therefore, it is likely that the pelvic lymph nodes have historically been inadequately treated with conventional radiotherapy in a large proportion of patients.

Recent advances in radiation treatment technology have the potential to overcome the limitations of previous techniques, thereby dramatically improving the likelihood of permanently eradicating bladder cancer and at the same time minimizing the risk of complications and preserving normal bladder function.

IMRT allows dose escalation to the primary bladder tumor and pelvic lymph nodes (see Figure 54.3) with the expectation of improved tumor and equal or reduced toxicity.[30] Tighter radiation treatment margins around the tumor imply the need for greater accuracy in tumor delineation at the time of treatment planning using high-definition imaging modalities such as MRI (see Figure 54.1), and an enhanced capacity to ensure that the radiotherapy is actually delivered as planned each day during a course of fractionated treatment. This can be accomplished through daily imaging of patients prior to treatment, with correction of individual radiation beams to account for variation in patient positioning and tumor movement. Radiation treatment units that incorporate volumetric imaging, such as cone-beam CT[42] (see Figure 54.2), coupled with fast and accurate software to automatically calculate beam corrections, are well suited to this application.

Overall, image-guided IMRT, coupled with advances in our understanding of tumor and normal tissue radiobiology, has the potential to revolutionize the treatment of bladder cancer. However, further development is necessary to assure its safe implementation in routine clinical practice. The success of IMRT in this setting will depend on the combined efforts of radiation oncologists, physicists, radiation therapists, and nurses. Coordination and communication among these professional groups is essential to ensure that important technical and patient-related issues are adequately addressed.

## MODERN CONCEPTS IN BLADDER CANCER RADIOBIOLOGY

Although radiation has proven efficacy in the treatment of muscle-invasive bladder cancer, there is the potential to significantly enhance the therapeutic effect by better understanding the molecular events that lead to radiation-induced cell death in tumors and normal tissues, and modulating the radiosensitivity of these tissues using molecularly targeted treatments.

The aim of clinical radiotherapy is to sterilize all malignant clonogenic cells that are capable of regrowing the tumor. Ionizing radiation leads to the rapid generation of reactive free radicals that randomly interact with the DNA, RNA, and proteins within the cell membrane and nucleus. Clustering of ionizations close to DNA leads to multiply damaged DNA sites consisting of DNA single- and double-strand breaks (DNA-ssb, DNA-dsb), DNA base damage, and DNA–DNA or DNA–protein crosslinks. The most lethal of these lesions is a non-repaired DNA-dsb.[68] Within seconds following irradiation, a cascade of signaling pathways is activated, which together control cell proliferation, DNA repair, and initiation of cell death. Many of these

signaling pathways, which are associated with activated oncogenes (H-ras, raf or EGFR mutations) or inactivated tumor suppressor proteins (mutated p53 or pRb-retinoblastoma), are abnormal in bladder cancer cells.[69-71]

Following a lethal dose of ionizing radiation, cells may: 1) undergo apoptosis; 2) proceed through up to four abortive mitotic cycles, and then undergo mitotic catastrophe and cell lysis; or 3) undergo permanent growth arrest such as that observed for irradiated fibroblasts.[72] Complex, inter-related molecular mechanisms that regulate the cell cycle and DNA repair determine whether or not cell death occurs following exposure to ionizing radiation, and which of these morphologic patterns dominates in a particular tumor. Figure 54.4 illustrates the molecular pathways involved in the cellular response to radiation, and Table 54.4 summarizes the molecular targets that might be used to radiosensitize bladder cancer.

## ALTERED CELL CYCLE DYNAMICS

Human cells respond to radiotherapy through altered cell cycle dynamics. Delayed progression through the G1, S, and G2 phases of the cell cycle (the G1, S, and G2 cell cycle checkpoints) potentially allows repair of DNA

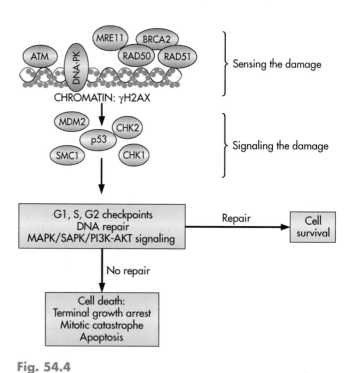

**Fig. 54.4**
Radiation-induced DNA breaks are sensed by a series of chromatin-binding kinases that mediate intracellular signaling within the cell. This activates a variety of downstream signaling pathways that ultimately result in either cell survival or cell death. Cell death occurs as a result of apoptosis, mitotic catastrophe or terminal growth arrest, the last two being the dominant mechanisms in the majority of human solid tumors.

**Table 54.4** Biomarkers of bladder cancer radioresistance

| Biomarker | Detection technique | Affected pathway | Treatment strategy |
|---|---|---|---|
| Mutant p53 | IHC DNA sequencing | Defective checkpoints and apoptosis Increased cell proliferation and metastasis | Increase radiation dose and radioprotect normal tissues Utilize pro-p53 gene therapy Convert abnormal p53 expression using pharmacologic manipulation |
| Decreased BAX:BCL2 ratio | IHC | Defective apoptotic response | Anti-BCL2 gene therapy or pro-BAX gene therapy |
| EGFR overexpression | IHC ELISA, FISH | Defective EGFR signaling and increased tumor cell proliferation, survival and angiogenesis | Target EGFR receptor (C225-Cetuximab) or abnormal tyrosine kinase activity (ZD1389-Iressa) |
| Mutation in RAS or PI3K/AKT pathway High expression of CAIX, HIF1α, GLUT1, or VEGF | IHC ELISA IHC | Increased tumor cell survival and proliferation Increased acute and chronic hypoxia and angiogenesis, leading to tumor cell resistance and increased metastases | Farnesyl transferase inhibitors or PI3K inhibitors ARCON radiotherapy Selective hypoxic cell toxins (tirapazamine) Antiangiogenesis (COX2 inhibitors) |
| Overexpression of Ki67, cyclins A and D Short tumor doubling time (Tpot or labeling index) | IHC Flow cytometry | Increased cell proliferation and tumor cell repopulation | Accelerated fractionation |

ARCON, accelerated radiotherapy and carbogen and nicotinamide; FISH, fluorescent in situ hybridization; IHC, immunohistochemistry.

and cellular damage to occur, thereby preventing cell death.[73] Central to these checkpoints is the activation of the ATM (ataxia telangiectasia mutated) protein kinase, which initiates the G1 checkpoint by stabilizing the p53 tumor suppressor protein. This in turn leads to an upregulation of the cyclin-kinase inhibitor, p21[WAF], hypophosphorylation of the RB protein, and inhibition of DNA replication.[74] The radiation-induced G1 arrest is lost in cells without functional p53 or RB proteins, and this may influence local tumor control and survival of patients with bladder cancer.[75,76]

The S-phase checkpoint following DNA damage is controlled though an ATM-mediated phosphorylation of the BRCA1, NBS1, and SMC1 proteins, which modify transcription factors and other proteins (RPA, PCNA) required during DNA replication.[77] The G2 delay occurs as a result of decreased expression, reduced stability, or nuclear accumulation of cyclin B complexes, which prevent the formation of active nuclear cyclin B-CDC2 complexes required for the transition from G2 to mitosis.[78] Radiosensitization theoretically may be achieved with drugs that abrogate the G2 checkpoint (caffeine, methylxanthines, UCN-01) leading to increased mitotic catastrophe. These agents are currently being tested, together with radiation in phase I–II clinical trials.[79–81]

## DNA REPAIR

Repair of DNA damage is an important determinant of malignant and normal tissue cellular response to ionizing radiation. Clinical radiotherapy endeavors to maximize the therapeutic ratio, so that maximal tumor cell killing occurs with minimal normal tissue toxicity. The utopian goal, therefore, is to completely inhibit DNA repair in malignant cells, while at the same time maximizing repair in normal tissue cells. The repair of DNA-dsb breaks has been correlated with bladder cancer cell survival following irradiation in vitro.[82–86]

Radiation-induced DNA breaks are initially sensed by the ATM, DNA-PK$_{CS}$ and RAD50 proteins, which in turn recruit other proteins involved in DNA repair and cell cycle control.[87] Two main pathways for DNA-dsb repair exist in human cells. The homologous recombination (HR) pathway includes the concerted actions of the RAD51, RAD50-57, RPA, and BRCA2 proteins, and dominates in the S and G2 phases of the cell cycle. In contrast, the nonhomologous end-joining (NHEJ) pathway includes the DNA-PK$_{CS}$, Ku70/Ku80, DNA ligase IV, and XRCC4 proteins, and is the preferred pathway for cells in the G1 phase of the cell cycle.[78,88] In addition, the HR and NHEJ repair pathways have recently been shown to influence the repair of platinum- and gemcitabine-induced DNA crosslinks and DNA-dsbs in bladder cancer cells.[89–92] This supported previous work in which the interaction of ionizing radiation and cisplatin was shown to be secondary to increased fixation of chemotherapy-induced DNA adducts by ionizing radiation.[92,93] This may in part explain the efficacy of combining radiation with cisplatin chemotherapy that has been demonstrated in randomized clinical studies of patients with bladder cancer.[58,94]

Taken together, the biologic responses outlined above interact to control the extent of cell death in malignant or normal tissues by recognizing whether the damage is sublethal or lethal, and whether sublethal damage can be effectively repaired. For each different type of tissue within the radiation volume, different mechanisms of cell death and cellular repair may be involved. In the context of clinical practice with fractionated radiotherapy, the factors that most prominently influence the response of a particular tissue may be summarized as the five Rs of radiotherapy:

- intrinsic *radiosensitivity*
- *redistribution* of cells within the cell cycle
- *reoxygenation* of cells during the course of radiotherapy
- *repopulation* of cells during radiotherapy
- cellular *repair* of tumor relative to normal tissue cells.[68]

## INTRINSIC RADIOSENSITIVITY

In many bladder cancer radiobiology studies, survival has been determined using a clonogenic assay that represents the total or cumulative cell death within an irradiated cell population as a result of all types of cell death.[82] The surviving fraction of cells following a dose of 2 Gy (SF2), which is in the clinically relevant range for fractionated radiotherapy, varies between 0.3 and 0.8 for most bladder cancer cell lines. The SF2 value of primary explanted patient biopsies has been shown to correlate with outcome following radiotherapy in cervical cancer, supporting the concept that intrinsic radiosensitivity is an important determinant of clinical response.[78,95] Unfortunately, human ex vivo clonogenic assays are unlikely to be clinically valuable as an indicator of bladder cancer radiocurability in individual patients because the results take 5–9 weeks to generate and the growth of bladder cancer biopsies ex vivo is poor. Surrogate tests of intrinsic radiosensitivity such as the relative repair of DNA breaks or DNA crosslinks in irradiated or chemotherapy-treated bladder biopsies show promise, but require further confirmatory studies.[84–86]

There have been reports of a correlation between increased pretreatment apoptosis and improved local control following radiotherapy in patients with bladder cancer.[96] This relationship between pretreatment apoptotic index and radioresponse relates to activation of the extrinsic, receptor-based (TNF or TRAIL family members) and intrinsic, mitochondrial-based (BAX, BCL2 family members) pathways.[97] The threshold for activation of apoptosis is controlled by p53 protein function and by the relative levels of the BAX and BCL2 proteins. Mutations of the p53 gene and decreased BAX:BCL2 ratio have been associated with increased

radioresistance in vitro and decreased bladder cancer clinical radioresponse.[96,98–110] This has led to a series of preclinical experiments pro-p53 or anti-BCL2 gene therapy to augment radiation-induced apoptosis.[74,111–113]

Although apoptosis is an important pathway leading to radiation-induced cell death, it is insufficient to account for the total therapeutic effect of anticancer agents in solid epithelial tumors. In fact, the level of radiation-induced apoptosis rarely correlates with eventual clonogenic cell survival as measured by colony-forming assays.[72,114] Other antiproliferative responses that directly impact on radiation clonogenic survival include mitotic catastrophe and terminal growth arrest.

Mitotic catastrophe is the failure of human tumor cells to undergo mitosis after DNA damage because of defective cell cycle checkpoint control and DNA repair. This leads to chromosomal abnormalities (tetraploidy or aneuploidy), which have been observed in bladder cancer cells.[115,116] Survivin is a member of the inhibitors of the apoptosis (IAP) protein family, and controls both apoptosis and mitosis. Increased levels of survivin have been observed in malignant relative to normal bladder.[117] Survivin may also be a powerful new biomarker of prognosis and local recurrence following radical cystectomy.[118,119] Ionizing radiation can activate transcriptional downregulation of survivin mRNA in a p53-dependent and PI3K/AKT-dependent manner. Early preclinical studies have shown that reduction in survivin expression using antisense or silencing RNA (siRNA) in bladder cancer cells leads to radiosensitization in vitro.[72,120,121]

Cellular senescence was originally linked to the observation that human diploid cells can undergo only a finite number of divisions before their growth is terminally arrested because of critical shortening of chromosome telomeres. The fact that tumor cell lines may also undergo accelerated senescence after irradiation in vitro explains the correlation between pretreatment or post-treatment expression of terminal growth arrest biomarkers (p53, p21$^{WAF}$, p16$^{INK4a}$, senescence-associated β-galactosidase) and clinical outcome following radiotherapy.[72,101,102,104,108,122] Agents that differentially increase terminal arrest in bladder cancer cells, such as retinoids or histone deacetylase (HDAC) inhibitors, might therefore be useful as radiosensitizers in patients with bladder cancer.[123,124]

## REDISTRIBUTION, REOXYGENATION, REPOPULATION AND REPAIR

The remaining four Rs of radiotherapy also modify bladder radioresponse. During the typical 24-hour interval between daily radiotherapy treatments, tumor cells can reoxygenate and also redistribute to more radiosensitive phases of the cell cycle. Radioresistant S-phase cells that survive a single radiation fraction will eventually cycle into the more radiosensitive G2, M, and G1 phases of the cell cycle by the time the next radiation treatment is administered. Fractionation also allows normal cells to undergo cellular repair and to repopulate in order to maintain organ function. Fractionation, therefore, results in relatively greater cell killing in tumor cells with tolerable normal tissue toxicity. An improved therapeutic ratio might be achieved in patients with bladder cancer by targeting radioresistant hypoxic subpopulations or using altered radiation fractionation schemes.

Most solid malignant tumors, including bladder cancer, have regions of hypoxia that arise largely because of abnormal vascular anatomy, distribution, organization, and functional dynamics.[125] Hypoxic cells are more resistant to the effects of radiation, are genetically unstable, and are more likely to metastasize.[126,127] High pretreatment levels of tumor hypoxia have been associated with decreased local control, disease-free survival, and overall survival following radiotherapy in a number of tumor types.[125] Hoskin et al[128] evaluated tumor hypoxia in 64 patients with bladder cancer using the intrinsic hypoxic markers carbonic anhydrase IX (CAIX) and glucose transporter-1 protein (GLUT1). There was no association between hypoxia and control of the primary bladder tumor following treatment with radiotherapy, carbogen, and nicotinamide. However, hypoxia was strongly predictive of both cause-specific and overall survival independent of clinical prognostic factors. This is consistent with the results in cervical cancer and other tumors, where hypoxia has been shown to have only a minimal effect on local control with radiotherapy, perhaps in part because of the effect of reoxygenation between radiation fractions, but a profound effect on the development of lymph node and distant metastases.[129,130] The combination of accelerated radiotherapy and the hypoxia-modifying agents carbogen and nicotinamide (ARCON) has shown promise in clinical studies of patients with bladder cancer.[131] Other agents that specifically target hypoxic cells or the abnormal tumor vasculature may be useful additions to bladder cancer radiotherapy.[126,132–134]

Laboratory and clinical studies have shown that tumor growth kinetics can increase during a course of fractionated radiotherapy relative to the pretreatment state as a result of changes in the balance between cellular proliferation and cell loss.[135] This may offset the beneficial effects of radiation, and decrease the probability of tumor eradication. Poorly differentiated urothelial carcinoma has been reported to have a high labeling index and short potential doubling time,[136–138] both indicators of rapid tumor growth and repopulation. In addition, high levels of the proliferative markers Ki67 and cyclins A and D have been correlated with decreased clinical radioresponse.[99,110,139] It has been estimated that

prolongation of bladder cancer radiotherapy by 20% or more will decrease local control by a factor of 5 to 10.[140]

Accelerated radiotherapy regimens are designed to deliver the same total dose of radiation in a shorter interval of time relative to conventionally fractionated regimens to offset tumor cell repopulation. At least six phase II studies of accelerated radiotherapy have reported encouraging locoregional control rates and acceptable toxicity.[141–146] Horwich et al[147] reported the results of a prospective study in which 229 patients with bladder cancer were randomly assigned to receive accelerated radiation consisting of 60.8 Gy in 32 fractions over 26 days or conventional radiation with 64 Gy in 32 fractions over 45 days. There was no difference in local control, time to metastases, or overall survival between the groups, and patients in the accelerated arm had a significantly higher rate of bowel injury.

Finally, the therapeutic ratio theoretically can be enhanced in patients with bladder cancer by exploiting differences in the intrinsic DNA repair capacity between tumor and normal tissue cells. Hyperfractionated regimens, defined as the delivery of a larger number of smaller fractions (usually 1.5 Gy or less) with no increase in overall treatment time, should allow an increase in radiation dose leading to a greater likelihood of tumor control with no increase in the risk of late bowel or bladder complications. There have been at least two phase III randomized studies of hyperfractionated versus conventional radiotherapy in patients with bladder cancer.[148,149] Clinical complete response and long-term local control were improved in the hyperfractionated arms relative to conventional fractionation. A meta-analysis based on the pooled data from these studies indicated a significant improvement in overall survival with hyperfractionated treatment.[150]

## FUTURE DIRECTIONS IN BLADDER CANCER RADIOBIOLOGY

Both tumors and patients are heterogeneous. Multiple genetic and microenvironmental factors must be assessed to accurately predict the response of the bladder cancer, normal bladder, and adjacent normal tissues to radiation. Genomic and proteomic analyses have shown that radiation-induced gene expression can be cell-type specific, dose dependent, and vary under in vitro versus in vivo conditions. This observation supports the concept that, in the future, 'molecular profiling' of an individual patient may predict the relevant radiation-associated stress responses within that patient.[151–153] Biopsies taken during radiotherapy may be required to optimize the patient profile, as they will better reflect radiation-associated stress responses than will the pretreatment state. These data will be required to fully utilize molecular-targeted agents in combination with radiotherapy and/or alternative radiotherapy fractionation protocols.

Noninvasive, molecular, and microenvironmental imaging has the potential to track changes in tumor and normal tissue biology over time during a course of fractionated radiotherapy, thereby allowing adaptation of treatment to optimize outcome. Imaging of cell death (apoptosis or necrosis), hypoxia, or the induction of radiation-induced signaling pathways (increased expression of $p21^{WAF}$ or cell proliferation genes) will become increasingly important as bladder-specific molecular biology is incorporated into clinic practice.[154-156]

In summary, future developments in our understanding of radiobiology will allow patients to be selected more accurately for either radical cystectomy or radiation at initial presentation. They will also greatly facilitate the use of modifiers of radiation response to increase tumor cell killing and yet protect normal tissues. Together with developments in anatomic imaging of bladder cancer and image-guided precision radiation treatment planning and delivery, the use of novel biomarkers and molecularly targeted agents has the potential to dramatically improve tumor control, organ preservation, and quality of life for patients with bladder cancer.

## REFERENCES

1. Gospodarowicz MK, Hawkins NV, Rawlings GA, et al. Radical radiotherapy for the muscle invasive transitional cell carcinoma of the bladder: failure analysis. J Urol 1989;142:1448–1454.
2. Greven KM, Solin LJ, Hanks GE. Prognostic factors in patients with bladder carcinoma treated with definitive irradiation. Cancer 1990;65:908–912.
3. Pollack A, Zagars GK, Swanson DA. Muscle-invasive bladder cancer treated with external beam radiotherapy: prognostic factors. Int J Radiat Oncol Biol Phys 1994;30:267–277.
4. Vale JA, A'Hern RP, Liu K, et al. Predicting the outcome of radical radiotherapy for invasive bladder cancer. Eur Urol 1993;24:48–51.
5. Duncan W, Quilty PM. The results of a series of 963 patients with transitional cell carcinoma of the urinary bladder primarily treated by radical megavoltage x-ray therapy. Radiother Oncol 1986;7:299–310.
6. Gospodarowicz MK, Rider WD, Keen CW, et al. Bladder cancer: long term follow-up results of patients treated with radical radiation. Clin Oncol 1991;3:155–161.
7. Rodel C, Grabenbauer G, Kuhn R, et al. Combined-modality treatment and selective organ preservation in invasive bladder cancer: long-term results. J Clin Oncol 2002;20:3061–3071.
8. Mameghan H, Fisher R, Mameghan J, Brook S. Analysis of failure following definitive radiotherapy for invasive transitional cell carcinoma of the bladder. Int J Radiat Oncol Biol Phys 1995;31:247–254.
9. Moonen L, vd Voet H, de Nijs R, Hart AA, Horenblas S, Bartelink H. Muscle-invasive bladder cancer treated with external beam radiotherapy: pretreatment prognostic factors and the predictive value of cystoscopic re-evaluation during treatment. Radiother Oncol 1998;49:149–155.
10. Shipley WU, Rose MA, Perrone TL, Mannix CM, Heney NM, Prout GR. Full-dose irradiation for patients with invasive bladder carcinoma: clinical and histologic factors prognostic of improved survival. J Urol 1985;134:679–683.
11. Blandy JP, Jenkins BJ, Fowler CG, et al. Radical radiotherapy and salvage cystectomy for T2/3 cancer of the bladder. Progr Clin Biol Res 1988;260:447–451.
12. Jenkins BJ, Caulfield MJ, Fowler, et al. Reappraisal of the role of radical radiotherapy and salvage cystectomy in the treatment of invasive (T2/T3) bladder cancer. Br J Urol 1988;62:342–346.
13. Smaaland R, Akslen L, Tonder B, Mehus A, Lote K, Albrektsen G. Radical radiation treatment of invasive and locally advanced bladder cancer in elderly patients. Br J Urol 1991;67:61–69.
14. Jahnson S, Pedersen J, Westman G. Bladder carcinoma—a 20-year review of radical irradiation therapy. Radiother Oncol 1991;22:111–117.
15. Shipley WU, Prout GR, Kaufman SD, Perrone TL. Invasive bladder carcinoma. The importance of initial transurethral surgery and other significant prognostic factors for improved survival with full-dose irradiation. Cancer 1987;60:514–520.
16. Timmer PR, Harlief HA, Hooijkaas JA. Bladder cancer: pattern of recurrence in 142 patients. Int J Radiat Oncol Biol Phys 1985;11:899–905.
17. Moonen L, vd Voet H, de Nijs R, Horenblas S, Hart AA, Bartelink. H. Muscle-invasive bladder cancer treated with external beam radiation: influence of total dose, overall treatment time, and treatment interruption on local control. Int J Radiat Oncol Biol Phys 1998;42:525–530.
18. Fung CY, Shipley WU, Young RH, et al. Prognostic factors in invasive bladder carcinoma in a prospective trial of preoperative adjuvant chemotherapy and radiotherapy. J Clin Oncol 1991;9:1533–1542.
19. Wolf H, Olsen PR, Hojgaard K. Urothelial dysplasia concomitant with bladder tumours: a determinant for future new occurrences in patients treated by full-course radiotherapy. Lancet 1985;1:1005–1008.
20. Zietman A, Grocela J, Zehr E, et al. Selective bladder conservation using transurethral resection, chemotherapy, and radiation: management and consequences of Ta, T1, and Tis recurrence within the retained bladder. Urology 2001;58:380–385.
21. Davidson SE, Symonds RP, Snee MP, Upadhyay S, Habeshaw T, Robertson AG. Assessment of factors influencing the outcome of radiotherapy for bladder cancer. Br J Urol 1990;66:288–293.
22. Fossa SD, Waehre H, Aass N, Jacobsen AB, Olsen DR, Ous S. Bladder cancer definitive radiation therapy of muscle-invasive bladder cancer. A retrospective analysis of 317 patients. Cancer 1993;72:3036–3043.
23. Goffinet DR, Schneider MJ, Glatstein EJ, et al. Bladder cancer: results of radiation therapy in 384 patients. Radiology 1975;117:149–153.
24. Yu WS, Sagerman RH, Chung CT, Dalal PS, King GA. Bladder carcinoma. Experience with radical and preoperative radiotherapy in 421 patients. Cancer 1985;56:1293–1299.
25. Goodman GB, Hislop TG, Elwood JM, Balfour J. Conservation of bladder function in patients with invasive bladder cancer treated by definitive irradiation and selective cystectomy. Int J Radiat Oncol Biol Phys 1981;7:569–573.
26. Lerner SP, Skinner DG, Lieskovsky G, et al. The rationale for en bloc pelvic lymph node dissection for bladder cancer patients with nodal metastases: long-term results. J Urol 1993;149:758–764.
27. Frazier HA, Robertson JE, Dodge RK, Paulson DF. The value of pathologic factors in predicting cancer-specific survival among patients treated with radical cystectomy for transitional cell carcinoma of the bladder and prostate. Cancer 1993;71:3993–4001.
28. Bassi P, Ferrante GD, Piazza N, et al. Prognostic factors of outcome after radical cystectomy for bladder cancer: a retrospective study of a homogeneous patient cohort. J Urol 1999;161:1494–1497.
29. Skinner DG, Tift JP, Kaufman JJ. High dose, short course preoperative radiation therapy and immediate single stage radical cystectomy with pelvic node dissection in the management of bladder cancer. J Urol 1982;127:671–674.
30. Milosevic M, Gospodarowicz M, Jewett M, Bristow R, Haycocks T. Intensity-modulated radiation therapy (IMRT) for lymph node metastases in bladder cancer. In Gregoire V, Scalliet P, Ang K (eds): Clinical Target Volumes in Conformal and Intensity Modulated Radiation Therapy. New York: Springer-Verlag, 2003, pp 157–169.
31. Agranovich A, Czaykowski P, Hui D, Pickles T, Kwan W. Radiotherapy for muscle-invasive urinary bladder cancer in elderly patients. Can J Urol 2003;10:2056–2061.

32. Borgaonkar S, Jain A, Bollina P, et al. Radical radiotherapy and salvage cystectomy as the primary management of transitional cell carcinoma of the bladder. Results following the introduction of a CT planning technique. Clin Oncol 2002;14:141–147.

33. Larsen LE, Engelholm SA. The value of three-dimensional radiotherapy planning in advanced carcinoma of the urinary bladder based on computed tomography. Acta Oncol 1994;33:655–659.

34. Bentzen SM, Jessen KA, Jorgensen J, Sell A. Impact of CT-based treatment planning on radiation therapy of carcinoma of the bladder. Acta Radiol Oncol 1984;23:199–203.

35. Rothwell RI, Ash DV, Jones WG. Radiation treatment planning for bladder cancer: a comparison of cystogram localisation with computed tomography. Clin Radiol 1983;34:103–111.

36. Logue JP, Sharrock CL, Cowan RA, Read G, Marrs J, Mott D. Clinical variability of target volume description in conformal radiotherapy planning. Int J Radiat Oncol Biol Phys 1998;41:929–931.

37. Meijer G, Rasch C, Remeijer P, Lebesque J. Three-dimensional analysis of delineation errors, setup errors, and organ motion during radiotherapy of bladder cancer. Int J Radiat Oncol Biol Phys 2003;55:1277–1287.

38. Cowan R, McBain C, Ryder W, et al. Radiotherapy for muscle-invasive carcinoma of the bladder: results of a randomized trial comparing conventional whole bladder with dose-escalated partial bladder radiotherapy. Int J Radiat Oncol Biol Phys 2004;59:197–207.

39. Turner SL, Swindell SL, Bowl N, et al. Bladder movement during radiation therapy for bladder cancer: implications for treatment planning. Int J Radiat Oncol Biol Phys 1997;39:355–360.

40. Muren L, Smaaland R, Dahl O. Organ motion, set-up variation and treatment margins in radical radiotherapy of urinary bladder cancer. Radiother Oncol 2003;69:291–304.

41. Muren L, Redpath A, McLaren D. Treatment margins and treatment fractionation in conformal radiotherapy of muscle-invading urinary bladder cancer. Radiother Oncol 2004;71:65–71.

42. Jaffray DA, Siewerdsen JH, Wong JW, Martinez AA. Flat-panel cone-beam computed tomography for image-guided radiation therapy. Int J Radiat Oncol Biol Phys 2002;53:1337–1349.

43. Turner WH, Markwalder R, Perrig S, Studer UE. Meticulous pelvic lymphadenectomy in surgical treatment of the invasive bladder cancer: an option or a must? Eur Urol 1998;33 (Suppl 4):21–22.

44. Vieweg J, Gschwend JE, Herr HW, Fair WR. Pelvic lymph node dissection can be curative in patients with node positive bladder cancer. J Urol 1999;161:449–454.

45. Stein JP, Lieskovsky G, Cote R, et al. Radical cystectomy in the treatment of invasive bladder cancer: long-term results in 1,054 patients. J Clin Oncol 2001;19:666–675.

46. Smith JA, Whitmore WF. Regional lymph node metastases from bladder cancer. J Urol 1981;126:591–593.

47. Zincke H, Patterson DE, Utz DC, Benson RC. Pelvic lymphadenectomy and radical cystectomy for transitional cell carcinoma of the bladder with pelvic lymph node disease. Br J Urol 1985;57:156–159.

48. Poulson AL, Horn T, Steven K. Radical cystectomy: extending the limits of pelvic lymph node dissection improves survival for patients with bladder cancer confined to the bladder wall. J Urol 1998;160:2015–2021.

49. Bretheau D, Ponthieu A. Results of radical cystectomy and pelvic lymphadenectomy for bladder cancer with pelvic node metastases. Urol Int 1996;57:27–31.

50. Quilty PM, Kerr GR, Duncan W. Prognostic indices for bladder cancer: an analysis of patients with transitional cell carcinoma of the bladder primarily treated by radical megavoltage x-ray therapy. Radiother Oncol 1986;7:311–321.

51. Sell A, Jakobsen A, Nerstrom B, Sorensen B, Steven K, Barlebo H. Treatment of advanced bladder cancer category T2, T3 and T4a. Scand J Urol Nephrol 1991;138:193–201.

52. Pisters LL, Tykochinsky G, Wajsman Z. Intravesical bacillus Calmette–Guérin or mitomycin C in the treatment of carcinoma in situ of the bladder following prior pelvic radiation therapy. J Urol 1991;146:1514–1517.

53. Palou J, Sanchez-Martin FM, Rosales A, Salvador J, Algaba F, Vicente J. Intravesical bacille Calmette–Guérin in the treatment of carcinoma in situ or high-grade superficial bladder carcinoma after radiotherapy for bladder carcinoma. BJU Int 1999;83:429–431.

54. Quilty PM, Duncan W, Chisholm GD, et al. Results of surgery following radical radiotherapy for invasive bladder cancer. Br J Urol 1986;58:396–405.

55. Bloom HJ, Hendry WF, Wallace DM, Skeet RG. Treatment of T3 bladder cancer: controlled trial of pre-operative radiotherapy and radical cystectomy versus radical radiotherapy. Br J Urol 1982;54:136–151.

56. Shipley W, Kaufman D, Zehr E, et al. Selective bladder preservation by combined modality protocol treatment: long-term outcomes of 190 patients with invasive bladder cancer. Urology 2002;60:62–67.

57. Zietman A, Sacco D, Skowronski U, et al. Organ conservation in invasive bladder cancer by transurethral resection, chemotherapy and radiation: results of a urodynamic and quality of life study on long-term survivors. J Urol 2003;170:1772–1776.

58. Coppin C, Gospodarowicz M, James K, et al. The NCI-Canada trial of concurrent cisplatin and radiotherapy for muscle invasive bladder cancer. J Clin Oncol 1996;14:2901–2907.

59. Shearer RJ, Chilvers CED, Bloom HJG, et al. Adjuvant chemotherapy in T3 carcinoma of the bladder. A prospective trial: preliminary report. Br J Urol 1988;62:558–564.

60. Wallace DMA, Raghavan D, Kelly KA, et al. Neo-adjuvant (pre-emptive) cisplatin therapy in invasive transitional cell carcinoma of the bladder. Br J Urol 1991;67:608–615.

61. Shipley WU, Winter KA, Kaufman DS, et al. Phase III trial of neoadjuvant chemotherapy in patients with invasive bladder cancer treated with selective bladder preservation by combined radiation therapy and chemotherapy: initial results of Radiation Therapy Oncology Group 89-03. J Clin Oncol 1998;16:3576–3583.

62. Sengelov L, von der Maase H, Lundbeck F, et al. Neoadjuvant chemotherapy with cisplatin and methotrexate in patients with muscle-invasive bladder tumours. Acta Oncol 2002;41:447–456.

63. Ghersi D, Stewart LA, Parmar KMB, et al. Neoadjuvant cisplatin, methotrexate, and vinblastine chemotherapy for muscle-invasive bladder cancer: a randomized controlled trial. Lancet 1999;354:533–540.

64. Farah R, Chodak GW, Vogelzang NJ, et al. Curative radiotherapy following chemotherapy for invasive bladder carcinoma (a preliminary report). Int J Radiat Oncol Biol Phys 1991;20:413–417.

65. Tester W, Caplan R, Heaney J, et al. Neoadjuvant combined modality program with selective organ preservation for invasive bladder cancer. results of Radiation Therapy Oncology Group phase II trial 8802. J Clin Oncol 1996;14:119–126.

66. Wajsman Z, Marino R, Parsons J, Oblon D, McCarley D. Bladder-sparing approach in the treatment of invasive bladder cancer. Semin Urol 1990;8(3):210–215.

67. Advanced Bladder Cancer Meta-analysis Collaboration. Neoadjuvant chemotherapy in invasive bladder cancer: a systematic review and meta-analysis. Lancet 2003;361:1927–1934.

68. Bristow RG, Hill RP. Molecular and cellular radiobiology. In Tannock IF, Hill RP, Harrington L, Bristow RG (eds): Basic Science of Oncology, 4th ed. New York: McGraw-Hill, 2005, Ch. 14.

69. Oxford G, Theodorescu D. The role of Ras superfamily proteins in bladder cancer progression. J Urol 2003;170:1987–1993.

70. Raghavan D. Molecular targeting and pharmacogenomics in the management of advanced bladder cancer. Cancer 2003;97:2083–2089.

71. Al-Sukhun S, Hussain M. Molecular biology of transitional cell carcinoma. Crit Rev Oncol Hematol 2003;47:181–193.

72. Faulhaber O, Bristow RG. Basis of cell kill following clinical radiotherapy. In Sluyser M (ed): Application of Apoptosis to Cancer Treatment. New York: Springer, 2005.

73. Wilson GD. Radiation and the cell cycle, revisited. Cancer Metastasis Rev 2004;23:209–225.

74. Cuddihy AR, Bristow RG. The p53 protein family and radiation sensitivity: Yes or no? Cancer Metastasis Rev 2004;23:237–257.

75. Doherty SC, McKeown SR, McKelvey-Martin V, et al. Cell cycle checkpoint function in bladder cancer. J Natl Cancer Inst 2003;95:1859–1868.

76. Pollack A, Wu CS, Czerniak B, Zagars GK, Benedict WF, McDonnell TJ. Abnormal bcl-2 and pRb expression are independent correlates of radiation response in muscle-invasive bladder cancer. Clin Cancer Res 1997;3:1823–1829.

77. Bakkenist CJ, Kastan MB. Initiating cellular stress responses. Cell 2004;118:9–17.

78. Bristow RG, Hill RP. The scientific basis of clinical radiotherapy. In Tannock IF, Hill RP, Harrington L, Bristow RG (eds): Basic Science of Oncology, 4th ed. New York: McGraw-Hill, 2005, Ch. 15.

79. Mack PC, Gandara DR, Bowen C, et al. RB status as a determinant of response to UCN-01 in non-small cell lung carcinoma. Clin Cancer Res 1999;5:2596–2604.

80. Chien M, Astumian M, Liebowitz D, Rinker-Schaeffer C, Stadler WM. In vitro evaluation of flavopiridol, a novel cell cycle inhibitor, in bladder cancer. Cancer Chemother Pharmacol 1999;44:81–87.

81. Bohm L, Roos WP, Serafin AM. Inhibition of DNA repair by pentoxifylline and related methylxanthine derivatives. Toxicology 2003;193:153–160.

82. Jones LA, Clegg S, Bush C, McMillan TJ, Peacock JH. Relationship between chromosome aberrations, micronuclei and cell kill in two human tumour cell lines of widely differing radiosensitivity. Int J Radiat Biol 1994;66:639–642.

83. Woudstra EC, Roesink JM, Rosemann M, et al. Chromatin structure and cellular radiosensitivity: a comparison of two human tumour cell lines. Int J Radiat Biol 1996;70:693–703.

84. Collis SJ, Sangar VK, Tighe A, et al. Development of a novel rapid assay to assess the fidelity of DNA double-strand-break repair in human tumour cells. Nucleic Acids Res 2002;30:E1.

85. McKeown SR, Robson T, Price ME, Ho ET, Hirst DG, McKelvey-Martin VJ. Potential use of the alkaline comet assay as a predictor of bladder tumour response to radiation. Br J Cancer 2003;89:2264–2270.

86. Moneef MA, Sherwood BT, Bowman KJ, et al. Measurements using the alkaline comet assay predict bladder cancer cell radiosensitivity. Br J Cancer 2003;89:2271–2276.

87. Abraham RT. PI 3-kinase related kinases: 'big' players in stress-induced signaling pathways. DNA Repair 2004;3:883–887.

88. van Gent DC, Hoeijmakers JH, Kanaar R. Chromosomal stability and the DNA double-stranded break connection. Nat Rev Genet 2001;2:196–206.

89. Ortiz T, Lopez S, Burguillos MA, Edreira A, Pinero J. Radiosensitizer effect of wortmannin in radioresistant bladder tumoral cell lines. Int J Oncol 2004;24:169–175.

90. Siddik ZH. Cisplatin: mode of cytotoxic action and molecular basis of resistance. Oncogene 2003;22:7265–7279.

91. Begg AC, Stewart FA, Dewit L, Bartelink H. Interactions between cisplatin and radiation in experimental rodent tumors and normal tissues. In Hill BT, Bellamy AS (eds): Antitumor Drug-Radiation Interactions. Boca Raton, FL: CRC Press, 2000, pp 153–170.

92. Wachters FM, van Putten JW, Maring JG, Zdzienicka MZ, Groen HJ, Kampinga HH. Selective targeting of homologous DNA recombination repair by gemcitabine. Int J Radiat Oncol Biol Phys 2003;57:553–562.

93. Pauwels B, Korst AE, Pattyn GG, et al. Cell cycle effect of gemcitabine and its role in the radiosensitizing mechanism in vitro. Int J Radiat Oncol Biol Phys 2003;57:1075–1083.

94. Sangar VK, Cowan R, Margison GP, Hendry JH, Clarke NW. An evaluation of gemcitabine's differential radiosensitising effect in related bladder cancer cell lines. Br J Cancer 2004;90:542–548.

95. West CM. Invited review: intrinsic radiosensitivity as a predictor of patient response to radiotherapy. Br J Radiol 1995;68:827–837.

96. Moonen L, Ong F, Gallee M, et al. Apoptosis, proliferation and p53, cyclin D1, and retinoblastoma gene expression in relation to radiation response in transitional cell carcinoma of the bladder. Int J Radiat Oncol Biol Phys 2001;49:1305–1310.

97. Wang S, El-Deiry WS. TRAIL and apoptosis induction by TNF-family death receptors. Oncogene 2003;22:8628–8633.

98. Hussain SA, Ganesan R, Hiller L, et al. BCL2 expression predicts survival in patients receiving synchronous chemoradiotherapy in advanced transitional cell carcinoma of the bladder. Oncol Rep 2003;10:571–576.

99. Matsumoto H, Wada T, Fukunaga K, Yoshihiro S, Matsuyama H, Naito K. Bax to Bcl-2 ratio and Ki-67 index are useful predictors of neoadjuvant chemoradiation therapy in bladder cancer. Jpn J Clin Oncol 2004;34:124–130.

100. Ong F, Moonen LM, Gallee MP, et al. Prognostic factors in transitional cell cancer of the bladder: an emerging role for Bcl-2 and p53. Radiother Oncol 2001;61:169–175.

101. Qureshi KN, Griffiths TR, Robinson MC, et al. Combined p21WAF1/CIP1 and p53 overexpression predict improved survival in muscle-invasive bladder cancer treated by radical radiotherapy. Int J Radiat Oncol Biol Phys 2001;51:1234–1240.

102. Rotterud R, Berner A, Holm R, Skovlund E, Fossa SD. p53, p21 and mdm2 expression vs the response to radiotherapy in transitional cell carcinoma of the bladder. BJU Int 2001;88:202–208.

103. Ribeiro JC, Barnetson AR, Fisher RJ, Mameghan H, Russell PJ. Relationship between radiation response and p53 status in human bladder cancer cells. Int J Radiat Biol 1997;72:11–20.

104. Rotterud R, Skomedal H, Berner A, Danielsen HE, Skovlund E, Fossa SD. TP53 and p21WAF1/CIP1 behave differently in euploid versus aneuploid bladder tumours treated with radiotherapy. Acta Oncol 2001;40:644–652.

105. Fechner G, Perabo FG, Schmidt DH, et al. Preclinical evaluation of a radiosensitizing effect of gemcitabine in p53 mutant and p53 wild type bladder cancer cells. Urology 2003;61:468–473.

106. Hinata N, Shirakawa T, Zhang Z, et al. Radiation induces p53-dependent cell apoptosis in bladder cancer cells with wild-type-p53 but not in p53-mutated bladder cancer cells. Urol Res 2003;31:387–396.

107. Pollack A, Czerniak B, Zagars GK, et al. Retinoblastoma protein expression and radiation response in muscle-invasive bladder cancer. Int J Radiat Oncol Biol Phys 1997;39:687–695.

108. Muro XGd, Condom E, Vigues F, et al. p53 and p21 Expression levels predict organ preservation and survival in invasive bladder carcinoma treated with a combined-modality approach. Cancer 2004;100:1859–1867.

109. Wu CS, Pollack A, Czerniak B, et al. Prognostic value of p53 in muscle-invasive bladder cancer treated with preoperative radiotherapy. Urology 1996;47:305–310.

110. Rodel C, Grabenbauer GG, Rodel F, et al. Apoptosis, p53, bcl-2, and KI-67 in invasive bladder carcinoma: possible predictors for response to radiochemotherapy and successful bladder preservation. Int J Radiat Oncol Biol Phys 2000;46:1213–1221.

111. Duggan BJ, Maxwell P, Kelly JD, et al. The effect of antisense Bcl-2 oligonucleotides on Bcl-2 protein expression and apoptosis in human bladder transitional cell carcinoma. J Urol 2001;166:1098–1105.

112. Pagliaro LC, Keyhani A, Williams D, et al. Repeated intravesical instillations of an adenoviral vector in patients with locally advanced bladder cancer: a phase I study of p53 gene therapy. J Clin Oncol 2003;21:2247–2253.

113. Slaton JW, Benedict WF, Dinney CP. P53 in bladder cancer: mechanism of action, prognostic value, and target for therapy. Urology 2001;57:852–859.

114. Bromfield GP, Meng A, Warde P, Bristow RG. Cell death in irradiated prostate epithelial cells: role of apoptotic and clonogenic cell kill. Prostate Cancer Prostatic Dis 2003;6:73–85.

115. Okada H, Mak TW. Pathways of apoptotic and non-apoptotic death in tumour cells. Nat Rev Cancer 2004;4:592–603.

116. Nakahata K, Miyakoda M, Suzuki K, Kodama S, Watanabe M. Heat shock induces centrosomal dysfunction, and causes non-apoptotic mitotic catastrophe in human tumour cells. Int J Hyperthermia 2002;18:332–343.

117. Altieri DC. Survivin, versatile modulation of cell division and apoptosis in cancer. Oncogene 2003;22:8581–8589.

118. Schultz IJ, Kiemeney LA, Karthaus HF, et al. Survivin mRNA copy number in bladder washings predicts tumor recurrence in patients with superficial urothelial cell carcinomas. Clin Chem 2004;50:1425–1428.

119. Swana HS, Grossman D, Anthony JN, Weiss RM, Altieri DC. Tumor content of the antiapoptosis molecule survivin and recurrence of bladder cancer. N Engl J Med 1999;341:452–453.

120. Ning S, Fuessel S, Kotzsch M, et al. siRNA-mediated down-regulation of survivin inhibits bladder cancer cell growth. Int J Oncol 2004;25:1065–1071.

121. Fuessel S, Kueppers B, Ning S, et al. Systematic in vitro evaluation of survivin directed antisense oligodeoxynucleotides in bladder cancer cells. J Urol 2004;171:2471–2476.

122. Glaser KB, Staver MJ, Waring JF, Stender J, Ulrich RG, Davidsen SK. Gene expression profiling of multiple histone deacetylase (HDAC) inhibitors: defining a common gene set produced by HDAC inhibition in T24 and MDA carcinoma cell lines. Mol Cancer Ther 2003;2:151–163.

123. Richon VM, Sandhoff TW, Rifkind RA, Marks PA. Histone deacetylase inhibitor selectively induces p21WAF1 expression and gene-associated histone acetylation. Proc Natl Acad Sci USA 2000;97:10014–10019.

124. Duchesne GM, Hutchinson LK. Reversible changes in radiation response induced by all-trans retinoic acid. Int J Radiat Oncol Biol Phys 1995;33:875–880.

125. Milosevic M, Fyles A, Hedley D, Hill R. The human tumor microenvironment: invasive (needle) measurements of oxygen and interstitial fluid pressure. Semin Radiat Oncol 2004;14:249–258.

126. Brown JM, Wilson WR. Exploiting tumour hypoxia in cancer treatment. Nat Rev Cancer 2004;4:437–447.

127. Subarsky P, Hill RP. The hypoxic tumour microenvironment and metastatic progression. Clin Exp Metastasis 2003;20:237–250.

128. Hoskin P, Sibtain A, Daley F, Wilson G. GLUT1 and CAIX as intrinsic markers of hypoxia in bladder cancer: relationship with vascularity and proliferation as predictors of outcome of ARCON. Br J Cancer 2003;89:1290–1297.

129. Fyles A, Milosevic M, Hedley D, et al Tumor hypoxia has independent predictor impact only in patients with node-negative cervix cancer. J Clin Oncol 2002;20:680–687.

130. Brizel DM, Scully SP, Harrelson JM, et al. Tumor oxygenation predicts for likelihood of distant metastases in human soft tissue sarcoma. Cancer Res 1996;56:941–943.

131. Kaanders JH, Bussink J, van der Kogel AJ. ARCON: a novel biology-based approach in radiotherapy. Lancet Oncol 2002;3:728–737.

132. Chaudhary R, Bromley M, Clarke NW, et al. Prognostic relevance of micro-vessel density in cancer of the urinary bladder. Anticancer Res 1999;19:3479–3484.

133. Sabichi AL, Lippman SM. COX-2 inhibitors and other nonsteroidal anti-inflammatory drugs in genitourinary cancer. Semin Oncol 2004;31:36–44.

134. Ma BB, Bristow RG, Kim J, Siu LL. Combined-modality treatment of solid tumors using radiotherapy and molecular targeted agents. J Clin Oncol 2003;21:2760–2776.

135. Thames HD, Hendry JH. Fractionation in radiotherapy. London: Taylor and Francis, 1987, p 297.

136. Trott KR, Kummermehr J. What is known about tumour proliferation rates to choose between accelerated fractionation or hyperfractionation? Radiother Oncol 1985;3:1–9.

137. Hainau B, Dombernowsky P. Histology and cell proliferation in human bladder tumors. Cancer 1974;33:115–126.

138. Rew DA, Thomas DJ, Coptcoat M, Wilson GD. Measurement of in vivo urological tumour cell kinetics using multiplanar flow cytometry. Preliminary study. Br J Urol 1991;68:44–48.

139. Subarsky P, Hill R. The hypoxic tumour microenvironment and metastatic progression. Clin. Exp Metastasis 2003;20:237–250.

140. Majewski W, Maciejewski B, Majewski S, Suwinski R, Miszczyk L, Tarnawski R. Clinical radiobiology of stage T2-T3 bladder cancer. Int J Radiat Oncol Biol Phys 2004;60:60–70.

141. Cole DJ, Durrant KR, Roberts JT, Dawes PJ, Yosef H, Hopewell JW. A pilot study of accelerated fractionation in the radiotherapy of invasive carcinoma of the bladder. Br J Radiol 1992;65:792–798.

142. Pos F, Tienhoven Gv, Hulshof M, Koedooder K, Gonzalez DG. Concomitant boost radiotherapy for muscle invasive bladder cancer. Radiother Oncol 2003;68:75–80.

143. Yavuz A, Yavuz M, Ozgur G, et al. Accelerated superfractionated radiotherapy with concomitant boost for invasive bladder cancer. Int J Radiat Oncol Biol Phys 2003;56:734–745.

144. Zouhair A, Ozsahin M, Schneider D, et al. Invasive bladder carcinoma: a pilot study of conservative treatment with accelerated radiotherapy and concomitant cisplatin. Int J Cancer 2001;96:350–355.

145. Moonen L, van der Voet H, Horenblas S, Bartelink H. A feasibility study of accelerated fractionation in radiotherapy of carcinoma of the urinary bladder. Int J Radiat Oncol Biol Phys 1997;37:537–542.

146. Plataniotis G, Michalopoulos E, Kouvaris J, Vlahos L, Papavasiliou C. A feasibility study of partially accelerated radiotherapy for invasive bladder cancer. Radiother Oncol 1994;33:84–87.

147. Horwich A, Dearnaley D, Huddart R, et al. A trial of accelerated fractionation (AF) in T2/3 bladder cancer [abstract]. Eur J Cancer 1999;35(Suppl 4):S342.

148. Naslund I, Nilsson B, Littbrand B. Hyperfractionated radiotherapy of bladder cancer. A ten-year follow-up of a randomized clinical trial. Acta Oncol 1994;33:397–402.

149. Goldobenko G, Matveev B, Shipilov V, Klimakov B, Tkachev S. Radiation treatment of bladder cancer using different fractionation regimens. Med Radiol (Mosk) 1991;36:14–16.

150. Stuschke M, Thames HD. Hyperfractionated radiotherapy of human tumors: overview of the randomized clinical trials. Int J Radiat Oncol Biol Phys 1997;37:259–267.

151. Dyrskjot L. Classification of bladder cancer by microarray expression profiling: towards a general clinical use of microarrays in cancer diagnostics. Expert Rev Mol Diagn 2003;3:635–647.

152. Ferguson RE, Selby PJ, Banks RE. Proteomic studies in urological malignancies. Contrib Nephrol 2004;141:257–279.

153. Sanchez-Carbayo M, Cordon-Cardo C. Applications of array technology: identification of molecular targets in bladder cancer. Br J Cancer 2003;89:2172–2177.

154. Blankenberg FG. Recent advances in the imaging of programmed cell death. Curr Pharm Des 2004;10:1457–1467.

155. Shah R, El-Deiry WS. p53-Dependent activation of a molecular beacon in tumor cells following exposure to doxorubicin chemotherapy. Cancer Biol Ther 2004;3(9):871–875.

156. Lewis JS, Welch MJ. PET imaging of hypoxia. Q J Nucl Med 2001;45:183–188.

# Urinary tract reconstruction

# Trimodality therapy in the management of muscle-invasive bladder cancer: a selective organ-preserving approach

55

*John J Coen, Anthony L Zietman, Donald S Kaufman, Niall M Heney,*
*Alex F Althausen, William U Shipley*

## OVERVIEW

Combined modality therapy with organ preservation has become standard therapy for a variety of solid tumors. Although radical cystectomy continues to be standard therapy for invasive bladder cancer, there is evidence to suggest that selective bladder preservation results in similar outcome with the opportunity to retain the native bladder. Older randomized trials have failed to demonstrate a survival advantage for immediate cystectomy as opposed to salvage cystectomy for recurrent disease in patients receiving radiation therapy. Selective bladder preservation using a trimodality approach, as commonly practiced in the US, affords an early cystectomy for patients who fail to respond to chemoradiation. Using this approach, a complete transurethral resection is performed. Following an induction course of concurrent chemotherapy and radiation, histologic response is evaluated by cystoscopy and rebiopsy. Clinical 'complete responders' (tumor site biopsy and urine cytology negative) continue with a consolidation course of chemotherapy and radiation, while others are encouraged to have an immediate cystectomy. Complete response rates of 65% to 80% can be achieved. Conserved bladders are closely followed by a urologist who will perform a prompt cystectomy if there is an invasive recurrence. Noninvasive recurrences can be managed by more conservative measures in a manner similar to a de novo tumor. Bladder conservation trials using this approach report 5-year survival rates of approximately 50%, with 80% of surviving patients retaining their bladder. Quality of

life and urodynamic studies reveal good functional outcomes for patients with preserved bladders.

## INTRODUCTION

The treatment options for muscle-invasive bladder cancer can be broadly divided into organ-sparing regimens and those that require immediate removal of the bladder. Radical cystectomy with surgical removal of the bladder, its adnexae, and the regional lymph nodes represents the most prevalent treatment offered in the US. Radiation therapy, the traditional bladder-sparing approach, has only been recommended for patients deemed 'unfit' for surgery secondary to advanced age, comorbidities or disease extent. Consequently, when comparisons of retrospective radiation and surgical series have been made, better outcomes for patients undergoing cystectomy are reported. This comparison is further confounded as an additional 15% of patients are excluded from cystectomy series secondary to intraoperative discovery of extravesical tumor extension, prompting abortion of the procedure. In contrast to historic series, modern bladder-sparing regimens do not consist of radiation monotherapy but are typified by a multimodality approach.

Nevertheless, radical cystectomy represents the standard against which bladder-conserving regimens must be measured. Pelvic recurrence rates between 5% and 30%, and overall 5-year survival between 45% and 60%, have been reported after cystectomy.[1-4] Following a radical cystectomy, a urinary diversion must be created which may be an incontinent or continent diversion. The ileal loop procedure allows urine to drain into an isolated segment of ileum which acts as a conduit to a stoma created at the skin surface. An appliance acts as an external reservoir to collect urine. Recent surgical advances offer the potential to make the loss of the native bladder more acceptable to the patient. For continent diversions, bowel segments are used to create internal reservoirs that are either intermittently catheterized by the patient through an abdominal wall stoma, or are anastomosed to the urethra (an orthotopic neobladder), allowing the patient to void more naturally. Although continent diversions are becoming more popular, they are still performed on less than half of patients undergoing radical cystectomy. They are also not without problems including enuresis, stenosis, mucosuria, alkalosis, and progressive renal impairment. Revision procedures may be required to resolve one or more of these problems. Despite the enthusiasm of the surgical community, the largest reported series looking at quality of life reported no increase in patient satisfaction with continent diversions as compared to an ileal conduit.[5] Although surgical advances are likely to continue, for the foreseeable future it is not expected that any internal reservoir will be created that functions as well as a preserved native bladder.

Multimodality organ-sparing treatment has become standard therapy for many solid malignancies, including those of the breast, anus, esophagus, and head and neck. Similar advances have been made in the treatment of muscle-invasive bladder cancer evolving into a trimodality approach involving cooperation between urologists, radiation oncologists, and medical oncologists. Modern bladder-sparing represents a selective bladder-preserving regimen where the primary goal is to cure the patient, using early cystectomy when necessary, with a secondary goal of conserving a well-functioning, tumor-free bladder in patients in whom avoidance of cystectomy does not compromise survival.

# EVOLUTION OF THE MODERN BLADDER-PRESERVING APPROACH

## RANDOMIZED COMPARISONS OF EXTERNAL BEAM RADIATION WITH RADICAL CYSTECTOMY

External beam radiation therapy represents the traditional alternative to radical cystectomy, with surgery reserved for salvage should there be any recurrence within the bladder. Urologists have feared that the delay of definitive surgery may compromise survival as the recurrent cancer has a second opportunity to metastasize.

By 1985, four randomized trials had been completed comparing external beam radiation with cystectomy reserved for salvage, with preoperative radiation plus immediate radical cystectomy[6-9] (Table 55.1) Miller et al reported the results of a randomized trial from the University of Texas M.D. Anderson Cancer Center for patients with clinical stage T3 tumors, demonstrating improved overall survival at 5 years for patients randomized to cystectomy as compared to radiation, 45% versus 22%.[6] This is the only trial that demonstrates a statistically significant benefit to early cystectomy; however; it included large T3 tumors unlikely to be adequately managed with radiation alone.

The Urologic Cooperative Group from the UK reported a larger randomized trial of 189 patients comparing radiation with cystectomy reserved for salvage with radiation plus immediate cystectomy.[7] The 5- and 10-year overall survival was 39% and 19% for patients randomized to immediate cystectomy, respectively. In patients randomized to radiation with salvage cystectomy, the 5- and 10-year overall survival was 28% and 15%, respectively. These differences were not statistically significant.

The Danish National Cancer Group also failed to demonstrate a significant overall survival difference at 5

**Table 55.1** Randomized trials of irradiation that did or did not defer radical cystectomy for salvage of recurrence

| Treatment | No. pts | Clinical stage | 5-year survival (%) | 10-year survival (%) | Distant metastases (%) |
|---|---|---|---|---|---|
| M.D. Anderson Hospital[6] | | | | | |
| 50 Gy + cystectomy | 35 | T3 | 46 | – | – |
| 60 Gy + salvage cystectomy | 32 | T3 | 22 | – | – |
| UK Coop Group[7] | | | | | |
| 40 Gy + radical cystectomy | 98 | T3 | 39 | 19 | – |
| 60 Gy + salvage cystectomy | 91 | T3 | 28 | 15 | – |
| National Danish Trial[8] | | | | | |
| 40 Gy + radical cystectomy | 88 | T3 | 29 | – | 34 |
| 60 Gy + salvage cystectomy | 95 | T3 | 23 | – | 32 |
| National Bladder Cancer Group[9] | | | | | |
| 40 Gy + radical cystectomy | 37 | T2–4a | 27 | – | 38 |
| S60 Gy + salvage cystectomy | 35 | T2–4a | 40 | – | 31 |

years: 29% for cystectomy versus 23% for radiation and salvage cystectomy.[8] The local or pelvic failure was lower in patients randomized to immediate cystectomy as compared to radiation alone: 7% versus 35%, respectively. However, the incidence of metastatic disease was similar in both groups: 34% and 32% at 5 years, respectively.

The National Bladder Cancer Group performed a randomized trial of 72 patients.[9] There was no difference in the 5-year overall survival or distant metastasis rate in patients randomized to immediate cystectomy (27% and 38%, respectively) as compared to primary radiation and salvage cystectomy (40% and 31%, respectively).

These trials suggest that deferral of cystectomy until the time of local recurrence does not adversely influence overall survival or the incidence of metastatic disease after external beam radiation. Similarly, the Memorial Sloan-Kettering Cancer Center reported that deferring cystectomy in patients receiving neoadjuvant MVAC (methotrexate, vinblastine, doxorubicin [adriamycin], cisplatin) chemotherapy did not decrease overall survival at 5 years.[10] Thus, selective bladder preservation approaches with cystectomy offered for local tumor recurrence or persistence may be a safe alternative to radical cystectomy for invasive bladder cancer.

## MONOTHERAPY

Transurethral resection and chemotherapy provide a durable local control rate of less than 20% when used as monotherapy (Table 55.2). Although external beam radiation results in a higher local control rate, salvage cystectomy is still required for many of these patients. Compelled by the success of combined modality treatment as organ-preserving therapy in anal and breast cancer, efforts were made to establish a similar treatment approach in invasive bladder cancer. The complete response rate to transurethral resection followed by chemotherapy is nearly twice that achieved by chemotherapy alone, and is slightly greater than that achieved by radiation alone. Trimodality therapy achieves a complete response rate of more than 70%, far greater than that achieved with monotherapy (Table 55.3).

## TRIMODALITY THERAPY

The combination of transurethral resection, chemotherapy, and radiation therapy may serve two purposes: 1) local control is enhanced as surgical debulking provides cytoreduction prior to radiation therapy; 2) concurrent chemotherapy with radiation-sensitizing agents such as cisplatin, 5-fluorouracil (5-FU) or taxol, increases cell death during radiation in a synergistic fashion. Thus, the probability of complete tumor eradication following radiation is maximized. Cytotoxic chemotherapy may also address micro-metastatic disease present at the time of local treatment.

The success of a bladder-preserving treatment approach rests on the ability to select patients for organ conservation based on the initial tumor response. This

**Table 55.2** Success rates of bladder preservation with monotherapy

| Treatment | No. of evaluated series | No. pts | % with bladder free of invasive recurrence |
|---|---|---|---|
| Transurethral resection alone*[35,36] | 2 | 331 | 20‡ |
| Radiation therapy alone†[37–41] | 5 | 949 | 41 |
| Chemotherapy alone†[42] (cisplatin + methotrexate) | 1 | 27 | 19 |

\* Used selectively as monotherapy, most patients at these centers had cystectomy.
†No transurethral resection of tumor.
‡ Intravesical drug therapy often used for noninvasive recurrent tumors.

**Table 55.3** Complete response rates after monotherapies and combined modality therapies

| Treatment | No. of evaluated series | No. pts | Complete responses (%) |
|---|---|---|---|
| Radiation therapy alone[38,39,43,44] | 4 | 721 | 45 |
| Chemotherapy alone[45–50] | 6 | 301 | 27 |
| TURBT plus chemotherapy[51–55] | 5 | 336 | 52 |
| TURBT plus chemoradiotherapy [17,18,56,57] | 4 | 218 | 71 |

TURBT, transurethral resection of bladder tumor.

requires close cooperation with a urologist who is integral to the assessment of therapeutic response and who will perform a radical cystectomy if required. Commonly in the US, bladder conservation is reserved for patients found to have a complete clinical response mid-therapy[11,12] (Figure 55.1). Responders, who comprise more than two-thirds of patients, receive consolidation chemoradiation, and are followed indefinitely with regular cystoscopic examinations. Incomplete responders are encouraged to have an immediate cystectomy, thus averting further pelvic radiation which may complicate urinary diversion surgery. Prompt cystectomy is also recommended at the first sign of invasive recurrence for patients who have completed chemoradiation. Trimodality therapy with cystectomy when necessary results in overall survival rates comparable to radical cystectomy series when matched for age and clinical stage (49–63% at 5 years) (Table 55.4).

The potential success of trimodality therapy was exemplified in a study from the University of Paris. Transurethral resection of bladder tumor (TURBT) followed by concurrent cisplatin, 5-FU, and accelerated radiation was used initially as a precystectomy regimen. The first 18 patients demonstrated no residual tumor on cystoscopic examination and rebiopsy, but all underwent cystectomy as planned.[13] No patient had residual tumor identified in the cystectomy specimen. Subsequently, patients with a clinical complete response were selected for bladder preservation.[13] Radical cystectomy was reserved for patients with a lesser response. In a series of 120 patients, they reported a complete response rate of 77% and a 5-year survival of 63%. A study of 93 patients treated with trimodality therapy at the University of Erlangen reported a clinical complete response rate of 85%. The 5-year overall survival was 61%, with 47% surviving with their native bladder.[14] An update of the Erlangen experience using combined modality treatment reported a clinical complete response rate of 72% in 415 treated patients (126 with radiation alone, 289 with chemoradiation).[15] The 10-year disease-specific survival was 42%, with 80% of survivors retaining their bladder. There was no decrement in survival for patients requiring a salvage cystectomy.

In the US, the Radiation Therapy Oncology Group (RTOG) has studied combined modality therapy in a multi-institutional setting, enrolling 415 patients on six prospective protocols over the last 15 years. Five of these protocols were phase I–II trials of concurrent chemoradiation, and one was a phase III trial that tested the efficacy of neoadjuvant chemotherapy with methotrexate, cisplatin, and vinblastine (MCV). These trials have shaped the manner in which combined modality therapy is administered in the US. Encouraged by the results reported by the National Bladder Cancer Group, the RTOG opened 85-12 which defined the RTOG paradigm for selective bladder preservation.[16] It evaluated trimodality therapy with cystectomy reserved for patients who failed to respond completely to 40 Gy with concurrent cisplatin.[17] Complete responders

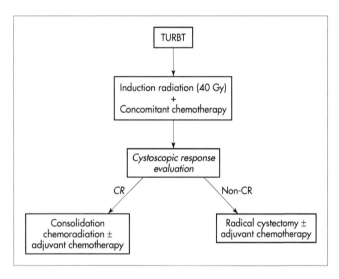

**Fig. 55.1**
Selective bladder preservation treatment algorithm using trimodality therapy. (CR, complete response; TURBT, transurethral resection of bladder tumor.)

**Table 55.4** Recent results of TURBT and chemotherapy concurrent with radiation

| Series (year) | Induction treatment | No. pts | 5-year survival (%) | 5-year survival with bladder preservation (%) |
|---|---|---|---|---|
| Dunst (1994)[57] | TURBT, cisplatin and XRT | 79 | 52 | 41 |
| RTOG (1993)[17] | Cisplatin and XRT | 42 | 52 | 42 |
| Shipley (2002)[11] | TURBT, MCV, cisplatin and XRT | 190 | 54 | 46 |
| RTOG (1998)[19] | TURBT, ± MCV, cisplatin and XRT | 123 | 49 | 38 |
| Paris (1997)[58] | TURBT, 5-fluorouracil, cisplatin and XRT | 120 | 63 | – |

MCV, methotrexate, cisplatin, vinblastine; TURBT, transurethral resection of bladder tumor, XRT, external beam irradiation.

received consolidation therapy, with an additional 24 Gy delivered with concurrent cisplatin. The safety and efficacy of the regimen were demonstrated with a complete response rate of 66% and a 3-year survival rate of 64%. The subsequent protocol, RTOG 88-02, was a phase I–II trial which demonstrated that the addition of neoadjuvant MCV was well tolerated. It yielded a 75% response rate and a 62% 4-year survival rate in 91 entered patients.[18] This was followed by RTOG 89-03, a phase III trial to assess the efficacy of neoadjuvant MCV chemotherapy. It fell short of its accrual goals secondary to poor patient tolerance of the regimen. Toxicities consisted of severe leukopenia and sepsis. The 5-year overall survival rate in the 123 entered patients was 49% with no difference between treatment arms.[19] There was also no difference in the rate of distant metastasis or bladder preservation. Neoadjuvant chemotherapy was abandoned in future studies due to the toxicity and lack of therapeutic efficacy in this trial.

Beginning in 1995, the RTOG began a series of phase I–II protocols to evaluate accelerated radiation fractionation schemes in combination with concurrent outpatient chemotherapy. Protocol RTOG 95-06 evaluated the regimen piloted by the University of Paris using an outpatient regimen of 5-FU and cisplatin, concurrent with accelerated but hypofractionated radiation delivered over 17 days.[20] The eligibility criteria of this protocol were more stringent than prior RTOG studies. Patients with tumor-associated hydronephrosis were excluded because they were found to have lower complete response rates on previous trials. Among 34 evaluable patients, the complete response rate was 67% and overall survival was 83% at 3 years; however, there was a 21% rate of grade 3–4 hematologic toxicity. Subsequent trials included adjuvant chemotherapy after either selective bladder preservation or cystectomy. In RTOG 97-06, induction and consolidation chemoradiation included twice-daily radiation and outpatient cisplatin (30 mg/m$^2$) given on the first three days of each week. Radiation doses of 1.8 Gy to the pelvis and 1.6 Gy to the tumor were given daily, with a 4–6 hour interval between treatments. After consolidation chemoradiation or cystectomy (depending on response), each patient received three cycles of MCV chemotherapy. Only 11% of patients experienced grade 3–4 toxicity during induction and consolidation chemoradiation.[21] The complete response rate was 71%. Only 40% of patients received a full three cycles of adjuvant MCV, and 35% of patients developed grade 3 toxicity. The development of metastasis may have been decreased by this regimen. The 2-year incidence of metastasis was 18%, which compares favorably to the arm of RTOG 89-03 that did not receive adjuvant chemotherapy. In the subgroup that did not have tumor-associated hydronephrosis, the 2-year incidence of distant metastasis was 31%. RTOG 99-06 included two innovative changes:

- the inclusion of an adjuvant chemotherapy regimen of cisplatin and gemcitabine. In the metastatic setting, this regimen has demonstrated efficacy with lesser toxicity than MVAC.[22–24]
- the inclusion of paclitaxel as a radiation-sensitizing agent during the induction and consolidation schedules.[25,26]

The trial has been closed, but the outcomes have not yet been reported.

In addition to the efforts made refining the combined modality regimen, the RTOG, through the Genitourinary Translational Research Group, has also made efforts to better delineate the molecular biology of bladder cancer and its response to therapy. They have assessed the significance of overexpression of p53, p21, pRb, p16, Erb1 (EGFR), and Erb2 (Her2) as measured by immunohistochemical staining in 73 patients treated on protocols RTOG 88-02, 89-03, 95-06, and 97-06.[27] Multivariate analysis revealed that p53, p21, pRb, and p16 fail to predict complete response rate, overall survival or disease-specific survival. Overexpression of Her2 was associated with a reduced complete response rate (50% versus 81%, p=0.026). EGFR positivity was associated with improved disease-specific survival. These preliminary data will need to be confirmed in larger data sets and evaluated on prospective trials. Delineation of the role of individual markers in the biology of bladder cancer and its response to therapy may lead to the rational development of targeted therapies.

The RTOG has refined the selective bladder-preserving approach as it is currently practiced in the US. These trials will continue to optimize radiation and chemotherapy schedules to maximize response to therapy and make bladder preservation more likely. The study of adjuvant chemotherapy regimens may also increase the survival rate of all patients with invasive bladder cancer regardless of local therapy.

# UROLOGIC CONCERNS ABOUT BLADDER-SPARING APPROACH

Despite the success of selective bladder preservation reported in retrospective series and phase II trials, its acceptance in the urologic community has been limited. Urologists have several concerns regarding leaving the diseased bladder in situ.

## DOES AN INCOMPLETE TURBT PRECLUDE BLADDER PRESERVATION?

While it is evident that a complete TURBT improves the complete response rate after chemoradiation, inability to perform a complete TURBT is not a contraindication to selective bladder preservation. The Erlangen experience revealed that completeness of TURBT and early tumor stage were the most important factors predicting complete response and overall survival.[15] They reported complete response rates of 90%, 77%, and 54% for visibly and microscopically complete (R0), visibly but not microscopically complete (R1), and visibly incomplete (R2) responses, respectively. The 10-year overall survival rates were 76%, 52%, and 34%, respectively. Although this series demonstrated TURBT extent as independent from tumor stage as a prognostic indicator for survival, it included superficial tumors whose clinical stage is more reliable and which are more apt to have R0 resections. Less complete TURBT may still serve as a marker for more advanced disease in the muscle-invasive tumors. It cannot be concluded that patients with incomplete TURBT gain a survival benefit from immediate cystectomy. In the Massachusetts General Hospital (MGH) experience, which included only muscle-invasive disease, there is no significant disease-specific survival detriment in patients with less than a visibly complete TURBT.[28] At 5 years, the rates were 69% and 58% for visibly complete and less than complete resections, respectively (log-rank, p=0.24). Furthermore, there was no demonstrated survival detriment for salvage as compared to immediate cystectomy in the series as a whole or in patients with lesser resections. However, the crude rate of cystectomy by last follow-up was higher for less than complete resections as compared to visibly complete resections, 50% versus 29%, respectively. For muscle-invasive bladder cancer, visibly complete TURBT increases the likelihood of bladder preservation, but inability to obtain a complete resection does not preclude selective bladder preservation. At MGH, the complete response rate for patients with less than a complete resection was 63%, and 74% of responders maintained their native bladder at 5 years.

## IS CYSTECTOMY FREQUENTLY REQUIRED FOR SUPERFICIAL RELAPSE?

Bladder cancer is often associated with a field change which leaves the conservatively treated patient at risk for a superficial relapse. A risk of 9% to 28% at 5 years has been reported. Zietman et al reported a 26% (32 recurrences in 121 patients) rate of superficial recurrence among complete responders to trimodality therapy.[29] Of the 32 recurrences, 27 patients were managed with transurethral resection and intravesical therapy and tolerated it well. Cystectomy was ultimately required in 31% (10 of 32 cases), for additional superficial recurrence in seven patients and invasive recurrence in three. There was no survival decrement associated with superficial relapse. With routine urologic surveillance,

superficial recurrences can be detected promptly, and salvage cystectomy averted in the majority of cases.

## IS BLADDER FUNCTION POOR AFTER TRIMODALITY THERAPY?

Many urologists believe that an irradiated bladder is functionally worthless as it is prone to bleeding and contracture. Recent reports contradict this assumption for patients receiving modern radiation therapy. In the Erlangen experience, only three cystectomies were required for bladder contracture in 186 preserved bladders for an incidence of 2%.[15] In that series, 3% of patients had a reduced bladder capacity and 10% reported mild urinary symptoms including frequency, urgency, and dysuria. In the MGH experience, none of the 190 patients treated on selective bladder preservation protocols has required a cystectomy because of bladder morbidity.[11] A British quality of life analysis of 72 patients treated to 60 Gy in 30 fractions reported no difference in urinary and rectal function as compared to an age- and sex-matched control group.[30] More recently, Zietman et al reported the results of an urodynamic and quality of life study performed on 49 patients with preserved bladders several years after treatment at MGH.[31] Urodynamic studies demonstrated that 77% (24/31) of patients had normal bladder function by sex and age. Bladder outlet obstruction was demonstrated in 33% of men, and 30% of the studied women had involuntary detrusor contractions. Bladder symptoms were uncommon with the exception of urinary control. Overall, 19% of patients reported control problems, with 11% wearing pads. All pad wearers were women. Only 6% of patients reported moderate or higher urinary distress, and 14% reported distress over bowel urgency. Sexual function was maintained in the majority of the men studied, with 54% reporting satisfactory erections. Comparative quality of life studies from Denmark and Italy suggest an advantage to bladder preservation using chemoradiation over cystectomy with regards to urinary and sexual function.[32,33] Trimodality therapy, as practiced today, results in a well-functioning bladder and maintenance of sexual function in the majority of patients.

## IS UNCONTROLLED PELVIC DISEASE COMMON AFTER TRIMODALITY THERAPY?

Local control rates of 40% achieved in radiation monotherapy series are inferior to those obtained with radical cystectomy. The poor results do not apply to patients treated with trimodality therapy if a prompt cystectomy is performed in less than complete responders. Invasive relapse rates of 9% to 17% have been reported after trimodality therapy. At MGH, 66 of 190 patients treated on selective bladder preservation protocols (35%) required a cystectomy: 41 for a less than complete response and 25 for recurrent tumors.[11] In this series, the rate of pelvic recurrence was 8.4%. A rate of 12% was reported by the RTOG for 123 patients treated on multi-institutional selective bladder preservation protocols. These rates compare favorably to the 9% pelvic recurrence rate reported for patients receiving a contemporary radical cystectomy for bladder cancer at the University of Southern California.[34] Chemoradiation does not result in a high rate of pelvic recurrence; however, close urologic surveillance should be pursued in order to detect invasive recurrences while they are still confined to the bladder.

## DOES DELAYING CYSTECTOMY DECREASE SURVIVAL?

Multiple randomized trials demonstrate that delayed cystectomy does not result in inferior survival after radiation as compared to immediate surgery. Comparison of modern cystectomy and modern trimodality series demonstrate that, when matched for tumor stage, selective preservation results in comparable survival rates while preserving the bladder in the majority of patients. For T2–4a bladder cancer, 5-year overall survival rates of 45% to 50% have been reported after selective bladder preservation as compared to 36% to 58% after contemporary radical cystectomy (Table 55.5).

Care must be taken when comparing surgical series to bladder preservation series as several biases exist. Cystectomy series do not report by 'intention to treat', and exclude patients where the procedure is abandoned secondary to intraoperative findings such as node positivity or unresectable disease. Conversely, trimodality series include patients that fail to respond to chemoradiation and require cystectomy. Also, many surgical series do not have preoperative proof of muscle-invasive disease. Cystectomy series commonly include less than P2 stage tumors in 25% to 40% of patients.

## CONCLUSION

Bladder preserving treatment for invasive bladder cancer in patients selected on the basis of their response to transurethral resection, concurrent chemotherapy, and radiation results in overall survival and freedom from disease comparable to radical cystectomy. This approach results in 5-year survival of approximately 50%, with 80% of these patients retaining their native bladder. Despite these results, the acceptance of this approach in the urologic community has been limited due to the following concerns addressed in this chapter:

1. The inability to obtain a visibly complete transurethral resection, which does result in a higher cystectomy rate, has a 63% complete response rate, and does not preclude selective bladder preservation.
2. Superficial relapse, which may occur in 26% of patients after bladder preservation, is adequately managed by transurethral resection and intravesical therapy in the majority of patients.
3. Quality of life and urodynamic studies demonstrate that preserved bladders function well.
4. Pelvic recurrence rates after selective bladder preservation are comparable to rates seen after cystectomy.
5. Several randomized trials demonstrate no survival detriment to delayed cystectomy for patients receiving radiation therapy.

Selective bladder preservation using trimodality therapy represents a cooperative effort between the treating urologist, radiation oncologist, and medical oncologist. Bladder conservation trials have demonstrated results comparable to radical cystectomy with a high rate of bladder preservation.

### REFERENCES

1. McDougal WS. Continent urinary diversion. In Osterling JE, Richie JP (eds): Urologic Oncology. Philadelphia: WB Saunders, 1997, pp 336–340.
2. Greven KM, Spera JA, Solin LJ, Morgan T, Hanks GE. Local recurrence after cystectomy alone for bladder carcinoma. Cancer 1992;69:2767–2770.

**Table 55.5** Survival in contemporary cystectomy and selective bladder preservation series

| Series (year) | Stages | No. pts | 5-year survival (%) | 10-year survival (%) |
|---|---|---|---|---|
| Cystectomy | | | | |
| USC (2001)[59] | P2–4A | 633 | 48 | 32 |
| MSKCC (2001)[60] | P2–4A | 181 | 36 | 27 |
| Selective bladder preservation | | | | |
| Erlangen (2002)[15] | cT2–4 | 326 | 45 | 29 |
| MGH (2002)[11] | cT2–4a | 190 | 54 | 36 |
| RTOG (1998)[19] | cT2–4a | 123 | 49 | – |

3. Martinez-Pineiro JA, Gonzalez Martin M, Arocena F, et al. Neoadjuvant cisplatin chemotherapy before radical cystectomy in invasive transitional cell carcinoma of the bladder: a prospective randomized phase III study. J Urol 1995;153:964–973.

4. Pressler LB, Petrylak DP, Olsson CA. Invasive transitional cell carcinoma of the bladder: prognosis and management. In Osterling JE, Richie JP (eds): Urologic Oncology. Philadelphia: WB Saunders, 1997, pp 275–291.

5. Hart S, Skinner EC, Meyerowitz BE, Boyd S, Lieskovsky G, Skinner DG. Quality of life after radical cystectomy for bladder cancer in patients with an ileal conduit, cutaneous or urethral Kock pouch [comment]. J Urol 1999;162:77–81.

6. Miller LS. Bladder cancer: superiority of preoperative irradiation and cystectomy in clinical stages B2 and C. Cancer 1977;39:973–980.

7. Bloom HJ, Hendry WF, Wallace DM, Skeet RG. Treatment of T3 bladder cancer: controlled trial of pre-operative radiotherapy and radical cystectomy versus radical radiotherapy. Br J Urol 1982;54:136–151.

8. Sell A, Jakobsen A, Nerstrom B, Sorensen BL, Steven K, Barlebo H. Treatment of advanced bladder cancer category T2, T3 and T4a. A randomized multicenter study of preoperative irradiation and cystectomy versus radical irradiation and early salvage cystectomy for residual tumor. DAVECA protocol 8201. Danish Vesical Cancer Group. Scand J Urol Nephrol 1991;138(Suppl):193–201.

9. Cutler SD. National Cancer Institute, unpublished observations, 1983.

10. Schultz PK, Herr HW, Zhang ZF, et al. Neoadjuvant chemotherapy for invasive bladder cancer: prognostic factors for survival of patients treated with M-VAC with 5-year follow-up [comment]. J Clin Oncol 1994;12:1394–1401.

11. Shipley WU, Kaufman DS, Zehr E, et al. Selective bladder preservation by combined modality protocol treatment: long-term outcomes of 190 patients with invasive bladder cancer. Urology 2002;60:62–67; discussion 67–68.

12. Shipley WU, Kaufman DS, Tester WJ, et al. Overview of bladder cancer trials in the Radiation Therapy Oncology Group. Cancer 2003;97:2115–2119.

13. Housset M, Maulard C, Chretien Y, et al. Combined radiation and chemotherapy for invasive transitional-cell carcinoma of the bladder: a prospective study. J Clin Oncol 1993;11:2150–2157.

14. Sauer R, Birkenhake S, Kuhn R, Wittekind C, Schrott KM, Martus P. Efficacy of radiochemotherapy with platin derivatives compared to radiotherapy alone in organ-sparing treatment of bladder cancer. Int J Radiat Oncol Biol Phys 1998;40:121–127.

15. Rodel C, Grabenbauer GG, Kuhn R, et al. Combined-modality treatment and selective organ preservation in invasive bladder cancer: long-term results [comment]. J Clin Oncol 2002;20:3061–3071.

16. Shipley WU, Prout GR Jr, Einstein AB, et al. Treatment of invasive bladder cancer by cisplatin and radiation in patients unsuited for surgery. JAMA 1987;258(7):931–935.

17. Tester W, Porter A, Asbell S, et al. Combined modality program with possible organ preservation for invasive bladder carcinoma: results of RTOG protocol 85-12. Int J Radiat Oncol Biol Phys 1993;25:783–790.

18. Tester W, Caplan R, Heaney J, et al. Neoadjuvant combined modality program with selective organ preservation for invasive bladder cancer: results of Radiation Therapy Oncology Group phase II trial 8802. J Clin Oncol 1996;14:119–126.

19. Shipley WU, Winter KA, Kaufman DS, et al. Phase III trial of neoadjuvant chemotherapy in patients with invasive bladder cancer treated with selective bladder preservation by combined radiation therapy and chemotherapy: initial results of Radiation Therapy Oncology Group 89-03 [comment]. J Clin Oncol 1998;16:3576–3583.

20. Kaufman DS, Winter KA, Shipley WU, et al. The initial results in muscle-invading bladder cancer of RTOG 95-06: phase I/II trial of transurethral surgery plus radiation therapy with concurrent cisplatin and 5-fluorouracil followed by selective bladder preservation or cystectomy depending on the initial response. Oncologist 2000;5:471–476.

21. Hagan MP, Winter KA, Kaufman DS, et al. RTOG 9706: initial report of a phase I/II trial of bladder-conservation employing TURB, twice daily accelerated irradiation sensitized with cisplatin followed by

22. adjuvant MCV combination chemotherapy. Int J Radiat Oncol Biol Phys 2003;57:665–672.

22. Moore MJ, Winquist EW, Murray N, et al. Gemcitabine plus cisplatin, an active regimen in advanced urothelial cancer: a phase II trial of the National Cancer Institute of Canada Clinical Trials Group. J Clin Oncol 1999;17:2876–2881.

23. Kaufman D, Raghavan D, Carducci M, et al. Phase II trial of gemcitabine plus cisplatin in patients with metastatic urothelial cancer. J Clin Oncol 2000;18:1921–1927.

24. von der Maase H, Hansen SW, Roberts JI, et al. Gemcitabine and cisplatin versus methotrexate, vinblastine, doxorubicin, and cisplatin in advanced or metastatic bladder cancer: results of a large, randomized, multinational, multicenter, phase III study [comment]. J Clin Oncol 2000;18:3068–3077.

25. Roth BJ. The role of paclitaxel in the therapy of bladder cancer. Semin Oncol 1995;22:33–40.

26. Dreicer R, Manola J, Roth BJ, Cohen MB, Hatfield AK, Wilding G. Phase II study of cisplatin and paclitaxel in advanced carcinoma of the urothelium: an Eastern Cooperative Oncology Group Study. J Clin Oncol 2000;18:1058–1061.

27. Chakravarti A, Winter K, Wu CL. Expression of EGFR is associated with improved outcome in muscle invading bladder cancer: An RTOG study. Proceedings of the American Society of Clinical Oncology (ASCO) Meeting, Orlando, FL. J Clin Oncol 2002;179a:Abstract 713.

28. Coen JJ, Heney NM, Althausen AF, Zietman AL, Kaufman DS, Shipley WU. An update of selective bladder preservation using combined modality treatment in invasive bladder cancer: long term outcome reveals a low risk of invasive recurrence and a high probability of bladder preservation, American Urologic Association, San Francisco, 2004.

29. Zietman AL, Grocela J, Zehr E, et al. Selective bladder conservation using transurethral resection, chemotherapy, and radiation: management and consequences of Ta, T1, and Tis recurrence within the retained bladder. Urology 2001;58:380–385.

30. Lynch WJ, Jenkins BJ, Fowler CG, Hope-Stone HF, Blandy JP. The quality of life after radical radiotherapy for bladder cancer. Br J Urol 1992;70:519–521.

31. Zietman AL, Sacco D, Skowronski U, et al. Organ-conservation in invasive bladder cancer by transurethral resection, chemotherapy, and radiation: results of a urodynamic and quality of life study on long-term survivors. J Urol 2003;170(5):1772–1776.

32. Caffo O, Fellin G, Graffer U, Luciani L. Assessment of quality of life after cystectomy or conservative therapy for patients with infiltrating bladder carcinoma. A survey by a self-administered questionnaire [erratum appears in Cancer 1996;78(5):2037]. Cancer 1996;76(9):1089–1097.

33. Henningsohn L, Steven K, Kallestrup EB, Steineck G. Distressful symptoms and well-being after radical cystectomy and orthotopic bladder substitution compared with a matched control population. J Urol 2002;168:168–174; discussion 174–175.

34. Stein JP, Lieskovsky G, Cote R, et al. Radical cystectomy in the treatment of invasive bladder cancer: long-term results in 1,054 patients. J Clin Oncol 2001;19:666–675.

35. Henry K, Miller J, Mori M, Loening S, Fallon B. Comparison of transurethral resection to radical therapies for stage B bladder tumors. J Urol 1988;140:964–967.

36. Herr HW. Conservative management of muscle-infiltrating bladder cancer: prospective experience. J Urol 1987;138:1162–1163.

37. De Neve W, Lybeert ML, Goor C, Crommelin MA, Ribot JG. Radiotherapy for T2 and T3 carcinoma of the bladder: the influence of overall treatment time. Radiother Oncol 1995;36:183–188.

38. Gospodarowicz MK, Hawkins NV, Rawlings GA, et al. Radical radiotherapy for muscle invasive transitional cell carcinoma of the bladder: failure analysis. J Urol 1989;142:1448–1453; discussion 1453–1454.

39. Jenkins BJ, Caulfield MJ, Fowler CG, et al. Reappraisal of the role of radical radiotherapy and salvage cystectomy in the treatment of invasive (T2/T3) bladder cancer. Br J Urol 1988;62:343–346.

40. Mameghan H, Fisher R, Mameghan J, Brook S. Analysis of failure following definitive radiotherapy for invasive transitional cell carcinoma of the bladder. Int J Radiat Oncol Biol Phys 1995;31:247–254.

41. Shearer RJ, Chilvers CE, Bloom HJ, Bliss JM, Horwich A, Babiker A. Adjuvant chemotherapy in T3 carcinoma of the bladder. A prospective trial: preliminary report. Br J Urol 1988;62:558–564.

42. Hall RR. Transurethral resection for transitional cell carcinoma. Prob Urol 1992;6:460–470.

43. Quilty PM, Duncan W. Primary radical radiotherapy for T3 transitional cell cancer of the bladder: an analysis of survival and control. Int J Radiat Oncol Biol Phys 1986;12:853–860.

44. Smaaland R, Akslen LA, Tonder B, Mehus A, Lote K, Albrektsen G. Radical radiation treatment of invasive and locally advanced bladder carcinoma in elderly patients. Br J Urol 1991;67:61–69.

45. Farah R, Chodak GW, Vogelzang NJ, et al. Curative radiotherapy following chemotherapy for invasive bladder carcinoma (a preliminary report). Int J Radiat Oncol Biol Phys 1991;20:413–417.

46. Hall RR, Roberts JT. Neoadjuvant chemotherapy, a method to conserve the bladder? Proceedings of the 6th European Cancer Conference on Oncology and Cancer Nursing, Florence, Italy, 1991. Eur J Cancer 1991;27(Suppl 2):Abstract 144.

47. Keating JP, Zincke H, Hahn RG, Morgan WR. Extended experience of neo-adjuvant M-VAC chemotherapy for T1–4 N0 M0 transitional cell carcinoma of the urinary bladder. Progr Clin Biol Res 1990;353:119–127.

48. Kurth KH, Splinter TA, Jacqmin D. Transitional cell carcinoma of the bladder: a phase II study of chemotherapy in T3–4 N0 M0 of the EORTC GU group. In Alderson AR, Oliver RT, Hanham IW, Bloom HJ (eds): Urologic Oncology Dilemmas and Developments. New York: Wiley-Liss, 1991, pp 115–128.

49. Maffezzini M, Torelli T, Villa E, et al. Systemic preoperative chemotherapy with cisplatin, methotrexate and vinblastine for locally advanced bladder cancer: local tumor response and early followup results. J Urol 1991;145:741–743.

50. Roberts JT, Fossa SD, Richards B, et al. Results of Medical Research Council phase II study of low dose cisplatin and methotrexate in the primary treatment of locally advanced (T3 and T4) transitional cell carcinoma of the bladder. Br J Urol 1991;68:162–168.

51. Hall RR, Newling DW, Ramsden PD, Richards B, Robinson MR, Smith PH. Treatment of invasive bladder cancer by local resection and high dose methotrexate. Br J Urol 1984;56:668–672.

52. Parsons JT, Million RR. Bladder cancer. In: Perez CA, Brady IW (eds): Principles and Practice of Radiation Oncology. Philadelphia: Lippincott, 1991, pp 1036–1058.

53. Prout GR Jr, Shipley WU, Kaufman DS, et al. Preliminary results in invasive bladder cancer with transurethral resection, neoadjuvant chemotherapy and combined pelvic irradiation plus cisplatin chemotherapy. J Urol 1990;144:1128–1134; discussion 1134–1136.

54. Scher HI, Herr HW, Sternberg C, Fair W, Bosl G, Sogani P. Neoadjuvant chemotherapy for invasive bladder cancer: experience with the MVAC regimen. Br J Urol 1989;64:250–256.

55. Herr HW, Bajorin DF, Scher HI. Neoadjuvant chemotherapy and bladder-sparing surgery for invasive bladder cancer: ten-year outcome. J Clin Oncol 1998;16(4):1298–1301.

56. Cervak J, Cufer T, Marolt F. Combined chemotherapy and radiotherapy in muscle-invasive bladder carcinoma. Complete remission results. Proceedings of the 6th European Conference on Oncology and Cancer Nursing, Florence, Italy, 1991. Eur J Cancer 1991;27(Suppl 2):Abstract 561.

57. Dunst J, Sauer R, Schrott KM, Kuhn R, Wittekind C, Altendorf-Hofmann A. Organ-sparing treatment of advanced bladder cancer: a 10-year experience. Int J Radiat Oncol Biol Phys 1994;30:261–266.

58. Housset M, Dufour B, Maulard C. Concomitant 5-fluorouracil–cisplatin and bifractionated split course radiation therapy for invasive bladder cancer. Proc Am Soc Clin Oncol 1997;16:319a.

59. Stein JP, Lieskovsky G, Cote R, et al. Radical cystectomy in the treatment of invasive bladder cancer: long-term results in 1,054 patients. J Clin Oncol 2001;19:666–675.

60. Dalbagni G, Genega E, Hashibe M, et al. Cystectomy for bladder cancer: a contemporary series. J Urol 2001;165:1111–1116.

*Richard E Hautmann*

## INTRODUCTION

Urinary diversion has reached a new level. The ultimate goal of urinary reconstruction has become not only to create a means to divert urine and protect the upper urinary tract, but also to provide patients with a continent means to store urine and allow for volitional voiding through the native urethra. These advances in urinary diversion have been made in an effort to give patients a normal lifestyle with a positive self-image following removal of the bladder. We and others have been dedicated to the continued improvement of lower urinary tract reconstruction, and believe that the neobladder represents the most ideal form of urinary diversion.[1-4] Orthotopic reconstruction was proposed by Tizzoni and Foggi in 1888.[5] They replaced the bladder in one female dog by an isoperistaltic ileal segment. In 1951 Couvelaire reactivated this idea.[6]

During the past 15 years orthotopic reconstruction has evolved from 'experimental surgery' to 'standard of care at larger medical centers' and to the 'preferred method of urinary diversion' in both sexes. The ileal conduit was described 1950 by Bricker and has remained the standard urinary diversion against which others have to be judged.[7] During the last decade, use of the time-honored conduit has given way to the increasingly frequent use of orthotopic reconstruction.

## INDICATION: SUBSTANTIAL CHANGE IN PARADIGM FOR URINARY DIVERSION

The goal of patient counseling about urinary diversion should be to find the method that would be the safest for cancer control, has the fewest complications in both the short and long term, and provides the easiest adjustment for the patient's lifestyle, i.e. supporting the best quality of life. The paradigm for choosing a urinary diversion has changed substantially. Today, all cystectomy patients are candidates for a neobladder, and we should identify patients in whom orthotopic reconstruction may be less than ideal. The proportion of cystectomy patients receiving a neobladder has increased at medical centers from 50% to 90%.[8-11]

## PATIENT SELECTION CRITERIA

### ABSOLUTE AND RELATIVE CONTRAINDICATIONS

Absolute contraindications to continent diversion of any type are compromised renal function as a result of long-standing obstruction or chronic renal failure, with serum creatinine >150–200 µmol/l. Severe hepatic dysfunction is also a contraindication to continent diversion. Patients with compromised intestinal function, particularly inflammatory bowel disease, may be better served by a bowel conduit. Orthotopic reconstruction is absolutely contraindicated in all patients that are candidates for simultaneous urethrectomy because of their primary tumor.[12,13]

The role of relative contraindications and comorbidity is steadily decreasing. However, mental impairment, external sphincter dysfunction, or recurrent urethral strictures deserve serious consideration.

## PATIENT FACTORS: PROS

The primary patient factor is the 'patient's desire for a neobladder'. The patient needs a certain motivation to tolerate the initial and sometimes lasting inconveniences of nocturnal incontinence associated with a neobladder. Most patients readily accept some degree of nocturnal incontinence for the benefit of avoiding an external stoma and pouch. However, not all patients do, and realistic expectations of the functional outcome are essential for both the surgeon and the patient. The psychological damaging stigma to the patient who enters surgery expecting a neobladder, but awakens with a stoma, plays an increasing role. It should always be remembered that in many parts of the world a bag may be either socially unacceptable or economically unrealistic as a long-term solution. These pressures may drive the urologist toward some form of continent urinary diversion, and although rectal pouches have been utilized widely as an alternative to conduits, continent catheterizable reservoirs, and orthotopic bladder substitutes in particular, represent attractive alternative options.

## PATIENT FACTORS: CONS

There are still patients that are better served with a conduit. Patient factors arguing against a neobladder include the following:

- If the patient's main motivation is to 'get out of the hospital as soon as possible' and resume normal, rather sedentary activities. Many frail patients undergoing cystectomy will have less disruption of normal activities with a well-functioning conduit than with an orthotopic reservoir associated with less than ideal continence.
- If the patient is an elderly person.
- If the patient is not concerned about body image. Most older patients do not have the same 'body image' concerns that a younger patient might have, and their main goal is returning to their previous lifestyle, which is often quite sedentary.[14]

## ONCOLOGIC FACTORS

Following cystectomy the rhabdosphincter must remain intact. Nevertheless, the cancer operation must not be compromised. This concern applies to urethral tumor recurrence in men and the use of orthotopic replacement in women. One of the initial deterrents to orthotopic diversion is the risk for urethral recurrence of cancer. Historically this risk following cystectomy was 10%.[15] The best predictor of the risk for urethral disease is the presence and extent of carcinoma in situ (CIS) in the prostatic urethra, ducts, or stroma. If there is diffuse CIS in the ducts and invasion of the stroma, the risk for urethral disease historically has been 25% to 35%,[16] a risk that discouraged use of the urethra. Lesser amounts of CIS confer a lesser degree of risk. Our aggressive approach to neobladder diversion relies only on a frozen section of the urethral margin at the time of surgery. A conservative approach would disqualify a patient with any prostatic involvement. In our view, neither multifocal bladder tumors nor CIS of the bladder are indications for urethrectomy. The frequency of urethral recurrence after orthotopic diversions is much less than anticipated. Freeman et al[15] and others[8,9] provide data on a 2% to 4% frequency of urethral recurrence after orthotopic diversion.

Orthotopic bladder substitution for women with invasive bladder cancer has recently become popular.[17-19] Analysis of pathologic specimens has supported its use in women who have no evidence of tumor at the bladder neck.[20,21] Indeed, the majority of the invasive cancers are located in the area of the trigone, making a wide excision—together with the anterosuperior part of the vagina and the dorsomedial bladder pedicle in the paravaginal region—necessary.

Increasing experience with orthotopic reconstruction has fostered less restrictiveness for patient selection based on tumor stage. Should extensive pelvic disease, a palpable mass, or positive but resectable lymph nodes preclude a neobladder because of the high propensity for a pelvic recurrence or distant relapse?

We have studied local recurrence and diversion-related complications in a series of 435 patients. The local recurrence rate was the expected 10%. Interference of a local recurrence with the neobladder occurred in 11 patients only: infiltration of the neobladder occurred in 6 patients and obstruction was the problem in the remaining 5. There is no convincing evidence that a patient with an orthotopic diversion tolerates adjuvant chemotherapy less well or that a pelvic recurrence is any more difficult to manage with a neobladder than after an ileal conduit. Patients can anticipate normal neobladder function until the time of death.[22]

Adjuvant chemotherapy may substantially weaken the patient and prolong the time for neobladder maturation. Nevertheless, our philosophy respects the patient's desire for a neobladder if the patient is strongly motivated. Even though the patient has a poor prognosis and relapse is likely to occur, we still try to construct the diversion they want. Previous radiation therapy, especially with an advanced cancer, usually mitigates against an orthotopic diversion but does not absolutely preclude it. However, all patients should be informed that diversion to the skin, either by a continent reservoir or an ileal conduit, may be necessary because of unexpected tumor extent, and there should be an appropriate stoma site marked on the abdominal wall beforehand.

# CURRENT PRACTICE

Despite the fact that orthotopic bladder replacement provides the ideal method of urinary diversion after cystectomy, many patients treated outside of centers that are dedicated to neobladder reconstruction receive an ileal conduit. In addition, patients selected for a conduit are frequently older patients with more comorbidity, and more previous cancer therapy, including patients with previously deemed unresectable cancers undergoing desperation cystectomy or after failed previously combined radiation therapy and chemotherapy regimens.[14]

Thus, despite our strong desire to offer orthotopic diversion whenever possible, some patients do not qualify on the basis of current clinical judgment. An ileal conduit remains an expedient, safe, and appropriate method of diversion in these patients. Many factors go into the decision to perform a urinary diversion and must be kept paramount in discussing the pros and cons of each method with the patient and the family.

## COMPARISON OF ILEAL, ILEOCOLIC, RIGHT COLIC AND SIGMOID RESERVOIRS

There are clear differences between ileum and colon in regard to metabolic consequences (see section 'Gut mucosa as a substitute for urothelium'). But this is only one consideration when planning orthotopic reconstruction. Because of the reduced absorption of electrolytes in ileal urinary reservoirs, ileum seems to be preferable to large bowel for storing urine, at least in patients with decreased kidney function and increased risk for metabolic disorders.[23,24]

An obvious advantage of the sigmoid reservoir is its ease of accessibility. However, there is the substantial disadvantage of high reservoir pressures as compared to cecum or ileum that is confirmed by most urodynamic studies.[25--27] We, like others, use a sigmoid reservoir only in cases in which ileum or right colon is not available.[11] An advantage of the ileocolonic reservoir is its initial volume. However, it requires mobilization of the entire right colon and is potentially the most tedious procedure to perform.[28] The greatest disadvantage of the procedure is the loss of the ileocecal valve. There is also a greater risk of vitamin $B_{12}$ deficiency secondary to resection of terminal ileum and the ileocecal valve. Most investigators have reported on one single type of diversion. Santucci et al performed six different continent urinary reservoir operations and revealed remarkably different continence rates and urodynamic data. Their experience suggests that neobladders composed of stomach or sigmoid should be used only under unusual circumstances because of the high rates of incontinence.[27]

Ileal reservoirs are the most common form of neobladders used worldwide. There are three major categories:

- The Hemi Kock was originally developed by Kock and popularized by Skinner and associates.[29,30] The most recent modification (T pouch) is technically complex, unnecessarily time consuming, and has yet to be widely adopted.[10]
- The ileal reservoir initially described by Studer et al has the advantage of an afferent limb that facilitates placement of the ileoureterostomies but without any valve formation.[3]
- The ileal neobladder is a W-shaped reservoir described by Hautmann and coworkers.[1,2,31] Its obvious advantage is the high continence rates as a consequence of having the greatest volume of all reservoirs. Both the incorporation of an afferent or efferent limb for ureteral anastomosis, and orthotopic anastomosis of the ureters directly into the reservoir, with or without antireflux technique, is feasible.[11,31-33] In our experience, difficulty reaching the urethral remnant occurs less often with this type of reservoir.

Of course, other patient and surgeon issues might supersede these guidelines. Surgeon's preference, length of surgery, ease of construction, potential need for revision, differences in body image, and other patient characteristics are among the many factors that must be considered when choosing which type of orthotopic reconstruction to provide for each individual patient.

## REFLUX PREVENTION IN NEOBLADDERS

Controversy exists about the importance of an antireflux mechanism,[7,10,13,34] and the benefits are not easy to define. It is clear that the need for reflux prevention is not the same as in ureterosigmoidostomy conduit or continent diversion. Many reports have revealed a high incidence (13–41%) of renal deterioration associated with a refluxing ileal conduit, as evaluated using serum creatinine and urography.[35,36] After long-term follow-up (mean 13 years) in patients with colonic conduits, significantly more renal units not showing reflux on the loopogram remained normal on urography than did units with reflux.[37]

Conduits are not low-pressure systems[38] because of distal obstruction at the level of the fascia immediately superficial to the external oblique muscle. This, coupled with the very frequent presence of infected urine, means that high-pressure reflux may occur. This reflux, or alternatively, ureteroileal obstruction, may contribute to the gradual deterioration in renal function in these patients that has become apparent over the past two decades.

The rationale for implanting the ureters in an antireflux fashion into orthotopic bladder substitutes or continent reservoirs is to prevent the upper urinary tract from retrograde hydrodynamically transmitted pressure peaks and from ascending bacteriuria. However, the routine of antireflux ureter implantation into intestinal urinary reservoirs was born in the era before creation of designated low-pressure reservoirs.

Glomerular filtration pressure is calculated to 25–30 cm of water, and the amplitude of the peristaltic waves in the ureters is normally less than 10 cm. In view of these figures, long-lasting periods with pressure exceeding about 25 cm of water in the urinary receptacle, in the long run, will probably impair renal function by impeding the urine flow. Patients with a continent ileal reservoir for urinary diversion utilize approximately 60% of the maximal volume capacity during the daytime, i.e. about 300–500 ml. At this reservoir volume, the pressure exceeds zero by more than 25 cm water only during about 2 min/hour.[39]

Reflux prevention in neobladders is even less important than in a normal bladder: 1) there are no coordinated contractions during micturition; 2) a simultaneous pressure increase in neobladder, abdomen, and kidney pelvis during the Valsalva maneuver; and 3) the ileourethrostomy provides a true leak point. When nonrefluxing techniques are used, the risk of obstruction is at least twice that of a direct anastomosis, irrespective of the type of bowel segment used. Half of these strictures require secondary procedures.[9]

In a recent study, the reported obstruction rate following direct anastomoses was 1.7%, and was significantly lower than the 13% rate for nonrefluxing techniques.[40] Of the latter techniques, the LeDuc is associated with the highest postoperative stricture rate. Studer et al reported a 3% obstruction rate using ureteral direct anastomoses as opposed to 13% postoperative strictures in patients in whom Coffey flap valves were used.[40]

Roth et al reported 3.6% and 20.4% obstruction rates respectively when ureteral direct anastomoses to an afferent loop were compared with the LeDuc antireflux anastomoses.[41] Moreover, the reported obstruction rate was 3.8% for the nipple valve of the Kock pouch,[42] but 9.3% for the LeDuc antireflux anastomoses of the Hautmann neobladder.[9] For the latter antireflux technique, an obstruction rate of up to 29% has been reported.[43]

We conclude that obstruction from anastomotic strictures is a greater potential source of short- and long-term morbidity than reflux. Direct techniques are easier to use and preserve renal function equally as well as nonrefluxing methods. We see no justification for any antireflux mechanism in neobladders.

Since 1996 we have been using a freely refluxing open end-to-side ureteroileal anastomosis which is the simplest small bowel surgery (Fig. 56.1).[31] Our 9.5% stenosis rate associated with LeDuc (first 363 patients) went down to 1.0% (patient numbers 364–558).

Further advantages of this chimney modification are:[7]

- extra length to reach the ureteral stump
- ease of surgery far outside the pelvic cavity
- a tension-free anastomosis
- no risk of ureteral angulation with neobladder filling
- a simplified flank access for revisional surgery.[31–33]

## INTESTINAL TISSUES AS A SUBSTITUTE FOR THE BLADDER

It would be ideal if, over time, the transposed gut segment lost its own organization and intrinsic control, and the smooth muscle changed properties to become more like normal detrusor, being reinnervated through the sacral parasympathetic micturition pathway so that it could contribute to bladder emptying.

Potentially the greatest difference between conduit and neobladder is that the conduit functions as a

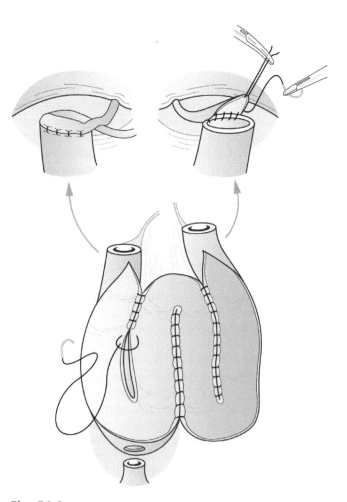

**Fig. 56.1**
Refluxing ileoureteral anastomosis using chimneys of a 3–5 cm afferent limb on each side.

somewhat longer ureter, whereas a neobladder is a substitute for the detrusor. Understanding orthotopic bladder replacement in full means understanding the phenomenon of maturation, i.e. unlike a conduit, the motor and pharmacologic responses of a neobladder change dramatically towards that of the original bladder. Maturation of a neobladder takes anywhere from a few weeks to over several months up to 8 years.[7] Approximately 4–6 weeks after surgery conduit patients are usually into a well-established routine.

## GUT AS A SUBSTITUTE FOR THE DETRUSOR

### Structural changes

Interstitial cells of Cajal (ICC), so named for their identification with the interstitial cells observed by Cajal in the mammalian small intestine,[44] possess a morphology and location specific for each of the specialized regions of the gastrointestinal tract.[45,46] ICC are considered of primary importance for gastrointestinal motility, and are accepted as the intestinal pacemaker cells. In the small intestines of humans, ICC are located at two different muscle coat areas.[47] One population (the ICC-MP) is located between the longitudinal and circular muscle layers and has a relationship to the myenteric plexus (MP). The presence of this cell type has been correlated with slow-wave activity, and found to be of fundamental importance for the occurrence of normal peristalsis.[48] The second ICC population (the ICC-DMP) is specific for the small intestine. It is located between the innermost inner circular muscle layer (ICL) and outermost subdivisions of the circular muscle layer, in association with the deep muscular plexus (DMP), and its role might be related to motility that is specific to this gut area.

Faussone-Pellegrini and coworkers[49] have studied motor patterns, intraluminal pressures, volume capacity, and histoanatomic characteristics in full-thickness specimens from orthotopic ileal bladders removed during corrective surgery. The ICC-MP were scarce in the detubularized segments 1–6 years after reconstruction, and intact ICC-DMP cells and DMP nerve fibers were not seen. Furthermore, the innermost circular muscular layer could not be identified. This loss of structural organization was associated with a better functional outcome. In contrast, the tubular segments (the ICC-MP, ICC-DMP, and circular muscle layer) retained normal features for up to 3 years. After this, ICC-DMP was lost, DMP nerve fibers were scant, the circular muscle layer appeared to degenerate but the ICC-MP remained intact. It was apparent that those reservoirs maintaining a normal ICC-MP population developed pressure waves and those segments with intact ICC-DMP had a contractile response to distension. Whether these physiologic changes are a result of the ileal segment chronically functioning as a reservoir, or are the product of the surgical interruption of myoneural networks and the ICC syncytium, is unclear (Table 56.1).[49]

### Pharmacologic changes

In experimental animals, it has been possible to follow the changes in function of implanted segments after their incorporation into the bladder, to see if they do indeed become more like detrusor in their function. Batra et al[50] have looked in detail at the changes in the pharmacologic properties of muscle strips taken from the ileal segment of augmentation cystoplasty in rabbit models. The contractile response of the ileal segment changed from the response typical of normal ileum to a phasic response more characteristic of detrusor. Furthermore, the normal ileal relaxation reverses to a

**Table 56.1** Distribution of ICC in ileal reservoirs (humans) and motor response characteristics

|  | Tubular | | Detubularized |
|---|---|---|---|
|  | Early (<3 years) | Late (3–8 years) | Early + late |
| ICC-MP | Retained | Retained | Scarce |
| ICC-DMP | Retained | Lost | Lost |
| DMP nerve fibers | Retained | Scant | Disappeared |
| Inner circular muscle layer | Retained | Scant | Disappeared |
| Pressure | High | High | Low |
| Peristaltic activity | Normal | Normal | Absent |
| Contractile activity<br>Low filling<br>Increased filling | Present | Present |  |
| Capacity | Low | Increased | High |

Based on data from Faussone-Pellegrini et al.[49]
DMP, deep muscular plexus; ICC, interstitial cells of Cabal; MP, myenteric plexus.

contractile response similar to that seen in the detrusor, after incorporation into the cystoplasty. The number of muscarinic receptors in the ileal segment decreased after incorporation. Further experiments comparing strip responses from tubular and detubularized segments showed that these changes were more profound in detubularized cystoplasties. This observation was compatible with the concept that the surgical interruption of myoneural networks is the primary signal for the transformation from ileal-type to detrusor-type responses, as opposed to exposure to urine or chronic functioning as a reservoir.

## DETUBULARIZATION

Although it would be ideal if the bowel segment could contribute to voluntary voiding, in reality this does not seem to happen, and a highly compliant neobladder is the desired outcome.[51] Detubularized bowel segments provide greater capacity at lower pressure and require a shorter length of intestine than do intact segments. Four factors account for their superiority:

- their configuration takes advantage of the geometric fact that volume increases by the square of the radius so that a pouch has a larger diameter than a tube
- they accommodate to filling more readily because, as Laplace's law states, the container with the greater radius—and, thus, the lower mural tension—will hold larger volumes at lower pressure
- compliance is superior to that of the tubular bowel
- contractile ability is blunted by the failure of contractions to encompass the entire circumference.[52]

These theoretical considerations are consistent with clinical observations showing that detubularization substantially increases reservoir capacity and delays the onset and reduces the amplitude of the pressure rise produced by contractions. These findings account for the markedly improved initial nocturnal incontinence (80% versus 17% at 2 years), the longer voiding intervals (2.5 hours initial versus 4 hours at 1 year), and the predisposition to urinary retention (0% initial versus 25% at 1 year) with detubularized bladder substitution. Altering the shape of a reservoir from spherical to ellipsoid is calculated to have only a slight effect on its mechanical characteristics. Consequently, the essence of detubularization is to create a reservoir with high capacity, while shape is of secondary importance.[53]

## CAPACITY AND PRESSURE CHARACTERISTICS OF RESERVOIRS (Table 56.2)[39,53–55]

Berglund et al have studied the volume capacity and the pressure characteristics of three types of intestinal reservoir—the continent ileostomy, the continent ileal urostomy, and the continent cecostomy—in patients at intervals after surgical construction of the reservoirs. The volume increases of the ileostomy and the urostomy reservoirs were almost identical but were significantly greater than those of the cecal reservoir. The basal pressure was low in all types of reservoir, although somewhat higher in the cecal reservoir at greater filling volumes. In the ileal reservoirs, motor activity appeared at a filling volume of about 40% of the maximal capacity, whereas in the cecal reservoir motor activity was recorded at all filling levels. The motor activity increased with greater volumes. The amplitude of the highest pressure wave in the cecal reservoir was twice as high as that of the ileal reservoirs. The motor activity of the cecal reservoir, calculated in two different ways, was 10–20 times greater than in the ileal reservoirs.[39]

**Table 56.2** Capacity and pressure characteristics of reservoirs

| | Ileum | Colon |
|---|---|---|
| Volume increase | | |
| Initially | | Advantage |
| Late | Advantage | |
| Capacity | | |
| First contraction | Advantage | |
| Maximum contraction | Advantage | |
| Involuntary contractions: maximum amplitude | Advantage | |
| Motor activity (calculated) | | 10–20× higher |
| Distensibility: ileum (ICL) >colon (CCL) >ileum (ILL) >colon (CLL) | Advantage | |
| Compliance | Advantage | |

Based on data from Berglund et al,[39] Colding-Jørgensen et al,[53] Hohenfellner et al,[54] Goldwasser et al.[55]
CCL, colonic circular layer; CLL, colonic longitudinal layer; ICL, ileal circular layer; ILL, ileal longitudinal layer.

An interesting comparison of the properties of different gut smooth muscles was made by Hohenfellner et al who examined the ileal and cecal segments incorporated into a canine model of the Mainz bladder substitution. Sonomicrometry transducers were implanted in the circular and longitudinal muscular layers to allow measurements of their properties. It was found that the circular ileal layer was most distensible, followed by the colonic circular and longitudinal ileal layers. The longitudinal layer of the colonic segment was relatively indistensible.[54]

Clinically significant cystoplasty contractions are arbitrarily defined as those 40 cmH$_2$O in amplitude or higher that begin to occur at low volumes (<200 ml). The incidence of such contractions was 70% for tubular ileocystoplasties, 36% for tubular right colon, 10% for detubularized colon, and none in patients with detubularized ileocystoplasties.[55]

The detubularized ileal reservoir for either continent stomal diversion or bladder replacement would seem to constitute the ideal low-pressure reservoir.

## GUT MUCOSA AS A SUBSTITUTE FOR UROTHELIUM

Most research on transposed gut segments has focused on the potential for malignancy arising in the reconstructed bladder substitute, a contingency that will not be discussed here.

## STRUCTURAL/ULTRASTRUCTURAL CHANGES IN NEOBLADDER MUCOSA

Systematic follow-up of the effects of the ileal mucosa in patients with continent reservoirs results in constant and homogeneous changes. They seem to be directly related to the time from surgery and can be subdivided into early and late. From these observations and those published previously, it seems evident that when the ileum is removed from its absorptive function and must respond to a chronic irritative stimulus, the result is biphasic; the first inflammatory phase is followed by a second regressive phase in which the epithelium tends to assume a morphology similar to that of the urothelium, better adapted for coating and protective functions than for absorption. Therefore, it is not surprising that it should be the structures responsible for absorption (brush border and villi) that suffer the most damage. Considering that in a normal ileum the villi increase the absorptive surface eightfold in comparison to a flat surface, their atrophy greatly reduces the area of absorption and, consequently, the risk of metabolic alterations. Paneth's cells (which produce digestive enzymes) and goblet cells seem more tolerant of the prolonged contact with urine, and the regressive phenomena appear significantly later. Because the villi

and crypta are markedly shorter, the ileal mucosa tends to become linear (Box 56.1).[56] This also explains the alternation of areas in which cells with few microvilli (corresponding to the primitive surface epithelium) are predominant, with others in which goblet cells (corresponding to the primitive glandular epithelium) are predominant.

After 4 years of follow-up, the areas of villous atrophy predominate; Paneth's and goblet cells are scanty, and only few residual glands are visible. The resulting epithelium has lost its absorptive and secretive functions to acquire the function of a urinary reservoir. Electron microscopy and enzyme histochemistry in the epithelial cells also showed that there was a reduction in the number of cell organelles and also a decreased metabolic activity.[57]

Progressive mucosal atrophy has been observed in continent colonic reservoirs. They show similar, although much less severe, changes of the microvilli.[56,58] Follow-up studies in patients with ileal conduit also showed atrophic changes with reduction of the villous height, although there are wide variations between different authors and individual patients.[59]

## BIOLOGIC CONSEQUENCES OF EXPOSING GUT MUCOSA TO URINE

Intestinal segments vary in handling of solutes. Length of bowel segment, surface area, duration of urinary exposure, solute concentration, pH, renal function, and urine osmolality all play a role. The reservoir surface is exceedingly difficult to estimate. There is no difference between ileal and colonic mucosa in regard to sodium-absorbing capacity. However, in the colon, chloride absorption and bicarbonate excretion are more pronounced, and there is increasing evidence to suggest that inherent chloride absorption is maintained when in

---

**Box 56.1** Structural and ultrastructural changes in ileal neobladder mucosa

1. Early (<1 year): inflammatory
   - Infiltration of lamina propria
   - Rarefaction of terminal web
   - Goblet cell hyperplasia
   - Reduction of microvilli:
     a. Toxic effect of urine
     b. Low pH
     c. Ischemia
     d. Lack of contact with intestinal content
2. Late (1–4 years): regressive
   - Villous atrophy
   - Shortening of crypts
   - Goblet cells decreased (>4 years)
   - Flat mucosa
   - Stratified epithelium

Based on data from Aragona et al.[56]

contact with urine.[23,57] Therefore, it may be preferable to use ileum rather than colon for bladder reconstruction to reduce the risk of hyperchloremic acidosis, particularly in the presence of renal impairment.

The final result of the process of maturation can be summarized as follows:

- Structure and pharmacologic response of the implanted ileum (not colon) change to detrusor-like responses.
- Structural and ultrastructural changes in ileal (not colonic) mucosa lead to a primitive surface and glandular epithelium similar to urothelium.
- The transformation of the ileal mucosa minimizes the risk of metabolic complications.

Consequently, Mother Nature has engineered a new bladder almost as good as the one given initially.

## UPPER URINARY TRACT PRESERVATION

In a prospective, randomized study of patients undergoing conduit or continent reservoir diversion, renal function was evaluated after a mean follow-up of 10 years.[60] Patients scheduled for conduit diversion were randomized as to the type of intestinal segment and technique for ureterointestinal anastomosis. There was a moderate decrease in the preoperative total glomerular filtration rate (GFR) in the ileal and colonic conduit groups (17 and 19 ml/min, respectively).

Part of the change in GFR is probably a normal age-related decrease, which has been estimated to be about 1 ml/min/year at ages >50 and 0.5 ml/min/year in younger people.[61] If ≥25% fall in GFR is defined as renal deterioration, then this occurred in 34% of patients after a conduit diversion (40% colonic, 28% ileal) and in 28% of those with a continent cecal reservoir. Similar results were reported in patients with a Kock pouch observed for 5–11 years and in patients with an ileal bladder substitute.[8,62]

In a recent report on upper tract preservation, Jonsson et al describe 25 years of follow-up on kidney function in 126 patients with a Kock reservoir.[63] They reach two significant conclusions: kidney function is not impaired by the diversion per se, provided stenosis is recognized and managed; the patient's health status is influenced more by the underlying disease than by the diversion.

## VOIDING DYSFUNCTION

When voiding dysfunction occurs after orthotopic bladder substitution, quality of life is no better than after failure of alternative forms of diversion. Functional results should be reported in accordance with the International Continence Society standards established for intestinal urinary reservoirs.[64]

A comparison of the severity and prevalence of voiding dysfunction in many surgical series is confounded by variability in endpoints, definitions, length of follow-up, patient age and sex, and surgical technique. Moreover, lower urinary tract symptoms, incontinence, or retention rarely have been assessed with validated outcome instruments and/or voiding diaries. Despite these obvious limitations, some general observations can be made and are reviewed in this report.

## FAILURE TO STORE

### Daytime incontinence

In a review of 2238 patients, with a follow-up of $26 \pm 18$ months, daytime incontinence occurs in $13.3 \pm 13.6\%$ of patients.[65] Functional urethral length does not correlate with daytime urinary incontinence. Rather, there is a trend for a lower maximal urethral closure pressure in patients that complain of stress urinary incontinence. More importantly, a suboptimal neobladder capacity is found in many patients with incontinence. Because the neobladder enlarges over time, these patients may become continent 6 months to a year after surgery. Evaluation should be postponed until after this period.

Risk factors for the development of daytime urinary incontinence include advanced patient age, the use of colonic segments, and, in some series, a lack of nerve-sparing techniques.[66,67]

Daytime continence rates decreased gradually 4–5 years after bladder substitution.[68] One factor is a declining external urethral sphincter function with age.[68] The importance of age is underlined by the fact that, at 5 and 10 years after surgery, the mean age of the patients was 68 years and 73 years, respectively. It is noteworthy that in this age group 10% to 15% of healthy men already report urinary incontinence.[69] Urethral sensitivity, which generally decreases after radical cystectomy, might be an additional factor. Hugonnet et al demonstrated that the sensory threshold in the membranous urethra was lower in incontinent patients.[70] It was suggested that the conscious or unconscious sensation of urine leakage in the membranous urethra, which normally produces either a reflex or voluntary contraction or increased tonus of the external urethral sphincter, is impaired.

### Nocturnal leakage

Some degree of nocturnal leakage is a constant finding in most reports, even despite a technically sound operation. Nocturnal incontinence following replacement cystoplasty, which is more common and lasts longer than daytime incontinence, is a feature shared by all forms of neobladders. Nocturnal enuresis plagues nearly 28% (range 0–67%) of patients.[65] Similar to daytime incontinence, night-time incontinence resolves as the functional capacity increases over time. Unlike patients after radical prostatectomy, those with an orthotopic bladder substitute have no detrusor–sphincteric reflex that increases urethral closure pressure as bladder pressure increases. Also, unlike a normal bladder, there are no sensory vesical fibers allowing feedback to the brain to alert the patient when the reservoir is full, particularly at night (overflow incontinence). As long as the functional capacity is lower than the (increased) nocturnal urinary output, the use of an alarm clock at night is recommended until the patient has learned to be awaked by the new sensation of bladder fullness. Apart from the same mechanisms responsible for the gradual decline in daytime continence with age, increased nighttime diuresis and shift of free water into the concentrated urine are additional factors.[54,71] Nocturnal incontinence may be related to the physiologic circadian rhythm of arginine vasopressin (AVP) secretion and an inter-dependence among urine osmolality, distensibility, and peristaltic contractions of the intestinal segments of a pouch, and the generation of pressure waves. Nocturnal antidiuresis with subsequently increased urine osmolality may reduce compliance and increase pressure waves, a phenomenon that may be reversed by the topical application of oxybutynin.[54]

Sensory innervation of the urethra from the intrapelvic branches of the pudendal nerve or branches of the pelvic plexus may also have a role in preventing urinary leakage. Division of these nerves may result in loss of the afferent innervation of the external sphincter guarding reflex stimulated by urinary leakage into the proximal urethra.[72]

## FAILURE TO EMPTY

From 4% to 25% of male patients must perform intermittent self-catheterization for incomplete emptying of the neobladder.[65] The reported functional outcome in female patients differs among series, particularly in regard to voiding ability. Some reported a 53%[19] and 41%[73] rate of intermittent catheterization, whereas others noted a much lower rate of 0%[74] and 3%.[75] The precise pathogenesis of urinary retention, or elevated residual urine requiring intermittent self-catheterization, remains uncertain. Angulation of the urethra is the most common basis for obstruction.[76,77] An attempt to preserve continence by lengthening the bladder neck anastomosed to the urethra can cause obstruction.[78] The angle of the reservoir with the urethra and the supporting system is highly important for emptying of the neobladder. Comparing good voiders with poor voiders, Mikuma et al found no differences of intrareservoir pressure. Instead, they demonstrated two findings in poor voiders: 1) the neobladder outlet was not located at the bottom of the pouch; and 2) funneling of the bladder outlet was not seen even on abdominal straining.[79] A preserved but dysfunctional

bladder neck may result in obstructed voiding; a denervated floppy proximal urethra may lead to ineffective active relaxation, or simply kinking, during voiding, and, thus, incomplete emptying.[80,81]

In the postoperative period, voiding re-education is of paramount importance. Patients must clearly understand the principle that lowering outlet resistance is the key to success. Increasing intra-abdominal pressure alone does not allow voiding. Instruction on pelvic floor relaxation, regular voiding to prevent overdistension, and regular follow-up are essential.[82] In some patients, incomplete voiding is associated with an inability to sustain abdominal straining.

## COMPLICATIONS

The complications of both continent catheterizable reservoirs and orthotopic bladder substitutes in the hands of the most experienced surgeons have been considered in detail.[83] Reoperation for early complications overall occurred in 3% of continent catheterizable reservoirs and 7% of orthotopic bladder substitutions. Reoperation for late complications overall occurred in about 30% of continent catheterizable reservoirs and 13% of orthotopic bladder substitutions. We believe that the morbidity of orthotopic bladder substitutes is actually similar to, or lower than, the true rates of morbidity after conduit formation, contrary to the popular view that conduits are simple and safe.[84–87]

There are several new complications unknown during the conduit era: incisional hernias as a consequence of the Valsalva maneuver, neobladder–intestinal and neobladder–cutaneous fistulas, mucus formation, and neobladder rupture. The secretion of mucus can be dramatically increased.[88] The constant exposure of the neobladder to urine is a chronic irritation and leads to morphologic changes in the reservoir mucosa (see section 'Intestinal tissues as a substitute for the bladder. Gut mucosa as a substitute for urothelium'). A relative increase in goblet cell number was evident after 6 months, continued in the following 8 years, and stopped thereafter. This confirms the clinical observation that, on long-term follow-up, mucus secretion tends to be constant. The increase of goblet cells results in a shift in the secretive pattern towards sialomucins.[89] Probably this shift makes the mucus less viscous and therefore N-acetyl-L-cystein is not necessary for most of the patients after 6–18 months.

Spontaneous late rupture of neobladders is a rare, but potentially life-threatening, complication. In the majority of cases it is secondary to acute or chronic overdistension and bacterial infection. Other factors are minor blunt abdominal trauma or urethral occlusion. Chronic ischemic changes of the neobladder wall, possibly facilitated by detubularization and the variability of the mesenteric circulation, are additional factors that lead to perforation. The rupture site is typically the upper part of the right side of the reservoir. This is the most mobile part of the reservoir, and it undergoes the most marked distension during overfilling, which may constitute an additional factor for perforation in this location.[7]

There is no reliable procedure to establish the diagnosis. Cystography is misleading in three out of four patients with neobladder rupture. A high index of suspicion and early aggressive operative treatment in patients suspected of having a neobladder rupture are instrumental in providing a successful outcome. (*Editor's note*: We have managed three patients with neobladder rupture, and no evidence of an acute abdomen, conservatively with Foley catheter drainage without surgical intervention.) Prevention of neobladder rupture requires careful monitoring of neobladder emptying.[90] Physicians must be aware of the risk of rupture. Patients must be encouraged to void regularly, especially at bedtime, and to perform clean intermittent self-catheterization to avoid chronic reservoir overdistension. In the event that an anesthetic is required, proper bladder drainage should be performed.

## MEDICAL ADVANTAGES OF NEOBLADDER URINARY DIVERSION VERSUS CONDUIT DIVERSION

Orthotopic bladder replacement stimulates earlier cystectomy at a time when the potential for cure is highest. When orthotopic reconstruction was considered experimental surgery, we offered cystectomy patients the choice of a neobladder versus a conduit. We evaluated the intervals from the primary diagnosis of bladder cancer, the diagnosis of invasive cancer, and the recommendation of cystectomy to cystectomy, as well as the number of previous transurethral resections of bladder tumor. Our data clearly suggest that the option of the neobladder may decrease physician and patient reluctance early in the disease process, thus increasing the survival rate significantly.[91]

The overall incidence and impact of ureterointestinal leakage remains rather constant, regardless of the form of urinary diversion used. However, if a bag leaks, it does so to a substantial degree that cannot be easily disguised. This contrasts with leakage of orthotopic bladder substitutes, which tend to be a little more than a few drops or milliliters, and thus can be controlled with a pad.

### UPPER TRACT SAFETY

See section 'Reflux prevention in neobladders'.

### METABOLIC SAFETY

Metabolic and nutritional complications of urinary diversions through bowel segments are common but, fortunately, not often severe. When metabolic abnormalities are problematic, deterioration or baseline insufficiency in renal function is the most likely cause. Deterioration is most commonly associated with obstruction or infection.[24,92–94] The urologist should be acutely aware of the potential for metabolic derangements when the prediversion creatinine is greater than 2.0 mg/dl. The more ileum used for reservoir construction, the higher the incidence of postoperative metabolic acidosis. This leads to the greatest advantage a conduit has over a neobladder.

### QUALITY OF LIFE

Some quality of life studies suggest that patients tolerate the orthotopic bladder better than an ileal conduit.[95] However, other outcome studies have pointed out that the orthotopic neobladder fails to provide increased quality of life compared to an ileal conduit when patients experience voiding dysfunction. The patient satisfaction rate is high with either type of diversion, thus requiring the surgeon to provide a full and informed consent regarding all of the diversion options.[96–98]

In fact, ileal conduit patients may find life with an ileal conduit better than anticipated in terms of satisfaction, whereas continent diversion patients, if they anticipated their internal reservoir to work as well as their original bladder, may be dissatisfied. Patient satisfaction depends on the anticipated results—this is largely a function of informed consent and a realistic preparation by the clinician and enterostomal therapist in explaining, before surgery, the physical and lifestyle changes required postoperatively.

The effects on sexual function of radical cystectomy and the accompanying urinary diversion may be difficult to separate. The presence of an external appliance may impose additional barriers to sexual function for both men and women and their partners.

Other advantages of a neobladder are superior cosmetic appearance, and the potential for normal voiding function and continence. There is no need for an abdominal stoma, and therefore no need for a stomal appliance.

### CONCLUSION

The disadvantages of conduits stimulated the development of orthotopic bladder substitutes. The early and late complication rates of orthotopic bladder substitutes are actually similar to, or lower than, the true rates of morbidity after conduit formation, contrary to the popular view that conduits are simple and safe. The experience with orthotopic bladder substitution has shown that patients who are well motivated and carefully selected can obtain outstanding outcomes.[7,9,10,11,89,99] For these patients, life is similar to that with a native lower urinary tract. Enthusiasm for the use of orthotopic reconstruction, however, should be tempered by an understanding of its indications and how not to contravene them.

## REFERENCES

1. Hautmann RE, Egghart G, Frohneberg D, et al. The ileal neobladder. J Urol 1988;139:39–42.
2. Hautmann RE. The ileal neobladder to the female urethra. Urol Clin North Am 1997;24:827–835.
3. Studer UE, Danuser H, Merz VW, et al. Experience in 100 patients with an ileal low pressure bladder substitute combined with an afferent tubular isoperistaltic segment. J Urol 1995;154:49–56.
4. Stein JP, Grossfeld GD, Freeman JA, et al. Orthotopic lower urinary tract reconstruction in women using the Kock ileal neobladder: updated experience in 34 patients. J Urol 1997;158:400–405.
5. Tizzoni G, Foggi A. Die Wiederherstellung der Harnblase. Zentralbl Chir 1888;15:921–924.
6. Couvelaire R. Le réservoir iléale de substitution après la cystectomie totale chez l'homme. J Urol (Paris) 1951;57:408–417.
7. Hautmann RE. Review article: Urinary diversion: ileal conduit to neobladder. J Urol 2003;169:834–842.
8. Studer UE, Zingg EJ. Ileal orthotopic bladder substitutes. What we have learned from 12 years' experience with 200 patients. Urol Clin North Am 1997;24:781–793.
9. Hautmann RE, Petriconi de R, Gottfried HW, et al. The ileal neobladder: complications and functional results in 363 patients after 11 years of followup. J Urol 1999;161:422–428.
10. Stein JP, Skinner DG. Application of the T-mechanism to an orthotopic (T-pouch) neobladder: a new era of urinary diversion. World J Urol 2000;18:315–323.
11. Montie JE, Wei JT. Formation of an orthotopic neobladder following radical cystectomy: historical perspective, patient selection and contemporary outcomes. J Pelvic Surg 2002;8:141–147.
12. Skinner DG, Studer UE, Okada K, et al. Which are suitable for continent diversion or bladder substitution following cystectomy or other definitive local treatment? Int J Urol 1995;2(Suppl 2):105–112.
13. Studer UE, Hautmann RE, Hohenfellner M, et al. Indications for continent diversion after cystectomy and factors affecting long-term results. Urol Oncol 1998;4:172–182.
14. Montie JE. Ileal conduit diversion after radical cystectomy. Pro Urology 1997;49:659–662.
15. Freeman JA, Tarter TA, Esrig D, et al. Urethral recurrence in patients with orthotopic ileal neobladders. J Urol 1996;156:1615–1619.
16. Hardeman SW, Soloway MS. Urethral recurrence following radical cystectomy. J Urol 1990;144:666–669.
17. Stein JP, Stenzl A, Esrig D, et al. Lower urinary tract reconstruction following cystectomy in women using the Kock ileal reservoir with bilateral ureteroileal urethrostomy: initial clinical experience. J Urol 1994;152:1404–1408.
18. Stenzl A, Draxl H, Posch K, et al. The risk of urethral tumors in female bladder cancer: can the urethra be used for orthotopic reconstruction of the lower urinary tract? J Urol 1995;153:950–955.
19. Hautmann RE, Paiss T, Petriconi de R. The ileal neobladder in women: 9 years of experience with 18 patients. J Urol 1996;155:76–81.
20. Groshen S, Skinner EC, Boyd SD, et al. Indications for lower urinary tract reconstruction in women after cystectomy for bladder cancer: a pathological review of female cystectomy specimens. J Urol 1995;154:1329–1333.
21. Coloby PJ, Kakizoe T, Tobisu K, et al. Urethral involvement in female bladder cancer patients: mapping of 47 consecutive cystourethrectomy specimens. J Urol 1994;152:1438–1442.
22. Hautmann RE, Simon J. Ileal neobladder and local recurrence of bladder cancer: patterns of failure and impact on function in men. J Urol 1999;162:1963–1966.
23. Åkerlund S, Forssell-Aronsson E, Jonsson O, et al. Decreased absorption of 22Na and 36Cl in ileal reservoirs after exposure to urine. An experimental study in patients with continent ileal reservoirs for urinary and fecal diversion. Urol Res 1991;19:249–252.
24. Mills RD, Studer UE. Metabolic consequences of continent urinary diversion. J Urol 1999;161:1057–1066.
25. Lytton B, Green DF. Urodynamic studies in patients undergoing bladder replacement surgery. J Urol 1989;141:1394–1397.
26. Koraitim MM, Atta MA, Foda MK. Early and late cystometry of detubularized and nondetubularized intestinal neobladders: new observations and physiological correlates. J Urol 1995;154:1700–1702; discussion 1702–1703.
27. Santucci RA, Park CH, Mayo ME, et al. Continence and urodynamic parameters of continent urinary reservoirs: comparison of gastric, ileal, ileocolic, right colon, and sigmoid segments. Urology 1999;54:252–252.
28. Kolettis PN, Klein EA, Novick AC, et al. The Le Bag orthotopic urinary diversion. J Urol 1996;156:926–930.
29. Skinner DG, Boyd SD, Lieskovsky G, et al. Lower urinary tract reconstruction following cystectomy: experience and results in 126 patients using the Kock ileal reservoir with bilateral ureteroileal urethrostomy. J Urol 1991;146:756–760.
30. Stein JP, Lieskovsky G, Ginsberg DA, et al. The T pouch: an orthotopic ileal neobladder incorporating a serosal lined ileal antireflux technique. J Urol 1998;159:1836–1842.
31. Hautmann RE. The ileal neobladder. Atlas Urol Clin North Am 2001;9:85.
32. Hollowell CMP, Christiano AP, Steinberg GD. Technique of Hautmann ileal neobladder with chimney modification: interim results in 50 patients. J Urol 2000;163:47–51.
33. Lippert MC, Theodorescu D. The Hautmann neobladder with a chimney: a versatile modification. J Urol 1997;158:1510–1512.
34. Studer UE, Spiegel T, Casanova GA, et al. Ileal bladder substitute: antireflux nipple or afferent tubular segment? Eur Urol 1991;20:315–326.
35. Pernet FP, Jonas U. Ileal conduit urinary diversion: early and late results of 132 cases in a 25-year period. World J Urol 1985;3:140–144.
36. Orr JD, Shand JE, Watters DA, Kirkland IS. Ileal conduit urinary diversion in children. An assessment of long-term results. Br J Urol 1981;53:424–427.
37. Elder DD, Moisey CU, Rees RW. A long-term follow-up of the colonic conduit operation in children. Br J Urol 1979;51:462–465.
38. Dybner R, Jeter K, Lattimer JK. Comparison of intraluminal pressures in ileal and colonic conduits in children. J Urol 1972;108:477–479.
39. Berglund B, Kock NG. Volume capacity and pressure characteristics of various types of intestinal reservoirs. World J Surg 1987;11:798–803.
40. Pantuck AJ, Han KR, Perrotti M. Ureteroenteric anastomosis in continent urinary diversion: long-term results and complications of direct versus nonrefluxing techniques. J Urol 2000;163:450–455.
41. Roth S, Ahlen van H, Semjonow A, et al. Does the success of ureterointestinal implantation in orthotopic bladder substitution depend more on surgeon level of experience or choice of technique? J Urol 1997;157:56–60.
42. Elmajian DA, Stein JP, Esrig D, et al. The Kock ileal neobladder: updated experience in 295 male patients. J Urol 1996;156:920–925.
43. Shaaban AA, Gaballah MA, el-Diasty TA, Ghoneim MA. Urethral controlled bladder substitution: a comparison between the intussuscepted nipple valve and the technique of Le Duc as antireflux procedures. J Urol 1992;148:1156–1161.
44. Cajal SR. Los Gangliosy Plexos Nerviosos del intestino de las Mammiferos. Madrid Moya 1893;1.

45. Faussone-Pellegrini MS. Histogenesis, structure and relationship of interstitial cells of Cajal (ICC): from morphology to functional interpretation. Eur J Morphol 1992;30:137–148.

46. Thuneberg L. Interstitial cells of Cajal. In Handbook of Physiology. The Gastrointestinal System. Motility and Circulation. Bethesda: American Physiological Society, 1989, Sect. 5, 1:349.

47. Rumessen JJ, Mikkelsen HB, Thuneberg L. Ultrastructure of interstitial cells of Cajal associated with deep muscular plexus of human small intestine. Gastroenterology 1992;102:56–68.

48. Huizinga JD, Thuneberg L, Kluppel M, et al. Gene acquired for interstitial cells of Cajal and for intestinal pacemaker activity. Nature 1995;373:347–349.

49. Faussone-Pellegrini MS, Serni S, Carini M. Distribution of ICC and motor response characteristics in urinary bladders reconstructed from human ileum. Am J Physiol 1997;273:G147–157.

50. Batra AK, Hanno PM, Ruggieri MR. Detubularization-induced contractile response change of the ileum following ileocystoplasty. J Urol 1992;148:195–199.

51. Moore JA, Brading AF. Gastrointestinal tissue as a substitute for the detrusor. World J Urol 2000;18:305–314.

52. Hinman F Jr. Selection of intestinal segments for bladder substitution: physical and physiological characteristics. J Urol 1988;139:519–523.

53. Colding-Jørgensen M, Poulsen AL, Steven K. Mechanical characteristics of tubular and detubularised bowel for bladder substitution: theory, urodynamics and clinical results. Br J Urol 1993;72:586–593.

54. Hohenfellner M, Burger R, Schad H. Reservoir characteristics of Mainz pouch studied in animal model. Osmolality of filling solution: an effect of oxybutinin. Urology 1993;42:741–746.

55. Goldwasser B, Madgar I, Hanani Y. Urodynamic aspects of continent urinary diversion, Review Scand J Urol Nephrol 1987;21:245–253.

56. Aragona F, De Caro R, Parenti A. Structural and ultrastructural changes in ileal neobladder mucosa: a 7-year follow up. Br J Urol 1998;81:55–61.

57. Philipson B, Hockenstrom T, Akerlund S. Biological consequences of exposing ileal mucosa to urine. World J Surg 1987;11:790–797.

58. Carlén B, Willen R, Mansson W. Mucosal ultrastructure of continent cecal reservoir for urine and its ileal nipple valve 2–9 years after construction. J Urol 1990;143:372–376.

59. Deane AM, Woodhouse CR, Parkinson MC. Histological changes in ileal conduits. J Urol 1984;132:1108–1111.

60. Kristiánsson A, Wallin L, Månsson W. Renal function up to 16 years after conduit (refluxing or anti-reflux anastomosis) or continent urinary diversion. 1. Glomerular filtration rate and patency of uretero-intestinal anastomosis. Br J Urol 1995;76:539–545.

61. Granerus G, Aurell M. Reference values for 51Cr-EDTA clearance as a measure of glomerular filtration rate. Scand J Clin Lab Invest 1981;41:611–616.

62. Studer UE, Danuser H, Möhrle K, et al. Results in the upper urinary tract in 220 patients with an ileal low pressure bladder substitute combined with an afferent tubular segment. J Urol 1999;161:91.

63. Jonsson O, Olofsson G, Lindholm E, et al. Long-time experience with the Kock ileal reservoir for continent urinary diversion. Eur Urol 2001;40:632–640.

64. Thüroff JW, Mattiasson A, Andersen JT, et al. The standardization of terminology and assessment of functional characteristics of intestinal urinary reservoirs. Br J Urol 1996;78:516–523.

65. Steers WD. Voiding dysfunction in the orthotopic neobladder. World J Urol 2000;18:330–337.

66. Park JM, Montie JE. Mechanisms of incontinence and retention after orthotopic neobladder diversion. Urology 1998;51(4):601–609.

67. Porru D, Madeddu G, Campus G. et al. Urodynamic analysis of voiding dysfunction in orthotopic ileal neobladder. World J Urol 1999;17(5):285–289.

68. Hammerer P, Michl U, Meyer-Moldenhauer WH, et al. Urethral closure pressure changes with age in men. J Urol 1996;156:1741–1743.

69. Temml C, Haidinger G, Schmidbauer J, et al. Urinary incontinence in both sexes: prevalence rates and impact on quality of life and sexual life. Neurourol Urodyn 2000;19:259–271.

70. Hugonnet, CL, Danuser H, Springer JP, et al. Decreased sensitivity in the membranous urethra after orthotopic ileal bladder substitute. J Urol 1999;161:418–421.

71. Jagenburg R, Kock NG, Norlen L, et al. Clinical significance of changes in composition of urine during collection and storage in continent ileum reservoir urinary diversion. Scand J Urol Nephrol 1978;49:43–48.

72. Garry RC, Roberts TD, Todd JK. Reflexes involving the external urethral sphincter in the cat. J Physiol 1953;149:653.

73. Linn JF, Hohenfellner M, Roth S, et al. Treatment of interstitial cystitis: comparison of subtrigonal and supratrigonal cystectomy combined with orthotopic bladder substitution. J Urol 1998;159:774–778.

74. Ghoneim MA. Orthotopic bladder substitution in women following cystectomy for bladder cancer. Urol Clin North Am 1997;24:225–239.

75. Stenzl A, Colleselli K, Bartsch G. Update for urethra-sparing approaches in cystectomy in women. World J Urol 1997;15:134–138.

76. Ali-El-Dein B, El-Sobky E, Hohenfellner M, et al. Orthotopic bladder substitution in women: functional evaluation. J Urol 1999;161:1875–1880.

77. Fujisawa M, Isotani S, Gotoh A, et al. Voiding dysfunction of sigmoid neobladder in women: a comparative study with men. Eur Urol 2001;40:191–195.

78. Smith E, Yoon J, Theodorescu D. Evaluation of urinary continence and voiding function: early results in men with neo-urethral modification of the Hautmann orthotopic neobladder. J Urol 2001;166:1346–1349.

79. Mikuma M, Hirose T, Yokoo A, et al. Voiding dysfunction in ileal neobladder. J Urol 1997;158:1365–1368.

80. Aboseif SR, Borirakchanyavat S, Lue TF, et al. Continence mechanism of the ileal neobladder in women: a urodynamic study. World J Urol 1998;16:400–404.

81. Arai Y, Okubo K, Konami T, et al. Voiding function of orthotopic ileal neobladder in women. Urology 1999;54:44–49.

82. Mills RD, Studer UE, Female orthotopic bladder substitution: a good operation in the right circumstances. J Urol 2000;163:1501–1504.

83. Rowland RG. Complications of continent cutaneous reservoirs and neobladders—series using contemporary technique. AUA Update Ser 1995;14(Lesson 25):201.

84. Turner WH, Bitton A, Studer UE. Reconstruction of the urinary tract after radical cystectomy: the case for continent urinary diversion [editorial]. Urology 1997;49:663–667.

85. Benson MC, Slawin KM, Wechsler MH, Olsson CA. Analysis of continent versus standard urinary diversion. Br J Urol 1992;69:156–162.

86. Gburek BM, Lieber MM, Blute ML. Comparison of Studer ileal conduit diversion with respect to perioperative outcome and late complications. J Urol 1998;160:721–723.

87. Jahnson S, Pedersen J. Cystectomy and urinary diversion during twenty years—complications and metabolic implications. Eur Urol 1993;24:343–349.

88. Leibovitch IJ, Ramon J, Chaim JB, et al. Increased urinary mucus production: a sequela of cystography following enterocystoplasty. J Urol 1991;145:736–737.

89. Gatti R, Ferretti S, Bucci G, et al. Histological adaptation of orthotopic ileal neobladder mucosa: 4-year follow-up of 30 patients. Eur Urol 1999;36:588–594.

90. Nippgen JBW, Hakenberg OW, Manseck A, et al. Spontaneous late rupture of orthotopic detubularized ileal neobladders: report of five cases. Urology 2001;58:43–46.

91. Hautmann RE, Paiss T. Does the option of the ileal neobladder stimulate patient and physician decision towards earlier cystectomy? [abstract]. J Urol 1996;155(Suppl):437A.

92. Stampfer DS, McDougal WS, McGovern FJ. Metabolic and nutritional complications. Urol Clin North Am 1997;24:715–722.

93. Kristjánsson A, Davidsson T, Månsson W. Metabolic alterations at different levels of renal function following continent urinary diversion through colonic segments. J Urol 1997;157:2099–2103.

94. Chang SS, Koch MO. Metabolic complications of urinary diversion. Urol Oncol 2000;5:60–70.

95. Hobisch A, Tosun K, Kinzl J, et al. Quality of life after cystectomy and orthotopic neobladder versus ileal conduit urinary diversion. World J Urol 2000;18:338–344.

96. Hart S, Skinner EC, Meyerowitz BE, et al. Quality of life after radical cystectomy for bladder cancer in patients with an ileal conduit, or cutaneous or urethral Kock pouch. J Urol 1999;162:77–81.

97. Månsson Å, Johnson G, Månsson W. Quality of life after cystectomy. Comparison between patients with conduit and those with continent caecal reservoir urinary diversion. Br J Urol 1988;62:240–245.

98. Henningsohn L, Wijkström H, Dickman PW, et al. Distressful symptoms after radical cystectomy with urinary diversion for urinary bladder cancer: a Swedish population-based study. Eur Urol 2001;40:151–162.

99. Abol-Enein H, Ghoneim MA. Functional results of orthotopic ileal neobladder with serous-lined extramural ureteral reimplantation: experience with 450 patients. J Urol 2001;165:1427–1432.

# Continent cutaneous diversion 57

Christoph Wiesner, Randall G Rowland, Joachim W Thüroff

## INTRODUCTION

Kock devised the first continent ileostomy reservoir for proctocolectomized patients in 1969. It was used first in 1975 for continent cutaneous urinary diversion.[1] Since that time, several surgical procedures for continent cutaneous diversion have been developed using different bowel segments for reservoir construction. Numerous modifications of reservoir construction have been established as well as surgical techniques for ureteral implantation and for construction of a continence mechanism.

In bladder cancer patients, in whom orthotopic diversion is not feasible, continent cutaneous diversion provides a catheterizable low-pressure reservoir, which contributes to an increased quality of life and body image.

## INDICATIONS AND PATIENT SELECTION

Indications for continent cutaneous diversion are cystourethrectomy for bladder cancer, when preservation of the sphincter and urethra are not possible due, for example, to positive urethral biopsies or positive intraoperative surgical margins. In addition, orthotopic bladder substitution should not be recommended for patients with incontinence due to urethral sphincter incompetence.

Careful patient selection for motivation, compliance and manual dexterity to perform self-catheterization is necessary to ensure success of the continent diversion in the long term. Patients with previous irradiation encompassing bowel segments required to construct the reservoir, bowel resection, and chronic inflammatory bowel disease (Crohn's disease, ulcerative colitis) should be excluded.

Contraindications for continent cutaneous diversion are inadequate manual dexterity to perform self-catheterization and reduced intellectual capacity of understanding the reservoir and its function. Furthermore, renal function must be adequate to compensate for reabsorption of acids and liquids from the intestinal reservoir (clearance >50% of age-specific norm, serum creatinine <2.0 mg/dl).

## PREOPERATIVE PREPARATION

Preoperative radiographic imaging includes intravenous pyelography (IVP) for exclusion of upper tract urothelial cancer. If upper tract dilation is present, a radioisotope study should be performed to ensure adequate renal function. If large bowel is used for reservoir construction, a colonic contrast study or colonoscopy to check for bowel polyps and diverticulosis is recommended.

For bowel preparation a liquid diet is given the day before surgery. For bowel cleansing, 3–4 liters of hyperosmotic solution are administered. Subcutaneous prophylaxis for deep vein thrombosis is started the evening before surgery and antithrombotic stockings are used perioperatively. Patients are shaved just before surgery. Patient positioning for surgery is supine with some hyperextension.

## POSTOPERATIVE CARE

Full parenteral nutrition is administered until regular bowel movements are encountered. Antibiotic therapy includes metronidazole for 5 days and amoxicillin until removal of the ureteral stents. The reservoir is irrigated twice a day with saline to avoid mucus formation and catheter blockage. The ureteral stents are usually removed between days 8 and 10 after surgery. After removal of the ureteral stents, drainage of the upper urinary tract is studied by ultrasound or IVP. Before removal of the indwelling catheter, 3 weeks postoperatively, a pouchogram is performed to check for extravasation and ureteral reflux. Patients are then instructed to perform intermittent self-catheterization. The interval between catheterization should not exceed 2 hours initially, and is to be stepwise increased until the pouch capacity reaches 500–600 ml.

## FOLLOW-UP

When the indwelling pouch catheter is removed about 3 weeks postoperatively, and urine storage is initiated in an intestinal urinary reservoir, patients are at risk of developing metabolic acidosis. Close follow-up of the acid–base balance from capillary blood gas analysis is required. Acid–base balance may vary between −2.5 and +2.5 mmol/l; acid–base balance below −2.5 mmol/l should be corrected by alkali substitution.

Serum creatinine and electrolytes should be obtained every 3 months in the first postoperative year.

Renal ultrasound is essential to check for postoperative hydronephrosis and should be obtained every 3 months within the first year after surgery. The interval can be prolonged to every 6 months in the second year and to once a year after 3 years. If hydronephrosis is diagnosed, diuretic radioisotope studies (e.g. MAG-III clearance) are recommended for differentiation between dilation and obstruction.

Patients with continent urinary diversion are at theoretical risk of developing cancer at the site of the ureteral implantation. Hence pouchoscopy starting 5 years postoperatively is recommended once a year.

## SURGERY

The basic principles of continent cutaneous diversion focus on creation of a high-capacity and low-pressure reservoir, which can easily be emptied by intermittent self-catheterization, preserves the upper urinary tract, and provides continence by its specific outlet. A variety of surgical techniques using different bowel segments have been established. Numerous variants of pouch formation, ureteral implantation, and outlet construction have been introduced and combined in modifications of original techniques to reduce the risk of complications and to optimize clinical outcome.

## KOCK POUCH

Kock was the first to present a continent ileal reservoir for urinary diversion using 60–70 cm of ileum for pouch formation and construction of two valves (Figure 57.1). At the proximal and distal ends of the ileum, which has been excluded from the fecal stream for pouch formation, 10–12 cm of bowel each are left intact for creation of the afferent and efferent valves. The remaining 40 cm of ileum is incised antimesenterically, sutured side-to-side in a U-shape, folded over, and closed to a spherical pouch (Figures 57.2, 57.3). For the final position, the reservoir is rotated in such a manner that the posterior aspect is brought anteriorly (Figure 57.4). Strips of fascia from the anterior rectus sheath or of Marlex mesh are used around the base of the intussusception to secure the afferent antirefluxing valve and the efferent continence valve. The ureters are implanted end-to-side into the afferent ileum. The nipple valves are intussuscepted over a length of 5 cm and fixed by four rows of staples (Figure 57.5). The technique was later modified with a longer ileal intussusception by placing three staple rows at the 6, 10 and 2 o'clock positions and fixation of the nipple by inserting fibrin glue and several sutures at the intussusception.[2]

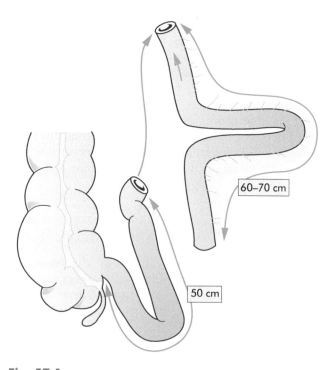

**Fig. 57.1**

Kock pouch cutaneous diversion. 60–70 cm of ileum are isolated approximately 50 cm above the ileocecal valve. The bowel is positioned in a U-shape. Adapted from Kock NG, Nilson LD, Nilson LJ, Philipson BM. Urinary diversion via a continent ileal reservoir: Clinical results in 12 patients. J. Urol 1982;128:469–475.

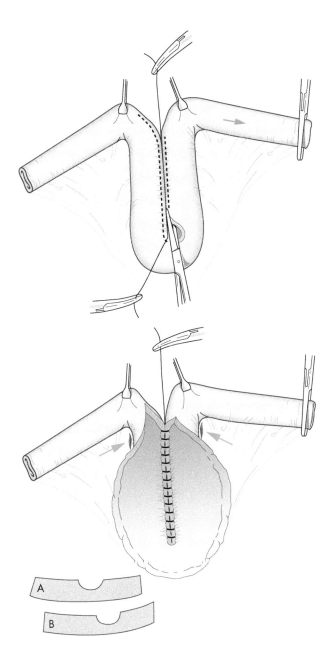

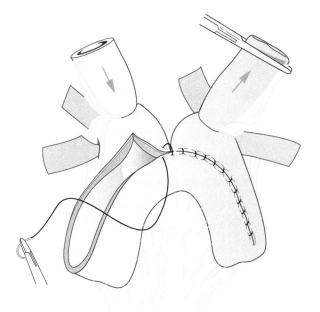

## Fig. 57.3

Kock pouch cutaneous diversion. Closure of the reservoir is performed by two inverting running sutures. Adapted from Kock NG, Nilson LD, Nilson LJ, Philipson BM. Urinary diversion via a continent ileal reservoir: Clinical results in 12 patients. J. Urol 1982;128:469–475.

## Fig. 57.2

Kock pouch cutaneous diversion. The ileum is incised along its antimesenteric border and sutured side-to-side in a U-shape. Adapted from Kock NG, Nilson LD, Nilson LJ, Philipson BM. Urinary diversion via a continent ileal reservoir: Clinical results in 12 patients. J. Urol 1982;128:469–475.

## COMPLICATION RATES

Complications with the need for surgical reintervention range between 32% and 53%.[2-8] In a series of 40 patients with Kock pouch diversion, early pouch-related complications were encountered in 25%, including two patients with reoperation for pouch rupture and pinhole fistula at the efferent segment.[2] Eight patients were re-hospitalized, seven because of pouch sepsis, which was associated with transient acidosis, and one with a pelvic abscess.

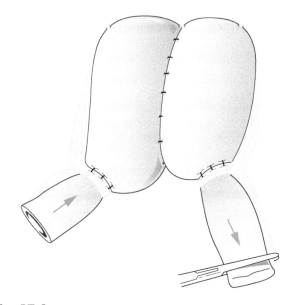

## Fig. 57.4

Kock pouch cutaneous diversion. For the final positioning, the reservoir is rotated in such a manner that the posterior aspect is brought anteriorly. Adapted from Kock NG, Nilson LD, Nilson LJ, Philipson BM. Urinary diversion via a continent ileal reservoir: Clinical results in 12 patients. J. Urol 1982;128:469–475.

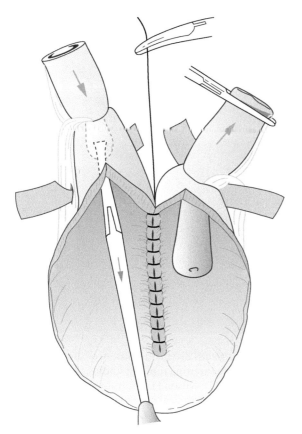

**Fig. 57.5**
Kock pouch cutaneous diversion. The nipple valves are fixed by ileal intussusception with three rows of staples. The afferent valve serves as antireflux mechanism to ureteral implantation, the efferent valve as the continent outlet. The valves are secured by strips of fascia or Marlex mesh, which are positioned around the base of each valve. Adapted from Kock NG, Nilson LD, Nilson LJ, Philipson BM. Urinary diversion via a continent ileal reservoir: Clinical results in 12 patients. J. Urol 1982;128:469–475.

Late complications were most frequently associated with dysfunction of the efferent segment including stomal incontinence (17–23%), nipple prolapse/nipple gliding (7–10%), stomal stenosis (0–10%), or calculus formation (8–15%). Complications of the afferent segment are rare and comprise mostly strictures of the ureteroileal anastomosis (2–5%), ureteral reflux (2–13%), afferent nipple stones (5.2%), or afferent limb stenosis in 4.3%.[8] Continence rates vary between 78% and 94%.

## MAINZ POUCH AND ALTERNATIVE/MODIFIED PROCEDURES

The Mainz pouch I procedure was established in 1983 using 10–15 cm of cecum and ascending colon and two terminal ileal segments of equal length for reservoir construction (Figure 57.6).[9] The surgical procedure

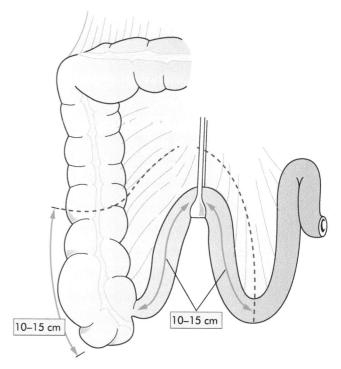

**Fig. 57.6**
Mainz pouch diversion. 10–15 cm of cecum and ascending colon and two ileal segments of the same length are used for reservoir construction.

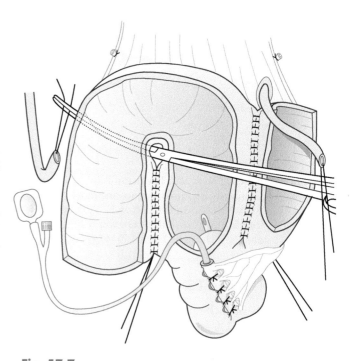

**Fig. 57.7**
Implantation of the ureters by extramural serosa lined tunnel technique. The serosa of the adjacent bowel segments is sutured approximately 2 cm from the margins by a nonabsorbable running suture for construction of the bed of the tunnel.

comprises antimesenteric incision of ileum, cecum, and ascending colon, and side-to-side anastomosis of the ascending colon with the terminal ileal loop, and of the latter with the proximal ileal loop. The anterior wall of the pouch is closed by a single row of running sutures.

Both ureters are implanted in an antirefluxing manner into the large bowel using the submucosal tunnel technique described by Goodwin et al.[10] Alternatively, the Aboul-Enein technique is performed for preoperatively dilated ureters in order to avoid postoperative obstruction (Figures 57.7–57.9).[11] The technique entails fashioning of two serosa lined extramural tunnels, and was first applied to the W-shaped ileal neobladder. The 'buttonhole' technique implies direct refluxing ureteral implantation.[12]

Originally, the continent outlet was created using 12–15 cm of terminal ileum, which was left intact and was intussuscepted isoperistaltically over a length of

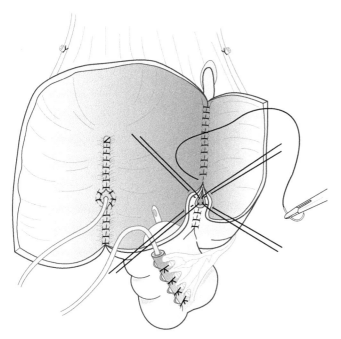

**Fig. 57.8**
Extramural serosa lined tunnel. After the ureters have been positioned into the serosa bed, the tunnel is closed by closing the bowel margins over it using a running absorbable suture.

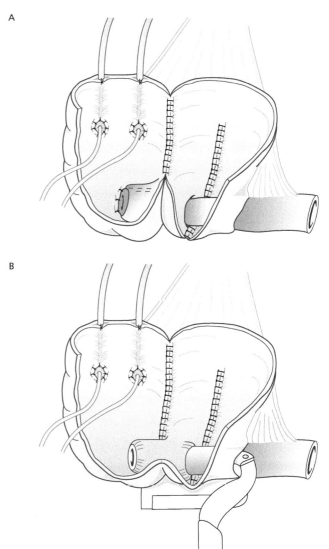

A

B

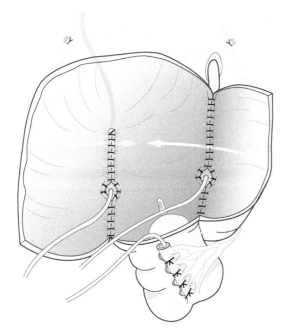

**Fig. 57.9**
Extramural serosa lined tunnel. The neo-orifices are created by 6-0 sutures of the ureter with the intestinal mucosa.

**Fig. 57.10**
Intussuscepted ileal nipple. **A** 12–15 cm of terminal ileum are used for construction of the intussuscepted ileal nipple valve. The ileum is left tubularized and intussuscepted isoperistaltically through the ileocecal valve and secured by three rows of metal staples. **B** One row of staples fixes the nipple to the reservoir wall.

about 5 cm through the ileocecal valve. Fixation of the segment was performed by three rows of metal staples, one of which fixed the nipple to the reservoir wall (Figure 57.10). Since 1990, the submucosally embedded in-situ appendix is increasingly used for construction of the continent outlet.[13] The submucosal tunnel is created by seromuscular incision of the tenia libra (Figure 57.11). The appendix is flipped over into the submucosal bed and the seromuscularis layer is closed over it (Figure 57.12).

The seromuscular and full-thickness bowel flap tubes were presented in 1995 as an alternative procedure for patients in whom the appendix was not available.[14] For the seromuscularis bowel flap tube, a 3 × 5 cm pedicled flap is created by an inverted U-shaped incision along the tenia libra and then tubularized. The bowel flap tube is embedded submucosally by closing the lateral margins of the seromuscular incisions over it. In the full-thickness bowel flap tube technique, the pedicled bowel flap is excised from the anterior tenia and embedded into a submucosal tunnel at the tenia omentalis (Figures 57.13 and 57.14).

The transverse colonic pouch (Mainz pouch III, transverse ascending or transverse descending pouch) was created for continent urinary diversion in patients with previous pelvic irradiation.[15] A total of 15–17 cm of transverse colon and either ascending or descending

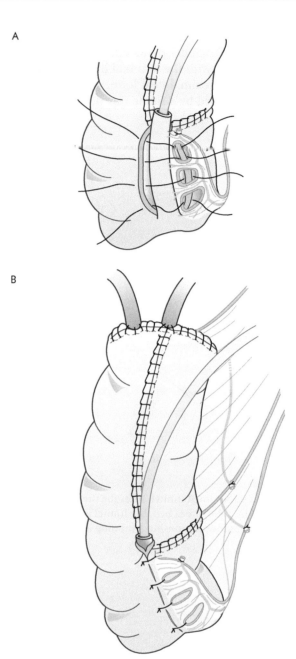

A

B

**Fig. 57.12**
Appendiceal stoma. **A** The appendix is flipped over into the submucosal bed. **B** The tunnel is finished by closure of the seromuscularis over the appendix.

colon are used (Figure 57.15). The outlet is created by tapering a 5–7 cm tubular colonic segment into a tube, which is embedded into a serosal or submucosal tunnel (Figure 57.16). The ureteral implantation follows the Goodwin technique or the serosal extramural tunnel technique (Figure 57.17).

## COMPLICATION RATES

Since the creation of the Mainz pouch, several techniques for outlet construction and ureteral

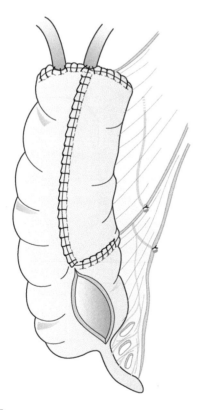

**Fig. 57.11**
Appendiceal stoma. The seromuscularis is incised along the tenia libra.

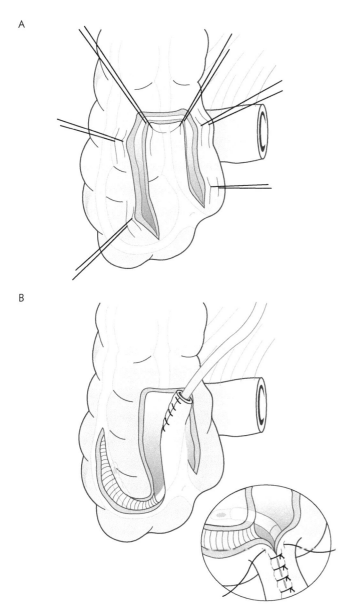

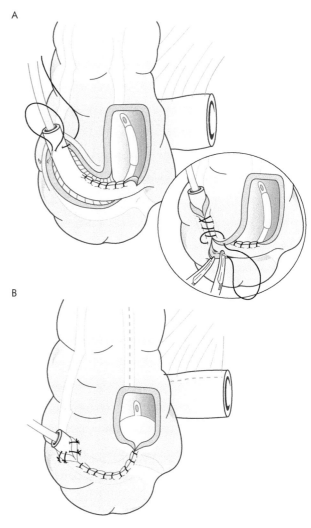

**Fig. 57.14**
Full-thickness bowel flap tube. **A** The tube is embedded into a submucosal tunnel at the tenia omentalis. **B** The tunnel is finished by closing the lateral margins of the seromuscularis.

**Fig. 57.13**
Full-thickness bowel flap tube. **A** A flap is created by an inverted U-shaped incision along the tenia libra of the cecum and tubularized (**B**).

implantation have been developed. The initial complication rates for sutured and stapled ileoileal intussusception nipples of 45% decreased to 10% for nipples with additional fixation to the ileocecal valve.[16,17] Minor complications of the intussuscepted ileal nipple are calculus formation (3–5.5%) and stoma stenosis (1.9–11.7%)[18,19]; major complications were nipple necrosis (3.8%) and nipple prolapse/nipple gliding (6.6%).[18]

Stoma stenosis is the most frequent complication of the appendix outlet, ranging from 14.6% to 21%.[17–20] Development of calculi is rare. Major complications

were appendiceal necrosis (2.1–2.5%) with the consequence of surgical revision and replacement by an ileal nipple.[18,20] Continence rates of the appendix outlet range between 98% and 100%.[18–20]

Stoma stenoses were seen in 11% of patients with a full-thickness bowel flap tube.[21] Antirefluxing ureteral implantation with a submucosal tunnel was associated with a 5.7% ureteral obstruction rate for preoperatively nondilated ureters, and a 16% obstruction rate for preoperatively dilated systems at long-term follow-up.[22] Direct ureterointestinal implantation was performed in 30 patients with Mainz pouch diversion.[12] The technique was used for primary anastomosis in 20 patients, and for reimplantation in cases of stenosis of the ureterointestinal anastomosis in another 10 patients. At follow-up there was no deterioration of kidney function and no evidence of obstruction; reflux occurred

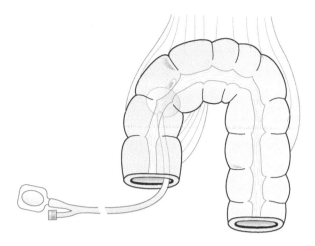

**Fig. 57.15**
Transverse colon pouch diversion (Mainz III). The colonic
pouch (Mainz III) is constructed by a 15–17 cm segment of
transverse colon and either ascending or descending colon.
Adapted from Leissner J, Black P, Fisch M, Hockel M,
Hohenfellner R. Colon pouch (Mainz pouch III) for continent
urinary diversion after pelvic irradiation. Urology
2000;56:798–802.

in one renal unit only without necessity for
intervention.

Complication rates (18%) of the transverse colonic
pouch (Mainz III) were related to the tapered colonic
efferent segment with stoma incontinence in 5% and
stoma stenosis in 14%.[15] Stoma incontinence required
surgical revision by creating a new outlet. Patients with
stoma stenosis were treated by endoscopic scar incision
(67%) or by open surgical YV-plasty (33%).

## INDIANA POUCH

The Indiana pouch was developed in 1984 as a
modification of the Gilchrist procedure.[23] Up to
8–10 cm of terminal ileum and 25–30 cm of cecum and
ascending colon are isolated and opened along the
antimesenteric border (Figure 57.18A). The distal end of
the opened colon is folded down to the apex of the
incision. The reservoir is closed with a single layer of
sutures (Figure 57.18B,C). If the reservoir was to be
constructed by mechanical stapling, a 2–3 cm incision at
the antimesenteric border of the cecum opposite to the
ileocecal valve is performed. The distal end of the
colonic segment is folded down to the cecal incision,
fixed by holding sutures, cut open and stapled between
the holding sutures using the GIA stapler with
absorbable staples until complete detubularization of
the colonic segment is achieved. The edges of the
opposing colonic segments are finally closed by
absorbable Ta 55 staples. Originally, ureteral

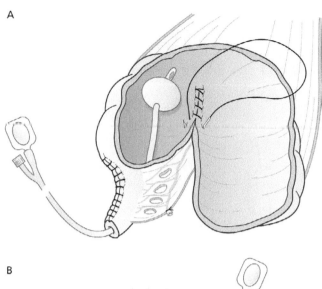

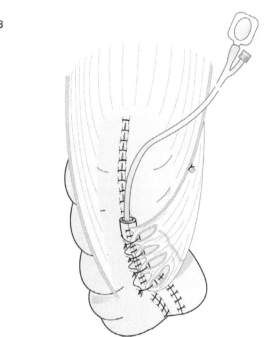

**Fig. 57.16**
Transverse colon pouch diversion (Mainz III). **A** The outlet is
created by tapering a 5–7 cm tubular colonic segment into a
tube, which is embedded into a serosal tunnel (**B**). Adapted
from Leissner J, Black P, Fisch M, Hockel M, Hohenfellner R.
Colon pouch (Mainz pouch III) for continent urinary
diversion after pelvic irradiation. Urology 2000;56:798–802.

implantation was performed through a T-shaped
incision of the colonic tenia, leaving the mucosa intact
(Figure 57.19A). The ureteral neo-orifice was established
after mucosal incision (Figure 57.19B), and the
submucosal tunnel was closed by a running suture
of the incised seromuscularis (Figure 57.19C, D).
Currently a refluxing end-to-side direct anastomosis is
used. The efferent segment is constructed by tapered
ileum. The antimesenteric portion of the terminal ileum
is tapered using metal GIA staples, leaving a residual

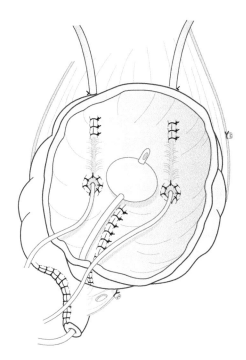

**Fig. 57.17**
Transverse colon pouch diversion (Mainz III). The ureters are implanted by the Goodwin technique, or by an extramural serosal tunnel. Adapted from Leissner J, Black P, Fisch M, Hockel M, Hohenfellner R. Colon pouch (Mainz pouch III) for continent urinary diversion after pelvic irradiation. Urology 2000;56:798–802.

caliber of ileum that allows easy passage of an 18 Fr. catheter. The outlet is imbricated and secured by sutures at the junction of ileum and cecum to create a functional continence mechanism (Figure 57.20).

The procedure was modified by Managadze, who embedded the tapered ileum segment into a submucosal tunnel by incision of the seromuscularis between the tenia libra and the tenia mesocolica of the cecum.[24]

## COMPLICATION RATES

Complication rates of urinary diversion using the Indiana pouch procedure were investigated in several studies and revealed a total rate of surgical reinterventions ranging between 10.8% and 52.0%.[25-27] Pouch-related complications were pouch rupture (2.5–3.2%) and calculus formation (3.7–10.5%). Complications of the efferent segment were stoma stenosis (3.7–15.2%) and stoma incontinence (1.2–28.2%). Obstruction of the ureteral anastomosis was recognized in 0% to 7.2%. Preoperative radiotherapy did influence postoperative outcome negatively.

Complication rates of 130 patients, including 34 (26%) patients with preoperative pelvic irradiation, were reported, in whom the Indiana pouch was performed for urinary diversion.[28] The overall

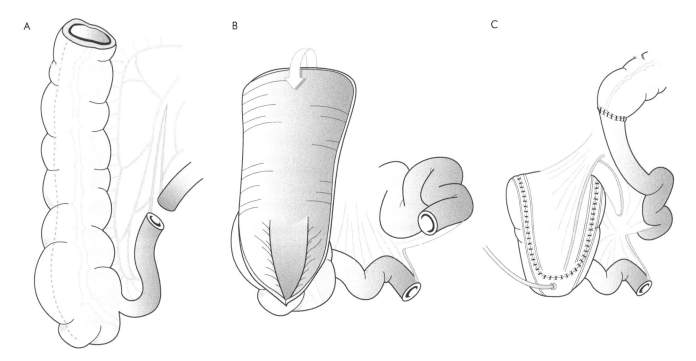

**Fig. 57.18**
Indiana pouch diversion. **A** 8–10 cm of terminal ileum and 25–30 cm of cecum and ascending colon are used for construction of the Indiana pouch and opened along the antimesenteric border. **B** The distal end of the opened colon is folded down to the apex of the incision, and closed with a single layer of sutures (**C**). Adapted from Rowland RG. Present experience with the Indiana Pouch. World J Urol 1986;14:92–98.

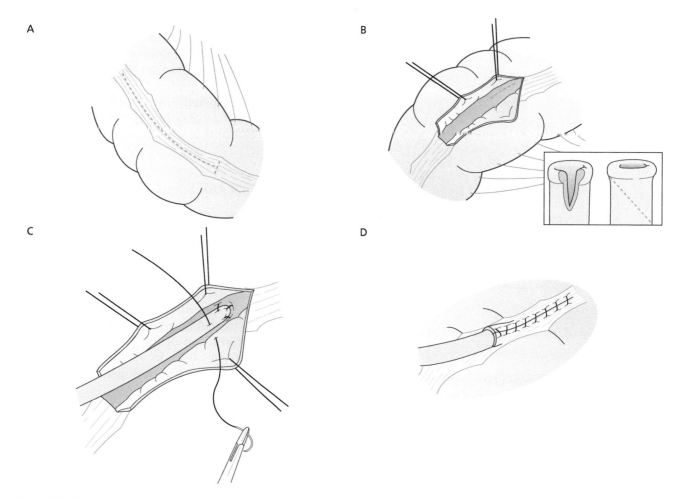

**Fig. 57.19**

Indiana pouch diversion. **A** Ureteral implantation is performed through a T-shaped incision of the colonic tenia leaving the mucosa intact. **B** The ureteral orifice is established after mucosal incision. **C** The spatulated ureter is anastomosed to the bowel mucosa by single sutures and **D** the seromuscularis is closed over it. As an alternative, a direct end-to-side anastomosis can be performed. Adapted from Rowland RG. Present experience with the Indiana Pouch. World J Urol 1986;14:92–98.

complication rate was 12%; ureteral obstruction was seen in 15% of the patients with preoperative irradiation and in 4% without preoperative irradiation. Stoma incontinence developed in 4% of the patients, all of whom had undergone preoperative radiotherapy.

## FLORIDA POUCH

In 1987 Lockhart described an alternative colonic reservoir (Florida pouch) that included cecum, ascending colon, one-third of the right transverse colon, and 10–12 cm of the terminal ileum for the outlet.[29] The colon is U-folded, fully detubularized, and closed by a locked running suture. Ureteral implantation was originally performed using the Le Duc antirefluxing ureteroileal implantation by ureteral fixation in a mucosal sulcus,[30] or by the Goodwin technique (described above).[10] It was later modified into a direct

anastomosis of the ureters to the colon, avoiding an antirefluxing implantation.[31] The ureteral adventitia is fixed to the seromuscularis of the bowel with four quadrant sutures, and the spatulated ureter is sutured to the bowel mucosa. The terminal ileum is used as the efferent segment. The ileum is left attached to the reservoir and plicated with two parallel rows of sutures, placed longitudinally into the ileum and ileocecal valve.

## COMPLICATION RATES

Complication rates of ureter implantation were evaluated concerning the ureteral implantation technique (tunneled by Le Duc/Goodwin or nontunneled end-to-side anastomosis).[31,32] Ureteral obstruction was noted in 13.3% with tunneled implantation, and in 4.9% with end-to-side implantation of the ureters; however, the rate of refluxing units was higher in the latter group (7.0%

Several techniques using only small bowel, small and large bowel segments, or large bowel only have been developed for creation of a high-capacity and low-pressure reservoir, which contribute to an increased quality of life and body image of the patients. Numerous surgical techniques and modifications referring to reservoir construction, ureteral implantation, and creation of the outlet have been established in the past. Variations of procedures and growing experience with bowel reservoirs have led to a reduction of their specific complication rates in the long run. Most of the complications are related to the reservoir outlet and can be treated by minor surgical interventions. Postoperatively, a close follow-up including acid–base balance, serum creatinine, serum electrolytes, and ultrasound of the upper urinary tract are essential. Pouchoscopy, starting 5 years postoperatively, is recommended once a year to check for tumor development.

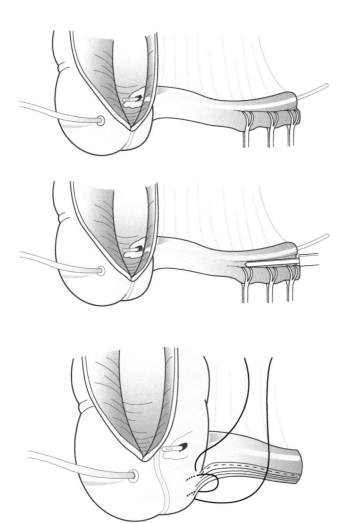

**Fig. 57.20**
Indiana pouch diversion. The efferent segment is established by tapering the terminal ileum using metal GIA staples leaving a caliber of ileum for passage of 18 Fr. catheter. The outlet is imbricated by sutures at the junction of the ileum and cecum to create the continence mechanism. Adapted from Rowland RG. Present experience with the Indiana Pouch. World J Urol 1986;14:92–98.

versus 3.3%). Complications of the efferent segment were stoma incontinence in 3.0% to 6.7%, and stoma stenosis in 4.0% to 10.0%.[17,30] Pouch stones were seen in 3.0% to 5.4%.[6,33]

## CONCLUSION

Continent cutaneous diversion with a catheterizable abdominal wall stoma is a reproducible and safe alternative for patients in whom orthotopic urinary diversion is not feasible. To ensure success of continent cutaneous diversion, careful patient selection is required prior to surgery.

## REFERENCES

1. Kock NG, Nilson AR, Norlen L, Sundin T, Trasti H. Urinary diversion via a continent ileum reservoir: clinical experience. Scand J Urol Nephrol Suppl 1978;49:23.
2. Soulie M, Seguin P, Martel P, Vazzoler N, Mouly P, Plante P. A modified intussuscepted nipple in the Kock pouch urinary diversion: assessment of perioperative complications and functional results. Br J Urol 2002;90:397–402.
3. Jonsson O, Olofsson G, Lindholm E, Törnquist H. Long time experience with Kock ileal reservoir for continent urinary diversion. Eur Urol 2001;40:632–640.
4. Skinner DG, Lieskovski G, Boyd S. Continent urinary diversion. J Urol 1989;141:1323–1327.
5. Okada Y, Shichiri Y, Terai A, et al. Management of late complications of continent urinary diversion using the Kock pouch and the Indiana pouch procedures. Int J Urol 1996;3:334–339.
6. Carr LK, Webster GD. Kock versus right colon continent urinary diversion: comparison of outcome and reoperation rate. Urology 1996;48:711–714.
7. Bander NH. Initial results with slightly modified Kock pouch. Urology 1991;37:100–105.
8. Stein JP, Freeman JA, Esrig D, et al. Complications of the afferent antireflux valve mechanism in the Kock ileal reservoir. J Urol 1996;155:1579–1584.
9. Thüroff JW, Alken P, Riedmiller H, Engelmann U, Jacobi GH, Hohenfellner R. The Mainz pouch (mixed augmentation ileum and cecum) for bladder augmentation and continent diversion. J Urol 1986;136:17–26.
10. Goodwin WE, Winter CC, Turner RD. Replacement of ureter by small intestine: clinical application and results of the 'ileal ureter'. J Urol 1959;81:406–418.
11. Aboul-Enein H, Ghoneim MA. A novel uretero-ileal re-implantation technique: the serous lined extramural tunnel. A preliminary report. J Urol 1994;151:1193–1198.
12. Hohenfellner R, Black P, Leissner J, Allhoff EP. Refluxing ureterointestinal anastomosis for continent cutaneous urinary diversion. J Urol 2002;168:1013–1017.
13. Riedmiller H, Bürger R, Müller S, Thüroff JW, Hohenfellner R. Continent appendix stoma: a modification of the Mainz pouch technique. J Urol 1990;143:1115–1116.
14. Lampel A, Hohenfellner M, Schultz-Lampel D, Thüroff JW. In situ tunneled bowel flap tubes: 2 new techniques of a continent outlet for Mainz pouch cutaneous diversion. J Urol 1995;153:308–315.
15. Leissner J, Black P, Fisch M, Höckel M, Hohenfellner R. Colon pouch (Mainz pouch III) for continent urinary diversion after pelvic irradiation. Urology 2000;56:798–802.

16. Thüroff JW, Alken P, Riedmiller H, Jacobi GH, Hohenfellner R. 100 cases of Mainz pouch: continuing experience and evolution. J Urol 1988;140:283–288.

17. Lampel A, Fisch M, Stein R, Schultz-Lampel D, Hohenfellner M, Thüroff JW. Continent diversion with the Mainz pouch. World J Urol 1996;14:85–91.

18. Gerharz EW, Köhl U, Weingärtner K, Melekos MD, Bonfig R, Riedmiller H. Complications related to different continence mechanisms in ileocecal reservoir. J Urol 1997;158:1709–1713.

19. Fichtner J, Fisch M, Hohenfellner R. Appendiceal continence mechanisms in continent urinary diversion. World J Urol 1996;14:105–107.

20. Gerharz EW, Köhl UN, Melekos MD, Bonfig R, Weingärtner K, Riedmiller H. Ten years' experience with the submucosally embedded in situ appendix in continent urinary diversion. Eur Urol 2001;40:625–631.

21. Roth S, Weining C, Hertle L. Continent cutaneous urinary diversion using the full thickened bowel flap tube as continence mechanism: a simplified tunnel technique. J Urol 1996;156:1922–1925.

22. Stein R, Pfitzenmaier J, Behringer M, Hohenfellner R, Thüroff JW. The long-term results (5–16 years) of Mainz pouch I technique at a single institution. J Urol 2001;165(Suppl):88.

23. Rowland RG, Mitchell ME, Bihrle R, Kahnoski RJ, Piser JE. Indiana continent urinary reservoir. J Urol 1987;137:1136–1139.

24. Chanturaia Z, Pertia A, Managadze G, Khvadagiani G, Chigogidze L, Managadze L. Right colonic reservoir with submucosally embedded tapered ileum—'Tiflis pouch'. Urol Int 1997;59:113–118.

25. Rowland RG. Present experiences with the Indiana pouch. World J Urol 1996;14:92–98.

26. Holmes DG, Trasher JB, Park GY, Kueker DC, Weigel JW. Long term complications related to the modified Indiana pouch. Urology 2002;60:603–606.

27. Aria Y, Kawakita M, Terachi T, et al. Long-term followup of the Kock and Indiana pouch procedures. J Urol 1993;150:51–55.

28. Wilson TG, Moreno JG, Weinberg A, Ahlering TE. Late complications of the modified Indiana pouch. J Urol 1994;151:331–334.

29. Lockhart JL. Remodeled right colon: an alternative urinary reservoir. J Urol 1987;138:730–734.

30. Le Duc A, Camey M, Teillac P, An original antireflux ureteroileal implantation technique: long term follow-up. J Urol 1987;137:1156–1158.

31. Helal M, Pow-Sang J, Sanford E, Figueroa E, Lockhart J. Direct (non tunneled) ureterocolonic reimplantation in association with continent reservoirs. J Urol 1993;150:835–837.

32. Lockhart JL, Pow-Sang JM, Persky L, Kahn P, Helal M, Sanford E. A continent colonic urinary reservoir: the Florida pouch. J Urol 1990;144:864–867.

33. Webster C, Bukkapatnam R, Seigne JD, et al. Continent colonic urinary reservoir (Florida pouch): long term surgical complications (greater than 11 years). J Urol 2003;169:174–176.

# Noncontinent urinary diversion 58

*Wiking Månsson, Fredrik Liedberg, Roland Dahlem, Margit Fisch*

## INTRODUCTION

Noncontinent urinary diversion remains the most commonly used method for reconstructing the lower urinary tract in conjunction with radical cystectomy. Thus, in 2002 in Sweden, 64% of all patients undergoing cystectomy within 3 months of diagnosis received a noncontinent form of reconstruction, while 13% got a continent cutaneous diversion and 21% an orthotopic bladder substitute. Data were missing for 3%.[1] This is not surprising considering the high age of the patients at cystectomy. It is our impression that older patients are, in general, little interested in continent reconstruction, although there are exceptions. Most of them want a simple system with low risk of early and late complications and a short hospital stay. We believe that 80 years of age is an arbitrary upper limit for recommending continent reconstruction. In fact, many patients above the age of 70 settle for an ileal conduit at the final counseling after having been informed about pros and cons, read some literature and, if possible, having met patients with different types of reconstruction. In addition, when a malignant disease is present, there seem to be no major differences in the quality of life when comparing patients with incontinent diversion and those with continent diversion.[2]

Other facts that contribute to a high incidence of noncontinent diversion are that a substantial number of patients turn out to have very advanced disease at laparotomy, and that a considerable number of cystectomies are performed outside major centers. Improvements in the quality of the appliances and the development of enterostomal therapy into a specific field of its own have been important for the acceptance of noncontinent diversion. Marking the site of the stoma and managing stomal complications are today carried out in close cooperation between the urologist and the stoma therapist.

## PATIENT PREPARATION

Together with the stoma therapist, the urologist should mark the site of the stoma prior to surgery. It should be placed in an area free of scars and skin folds, and most often it will be slightly below a line between the umbilicus and the anterior superior iliac spine. The adhesive portion of the appliance is usually a quadrant with the side 7–8 cm, which will influence position with regard to the umbilicus and the iliac spine. The patient should wear the appliance for a day or two preoperatively.

When a colonic conduit is planned, imaging with water-soluble contrast media should be performed in order to exclude polyps and diverticula. Bowel preparation is important in order to reduce infectious complications and for ease of working with the bowel intraoperatively. There are many suggestions as to how to prepare the bowel. Most common seems to be intake of polyethylene glycol or phospho-soda preparations. Alternatively, the intestine can be irrigated with 8–10 liters of Ringer's lactate solution via a gastric tube. Intraoperatively, broad-spectrum antibiotics such as cefoxitin or tetracycline together with metronidazole are usually given.

# SURGICAL TECHNIQUES

## CUTANEOUS URETEROSTOMY

This method of diversion is infrequently used today, and there are few reports in the literature during the past 10 years. The main indication has been palliation in advanced stages of bladder cancer. However, the current method of diversion of urine is usually through percutaneous nephrostomy tube. Cutaneous ureterostomy is associated with less risk of early complications than conduit diversion. Thus, Martinez-Pineiro et al[3] reported an incidence of 7% of such complications after cystectomy, whereas it was three times higher if a conduit was created. Stomal stenosis is a frequent problem, especially in nondilated ureters. However, high patency rates have been reported following primary plasty of the ureterocutaneous junction.[4,5] In addition, new materials allow for leaving indwelling single J-shaped stents in cases of ureterocutaneous obstruction for long periods of time with little tendency for infection and encrustation.

In certain cases cutaneous ureterostomy can be combined with a transureteroureterostomy with acceptable results. However, there is a risk with this procedure of urine pendulating from one ureter to the other—the 'yo-yo phenomenon'—due to disrupted ureteric peristalsis. In order to diminish this risk, the recipient ureter should be mobilized only to the level where the anastomosis will be performed.[6] The end of the nondilated donor ureter is cut obliquely and sutured without tension end-to-side to the recipient ureter, which is usually dilated.

## CONDUIT DIVERSION

Conduits can be constructed from stomach, jejunum, ileum, and colon, and there are specific indications for each conduit.

## ILEAL CONDUIT

This is the most common form of urinary diversion in conjunction with radical cystectomy. A 15–20 cm long distal ileal segment is isolated and the ureters implanted in the proximal end, most usually with a refluxing technique (Figure 58.1). There are many techniques described, the 'classical' ones being a Nesbit-like technique as used in Bricker's original publication[7] and the Wallace technique[8] (Figure 58.2). In Lund, the standard method is the open technique described by Sundin and Pettersson[9] (Figure 58.3). The stoma is usually below and to the right of the umbilicus.

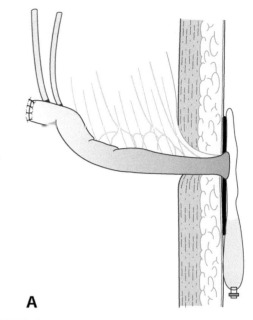

**A**

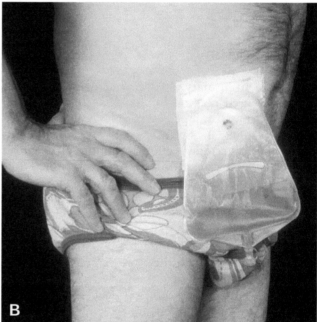

**B**

**Fig. 58.1**
**A** Ileal conduit. **B** Patient with ileal conduit diversion.

Although originally described in the early 1930s, the ileal conduit did not attain clinical popularity until 20 years later, after the publications by Eugene Bricker.[7,10,11] It quickly replaced ureterosigmoidostomy as the preferred method for urinary diversion with a lower incidence of metabolic disturbances, the most common being hyperchloremic acidosis. The technique has a low degree of complexity and a vast experience of ileal conduit has been gained. However, few publications have appeared during the last decade, when instead the focus has been on continent reconstruction.

Is radical cystectomy associated with fewer complications when combined with an ileal conduit

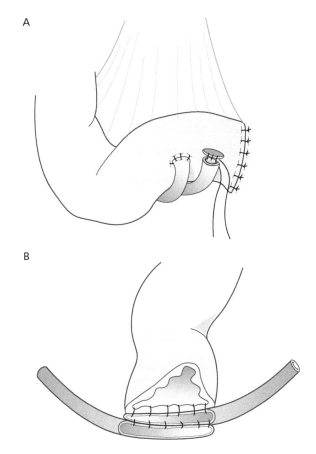

**Fig. 58.2**
A Nesbit type of ureteric implantation as used by Bricker.
B Ureteric implantation, 'head-to-tail', according to Wallace.[8]

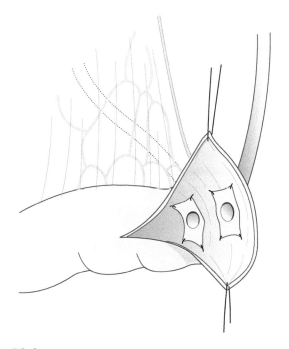

**Fig. 58.3**
Ureteric implantation according to Sundin and Pettersson.[9]

than in conjunction with continent reconstruction? Some studies have failed to find such differences when stratifying, according to the comorbidity index.[12–15] The authors are skeptical as to whether these findings have general applicability within this field: the more complicated the surgery, the higher the likelihood of complications, early as well as late. This should also be part of the preoperative information provided to the patient.

## JEJUNAL CONDUIT

The jejunal conduit received a bad reputation because of several reports in the 1970s on 'the jejunal conduit syndrome', characterized by hypochloremia, hyponatremia, and hyperkalemia and by acidosis, caused by the inherent absorptive characteristics of the jejunum. The clinical signs are dehydration and lethargy; treatment is by intravenous sodium chloride, which often has to be followed by oral salt supplementation for some period of time.[16,17] However, a recent report expressed satisfaction with this type of diversion and found a low incidence of electrolyte problems.[18] The authors stressed that a short conduit should be used. A possible indication is when the distal ileum cannot be used, as in radiation enteritis.

## GASTRIC CONDUIT

The gastric conduit can be used in exceptional cases. The good blood supply, relatively poorly absorbing mucosa, and acidification of urine have been considered advantageous.[19] In Lund, we have experience with four patients, three of whom had severely reduced renal function and required diversion. The conduit was created from the gastric antrum using the GIA instrument and we have seen no early or late complications. However, ulcer formation with perforation and subsequent death has been described.[20]

## COLONIC CONDUIT DIVERSION

In 1952, Übelhör described the use of a colonic segment for conduit urinary diversion.[21] Later reports by Mogg in 1967[22] and Morales and Golimbu in 1975[23] confirmed the usefulness of a sigmoid conduit. Today the sigmoid conduit is used mainly for intermediate diversion in children.[24,25] The transverse colonic conduit described by Hohenfellner and Wulff in 1970[26] has been increasingly used in patients with bladder cancer or gynecologic malignancies in whom radiotherapy has been given.[27,28] With its cranial position in the abdominal cavity, the transverse colon is outside the irradiation field used for pelvic malignancies, and the long mesentery enables individual adaptation.

Both the sigmoid and the transverse colon offer the possibility of antirefluxing ureteral implantation, and these segments are less prone to stomal stenosis than the ileum. A direct anastomosis of the conduit to the renal pelvis represents an option in patients with total damage to the ureters by irradiation or retroperitoneal fibrosis, and in patients with recurrent superficial urothelial tumor in a single kidney.[29]

### Sigmoid conduit

A 12–15 cm segment is isolated, respecting the blood supply. Bowel continuity is established using one-layer seromuscular single sutures. The ureters can be implanted directly (Nesbit technique) or via a submucous tunnel using an open end-to-side or 'buttonhole' technique. The conduit is usually placed lateral to the remaining sigmoid colon, probably with less risk of postoperative intra-abdominal complications (Figure 58.4).

### Transverse conduit

A more extensive bowel mobilization including the hepatic and splenic colon flexure is required for this type of diversion. The omentum should be dissected off the transverse colon. Subsequently, the desired segment is isolated. Ureteral implantation is identical to the techniques used for a sigmoid conduit (Figure 58.5). For the direct anastomosis of the renal pelvis to the ureters, the latter are divided at the ureteropelvic junction and the renal pelvis is spatulated longitudinally. The right renal pelvis is anastomosed end-to-end to the aboral end of the conduit, whereas an end-to-side technique is used for the left renal pelvis.

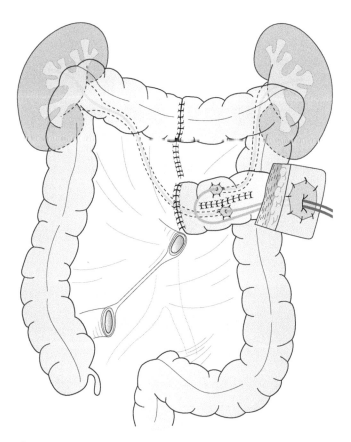

**Fig. 58.5**
Transverse colonic conduit.

## COMPLICATIONS

Long-term follow-up complications of ileal conduit diversion are frequent, the most common being stomal/peristomal problems, parastomal hernia, conduit stenosis, and upper tract deterioration. The incidence of these correlates with length of follow-up.[30]

### STOMAL AND PERISTOMAL COMPLICATIONS

These include erythematous/erosive, pseudoverrucous skin lesions, fungal infections, and stenosis, and retraction of the stoma. The skin lesions are often a consequence of inappropriate construction of the stoma, such as a flush stoma (Figure 58.6). Other causative factors may be allergic reaction to, or poor fit of, appliances and alkaline urine. These complications jeopardize adherence of the plate of the appliance to the skin and thus entail risk of urine leakage. It should be remembered that the stoma is the only part of the diversion that the patient can see and actively take care of. A spout at least 2 cm in length should be fashioned, which will decrease the risk of parastomal complications. The spout should protrude into the appliance bag. The appliance will fit much better and there will be less risk

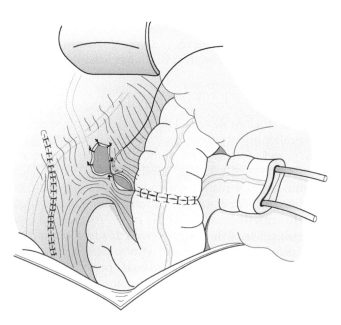

**Fig. 58.4**
Sigmoid conduit.

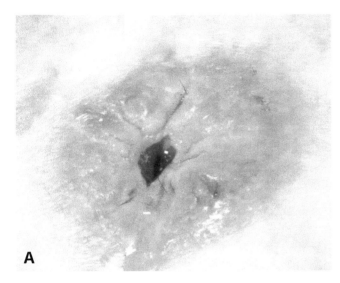

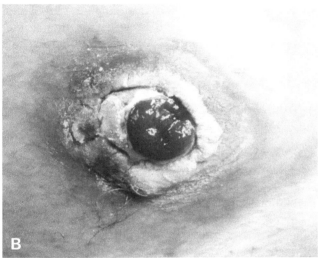

**Fig. 58.6**
**A** Parastomal pseudoverrucous skin lesion. **B** Parastomal Candida infection.

of urine leakage. Studies show that stomal and peristomal problems are common, being reported in up to 30%.[30,31] Such complications may secondarily affect the patient's lifestyle and also cause emotional and psychosocial problems, aspects of urinary diversion that have increasingly attracted interest. The quality of life issue is covered in Chapter 60.

## PARASTOMAL HERNIA

This occurs in 5% to 15% of patients.[30,32] Parastomal hernias are rather large, and although the majority of patients are asymptomatic, some need surgery (Figure 58.7). There is a high recurrence rate requiring reoperation if the repair is done in situ without relocating the stoma.[32] For first-time parastomal hernia repairs, stoma relocation is probably superior to fascial repair.[33] We have seen infections with erosions and

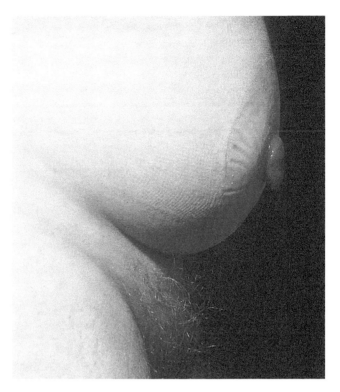

**Fig. 58.7**
Parastomal hernia.

fistulas using synthetic mesh, which usually is employed in recurrent hernia repair. Newer techniques with the incision placed lateral and far away from the stoma, with closure of the fascial defect and using mesh material as an onlay, have been reported to give good results.[34,35]

## CONDUIT STENOSIS

Conduit stenosis seems to be unique to ileal conduits. This condition has never been described in colonic conduits. The whole, or part, of the conduit is transformed into a thick-walled tube without peristaltic activity (Figure 58.8). The pathogenesis of this disorder, which usually manifests late after diversion, is obscure. Chronic inflammation and/or vascular insufficiency have been suggested. The clinical picture is colicky flank pain and/or fever and is produced by upper urinary tract obstruction. Treatment is by removal of the conduit or partial resection, with or without ureteric reimplantation.[36]

## UPPER URINARY TRACT DETERIORATION

Numerous retrospective studies during the 1970s and 1980s revealed a high incidence (13–41%) of renal deterioration associated with a refluxing ileal conduit.[37-40] These figures are not substantially different

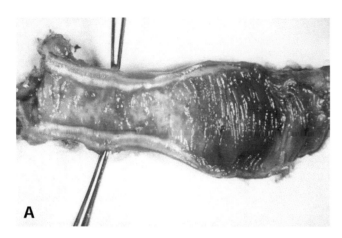

**A**

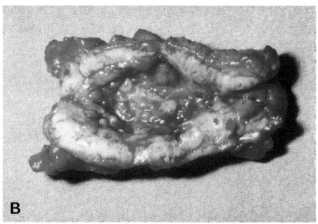

**B**

**Fig. 58.8**
**A** Stenosis of proximal part of ileal conduit. **B** Extensive ileal conduit stenosis.

from recent long-term follow-up reports,[30,32,41] although some study in patients with jejunal conduit gives more favorable results.[18] The generally dismal results provided the background for the recommendation of non-refluxing ureterointestinal anastomosis and a more favorable result was reported in nonrefluxing ileal conduit diversion.[42] It is, however, difficult to evaluate these different studies in relation to each other as they are all retrospective with differences regarding age, follow-up, underlying conditions, and pre- and postoperative techniques and routines.

Another problem relates to the methods of measuring renal function after urinary diversion. Most reports have relied upon serum creatinine and intravenous urography (IVP); however, both are imprecise for this purpose. In a prospective randomized study evaluating type of conduit (ileal versus colonic) and method of ureteric implantation (refluxing versus antirefluxing), total and separate glomerular filtration rate (GFR) was assessed using $^{51}$Cr-EDTA[43] and renal scarring was assessed using renal scintigraphy.[44] No statistically significant differences were found with regard to symptomatic urinary tract infection, number of ureterointestinal anastomotic strictures, and incidence

of GFR deterioration. With a mean follow-up of 10 years, mean GFR fell from 88 to 71 ml/min in ileal conduit patients and from 88 to 65 ml/min in colonic conduit patients. Corresponding figures for patients with continent diversion were 100 and 85 ml/min, respectively.

Scarring was more common in refluxing units than in antirefluxing units, supporting the role of reflux from the conduit in which pressure may be intermittently high.[45]

## FOLLOW-UP OF PATIENTS WITH CONDUIT DIVERSION

Due to the increasing incidence of complications seen with longer follow-up, it is essential that patients with urinary diversion are subjected to indefinite follow-up. This should include regular visits to the stomal therapist. In our opinion, follow-up should include periodic upper tract imaging studies. There are reasons to question the recommendations in the European Association of Urology guidelines,[46] in which follow-up is by ultrasonography and plain film. Ultrasonography can never be a substitute for IVP as obstruction can be present without gross dilation and vice versa. In addition, ultrasonography is user-dependent. In most cases serum creatinine can be used for following the patient's renal function. As tubular damage precedes glomerular damage from postrenal causes, estimation of $\alpha_1$-microglobulin in urine can be a suitable marker for tubular dysfunction.[47] If in doubt about true renal function, there is no substitute for estimation of GFR. Electrolytes should be assessed, particularly when renal function is affected.

## CONCLUSION

Even though several forms of continent urinary tract reconstruction are available today, urinary diversion via a conduit has a firm place in clinical urology. The low rate of surgical complexity, probably accompanied by less risk of complications compared to continent reconstruction, makes this type of diversion the most suitable for the majority of elderly patients undergoing radical cystectomy. Good quality appliances and access to a stoma therapist contribute to high patient acceptance.

## REFERENCES

1. National Bladder Cancer Registry in National Health Care Quality Registries in Sweden 2002, Information Dept. The Federation of Swedish County Councils, Stockholm, 2004, p 25.
2. Gerharz EW, Månsson Å, Hunt S, Månsson W. Is there any evidence that patients with continent reconstruction after radical cystectomy

have better quality of life than conduit patients? In: Dawson C, Muir G (eds): The Evidence for Urology. London: TFM Publishing, 2005.

3. Martinez-Pineiro L, Julve E, Garcia Cardoso JV, Madrid J, de la Pena J, Martinez-Pineiro JA. Review of complications of urinary diversions performed during a 6-year period in the era of orthotopic neobladders. Arch Esp Urol 1997;50:433–445.

4. Yoshimura K, Maekawa S, Ichioka K, Terada N, Matsuta Y, Okubo K, Arai Y. Tubeless cutaneous ureterostomy: the Toyoda method revisited. J Urol 2001;165:785–788.

5. Kearney GP, Docimo SG, Doyle CJ, Mahoney EM. Cutaneous ureterostomy in adults. Urology 1992;40:1–6.

6. Lindstedt E, Månsson W. Transureteroureterostomy with cutaneous ureterostomy for permanent urinary diversion. Scand J Urol Nephrol 1983;17:205–207.

7. Bricker EM. Bladder substitution after pelvic evisceration. Surg Clin North Am 1950;30:1511–1521.

8. Wallace DM. Uretero-ileostomy. Br J Urol 1970;42:529–534.

9. Sundin T, Pettersson S. Open technique for ureteric implantation in ileal conduits. Urol Int 1974;29:369–374.

10. Eiseman B, Bricker EM. Electrolyte absorption following bilateral ureteroenterostomy into an isolated intestinal segment. Ann Surg 1952;136:761–769.

11. Bricker EM, Butcher H, McAfee CA. Late results of bladder substitution with isolated ileal segments. Surg Gynec Obstet 1954;99:469–482.

12. Gburek BM, Lieber MM, Blute ML. Comparison of Studer ileal neobladder and ileal conduit urinary diversion with respect to perioperative outcome and late complications. J Urol 1998;160:721–723.

13. Parekh DJ, Gilbert WB, Koch MO, Smith JA Jr. Continent urinary reconstruction versus ileal conduit: a contemporary single-institution comparison of perioperative morbidity and mortality. Urology 2000;55:852–855.

14. Malavaud B, Vaessen C, Mouzin M, Rischmann P, Sarramon JP, Schulman C. Complications of radical cystectomy. Impact of the American Society of Anesthesiologists score. Eur Urol 2001;39:79–84.

15. Chang SS, Cookson MS, Baumgartner RG, Wells N, Smith JA. Analysis of early complications after radical cystectomy: results of a collaborative care pathway. J Urol 2002;167:2012–2016.

16. Golimbu M, Morales P. Electrolyte disturbances in jejunal urinary diversion. Urology 1973;1:432–438.

17. Månsson W, Lindstedt E. Electrolyte disturbances after jejunal conduit urinary diversion. Scand J Urol Nephrol 1978;12:17–21.

18. Fontaine E, Barthelemy Y, Houlgatte A, Chartier E, Beurton D. Twenty-year experience with jejunal conduits. Urology 1997;50:207–213.

19. Leong CH. Use of stomach for bladder replacement and urinary diversion. Ann R Coll Surg Engl 1978;60:283–289.

20. Tainio H, Kylmala T, Tammela TL. Ulcer perforation in gastric urinary conduit: never use a gastric segment in the urinary tract if there are other options available. Urol Int 2000;64:101–102.

21. Übelhör R. Die Darmblase. Langenbecks Arch Klein Chir 1952;271:202–205.

22. Mogg RA. Urinary diversion using the colonic conduit. Br J Urol 1967;39:687–692.

23. Morales P, Golimbu M. Colonic urinary diversion: 10 years of experience. J Urol 1975;113:302–307.

24. Skinner DG, Gottesmann JE, Ritchie JP. The isolated sigmoid segment: its value in temporary urinary diversion and reconstruction. J Urol 1975;113:614–618.

25. Hendren WH. Exstrophy of the bladder—an alternative method of management. J Urol 1975;115:195–202.

26. Hohenfellner R, Wulff HD. Zur Harnableitung mittels ausgeschalteter Dickdarmsegmente. Akt Urol 1970;1:18–27.

27. Alken P, Jacobi GH, Thüroff J, Walz P, Hohenfellner R. Transversumconduit, Bericht über das 7. Klinische Wochenende der Urologischen Universitätskliniken Mainz, Bern, Berlin-Charlottenburg 1984, pp 157–171.

28. Altwein JE, Hohenfellner R. Use of the colon as a conduit for urinary diversion. Surg Gynecol Obstet 1975;140:33–38.

29. Lindell O, Lethonen T. Rezidivierende urotheliale Tumoren in Einzelnieren mit Anschluss eines Kolonsegments an das Nierenbecken. Akt Urol 1988;19:130–133.

30. Madersbacher S, Schmidt J, Eberele JM, Thoeny HC, Burkhard F, Hochreiter W, Studer UE. Long-term outcome of ileal conduit diversion. J Urol 2003;169:985–990.

31. Nordström GM, Borglund E, Nyman CR. Local status of the urinary stoma—the relation to peristomal skin complications. Scand J Urol Nephrol 1990;24:117–122.

32. Singh G, Wilkinson JM, Thomas DG. Supravesical diversion for incontinence: a long-term follow-up. BJU Int 1997;79:348–353.

33. Rubin MS, Schoetz DJ Jr, Matthews JB. Parastomal hernia. Is stoma relocation superior to fascial repair? Arch Surg 1994;129:413–418.

34. Amin SN, Armitage NC, Abercrombie JF, Scholefield JH. Lateral repair of parastomal hernia. Ann R Coll Surg Engl 2001;83:206–209.

35. Franks ME, Hrebinko RL Jr. Technique of parastomal hernia repair using synthetic mesh. Urology 2001;57:551–553.

36. Magnusson B, Carlen B, Bak-Jensen E, Willen R, Mansson W. Ileal conduit stenosis—an enigma. Scand J Urol Nephrol 1996;30:193–197.

37. Schmidt JD, Hawtrey CE, Flocks RH, Culp DA. Complications, results and problems of ileal conduit diversion. J Urol 1973;109:210–216.

38. Pitts WR, Muecke A. A 20-year experience with ileal conduits: the fate of the kidneys. J Urol 1979;122:154–157.

39. Philip NH, Williams JL, Byers CE. Ileal conduit urinary diversion: long-term follow-up in adults. Br J Urol 1980;52:515–519.

40. Pernet FP, Jonas U. Ileal conduit urinary diversion: early and late results in 132 cases in a 25-year period. World J Urol 1985;3:140–144.

41. Iborra I, Casanova JL, Solsona E, Ricos JV, Monros J, Rubio J, Dumont R. Tolerance of external urinary diversion (Bricker) followed for more than 10 years. Eur Urol 2001;39(Suppl 5):146.

42. Starr A, Rose DH, Cooper JF. Antireflux ureteroileal anastomoses in humans. J Urol 1975;113:170–174.

43. Kristjánsson A, Wallin L, Mansson W. Renal function up to 16 years after conduit (refluxing or anti-reflux anastomosis) or continent urinary diversion 1. Glomerular filtration rate and patency of uretero-intestinal anastomosis. Br J Urol 1995;76:539–545.

44. Kristjánsson A, Bajc M, Wallin L, Willner J, Mansson W. Renal function up to 16 years after conduit (refluxing or anti-reflux anastomosis) or continent urinary diversion. Renal scarring and location of bacteriuria. Br J Urol 1995;76:546–550.

45. Neal DE. Urodynamic investigation of the ileal conduit: upper tract dilatation and the effects of revision of the conduit. J Urol 1989;142:97–100.

46. Oosterlinck W, Lobel B, Jakse G, Malmström P-U, Stockle M, Sternberg C. Guidelines on bladder cancer of the European Association of Urology. Eur Urol 2002;41:105–112.

47. Kristjansson A, Grubb A, Månsson W. Renal tubular dysfunction after urinary diversion. Scand J Urol Nephrol 1995;29:407–412.

# Metabolic aspects of diversion 59

*Robert D Mills, Urs E Studer*

## INTRODUCTION

Bowel segments are used frequently for a variety of forms of urinary tract reconstruction. Despite its versatility, bowel is not an ideal material to be incorporated into the urinary tract. As a result, there are numerous potential complications. Metabolic complications may also be encountered as a result of the structural and functional aspects of the reconstructed urinary tract. In this chapter, under four headings, we will cover the metabolic complications of using bowel in the urinary tract: 1) consequences of bowel loss; 2) consequences of urine contact with bowel; 3) effect on bone metabolism; and 4) effect on renal function.

## CONSEQUENCES OF BOWEL LOSS

The main metabolic effects of bowel resection are malabsorptive. The site of the removal and the length of bowel removed dictate the potential complications. Table 59.1 illustrates sites of absorption of various substances throughout the intestine. After small bowel resection, remaining small bowel is able to compensate to some degree by dilation, elongation, and brush border hypertrophy as well as alterations in membrane fluidity and permeability, and up- or downregulation of carrier-mediated transport.[1,2] Length for length, it is possible to compensate more easily for the loss of proximal than for distal small bowel.[3] Following radiotherapy, bowel may be less able to compensate, and transit time may be shortened, thus increasing the risk of malabsorption.[4] We will discuss each section of the bowel in order.

## GASTRIC RESECTION

Stomach has largely been used in the urinary tract for augmentation in children and young adults. It may be difficult to attain a sufficient reservoir for bladder replacement, but some surgeons have reported success.[5] As stomach has not been widely used in the urinary tract, data for malabsorptive sequelae are scarce. Although useful information can be gained from the general surgical literature, caution must be exercised when applying partial gastrectomy data to urologic practice, as relatively small sections of stomach are harvested for urinary tract reconstruction. For example, secondary osteoporosis and osteomalacia, as well as vitamin D deficiency, have been reported with long-term follow-up after partial gastrectomy.[6-9] An increased incidence of vertebral fracture has also been reported after partial gastrectomy.[10] Whether these problems are likely to be seen with urinary tract reconstruction remains to be seen.

Other potential consequences of removing part of the stomach for use in the urinary tract include vitamin $B_{12}$ deficiency, reduced hydrochloric acid secretion into the gut, hypergastrinemia, hematuria–dysuria syndrome, and hypochloremic, hypokalemic metabolic alkalosis.[5,11,12] The parietal cells of the body and fundus of the stomach produce intrinsic factor, a protein required for vitamin $B_{12}$ absorption. Intrinsic factor forms a complex with vitamin $B_{12}$ that is absorbed in the terminal ileum.[13] Loss of parietal cell mass may interfere with vitamin $B_{12}$ absorption. Parietal cells also produce hydrochloric acid, without which there may be maldigestion of protein and diminished release of calcium and iron from food, with resultant hypocalcemia and iron deficiency anemia. These

**Table 59.1** Sites of absorption of various substances throughout the gastrointestinal tract

|  | Stomach | Duodenum | Jejunum | Ileum | Terminal ileum | Colon |
|---|---|---|---|---|---|---|
| Carbohydrates | X | X | X | X |  |  |
| Protein |  | X | X | X |  |  |
| Lipids |  | X | X | X | (X) |  |
| Calcium |  | (X) | (X) |  |  |  |
| Iron |  | (X) | (X) |  |  |  |
| Water soluble vitamins |  |  | X | X |  |  |
| Fat-soluble vitamins |  |  | X | X |  |  |
| Vitamin B12 |  |  |  | ((X)) | X |  |
| Bile acids |  |  |  | (X) | X |  |
| Sodium, chloride, water |  |  |  | X | X | X |

X, absorption; (X), limited absorption; ((X)), very limited absorption.

problems have not, however, been reported as a result of urologic procedures.

The etiology of hypergastrinemia, hematuria–dysuria syndrome, and hypochloremic, hypokalemic metabolic alkalosis may all be linked. In animal studies, hypergastrinemia has been shown to be a result of resection rather than of contact with urine.[14] Hydrochloric acid production is partly stimulated by gastrin released from G cells in the antrum and duodenum. Normally, hydrochloric acid exerts a local negative feedback on gastrin release. If hydrochloric acid secretion into the stomach is reduced as a consequence of removing part of the body of the stomach for use in the urinary tract, hypergastrinemia may ensue, with continued stimulation of the relocated stomach segment. This may lead to excess acid and pepsinogen secretion into the urinary tract from parietal and chief cells, respectively, with subsequent ulceration in the urinary tract or peristomal skin, namely the hematuria–dysuria syndrome.[3,12] Once urine pH falls below 3.5, pepsin has increased activity and, therefore, ulceration is increasingly likely. Excess excretion of hydrochloric acid into the urinary tract may result in hypochloremic alkalosis. Proton pump inhibitors may be used in an attempt to stabilize urinary pH above 4. This is not always successful, however, and an alternative form of reconstruction may be necessary.[12]

## JEJUNAL RESECTION

The jejunum has no specific absorptive functions that cannot be performed by other parts of the intestine. Therefore, in the presence of a normal intestine, resection of the lengths required for urinary tract reconstruction would not lead to significant malabsorptive sequelae. However, due to the severe electrolyte and acid–base disturbance seen when jejunum is in prolonged contact with urine, jejunum should not be used for continent urinary diversion.

## ILEAL RESECTION

Ileum, together with cecum and ascending colon, has been widely used for urinary tract reconstruction. Two important absorptive functions are compromised by its removal, namely bile acid and vitamin $B_{12}$ absorption, for which the ileum is the sole site.[15,16] The terminal ileum is particularly important and will be discussed together with vitamin $B_{12}$ in the following section.

The length of resected ileum is the key factor determining the degree of absorptive dysfunction. Resection of up to 60 cm of ileum does not normally result in malabsorptive sequelae if the terminal ileum and ileocecal valve are preserved.[17,18] Hyper-triglyceridemia has been reported with resections of this length.[19,20] Whether this has any clinical significance is unclear. In addition, increased stool frequency has been reported with relatively short ileal resections.[21] The possible etiologies for the latter are discussed below. For ileal resections between 60 and 100 cm, serum cholesterol falls with a corresponding rise in triglycerides.[18] Neither the mechanism nor the long-term effect of these alterations in lipid metabolism is clear.

Bile acids are essential for normal fat digestion and absorption, as well as for absorption of fat-soluble vitamins. Normally bile acids pass through the enterohepatic circulation six to eight times daily. This maintains a relatively constant amount, between 2.5 and 5 g, with 300–600 mg excreted in the feces each day. Following ileal resections of up to 100 cm, bile acids are lost into the colon. However, increased hepatic synthesis is usually able to maintain the bile acid pool at a level sufficient to prevent significant fat malabsorption.[22–24] The bile acids lost into the colon may, however, have a cathartic effect, reducing sodium and water absorption, and increasing stool frequency.[17]

Bile acids also directly stimulate adenylate cyclase, leading to active chloride and water secretion and compounding diarrhea.[25] Increased stool concentration of bile acids increases colonic motility, reduces functional rectal capacity, and leads to urgent defecation, further increasing stool frequency.[17,26] Anion-exchange resins may be given to form an insoluble complex with bile salts and prevent diarrhea. They may, however, aggravate hypertriglyceridemia, interfere with absorption of a number of drugs, and exacerbate malabsorption of fat-soluble vitamins.[27] Long-term continuous use should, therefore, be avoided; however, anion-exchange resins may be useful in the short term because the remaining bowel adapts, and intermittent use may be beneficial. Loperamide or other antimotility agents may also be useful.

Theoretically, one could attempt to predict those at increased risk of bowel dysfunction following urinary diversion. Preoperative screening with selenium-75 labeled tauroselcholic acid (SeHCAT) may help identify those patients at risk for diarrhea related to bile acid load.[28] Normal bile acid retention at 1 week is greater than 19%.[29] This technique is expensive and not widely available; however, it might perhaps be considered in those with frequent loose stools preoperatively with a view to offering an alternative form of diversion when SeHCAT retention is below normal.

It should be recognized that side effects, as a result of lengths of resected ileum, are not absolute. Resection of lengths of less than 60 or 100 cm ileum does not exclude the possibility of malabsorptive sequelae in individual cases. Bowel dysfunction has been recognized as a frequent problem following bowel resection for urologic purposes. Durrans and colleagues were the first to report this problem with an increase in stool frequency from a mean of 1.3/day to a mean of 3/day following formation of an ileal conduit.[24] N'Dow et al more recently reported that 11 of 71 (15%) and 4 of 28 (14%) patients reported new bowel symptoms including flatus leakage, fecal urgency, and fecal leakage following ileal conduit formation and bladder reconstruction for non-neuropathic bladder, respectively.[21] Possible mechanisms for these findings include altered bile acid metabolism, reduced transit time, prior radiotherapy, preexisting abnormalities of smooth muscle that may be exacerbated following surgery, or even different levels of expectations of surgery.[21,30,31]

If ileal resection of greater than 100 cm is carried out, then hepatic synthesis will no longer be able to compensate for the bile acid loss, and fat maldigestion will result even in the presence of intact terminal ileum and ileocecal valve.[32] In the presence of normal bowel this problem is not encountered in urologic practice as such long segments are not required. However, following prior resection or radiotherapy this problem may be encountered. The resultant fat malabsorption usually results in moderate steatorrhea (fecal fat >20 g/day). The lipid content of stool has been shown to correlate with the length of resected ileum.[33] Normally less than 7% of ingested fat is present in the stool. Hydroxylated fatty acids presented to the colon also reduce its absorptive capacity, and cause active secretion of water and electrolytes.[34–36] Impaired uptake of essential fat-soluble vitamins (A, D, E, and K) and related deficiency syndromes are associated with fat malabsorption.[37] These problems are unlikely to be seen as a result of urologic reconstructive procedures.

Alterations in bile acid and lipid metabolism as a result of ileal resection may increase the risk of gallstone formation. Up to 35% of patients with loss of ≥100 cm ileum may form gallstones.[38] Data regarding the true incidence following the incorporation of bowel in the urinary tract are scarce. Holmes and colleagues reported an incidence of 18.4% following modified Indiana pouch formation at a mean of 41 months' follow-up.[39] Recently, Pfitzenmaier et al reported cholelithiasis in 9% of patients at a mean of 9 years following a Mainz pouch I procedure.[40] The real risk of cholelithiasis following urinary tract reconstruction is not clear because most patients are not screened, most data are retrospective, and 80% of patients are asymptomatic.[41] The etiology of lithogenic bile following ileal resection is unclear. Cholesterol is the major constituent of most gallstones and normally is kept in solution by mixed micelles of bile salts and phospholipids. A reduction in bile acids due to impaired ileal reabsorption might be expected to increase the likelihood of cholesterol to precipitate. Conversely, bile salt depletion increases hepatic conversion of cholesterol into bile salts, reducing serum low density lipoprotein cholesterol.[42] Furthermore, gallstone analysis following major ileal resection has demonstrated pigment rather than cholesterol as the major constituent.[43]

In contrast, calculi in urinary reservoirs following continent diversion, particularly in cutaneous pouches, are related to the presence of foreign material, mucous production, and bacteriuria.[44] Stones are usually of mixed composition, but analysis in one series revealed struvite stones in all but one of 64 patients with reservoir stones following a Kock pouch.[45]

Increased frequency of renal stones has been reported following urinary diversion.[40] These stones are usually of mixed composition. Reported metabolic alterations that increase the potential for upper tract stones following urinary tract reconstruction with bowel include increased urinary calcium, phosphate, sulfate, and oxalate, and decreased citrate.[46–48] Chronic acidosis leads to hypercalciuria resulting from buffering by carbonate in the bone, leading to calcium release into the circulation.[49–51] In addition, the ability of the renal tubule to reabsorb calcium is reduced in the presence of acidic urine and increased urinary sulfate.[47]

Hyperoxaluria may be seen in association with fat malabsorption following ileal resection. This is due to intraluminal binding of calcium by undigested fats, leaving free oxalate to form more soluble salts that may be reabsorbed in the colon. Normally the colon absorbs little oxalate, as most is precipitated before reaching it. There is a direct correlation between dietary fat malabsorption and urinary oxalate excretion.[52] Oxalate absorption in the colon is facilitated by increased permeability in the presence of fatty and bile acids.[53] As stomach may act as a powerful site for oxalate absorption with prolonged contact, so hyperoxaluria is also a potential risk of gastric reservoirs.[54] Hyper-sulfaturia is seen as a result of increased ammonium absorption.[47] Hypocitruria, a known risk factor for stone disease, is induced by acidosis,[55] and may also be seen as a result of bacterial degradation of urinary citrate.[56]

Pfitzenmaier and colleagues reported a 14% rate of upper tract stone formation at a median of 9 years after a Mainz pouch I procedure.[40] This is higher than the estimated life-long risk of one in eight white males of developing urinary tract stone disease.[57] In their study, however, it seems that the patients who developed upper tract stones were those that had a heterotopic cutaneous diversion rather than an orthotopic reconstruction, indicating that other etiologic factors such as infection, dehydration, and obstruction are likely to be important as well.

Patients should be encouraged to maintain a high fluid intake and avoid oxalate-rich food and beverages. Oral calcium citrate may be given to bind intraluminal oxalate, in order to reduce absorption. A low-fat diet will leave more free calcium to bind oxalate. Urinary infection in orthotopic reservoirs should be treated, and symptomatic infections treated in all. Frequent voiding to completion should be encouraged for all with continent reservoirs.

## TERMINAL ILEAL RESECTION

This region has particular significance for the absorption of vitamin $B_{12}$ and bile acids. Vitamin $B_{12}$ belongs to the family of cobalamins, which contain a nucleotide with a unique base, 5,6-dimethylbenzimidazole, and a corrin nucleus with four reduced pyrrole rings.[58] Cobalamins cannot be synthesized by mammalian tissues and so we rely solely on dietary sources. Vitamin $B_{12}$ digestion begins in the stomach where it is released from ingested food by the action of hydrochloric acid and digestive enzymes. Intrinsic factor from parietal cells binds free vitamin $B_{12}$ in the duodenum, where it has a high affinity at pH 8 in the presence of trypsin. This complex binds to specific receptors in the distal three-fifths of the ileum.[59] There are relatively small numbers of receptors on each cell (300–400, or one for each microvillus) which may explain the limited absorptive capacity for vitamin $B_{12}$ (1–2 μg/day). Binding requires a pH greater than 5.4, as well as calcium and magnesium, but is not energy dependent.[60] Cobalamin is transported in the circulation bound mainly to transcobalamin I. The total body store of cobalamin is 2–5 mg, with the liver as the predominant storage site. There is an obligatory daily loss of 0.1% of body stores regardless of the size of the body pool. Therefore, from a normal starting point, complete depletion in the absence of absorption will take 3–4 years. Partial malabsorption may take up to 30 years to become clinically manifest.[61]

Vitamin $B_{12}$ is required for synthesis of thymidylate, which is subsequently incorporated into DNA. Deficiency, therefore, leads to the typical megaloblastic changes in red cells and other rapidly proliferating cell lines. Vitamin $B_{12}$ is also required as a coenzyme for hydrogen transfer during conversion of methylmalonate to succinate; consequently, it is vital for fat and carbohydrate metabolism. Impaired myelin production is thought to be the cause of the typical neurologic manifestations of vitamin $B_{12}$ deficiency.[25] The neuro-logic sequelae (peripheral neuropathy, optic atrophy, subacute combined degeneration of the spinal cord, and dementia) may occur in isolation and be irreversible.

In a clinical context, resection of 60 cm or more of terminal ileum results in a sharply increased likelihood of vitamin $B_{12}$ malabsorption.[62–64] However, when some terminal ileum is spared, the degree of vitamin $B_{12}$ malabsorption is less than might be expected, suggesting the final few centimeters of ileum are of particular importance.[62] This has some support from radioactive $B_{12}$ uptake studies.[65] Retention of the distal 35–50 cm of terminal ileum has been shown to prevent $B_{12}$ malabsorption and bile acid loss, even in the absence of proximal ileum.[18]

In follow-up studies of the Kock pouch, which utilizes 60–70 cm of ileum, up to 35% of patients require vitamin $B_{12}$ supplementation.[66] Recent follow-up with the Mainz pouch I—which utilizes the ileocecal valve, the distal 24–36 cm of ileum, and only 12 cm of ascending colon—reported that 43% of 94 patients at a median follow-up of 9 years were either on $B_{12}$ supplementation or had a vitamin $B_{12}$ level below normal.[40] In contrast, if the terminal 25 cm of ileum are preserved, then $B_{12}$ deficiency is rare. Studer and Zingg reported only one patient in 200 that required vitamin $B_{12}$ supplementation with follow-up from 12 to 18 years after an ileal afferent limb orthotopic reconstruction in which 54–60 cm of ileum, 25 cm proximal to the ileocecal valve, was used.[67] Racioppi and colleagues reported no vitamin $B_{12}$ deficiency with their ileocecal orthotopic reservoir using only 5–6 cm of terminal ileum in 34 patients with a mean follow-up of 65 months.[68]

All patients should be monitored regularly for vitamin $B_{12}$ deficiency following the use of ileum in continent urinary diversion. If deficiency is confirmed, life-long supplementation with monthly intramuscular injection is required thereafter.

In addition to the specific absorptive functions, the terminal ileum also has an effect on small-bowel transit time, being responsible for the ileal brake mechanism.[69] Patients with ileostomies have been shown to have a significantly faster small-bowel transit time in the absence of the terminal 50–70 cm of terminal ileum, which may further contribute to malabsorption.[70]

## ILEOCECAL VALVE RESECTION

It is difficult functionally to separate the ileocecal valve from the terminal ileum and right colon. However there appear to be two main functions: additional control on small bowel transit time, and limitation of reflux of colonic contents into the terminal ileum.

### ADDITIONAL CONTROL ON SMALL BOWEL TRANSIT TIME

Preservation of the ileocecal valve and right colon following small bowel resection results in significantly less diarrhea and fewer malabsorptive complications.[3,33,35] Experimental data show that the ileocecal valve may increase intestinal transit time from 0.8 to 2.5 hours in humans.[71] Resection of the ileocecal valve in association with either the adjacent ileum or colon may enhance the effect of either resection in isolation.[33,72]

Roth and colleagues found the incidence of diarrhea after ileocecal resection to be twice that after ileal resection alone.[31] With this in mind, ileocecal valve reconstruction has been performed following continent diversion with an ileocecal pouch. Early results have shown some success, with 5 of 11 patients reporting decreased stool frequency after neovalve formation.[73] In a more recent paper from the same group, none of eight patients that had an ileocecal valve reconstruction had stool frequency.[40]

The postoperative intestinal transit time following a Mainz pouch I procedure with ileocecal valve reconstruction has been shown to be equal to that found preoperatively, whereas those without a reconstructed valve have been reported to have a significantly shorter transit time.[74] In contrast, N'Dow and colleagues recently reported no significant difference in new bowel symptoms between patients having an ileal conduit and those having bladder reconstruction using an ileocecal segment.[21] They assessed a number of other symptoms in addition to stool frequency. A prospective study would be interesting because it would provide good baseline bowel function to compare with postoperative outcome.

### LIMITATION OF REFLUX OF COLONIC CONTENTS INTO THE TERMINAL ILEUM

Under normal circumstances the ileal flora resembles the colonic flora qualitatively, but quantitatively the counts are lower by several logarithms. Following loss of the ileocecal valve, colonic organisms may proliferate in the distal small bowel. Species such as Bacteroides are able to cleave bile acids from their conjugates. Free bile acids are poor at emulsifying fats and are absorbed passively, reducing the availability for micellar formation and subsequent fat absorption, resulting in steatorrhea.[75-78] Experimental animal studies have shown vastly reduced anaerobic bacteria counts in the distal small bowel following the use of nipple valve substitutes.[79]

## COLONIC RESECTION

Resection of a considerable length of colon in isolation is possible without detrimental effect on absorption as long as the right colon remains intact. Explanation for this phenomenon comes from radioisotope studies, which demonstrate that the right and transverse colon appear to be sites of storage. Solid residue is retained in the right colon for up to 8 hours, whereas the left and rectosigmoid colon function mainly as conduits.[80] The absorptive role of the colon is mainly in recovery of salt and water. There is a large potential reserve capacity: up to 6 liters of water and 800 mEq of sodium can be absorbed when infused into the cecum over 24 hours.[81] Rapid infusion of smaller volumes produces diarrhea, demonstrating the importance of the ileocecal valve in controlling rate of delivery of ileal contents to the colon. The right colon is of particular importance in patients with ileal resection in whom the severity of diarrhea increases as the length of any associated colonic resection increases.[33,35] Indeed, the severity of diarrhea has been shown to depend more on the length of contiguous colonic resection than ileal resection.[35] It may therefore be best to avoid contiguous colonic and distal ileal resection in the formation of a continent urinary reservoir. The ileocecal valve should be preserved if possible, or consideration given to reconstruction.

## CONSEQUENCES OF URINE CONTACT WITH BOWEL

When considering the complications of urinary contact with bowel, not only are the type and length of segment used and the preoperative health of the patient important, but also the length of time the urine is retained, the concentration of urinary solutes, urinary pH and osmolality. The absorptive properties of the intestinal segment in contact with urine may change with time.[82,83] Histologically, areas of mucosal atrophy and decreased villous height are seen,[84,85] and these changes have been reputed to offer the advantage of reducing absorptive capacity.[86,87] Although most studies report a decreased absorptive capacity, with time others have shown the absorptive capacity for urinary solutes to be unchanged despite mucosal atrophy.[88] Similarly, most studies report a reduced requirement for treatment of acidosis with time following continent urinary diversion with ileum and colon.[89] However, some patients continue to have significant electrolyte problems many years after urinary diversion, indicating that mucosal transport properties are still functioning.[90]

Recent study of ileocystoplasty in dogs has shown a reduction in the number of ileal transporters for ammonium at the brush border after chronic exposure to urine.[83] However, those remaining appeared active, and the effect on the basolateral membrane enzyme activity appeared to be less detrimental. If transporters are so numerous that they are not normally saturated, significant metabolic disturbance may be seen despite a reduction in number. It is clear that histologic changes are not necessarily paralleled by a significant protective effect against reabsorption with urinary reservoirs.

## WATER AND SOLUTE TRANSPORT

The possible abnormalities found with each segment of bowel, when used for a urinary reservoir, are best understood by considering the transport of water and solutes across intestinal epithelium. The lateral borders of epithelial cells are firmly connected to each other by cell junctions. At the luminal surface they form a continuous tight belt around the cell (tight junction). This isolates the intercellular space from the lumen. Paracellular transport is through these tight junctions. The movement of water is dependent on its osmotic gradient and the efficiency of tight junctions at each level of the intestine. The least net water movement occurs with stomach. At the most proximal section of the small gut, jejunum has a relatively loose membrane adapted for rapid equilibration of its contents with body fluids in order that digestive processes may take place. Therefore, large water shifts may be seen with jejunal urinary diversion, particularly when exposure to urine is prolonged. Ileal tight junctions are more efficient than jejunal, and colonic are more efficient than ileal. An osmotic gradient is therefore maintained longer with colon than with ileum, leading to better water preservation. However, if urine remains in contact for prolonged periods, re-equilibration towards iso-osmolarity will occur no matter what type of intestinal segment is used. This will result in water reabsorption or loss depending on the initial concentration of the urine. The final concentration of particular solutes will depend on the type of bowel segment used. This law of equilibration leads to increased night-time urine production, which equals that during the day.[91] Water

may also move transcellularly to maintain intracellular isotonicity, but quantitatively this is of less importance.

Ions and solutes cross epithelia by either active or passive transport: active transport, against a chemical or an electrical gradient, is transcellular and requires energy; passive transport proceeds down an electrochemical gradient, does not consume energy, and may be transcellular or paracellular. The presence of a gradient does not by itself ensure effective movement of a solute or ion as the cell membrane and tight junctions present a barrier to diffusion. Specialized membrane proteins—termed channels, carriers, and pumps—control the movement of ions and solutes across cell membranes. The specific properties of the tight junctions within a segment of the gut will largely determine the relative contribution of paracellular fluxes to overall transport. There is a sodium–potassium energy-dependent exchange on the basolateral membrane ($Na^+$, $K^+$ ATPase) exchanging three intracellular sodium ions for two extracellular potassium ions. This directly affects the movement of ions on the luminal side by altering intracellular solute concentration and is the ultimate source of energy for the active transport of monovalent ions (secondary active transport). Under normal circumstances the intestine is an avid conserver of sodium. In the jejunum there is a $Na^+ \leftrightarrow H^+$ exchange mechanism, whereas in the ileum and colon there is a double exchange mechanism at the luminal border involving both $Na^+ \leftrightarrow H^+$ and $Cl^- \leftrightarrow HCO_3^-$ exchange (antiports).[92,93] They may work in either direction depending on circumstances but, normally, hydrogen is secreted into the lumen in exchange for sodium, whereas bicarbonate is secreted into the lumen in exchange for chloride. Thus, the system is electroneutral.

In the ileum and colon there is also an electrogenic sodium transport system.[94] Sodium enters the epithelial cell down an electrochemical gradient. The $Na^+$, $K^+$ ATPase pump then transports it to the serosal surface. In the ileum, chloride is mainly absorbed passively through the paracellular route down an electrochemical gradient. As the colonic mucosa is tighter, passive ion flux is less than through ileal mucosa. The colonic mucosa has a major conserving function with regard to sodium and chloride, and these ions can be absorbed against large concentration gradients.[95] Under normal circumstances and with equal luminal concentrations of sodium and chloride, the absorption of chloride exceeds that of sodium in both ileum and colon.[93,95,96]

The bulk of potassium movement is thought to be passive. Many solutes such as potassium, ammonia, urea, creatinine, and inulin move along their concentration gradients. The movement of urea, creatinine, and inulin makes measurement of renal function using these solutes inaccurate in patients with intestinal urinary reservoirs, particularly in the absence of continuous drainage. This problem can be overcome using $^{51}Cr$ EDTA that crosses the intestinal mucosa in negligible quantities.[97]

## STOMACH

Although there are potential complications of gastric resection as discussed earlier, the use of stomach does have potential advantages over other bowel segments with regard to urine contact. Gastric mucosa is impermeable to most ions and allows little flux of water. Therefore, as ammonium chloride is not absorbed, hyperchloremic acidosis that may be seen with ileum and colon is avoided.[98] As discussed earlier, there is a tendency to metabolic alkalosis rather than acidosis. Aciduria may have a potential benefit of reducing the incidence of urinary tract infection.[99] This may reduce the long-term risk of carcinogenesis if nitrosamine production is reduced. It has been suggested that a composite reservoir of stomach combined with either ileum or colon may balance out some of the detrimental effects that each segment has individually.[100] This may be of particular interest for patients with preoperative acidosis, short bowel syndrome, diarrhea, or a history of pelvic radiotherapy.

## JEJUNUM

The use of jejunum in urinary diversion leads to hyponatremic, hypochloremic, hyperkalemic metabolic acidosis. The more proximal the segment, the greater the chance of electrolyte disturbance, which is often severe because of the large jejunal surface area (high villi). This condition occurs in response to sodium and chloride secretion and increased reabsorption of potassium and hydrogen ions. In contrast to the kidney, which will preserve salt when serum sodium and chloride fall, a jejunal urinary reservoir will continue to lose large amounts as long as the serum concentrations of sodium and chloride are greater than the urinary levels.[101,102] Jejunal sodium absorption is only able to take place against a weak concentration gradient, and is markedly influenced by water movement, which is linearly related to osmolality.[93] Therefore, with normal serum osmolality (280–295 mOsm/kg), and urine of normal osmolality (>350 mOsm/kg) and sodium concentration (100–250 mmol/24 hour), salt and water will be lost. The decrease in extracellular fluid volume, as well as hyperkalemia, stimulates aldosterone production. This facilitates sodium reabsorption in the distal tubule and collecting duct in exchange for potassium and protons, although excretion of protons is reduced in the presence of hyponatremia and hyperkalemia and so contributes to acidosis. The resulting potassium diuresis with low urinary sodium concentration in the reservoir is favorable for sodium loss in exchange for hydrogen ions

and increased potassium absorption, and perpetuates the abnormality. There is a shift of intracellular potassium in exchange for hydrogen ions as a result of the acidosis.

## ILEUM

Although ileal tight junctions are more secure and ileum is able to actively absorb sodium against a much greater gradient than jejunum, the same pathophysiologic mechanisms seen with jejunum may apply to ileal reservoirs, albeit in a more protracted fashion. Electrolyte disturbances are influenced by the constituents of the urine in the reservoir, which in turn depend on many factors including fluid intake and diet, which may be particularly important during times of illness such as gastroenteritis or other causes of dehydration. In the presence of a dilute urine, seen in the early postoperative period due to low salt intake, particularly when patients are switched from intravenous supplementation to oral intake, a hypovolemic salt-losing state with subsequent acidosis, hypochloremia, and hyperkalemia may be seen (Figure 59.1). Clinically, the metabolic disturbances may result in lethargy, nausea, abdominal pain, vomiting, dehydration, and muscular weakness. These symptoms may develop very soon after catheter removal. Treatment is by catheter drainage of the reservoir and saline infusion in the acute stage. Acidosis may be corrected with sodium bicarbonate, which may also be required in the long term.

Hyperchloremic acidosis may also be seen in patients with ileal reservoirs as sodium chloride absorption by normal ileum may proceed against a strong electrochemical gradient and is less influenced by water movement than in jejunum.[93] Saline test solutions instilled into balloon-isolated ileum equilibrate with an alkaline pH, a high concentration of bicarbonate, and a low chloride concentration. These changes become more pronounced as the ileocecal valve is approached.[103]

Mild metabolic acidosis may be expected in up to 15% to 20% of patients after ileal conduit diversion,[104,105] with persistent acidosis requiring treatment reported in up to 10%.[106] Due to increased urine contact time, the incidence of metabolic complications is greater following continent diversion, with up to 50% of patients reported to have metabolic acidosis after bladder substitution by continent diversion using an ileal segment,[107] and may furthermore depend on renal function. Ileal reservoirs constructed from a 60 cm length have been shown to be associated with a significantly increased incidence of metabolic acidosis compared with the use of 40 cm.[108] This result has to be balanced against the lesser capacity achieved with a shorter length and the resulting increase in early postoperative incontinence.

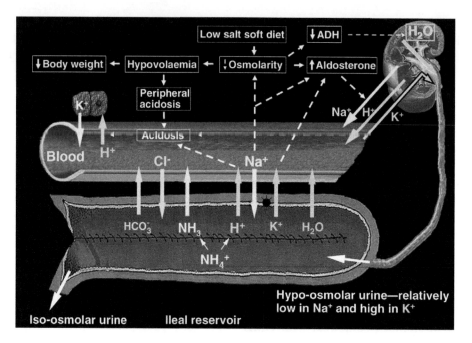

**Fig. 59.1**
Mechanism for hypochloremic acidosis (salt loss syndrome) seen with jejunal and ileal continent urinary reservoirs. (ADH, antidiuretic hormone; Cl⁻, chloride; H⁺, hydrogen; H₂O, water; HCO₃, bicarbonate; K⁺, potassium; Na⁺, sodium; NH₃, ammonia; NH₄⁺, ammonium.) (Based on Figure 1 in Mills RD, Studer UE. Metabolic consequences of continent urinary diversion. J Urol 1999;161:1061.)

## COLON

Colonic tight junctions are more efficient than ileal, thus equilibration is slower and water losses are less than with ileal reservoirs. Indeed, the main absorptive function of the normal colon is water recovery through active sodium and chloride reabsorption. In the normal situation, sodium can be absorbed from iso-osmolar solutions with as little as 25 mmol sodium. Chloride is absorbed even more effectively, and absorption of both ions increases significantly as luminal concentration increases. Normal stool concentrations for sodium and chloride average 40 and 16 mmol/l, respectively. In patients with colonic urinary reservoirs this may lead to serum hyperosmolarity and subsequent decreased aldosterone release with increased antidiuretic hormone release (Figure 59.2). This results in highly concentrated urine from which the colonic mucosa will absorb further sodium and chloride. Following continent urinary reconstruction with a colonic reservoir, acidosis has been reported in all patients, even if only to a mild degree.[109]

## ACIDOSIS

The principal mechanism leading to the production of acidosis is thought to be ammonium reabsorption (Figures 59.1, 59.2). It has been shown that ammonia,

ionized ammonium, and chloride are reabsorbed when ileum or colon is exposed to urine.[110,111] The acid load comes mainly from the reabsorption of ammonium chloride. Quantitatively, hydrogen reabsorption is minimal and bicarbonate secretion is exceeded many times by ammonium reabsorption.[112] Ammonia may diffuse freely across the bowel mucosa, and, as urinary pH increases, absorption will increase. There is evidence, however, that reabsorption of ionized ammonium takes place, and this can be seen at a luminal pH of 5 when non-ionized ammonia is present in only small amounts. Moreover, in brush border membrane vesicle studies, ammonium transport can be demonstrated against an ammonia concentration gradient.[113] If the sodium concentration within a urinary reservoir is increased, ammonium absorption is decreased, one of the reasons why patients with ileal reservoirs must be advised to have an increased salt intake in the first postoperative months. It is thought that ammonium is absorbed principally by substitution for sodium in the sodium–hydrogen antiport,[114] the ammonium ion acting as a competitive inhibitor of sodium uptake. There is also evidence for ionized ammonium absorption through potassium channels,[115] although this is not thought to contribute significantly to acidosis.[113]

The mainstay of management for metabolic acidosis secondary to urinary tract reconstruction is with alkalinizing agents, of which sodium bicarbonate is most widely used. Inhibitors of chloride transport

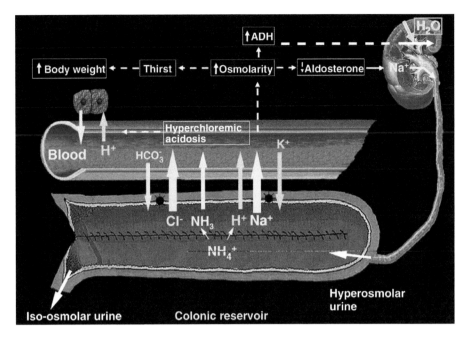

**Fig. 59.2**
Proposed mechanism for hyperchloremic acidosis following colonic continent urinary diversion. If urine is instilled into isolated colon, chloride and sodium are absorbed, pH in reservoir increases, and volume decreases. Although the mechanism is not fully elucidated, absorption of ammonium chloride leads to production of acidosis. (ADH, antidiuretic hormone; Cl⁻, chloride; H⁺, hydrogen; $H_2O$, water; $HCO_3$, bicarbonate; K⁺, potassium; Na⁺, sodium; $NH_3$, ammonia; $NH_4^+$, ammonium.) (Based on Figure 2 in Mills RD, Studer UE. Metabolic consequences of continent urinary diversion. J Urol 1999;161:1061.)

(chlorpromazine or nicotinic acid) may, particularly for patients with small bowel reservoirs, occasionally be used in addition. Oral sodium bicarbonate is effective in restoring normal acid–base status. However, intestinal gas formation can be a problem and the dose required to correct acidosis is unpredictable. Sodium supplements may increase blood pressure or cause fluid retention and pulmonary edema in those at risk. If excessive sodium loads are undesirable, chlorpromazine or nicotinic acid may be used, although they also are not without significant side effects. They act through inhibition of cyclic adenosine monophosphate, thereby impeding chloride transport. They will not correct acidosis alone but will alleviate the situation, allowing a reduced dose of alkalizing agent.[90]

Hypokalemia and total body depletion of potassium may be seen with both ileal and colonic urinary intestinal diversion, although more frequently with colonic, as ileal segments absorb more potassium than colonic.[111] In one study, patients with ureterocolonic diversion were found to have a 30% decrease in total body potassium and those with ileal conduit up to a 14% decrease.[116] Therefore, treatment with potassium citrate may be appropriate, particularly for patients with colonic reservoirs.

Acid–base balance should be monitored regularly in patients with continent diversions, particularly in the early postoperative period. One should have a high index of suspicion if patients become nonspecifically

unwell, and complain about stomach burning or of vomiting following urinary tract reconstruction of any form. Acidosis and electrolyte disturbance should be excluded early. It is important to be aware that normal serum pH and bicarbonate do not exclude a compensated metabolic acidosis, and venous blood gas analysis and body weight measurements are required. For most closely followed patients, with normal renal function, metabolic acidosis is usually mild and relatively easily corrected, although long-term treatment may be required. There are, however, a number of case reports of severe metabolic disturbance, but on reviewing these cases additional problems—such as poor reservoir emptying, a large surface area of bowel in contact with urine, poor renal function, or other illness resulting in dehydration—are usually found.[117]

There are theoretical differences between ileum and colon in terms of the potential metabolic consequences following urinary tract reconstruction with bowel. As discussed, the colon has a more powerful mechanism for the reabsorption of sodium and chloride, and, as a result, there is a greater tendency to hyperchloremic acidosis with colonic than with ileal reservoirs. There is evidence to suggest that inherent chloride absorption from colonic reservoirs is maintained when in contact with urine.[118] The incidence of hyperchloremic acidosis is most prevalent after ureterosigmoidostomy as the urine may come in contact with the whole colonic mucosa.[119,120] Comparative studies of ileal and colonic pouches are perhaps limited, as absorptive surface areas are difficult to calculate. In clinical practice, however, differences have been reported. In the recent publication by Pfitzenmaier and colleagues, 37% of 94 patients with an ileocecal reservoir were taking long-term alkali at a mean of 9 years to prevent metabolic acidosis, although only three patients had a history of significant acidosis.[40] In contrast, 3 months after ileal afferent limb orthotopic bladder substitution, only three of 200 patients required continued oral alkalinization.[67] In one of the few comparative studies from a single institution, Racioppi and colleagues reported a 31% incidence of hypochloremia following ileocecal reservoir and 22% with an ileal reservoir.[121] The difference was not statistically significant although the numbers were small, with just 18 in the ileal group. They did find a statistically significant difference in the incidence of hypokalemia.

Providing the length of bowel harvested is not too long, then other factors such as contact time, renal function, the concentration of solutes in the urine, and voiding frequency and efficiency seem to play a more important part in the metabolic outcome than the type of bowel used. It may be preferable to use ileum rather than colon in patients with renal impairment in order to reduce the risk of metabolic acidosis. Whatever segment of bowel is used, regular voiding or drainage to completion is of great importance. There are also many nonmetabolic factors, such as surgical experience, and therefore preference, comorbidity, and prior radiotherapy need to be considered when choosing an appropriate bowel segment.

## HYPOMAGNESEMIA

Hypomagnesemia may rarely be seen following urinary diversion and may be due to both malabsorption and renal loss as renal tubular reabsorption is reduced in the presence of acidosis. Often hypomagnesemia is found with hypocalcemia as they share many of the same transport processes in the renal tubule. Hypomagnesemia causes symptoms of nausea, vomiting, and fatigue, as well neuromuscular symptoms, such as muscle fasciculation, tremor, tetany, personality change, and seizures.[122]

Venous return from intestinal segments is to the liver, which metabolizes ammonium through the ornithine cycle to urea. Under normal circumstances the increased ammonia load is compensated for by hepatic enzyme induction.[123] In the presence of hepatic insufficiency the liver may not be able to cope with this increased load, and hyperammonemia and hepatic coma may result. Although rare, this syndrome is most commonly seen with ureterosigmoidostomy as intestinal bacteria split urea with urease to produce ammonia. It may also be seen in patients with normal hepatic function in the presence of a urinary tract infection with urea-splitting organisms.[124] It would be expected to occur more often in patients with catheterizable reservoirs, as they are more frequently chronically infected, than in patients with orthotopic bladder substitutes, which usually contain sterile urine.[67] The treatment is to drain the reservoir and treat the infection with antibiotics. Lactulose may be given orally and protein intake restricted until ammonia levels return to normal. Following recovery, a source for infection should be actively sought.

## DRUG TOXICITY

Absorption of drugs from bowel segments in the urinary tract may lead to toxic effects. Those drugs secreted unchanged in the urine and absorbed by the intestinal tract are most likely to lead to problems. Of particular interest are chemotherapeutic agents used in the treatment of bladder cancer. Methotrexate toxicity in patients with ileal conduits is well recognized.[125,126] Patients with continent diversion receiving chemotherapy should be monitored closely, be well hydrated, and have their reservoir drained during treatment. Other drugs that have been reported to be absorbed from intestinal segments in the urinary tract are phenytoin, theophylline, and antibiotics.[97,127,128] Diabetics appear to have an enhanced ability to absorb glucose from intestinal reservoirs. Screening with urine tests may therefore be inaccurate, and surveillance of known diabetics should rely on blood tests.[129] It is also interesting and important to remember that false-positive pregnancy tests may occur in patients with enterocystoplasties.[130]

## EFFECT ON BONE METABOLISM

The risk of abnormal bone mineralization and metabolism following urinary tract reconstruction has been recognized ever since the reports of children with rickets and adults with osteomalacia following ureterosigmoidostomy.[131-135] Chronic acidosis is likely to be the main factor affecting bone metabolism, although there may also be reduced intestinal absorption of calcium and vitamin D following ileal resection.

Chronic acidosis may affect bone metabolism in a number of ways. Bone minerals, including calcium, carbonate, and sodium, may act as buffers in exchange for hydrogen ions, thus decreasing the skeletal calcium content.[136-138] Acidosis impairs $\alpha_1$-hydroxylation of 25-hydroxycholecalciferol in the kidney. This reduction in activated vitamin D level results in bone mineralization defects.[139] Acidosis also activates osteoclasts and results in bone resorption.[140] Patients with preexisting renal disease will be more prone to acidosis; they may also have impaired activated vitamin D production secondary to tubular cell damage and so are at particular risk. Campanello and colleagues have reported a significant correlation between glomerular filtration rate and change in bone mineral density measurements taken 3 years apart.[141]

The changes in acid–base balance may be very subtle, and experiments in animals with urinary diversion have shown that oral supplementation with bicarbonate can prevent demineralization in the absence of significant systemic acidosis.[138] Oral intake of sodium bicarbonate has therefore been recommended when the base excess falls below –2.5 mmol/l.[40]

Patients with bone demineralization may be asymptomatic, complain of pain in weight-bearing joints, or present with fractures. Laboratory tests may be normal despite symptoms,[137] although there may be reduced serum calcium and phosphate with an elevated alkaline phosphatase.[134] Parathormone levels are usually not raised and serum levels of activated vitamin D may be normal. Radiologic appearances are usually normal also. Bone densitometry is useful but may not detect subtle changes without repeat testing. Bone biopsy may be the only way to confirm the diagnosis. Analysis of urinary markers of bone turnover such as collagen type I crosslinked N-telopeptide has not been widely reported in this group of patients.[142]

Long-term follow-up of myelomeningocele patients with intestine in the urinary tract has shown a greater number of fractures and higher intervention rate for spinal curvature with increased incidence of non-union and delayed healing than in a control group managed with intermittent catheterization.[143] Chronic acidosis is likely to have the greatest impact on young adults who may be exposed for a longer period of time and also on children in whom bone growth may be reduced.[144] Reduction in growth potential was reported following both ileocystoplasty and colocystoplasty[145,146] in two studies of enterocystoplasty that were small and retrospective. In a more recent, larger (242 patients), prospective study of enterocystoplasty in children with longer follow-up (mean 8.3 years), loss of preoperative percentile position on the growth curve was thought unlikely to be related to surgery.[147] This perhaps emphasizes that close follow-up and early treatment with oral bicarbonate may reduce bone complications as a result of urinary reconstructive procedures.

In adult urologic practice, many investigators have found that effects on bone metabolism do not seem to be a clinically relevant problem up to 10 years after continent reconstruction[40,148–151]; however, others have reported a decrease in bone mineral density in association with metabolic acidosis following orthotopic reconstruction.[142,152–154] Urinary diversion with the ileal Kock reservoir has been reported to reduce

bone mineral density of the spine and total skeleton in comparison to normal aged-matched controls.[155]

Patients with osteomalacia should have their acid–base abnormalities corrected first. This alone may relieve symptoms and lead to remineralization.[134,156,157] If remineralization does not occur, further treatment should be given with activated vitamin D and calcium supplements,[133] although this does not guarantee resolution.[158]

In summary, chronic acidosis may cause bone demineralization with subsequent pain and increased fracture risk. The length of exposure and the severity of acidosis are important. For most adult patients with normal renal function followed closely after surgery, significant bone sequelae can be avoided following ileal or colonic continent reservoir formation.

## EFFECT ON RENAL FUNCTION

Long-term safety of the upper tracts is an essential requirement for successful lower urinary tract reconstruction. There are many potential reasons for deterioration in renal function, including transmission of high bladder pressure to the upper urinary tract (reflux or functional obstruction), stone formation, infection, and physical obstruction at any site (ureteroileal being the most common). The pathologic changes seen with varying etiologies are the same, and thus the cause at the time of detection may not be obvious. In addition to an age-related decline, there may be many nonurologic causes for declining renal function, with hypertension, diabetes, and drugs being frequently implicated.

A number of retrospective studies have reported renal functional/morphologic deterioration ranging from 13% to 41% after ileal conduit diversion.[159–161]

Following continent cutaneous diversion, Kristjansson and colleagues reported a decrease in renal function in 28% of patients 11 years after cecal reservoir formation.[162] Akerlund and colleagues at a mean of 6.6 years after creation of a Kock pouch reported upper tract dilation in five of 17 patients (29%), which was associated with scarring in two.[66] Only one (6%) patient had an abnormal creatinine at the last follow-up, but four had a low age-adjusted glomerular filtration rate (GFR), three of whom had a low GFR preoperatively. Jonsson and colleagues recently reported follow-up of 126 patients up to 25 years after Kock pouch.[163] They found a significant reduction in glomerular filtration from 6 years onwards, but this was of a magnitude expected with ageing. Renal function was not affected by the diversion as long as obstruction was recognized and managed.

There are few long-term reports of renal function following orthotopic reconstruction. In addition, reported methods of measuring renal function usually rely on serum creatinine or radiologic studies, both of which have limitations. Serum creatinine begins to rise only after a significant reduction in glomerular filtration, and the presence of upper tract dilation does not necessarily equate to a reduction in renal function. Many studies are also retrospective with incomplete preoperative data. Measurement of pre and postoperative renal function using radioisotope studies would provide the best information on upper tract safety.

Thoeny and colleagues recently reported a prospective analysis of renal morphology and function in 76 patients with a median follow-up of 84 months (range 60–155 months) after a low-pressure ileal afferent limb bladder substitute.[164] Serum creatinine and excretory intravenous pyelogram were performed preoperatively and at regular intervals postoperatively. Of 148 ureterorenal units, 141 (95%) showed no significant change in size or parenchymal thickness. In six (4%), renal size and parenchymal thickness decreased, and, in one, parenchymal thickness alone was reduced. However, the majority (five) of these ureterorenal units had preoperative renal pathology such as dilation, obstruction, or scarring. Loss of parenchyma from kidneys that were normal preoperatively was seen in only two ureterorenal units (1%), associated with ureteroileal stenosis. In this prospective study, renal deterioration was seen only in the presence of preexisting renal pathology or postoperative obstruction. Renal deterioration following an ileal afferent limb bladder substitute with a simple end-to-side, freely refluxing ureteroileal anastomosis is minimal at 10 years' follow-up. It seems widely accepted now that the potential benefit of 'conventional' antireflux procedures in combination with orthotopic reconstruction is outweighed by the higher complication and associated reoperation rate.[165] Close follow-up is required in order to identify correctable causes early, in particular ureteroileal stenosis. Those with preexisting renal pathology prior to surgery seem to be at greatest risk of postoperative renal deterioration.

## CONCLUSION

Bowel is not the ideal material for urinary tract reconstruction. Unfortunately, despite advances in biotechnology, the use of bowel will be widespread for the foreseeable future. All patients that have had bowel transposed into the urinary tract require life-long follow-up by healthcare workers with a genuine understanding of the potential complications. As long as patients are selected judiciously, then malabsorptive sequelae should not often be problematic. Low-grade acidosis is almost uniform in patients that have a urinary reservoir created from bowel. If, however, these patients are followed closely and managed appropriately, significant absorptive complications should be rare.

## ACKNOWLEDGMENT

Figures 59.1 and 59.2 are based on those from our review in the *Journal of Urology* (1999;161:1057–1066). The text for this chapter, although extensively revised and updated, has also been adapted from that review article.

## REFERENCES

1. Mackenzie GW, Boileau MD, St Clair WR. Short-gut syndrome: a review with a case report. Can J Surg 1973;16:3–11.
2. Thiesen A, Drozdowski L, Iordache C, et al. Adaptation following intestinal resection: mechanisms and signals. Best Pract Res Clin Gastroenterol 2003;17:981–995.
3. Cosnes J, Gendre JP, Le Quintrec Y. Role of the ileocecal valve and sites of intestinal resection in malabsorption after extensive small bowel resection. Digestion 1978;18:359–366.
4. Berthrong JB, Fajardo LF. Radiation injury in surgical pathology. Part II. Am J Surg Pathol 1981;5:153–178.
5. Hauri D. Can gastric pouch as orthotopic bladder replacement be used in adults? J Urol 1996;156:931–935.
6. Riggs BL, Melton LJ. Involutional osteoporosis. N Engl J Med 1986;26:1676–1685.
7. Hoikka V, Alhava EM, Savolainen K, Karjalainen P, Parviainen M. The effect of partial gastrectomy on bone mineral metabolism. Scand J Gastroenterol 1982;17:257–261.
8. Morgan DB, Paterson CR, Woods CG, Pulvertaft CN, Fourmau P. Osteomalacia after gastrectomy: a response to very small doses of vitamin D. Lancet 1965;ii:1089–1091.
9. Eddy RL. Metabolic bone disease after gastrectomy. Am J Med 1971;50:442–449.
10. Mellstrom D, Johansson C, Johnell O, et al. Osteoporosis, metabolic aberrations, and increased risk for vertebral fractures after partial gastrectomy. Calcif Tissue Int 1993;53:370–377.
11. Nguyen DH, Bain MA, Salmonson KL, Ganesan GS, Burns MW, Mitchell ME. The syndrome of dysuria and hematuria in pediatric urinary tract reconstruction with stomach. J Urol 1993;150:707–709.
12. Leonard MP, Dharamsi N, Williot PE. Outcome of gastrocystoplasty in tertiary pediatric urology practice. J Urol 2000;164:947–950.
13. Hagedorn CH, Alpers DH. Distribution of intrinsic factor-vitamin B12 receptors in human intestine. Gastroenterology 1977;73:1019–1022.
14. Ortiz V, Goldenberg S. Hypergastrinemia following gastrocystoplasty in rats. Urol Res 1995;23:361–363.
15. Borgstrom B, Lundh G, Hofmann A. The site of absorption of conjugated bile salts in man. Gastroenterology 1963;45:229–238.
16. Weiner IM, Lack L. Absorption of bile salts from the small intestine in vivo. Am J Physiol 1962;202:155–157.
17. Alpers D, Wessler S, Avioli LV. Ileal resection and bile salt metabolism. JAMA 1971;215:101–104.
18. Miettinen TA. Relationship between fecal bile acids, absorption of fat and vitamin B12 and serum lipids in patients with ileal resections. Eur J Clin Invest 1971;1:452–460.
19. Weise ES, Fleischmann A, Studer UE. Persistent hypertriglyceridaemia in patients after construction of a low pressure ileal orthotopic reservoir. J Urol 1997;Abstract 932:238.
20. Salomon L, Lugagne PM, Herve JM, Barre P, Lebret T, Botto H. No evidence of metabolic disorders 10 to 22 years after Camey type I ileal enterocystoplasty. J Urol 1997;157:2104–2106.

21. N'Dow J, Leung HY, Marshall C, Neal DE. Bowel dysfunction after bladder reconstruction. J Urol 1998;159:1470–1474.

22. Aldini R, Roda A, Festi D. Bile acid malabsorption and bile acid diarrhea in intestinal resection. Dig Dis Sci 1982;27:495–502.

23. Cummings JH, James WP, Wiggins HS. Role of the colon in ileal-resection diarrhea. Lancet 1973;1:344–347.

24. Durrans D, Wujanto R, Carroll RN, Torrance HB. Bile acid malabsorption: a complication of conduit surgery. Br J Urol 1989;64:485–488.

25. Steiner MS, Morton RA. Nutritional and gastrointestinal complications of the use of bowel segments in the lower urinary tract. Urol Clin North Am 1991;18:743–754.

26. Edwards CA, Brown S, Baxter AJ, Bannister JJ, Read NW. Effect of bile acid on anorectal function in man. Gut 1989;30:383–386.

27. Vroonhof K, van Rijn HJ, van Hattum J. Vitamin K deficiency and bleeding after long-term use of cholestyramine. Neth J Med 2003;61:19–21.

28. Olofsson G, Fjalling M, Kilander A, Ung KA, Jonsson O. Bile acid malabsorption after continent urinary diversion with an ileal reservoir J Urol 1998;160:724–727.

29. Nyhlin H, Merrick MV, Eastwood MA, Brydon WG. Evaluation of ileal function using 23-selena-25-homotaurocholate, a gamma labeled conjugated bile acid. Gastroenterology 1983;84:63–68.

30. Barrington JW, Fern-Davies H, Adams RJ, Evans WD, Woodcock JP. Bile acid dysfunction after clam enterocystoplasty. Br J Urol 1993;76:169–171.

31. Roth S, Semjonow A, Waldner M, Hertle L. Risk of bowel dysfunction with diarrhea after continent urinary diversion with ileal and ileocecal segments. J Urol 1995;154:1696–1699.

32. Hofmann AF. Bile acid malabsorption caused by ileal resection. Arch Intern Med 1972;130:597–605.

33. Mitchell JE, Breuer RI, Zuckermann L, Berlin J, Schilli R, Dunn JK. The colon influences ileal resection diarrhea. Digest Dis Sci 1980;25:33–41.

34. Aldini R, Roda A, Festi D, et al. Bile acid malabsorption and bile acid diarrhea in intestinal resection. Dig Dis Sci 1982;27:495–502.

35. Cummings JH, James WP, Wiggins HS. Role of the colon in ileal-resection diarrhea. Lancet 1973;1:344–347.

36. Mekjian HS, Phillips SF, Hofmann AF. Colonic secretion of water and electrolytes induced by bile acids: perfusion studies in man. J Clin Invest 1971;50:1569–1577.

37. Bertoni JM, Abraham FA, Falls HF, Itabashi HH. Small bowel resection with vitamin E deficiency and progressive spinocerebellar syndrome. Neurology 1984;34:1046–1052.

38. Andersson H, Bosaeus I, Fasth S, Hellberg R, Hulten L. Cholelithiasis and urolithiasis in Crohn's disease. Scand J Urol 1987;22:253–256.

39. Holmes DG, Park GY, Thrasher JB, Kueker D, Weigel JW. Incidence of cholelithiasis in 125 continent urinary diversions. J Urol 2001;165:1897–1899.

40. Pfitzenmaier J, Lotz J, Faldum A, Beringer M, Stein R, Thuroff JW. Metabolic evaluation of 94 patients 5 to 16 years after ileocecal pouch (Mainz pouch I) continent urinary diversion. J Urol 2003;170:1884–1887.

41. Hill GL, Mair WS, Goligher JC. Gallstones after ileostomy and ileal resection. Gut 1975;16:932–936.

42. Kern F. Consequences of intestinal resection. N Engl J Med 1969;281:440–441.

43. Pitt HA, Lewinski MA, Muller EL. Ileal resection-induced gallstones: altered bilirubin or cholesterol metabolism? Surgery 1984;96:154–162.

44. Arai Y, Kawakita M, Terachi T, et al. Long-term follow-up of the Kock and Indiana pouch procedures. J Urol 1993;150:51–55.

45. Ginsberg D, Huffman JL, Lieskovsky G, Boyd S, Skinner DG. Urinary tract stones: a complication of the Kock pouch continent urinary diversion. J Urol 1991;145:956–959.

46. Terai A, Arai Y, Kawakita M, Okada Y, Yoshida O. Effect of urinary intestinal diversion on urinary risk factors for urolithiasis. J Urol 1995;153:37–41.

47. McDougal WS, Koch MO. Effect of sulphate on calcium and magnesium homeostasis following urinary diversion. Kid Int 1989;35:105–115.

48. Dobbins JW, Binder HJ. Importance of the colon in enteric hyperoxaluria. N Engl J Med 1977;296:298–301.

49. Lemann J, Litzow JR, Lennon EJ. The effects of chronic acid loads in normal man. Further evidence for participation of bone mineral in the defense against chronic metabolic acidosis. J Clin Invest 1966;45:1608–1614.

50. Lemann J, Litzow JR, Lennon EJ. Studies of the mechanism by which chronic metabolic acidosis augments urinary calcium excretion in man. J Clin Invest 1967;46:1318–1328.

51. Drettler SP. The pathogenesis of urinary tract calculi occurring after ileal conduit diversion: I. Clinical study. II. Conduit study. III. Prevention. J Urol 1973;109:204–209.

52. Earnest DL, Johnson G, Williams HE, Admirand WH. Hyperoxaluria in patients with ileal resection: an abnormality in dietary oxalate absorption. Gastroenterology 1974;66(6):1114–1122.

53. Adibi SA, Stanko RT. Perspectives on gastrointestinal surgery for the treatment of morbid obesity: the lesson learned. Gastroenterology 1984;87:1381–1391.

54. Hautmann R. The stomach. A new and powerful oxalate absorption site in man. J Urol 1993;149:1401–1404.

55. Assimos DG. Editorial: Nephrolithiasis in patients with urinary diversion. J Urol 1996;155:69–70.

56. Graef V, Schmidtmann H, Jarrarr K. On the preservation of urines for the determination of citrate. In Schwille PO (ed): Urolithiasis and Related Clinical Research. New York: Plenum Press, 1985, pp 689–692.

57. Menon M, Parulkar BG, Drach GW. In Walsh PC, Retik AB, Vaughn ED, Wein AJ (eds): Campbell's Urology, 7th ed. Philadelphia: WB Saunders, 1998, Chapter 91.

58. Selub SE. Water, electrolyte and vitamin transport. In Haubrich WS, Schaffner F, Berk JE (eds): Gastroenterology. Philadelphia: WB Saunders, 1991, pp 947–950.

59. Hagedorn CH, Alpers DH. Distribution of intrinsic factor-vitamin B12 receptors in human intestine. Gastroenterology 1977;73:1019–1022.

60. MacKenzie IL, Donaldson RM. Effect of divalent cations and pH on intrinsic factor mediated attachment of vitamin B12 to intestinal microvillus membranes. J Clin Invest 1972;51:2465–2471.

61. Herbert VD, Colman N. Folic acid and vitamin B12. In: Shils ME, Young VR (eds): Modern Nutrition in Health and Disease. Philadelphia: Lea & Febiger, 1988, pp 388–416.

62. Thompson WG, Wrathell E. The relation between ileal resection and vitamin B12 absorption. Can J Surg 1977;20:461–464.

63. Fromm H, Thomas PJ, Hofmann AF. Sensitivity and specificity in tests of distal ileal function: prospective comparison of bile acid and vitamin B12 absorption in ileal resection patients. Gastroenterology 1973;64:1077–1090.

64. Filipsson S, Hulten L, Lindstedt G. Malabsorption of fat and vitamin B12 before and after intestinal resection for Crohn's disease. Scand J Gastroenterol 1978;13:529–536.

65. Booth CC, Mollin DL. Site of absorption of vitamin B12 in man. Lancet 1959;1:18–21.

66. Akerlund S, Delin K, Kock NG, Lycke G, Philipson BM, Volkmann R. Renal function and upper urinary tract configuration following urinary diversion to a continent ileal reservoir (Kock pouch): a prospective 5 to 11 year follow-up after reservoir construction. J Urol 1989;142:964–968.

67. Studer UE, Zingg EJ. Ileal orthotopic bladder substitutes. What we have learned from 12 years experience with 200 patients. Urol Clin North Am 1997;24(4):781–793.

68. Racioppi M, D'Addessi A, Fanasca A, et al. Vitamin B12 and folic acid plasma levels after ileocecal and ileal neobladder reconstruction. Urology 1997;50(6):888–892.

69. Spiller RC, Trotman IF, Adrian TE, Bloom SR, Misiewicz JJ, Silk DB. Further characterization of the 'ileal brake' reflex in man—effect of ileal infusion of partial digests of fat, protein and starch on jejunal motility and release of neurotensin, enteroglucagon and peptide YY. Gut 1988;29:1042–1051.

70. Neal DE, Williams NS, Barker MCJ, King RFGJ. The effect of resection of the distal ileum on gastric emptying, small bowel transit and absorption after proctocolectomy. Br J Surg 1984;71:666–670.

71. Mojaverian P, Chan K, Desai A, John V. Gastrointestinal transit of solid indigestible capsule as measured by radiotelemetry and dual gamma scintigraphy. Pharm Res 1989;6:719–724.

72. Gazet JC. The surgical significance of the ileo-caecal junction. Ann R Coll Surg Engl 1968;43:19–38.

73. Fisch M, Wammack R, Spies F, et al. Ileocecal valve reconstruction during continent urinary diversion. J Urol 1994;151:861–865.

74. Stein R, Fisch M, Beetz Y, et al. Urinary diversion in children and young adults using the Mainz Pouch I technique. Br J Urol 1997;79:354–361.

75. Donaldson RM. Malabsorption of CO 60-labeled cyanocobalamin in rats with intestinal diverticula. Evaluation of the possible mechanisms. Gastroenterology 1962;43:271–281.

76. Kim YS, Spring H, Bloom H, Terz G, Sherlop P. The role of altered bile acid metabolism in steatorrhea of experimental blind loop. J Clin Invest 1966;45:956–962.

77. Panish JF. Experimental blind loop steatorrhea. Gastroenterology 1963;45:394–399.

78. Tilson MD. Pathophysiology and treatment of short bowel syndrome. Surg Clin North Am 1980;60(5):1273–1284.

79. Myrvold H, Tindel MS, Isenberg HD, Stein TA, Scherer J, Wise L. The nipple valve as a sphincter substitute for the ileocecal valve: prevention of bacterial overgrowth in the small bowel. Surgery 1984;96:42–47.

80. Proano M, Camilleri M, Phillips SF, Brown ML, Thomforde GM. Transit of solids through the human colon: regional quantification in the unprepared bowel. Am J Physiol 1990;258:G856–G862.

81. Debongnie JC, Phillips SF. Capacity of the human colon to absorb fluid. Gastroenterology 1978;74:698–703.

82. Filipas D, Fisch M, Abol Enein H, Fichtner J, Bocckisch A, Hohenfellner R. Chloride absorption in patients with a continent ileocecal reservoir (Mainz pouch I). Br J Urol 1997;79:588–591.

83. Grocela JA, McDougal WS. Ammonium transport in the intestine chronically exposed to urine: is it reduced over time? Urology 1999;54:373–376.

84. Deane AM, Woodhouse CRJ, Parkinson MC. Histological changes in ileal conduits. J Urol 1984;132:1108–1111.

85. Kojima Y, Asaka H, Ando Y, Takanashi R, Kohri K. Mucosal morphological changes in the ileal neobladder. Br J Urol 1998;82:114–117.

86. Akerlund S, Jagenburg R, Kock NG, Philipson BM. Absorption of L phenylalanine in human ileal reservoirs exposed to urine. Urol Res 1988;16:321–323.

87. Akerlund S, Forssell-Aronsson E, Jonsson O, Kock NG. Decreased absorption of $^{22}$Na and $^{36}$Cl in ileal reservoirs after exposure to urine. An experimental study in patients with continent ileal reservoirs for urinary or fecal diversion. Urol Res 1991;19:249–252.

88. Hall MC, Kock MO, Halter SA, Dahlstedt SM. Morphological and functional alterations of intestinal segments following urinary diversion. J Urol 1993;149:664–666.

89. Thuroff JW, Alken P, Riedmiller H, Jacobi GH, Hohenfellner R. 100 cases of Mainz pouch: continuing experience and evolution. J Urol 1988;140:283–288.

90. McDougal WS. Metabolic complications of urinary diversion. J Urol 1992;147:1199–1208.

91. Studer UE, Gerber E, Springer J, Zingg EJ. Bladder reconstruction with bowel after radical cystectomy. World J Urol 1992;10:11–19.

92. Turnberg LA, Biederdorf FA, Morawski SG, Fordtran JS. Interrelationships of chloride, bicarbonate, sodium and hydrogen transport in the human ileum. J Clin Invest 1970;49:557–567.

93. Fordtran JS, Rector FC, Carter NW. The mechanism of sodium absorption in the human small intestine. J Clin Invest 1968;47:884–900.

94. Grady GF, Duhamel RC, Moore EW. Active transport of sodium by human colon in vitro. Gastroenterology 1970;59:583–588.

95. Devroede GJ, Phillips SF. Conservation of sodium, chloride and water by the human colon. Gastroenterology 1969;56:101–109.

96. Parsons FM, Powell FJN, Pyrah LN. Chemical imbalance following ureterocolic anastomosis. Lancet 1952;2:599–602.

97. Davidsson T, Akerlund S, White T, Olaisson G, Mansson W. Mucosal permeability of ileal and colonic reservoirs for urine. Br J Urol 1996;78:64–68.

98. Adams MC, Mitchell ME, Rink RC. Gastrocystoplasty: an alternative solution to the problem of urological reconstruction in the severely compromised patients. J Urol 1988;140:1152–1156.

99. Nguyen DH, Mitchell ME. Gastric bladder reconstruction. Urol Clin North Am 1991;18:649–657.

100. Austin PF, DeLeary G, Homsy YL, Persky L, Lockhart JL. Long-term metabolic advantages of a gastrointestinal composite urinary reservoir. J Urol 1997;158:1704–1708.

101. Golimbu M, Morales P. Electrolyte disturbances in jejunal urinary diversion. Urology 1973;1:432–438.

102. Mansson W, Lindstedt E. Electrolyte disturbances after jejunal conduit urinary diversion. Scand J Urol Nephrol 1978;12:17–21.

103. Bucher GR, Flynn JC, Robinson CS. The action of the human small intestine in altering the composition of physiologic saline. J Biol Chem 1944;155:305–313.

104. Bowels WT, Tail BA. Urinary diversion in children. J Urol 1967;98:597–605.

105. Allen TD, Roehrborn CG, Peters PC. Long-term follow-up of patients after cystectomy and urinary diversion via ileal loop (IL) versus ureterosigmoidostomy (US). J Urol 1989;141:350A.

106. Schmidt JD, Hawtrey CE, Flocks RH, Culp DA. Complications, results and problems of ileal conduit diversions. J Urol 1973;109:210–216.

107. Poulsen AL, Steven K. Acid–base metabolism following bladder substitution with the ileal urethral Kock reservoir. Br J Urol 1996;78:47–53.

108. Studer UE, Springer J, Casanova GA, Gurtner F, Zingg EJ. Correlation between the length of ileum used for a bladder substitute and metabolic acidosis, functional capacity and urinary incontinence. J Urol 1991;145:423(abstract 318).

109. Kock MO, McDougal WS, Reddy PK, Lange PH. Metabolic alterations following continent urinary diversion through colonic segments. J Urol 1991;145:270–273.

110. Koch MO, McDougal WS, Thompson CO. Mechanisms of solute transport following urinary diversion through intestinal segments: an experimental study with rats. J Urol 1991;146:1390–1394.

111. Koch MO, Gurevitch E, Hill DE, McDougal WS. Urinary solute transport by intestinal segments: a comparative study of ileum and colon in rats. J Urol 1990;143:1275–1279.

112. Davidsson T. Urinary diversion by intestinal segments [thesis]. Lund, Sweden: Lund University, 1995, pp 19–22.

113. McDougal, Stampfer DS, Kirley S, Bennett PM, Lin CW. Intestinal ammonium transport by ammonium and hydrogen exchange. J Am Coll Surg 1995;181:241–248.

114. Stampfer DS, Mc Dougal WS. Inhibition of the sodium/hydrogen antiport by ammonium ion. J Urol 1997;157:362–365.

115. McDougal WS, Stampfer DS, Kirley S, Bennett PM, Lin CW. Intestinal ammonium transport by ammonium hydrogen exchange. J Am Coll Surg 1995;181:241–248.

116. Williams RE, Davenport TJ, Burkinshaw L, Hughes D. Changes in whole body potassium associated with uretero-intestinal anastomosis. Br J Urol 1967;39:676–680.

117. Dunn SR, Farnsworth TA, Karunaratne WU. Hypokalaemic, hyperchloraemic metabolic acidosis requiring ventilation. Anaesthesia 1999;54:564–574.

118. Davidsson T, Akerlund S, Forssell-Aronsson E, Kock NG, Mansson W. Absorption of sodium and chloride in continent reservoirs for urine: comparison of ileal and colonic reservoirs. J Urol 1994;151:335–337.

119. Ferris DO, Odel HM. Electrolyte pattern of the blood after bilateral ureterosigmoidostomy. JAMA 1950;142:634–640.

120. Caprilli R, Frieri G, Latella G, Gallucci M, Bracci U. Electrolyte and acid base imbalance in patients with rectosigmoid bladder. J Urol 1986;135:148–150.

121. Racioppi M, D'Addessi A, Fanasca A, et al. Acid–base and electrolyte balance in urinary intestinal orthotopic reservoir: ileocecal neobladder compared with ileal neobladder. Urol 1999;54:629–635.

122. Fagan C, Phelan D. Severe convulsant hypomagnesaemia and short bowel syndrome. Anaesth Intensive Care 2001;29:281–283.

123. Koch MO, McDougal WS. The pathophysiology of hyperchloremic metabolic acidosis after urinary diversion through intestinal segments. Surgery 1985;98:561–570.

124. Gabra HO, Fenton PA, Bonham JR, Mackinnon AE. Hyperammonemia with complex urinary tract anomaly: a case report. J Pediatr Surg 2003;38:E16–E17.

125. Fossa SD, Heilo A, Bormer O. Unexpectedly high serum methotrexate levels in cystectomized bladder cancer patients with an ileal conduit treated with intermediate doses of the drug. J Urol 1990;143:498–501.

126. Bowyer GW, Davies TW. Methotrexate toxicity associated with an ileal conduit. Br J Urol 1987;60:592–596.

127. Savarirayan F, Dixey GM. Syncope following ureterosigmoidostomy. J Urol 1969;101:844–845.

128. Ekman I, Mansson W, Nyberg L. Absorption of drugs from continent cecal reservoir for urine. Br J Urol 1989;64:412–416.

129. Sridhar KN, Samuell CT, Woodhouse CRJ. Absorption of glucose from urinary conduits in diabetics and non-diabetics. Br Med J 1983;287:1327–1329.

130. Nethercliffe J, Trewick A, Samuell C, Leaver R, Woodhouse CR. False-positive pregnancy tests in patients with enterocystoplasties. BJU Int 2001;87:780–782.

131. Boyd JD. Chronic acidosis secondary to ureteral transplantation. Am J Dis Child 1931;42:366–371.

132. Specht EE. Rickets following ureterosigmoidostomy and chronic hypochloremia. J Bone Joint Surg 1969;49:1422–1430.

133. Perry W, Allen LN, Stamp TC, Walker PG. Vitamin D resistance in osteomalacia after ureterosigmoidostomy. N Engl J Med 1977;297:1110–1112.

134. Siklos P, Davie M, Jung RT, Chalmers TM. Osetomalacia in ureterosigmoidostomy: healing by correction of the acidosis. Br J Urol 1980;52:61–62.

135. Leite CA, Frame B, Frost HM, Arnstein AR. Osteomalacia following ureterosigmoidostomy. Clin Orthop 1966;49:103–108.

136. Bettice JA, Gamble JL. Skeletal buffering of acute metabolic acidosis. Am J Physiol 1975;229:1618–1623.

137. Bushinsky DA, Krieger NS, Geisser DI, Grossman EB, Coe FL. Effects of pH on bone calcium and proton fluxes in vitro. Am J Physiol 1983;245:F204.

138. McDougal WS, Koch MO, Shands C, Price RR. Bony demineralization following urinary intestinal diversion. J Urol 1988;140:853–855.

139. Lee SW, Russell J, Avioli LV. 25-hydroxycholecalciferol to 1,25-dihydroxycholecalciferol: conversion impaired by systemic metabolic acidosis. Science 1977;195:994–996.

140. Arnett TR, Dempster DW. Effect of pH on bone resorption by rat osteoclasts in vitro. Endocrinology 1986;119:119–124.

141. Campanello M, Herlitz H, Lindstedt G, et al. Determinants of bone loss in patients with Kock ileal urinary reservoir. Scand J Urol Nephrol 1999;33:312–317.

142. Fujisawa M, Nakamura I, Yamanaka N, et al. Changes in calcium metabolism and bone demineralization after orthotopic intestinal neobladder creation. J Urol 2000;163:1108–1111.

143. Koch MO, McDougal WS, Hall MC, Hill DE, Braren HV, Donofrio MN. Long-term metabolic effects of urinary diversion: a comparison of myelomeningocele patients managed by clean intermittent catheterization and urinary diversion. J Urol 1992;147:1343–1347.

144. Hafez AT, Elsherbiny MT, Dawaba MS, Abol-Enein H, Ghoneim MA. Long-term outcome analysis of low-pressure rectal reservoirs in 33 children with bladder exstrophy. J Urol 2001;165:2414–2417.

145. Wagstaff KE, Woodhouse CRJ, Rose GA, Duffy PG, Ransley PG. Blood and urine analysis in patients with intestinal bladders. Br J Urol 1991;68:311–316.

146. Mundy AR, Nurse DE. Calcium balance, growth and skeletal mineralization in patients with cystoplasties. Br J Urol 1992;69:257–259.

147. Gerharz EW, Preece M, Duffy PG, Ransley PG, Leaver R, Woodhouse CRJ. Enterocystoplasty in childhood: a second look at the effect on growth. BJU Int 2003;91:79–83.

148. Tschopp ABS, Lippuner K, Jaeger P, Merz VW, Danuser H, Studer UE. No evidence of osteopenia 5 to 8 years after ileal orthotopic bladder substitution. J Urol 1996;155:71–75.

149. Campanello M, Herlitz H, Lindstedt G, et al. Bone mineral and related biochemical variables in patients with Kock ileal reservoir or Bricker conduit for urinary diversion. J Urol 1996;155:1209–1213.

150. Davidsson T, Lindergard B, Obrant K, Mansson W. Long-term metabolic effects of urinary diversion on skeletal bone: histomorphometric and mineralogic analysis. Urology 1995;46:328–333.

151. Stein R, Fisch M, Andreas J, Bockisch A, Hohenfellner R, Thuroff JW. Whole body potassium and bone mineral density up to 30 years after urinary diversion. Br J Urol 1998;82:798–803.

152. Kawakita M, Arai Y, Shigeno C, et al. Bone demineralization following urinary intestinal diversion assessed by urinary pyrinidium cross-links and dual energy x-ray absorptiometry. J Urol 1996;156:355–359.

153. Giannini S, Nobile M, Sartori L, et al. Bone density and skeletal metabolism in patients with orthotopic ileal neobladder. J Am Soc Nephrol 1997;8:1553–1559.

154. Sevin G, Kosar A, Perk H, Serel TA, Gurbuz G. Bone mineral content and related biochemical variables in patients with ileal bladder substitution and colonic Indiana pouch. Eur Urol 2002;41:655–659.

155. Poulsen AL, Overgaard C, Christiansen C, Thode J, Steven K. Bone mineral status following urinary diversion with the ileal Kock reservoir. Scand J Urol Nephrol 1992;142(Suppl):136.

156. Hossain M. The osteomalacia syndrome after colocystoplasty. A cure with sodium bicarbonate alone. Br J Urol 1970;42:243–245.

157. Bailey RR. Chronic acidosis with metabolic bone disease. N Z Med J 1985;98:483–484.

158. Salahudeen AK, Elliott RW, Ellis HA. Osteomalacia due to ileal replacement of ureters: report of 2 cases. J Urol 1983;131:335–337.

159. Madersbacher S, Schmidt J, Eberele JM, Thoeny H, Burkhard F, Hochreiter W, Studer UE. Long term outcome of ileal conduit diversion. J Urol 2003;169:985–990.

160. Schmidt JD, Hawtrey CE, Flocks RH, Culp DA. Complications, results and problems of ileal conduit diversion. J Urol 1973;109:210–216.

161. Pitts WR Jr, Muecke EC. A 20 year experience with ileal conduits: the fate of the kidneys. J Urol 1979;122:154–157.

162. Kristjansson A, Wallin L, Mansson W. Renal function up to 16 years after conduit (refluxing or antireflux anastomosis) or continent urinary diversion. 1. Glomerular filtration rate and patency of uretero-intestinal anastomosis. Br J Urol 1995;76:539–545.

163. Jonsson O, Olofsson G, Lindholm E, Tornqvist H. Long-time experience with the Kock ileal reservoir for continent urinary diversion. Eur Urol 2001;40:632–640.

164. Thoeny HC, Sonnenschein MJ, Madersbacher S, Vock, P, Studer UE. Is ileal orthotopic bladder substitution with an afferent tubular segment detrimental to the upper urinary tract in the long term? J Urol 2002;168:2030–2034.

165. Hautmann RE. Urinary diversion: ileal conduit to neobladder. J Urol 2003;169:834–842.

# Psychosocial and quality-of-life issues

60

*Åsa Månsson, Eila C Skinner*

## INTRODUCTION

### THE CONCEPT AND THE PROBLEM

Over the last two decades, increasing attention has been focused on the psychosocial problems and needs of patients undergoing treatment for cancer. It is now understood and accepted that cancer management implies efforts not only to cure or control the malignancy, but also to help the patient cope with social, psychological, and sexual issues. Intensive clinical research has led to the current awareness regarding psychological and social consequences of cancer. Furthermore, quality of life (QoL) is now a well-established concept in clinical medicine and is increasingly used in the evaluation of new surgical and medical methods.

A major problem for all researchers in this field is the lack of a universally accepted definition of 'quality of life'. The meaning of the term can differ between cultures, countries, and study groups, and it often covers a wide array of human experiences, ranging from daily living, relationships with partners or family members and friends, to general activities and personal happiness. The concept is far from new. As early as 1958, the American social psychologist Marie Jahoda stated that provision of the conditions necessary for good mental health will also enhance 'quality of living' for the individual. However, definitions of QoL have varied within the realm of medicine. According to Cella and Cherin, QoL refers to 'patients' appraisal of and satisfaction with their current level of functioning compared to what they perceived to be possible or ideal'.[1] By comparison, Lewis offered the following definition: 'the degree to which one has self-esteem, a purpose in life, and minimal anxiety'.[2] Aaronson considered QoL in a health-related framework and called it 'a multidimensional construct composed minimally of...functional status, disease-related and treatment-related symptoms, psychological functioning and social functioning'.[3] The World Health Organization has explained QoL as the way that individuals perceive their position in life in the context of their own culture and system of values and in relation to their goals, expectations, standards, and concerns.[4] This definition implies that QoL is intricately affected by people's physical health, mental state, level of independence, social relationships, and personal beliefs, as well as their associations with salient features of their environment.

QoL is obviously a hypothetical construct, and it is doubtful whether introduction of the term 'health-related quality of life' (HRQoL) has made it easier to decide what should be included or excluded, since it is probably difficult to distinguish between components that are and are not associated with health.[5] QoL may be existential in nature, which, of course, would make it very difficult to measure. Indeed, probably to the disappointment of many clinicians, it must be recognized that QoL seems to have little to do with health status. A possible danger in not accepting that assumption, is that patients physically affected by diseases or 'older' surgical procedures will be considered to have a lower QoL than patients that have undergone a more 'modern' type of reconstruction, or individuals that are looked upon as average or 'normal'. Such reasoning could lead to serious ethical consequences in the way that we perceive the disabled. It has even been suggested that measuring QoL is counterproductive, and that it would be better to employ a more easily understood assessment of common features of the observed health status.[6] Nevertheless, it is important to study health-related aspects of malignant disorders and the different methods of treating such conditions, although greater caution should be used when applying the term QoL.

The conceptual vagueness of QoL is clearly reflected by the host of measurement modalities that are now in use: open-ended, face-to-face interviews, telephone interviews, proxy rating, and self-reporting, along with a countless number of questionnaires. In most cases QoL/HRQoL is evaluated by use of questionnaires. These tools can be divided into two main categories:

- psychometrically-based instruments that provide a 'profile' of different dimensions (psychometrics is the science of assessing the measurement characteristics of scales)
- other types of instruments based on a utility or preference measure.

These have arisen from the discipline of health economics, and have so far been used very little to assess QoL in patients with urologic disorders.

Most investigators involved in the early research on QoL employed ad hoc instruments without proper psychometric evaluation, and, unfortunately, this is a practice still all too common. Members of the urologic community have adopted the concept of QoL in a rather uncritical manner, and many enthusiastic urologists lack the necessary knowledge in epidemiology, psychology, and social medicine. A recent survey of studies of QoL in patients that had undergone radical cystectomy for bladder cancer showed that half of the publications were written solely by urologists.[7]

## REQUISITE FEATURES OF QOL INSTRUMENTS

It is now understood that clinical and laboratory measures alone are inadequate for evaluating the results of a particular medical or surgical treatment. Hence, they must be complemented by patient-based outcome measures. However, assessments of QoL cannot be conducted according to whim or convenience, but must instead be guided by strict criteria that should be considered very carefully in the choice of a suitable instrument for evaluating patient-based outcome measures.[8] Homemade, ad hoc tools should be banned. The properties for which an instrument should be evaluated include reliability, validity, and responsiveness.

### Reliability

Reliability is a measure of the extent to which an instrument is devoid when measuring errors or, in other words, the degree to which the same results are obtained in repeated measurements of the same subjects. This is checked by studying the same individuals in test–retest situations, including the same individuals under the same conditions at different points in time.

Another form of reliability is internal consistency. This feature is an expression of the homogeneity of the instrument in question, measured using Cronbach's coefficient alpha, which represents the degree of interaction between items within a single scale. A Cronbach's alpha above 0.85 indicates that a scale is internally consistent, although a lower limit of 0.70 is often accepted.

### Validity

Validity indicates how well an instrument actually measures what it is supposed to measure. Two criteria have to be met: content validity, which assesses the adequacy of the defining and sampling of a domain, and construct validity, which is more complex and involves testing both the underlying theory and the method used.

### Responsiveness

Responsiveness (also called sensitivity) is related to the ability of an instrument to detect true changes that occur over time and requires correlation with other methods.

Obviously, appropriate background knowledge and much time and effort are required to perform scientifically sound research on QoL. Comprehensive studies of the problems that are involved in measuring QoL have been described recently by Staquet and colleagues and Bowling.[9,10]

## INSTRUMENTS

Psychometrically-based instruments can be classified as generic, domain-specific, generally cancer-specific, and specific to a certain type of cancer. Some of the most widely used instruments are listed in Box 60.1.

An example of patient-preference measurement, i.e. the attempt to weigh the dimensions of health and to obtain a global index or utility score of health status, is the concept of quality-adjusted life year (QUALY), in which the underlying assumption is that, offered a choice, an individual will prefer a life that is shorter but offers a satisfactory health status to a life that is longer but entails severe handicap or discomfort. Of the different utility measures that are available today, time trade-off is used most often, although that strategy has been severely criticized. Thus, patients with a chronic condition often adapt and adjust their lives to the disease. Further, the model has not been adequately tested for validity and reliability.[5,10]

An alternative to allowing patients themselves to fill in questionnaires is to conduct qualitative research,

1. Generic instruments
   - SF-36 (Short Form 36)
   - SIP (Sickness Impact Profile)
   - NHP (Nottingham Health Profile)
   - EQ (EuroQol)
2. Domain-specific instruments, such as those focused on mental issues
   - HADS (Hospital Anxiety and Depression Scale)
   - POMS (Profile of Moods States)
   - PAIS (Psychosocial Adjustment to Illness Scale)
   - BDI (Beck Depression Inventory)
   - BSI (Brief Symptom Inventory)
3. Cancer-specific instruments
   - QLQ-C30 (EORTC Quality of Life Core Questionnaire)
   - FLIC (Functional Living Index for Cancer)
   - FACT-G (Functional Assessment of Cancer Therapy—General)
   - CARES-SF (Cancer Rehabilitation Evaluation System—Short Form)
4. Bladder cancer-specific instruments
   - QLQ-BLS-24 (EORTC module for superficial bladder cancer)
   - QLQ-BLM-30 (EORTC module for muscle-invasive bladder cancer)
   - FACT-Bl (Functional Assessment of Cancer Therapy—Bladder Cancer)
5. Cystectomy for bladder cancer-specific instrument
   - FACT-VCI (Functional Assessment of Cancer Therapy—Vanderbilt Cystectomy Index)

usually in the form of in-depth interviews followed by step-by-step analysis of the collected data.[11] Such studies have the drawback of being costly and time consuming, but they offer the advantages of providing a better understanding and knowledge about the experiences of individual patients and how they perceive different phenomena.

## FURTHER CONSIDERATIONS

Even well-established and tested questionnaires, such as those mentioned above, measure diverse aspects of the experiences of a patient. Some of these instruments (e.g. SF-36 and QLQ-C30, see Box 60.1) assess several distinct factors that are assumed to be associated with QoL, including physical limitations, mental distress, social interaction, and symptoms. A serious problem is that each of these components can be viewed differently by different people. Also, when subscales are used, the outcome can be negative for one item but positive for another. Since there is no model that can predict how these different items contribute to QoL, it may be difficult to draw reliable conclusions.

Instruments may also vary in the care with which they have been developed in terms of reliability and validity, and for the rationale underlying their claim to measure QoL. Several studies have shown that patients adapt to almost any circumstances after reassessing their life situation. Because values associated with life and various activities can change, timing is crucial when studying a

'before and after' situation or comparing different groups. For example, Kulaksizoglu and coworkers studied patients that had undergone radical cystectomies for bladder cancer, and noted that psychological and health-related QoL measurements had stabilized 12 months after the procedure.[12]

It is equally important to consider the surroundings in which subjects fill in a questionnaire. Standardization is essential, and results will not be comparable if patients in one group complete the questionnaire in the hospital and those in another answer it at home, possibly in the presence of (and influenced by) members of their family. Similarly, if a pretreatment questionnaire is completed in the hospital and a post-treatment questionnaire is sent by mail, it may be difficult to compare the collected data. Other problems in this context are missing data and low response rates. Far too many studies have response rates of less than 80%, which could seriously impair the validity of the results.[13]

Proponents for evidence-based medicine have also pointed out the importance of including a neutral third party to assess outcome.[13] So far, questionnaires employed to study QoL in bladder cancer patients have been administered and evaluated by doctors and/or institutions providing the treatment, and it is certainly possible that such an approach can introduce bias.[14]

## QUALITY-OF-LIFE STUDIES IN CYSTECTOMY PATIENTS

A number of studies have now been completed in patients undergoing a radical cystectomy. The majority of these have been undertaken in patients that are at least 1 year out from surgery, and many have been limited to patients that are free from disease recurrence. The conclusion of these studies is that patients that have recovered from a radical cystectomy have a generally high quality of life, not significantly different from that of people of similar age in the general population.[15–17] Severe emotional and physical problems appear to be rare, and general emotional well-being is high.[18] The primary negative effect of a cystectomy has been on sexual function and, in some studies, on social function and autonomy.[19,20] However, in spite of the magnitude of the surgery and the degree of change in the function of a major organ, patients that recover from surgery and are cured appear to be able to live a full and happy life.

It has been much more problematic to use the available validated QoL instruments to try to understand the impact of the different types of urinary diversion on patients' quality of life. There is a general assumption by many of us that a continent diversion provides better QoL than an ileal conduit, and that the best results will be obtained with a neobladder replacement. This fits with the general notion that most patients faced with a cystectomy tend to prefer the idea of a 'natural' bladder replacement that makes them feel as close to normal as possible. However, it has been very difficult to document such an advantage in patients that have undergone these surgeries. This may in part be due to the fact that there is basically good overall QoL among ileal conduit patients, so an incremental improvement will be hard to measure. In addition, the types of diversion are not randomly assigned, and individuals tend to adapt well to the type of diversion they receive. Finally, the instruments simply may be insensitive to subtle differences.

There have now been a number of studies comparing various types of diversion using standardized questionnaires.[14,16–18,20–23] Most of these have been single-institution studies that include relatively small numbers of patients—most less than 50 patients per group, and some as few as 20. Many have serious methodologic problems, as noted earlier. For example, often the ileal conduit patients are older, have more comorbidities, and have had their surgery longer ago than the patients with continent diversion. Age and gender are especially important variables that influence QoL, but they are not always considered. All studies contain very few women by virtue of the nature of the disease, which is much more common in men. Socioeconomic and racial or ethnic differences have not been addressed in any of these small studies.

We published one of the larger studies in 1999.[20] We sent a battery of four comprehensive questionnaires to 287 men and 81 women that were at least 1 year out from surgery. Approximately 61% of patients returned the questionnaires, a fairly typical participation rate for such studies. We used both standardized questionnaires (for depression, overall quality of life, and sexual function) and some others that were adapted to try to capture issues related to side effects of the urinary diversion. There were 25 patients with ileal conduits, 93 with cutaneous continent diversion, and 103 with Kock neobladders (almost all of the latter were men, since we were not doing neobladders in women at that time). Once we controlled for age and gender differences in the three groups, we were not able to demonstrate any convincing differences in QoL based on the type of diversion performed. When the problems of urinary diversion were grouped in subscales (e.g. including an item related to urinary leakage with one related to difficulty catheterizing, without any judgment about which might be worse), the differences between the groups disappeared.

A study by Gerharz and colleagues in Germany evaluated questionnaires from 192 patients (130 with ileal conduits and 62 with continent cutaneous diversion). Their patient groups were well matched in age and social and educational background. They did find a significant advantage for continent diversion in several domains of QoL, including global overall quality of life.[22] Hobisch and colleagues found an improved QoL in orthotopic neobladder patients,[16] and Dutta and colleagues found an advantage in patients with a similar reconstruction, but their study illustrates the difficulties in carrying out such research. There were only 23 conduit patients and 49 neobladder patients in the study. The conduit patients were older (64 versus 74 years) and more likely to have recurrent disease (20% versus 2%). Although the investigators tried statistically to control for such differences, the conclusion that the neobladder patients scored better in a number of domains of QoL could certainly have been biased by these important differences in the groups.[21]

It has been even more difficult to sort out any difference between patients with continent cutaneous diversion and those with continent orthotopic diversion to the urethra. These patients tend to be similar in age and in time since surgery. However, the currently available instruments are almost certainly not sensitive enough to detect differences between these groups. Månsson and colleagues completed a study using the FACT-Bl and the HADS instruments (see Box 60.1) in 80 patients, and could not demonstrate a clear difference between the two groups.[24] It is not surprising that differences in QoL associated with diversion type are difficult to demonstrate, since no diversion is completely without problems (and in fact, native bladders cause significant problems in patients in this age group). For example, one patient may have anxiety about difficulty catheterizing the pouch, while another has concern about urethral leakage. Similar problems have different impacts on different patients as well. It is likely to be equally difficult to try to assess, for example, the outcomes of cystectomy versus bladder salvage procedures. Such studies will require large groups of similar patients and use of new instruments that capture all of the potential problems that affect patients undergoing these treatments.[25]

Better instruments will allow us to study patients in more detail, and perhaps to advise patients more wisely in the future. Today it appears that the most honest approach is to offer the cystectomy patient the options that are medically reasonable, while trying to avoid any value judgment that one is clearly superior to the other in terms of quality of life. A clear understanding by the patient of the pros and cons of each type of diversion is probably most important to their ultimate satisfaction with the result.

## CONCLUSION

QoL research is a difficult and demanding field. Therefore, it is of concern that most studies have been retrospective and have had serious flaws with regard to patient selection, soundness of the instrument used, and the response rate. This finding clearly undermines QoL as a scientific concept in urology. In the future we need to move away from simply documenting the impact of our treatments toward identifying predictors of psychological and emotional distress, and testing ways in which we can intervene to minimize that distress.

## REFERENCES

1. Cella DF, Cherin EA. Quality of life during and after cancer treatment. Compr Ther 1988;14:69–75.

2. Lewis FM. Experienced personal control and quality of life in late-stage cancer patients. Nurs Res 1982;31:113–119.

3. Aaronson NK. Quality of life: what is it? How should it be measured? Oncology (Huntington) 1988;2:69–76.

4. World Health Organization. QOL. Measuring quality of life. Geneva: WHO, 1997 (MSA/MNH/PSF/97.4).

5. Hunt SM. The problem of quality of life. Qual Life Res 1997;6:205–212.

6. Smith KW, Avis NE, Assman SF. Distinguishing between quality of life and health status in quality of life research: a meta-analysis. Qual Life Res 1999;8:447–459.

7. Gerharz EW, Månsson Å, Hunt S, Månsson W. Is there any evidence that patients with continent reconstruction after radical cystectomy have better quality of life than conduit patients? In Dawson C, Muir G (eds): The Evidence for Urology. London: TFM Publishing, 2005.

8. Fitzpatrick R, Davey C, Buxton MJ, Jones DR. Evaluating patient-based outcome measures for use in clinical trials. Health Technol Assess 1998;2:1–74.

9. Staquet MJ, Hays RD, Fayers PM. Quality of Life Assessment in Clinical Trials, Methods and Practice. Oxford: Oxford University Press, 1999.

10. Bowling A. Measuring Health. A Review of Quality of Life Measurement Scales, 2nd ed. Buckingham: Open University Press, 2001.

11. Burnard P. A method of analysing interview transcripts in qualitative research. Nurse Educ Today 1991;11:461–466.

12. Kulaksizoglu H, Toktas G, Kulaksizoglu IB, Aglamis E, Unluer E. When should quality of life be measured after radical cystectomy? Eur Urol 2002;42:350–355.

13. McCulloch P, Taylor I, Sasako M, Lovett B, Griffin D. Randomised trials in surgery: problems and possible solutions. BMJ 2002;342:1448–1451.

14. Månsson Å, Henningsohn L, Steineck G, Månsson W. Neutral third party versus treating institution for evaluating quality of life after radical cystectomy. Eur Urol 2004;46(2):195–199.

15. Boyd SD, Feinberg SM, Skinner DG, Lieskovsky G, Baron D, Richardson J. Quality of life survey of urinary diversion patients: comparison of ileal conduits versus continent Kock ileal reservoirs. J Urol 1987;138:1380–1389.

16. Hobisch A, Tosun K, Kinzl J, et al. Life after cystectomy and orthotopic neobladder versus ileal conduit urinary diversion. Semin Urol Oncol 2001;19:18–23.

17. Hardt J, Filipas D, Hohenfellner R, Egle UT. Quality of life with bladder carcinoma after cystectomy: first results of a prospective study. Quality of Life Res 2000;9:1–12.

18. Henningsohn L, Steven K, Kallestrup EB, Steineck G. Distressful symptoms and well-being after radical cystectomy and orthotopic bladder substitution compared with a matched control population. J Urol 2002;168:168–174.

19. Matsuda T, Aptel I, Exbrayat C, Grosclaude P. Determinants of quality of life of bladder cancer survivors five years after treatment in France. Int J Urol 2003;10:423–429.

20. Hart S, Skinner EC, Meyerowitz, BE, Boyd S, Lieskovsky G, Skinner DG. Quality of life after radical cystectomy for bladder cancer in patients with an ileal conduit or cutaneous or urethral Kock pouch. J Urol 1999;162:77–81.

21. Dutta SC, Chang SS, Coffey CS, Smith JA Jr, Gregory J, Cookson MS. Health related quality of life assessment after radical cystectomy: comparison of ileal conduit with continent orthotopic neobladder. J Urol 2002;168:164–167.

22. Gerharz EW, Weingartner K, Dopatka T, Kohl UN, Basler H-D, Riedmiller HN. Quality of life and urinary diversion: results of a retrospective interdisciplinary study. J Urol 1997;158:778–785.

23. Hara I, Miyake H, Hara S, et al. Health-related quality of life after radical cystectomy for bladder cancer: a comparison of ileal conduit and orthotopic bladder replacement. BJU Int 2002;89:10–13.

24. Månsson Å, Davidsson T, Hunt S, Månsson W. The quality of life in men after radical cystectomy with a continent cutaneous diversion or orthotopic bladder substitution: is there a difference? BJU Int 2002;90:386–390.

25. Cookson MS, Dutta SC, Chang SS, Clark T, Smith JA Jr, Wells N. Health related quality of life in patients treated with radical cystectomy and urinary diversion for urothelial carcinoma of the bladder: development and validation of a new disease-specific questionnaire. J Urol 2003;170:1926–1930.

# Treatment of regionally advanced and metastatic bladder cancer

# Tissue engineering of the bladder 61

Gilad E Amiel, Anthony Atala, Donald P Griffith

## INTRODUCTION

Individuals are exposed to a variety of disorders in the genitourinary system that may require reconstruction: maldevelopment may occur during fetal life, and trauma, malignancy, infection, and iatrogenic injuries may result in loss or damage to tissue that may require reconstruction. However, because native tissue in the genitourinary system is limited, current modalities of reconstruction necessitate recruiting nonurologic tissue such as skin, buccal mucosa, small or large bowel, or stomach as replacement for the lost or damaged tissue. The use of gastrointestinal segments is widespread in genitourinary reconstruction due to lack of alternatives. Nonetheless, occurrence of adverse effects such as metabolic abnormalities, infection, perforation, urolithiasis, increased mucus production, and malignancy, are well documented.[1] These complications are especially pronounced in patients undergoing radical cystectomy and bladder substitution or diversion because of the relatively large segments of bowel that are needed. The use of bowel as replacement for urothelial-lined tissue was first proposed over 100 years ago, and, despite all the potential complications involved, it is still the gold standard for the replacement of urothelial tissue, whether ureter or bladder.

An artificial bladder was proposed as a viable replacement for a diseased bladder, and its required characteristics were outlined.[2] It should provide adequate urine storage, allow volitional complete evacuation of urine, and preserve renal function. Its structure would have to be biocompatible, resistant to urinary encrustation, and tolerant of bacterial infection. Despite numerous attempts over the last 50 years, the published prototypes have not advanced beyond the stage of a preliminary report of experimental data. Most noteworthy models were described by O'Sullivan and Barrett,[3] Barrett and Donovan,[4] and Barrett et al[5] (e.g. the Mayo Clinic model), and Rohrman et al (e.g. the Aachen, Germany, model).[6] These were abandoned and a new concept of tissue engineering was introduced in the 1990s.

The emerging concept of engineering replacement tissue is that cells and support matrices will carry cells to the site of the implant and maintain them there. Many researchers attempted to implant matrices without cells, on the assumption that native cells would migrate and populate these matrices. This approach achieved limited success, and is suitable mainly for a small surface area of implanted matrix, such as that for urethral reconstruction, especially onlay flaps. More complex or larger structures require a confluent layer of cells attached to the matrix before implantation. Although great strides have been made in recruiting stem and progenitor cells for reconstructive purposes, most of the published data on tissue engineering of urologic segments rely on a common basic paradigm in which donor tissue harvested via biopsy is dissociated into individual cells, which are expanded in vitro, seeded onto a support matrix, and further grown ex vivo on the matrix until confluence is achieved. The cell-seeded construct is then returned as autologous tissue to the patient (Figure 61.1). Key factors to success are the cell source, cell expansion, the ability to produce balanced co-cultures, and a supporting matrix that can allow diffusion of nutrients in the short term and vascularization in the long term to maintain cell viability in vivo.

Although theoretically the source of the cells could be heterologous, allogenic, or autologous, a large body of

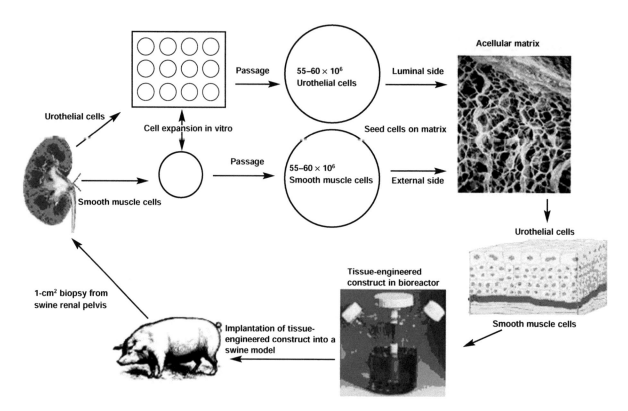

**Fig. 61.1**

Tissue-engineered approach to genitourinary regeneration utilizing autologous cells in a swine model.

the published literature reports adoption of a model of autologous cells as an ideal source that avoids the need to deal with immunocompatability and rejection.[7–15] This approach is not without difficulties. Success depends upon the ability to use the donor tissue efficiently and to supply nutrition and blood to the reconstructed tissue that will allow long-term survival, differentiation, and growth. This may involve optimization of cell proliferation in vitro and in vivo by optimizing the utilization of media and growth factors. Furthermore, the support matrix, whether synthetic or biologically derived, should possess qualities that allow for cell migration and proliferation, diffusion of nutrients in vivo, and, ultimately, vascularization in concert with cell expansion to allow the tissue-engineered construct to maintain its viability.

This chapter summarizes the importance of the building blocks of tissue-engineered constructs, as they relate to the bladder, and discusses recently reported advances in tissue engineering.

## SELECTIVE CELL TRANSPLANTATION

As initially described by Judah Folkman in 1973, neither cells nor tissues can be implanted in volumes exceeding 3 mm.[3,16] Nutrition and gas exchange is limited by this maximal diffusion distance. If cells were implanted in volumes exceeding 3 mm,[3] only the cells on the surface

would survive, and the central cell core would undergo necrosis resulting from a lack of vascularity. Therefore, the implantation of viable tissue larger than a few millimeters without a supply of nutrients via a vascular system is not feasible.

The concept of utilizing a selective set of cells for transplantation has been applied clinically for many disorders. A few of these are the use of engineered skin for burn patients, replacement of opaque cornea with engineered epithelial cells, engineered cartilage for replacement of knee components, and engineered injectable chondrocytes for vesicoureteral reflux and urinary incontinence.[10,13,17,18]

## EXPANSION OF UROTHELIAL AND SMOOTH MUSCLE CELLS

Currently, methods of growing urothelial cells in the culture dish involve utilization of serum-free media combined with growth factors. It has been demonstrated previously that it is possible, using appropriate methods of cell expansion, to isolate cells from a 1-cm[2] biopsy of urothelium and to expand the cells at a rate that will allow covering a surface area of 4202 m[2] (an area equivalent to that of one football field) within 8 weeks.[12] The deeper, smooth-muscle cell layer of the same biopsy can be processed concurrently, and, if the cells are placed in serum-rich media, the smooth muscle cells can be expanded at a similar, if not faster, rate. The differentiation characteristics, growth requirements, and other biologic properties of normal human bladder epithelial and muscle cells have been studied extensively.[7,12,19–32]

# EXTRACELLULAR MATRIX

In tissue engineering, the extracellular matrix (ECM) serves as a support system for the cells and elicits biologic and mechanical functions of native ECM in the body. These functions include bringing cells together into tissue, controlling tissue structure, and regulating cell phenotype.[33] Biologic or synthetic biomaterials may facilitate the capture of cells, cell-adhesion peptides, and growth factors and transportation to predetermined areas in the body, delineation of a three-dimensional formation of new structures, and direct the development of a desired function.[34] Direct injection of cell suspensions without the support system of biomaterial matrices has been performed in the past, but with limited success because of difficulty in controlling the localization of transplanted cells.[10,35]

## DESIGN AND SELECTION OF BIOMATERIALS

Any biomaterial for tissue-engineering purposes must possess the qualities of controlling the three-dimensional structure and function of the engineered tissue, interacting with transplanted cells, and accommodating migrating host cells. The ideal biomaterial should be biocompatible, promote cellular interaction and tissue development, and retain proper mechanical and physical properties. A biodegradable and bioresorbable material would be useful to support the reconstruction of native tissue without foreign body reaction and inflammation. Because mechanical support of the biomaterials is best retained until the engineered tissue has sufficient mechanical strength to support itself, the rate of degradation should be predetermined and is of crucial importance.[36] In order to allow the delivery of cells at a high density, a high ratio of surface-area-to-volume is mandatory. A high degree of porosity, interconnected pore structures, and specific pore sizes promote a high initial cell seeding density and host tissue ingrowth. Current techniques allow the control of porosity, pore size, and pore structure in synthetic matrices.[34] Degradation rate and concentration of degradation products locally and systemically should be at a rate that would not cause overburden on the liver or kidneys, and would avoid accumulation of toxic products in the body.[37,38] Controlled release of growth factors and other bioactive agents from the biomaterial can also induce cell adhesion, proliferation, migration, differentiation, and tissue-specific gene expression in the cells.[38]

## TYPES OF BIOMATERIAL

Three classes of biomaterial have been used for engineering of genitourinary tissues:

- naturally derived materials, such as collagen and alginate
- decellularized tissue matrices, such as bladder submucosa and small intestinal submucosa (SIS)
- synthetic polymers, such as polyglycolic acid (PGA), polylactic acid (PLA), and poly(lactic-co-glycolic acid) (PLGA).

Each of these groups of materials has specific advantages for tissue-engineering applications. Cells may respond to naturally derived biologic materials and decellularized tissue matrices. Synthetic polymers can be manufactured on a large scale with high precision and reproducibly. Additionally, they possess the advantage of predetermined properties of strength, degradation rate, and microstructure that can be controlled.

### Collagen

Collagen, the most abundant and ubiquitous structural protein in the body, can be readily purified from animal and human tissues alike,[39] and induces minimal inflammatory or antigenic response.[40] Collagen has been approved by the United States Food and Drug Administration (FDA) for many types of medical applications, including wound dressings and artificial skin.[41] When implanted, it may undergo degradation by lysosomal enzymes. The density of the implant and the extent of intermolecular crosslinking determine the in vivo resorption rate. There is a caveat with cell seeding, however, since the lower the density of collagen matrix, the greater the interstitial space and, generally, the larger the pores. (Low-density collagen matrix has larger pore sizes and thereby greater interstitial spaces.) Although this allows for increased cell infiltration, it also leads to a higher rate of collagen implant degradation. Collagen demonstrates high tensile strength and flexibility, and it can be processed into a wide assortment of structures.[39,42,43]

### Alginate

Alginate is a polysaccharide isolated from seaweed. It has been used as an injectable cell-delivery vehicle[44] and as a cell-stabilizing matrix.[45] In the presence of divalent ions such as calcium, it demonstrates gentle gelling properties that are hospitable to cells. Alginate is a biocompatible series of copolymers of D-mannuronate and L-glucuronate which has been approved by the FDA as a wound-dressing material for humans. Alginate does not possess a biologic recognition domain (i.e. cells do not line up or assume any organized spatial arrangement on alginate), and mechanical properties of alginate hydrogels are limited.

## Decellularized tissue matrices

These matrices are collagen-based materials. They are tissue components that are processed mechanically or chemically to remove all cellular components from the tissue, without affecting its principal mechanical properties. Examples of this process are the decellularization of a segment of bladder tissue or SIS.[14,46-48] Upon implantation, these matrices slowly degrade and are replaced and remodeled by ECM proteins synthesized and secreted by transplanted or migrating cells into the matrix. With a well-controlled cleaning sequence, the structure of the proteins (e.g. collagen and elastin) can be retained, and one can achieve a well-conserved and normally arranged decellularized matrix.[49] Decellularized tissue matrices have been proven to support cell ingrowth and regeneration of genitourinary tissues, including urethra and bladder tissues, with no evidence of immunogenic rejection.[14,46] However, shrinkage of the matrices is a major problem, and shrinkage of the implanted matrix is especially problematic in the absence of preimplantation cell seeding of the matrix.

SIS is a biodegradable, acellular, xenogeneic collagen-based tissue-matrix graft. This is the most extensively studied decellularized, naturally derived matrix to date. The matrix is derived from porcine small intestine, which undergoes a fully mechanical process whereby the mucosa is removed from the inner surface, and the serosa and muscular layer from the outer surface. SIS has been shown to promote regeneration of a variety of host tissues, including blood vessels, ligaments, and bladder, which will be described later in the chapter. The FDA has approved clinical use of SIS in its application as a sling material.

## Polyesters

Polyesters have been widely studied for tissue-engineering applications. The most popular are the α-hydroxy acids, which include PGA, PLA, and PLGA. Currently, these materials are widely used as absorbable sutures.[50] These polymers readily degrade by nonenzymatic hydrolysis because of their hydrolytically labile ester bonds. The degradation products of α-hydroxy acids are nontoxic, natural metabolites that are eventually eliminated from the body in the form of carbon dioxide and water.[12,50] Alteration of the initial molecular weight, crystallinity, and the copolymer ratio of lactic to glycolic acid allows customization of the degradation rate of these polymers from several weeks to several years. Due to their thermoplastic characteristics, they can be formed into a desired three-dimensional shape by various techniques, including molding, extrusion,[51] solvent casting,[52] phase-separation

techniques,[53] and a gas-foaming technique.[54] In the genitourinary tract there are many applications for a polyester scaffold that has high porosity and a high ratio of surface-area-to-volume.

## BIOCOMPATIBILITY

The biocompatibility of biologic and synthetic materials is of extreme importance. Tissue compatibility was rarely studied in the context of genitourinary problems. However, two studies assessed the cytotoxic and bioactive effects of naturally derived SIS, bladder submucosa, collagen, and the synthetically derived alginate, PGA, PLGA, and poly(L-lactic acid) (PLLA). Compatibility was measured by assessing human urothelial cell[55] and smooth muscle cell[56] viability, metabolic activity, apoptotic properties, and DNA synthesis activity on the matrices. All but alginate exhibited nontoxic and bioactive effects on the cells in vitro.

The current strategy for tissue engineering relies heavily on incorporating a material (biologic or synthetic) that is called a matrix into the dysfunctional area, with or without autologous cells attached to it. A great deal of effort has been devoted to the implantation of various matrices without cells attached, with the hope that migrating cells will repopulate the matrix and produce/result in a functional segment. However, in recent years it has become evident that matrices become more functional when seeded in vitro with autologous cells prior to implantation. This is especially true in the bladder. A summary of the significant steps toward bladder tissue regeneration follows; it is organized by the type of matrix utilized.

## SIGNIFICANT STEPS IN TISSUE ENGINEERING OF THE BLADDER

Neuhoff reported the first application of a free tissue graft for bladder replacement in 1917. He used fascia to augment bladders in dogs.[57] Since then, numerous publications have reported utilization of free grafts in experimental and clinical settings. Natural materials included bladder allografts, pericardium, dura, and placenta.[28,58-60] Synthetic materials included polyvinyl sponge, tetrafluoroethylene (Teflon), collagen matrices, Vicryl matrices, and silicone.[6,61-63] Most of these attempts were unsuccessful because of mechanical, structural, functional, or biocompatibility failure. A review of results of decades of research indicates that nondegradable synthetic materials are compromised by mechanical failure and urinary stone formation. Within time, however, degradable materials without cells succumb to fibroblast deposition, scarring, graft shrinkage, and insufficient reservoir volume.

Collagen-based matrices for tissue regeneration have been popularized in recent years, but results were inconsistent. Newly harvested placental membranes[58] and biodegradable pericardial implants[59] have been used in dogs for bladder augmentation. Functionally, in urodynamic studies these implanted bladders demonstrated acceptable capacity for up to 36 months. However, grossly, they underwent graft shrinkage. Interestingly, the histology demonstrated an abundant epithelial layer, but the muscular layer was almost undetectable. Similar results were also observed in many other studies that utilized bladder grafts.[14,28,30,64] Acellular grafts used for cystoplasty repeatedly regenerated a near-normal urothelial layer, but failed to produce a fully developed muscle layer.[14,30,64,65]

## SMALL INTESTINAL SUBMUCOSA (SIS)

SIS was initially introduced more than a decade ago as a vascular graft.[66] In the mid 1990s, assessments of its regenerative potential in the bladder were published.[67–70] Currently, SIS is commercially available, mainly to use as a sling in a procedure and not for regenerative purposes. In one study utilizing SIS for augmentation cystoplasty in a dog model (n=8; maximal follow-up 15 months), the pre- and postoperative mean bladder capacities were 51 and 55 ml, respectively.[65] Mean maximal voiding pressures were 52 and 45 $cmH_2O$, respectively. Histologic analysis confirmed that the transitional cell layer resembled that of the native bladder tissue. However, the muscle layer was only partially developed. A pathologically increased amount of collagen was intermingled within the small amount of muscle fibers. A computed tomography scan image analysis confirmed the decreased muscle-to-collagen ratio and the loss of the normal architecture in the portion of the bladder that was regenerated by the SIS. In vitro contractility studies performed on strips from the SIS-regenerated dog bladders demonstrated a decrease of more than 50% in maximal contractile response compared to that of normal bladder tissues. Immunohistochemistry studies demonstrated the expression of various receptors in the matrix, including muscarinic, purinergic, and β-adrenergic receptors in addition to functional cholinergic and purinergic innervation.[65]

A rabbit model was used to compare SIS and a biochemically reconstructed collagen-based matrix for bladder tissue regeneration. Rabbits underwent partial cystectomy and cystoplasty with a patch graft. Although both matrices demonstrated good epithelialization and ingrowth of smooth muscle cells, considerable encrustation was noted, especially in the shorter time periods.[71]

The feasibility of augmenting the bladder laparoscopically with a multilayered SIS compared with the feasibility of using an ileal segment was assessed in a porcine model.[72] Within 3 months the multilayered SIS has shrunk, and by the sixth month it was replaced by dense calcified scar tissue. At 12 months, the bladder capacity of the SIS-augmented bladders was less than half that of bladders receiving an ileal supplement (431 versus 825 cc, p=0.016).

In a recent laparoscopic model, hemicystectomy and bladder reconstruction with SIS and ureteral reimplantation into the SIS material was evaluated.[73] Six mini-pigs underwent bladder reconstruction with SIS, and six control pigs underwent hemicystectomy and primary bladder closure with ipsilateral nephro-ureterectomy. Bladder capacity and bladder compliance were found to be similar in the two groups at all time points. Histology after 1 year revealed muscle at the graft periphery and center but this consisted of small fused bundles with significant fibrosis. Comparison showed no advantage in bladder capacity or compliance.

In order to improve the results with SIS, an attempt was made to compare use of porcine SIS from the proximal jejunum to the use of SIS from the distal ileum as an unseeded bladder patch.[74] Investigators reported that only distal ileum SIS in a sow older than 3 years of age produced consistent bladder regeneration without bone formation and severe shrinkage. They also stated that before clinical bladder augmentation with SIS can be implemented, further investigation is needed to identify the regenerative potential of specific SIS segments.

In an attempt to demonstrate the potential for cell-seeded SIS to induce organized bladder regeneration in vivo, human smooth muscle cells and urothelial cells were seeded in a layered co culture fashion on SIS, utilizing a nude mouse model. Grafts of 1 cm$^2$ were implanted subcutaneously in the flanks of the nude mice, and unseeded SIS grafts were implanted in the contralateral flanks of these mice as controls. After 12 weeks, layered urothelium and early smooth muscle bundle formation were noted only in the groups with seeded grafts.[75]

In a recent article, a German group presented a novel approach to retain the vasculature of porcine decellularized small bowel segments, preserving the jejunal arteriovenous pedicles.[76] The matrix was reseeded with primary bladder smooth muscle cells and urothelial cells, and its vascular structures were resurfaced with endothelial progenitor cells. Perfusion stagnation and implant thrombosis occurred within 30 minutes after the implantation of acellular scaffolds not seeded with endothelial cells. The reseeded group demonstrated intact perfusion into the vascular system and no relevant thrombus formation after 1 or 3 hours. Although these results are short-term only, they represent a promising initial step for incorporating vascular structures into genitourinary tissue-engineered constructs in vivo.

## ACELLULAR MATRIX FROM BLADDER

Utilization of allogenic bladder submucosa for genitourinary reconstruction was first described by Dr Anthony Atala's group in a canine model.[30] The regenerated bladder tissues contained a normal cellular organization consisting of urothelium and smooth muscle, and exhibited normal compliance. Biomaterials preloaded with cells before their implantation exhibited better tissue regeneration than the controls implanted without cells. The bladders showed a significant increase (100%) in capacity when augmented with scaffolds seeded with cells as compared with scaffolds without cells (30%). Subsequently, the same group demonstrated that porcine acellular bladder submucosa can serve as an 'off the shelf' biomaterial for urethral repair in a rabbit model.[46]

In another study, the allogenic acellular bladder matrix served as a scaffold for the ingrowth of host bladder wall components in rats. The matrix was prepared by mechanical and chemical removal of all cellular components from bladder tissue.[14] Partial cystectomy (25% ± 50%) was performed, followed by augmentation cystoplasty using acellular bladder matrices. The mucosal lining was complete within 10 days. After 4 weeks, muscular and vascular regeneration were complete. Nerve regeneration continued to improve until week 20.[14,64] The grafted bladders had significantly better capacity and compliance than did the autoregenerated bladders after partial cystectomy alone. The bladders regenerated with acellular matrix grafts exhibited contractile activity in response to electric and carbachol stimulation.[48] Clinically relevant antigenicity was not evident.[14] However, there was a high incidence of bladder stone formation.[14,64]

A Japanese group investigated the use of bladder acellular matrix (BAM) as a carrier of exogenous basic fibroblast growth factor (bFGF).[77] The growth factor was loaded in a lyophilized BAM by rehydrating the matrix with the growth factor solution. To assess the biologic effect of the released bFGF, BAMs incorporating bFGF were implanted in the subcutaneous space of mice, and vascular endothelial growth factor levels in the local tissue were evaluated. Additionally, bladder augmentation was performed in rats with BAM grafts containing various concentrations of bFGF. The authors demonstrated a preserved biologic activity of bFGF in BAM for more than 3 weeks. In the bladder augmentation model, angiogenesis into the matrix was increased and shrinkage was significantly inhibited in matrices containing bFGF.

## COLLAGEN

Collagen/Vicryl (PGA/PLA) composite membranes have been used as a scaffold for tissue ingrowth to repair a full-thickness defect in the bladder of rabbits. The collagen membranes were reinforced with meshes of Vicryl, a biodegradable polymer composed of PLGA, to strengthen the collagen membranes, which are too soft for reliable suturing. The results of the initial study were not encouraging because of the occurrence of severe infection.[63] However, a later study obtained a high success rate when the experiments were repeated using purification and gamma-irradiation of collagen and postoperative administration of antibiotics. After 3 weeks, normal urothelium was noted. At 6 weeks, no implanted biomaterial was identified. After 35 weeks, smooth muscle regeneration was evident. During this period there was no evidence of urinary leakage, infection, or bladder calculi.[78]

## PGA/PLGA

Dr Atala's group introduced the most complete and successful attempt to date for constructing a viable bladder substitute by transplantation into dogs of autologous smooth muscle cells and urothelial cells on biodegradable polymer scaffolds.[25] PGA-fiber-based scaffolds were configured into a bladder-shaped mold and then coated with a 50:50 copolymer of glycolide and lactide. Urothelial and smooth muscle cells were isolated from 1-cm² bladder biopsies, expanded in vitro, and seeded on the scaffolds. These neobladders were implanted in dogs that had had the majority of their native bladders excised. In functional evaluations carried out for up to 11 months, the bladder neo-organs demonstrated a normal capacity for retention of urine, normal compliance, ingrowth of neural structures, and a normal histologic architecture, including a normal concentration of urothelium, submucosa, and muscle. The control group, which consisted of bladder-shaped molds implanted alone (without cells) were fibrotic, displayed a paucity of muscle, and collapsed over time.[25]

## CONCLUSION

Multiple tissue engineering approaches are being intensely investigated. Each approach has its own inherent advantages, disadvantages, and limitations. However, a common strategy has emerged over the past decade that should lead to more successful outcomes in in vivo models (see Figure 61.1). This strategy requires a biodegradable matrix, whether naturally derived or synthetic and autologous cells that are harvested via a biopsy, separated and expanded in vitro, and seeded on the matrix to confluence before implantation. Furthermore, enhanced vascularization and neoinnervation in vivo are required to allow the implanted constructs to maintain long-term function.

Although great strides have been made, a significant body of research and development is still required to achieve the holy grail of genitourinary reconstruction, namely a reproducible and reliable tissue-engineered bladder.

## REFERENCES

1. Krane RJ, Siroky MB, Fitzpatrick JM. Clinical Urology. Philadelphia: Lippincott, 1994, xxiii, p 1360.
2. Desgrandchamps F, Griffith DP. The artificial bladder. Eur Urol 1999;35:257–266.
3. O'Sullivan DC, Barrett DM. Prosthetic bladder: in vivo studies on an active negative-pressure-driven device. J Urol 1994;151:776–780.
4. Barrett DM, Donovan MG. Prosthetic bladder augmentation and replacement. Semin Urol 1984;2:167–175.
5. Barrett DM, O'Sullivan DC, Parulkar BG, Donovan MG. Artificial bladder replacement: a new design concept [see comment]. Mayo Clin Proc 1992;67:215–220.
6. Rohrmann D, Albrecht D, Hannappel J, Gerlach R, Schwarzkopp G, Lutzeyer W. Alloplastic replacement of the urinary bladder. J Urol 1996;156:2094–2097.
7. Amiel GE, Atala A. Current and future modalities for functional renal replacement. Urol Clin North Am 1999;26:235–246, xi.
8. Atala A. Autologous cell transplantation for urologic reconstruction. J Urol 1998;159:2–3.
9. Atala A, Vacanti JP, Peters CA, Mandell J, Retik AB, Freeman MR. Formation of urothelial structures in vivo from dissociated cells attached to biodegradable polymer scaffolds in vitro. J Urol 1992;148:658–662.
10. Brittberg M, Lindahl A, Nilsson A, Ohlsson C, Isaksson O, Peterson L. Treatment of deep cartilage defects in the knee with autologous chondrocyte transplantation. N Engl J Med 1994;331:889–895.
11. Cartwright PC, Snow BW. Bladder autoaugmentation: partial detrusor excision to augment the bladder without use of bowel. J Urol 1989;142:1050–1053.
12. Cilento BG, Freeman MR, Schneck FX, Retik AB, Atala A. Phenotypic and cytogenetic characterization of human bladder urothelia expanded in vitro. J Urol 1994;152:665–670.
13. Gallico GG III, O'Connor NE, Compton CC, Kehinde O, Green H. Permanent coverage of large burn wounds with autologous cultured human epithelium. N Engl J Med 1984;311:448–451.
14. Probst M, Dahiya R, Carrier S, Tanagho EA. Reproduction of functional smooth muscle tissue and partial bladder replacement. Br J Urol 1997;79:505–515.
15. Machluff M, Atala A. Emerging concepts for tissues and organ transplantation. Graft 1998;1:31.
16. Folkman J, Hochberg M. Self-regulation of growth in three dimensions. J Exp Med 1973;138:745–753.
17. Atala A, Cima LG, Kim W, et al. Injectable alginate seeded with chondrocytes as a potential treatment for vesicoureteral reflux. J Urol 1993;150:745–747.
18. Atala A, Kim W, Paige KT, Vacanti CA, Retik AB. Endoscopic treatment of vesicoureteral reflux with a chondrocyte–alginate suspension. J Urol 1994;152:641–643; discussion 644.
19. Atala A. Future perspectives in reconstructive surgery using tissue engineering. Urol Clin North Am 1999;26:157–165, ix–x.
20. Atala A. Tissue engineering techniques for closure of bladder exstrophy: an experimental animal model. In Gearhart J, Matthews G (eds): The exstrophy–epispadias complex. New York: Plenum, 1999, pp 63–64.
21. Fauza DO, Fishman SJ, Mehegan K, Atala A. Videofetoscopically assisted fetal tissue engineering: bladder augmentation. J Pediatr Surg 1998;33:7–12.
22. Fauza DO, Fishman SJ, Mehegan K, Atala A. Videofetoscopically assisted fetal tissue engineering: skin replacement. J Pediatr Surg 1998;33:357–361.
23. Freeman MR, Yoo JJ, Raab G, et al. Heparin-binding EGF-like growth factor is an autocrine factor for human urothelial cells and is synthesized by epithelial and smooth muscle cells in the human bladder. J Clin Invest 1997;99:1028–1036.
24. Nguyen HT, Park JM, Peters CA, et al. Cell-specific activation of the HB-EGF and ErbB1 genes by stretch in primary human bladder cells. In Vitro Cell Dev Biol Anim 1999;35:371–375.
25. Oberpenning F, Meng J, Yoo JJ, Atala A. De novo reconstitution of a functional mammalian urinary bladder by tissue engineering. Nat Biotechnol 1999;17:149–155.
26. Park HJ, Yoo JJ, Kershen RT, Moreland R, Atala A. Reconstitution of human corporal smooth muscle and endothelial cells in vivo. J Urol 1999;162:1106–1109.
27. Tobin MS, Freeman MR, Atala A. Maturational response of normal human urothelial cells in culture is dependent on extracellular matrix and serum additives. Surg Forum 1994;45:786–789.
28. Tsuji I, Ishida H, Fujieda J. Experimental cystoplasty using preserved bladder graft. J Urol 1961;85:42–44.
29. Yoo JJ, Atala A. A novel gene delivery system using urothelial tissue engineered neo-organs. J Urol 1997;158:1066–1070.
30. Yoo JJ, Meng J, Oberpenning F, Atala A. Bladder augmentation using allogenic bladder submucosa seeded with cells. Urology 1998;51:221–225.
31. Yoo JJ, Lee I, Atala A. Cartilage rods as a potential material for penile reconstruction. J Urol 1998;160:1164–1168; discussion 1178.
32. Yoo JJ, Park HJ, Lee I, Atala A. Autologous engineered cartilage rods for penile reconstruction. J Urol 1999;162:1119–1121.
33. Alberts B, Bray D, Lewis J, Raff M, Roberts K, Watson JD (eds). Molecular Biology of the Cell. New York: Garland, 1994, pp 971–995.
34. Kim BS, Mooney DJ. Development of biocompatible synthetic extracellular matrices for tissue engineering. Trends Biotechnol 1998;16:224–230.
35. Ponder KP, Gupta S, Leland F, et al. Mouse hepatocytes migrate to liver parenchyma and function indefinitely after intrasplenic transplantation. Proc Natl Acad Sci USA 1991;88:1217–1221.
36. Kim BS, Mooney DJ. Engineering smooth muscle tissue with a predefined structure. J Biomed Mater Res 1998;41:322–332.
37. Bergsma JE, Rozema FR, Bos RRM, et al. Biocompatibility and degradation mechanism of predegraded and non-degraded poly(lactide) implants: an animal study. Mater Med 1995;6:715–724.
38. Peters MC, Isenberg BC, Rowley JA, Mooney DJ. Release from alginate enhances the biological activity of vascular endothelial growth factor. J Biomater Sci Polym Ed 1998;9:1267–1278.
39. Li ST. Biologic biomaterials: tissue-derived biomaterials (collagen). In: Bronzino JD (ed): The Biomedical Engineering Handbook, vol xxxii, 2862. Boca Raton: CRC Press/IEEE Press, 1995, pp 627–647.
40. Furthmayr H, Timpl R. Immunochemistry of collagens and procollagens. Int Rev Connect Tissue Res 1976;7:61–99.
41. Pachence JM. Collagen-based devices for soft tissue repair. J Biomed Mater Res 1996;33:35–40.
42. Cavallaro JF, Kemp PD, Kraus KH. Collagen fabrics as biomaterials. Biotechnol Bioeng 1994;43:781–791.
43. Yannas IV, Burke JF. Design of an artificial skin. I. Basic design principles. J Biomed Mater Res 1980;14:65–81.
44. Smidsrod O, Skjak-Braek G. Alginate as immobilization matrix for cells. Trends Biotechnol 1990;8:71–78.
45. Lim F, Sun AM. Microencapsulated islets as bioartificial endocrine pancreas. Science 1980;210:908–910.
46. Chen F, Yoo JJ, Atala A. Acellular collagen matrix as a possible 'off the shelf' biomaterial for urethral repair. Urology 1999;54:407–410.
47. Dahms SE, Piechota HJ, Nunes L, Dahiya R, Lue TF, Tanagho EA. Free ureteral replacement in rats: regeneration of ureteral wall components in the acellular matrix graft. Urology 1997;50:818–825.
48. Piechota HJ, Dahms SE, Nunes LS, Dahiya R, Lue TF, Tanagho EA. In vitro functional properties of the rat bladder regenerated by the bladder acellular matrix graft. J Urol 1998;159:1717–1724.
49. Dahms SE, Piechota HJ, Dahiya R, Lue TF, Tanagho EA. Composition and biomechanical properties of the bladder acellular matrix graft: comparative analysis in rat, pig and human. Br J Urol 1998;82:411–419.

50. Gilding DK. Biodegradable polymers. In Williams DF (ed): Biocompatibility of clinical implant materials, vol 2. Boca Raton: CRC Press, 1981, pp 209–232.

51. Freed LE, Vunjak-Novakovic G, Biron RJ, et al. Biodegradable polymer scaffolds for tissue engineering. Biotechnology 1994;12:689–693.

52. Mikos AG, Thorsen AJ, Czerwonka LA, et al. Preparation and characterization of poly(L-lactic acid) foams. Polymer 1994;35:1068–1077.

53. Nam YS, Park TG. Porous biodegradable polymeric scaffolds prepared by thermally induced phase separation. J Biomed Mater Res 1999;47:8–17.

54. Harris LD, Kim BS, Mooney DJ. Open pore biodegradable matrices formed with gas foaming. J Biomed Mater Res 1998;42:396–402.

55. Goldstein MB, Dearden LC, Gualtieri V. Regeneration of subtotally cystectomized bladder patched with omentum: an experimental study in rabbits. J Urol 1967;97:664–668.

56. Bentz H, Schroeder JA, Estridge TD. Improved local delivery of TGF-beta2 by binding to injectable fibrillar collagen via difunctional polyethylene glycol. J Biomed Mater Res 1998;39:539–548.

57. Neuhof H. Fascial transplantation into visceral defects: an experimental and clinical study. Surg Gynecol Obstet 1917;25:383.

58. Fishman IJ, Flores FN, Scott FB, Spjut HJ, Morrow B. Use of fresh placental membranes for bladder reconstruction. J Urol 1987;138:1291–1294.

59. Kambic H, Kay R, Chen JF, Matsushita M, Harasaki H, Zilber S. Biodegradable pericardial implants for bladder augmentation: a 2.5-year study in dogs. J Urol 1992;148:539–543.

60. Kelami A, Ludtke-Handjery A, Korb G, Roll J, Schnell J, Danigel KH. Alloplastic replacement of the urinary bladder wall with lyophilized human dura. Eur Surg Res 1970;2:195–202.

61. Bona AV, De Gresti A. Partial substitution of urinary bladder with Teflon prosthesis. Minerva Urol 1996;18:43–47.

62. Gleeson MJ, Griffith DP. The use of alloplastic biomaterials in bladder substitution. J Urol 1992;148:1377–1382.

63. Monsour MJ, Mohammed R, Gorham SD, French DA, Scott R. An assessment of a collagen/vicryl composite membrane to repair defects of the urinary bladder in rabbits. Urol Res 1987;15:235–238.

64. Sutherland RS, Baskin LS, Hayward SW, Cunha GR. Regeneration of bladder urothelium, smooth muscle, blood vessels and nerves into an acellular tissue matrix. J Urol 1996;156:571–577.

65. Kropp BP, Rippy MK, Badylak SF, et al. Small intestinal submucosa: urodynamic and histopathologic evaluation in long term canine bladder augmentations. J Urol 1996;155:2098–2104.

66. Sandusky GE Jr, Badylak SF, Morff RJ, Johnson WD, Lantz G. Histologic findings after in vivo placement of small intestine submucosal vascular grafts and saphenous vein grafts in the carotid artery in dogs. Am J Pathol 1992;140:317–324.

67. Knapp PM, Lingeman JE, Siegel YI, Badylak SF, Demeter RJ. Biocompatibility of small-intestinal submucosa in urinary tract as augmentation cystoplasty graft and injectable suspension. J Endourol 1994;8:125–130.

68. Kropp BP, Badylak S, Thor KB. Regenerative bladder augmentation: a review of the initial preclinical studies with porcine small intestinal submucosa. Adv Exp Med Biol 1995;385:229–235.

69. Kropp BP, Eppley BL, Prevel CD, et al. Experimental assessment of small intestinal submucosa as a bladder wall substitute. Urology 1995;46:396–400.

70. Kropp BP, Rippy MK, Badylak SF, et al. Regenerative urinary bladder augmentation using small intestinal submucosa: urodynamic and histopathologic assessment in long-term canine bladder augmentations. J Urol 1996;155:2098–2104.

71. Nuininga JE, van Moerkerk H, Hanssen A, et al. A rabbit model to tissue engineer the bladder. Biomaterials 2004;25:1657–1661.

72. Paterson RF, Lifshitz DA, Beck SD, et al. Multilayered small intestinal submucosa is inferior to autologous bowel for laparoscopic bladder augmentation. J Urol 2002;168:2253–2257.

73. Landman J, Olweny E, Sundaram CP, et al. Laparoscopic mid sagittal hemicystectomy and bladder reconstruction with small intestinal submucosa and reimplantation of ureter into small intestinal submucosa: 1-year followup. J Urol 2004;171:2450–2455.

74. Kropp BP, Cheng EY, Lin HK, Zhang Y. Reliable and reproducible bladder regeneration using unseeded distal small intestinal submucosa. J Urol 2004;172:1710–1713.

75. Zhang Y, Kropp BP, Lin HK, Cowan R, Cheng EY. Bladder regeneration with cell-seeded small intestinal submucosa. Tissue Eng 2004;10:181–187.

76. Schultheiss D, Gabouev AI, Cebotari S, et al. Biological vascularized matrix for bladder tissue engineering: matrix preparation, reseeding technique and short-term implantation in a porcine model. J Urol 2005;173:276–280.

77. Kanematsu A, Yamamoto S, Noguchi T, Ozeki M, Tabata Y, Ogawa O. Bladder regeneration by bladder acellular matrix combined with sustained release of exogenous growth factor. J Urol 2003;170:1633–1638.

78. Scott R, Mohammed R, Gorham SD, et al. The evolution of a biodegradable membrane for use in urological surgery. A summary of 109 in vivo experiments. Br J Urol 1988;62:26–31.

# Clinical trial design

## 62

*Richard J Sylvester, Takuhiro Yamaguchi*

## INTRODUCTION

The importance of proper clinical trial design cannot be overemphasized. Even the most experienced statistician may not be able to draw valid conclusions at the end of a study that has serious flaws in its design. Thus a statistician should be involved in the development of a new study from the very beginning. At the design stage, the statistician's role is not simply limited to calculating the sample size, but should also involve discussions on the:

1. type of trial, its design and its objectives
2. prognostic factors and patient selection criteria
3. definition of endpoints
4. statistical considerations:
   - design—sample size, patient accrual rate, duration of patient entry and follow-up, trial feasibility
   - randomization/stratification—randomization procedure, stratification factors
   - statistical analysis techniques—statistical tests and procedures
5. number and timing of interim analyses and choice of early stopping rules.

The basic statistical principles of clinical trial design can be found in the International Conference on Harmonization (ICH) E9 guideline.[1]

In this chapter we will review the basic principles of clinical trial design for phase II and phase III studies and then consider the special cases of superficial, locally advanced, and metastatic bladder cancer. Phase I and phase IV studies will not be covered.

## PHASE II TRIALS

### INTRODUCTION

After determination of the maximum tolerated dose in phase I studies, the biologic antitumor activity of a new drug is assessed, first as a single agent in phase II trials and then later in combination with other drugs. Such trials are carried out in patients with metastatic disease, generally after having failed all other available treatment, although in some cases it may also be as first line therapy. A further aim of phase II trials is to obtain a more detailed description of the drug's toxicity, particularly cumulative toxicity. At the conclusion of the phase II trial, a decision is made whether or not to continue the drug's further clinical development.

The primary endpoint is generally the objective response rate. Secondary endpoints include the duration of response and the acute toxicity graded according to the 'Common Terminology Criteria for Adverse Events' (CTCAE) (http://ctep.cancer.gov/reporting/ctc.html).

### NONRANDOMIZED PHASE II TRIALS

Phase II trials are generally nonrandomized, with all patients receiving the same treatment. Both single-stage and multistage designs have been proposed. In order to reject an ineffective drug from further study as quickly as possible, two-stage designs are desirable from both a theoretical and an ethical point of view. An initial sample of $n_1$ patients is treated and if more than $r_1$ responses are observed, the trial continues in a second sample of $n_2$ patients. If more than $r = r_1 + r_2$ responses are observed in a total of $n = n_1 + n_2$ patients, then the drug is accepted for further study. Two-stage designs have the practical consequence that the trial may have to be temporarily closed to patient entry after the $n_1$ patients required for the first stage have been entered. It may not be known at that time whether the criteria for continuation to the second stage are met or not.

Some of the most popular designs for phase II studies are described below and include:

- Gehan two-stage design[2]
- Fleming one-stage and multistage designs[3]
- Simon optimal and minimax two-stage designs[4]
- Bryant and Day two-stage design.[5]

Based on some minimal response rate of interest, the Gehan design has the property that it will reject the drug from further study after the first stage only if no responses have been observed. Thus it minimizes the number of patients treated with a totally inactive drug. The second stage is based on the width of the confidence interval of the estimate of the response rate, and does not provide a decision rule for the acceptance or rejection of the drug. The Gehan rule should only be used for the first very early phase II trials of a new drug.

The Fleming and Simon hypothesis testing designs are also based on the response rate. One specifies:

- $P_0$: the highest response rate that investigators would like to reject with a high probability
- $P_1$: the lowest response rate greater than $P_0$ that investigators would like to accept with a high probability
- Alpha = size of the type I error = false-positive rate = probability (accept drug when $P=P_0$)
- Beta = size of the type II error = false-negative rate = probability (reject drug when $P=P_1$).

Since the most serious error in a phase II study is to reject an effective drug from further study, the false-negative rate should be strictly controlled. It should not be greater than 0.10 (0.05 is recommended), even at the expense of a slightly larger false-positive rate (maximum 0.20, preferably 0.10 or less).

If it is desired to formally take into account toxicity as well as activity, the two-stage Bryant and Day design may be used. Unacceptable and acceptable severe toxicity rates $T_0$ and $T_1$ ($T_0 > T_1$) and their corresponding error probabilities are also specified. Both the type I and type II error rates should generally be set to 0.10 or less. The drug is rejected from further study if either it is too toxic ($\geq s_1$ or $s = s_1 + s_2$ patients with severe toxicity) or has insufficient activity ($\leq r_1$ or $r = r_1 + r_2$ responses).

The Fleming, Simon, and Bryant and Day designs all provide formal decision rules for accepting or rejecting the drug for further study at the end of the trial. For given error rates, the Simon optimal design minimizes the number of patients to be treated if the drug is ineffective (response rate = $P_0$), whereas the Simon minimax design minimizes the maximum number of patients that are treated. The Fleming multistage design satisfies the error rate requirements, but does not necessarily satisfy any optimality criteria.

Phase II sample size tables for the Gehan two stage, Fleming one-stage, and Simon optimal and minimax two-stage designs can be found in *Sample Size Tables for Clinical Studies*.[6] The two-stage Simon and Bryant and Day designs can be calculated at biostats.upci.pitt.edu/biostats/index2.html.

## RANDOMIZED PHASE II TRIALS

Phase II trials are generally not randomized; however, randomized trials should be considered in the following situations:

- Different schedules of the same drug are to be tested.
- Two or more drugs are to be tested at the same time.
- An analog of an active drug is tested.
- A combination of two or more drugs is being tested.

Nonrandomized phase II trials of drug combinations are often meaningless, even misleading, due to the temptation to compare the results to previous, noncomparable series of patients treated with other regimens.[7] Randomized phase II trials should be viewed as a simultaneous screening of different regimens and not as comparative trials. They provide a concurrent control group and the possibility of continuing the trial as a phase III study if the phase II trial is positive.

For randomized phase II trials, the sample size calculations are carried out as described above by applying one of the nonrandomized designs to each arm. If several arms are found to be active at the conclusion of the randomized phase II trial, the trial may be continued as a randomized phase III trial by including the patients already randomized in the phase II part of the study. It must be decided whether the decision rule for continuing to phase III is applied to only one or both of the treatment arms, and whether some minimum difference in response rate is also required.

Multiple arm randomized phase II (or phase II/III) screening trials have also been designed based on selection procedure techniques; however, they should only be used if the error rates are adequately controlled.[8,9]

## FEASIBILITY STUDIES

Trials assessing the feasibility of a new therapeutic approach, for example bladder preservation trials involving combination treatment, are sometimes incorrectly labeled as phase II trials, or even as phase I or phase III trials. This is incorrect. The endpoint of a feasibility study is rarely the response rate alone and is based on other factors related to the goals of the study (percent of patients completing the treatment, treatment morbidity or toxicity profile, disease-free rate, etc.). Randomization is recommended in order that the trial can be continued as a randomized phase III trial if the feasibility of the experimental arm is shown.

## DESIGN OF PHASE II STUDIES IN SUPERFICIAL AND ADVANCED BLADDER CANCER

### Superficial bladder cancer (papillary tumors)

Although somewhat controversial, phase II marker lesion studies are carried out to determine the ablative effect of an intravesical treatment before it is used prophylactically after transurethral resection (TUR).[10] The complete response (CR) of a single marker lesion left after TUR is determined based on negative cystoscopy, biopsy, and cytology. A minimum CR rate of 50% or more is generally sought, based on the Fleming one-stage design. Sample sizes for such a design are given in Table 62.1. Marker lesion studies are considered in more detail elsewhere in this book.

### Superficial bladder cancer (carcinoma in situ)

The statistical design of phase II trials in patients with carcinoma in situ (CIS) is very similar to that of papillary marker lesion studies as described above. All visible papillary lesions, if any, are resected prior to starting intravesical treatment. A minimum CR of at least 50% to 60% is sought after one or two 6- or 8-weekly induction treatment cycles. Potential prognostic factors for CR include the extent of CIS (focal versus diffuse), the type of CIS (primary, secondary, or concomitant), involvement of the upper urinary tract or prostatic urethra, previous treatment failure (bacillus Calmette–Guérin (BCG), other), and molecular markers (p53, p21, e-cadherin). Table 62.1 also provides sample sizes that can be used for phase II studies in CIS.

### Inoperable locally advanced and metastatic bladder cancer

Response to treatment (measurement of antitumor activity) is assessed on the basis of objective criteria such as RECIST (www.eortc.be/recist/default.htm) which measures the decrease in size of prospectively selected target lesions.[11] Response is not a surrogate for therapeutic benefit; it is only an indicator of antitumor activity.

The minimal response rate of interest will depend on the patient's characteristics and prognostic factors.

**Table 62.1** Phase II sample sizes for the Fleming one-stage design in superficial bladder cancer (papillary marker lesion or CIS)

| $P_0$ | $P_1$ | n | r |
|-------|-------|-----|-----|
| 0.30 | 0.50 | 51 | 19 |
| 0.35 | 0.50 | 93 | 38 |
| 0.35 | 0.55 | 52 | 22 |
| 0.40 | 0.55 | 96 | 44 |
| 0.40 | 0.60 | 52 | 25 |
| 0.45 | 0.60 | 94 | 48 |
| 0.45 | 0.65 | 51 | 27 |
| 0.50 | 0.65 | 91 | 51 |
| 0.50 | 0.70 | 50 | 29 |

$\alpha=0.10$; $\beta=0.05$.
Reject if there are $\leq r$ responses in n patients.

Prognostic factors for response include the extent of disease (tumor, node, metastasis classification), the site, type and number of metastases, the patient's performance status, and the amount of previous treatment received.

More recently, the progression-free rate or progression-free survival has been proposed as the primary endpoint in phase II trials with noncytotoxic agents where an initial period of stabilization in progressive patients may be expected.[12,13]

Table 62.2 provides an example of sample size and decision rules for the Fleming one-stage and the Simon, and Bryant and Day two-stage designs where a minimal response rate of 30% is sought.

**Table 62.2** Phase II sample sizes for Fleming one-stage, Simon two-stage, and Bryant and Day two-stage designs in advanced bladder cancer

| | Fleming | Simon optimal | Simon minimax | Bryant and Day |
|-------|---------|---------------|---------------|----------------|
| $n_1$ | NA | 20 | 26 | 23 |
| $r_1$ | NA | 2 | 3 | 2 |
| $s_1$ | NA | NA | NA | 7 |
| n | 32 | 40 | 33 | 41 |
| r | 5 | 6 | 5 | 6 |
| s | NA | NA | NA | 9 |

$P_0=0.10$; $P_1=0.30$; $T_0=0.30$; $T_1=0.10$; $\alpha=0.10$; $\beta=0.05$.
Reject if there are: $\leq r_1$ responses in $n_1$ patients; $\geq s_1$ patients with unacceptable toxicity in $n_1$ patients; $\leq r$ responses in n patients; $\geq s$ patients with unacceptable toxicity in n patients.
NA, not applicable.

# PHASE III TRIALS

## OBJECTIVE

After a drug has been found to have at least some predefined minimal amount of activity in phase II trials, or a new therapeutic approach has been found to be feasible, the next step is to determine its relative efficacy in randomized phase III trials.

The objective of a phase III trial is generally to determine:

- the effectiveness of the new treatment regimen as compared to the best current standard therapy or no treatment (superiority study), *or*
- if a new treatment is as effective as the standard therapy but is associated with less severe toxicity or a better quality of life (noninferiority or equivalence study).

## RANDOMIZATION

In order to obtain the correct results and to be able to convince others of their validity, large randomized trials are required: randomized in order to reduce the possibility of systematic bias and large in order to have a high power to detect small but medically important differences and reduce the risk of random errors.

In order to improve the balance of both the number of patients and the distribution of the prognostic factors in the treatment groups, it is generally recommended to stratify at randomization by a small number (one or two) of the most important prognostic factors and also by institution in multicenter trials. The minimization technique, which attempts to dynamically balance the distribution of each factor separately, is generally to be preferred to the static system of randomized blocks.[14] Randomization software, which uses the minimization technique, is available at www.sghms.ac.uk/depts/phs/guide/minim.htm.

## DESIGN

In order to ensure the trial's feasibility, the design should be kept as simple as possible. Broad eligibility criteria are preferable to narrow ones except if there are good a priori reasons to believe that the treatment will be beneficial to only a subgroup of patients. In most cases, a simple randomization between just two treatments is recommended. Trials with more than two treatment groups require proportionally more patients (except for factorial trials), and may be more difficult to recruit because patients must agree to receive any of the possible treatments. Formal crossover trials are generally

to be avoided since the underlying assumptions for carrying out such trials are almost never valid in cancer studies. The frequency of follow-up should be the same in all treatment groups, otherwise patients may appear to recur earlier on one arm simply because they have been assessed more frequently.

The primary endpoint in phase III trials should be related to patient benefit, for example duration of survival or progression-free survival. Quality of life, symptom control supported by quality of life data, and toxicity may be secondary endpoints. Response to treatment, while an indicator of anticancer activity, is not a surrogate for endpoints quantifying patient benefit.

A distinction should be made between superiority trials, which attempt to show a difference in treatment effectiveness, and noninferiority (one-sided) or equivalence (two-sided) trials, which attempt to show that one treatment is not significantly worse than another treatment.[15,16] In trials designed to show a difference, the attempt is to reject the null hypothesis of no difference (d=0) in treatment efficacy versus the alternative of a difference (d >0). Two-sided significance tests are generally to be recommended since it is possible that the new treatment could have a negative effect, for example due to unexpected treatment-related deaths. A nonsignificant result does not imply that two treatments are equivalent since the P value by itself does not give any information about the possible size of the treatment effect.

In trials designed to show the noninferiority or equivalence of a new, more conservative treatment, the null hypothesis that the new treatment is worse than the standard treatment by some given amount, $\Delta$, is tested.[16,17] Since the null hypothesis is always the 'opposite' of what you are trying to prove, the null and alternative hypotheses are reversed in superiority and noninferiority trials. A confidence interval approach is generally used in the analysis of noninferiority and equivalence trials.[15]

## SAMPLE SIZE

Sufficient numbers of patients should be entered so that the trial has a high power to detect a difference in treatment effectiveness should it exist. The sample size depends on the primary endpoint of the trial and on the statistical analysis technique that will be used to analyze the data. The number of patients entered into a phase III trial (the sample size) is calculated to ensure a given power ($1 - \beta \geq 0.80$) of detecting a postulated treatment difference at a prespecified significance level ($\alpha \leq 0.05$).

Using the primary endpoint of interest, the number of *patients* for binary endpoints (response rate, percent with unacceptable toxicity) and the number of *events* for time-to-event endpoints (such as duration of survival) depend on the following factors:

- A realistic estimate for the primary endpoint of interest in the control group.
- Realistic estimates of the size of the plausible treatment effect and/or the medically worthwhile treatment effect.
- The size of the type I error $\alpha$ (false-positive rate $\leq 0.05$; generally two-sided except for noninferiority trials where it is recommended to take a one-sided $\alpha = 0.025$) and type II error $\beta$ (false-negative rate $\leq 0.20$). $1 - \beta$ is the power.
- The test statistic used to compare the treatment groups.

For example, to detect a difference in response rate, assuming a response rate of 50% in the control arm, the approximate number of patients required on each treatment for a two-sided test with type I and type II errors of 5% and 20%, respectively, is given in Table 62.3.

For time-to-event endpoints, such as time to recurrence or duration of survival, the power to detect treatment differences depends on the number of events observed, not on the number of patients entered.[18] A sufficiently large number of patients must be entered and followed for a sufficiently long time in order to observe the required number of events. Thus a large number of patients and a long follow-up will be required in an adjuvant trial if the primary therapy is curative in a large percentage of the patients entered.

The number of events required increases sharply when the size of the treatment difference of interest decreases. For example, the total number of deaths required in a phase III study may vary from 192 for a simple two-arm study trying to detect a 50% increase in the median duration of survival, to more than 13,000 trying to detect an increase of 5% (Table 62.4).

The number of patients in time-to-event studies depends on:

- the total number of events required
- the expected duration of patient entry, which in general should not exceed 5 years
- the duration of follow-up after closing the trial to patient entry.

**Table 62.3** Approximate number of patients on each treatment group required to detect a difference in response rate, assuming a response rate of 50% in the control arm, for a two-sided test with type I and type II errors of 5% and 20%, respectively

| Absolute difference (%) | Patients per group |
| --- | --- |
| 5 | 1565 |
| 10 | 390 |
| 15 | 170 |
| 20 | 95 |
| 25 | 60 |

**Table 62.4** Number of deaths on each treatment group required to detect a relative increase in median survival (median ratio) or relative decrease in the death rate (hazard ratio) for a two-sided test with type I and type II errors of 5% and 20%, respectively

| Median ratio | Hazard ratio | Deaths per group |
| --- | --- | --- |
| 1.05 | 0.952 | 6596 |
| 1.10 | 0.909 | 1729 |
| 1.15 | 0.870 | 804 |
| 1.20 | 0.833 | 473 |
| 1.25 | 0.800 | 316 |
| 1.30 | 0.769 | 229 |
| 1.35 | 0.741 | 175 |
| 1.40 | 0.714 | 139 |
| 1.45 | 0.690 | 114 |
| 1.50 | 0.667 | 96 |

In general, a compromise is made between the two extremes of entering only the same number of patients as the number of deaths that are required (minimizes the number of patients, maximizes the duration of the study), or continuing to enter patients until the required number of events is observed (minimizes the duration of the study, maximizes the number of patients). Thus the required number of patients is not unique and decreases as the duration of follow-up after the last patient has been entered increases (Table 62.5).

To account for possible loss to follow-up in studies requiring long-term follow-up, the required number of patients should either be increased by 5% in metastatic studies and 10% in adjuvant studies, or the duration of follow-up extended in order to ensure that the required number of events will be observed.

When calculating the sample size for time-to-event studies, it is important to ensure that the event rate does not greatly decrease over time, otherwise long-term follow-up will not necessarily yield the required number of events. For example, if nearly all events are expected to occur within the first 2 years, then follow-up beyond 2 years will not produce many additional events. In this

**Table 62.5** Number of patients on each treatment group needed to achieve the 458 deaths required to detect an increase in median survival from 5 years to 6.5 years (median ratio=1.30, hazard ratio=0.769) for a two-sided test with type I and type II errors of 5% and 20%, respectively, and an entry rate of 250 patients per year

| Duration of follow-up after entry of last patient | Patients per group |
| --- | --- |
| 1 year | 665 |
| 2 years | 578 |
| 3 years | 511 |
| 4 years | 459 |
| 5 years | 419 |
| 6 years | 387 |

case it is important that sufficient patients are entered to yield the required number of events, assuming a follow-up of just 2 years for each patient.

Noninferiority trials and equivalence studies require considerably more events and patients than superiority trials since the hypothesized difference between the new treatment and the control group in such trials should be no more than one third to one half of the benefit of the control group found in previous superiority studies.[17]

Except for four-arm 2 × 2 factorial design studies, trials with more than two arms require proportionally more patients on *each* treatment group for both an overall test and pairwise comparisons. If three pairwise comparisons are made in a three-arm trial, then in order to maintain the overall size of the type I error at 0.05, each comparison should be made at approximately the 0.05/3 = 0.0167 level (Bonferroni inequality), thus requiring more patients on each treatment group to maintain the same power.

It may be possible to use a 2 × 2 factorial design to answer two questions for the price of one.[19] For example, after TUR, investigators might randomize between full-dose and low-dose BCG, and between 1 year and 3 years of maintenance in patients with superficial bladder cancer. Although this results in four treatment groups, each of the two questions is analyzed separately, and there is no increase in sample size as compared to a trial with just two treatment groups. However, in the presence of an interaction, the hypotheses underlying the 2 × 2 factorial design are not satisfied and an analysis based on this design may yield meaningless results.

Phase III sample size tables can be found in *Sample Size Tables for Clinical Studies* by Machin et al[6] and the paper by Freedman,[18] or they may be calculated using commercial software such as nQuery Advisor (www.statsol.ie) or EAST (www.cytel.com).

## INTERIM ANALYSES AND EARLY STOPPING RULES

It should be specified in the protocol if there will be a formal interim analysis with early stopping rules, whether for treatment differences or because it is unlikely that a difference will ever be found (futility). The two most well-known group sequential designs are the Pocock design, which employs the same significance level at each analysis, and the O'Brien–Fleming design where the significance level to be used is proportional to the percentage of information (events) that is currently available and thus increases with each successive analysis.

Although the O'Brien–Fleming early stopping rule allows the final analysis to be carried out at close to the overall 5% significance level, it may be much too

conservative at the early interim analyses, especially when the total number of events required is large and thus the information fraction is low. It may be so conservative that it is very unlikely, nearly impossible, to reject the null hypothesis early on, even when a true treatment difference exists. The use of early stopping rules, which fall between the extremes of O'Brien Fleming and Pocock, should be investigated in order to reach a satisfactory compromise.

The design of phase III trials will now be considered for superficial, locally advanced, and metastatic bladder cancer.

## SUPERFICIAL BLADDER CANCER (PAPILLARY TUMORS)

After TUR to remove all visible tumors, trials are carried out to compare the prophylactic effect of different chemotherapeutic and/or immunologic agents in delaying or preventing tumor recurrence and/or progression. In order to tailor the treatment to the patient's prognosis, patients are divided into risk groups, and separate trials are generally carried out in good risk and intermediate or poor risk patients.[20,21]

Prognostic factors are different according to the primary endpoint of the study. The number of tumors prior to TUR and the prior recurrence rate are the most important prognostic factors for tumor recurrence, whereas the G grade, T category and the presence of CIS are the most important prognostic factors for progression to muscle-invasive disease.[20–22] Recurrence at the first follow-up cystoscopy and tumor size have also been found to be of prognostic importance. Thus the entry criteria for a study will often take into account one or more of these factors. However, the use of the T category and G grade as part of the eligibility criteria may be problematic due to possible inaccuracies in their assessment, as shown by discrepancies between local and review pathology.[23]

In poor prognosis patients, the goal is not only to delay or prevent recurrence, but also, and more specifically, to prevent progression to muscle-invasive disease. Unfortunately, the number of patients that can be expected to progress during follow-up is generally too small for time to progression to be used as the primary endpoint.[24,25] For this reason, time to first recurrence (disease-free interval or disease-free survival) is generally used as the primary endpoint even in this setting. Time to progression may be used as a secondary endpoint. Time to recurrence and time to progression are estimated using the Kaplan–Meier technique and compared using the logrank test.

The percent of patients that are recurrence-free at a fixed point in time, for example at 12 months, is not a good endpoint for the following reasons:

- A significant number of patients may still have their first recurrence after 12 months.
- Differences (or lack thereof) at 12 months may not be representative of differences at other time points.
- Comparisons at a fixed point in time usually have less power to detect differences than an analysis which takes into account the time of the recurrence, such as with the logrank test.
- There is the problem of censoring; for example, how should patients that have not been followed for at least 12 months be handled?

As witnessed by the large variability between institutions in the percent of patients that recur at the first follow-up cystoscopy,[26] the TUR at entry may have been incomplete. Prior to starting the (6-weekly) induction treatment after TUR, allowance should be made for the possibility of: 1) one immediate instillation of chemotherapy after TUR[27]; and 2) a second-look cystoscopy and TUR to remove any residual tumor that was originally missed or incompletely resected.[28]

Thus, when setting a maximum time delay for randomization and starting induction treatment after the TUR at entry on study, the possibility of a second TUR needs to be taken into account, i.e. the patient should be randomized only after the second TUR, if one is carried out.

The time to first recurrence (disease-free interval) is defined as the time from randomization to the first biopsy-proven recurrence. If no recurrence is observed, then it is censored at the date of the last follow-up cystoscopy. If a second-look cystoscopy and TUR are not mandatory, then any recurrence found at the first follow-up cystoscopy (e.g. at 3 months) may in fact be residual disease. For this reason, the recurrence rate, which takes into account additional recurrences over time after the first recurrence, is sometimes used as an endpoint.

Tables 62.4 and 62.5 provide sample sizes that may be appropriate in this setting. For example, assuming a patient entry rate of 250 patients per year and a follow-up of 3 years after the last patient has been entered, then in order to detect an increase in the median disease-free survival from 5 years to 6.5 years (median ratio=1.30, hazard ratio=0.769) at error rates $\alpha$=0.05 and $\beta$=0.20 based on a two sided logrank test, a total of 458 events and 1022 patients entered over 4.1 years will be required.

## SUPERFICIAL BLADDER CANCER (CARCINOMA IN SITU)

Since carcinoma in situ (CIS) may not be visible or detected during cystoscopy, it cannot be completely resected. Thus, in a patient with CIS, the treatment is used therapeutically rather than just prophylactically.

CIS patients, especially those with concomitant high-stage and/or high-grade papillary lesions (e.g. T1 G3), are at a particularly high risk of progression.

The main endpoint in CIS studies is generally the complete response rate as assessed by negative cystoscopy, biopsy, and cytology. Secondary endpoints may include disease-free survival or disease-free interval (equals zero for patients without a complete response), the time to progression to muscle-invasive disease, and the time to recurrence in complete responders.

Separate trials should be done in patients with CIS (whether concomitant, secondary or primary) or at least they should be assessed separately from patients with papillary lesions only. Any given treatment may not have the same efficacy in patients with only papillary lesions and in those with CIS.

In practice, phase III trials in CIS are difficult to carry out due the relative rarity of the disease. With several exceptions, CIS patients are typically included in trials in intermediate and high-risk superficial bladder cancer where most patients have only papillary lesions, resulting in underpowered treatment comparisons for CIS.

## LOCALLY ADVANCED BLADDER CANCER

The goal in patients with operable, locally advanced bladder cancer is cure. Hence overall survival should be the primary endpoint in both neoadjuvant and adjuvant studies of systemic chemotherapy.

A meta-analysis of neoadjuvant studies of combination chemotherapy in some 2100 patients has shown a 13% reduction in the relative risk of death and an absolute improvement of 5% in 5 year survival, going from 45% to 50%.[29] Based on a median follow-up of 6 years, 58% of the patients died. Any trial studying differences of this magnitude will need approximately 2500 patients to achieve the 1500 deaths that will be required.

Previous trials studying the role of adjuvant combination chemotherapy after cystectomy have had methodologic flaws and/or been seriously underpowered to detect differences in survival.[30] Recently, the European Organisation for Research and Treatment of Cancer (EORTC), in collaboration with the Global Genitourinary Group and other international research organizations, launched an adjuvant trial comparing immediate to delayed chemotherapy after cystectomy and bilateral lymphadenectomy in pT3–4 or pN+ patients. In order to detect an increase in 5-year survival from 30% to 40% (hazard ratio=0.76, median ratio=1.31), a total of 436 events are required and a total of 660 patients are required for the study.[30]

Potential prognostic factors include age, performance status, hemoglobin level, the clinical and pathologic T stage and N category, tumor size, lymph node density, the histologic grade and type, lymphatic/vascular involvement, presence of positive margins after cystectomy, hydronephrosis, EGF receptor, p53 mutation, and the retinoblastoma gene (Rb).

P53 is of particular interest as a predictive marker, as witnessed by a randomized intergroup trial of methotrexate, vinblastine, doxorubicin, and cisplatin (MVAC) versus observation after cystectomy in p53-altered, pT1–2, pN0 patients (www.uscnorris.com/p53/). It is foreseen that 190 p53-positive patients will be randomized in order to detect a difference of 20% in the recurrence-free survival rate at 3 years.

## METASTATIC BLADDER CANCER

Duration of survival or progression-free survival is recommended as the primary endpoint in phase III trials of metastatic bladder cancer. Quality of life and response to treatment may be included as secondary endpoints. Although treatment with combination chemotherapy such as MVAC or gemcitabine/cisplatin can produce response rates of more than 50%, the overall median survival is still short, on average only slightly more than 1 year. However, there are a small number of long-term survivors, and a patient's pretreatment characteristics play an important role in determining prognosis.

Bajorin et al[31] developed a risk group classification based on a patient's performance status and the presence of visceral metastases (lung, liver or bone) where the median survival varied from 9 to 13 to 33 months according to the number of risk factors present. Sengelov et al[32] identified performance status, alkaline phosphatase, and liver metastases as independent prognostic factors, and derived risk groups based on the first two factors. Molecular markers such as Ki67, p53, p21, and Rb have also received attention as possible prognostic factors.[33]

Due to a heterogeneous prognosis, metastatic patients should be stratified at randomization according to their risk group. The number of patients required in metastatic studies is considerably less than that for locally advanced disease since 80% of the patients can be expected to die within 2–3 years.[34,35] For example, to detect an increase in median survival from 14 months to 18 months (21 months) based on a two-sided logrank test at error rates $\alpha=0.05$ and $\beta=0.20$, a total of approximately 500 (200) deaths are required.

## CONCLUSION

The biggest obstacle to the proper assessment of new treatments has been the underestimation of the number of patients required to detect medically plausible treatment differences. This has, in large part, been due to

an overly optimistic estimate of the size of the treatment difference that can be expected. Meta-analyses of small, undersized clinical trials should not be used to replace well-conducted, large-scale randomized clinical trials. However, when individual trials cannot answer the question of interest, they do provide the best overall summary of a treatment's effectiveness, and an estimate of the size of treatment differences that may be expected when designing new studies.[24,25,27]

In order to achieve the large sample sizes that are required to detect small but realistic and medically important treatment differences, multicenter, multigroup, and even multinational collaborative efforts are required. Although their administrative obstacles may appear daunting, it is through the conduct of true large scale, international, intergroup studies that we will be able to enter the required number of patients and draw definitive conclusions in the shortest period of time. The Global Genitourinary Group (www.guglobal.org) has been instrumental in this regard by establishing and maintaining active communication and collaboration between the leaders of the clinical trials groups around the world.

## REFERENCES

1. International Conference on Harmonization (ICH). Topic E9: Statistical Principles for Clinical Trials, CPMP/ICH/363/96. 1998. Online. Available: www.ich.org/MediaServer.jser?@_ID=485&@_MODE=GLB.

2. Gehan E. The determination of the number of patients required in a preliminary and a follow-up trial of a new chemotherapeutic agent. J Chron Dis 1961;13:346–353.

3. Fleming T. One sample multiple testing procedure for phase ii clinical trials. Biometrics 1982;38:143–151.

4. Simon R. Optimal two-stage designs for phase ii clinical trials. Controlled Clin Trials 1989;10:1–10.

5. Bryant J, Day R. Incorporating toxicity considerations into the design of two-stage phase ii clinical trials. Biometrics 1995;51:1372–1383.

6. Machin D, Campbell M, Fayers P, Pinol A. Sample Size Tables for Clinical Studies. Ltd: Oxford: Blackwell, 1997.

7. Van Glabbeke M, Stewart W, Armand JP. Non-randomized phase II trials of drug combinations: often meaningless, sometimes misleading. Are there alternative strategies? Eur J Cancer 2002;38:635–638.

8. Simon R, Wittes R, Ellenberg S. Randomized phase II clinical trials. Cancer Treat Rep 1985;69:1375–1381.

9. Sargeant D, Goldberg R. A flexible design for multiple armed screening trials. Stat Med 2001;20:1051–1060.

10. van der Meijden APM, Hall RR, Kurth KH, Bouffioux C, Sylvester R and members of the EORTC Genitourinary Group. Phase II trials in Ta, T1 bladder cancer: the marker tumour concept. Br J Urol 1996;77:634–637.

11. Therasse P, Arbuck SG, Eisenhauer EA, et al. New guidelines to evaluate the response to treatment in solid tumors. J Natl Cancer Inst 2000;92:205–216.

12. Van Glabbeke M, Verweij J, Judson I, Nielsen OS on behalf of the EORTC Soft Tissue and Bone Sarcoma Group. Progression free rate as the principal endpoint for phase II trials in soft tissue sarcomas. Eur J Cancer 2002;38:543–549.

13. Mick R, Crowley J. Phase II clinical trial design for non-cytotoxic anticancer agents for which time to disease progression is the primary endpoint. Controlled Clin Trials 2000;21:343–359.

14. Freedman LS, White SJ, On the use of Pocock and Simon's method for balancing treatment numbers over prognostic factors in the controlled clinical trial. Biometrics 1976;32:691–694.

15. Committee for Proprietary Medicinal Products (CPMP). Points to consider on switching between superiority and non-inferiority, CPMP/EWP/482/9. 2000. Online. Available: www.emea.eu.int/pdfs/human/ewp/048299en.pdf.

16. Blackwelder W. Proving the null hypothesis in clinical trials. Controlled Clin Trials 1982;3:345–353.

17. Rothmann M, Li N, Chen G, Chi GY, Temple R, Tsou HH. Design and analysis of non-inferiority mortality trials in oncology. Stat Med 2003;22:239–264.

18. Freedman L. Tables of the number of patients required in clinical trials using the logrank test. Stat Med 1982;1:121–129.

19. Green S, Liu PY, O'Sullivan J. Factorial design considerations. J Clin Oncol 2002;20:3424–3430.

20. Kurth KH, Denis L, Bouffioux C, et al. Factors affecting recurrence and progression in superficial bladder tumors. Eur J Cancer 1995;31A:1840–1846.

21. Millan-Rodriguez F, Chechile-Toniolo G, Salvador-Bayarri J, Palou J, Algaba F, Vicente-Rodriquez J. Primary superficial bladder risk groups according to progression, mortality and recurrence. J Urol 2000;164:680–684.

22. Millan-Rodriguez F, Chechile-Toniolo G, Salvador-Bayarri J, Palou J, Vicente-Rodriquez J. Multivariate analysis of the prognostic factors of primary superficial bladder cancer. J Urol 2000;163:73–78.

23. van der Meijden A, Sylvester R, Collette L, Bono A, Ten Kate F. The role and impact of pathology review on stage and grade assessment of stages Ta and T1 bladder tumors: a combined analysis of 5 European Organisation for Research and Treatment of Cancer cancer trials. J Urol 2000;164:1533–1537.

24. Sylvester RJ, van der Meijden APM, Lamm DL. Intravesical bacillus Calmette–Guérin reduces the risk of progression in patients with superficial bladder cancer: a meta-analysis of the published results of randomized clinical trials. J Urol 2002;168:1964–1970.

25. Pawinski A, Sylvester R, Kurth KH, et al. A combined analysis of European Organisation for Research and Treatment of Cancer and Medical Research Council randomized clinical trials for the prophylactic treatment of stage Ta T1 bladder cancer. J Urol 1996;156:1934–1941.

26. Brausi M, Collette L, Kurth K, et al. Variability in the recurrence rate at first follow up cystoscopy after TUR in stage Ta T1 transitional cell carcinoma of the bladder: a combined analysis of seven EORTC studies. Eur Urol 2002;41:523–531.

27. Sylvester RJ, Oosterlinck W, van der Meijden APM. A single immediate postoperative instillation of chemotherapy decreases the risk of recurrence in patients with stage Ta T1 bladder cancer: a meta-analysis of published results of randomized clinical trials. J Urol 2004;171:2186–2190.

28. Jakse G, Algaba F, Malmstrom PU, Oosterlinck W. A second-look TUR in T1 transitional cell carcinoma: why ? Eur Urol 2004;45:539–546.

29. Advanced Bladder Cancer (ABC) Meta-Analysis Collaboration. Neoadjuvant chemotherapy in invasive bladder cancer: a systematic review and meta-analysis. Lancet 2003;361:1927–1934.

30. Sylvester R, Sternber C. The role of adjuvant combination chemotherapy after cystectomy in locally advanced bladder cancer: what we don't know and why. Ann Oncol 2000;11:851–856.

31. Bajorin D, Dodd P, Mazumdar M, et al. Long-term survival in metastatic transitional cell carcinoma and prognostic factors predicting outcome of therapy. J Clin Oncol 1999;17:3173–3181.

32. Sengelov L, Kamby C, von der Maase H. Metastatic urothelial cancer: evaluation of prognostic factors and change in prognosis during the last twenty years. Eur Urol 2001;39:634–642.

33. Kausch I, Bohle A. Molecular aspects of bladder cancer. III. Prognostic markers of bladder cancer. Eur Urol 2002;41:15–29.

34. Sternberg CN, de Mulder PHM, Schornagel JH, et al for the European Organisation for Research and Treatment of Cancer Genitourinary Tract Cancer Cooperative Group. Randomized phase III trial of high dose intensity methotrexate, vinblastine, doxorubicin, and cisplatin (MVAC) chemotherapy and recombinant human granulocyte colony stimulating factor versus classic MVAC in advanced urothelial tract tumors: European Organisation for Research and Treatment of Cancer protocol no. 30924. J Clin Oncol 2001;19:2638–2646.

35. von der Maase H, Hansen SW, Roberts JT, et al. Gemcitabine and cisplatin versus methotrexate, vinblastine, doxorubicin, and cisplatin in advanced or metastatic bladder cancer: results of a large, randomized, multinational, multicenter, phase III study. J Clin Oncol 2000;17:3068–3077.

# Neoadjuvant chemotherapy in the treatment of muscle-invasive bladder cancer

# 63

*Cora N Sternberg*

## INTRODUCTION

Bladder cancer is the second most common cancer of the genitourinary tract, with some 350,000 new cases worldwide,[1] in which one third are locally invasive or metastatic. There is a very high rate of early systemic dissemination. In patients with locally advanced bladder cancer infiltrating the musculature, 5-year survival is dependent upon pathologic stage, grade, and nodal status. As the stage advances, especially when there is cancer that extends outside of the bladder wall, the prognosis worsens. Local or metastatic failure is most often due to occult metastatic disease that was present at the time of initial diagnosis.

## CYSTECTOMY SERIES

Most physicians consider cystectomy as the gold standard of treatment for localized muscle-invasive bladder cancer. This idea has been fortressed by the widespread practice of performing orthotopic bladder substitutions. Five-year survival after cystectomy in major published series in patients with muscle-invasive bladder cancer (P2–4) from the University of Padua, Memorial Sloan-Kettering Cancer Center (MSKCC), and the University of Southern California varies from 36% to 48%.[2–5] High-risk patients with pathologic stage pT3–4 and/or pN+ M0 bladder cancer have the poorest 5-year survival which is somewhere between 25% and 35%.

## NEOADJUVANT CHEMOTHERAPY

### ADVANTAGES AND DISADVANTAGES

Neoadjuvant chemotherapy when given prior to cystectomy can reduce tumor volume, and can be effective in controlling metastatic disease when the volume of micrometastatic disease is small. Systemic chemotherapy is delivered early when the burden of metastatic disease is minimal. Patients may tolerate therapy better before they have received potentially debilitating local treatment with either surgery or radiation therapy (RT). Local therapy may also affect drug delivery by altering the blood supply to the tissues affected by the tumor.

Neoadjuvant chemotherapy was designed for patients with operable clinical stage cT2–4A muscle-invasive disease, and has been increasingly used with the intent of bladder preservation.[6] Neoadjuvant chemotherapy has the potential to deliver drugs at higher doses than in the adjuvant setting, and provides the opportunity to prospectively evaluate the response to chemotherapy. Toxicity is less than that seen in patients with metastatic disease, as subjects with localized disease usually have a better performance status.

Disadvantages to neoadjuvant chemotherapy are that patients treated with neoadjuvant chemotherapy are clinically staged which may lead to some difficulties in assessing response to therapy. A discrepancy between clinical and pathologic staging can be expected in some 30% of cases.[7,8] In addition, there is a delay in cystectomy or RT during the administration of neoadjuvant chemotherapy. This may be potentially harmful for those patients that do not respond to chemotherapy.

It is unknown whether three or four cycles of therapy are needed since this question has never been systematically evaluated. The mortality due to neoadjuvant chemotherapy can be assessed in two large cooperative group randomized trials. In the US Intergroup trial coordinated by the Southwest Oncology Group (SWOG), there were no deaths due to methotrexate, vinblastine, adriamycin, and cisplatin (MVAC) chemotherapy.[9] However, in the European Organisation for Research and Treatment of Cancer/Medical Research Council (EORTC/MRC) trial of neoadjuvant cisplatin, methotrexate, and vinblastine (CMV) chemotherapy, there was a 1% mortality rate due to CMV.[10]

## RANDOMIZED TRIALS

Neoadjuvant chemotherapy should theoretically have a similar benefit for patients whether they are definitively treated by cystectomy or by RT. In the US and in most of Europe, radical cystectomy is preferred for patients 70 years old or younger with a good performance status.

Several randomized trials, most of which have included cisplatin-based regimens, have been undertaken to investigate whether or not neoadjuvant chemotherapy improves survival. Older studies evaluated single agent cisplatin, but most recent trials have employed cisplatin-containing combination chemotherapy. These trials have been of modest size and have shown inconclusive results. Randomized trials in the literature can be found in Table 63.1.

Results from the Intergroup trial conducted by the SWOG have been published in the *New England Journal of Medicine*.[9] Patients with cT2–4A were randomized between three cycles of neoadjuvant MVAC chemotherapy and cystectomy or cystectomy alone. Enrolment took place over an 11-year period at 126 institutions. Patients were stratified according to age (<65 years or ≥65 years) and stage (cT2 versus cT3 or cT4A). Of the 317 patients entered, 307 were eligible; 82% in the MVAC group and 81% in the surgery group actually underwent the planned cystectomy.

Median survival was 77 months in patients that received neoadjuvant MVAC as compared to 46 months in patients that underwent cystectomy alone. The results when initially presented were not statistically significant. The results at present do not show a statistically significant improvement in overall survival (p=0.06, two-sided testing). However, the size of the study has only limited potential to discern a clinically meaningful difference and as such does not rule out the relevance of this approach. There was a trend towards improved survival in favor of MVAC-treated patients. The estimated risk of death was reduced by 25% (hazard ratio 1.33).[11]

An almost identical trial to the SWOG study was performed by an Italian cooperative group (GUONE). In this trial, 206 patients were randomized in a 6.5-year period to neoadjuvant MVAC prior to cystectomy versus cystectomy alone.[12] No clear difference in survival was demonstrated. In fact, 3-year survival was 62% for the MVAC-treated patients and 68% for the cystectomy alone arm.

The EORTC/MRC trial, performed at the same time as the SWOG trial, is the largest neoadjuvant randomized trial in the literature.[10] In this trial, 976 patients from 106 institutions were accrued over a shorter period (5.5 years) than in the SWOG trial. Patients with transitional cell bladder cancer <7 cm in size that were cT2 (G3), cT3,

**Table 63.1** Randomized phase III trials of neoadjuvant chemotherapy: study group neoadjuvant arm versus standard arm patients' survival

| Trial | Neoadjuvant arm | Standard arm | No. pts | Survival benefit |
|---|---|---|---|---|
| Aust/UK[66] | DDP/RT | RT | 255 | No difference |
| Canada/NCI[67] | DDP/RT or preop RT + Cyst | RT or preop RT + Cyst | 99 | No difference |
| Spain (CUETO)[68] | DDP/Cyst | Cyst | 121 | No difference |
| EORTC/MRC[10] | CMV/RT or Cyst | RT or Cyst | 976 | 5.5% difference in favor of CMV |
| SWOG Intergroup[11] | MVAC/Cyst | Cyst | 298 | Benefit with MVAC |
| Italy (GUONE)[12] | MVAC/Cyst | Cyst | 206 | No difference |
| Italy (GISTV)[69] | MVEC/Cyst | Cyst | 171 | No difference |
| Genoa[70] | DDP/5FU/RT/Cyst | Cyst | 104 | No difference |
| Nordic 1[14] | ADM/DDP/RT/Cyst | RT/Cyst | 311 | No difference, 15% benefit with ADM + DDP in T3–4a |
| Nordic 2[15] | MTX/DDP/Cyst | Cyst | 317 | No difference |
| Abol-Enein[71] | CarboMV/Cyst | Cyst | 194 | Benefit with CarboMV |

5FU, 5-fluorouracil; ADM, doxorubicin; CarboMV, carboplatin, methotrexate, vinblastine; CMV, cisplatin, methotrexate, vinblastine; Cyst, cystectomy; DDP or C, cisplatin; MTX, methotrexate; MVAC, methotrexate, vinblastine, adriamycin, cisplatin; MVEC, methotrexate, vinblastine, epirubicin, cisplatin; RT, cisplatin.

or cT4A, N0, NX, M0, were randomized between three cycles of neoadjuvant CMV chemotherapy and cystectomy or cystectomy alone. Definitive local therapy was left up to the choice of the investigators and included cystectomy and RT. When published in 1999, there was a nonsignificant trend towards improvement in survival in patients on the CMV arm.[10] In a 2002 ASCO update, with follow-up of 7.4 years, the data reached statistical significance (p=0.048). There was a 5.5% benefit in favor of patients treated with CMV chemotherapy.[13] Survival at 5 years was 50% compared to 44%, and at 8 years was 43% as opposed to 37% in the CMV arm. Although Hall concluded that there was no change in absolute benefit, patients treated with CMV had a consistent survival benefit that was maintained over time.

The Nordic Group, in their first randomized neoadjuvant trial, compared neoadjuvant adriamycin, cisplatin, and preoperative RT prior to cystectomy versus preoperative RT and cystectomy. In a subset analysis of patients with T3–4 disease, a 15% survival difference in favor of patients treated with chemoradiotherapy was seen.[14] These investigators were unable to confirm this survival advantage in a subsequent trial in which 317 patients were randomized between cystectomy or cystectomy preceded by methotrexate and cisplatin (without RT).[15] Nonetheless, when the two trials were combined in a subsequent analysis of 620 patients, the combined results were in favor of neoadjuvant chemotherapy.[16,17] The combined study results showed a hazard ratio (HR) of 0.80 (95% CI: 0.64–0.99) for overall survival in favor of neoadjuvant treatment. Survival was 56% at 5 years in the experimental group versus 48% in the control group, corresponding to an 8% absolute risk reduction after neoadjuvant chemotherapy. This was associated with a 20% reduction in the estimated risk of death.

What is the true value of neoadjuvant chemotherapy?[18] Although more than 3000 patients had been evaluated in neoadjuvant chemotherapy randomized trials, the real effect of neoadjuvant chemotherapy on survival was not clear. For this reason, two recent meta-analyses have combined the results of relevant randomized trials to obtain sufficient statistical power to reliably assess the value of neoadjuvant chemotherapy in invasive bladder cancer.[19,20]

The first meta-analysis was published by the MRC in *The Lancet*. Analysis of 10 neoadjuvant chemotherapy trials was performed, using individual patient data, which has many advantages in such an analysis.[21] Unfortunately, original data from the SWOG trial were not made available to the MRC.

Overall survival for the whole group and for a subgroup of patients treated with single agent cisplatin was not affected by neoadjuvant chemotherapy. In a subset of patients treated with cisplatin-containing combination chemotherapy, a 5% (p=0.17, 95% CI: 1–7%) difference in favor of neoadjuvant chemotherapy

was demonstrated. This reflected a change in survival from 45% to 50%, also consistent with a 1% to 7% difference in survival. The majority of patients were from the EORTC/MRC trial, and thus the results are similar to the results in that trial.

The second meta-analysis was performed in Canada.[22] This analysis did not include individual patient data, but rather obtained data from a thorough literature search and use of published meta-analyses. Sixteen eligible randomized clinical trials were identified. Trials that employed concomitant chemotherapy and radiotherapy were excluded. Of a potential 3315 patients, 2605 patients provided suitable data for the meta-analysis of overall survival. Eight trials used cisplatin-based combination chemotherapy and the pooled HR was 0.87 (95% CI: 0.78–0.96, p=0.006), consistent with an absolute overall survival benefit of 6.5% (95% CI: 2–11%) from 50% to 56.5%. Mortality due to combination chemotherapy was 1.1%.

A third meta-analysis included individual patient data from the SWOG trial. Based on 11 trials and 3005 patients a survival benefit was found with platinum-based neoadjuvant combination chemotherapy (HR=0.86, 95% CI 0.77–0.95, p=0.003); equivalent to a 5% absolute improvement in survival at 5 years. In addition, this was associated with a 9% absolute improvement in disease-free survival with combination chemotherapy (HR=0.78 95% CI 0.71–0.86, p <0.0001) at 5 years.[23]

It appears from these large meta-analyses of randomized trials that neoadjuvant cisplatin-based chemotherapy has some effect on improving overall survival in muscle-invasive bladder cancer, although the size of the effect is modest.

Combination chemotherapy can be administered safely without an adverse effect on the subsequent local therapy. These data are supported by the University of Texas M.D. Anderson Hospital trial of neoadjuvant and adjuvant MVAC chemotherapy,[24] the SWOG trial of neoadjuvant MVAC chemotherapy,[9] the EORTC/MRC trial of CMV neoadjuvant chemotherapy,[10] and our own data with neoadjuvant MVAC chemotherapy in Rome, Italy.[7]

Surgical factors were evaluated in 268 patients with muscle-invasive bladder cancer who underwent radical cystectomy in the SWOG Intergroup trial.[25] Cystectomies were performed by 106 surgeons in 109 institutions. Half of the patients received neoadjuvant MVAC. Five-year postcystectomy and local recurrence rates in all patients receiving cystectomy were 54% and 15%, respectively. Surgical variables associated with longer postcystectomy survival were negative margins (versus positive; HR, 0.37; p=0.0007), and ≥10 nodes removed (versus <10; HR, 0.51; p=0.0001). These associations did not differ by treatment arms (p>0.21 for all tests of interactions between treatment and surgical variables). Predictors of local recurrence were positive margins (versus negative; odds ratio [OR], 11.2;

p=0.0001) and <10 nodes removed (versus ≥10; OR, 5.1; p=0.002). The quality of surgery was an independent prognostic factor for outcome after adjustment for pathologic factors and neoadjuvant chemotherapy.

Available data suggest that for 'average risk' cT2 patients, there is at best a modest benefit of adding chemotherapy to definitive local therapy (cystectomy or RT). Likewise, available studies suggest a much more substantial benefit for patients with high-risk disease, such as cT3b cancers.

Newer agents are being introduced into the neoadjuvant setting. The SWOG is evaluating neoadjuvant gemcitabine, paclitaxel, and carboplatin followed by observation or immediate cystectomy. Molecular markers, recurrence rates, and cystectomy-free survival are evaluated. At this time, however, an optimal chemotherapy regimen has not been identified, and newer regimens have not been tested in the context of randomized controlled trials in the neoadjuvant setting. Efforts to identify the patients most likely to benefit from neoadjuvant therapy are necessary. Furthermore, in cases where there are small differences in survival it is unfortunate that there are few data available on quality of life.

## BLADDER PRESERVATION

Although mortality rates with radical cystectomy have decreased by half since the 1990s, survival rates with surgery alone have remained steady, with 5-year survival rates of 66% for pathologic stage T2, 35% for T3, and 27% for T4 disease.[2,3,9,26–37] In addition, up to 15% of patients with muscle-invasive disease will have no pathologic residual disease at the time of cystectomy, indicating the potential curability of select patients with transurethral resection of bladder tumor (TURBT) alone. The risk of clinical understaging in 30% to 50% of patients,[38–40] the limited effectiveness of surgery alone, and the advent of more effective combination chemotherapy has led to a multidisciplinary approach to bladder preservation.

Since the advent of orthotopic bladder substitutions, many urologists prefer early cystectomy with the creation of a continent urinary neobladder. Surgery alone will be successful in only a limited percentage of patients, and bladder preservation can be a viable option to radical cystectomy in selected patients. Bladder preservation influences quality of life as it means less surgery, no need for a urinary diversion, and normal sexual function. From phase II trials, bladder preservation may be possible in selected patients that respond to neoadjuvant chemotherapy.[7,41,42] The question is, can we preserve the bladder and achieve the same survival as with radical cystectomy?

TURBT plays an important role in multimodality bladder preservation strategies, and it is difficult to interpret the contribution to survival of each component in a multimodality bladder-sparing approach. As restaging TURBT has not been performed as standard practice in all combined modality series, it is hard to know the impact that TURBT alone may have had on survival in most series. One would expect patients that have been rendered clinical p0 by either TURBT alone or TURBT plus chemotherapy prior to radiation or cystectomy to have better long-term survival,[43] and this has been demonstrated in several prospective series.[41,44–48] Clinical factors in these studies associated with a better chance of a complete clinical response to TURBT alone or TURBT plus chemotherapy, and thus better survival, are clinical stage (organ-confined), tumor size less than 3–5 cm, no hydronephrosis, no palpable mass, and unifocal disease,[21,22,25–29,31–38,49] although this has not been prospectively verified in a randomized trial.

Response to chemotherapy is another important prognostic factor.[6,7,9,13] However, this too may reflect patient selection, as it is possible that patients that do well have characteristics that would make them survive longer whether or not they were treated with chemotherapy. In the SWOG trial, the pT0 rate in MVAC patients was 38% as compared to 15% for patients that underwent cystectomy alone (p<0.001). The pT0 rate after CMV in the EORTC/MRC trial was similarly 33%. Likewise, after two cycles of neoadjuvant MVAC chemotherapy, the pT0 rate was 40% in the M.D. Anderson trial of neoadjuvant and adjuvant versus adjuvant MVAC.[24] The Canadian meta-analysis found that a major pathologic response was associated with improved overall survival in four trials.[20] Improved survival has clearly been shown in patients that become pT0 at cystectomy. These may be the same patients that would benefit from a bladder-preservation strategy.

In Rome, 104 patients with clinical T2–4 N0 M0 of the bladder were treated with three cycles of neoadjuvant MVAC[7] followed by clinical restaging (computed tomography scan, TURBT, and biopsies). At the TURBT following MVAC, 49 (49%) patients were T0. Responding patients were placed in a bladder preservation protocol and underwent TURBT alone or partial cystectomy following chemotherapy. Of the 52 patients that underwent TURBT alone, 13 had a partial cystectomy, and 39 had a radical cystectomy. The median survival for the entire group was 7.49 years (95% CI: 4.86–10.0 years). Of the patients that had MVAC and TURBT alone, 60% were alive at a median follow-up of 56+ months (10–160+). Forty-four percent of the patients in this TURBT group maintained an intact bladder. Of the responding patients with monofocal lesions that underwent partial cystectomy, only one required salvage cystectomy, and 5-year survival was 69%.

Of note, in 77 patients that had downstaging to T0 or superficial disease, 5-year survival was 69%. This is in contrast to 5-year survival of only 26% in 27 patients that failed to respond and had muscle-invasive disease (T2 or greater) after chemotherapy. Additionally, the median survival for 27 elderly patients >70 years (median 73 years, range 70–82 years) was surprisingly long at 90 months (7.5 years). For elderly patients that underwent TURBT and partial cystectomy, 5-year survival was 67% with a median survival of 9 years; 47% preserved their bladders.

At MSKCC, 111 patients with T2–4 N0 M0 bladder cancer were treated with neoadjuvant MVAC. Downstaging was associated with improved survival. The 5-year survival rate was 54% for patients with downstaging versus 12% for those without downstaging.[50] Twenty-six patients underwent a partial cystectomy after neoadjuvant chemotherapy.[51] Of these 26 patients, 17 (65%) were alive beyond 5 years (median 6.9 years, range 4–8 years), including 14 (54%) with an intact, functioning bladder. Twelve patients (46%) developed bladder recurrences, which were invasive in five (19%) and superficial in seven (26%). Those patients without (p0) or noninvasive (pTis) tumor in their surgical specimens had a 5-year survival rate of 87%, compared with 30% in patients with residual invasive cancer.

Neoadjuvant MVAC chemotherapy permits bladder-sparing surgery in selected responding patients with invasive bladder cancer. The bladder remains at risk for new tumor development, but local recurrences can be treated successfully by local therapy or salvage cystectomy. Patients that undergo neoadjuvant chemotherapy and bladder preservation should be highly informed and willing to undergo frequent follow-up, multiple cystoscopies, and understand the possibility that cystectomy may become necessary.

## RADIATION THERAPY

Combining systemic chemotherapy with radiation therapy (RT) may preserve the bladder while sensitizing the tumor to radiation, while at the same time treating occult metastases. Trials of combined neoadjuvant chemotherapy and RT are shown in Table 63.2. This approach has been used in the Radiation Therapy Oncology Group (RTOG) at the Massachusetts General Hospital,[42] and by investigators in Erlangen and Paris.[52,53]

Most patients undergo TURBT, followed by chemoradiation. They then have a restaging TURBT, and consolidative RT is given to responding patients and nonresponders under cystectomy. Five-year survivals between 42% and 63%, with organ preservation in approximately 40% of patients, have been reported. Selection criteria for chemoradiation are similar to those which predict a good prognosis after cystectomy. Patients with small T2–3 lesions without hydronephrosis who undergo a thorough TURBT tend to have the best results. Although survival is similar to that in contemporary cystectomy series, the combined morbidity of chemotherapy and RT can be significant. As in the case of neoadjuvant chemotherapy alone, patients should be highly motivated to preserve their bladders and understand the possible side effects of combined therapy.

## BIOLOGIC AND MOLECULAR APPROACHES TO MUSCLE-INVASIVE BLADDER CANCER

Tumor formation and tumor progression are thought to result from an accumulation of several genetic alterations including the activation of oncogenes, loss of distinct chromosomal regions, and inactivation of tumor suppressor genes. Molecular markers are increasingly being used to predict survival and response to chemotherapy, with p53, pRb, and p21 being among the first evaluated as predictive markers in bladder cancer. In a landmark study, investigators at the

**Table 63.2** Trials of combined chemotherapy and radiotherapy

| Series | Year | No. pts | Chemotherapy | 5-year survival (%) | 5-year survival with intact bladder (%) |
|---|---|---|---|---|---|
| Radiation Therapy Oncology Group study 85-121[72] | 1993 | 42 | DDP | 52 | 42 |
| Radiation Therapy Oncology Group study 88-02[73] | 1996 | 91 | MCV + RT and DDP | 62* | 44 |
| Radiation Therapy Oncology Group study 89-03[74] | 1998 | 123 | MCV + RT and DDP | 48 | 36 |
| University of Erlangen[52,75] | 2001 | 199 | DDP, or Carbo | 52 | 41 |
| University of Paris[53,76] | 2001 | 120 | DDP/5FU | 63 | |
| Massachusetts General[77] | 2002 | 190 | MCV or DDP/5FU | 54 | 46 |

*Four-year survival data.
5FU, 5-fluorouracil; Carbo, carboplatin; DDP, cisplatin; MCV, methotrexate, cisplatin, vinblastine; RT, radiation therapy.

University of Southern California found that patients with altered p53 had a markedly higher chance of recurrence than patients that had normal p53.[54] Furthermore, patients with tumors expressing alterations in both p53 and pRb had significantly increased rates of recurrence and decreased survival compared to patients without alterations in pRb and p53.[55,56] Although these results have been questioned,[57,58] evaluation of these markers is important as molecular markers may be able to determine the outcome of patients with locally advanced bladder cancer.

At MSKCC, p53 status was evaluated in 60 (54%) patients that had a complete clinical response (T0) to MVAC chemotherapy. Ten-year outcome was recorded and patients were stratified by p53 status, stage of the primary tumor (T2 versus T3), and type of surgery (bladder sparing versus cystectomy).[59] These authors showed that in patients with stage T2 tumors that lacked detectable p53 and obtained a response to neoadjuvant chemotherapy, the bladder could be preserved for up to 10 years.

In a Spanish study, 82 patients with invasive bladder cancer treated on three different bladder-sparing studies were evaluated by immunohistochemistry (IHC) for p53, p21, and pRB expression.[60] Immunoreactivity for p53, p21, and pRB was observed in 47%, 52%, and 67% of patients, respectively. When combined expression of p53 and p21 was assessed, positive expression of both markers was a strong and unfavorable prognostic factor for survival for bladder preservation (p=0.006), disease-free survival (p=0.003), and overall survival (p=0.02). The authors concluded that, when simultaneously assessed, expression levels of p53 and p21 exhibited independent predictive value for long-term bladder preservation and survival in their patients treated with combined-modality therapy, and may be useful in selecting candidates for bladder-preserving treatments.

Two other recent studies have elucidated the role of these molecular markers in bladder cancer. At Baylor College of Medicine, IHC staining for p53, p21, pRB, and p16 was done on archival specimens from 80 patients that underwent bilateral pelvic lymphadenectomy and radical cystectomy for bladder cancer. The median follow-up was 101 months.[61] Alteration of each of the markers was independently associated with disease progression and disease-specific survival. When combined with pathologic prognostic factors such as lymph node positivity, the number of altered markers was associated with an increased risk of bladder cancer progression and mortality. P53 was the strongest molecular marker in this study, followed by p21, suggesting a more important role of the p53/p21 pathway in bladder cancer progression.

Another study from the University of Southern California sought to determine the predictive value of altered expression patterns of p53, p21, and pRb on progression of bladder cancer. P53, p21, and pRb expression was examined on archival radical cystectomy samples from 164 patients with invasive or high-grade recurrent superficial transitional cell carcinoma. The median follow-up was 8.6 years. Examined in combination after stratifying by stage, the authors concluded that the number of altered proteins significantly correlated with both time to progression and overall survival. This study again confirms that patients with bladder tumors with alterations in p53, p21, and pRb protein products are at high risk of recurrence and death.[62]

Other important markers such as BCL2, a protein fundamental in preventing apoptosis, are increasingly making their way into the clinic. In a small study from the UK, overexpression of BCL2 in patients receiving synchronous chemoradiotherapy was an independent indicator of poor survival in muscle-invasive bladder cancer.[63]

Most recently, microarray technology has permitted the study of expression of thousands of genes in tumor tissue. The new paradigm of treatment tailored to the individual patient could be realized in the very near future in bladder cancer patients where there are many opportunities to readily obtain tumor samples for microarray studies. Molecular profiling of samples should enable us to study the microevolution of tumors, to tailor existing treatment options, and to introduce new biologicals into the clinic.[64]

## CONCLUSION

For muscle-invasive bladder cancer, neoadjuvant chemotherapy followed by radical cystectomy has become one of the new standards of care. Molecular prognostication is now being incorporated into the design of clinical trials. The p53 phenotype seems to be the most important molecular predictive factor for bladder cancer outcome and death in patients that undergo radical cystectomy. Determinations of molecular pathways are likely to become useful in the selection of candidates for bladder-preserving treatments. Clinical protocols based on the integration of conventional clinical and anatomic information with molecular approaches, such as the University of Southern California international adjuvant p53 trial, should be supported.[65]

## REFERENCES

1. Parkin DM, Pisani P, Ferlay J. Global cancer statistics. CA Cancer J Clin 1999;49(81):33–64.
2. Stein JP, Lieskovsky G, Cote R, et al. Radical cystectomy in the treatment of invasive bladder cancer: long-term results in 1,054 patients. J Clin Oncol 2001;19(3):666–675.
3. Dalbagni G, Genega E, Hashibe M, et al. Cystectomy for bladder cancer: a contemporary series. J Urol 2001;165(4):1111–1116.

4. Bassi P, Ferrante GD, Piazza N, et al. Prognostic factors of outcome after radical cystectomy for bladder cancer: a retrospective study of a homogeneous patient cohort. J Urol 1999;161(5):1494–1497.

5. Ghoneim MA, el-Mekresh MM, el-Baz MA, el-Attar IA, Ashamallah A. Radical cystectomy for carcinoma of the bladder: critical evaluation of the results in 1,026 cases. J Urol 1997;158(2):393–399.

6. Sternberg CN. Current perspectives in muscle-invasive bladder cancer. Eur J Cancer 2002;38(4):460–467.

7. Sternberg CN, Pansadoro V, Calabrò F, et al. Can patient selection for bladder preservation be based on response to chemotherapy? Cancer 2003;97(7):1644–1652.

8. Herr HW, Scher HI. Surgery of invasive bladder cancer: is pathologic staging necessary? Semin Oncol 1990;17:590–597.

9. Grossman HB, Natale RB, Tangen CM, et al. Neoadjuvant chemotherapy plus cystectomy compared with cystectomy alone for locally advanced bladder cancer. N Engl J Med 2003;349(9):859–866.

10. International Collaboration of Trialists. Neoadjuvant cisplatin, methotrexate, and vinblastine chemotherapy for muscle-invasive bladder cancer: a randomised controlled trial. Lancet 1999;354(9178):533–540.

11. Grossman HB, Natale RB, Tangen CM, et al. Errata Corrige for: 'Neoadjuvant chemotherapy plus cystectomy compared with cystectomy alone for locally advanced bladder cancer' published in N Engl J Med 2003;349(9):859–866. N Engl J Med 2003;349(9):1880.

12. Bassi P, Pagano F, Pappagallo G, et al. Neoadjuvant M-VAC of invasive bladder cancer: The G.U.O.N.E. multicenter phase III trial. Eur Urol 1998;33(Suppl 1):142.

13. Hall RR. Updated results of a randomised controlled trial of neoadjuvant cisplatin (C), methotrexate (M) and vinblastine (V) chemotherapy for muscle-invasive bladder cancer. International Collaboration of Trialists of the MRC Advanced Bladder Cancer Group. Proc Annu Meet Am Soc Clin Oncol 2002;21(1):178a.

14. Malmstrom PU, Rintala E, Wahlqvist R, Hellstrom P, Hellsten S, Hannisdal E. Five year follow-up of a prospective trial of radical cystectomy and neoadjuvant chemotherapy. J Urol 1996;155:1903–1906.

15. Sherif A, Rintala E, Mestad O, et al. Neoadjuvant cisplatin–methotrexate chemotherapy of invasive bladder cancer—Nordic cystectomy trial 2. Scand J Urol Nephrol 2002;36(6):419–425.

16. Sherif A, Rintala E, Mestad O, Nilsson J, Holmberg L, Nilsson S, Malmstrom PU. Neoadjuvant platinum based combination chemotherapy improves overall survival in patients with locally advanced bladder cancer. A meta-analysis of two Nordic collaborative studies of 620 patients. J Urol 2003;169:307.

17. Sherif A, Holmberg L, Rintala E, et al. Neoadjuvant cisplatinum based combination chemotherapy in patients with invasive bladder cancer: a combined analysis of two Nordic studies. Nordic Urothelial Cancer Group. Eur Urol 2004;45(3):297–303.

18. Sternberg CN, Parmar MKB. Neoadjuvant chemotherapy is not (yet) standard treatment for muscle-invasive bladder cancer. J Clin Oncol 2001;19(Suppl 1):21S–26S.

19. Advanced Bladder Cancer Meta-analysis Collaboration. Neoadjuvant chemotherapy in invasive bladder cancer: a systematic review and meta-analysis. Lancet 2003;361:1927–1934.

20. Winquist E, Kirchner TS, Segal R, Chin J, Lukka H. Genitourinary Cancer Disease Site Group of Cancer Care Ontario Program in Evidence-based Care Practice Guidelines Initiative. Neoadjuvant chemotherapy for transitional cell carcinoma of the bladder: a systematic review and meta-analysis. J Urol 2004;171(2):561–569.

21. Stewart LA, Clarke M. Practical methodology of meta-analyses (overviews) using updated individual patient data. Cochrane Working Group. Stat Med 2004;124(19):2057–2079.

22. Winquist E, Kirchner TS, Segal R, Chin J, Lukka H. Neoadjuvant chemotherapy for transitional cell carcinoma of the bladder: a systematic review and meta-analysis. Genitourinary Cancer Disease Site Group, Cancer Care Ontario Program in Evidence-based Care Practice Guidelines Initiative. J Urol 2004;171(2 Pt 1):561–569.

23. Advanced Bladder Cancer (ABC) Meta-analysis Collaboration. Neoadjuvant Chemotherapy in Invasive Bladder Cancer: Update of a Systematic Review and Meta-Analysis of Individual Patient Data. European Urology; 2005;48:202–206.

24. Millikan R, Dinney C, Swanson D, et al. Integrated therapy for locally advanced bladder cancer: final report of a randomized trial of cystectomy plus adjuvant M-VAC versus cystectomy with both preoperative and postoperative M-VAC. J Clin Oncol 2001;19:4005–4013.

25. Herr HW, Faulkner JR, Grossman HB, et al. Surgical factors influence bladder cancer outcomes: a cooperative group report. J Clin Oncol 2004; 22(14):2781–2789.

26. Ritchie JP, Skinner DG, Kaufman JJ. Radical cystectomy for carcinoma of the bladder: 16 years of experience. J Urol 1975;113:186–189.

27. Bredael JJ, Croker BP, Glenn JF. The curability of invasive bladder cancer treated by radical cystectomy. Eur Urol 1980;6:206–208.

28. Mathur VK, Krahn HP, Ramsey EW. Total cystectomy for bladder cancer. J Urol 1981;125:784–786.

29. Skinner DG, Lieskovsky G. Contemporary cystectomy with pelvic node dissection compared to preoperative radiation therapy plus cystectomy in the management of invasive bladder cancer. J Urol 1984;131:1069–1072.

30. Montie JE, Straffon RA, Stewart BH. Radical cystectomy without radiation therapy for carcinoma of the bladder. J Urol 1984;131:477–482.

31. Giuliani L, Gilberti C, Martorrama G. Results of radical cystectomy for primary bladder cancer. Urology 1985;26(3):243–245.

32. Roehrborn CG, Sagalowsky AI, Peters PC. Long-term patient survival after cystectomy for regional metastatic transitional cell carcinoma of the bladder. J Urol 1991;146:36–39.

33. Pagano F, Bassi P, Galetti TP, et al. Results of contemporary radical cystectomy for invasive bladder cancer: a clinicopathological study with an emphasis on the inadequacy of the tumor, nodes and metastases classification. J Urol 1991;145:45–50.

34. Wishnow KI, Tenney DM. Will Rogers and the results of radical cystectomy for invasive bladder cancer. Urol Clin North Am 1991;18:529–537.

35. Waehre H, Ous S, Klevmark B, et al. A bladder cancer multi-institutional experience with total cystectomy for muscle-invasive bladder cancer. Cancer 1993;72(10):3044–3051.

36. Vieweg J, Gschwend JE, Herr HW, et al. The impact of primary stage on survival in patients with lymph node positive bladder cancer. J Urol 1999;161(1):72–76.

37. Mardersbacher S, Hochreiter W, Burkhard F, et al. Radical cystectomy for bladder cancer today—a homogenous series without neoadjuvant therapy. J Clin Oncol 2003;21(4):690–696.

38. Frazier HA, Robertson JE, Dodge RK, Paulson DF. The value of pathologic factors in predicting cancer-specific survival among patients treated with radical cystectomy for transitional cell carcinoma of the bladder and prostate. Cancer 1993;71:3993–4001.

39. Amling CL, Thrasher JB, Frazier HA, Dodge RK, Robertson JE, Paulson DF. Radical cystectomy for stages Ta, Tis and T1 transitional cell carcinoma of the bladder. J Urol 1994;151(1):31–35.

40. Stein JP. Indications for early cystectomy. Semin Urol Oncol 2000;18:289–295.

41. Herr HW, Bajorin DF, Scher HI. Neoadjuvant chemotherapy and bladder sparing surgery for invasive bladder cancer: ten-year outcome. J Clin Oncol 1998;16(4):1298–1301.

42. Shipley WU, Kaufman DS, Tester WJ, et al. Overview of bladder cancer trials in the Radiation Therapy Oncology Group. Cancer 2003;97(8 Suppl):2115–2119.

43. Herr HW. Uncertainty and outcome of invasive bladder tumors. Urol Oncol 1996;2:92–95.

44. Hall RR, Newling DW, Ramsden PD, Richards B, Robinson MR, Smith PH. Treatment of invasive bladder cancer by local resection and high dose methotrexate. B J Urol 1984;56:668–672.

45. Thomas DJ, Roberts JT, Hall RR, Reading J. Radical transurethral resection and chemotherapy in the treatment of muscle-invasive bladder cancer: a long-term follow-up. Br J Urol 1999;83:432–437.

46. Angulo JC, Sanchez-Chapado M, Lopez JI, Flores N. Primary cisplatin, methotrexate and vinblastine aiming at bladder preservation in invasive bladder cancer: multivariate analysis on prognostic factors. J Urol 1996;155(6):1897–1902.

47. Sternberg CN, Pansadoro V, Calabrò F, et al. Neoadjuvant chemotherapy and bladder preservation in locally advanced transitional cell carcinoma of the bladder. Ann Oncol 1999;10(11):1301–1305.

48. De la Rosa F, Garcia-Carbonero R, Passas J, Rosino A, Lianes P, Paz-Ares L. Primary cisplatin, methotrexate and vinblastine chemotherapy with selective bladder preservation for muscle-invasive carcinoma of the bladder: long-term followup of a prospective study. J Urol 2002;167:2413–2418.

49. Montie JE, Stratton RA, Stewart BH. Radical cystectomy without radiation therapy for carcinoma of the bladder. J Urol 1984;131:477–482.

50. Schultz PK, Herr HW, Zhang Z. Neoadjuvant chemotherapy for invasive bladder cancer: prognostic factors for survival of patients with M-VAC with 5 years follow-up. J Clin Oncol 1994;12(7):1394–1401.

51. Herr HW, Scher HI. Neoadjuvant chemotherapy and partial cystectomy for invasive bladder cancer. J Clin Oncol 1994;12(5):975–980.

52. Sauer R, Birkenhake S, Kühn R, et al. Muscle-invasive bladder cancer: transurethral resection and radiochemotherapy as an organ-sparing treatment option. In Petrovich Z, Baert L, Brady LW (eds): Carcinoma of the Bladder. New York: Springer, 1998, pp 205–214.

53. Housset M, Dufour B, Maulard-Durdux C, Chretien Y, Mejean A. Concomitant fluorouracil (5-FU)-cisplatin (CDDP) and bifractionated split course radiation therapy (BSCRT) for invasive bladder cancer. Proc Am Soc Clin Oncol 1997;16:319A.

54. Esrig D, Elmajian D, Groshen S, et al. Accumulation of nuclear p53 and tumor progression in bladder. N Engl J Med 1994;331(19):1259–1264.

55. Cote RJ, Esrig D, Groshen S, Jones PA, Skinner DG. p53 and treatment of bladder cancer. Nature 1997;385(6612):123–125.

56. Cote RJ, Dunn MD, Chatterjee SJ, et al. Elevated and absent pRb expression is associated with bladder cancer progression and has cooperative effects with p53. Cancer Res 1998;58(6):1090–1094.

57. Williams SG, Gandour-Edwards R, Deitch AD, et al. Differences in gene expression in muscle-invasive bladder cancer: a comparison of Italian and American patients. Eur Urol 2001;39(4):430–437.

58. McShane LM, Aamodt R, Cordon-Cardo C, et al. Reproducibility of p53 immunohistochemistry in bladder tumors. National Cancer Institute, Bladder Tumor Marker Network. Clin Cancer Res 2000;6(5):1854–1864.

59. Herr HW, Bajorin DF, Scher HI, Cordon-Cardo C, Reuter VE. Can p53 help select patients with invasive bladder cancer for bladder preservation? J Urol 1999;161(1):20–22.

60. Garcia del Muro X, Condom E, Vigues F, et al. p53 and p21 Expression levels predict organ preservation and survival in invasive bladder carcinoma treated with a combined-modality approach. Cancer 2004;100(9)1859–1867.

61. Shariat SF, Tokunaga H, Zhou J, et al. p53, p21, pRB, and p16 expression predict clinical outcome in cystectomy with bladder cancer. J Clin Oncol 2004;22(6):1014–1024.

62. Chatterjee SJ, Datar R, Youssefzadeh D, et al. Combined effects of p53, p21, and pRb expression in the progression of bladder transitional cell carcinoma. J Clin Oncol 2004;22(6):1007–1013.

63. Hussain SA, Ganesan R, Hiller L, et al. BCL2 expression predicts survival in patients receiving synchronous chemoradiotherapy in advanced transitional cell carcinoma of the bladder. Oncol Rep 2003;10(3):571–576.

64. Nawrocki S, Skacel T, Brodowicz T. From microarrays to new therapeutic approaches in bladder cancer. Pharmacogenomics 2003;4(2):179–189.

65. Cordon-Cardo C. p53 and RB: simple interesting correlates or tumor markers of critical predictive nature? J Clin Oncol 2004;22(6):975–977.

66. Wallace DM, Raghavan D, Kelly KA, et al. Neoadjuvant (pre-emptive) cisplatin therapy in invasive transitional cell carcinoma of the bladder. Br J Urol 1991;67:608–615.

67. Coppin CM, Gospodarowicz MK, James K, et al. Improved local control of invasive bladder cancer by concurrent cisplatin and preoperative or definitive radiation. The National Cancer Institute of Canada Clinical Trials Group. J Clin Oncol 1996;14(11):2901–2907.

68. Martinez Pineiro JA, Gonzalez Martin M, Arocena F. Neoadjuvant cisplatin chemotherapy before radical cystectomy in invasive transitional cell carcinoma of the bladder: prospective randomized phase III study. J Urol 1995;153:964–973.

69. GISTV (Italian Bladder Cancer Study Group). Neoadjuvant treatment for locally advanced bladder cancer: a randomized prospective clinical trial. J Chemother 1996;8:345–346.

70. Orsatti M, Curotto A, Canobbio L. Alternating chemo-radiotherapy in bladder cancer: a conservative approach. Int J Radiat Oncol Biol Phys 1995;33:173–178.

71. Abol-Enein H, El-Makresh M, El-Baz M, Ghoneim M. Neoadjuvant chemotherapy in treatment of invasive transitional bladder cancer: a controlled, prospective randomised study. Br J Urol 1997;80(Suppl 2):49.

72. Tester W, Porter A, Asbell S. Combined modality program with possible organ preservation for invasive bladder carcinoma: results of RTOG protocol 85-12. Int J Radiat Oncol Biol Phys 1993;25:783–790.

73. Tester W, Caplan R, Heaney J. Neoadjuvant combined modality program with selective organ preservation for invasive bladder cancer: results of Radiation Therapy Oncology Group phase II trial 88-02. J Clin Oncol 1996;14(1):119–126.

74. Shipley WU, Winter KA, Kaufman DS, et al. Phase III trial of neoadjuvant chemotherapy in patients with invasive bladder cancer treated with selective bladder preservation by combined radiation therapy and chemotherapy: initial results of Radiation Therapy Oncology Group 89-03. J Clin Oncol 1998;16(11):3576–3583.

75. Sauer R, Rodel C. Biological selection for organ conservation. Eur J Cancer 2001;37(Suppl 6):S286.

76. Durdux C, Housset M, Dufour B. Altered fractionation in chemoradiation for bladder cancer. Eur J Cancer 2001;37(Suppl 6):S286.

77. Shipley WU, Kaufman DS, Zehr E, et al. Selective bladder preservation by combined modality protocol treatment: long-term outcomes of 190 patients with invasive bladder cancer. Urology 2002;60(1):62–67.

# Adjuvant chemotherapy for invasive bladder cancer

# 64

*James O Jin, Michelle Boyar, Daniel P Petrylak, Walter M Stadler*

## INTRODUCTION

Approximately 15% to 20% of patients with bladder cancer presenting with locally invasive disease and 10% to 25% of patients with superficial disease will eventually develop muscle invasion. As discussed elsewhere in this book, the standard and most common definitive treatment for invasive bladder cancer is radical cystectomy. The 5-year disease-free survival rate is 50% to 80% for patients with muscle-invasive disease (pT2) and 20% to 50% for those with nonorgan-confined cancers (pT3–4).[1–8] For patients with node-positive disease, the 5-year disease-free survival rate is 7% to 36%.[2–8] Patients with metastatic bladder cancer can be treated with multiagent chemotherapy, with high objective response rates and improved survival, but long-term (>5 year) survival is unusual.[9–11] Improved long-term survival has been demonstrated with adjuvant chemotherapy in other solid tumors, such as breast and colon cancer, in which high response rates with cytotoxic chemotherapy are observed in the metastatic setting. This is likely due to a greater sensitivity to chemotherapy of micrometastases present in patients destined for clinical metastatic disease than to the larger tumors present once metastatic disease is diagnosed.

The use of perioperative chemotherapy to improve survival for patients with locally advanced bladder cancer is thus theoretically attractive. Randomized data from trials utilizing neoadjuvant chemotherapy, as discussed in Chapter 63, lend further support to this concept. Unfortunately, these data suggest that the absolute survival advantage with neoadjuvant chemotherapy is only 10%. The value of exposing all patients to the toxicity of combination chemotherapy

for such a modest effect is debatable. A major challenge is thus to identify patients most likely to benefit from perioperative chemotherapy as well as those that will not benefit and can at least avoid the chemotherapy toxicities.

In this context, adjuvant chemotherapy offers several advantages. First, definitive local therapy, for the large fraction of patients not benefiting from chemotherapy, is not delayed. There is some evidence that delay of cystectomy is clinically important.[12,13] Second, clinical staging of locally advanced bladder cancer is notoriously inaccurate (see Chapter 21), and cystectomy provides the definitive pathologic stage. This in turn provides the most useful information for the risk of recurrence. Under a traditional paradigm, patients with the highest risk of recurrence can then be offered chemotherapy.

It is important to recognize that offering chemotherapy to patients at the highest risk of recurrence is logical if the relative benefit of chemotherapy is the same in all patients. In other words, if chemotherapy provides a 30% improvement in relative survival, this translates into an improvement in absolute survival of 90% to 93% or 50% to 65%. Clinical studies of cytotoxic therapy in breast and colon cancer suggest that such an assumption is reasonable. On the other hand, it would be preferable to administer adjuvant chemotherapy only to patients whose tumors are sensitive to the chosen regimen. The improvements in understanding the molecular biology of bladder cancer and its therapeutic implications suggest that selection of patients for chemotherapy based on molecular markers may soon become a reality. In this context, adjuvant chemotherapy offers a further advantage over neoadjuvant therapy in that the heterogeneity of small specimens obtained by transurethral resection (TUR) is overcome by large pathologic specimens obtained at cystectomy. Thus, the molecular phenotypes of these patients can be more accurately assessed.

## COMPLETED CLINICAL TRIALS

Logothetis et al at the University of Texas M.D. Anderson Cancer Center first suggested a benefit for adjuvant chemotherapy in a retrospective study in 1988.[14] The study showed that cyclophosphamide, doxorubicin, and cisplatin (CISCA) chemotherapy prolonged the disease-free survival in patients with high-risk, invasive bladder cancer following cystectomy. Seventy-one patients with resected nodal metastases, extravesicular involvement of tumor, lymphatic/vascular permeation of the primary tumor, or pelvic visceral invasion received adjuvant CISCA chemotherapy. Sixty-two patients at a similar high risk for recurrence did not receive adjuvant CISCA chemotherapy because they refused, had medical contraindications, or were not referred for chemotherapy. An additional 206 patients that had none of these high-risk factors were not given adjuvant chemotherapy during the same study period. The 5-year disease-free survival was significantly better for high-risk patients that received adjuvant chemotherapy compared to those that did not (7% versus 37%, p=0.00012), and was very similar to that of the low-risk patients (70%, p=0.33). Although the findings are provocative, it is well recognized that multiple biases are introduced when patients and/or their physicians choose to undergo a potentially toxic therapy. In such a nonrandomized trial, it is unclear whether the differences in survival are due to the treatment received or to the selection process.

Since the 1990s, five randomized trials have been reported comparing adjuvant chemotherapy to observation after cystectomy (Table 64.1).[15-19] Skinner et al at the University of Southern California reported the first randomized trial in 1991.[15] Ninety-one patients with pT–4 or N+M0 transitional cell carcinoma (TCC) of the bladder were randomly assigned to four cycles of cisplatin, doxorubicin, and cyclophosphamide (CAP) or observation after radical cystectomy. This study demonstrated a significant 3-year disease-free survival (70% versus 46%, p= 0.0062) and median survival (4.4 versus 2.2 years, p=0.0010) advantage for the adjuvant chemotherapy arm. This study has been heavily criticized for problems in its statistical design, as well as treatment employed. Only a small number of patients (91 of a total 498 eligible patients) were enrolled in the trial. This led to a small sample size, which rendered the study underpowered to detect any significant difference in survival. This once again raises the issue of bias in patient and physician selection and whether the results are applicable to the more general locally advanced bladder cancer population.

The statistical methodology used in this study has also been scrutinized, particularly the use of Wilcoxon statistics, which give more weight to early differences in survival. Although the authors report that all three nodal subgroups had a benefit from chemotherapy, closer analysis of patients with two or more nodes involved suggests that this particular subgroup fared worse than the observation group. The authors have also been criticized for drawing conclusions from subgroup analyses.

The chemotherapeutic regimen administered in the Skinner trial was not uniform. During the initial 3 years of the study, 17 patients received individualized chemotherapy based on a clonogenic assay, and 16 patients received cisplatin either as monotherapy or in combination with doxorubicin, cyclophosphamide, fluorouracil, vinblastine and bleomycin. Of the 44 patients randomized to chemotherapy, 11 subsequently elected not to be treated and 33 received one or more courses of chemotherapy.

Despite these inconsistencies, this was the first randomized clinical trial that suggested a role of adjuvant chemotherapy for invasive bladder cancer after radical cystectomy. The authors updated their results in 2001 after a median follow-up of 14 years.[20] There was a continued improvement in time-to-recurrence and survival in the chemotherapy group, although the

**Table 64.1** Randomized trials of adjuvant chemotherapy

| Investigator | Accrual year | No. pts | Chemotherapy | Survival benefit |
|---|---|---|---|---|
| Skinner et al[15] | 1980–1988 | 91 | CAP | Yes |
| Stockle et al[16] | 1987–1991 | 49 | MVAC or MEVC | Yes |
| Studer et al[18] | 1984–1989 | 77 | C | No |
| Bono et al[19] | 1984–1987 | 83 | CM | No |
| Freiha et al[17] | 1986–1993 | 50 | CMV | In relapse-free survival but not in overall survival |

C, cisplatin; CAP, cyclophosphamide, doxorubicin, cisplatin; CM, cisplatin, methotrexate; CMV, cisplatin, methotrexate, vinblastine; MVAC, methotrexate, vinblastine, doxorubicin, cisplatin; MVEC, methotrexate, vinblastine, epirubicin, cisplatin.

difference in overall survival was not statistically significant. Data were also analyzed from 1054 patients at the University of Southern California treated with radical cystectomy, of which 255 (24%) received systemic chemotherapy either in the adjuvant or neoadjuvant setting in a nonrandomized fashion. Although the data were not presented, the investigators reported that only those patients with lymph node-positive disease had a significant benefit from adjuvant chemotherapy in terms of recurrence-free and overall survival.

The second randomized trial to assess the potential benefits of adjuvant chemotherapy following cystectomy was reported by Stockle et al at the University of Mainz, Germany, in 1992.[16] The initial design of this study was to recruit 100 patients powered to detect a 35% improvement in the recurrence-free survival. Forty-nine patients with pT3B, PT4A, and/or pelvic lymph node involvement of TCC were initially enrolled and randomly assigned to observation or three cycles of methotrexate, vinblastine, and cisplatin plus either doxorubicin (MVAC) or epirubicin (MVEC) after radical cystectomy. This is the only randomized trial using a standard MVAC-type regimen. Interim analysis revealed a dramatic improvement in 3-year disease-free survival in the adjuvant chemotherapy arm (63% versus 13%, p=0.0015). The study also demonstrated the significant survival benefit in patients with node-positive disease. A survival benefit in the entire randomized population was demonstrated in later publications.[21] The trial was terminated prematurely after the results of interim analysis. Unfortunately, the early termination and small trial size mean that there remains a significant risk for lack of balance between the two arms for important but unmeasured prognostic factors. In addition, patients in the observation arm that developed metastatic disease were not offered chemotherapy. As such, this trial is inadequate to definitively demonstrate the survival benefit of adjuvant chemotherapy in the context of how these patients are treated today.

Freiha et al at Stanford University published data in 1996 from another small randomized trial of 50 patients with pT3–4 or node-positive TCC who received four cycles of cisplatin, methotrexate, and vinblastine (CMV) after cystectomy or cystectomy alone.[17] The adjuvant chemotherapy group had superior disease-free survival (median 37 versus 12 months, p=0.01). However, the study was terminated prematurely because of poor accrual and the significant disease-free survival found at the first interim analysis. Not surprisingly given the small study, an overall survival benefit was not observed.

Two other small, randomized trials failed to show a survival benefit from adjuvant chemotherapy[18,19] (see Table 64.1). However, the majority of patients enrolled in these studies had organ-confined disease (N0). Given the better baseline prognosis, the power to detect a

statistically significant survival benefit of adjuvant chemotherapy requires a larger number of patients. In addition, the chemotherapy regimen(s) used in these studies were considered less effective.

## METHODOLOGIC PROBLEMS IN ADJUVANT TRIALS

Three of the randomized studies suggest that adjuvant chemotherapy improves disease-free survival; however, interpretation of the data is difficult due to several methodologic problems common to these early trials.[15–17] These design problems are summarized below.

### SAMPLE SIZE

In contrast to adjuvant chemotherapy trials performed in breast and colon cancer enrolling thousands of patients, small sample sizes and poor accrual rates have been a consistent problem in bladder cancer trials. Each of the randomized controlled trials of adjuvant chemotherapy following cystectomy reported to date has enrolled fewer than 100 patients. None of these studies was adequately powered to detect a small survival advantage in favor of adjuvant chemotherapy. A study designed to detect an improvement in 2-year survival of at least 10% (from 50% to 60%) would require an enrollment of 1000 patients. If the treatment effect to be detected is smaller, an even larger sample size is needed.

Several factors contribute to the poor accrual rates for bladder cancer trials. For example, bladder cancer is a less common entity than colon or breast cancer, making it difficult to enroll a large number of patients with muscle-invasive bladder cancer. In addition, patients that develop bladder cancer often have significant comorbid conditions related to age, smoking, and complications of the disease or local treatment, which can limit the administration and type of chemotherapy.

### TREATMENT REGIMEN

The published adjuvant treatment trials used a variety of chemotherapeutic regimens, most of which are no longer utilized for bladder cancer. Only one trial used MVAC, which has been shown to be more effective for metastatic bladder cancer than single-agent cisplatin or CISCA.[22,23] MVAC toxicity nevertheless remains a concern and may be one of the reasons that previous adjuvant trials have suffered from poor accrual. Gemcitabine, paclitaxel, and docetaxel all have promising single-agent activity in advanced TCC of the bladder.[24-32] The combination of gemcitabine and cisplatin has also been compared to MVAC in a phase III randomized trial.[33] Four hundred and five patients were randomly assigned to up to six cycles of gemcitabine and cisplatin or to MVAC. A similar response rate (49% versus 46%) and median survival (13.8 versus 14.8 months), but with fewer infectious complications and less mucositis, were observed in the gemcitabine and cisplatin arm. The trial was designed to detect a 20% improvement in survival, but the sample size was insufficient to detect true therapeutic equivalence. Although the lower toxicity of gemcitabine/cisplatin and the palliative nature of metastatic bladder cancer treatment has led to gemcitabine/cisplatin being accepted as a standard therapy in the metastatic setting, the lack of data for therapeutic equivalence, and the lack of data on gemcitabine/cisplatin in the adjuvant setting, make the use of this regimen in the adjuvant setting controversial.

Baseline renal insufficiency can limit the use of cisplatin in the adjuvant setting. This has led many practitioners to recommend or use taxanes and/or carboplatin, both of which can be administered more easily and safely in the setting of renal insufficiency.[34] The therapeutic equivalence of carboplatin compared to cisplatin remained a significant question. A randomized trial by the Hellenic Cooperative Oncology Group demonstrated improved toxicity of gemcitabine/carboplatin compared to gemcitabine/cisplatin, at the cost of a lower complete response rate in gemcitabine/carboplatin-treated patients.[35] A randomized trial of docetaxel/cisplatin versus MVAC in the metastatic setting demonstrated inferiority of the taxane regimen.[36] Thus, the use of carboplatin or taxane-based doublet therapy should be used in clinical trials, or if the patient is medically unfit to receive cisplatin-based therapy.

## PELVIC LYMPH NODE DISSECTION

Early studies of bladder cancer treated with total cystectomy found a significant decrease in local recurrence when pelvic lymphadenectomy was included.[2] The observation that pelvic nodal metastases could occur in the absence of distant metastatic spread further supported the rationale for including pelvic lymphadenectomy at the time of radical cystectomy, since the procedure can be curative for patients with a small volume of nodal disease. Retrospective studies have shown long-term survival of patients with grossly node-positive disease after pelvic lymph node dissection and radical cystectomy.[37] Bilateral pelvic iliac node dissection with en bloc radical and urinary diversion has been performed by Skinner and colleagues since 1971 on all patients undergoing radical cystectomy with the intent to cure. Preoperative clinical staging is often inaccurate, so a significant number of patients that appear to have localized tumors will have positive lymph nodes. Lymphadenectomy also enables accurate staging. Surgical technique, especially in regard to lymphadenectomy, introduces another variable into clinical trials of adjuvant chemotherapy. In the four randomized controlled trials, information regarding the technique used for lymphadenectomy is given in trials by Skinner[15] and Studer,[18] but no details are given in the Stockle[16] or Freiha[17] trials.

## TIMING OF ADJUVANT THERAPY

The timing of chemotherapy is another variable that can affect outcome in an adjuvant therapy trial. In the Skinner trial,[15] chemotherapy began 6 weeks after cystectomy; the Studer trial[18] started chemotherapy within 8 weeks after cystectomy; Stockle and Freiha did not report when chemotherapy commenced.[16,17] Starting therapy too quickly after cystectomy can lead to poor tolerance of the treatment regimen with subsequent treatment delays and dose reductions, which may affect the overall outcome. Conversely, starting adjuvant therapy too late may abrogate some of the theoretical advantages to adjuvant treatment.

## ONGOING ADJUVANT CLINICAL TRIALS

In order to address the deficits in previously published trials of adjuvant chemotherapy for bladder cancer, the European Organisation for Research and Treatment of Cancer (EORTC) has launched a large randomized clinical trial in which 660 patients with extravesical (pT3–4) or node-positive TCC will be randomly assigned either to immediate chemotherapy or to chemotherapy at the time of relapse. Given the above discussion on chemotherapy options, each participating institution can choose amongst MVAC, high-dose MVAC, or gemcitabine/cisplatin as the chemotherapeutic regimen to be used.

The Cancer and Leukemia Group B (CALGB), in collaboration with the Eastern Cooperative Oncology Group (ECOG), have taken a somewhat different approach. Taking into account both the reluctance of patients and physicians to participate in a 'no treatment' versus 'potentially toxic treatment' randomized study and the highly suggestive data noted above, these investigators have chosen to accept adjuvant therapy as the standard arm and a more aggressive approach as the experimental arm. The experimental arm is based on the Norton–Simon hypothesis in which a chemotherapy program of rapidly cycling sequential regimens is proposed to be more efficacious than a standard scheduled single regimen. Thus, 800 patients with extravesical (pT3–4) or node-positive TCC will be randomly assigned either to doxorubicin/gemcitabine followed by paclitaxel/cisplatin (sequenced doublet therapy), or to gemcitabine/cisplatin (conventional doublet therapy) after cystectomy. The choice of gemcitabine/cisplatin as the conventional arm was based on similar survival but less toxicity in a randomized trial versus MVAC in the metastatic setting. The sequential regimen is based on promising phase II data from investigators at the Memorial Sloan-Kettering Cancer Institute, who reported a much higher complete response to this regimen in the metastatic setting than expected in historical controls.

The final ongoing adjuvant study utilizes data on the molecular biology of bladder cancer. A number of studies have demonstrated that altered expression of p53, p21, pRB, and p16 act in cooperative or synergistic ways to promote bladder cancer progression.[38,39] Of these, p53 has been found to be the most consistent and strongest prognostic indicator[38] (see also Chapter 9). More importantly, investigators at the University of Southern California, using retrospective data from their randomized trial of adjuvant CISCA,[15] strongly suggested that patients with bladder tumors carrying p53 alterations are more likely to benefit from adjuvant chemotherapy than are patients with bladder tumors carrying a wild-type p53.[40] These observations have been supported by a number of laboratory studies, which demonstrate that p53 mutations confer sensitivity to DNA damaging agents such as cisplatin. These studies raise the intriguing possibility that p53 mutations not only define a population at high risk of recurrence, but also a population most likely to benefit from cisplatin-containing chemotherapy.

Thus, a multicenter, international randomized clinical trial testing this hypothesis has been initiated. Patients with organ-confined bladder cancers that carry a wild-type p53 have an overall good prognosis, with an estimated 5-year disease-free survival of 90%, and will be observed. Patients with organ-confined bladder cancer that carry an altered p53 have an approximately 40% 5-year disease-free survival and are predicted to benefit from chemotherapy.[41] Patients with p53 alterations will be randomly assigned to three cycles of MVAC or observation following their cystectomy. If this study is positive, it will define a molecularly-targeted therapy and usher in a new paradigm for bladder cancer treatment.

## CONCLUSION

Despite the methodologic flaws of the early trials of adjuvant chemotherapy for bladder cancer, the combination of chemotherapy and surgery in high-risk patients does appear to confer a survival advantage, and many physicians are administering adjuvant chemotherapy outside a protocol setting for patients with a high risk of recurrence.[42,43] However, the role of adjuvant chemotherapy still needs to be clearly defined. The three large multicenter-randomized trials should further define the role of adjuvant chemotherapy in the management of muscle-invasive bladder cancer. Thus, patients should be encouraged to enter in these studies.

REFERENCES

1. Wishnow KI, Levinson AK, Johnson DE, et al. Stage B (P2/3 A/N0) transitional cell carcinoma of bladder highly curable by radical cystectomy. Urology 1992;39:12–16.

2. Lerner SP, Skinner DG, Lieskovsky G, et al. The rationale for en bloc pelvic lymph node dissection for bladder cancer patients with nodal metastases: long-term results. J Urol 1993;149:758–764.

3. LaPlante M, Brice M III. The upper limits of hopeful application of radical cystectomy for vesical carcinoma: does nodal metastasis always indicate incurability? J Urol 1973;109:261–264.

4. Dretler SP, Ragsdale BD, Leadbetter WF. The value of pelvic lymphadenectomy in the surgical treatment of bladder cancer. J Urol 1973;109:414–416.

5. Smith JA Jr, Whitmore WF Jr. Regional lymph node metastasis from bladder cancer. J Urol 1981;126:591–593.

6. Skinner DG, Tift JP, Kaufman JJ. High dose, short course preoperative radiation therapy and immediate single stage radical cystectomy with pelvic node dissection in the management of bladder cancer. J Urol 1982;127:671–674.

7. Pagano F, Bassi P, Galetti TP, et al. Results of contemporary radical cystectomy for invasive bladder cancer: a clinicopathological study with an emphasis on the inadequacy of the tumor, nodes and metastases classification. J Urol 1991;145(1):45–50.

8. Schoenberg MP, Walsh PC, Breazeale DR, et al. Local recurrence and survival following nerve sparing radical cystoprostatectomy for bladder cancer: 10-year follow-up. J Urol 1996;155(2):490–494.

9. Loehrer P, Einhorn LH, Elson PJ, et al. A randomized comparison of cisplatin alone or in combination with methotrexate, vinblastine, and doxorubicin in patients with metastatic urothelial carcinoma: a Cooperative Group Study. J Clin Oncol 1992;10:1066–1073.

10. Sternberg CN, Yagoda A, Scher HI, et al. Methotrexate, vinblastine, doxorubicin and cisplatinum for advanced transitional cell carcinoma of the urothelium: efficacy and patterns of response and relapse. Cancer 1989;64:2448–2458.

11. Harker WG, Meyers FJ, Freiha FS, et al. Cisplatin, methotrexate, and vinblastine (CMV): an effective chemotherapy regimen for metastatic transitional cell carcinoma of the urinary tract. A Northern California Oncology Group study. J Clin Oncol 1985;3:1463–1470.

12. Chang SS, Hassan JM, Cookson MS, et al. Delaying radical cystectomy for muscle invasive bladder cancer results in worse pathological stage. J Urol 2003;170:1085–1087.

13. Sanchez-Ortiz RF, Huang WC, Mick R, et al. An interval longer than 12 weeks between the diagnosis of muscle invasion and cystectomy is associated with worse outcome in bladder carcinoma. J Urol 2003;169(1):110–115.

14. Logothetis C, Johnson D, Chong C, et al. Adjuvant cyclophosphamide, doxorubicin, and cisplatin chemotherapy for bladder cancer: an update. J Clin Oncol 1988;6:1590–1596.

15. Skinner DG, Daniels JR, Russell CA, et al. The role of adjuvant chemotherapy following cystectomy for invasive bladder cancer: a prospective comparative trial. J Urol 1991;145:459–464.

16. Stockle M, Meyenburg W, Wellek S, et al. Advanced bladder cancer (stages pT3b, pT4a, pN1 and pN2): improved survival after radical cystectomy and 3 adjuvant cycles of chemotherapy. Results of a controlled prospective study. J Urol 1992;148:302–306.

17. Freiha F, Reese J, Torti F. A randomized trial of radical cystectomy versus radical cystectomy plus cisplatin, vinblastine and methotrexate chemotherapy for muscle-invasive bladder cancer. J Urol 1996;155:495–499.

18. Studer U, Bacchi M, Biederman C, et al. Adjuvant cisplatin chemotherapy following cystectomy for bladder cancer: results of a prospective randomized trial. J Urol 1994;152:81–84.

19. Bono AV, Benvenuti C, Reali L, et al. Adjuvant chemotherapy in advanced bladder cancer. Italian Uro-Oncologic Cooperative Group. Prog Clin Biol Res 1989;303:533–540.

20. Stein JP, Lieskovsky G, Cote R, et al. Radical cystectomy in the treatment of invasive bladder cancer: long-term results in 1,054 patients. J Clin Oncol 2001;19(3):666–675.

21. Stockle M, Meyenburg W, Wellek S, et al. Adjuvant polychemotherapy of nonorgan-confined bladder cancer after radical cystectomy revisited: long-term results of a controlled prospective study and further clinical experience. J Urol 1995;153:47–52.

22. Loehrer PJ Sr, Einhorn LH, Elson PJ, et al. A randomized comparison of cisplatin alone or in combination with methotrexate, vinblastine, and doxorubicin in patients with metastatic urothelial carcinoma: a cooperative group study. J Clin Oncol 1992;10(7):1066–1073.

23. Logothetis CJ, Dexeus FH, Finn L, et al. A prospective randomized trial comparing MVAC and CISCA chemotherapy for patients with metastatic urothelial tumors. J Clin Oncol 1990;8(6):1050–1055.

24. Lorusso V, Pollera CF, Antimi M, et al. A phase II study of gemcitabine in patients with transitional cell carcinoma of the urinary tract previously treated with platinum. Italian Co-operative Group on Bladder Cancer. Eur J Cancer 1998;34:1208–1212.

25. Moore MJ, Tannock IF, Ernst DS, et al. Gemcitabine: a promising new agent in the treatment of advanced urothelial cancer. J Clin Oncol 1997;15:3441–3445.

26. Stadler WM, Kuzel T, Roth B, et al. Phase II study of single-agent gemcitabine in previously untreated patients with metastatic urothelial cancer. J Clin Oncol 1997;15:3394–3398.

27. Pollera CF, Ceribelli A, Crecco M, Calabresi F. Weekly gemcitabine in advanced bladder cancer: a preliminary report from a phase I study. Ann Oncol 1994;5:182–184.

28. Gebbia V, Testa A, Borsellino N, et al. Single agent 2′,2′-difluorodeoxycytidine in the treatment of metastatic urothelial carcinoma: a phase II study. Clin Ter 1999;150:11–15.

29. Roth BJ, Dreicer R, Einhorn LH, et al. Significant activity of paclitaxel in advanced transitional-cell carcinoma of the urothelium: a phase II trial of the Eastern Cooperative Oncology Group. J Clin Oncol 1994;12:2264–2270.

30. Dreicer R, Gustin DM, See WA, Williams RD. Paclitaxel in advanced urothelial carcinoma: its role in patients with renal insufficiency and as salvage therapy. J Urol 1996;156:1606–1608.

31. McCaffrey JA, Hilton S, Mazumdar M, et al. Phase II trial of docetaxel in patients with advanced or metastatic transitional-cell carcinoma. J Clin Oncol 1997;15(5):1853–1857.

32. de Wit R, Kruit WH, Stoter G, et al. Docetaxel (Taxotere): an active agent in metastatic urothelial cancer: results of a phase II study in non-chemotherapy-pretreated patients. Br J Cancer 1998;78:1342–1345.

33. von der Masse H, Hansen SW, Roberts JT, et al. Gemcitabine and cisplatin versus methotrexate, vinblastine, doxorubicin, and cisplatin in advanced or metastatic bladder cancer: results of a large, randomized, multinational, multicenter, phase III study. J Clin Oncol 2000;18:306–377.

34. Bamias A, Deliveliotis Ch, Aravantinos G, et al. Hellenic Cooperative Oncology Group. Adjuvant chemotherapy with paclitaxel and carboplatin in patients with advanced bladder cancer: a study by the Hellenic Cooperative Oncology Group. J Urol. 2004;171(4):1467–1470.

35. Carteni G, Dogliotti L, Crucitta E, et al. Phase II randomised trial of gemcitabine plus cisplatin and gemcitabine plus carboplatin in patients with advanced or metastatic transitional cell carcinoma of the urothelium [abstract]. Proc Am Soc Clin Oncol 2003;22:384, Abstract 1543.

36. Bamias A, Aravantinos G, Bafaloukos D, et al. Docetaxel plus cisplatin versus MVAC in advanced urothelial carcinoma: a multicenter, randomized phase III study conducted by the Hellenic Cooperative Oncology Group [abstract]. Proc Am Soc Clin Oncol 2003;22:384, Abstract 1541.

37. Herr HW, Donat SM. Outcome of patients with grossly node positive bladder cancer after pelvic lymph node dissection and radical cystectomy. J Urol 2001;16562–64.

38. Chatterjee SJ, Datar R, Youssefzadeh D, et al. Combined effects of p53, p21, and pRb expression in the progression of bladder transitional cell carcinoma. J Clin Oncol 2004;22(6):1007–1013.

39. Shariat SF, Tokunaga H, Zhou J, et al. p53, p21, pRB, and p16 expression predict clinical outcome in cystectomy with bladder cancer. J Clin Oncol 2004;22(6):1014–1024.

40. Cote R, Esrig D, Groshen S, et al. p53 and the treatment of bladder cancer. Nature 1997;385:123–125.

41. Esrig D, Elmajian D, Groshen S, et al. Accumulation of nuclear p53 and tumor progression in bladder cancer. N Engl J Med 1994;331(19):1259–1264.

42. Crawford ED, Wood DP, Petrylak DP, et al. Southwest Oncology Group studies in bladder cancer. Cancer 2003;97(Suppl 8):2099–2108.

43. Small EJ, Halabi S, Dalbagni G, et al. Overview of bladder cancer trials in the cancer and leukemia Group B. Cancer 2003;97(Suppl 8):2090–2098.

# Treatment of metastatic cancer

65

*Avishay Sella, Joaqim Bellmunt*

## INTRODUCTION

Transitional cell carcinoma (TCC) of the bladder is the fifth most common solid malignancy in the United States. It is diagnosed in approximately 57,400 patients and results in more than 12,500 deaths annually.[1] The standard treatment for invasive bladder cancer is radical cystectomy, whereas patients with metastatic or locally advanced urothelial cancer are usually treated with systemic chemotherapy. Notable advances have been developed during the last 20 years in the chemotherapeutic management of patients with advanced urothelial tumors.

## SINGLE AGENTS AND MVAC ERA

Studies in the 1970s identified the chemosensitivity of urothelial cancer to several agents: cisplatin, methotrexate, adriamycin, vinblastine, and 5-fluorouracil (5FU) were shown to be the most active.[2] Although these earlier trials led to a response rate of only 10% to 30% when used in monotherapy and with limited duration of responses, they established the foundation for combination chemotherapeutic trials which characterized the 1980s.[3] These trials were mainly cisplatin-based combination regimens such as cisplatin/methotrexate/vinblastine (CMV), cisplatin/adriamycin/cyclophosphamide (CISCA), and methotrexate/vinblastine/adriamycin/cisplatin (MVAC).[4-6] These combinations were reported initially as single-institution phase II studies with objective response rates as high as 65% to 75%, with approximately 20% to 35% of cases achieving complete remission (CR), and

median survival periods increasing from 3–4 months to 12–14 months.[3-7]

As a consequence, it became apparent that cisplatin was an essential component of combination chemotherapy regimens for patients with adequate renal function. A randomized study conducted in the UK comparing methotrexate and vinblastine (MV) with CMV demonstrated an absolute improvement in 1-year survival of 13% with the treatment containing cisplatin (29% for CMV and 16% for MV). The median survival for CMV was significantly longer than that for MV: 7 months compared with 4.5 months.[8] This study demonstrated the significant survival impact of cisplatin and has helped to justify the routine use of cisplatin-based combination chemotherapy. In addition, as more experience was gained with MVAC, it emerged as the preferred cisplatin-based combination therapy (Table 65.1).[9-13] In randomized trials, MVAC produced a modest, though significant, survival benefit when compared with cisplatin as a single agent, CISCA, or carboplatin-based regimens.[11,13,14] The tumor origin did not have an impact on response to MVAC.[2] Patients with CR appeared to gain survival benefits, and prognosis for those with nodal disease appeared more favorable.[2,9] Patients with nontransitional-cell histology and poor performance status had a poor prognosis and were unlikely to benefit significantly from MVAC chemotherapy.[15] In addition, long-term survival was low, with only 3.7% of patients experiencing more than 6 years of disease-free survival.[9,11-15]

Due to the toxicity that was reported with MVAC, with up to 25% incidence of neutropenic fever, 50% grade 2–3 stomatitis, and 3% drug-related mortality, the incorporation of granulocyte colony-stimulating factor (G-CSF) or granulocyte-macrophage colony-stimulating

**Table 65.1** Early global experience with MVAC

| Lead author | No. pts | Response rate (%) | Complete response (%) | Median survival (months) |
|---|---|---|---|---|
| Sternberg[9] | 121 | 72 | 36 | 13.4 |
| Tannock[10] | 30 | 40 | 13 | 10.0 |
| Logothetis[11] | 55 | 65 | 35 | 11.0 |
| Boutan-Laroze[12] | 67 | 57 | 57 | 13.0 |
| Loehrer[13] | 120 | 38 | 38 | 12.5 |

factor (GM-CSF) was added to the schedule. This was done both in an effort to reduce toxicity and to increase the dose density of the combination since, in the majority of patients, cycles were delivered every 5 weeks instead of every 4 weeks.[9-13] With the simultaneous use of G-CSF or GM-CSF, these toxicities can be reduced, allowing more patients to receive the dose originally planned in the conventional MVAC treatment, and even an intensified MVAC schedule. Unfortunately, dose intensification of the MVAC regimen has not translated into a clinical benefit in terms of improved survival.[16-22] A recent phase III study by the European Organisation for Research and Treatment of Cancer (EORTC), comparing classical MVAC to a high dose (HD) MVAC regimen every 2 weeks with G-CSF support, revealed significant differences in terms of complete response and overall response rates in favor of the HD-MVAC arm (25% and 72%, respectively), compared with the standard MVAC arm (11% and 58%, respectively). However, there was no statistically significant difference between the two treatment arms in terms of the primary endpoint: overall survival with a median survival of 15.5 months for the HD-MVAC arm and 14.1 months for the standard MVAC arm.[23]

The dismal long-term survival with the classical MVAC combination has led to the search for new treatment approaches aiming to improve outcome and treatment tolerance. Throughout the years, many phase III trials have evaluated new combinations, such as gemcitabine/cisplatin, carboplatin/paclitaxel, docetaxel/cisplatin, and interferon-$\alpha$/5-fluorouracil/cisplatin. Unfortunately, in all of these randomized trials, the new regimens have failed to demonstrate superiority in terms

of overall survival when compared with the classical MVAC.[22,24-26]

The experience of using MVAC chemotherapy has enabled the establishment of several prognostic factors that predict the benefits of chemotherapy. Investigators from the Memorial Sloan-Kettering Cancer Center (MSKCC) determined that two factors had an independent prognosis: Karnofsky performance status (KPS) less than 80%, and visceral (lung, liver, or bone) metastasis. Three risk categories were established on the basis of KPS and the presence or absence of visceral metastases. Median survival times for patients who had zero, one, or two risk factors were 33, 13.4, and 9.3 months, respectively ($p=0.0001$) (Table 65.2). Based on these data, it is clearly demonstrated that the median survival time of patient cohorts could vary from 9 to 26 months simply by altering the proportion of patients from different risk categories. This explains the divergent reported outcomes reported from different trials. Similar findings regarding prognostic factors, risk categories, and survival have been seen when using the triple combination of paclitaxel/cisplatin/gemcitabine reported by the Spanish Group (SOGUG).[27,28]

# NEW ACTIVE AGENTS AND COMBINATIONS: SINGLE AGENTS AND DOUBLETS

The efforts to improve the outcome of patients with metastatic TCC have focused on the identification of new drugs with single-agent activity and on their

**Table 65.2** Risk factors in metastatic bladder cancer

| No. risk factors | MVAC<br>Median survival<br>(months) | Paclitaxel/gemcitabine/cisplatin<br>Median survival<br>(months) |
|---|---|---|
| 0 | 33.0 | 32.8 |
| 1 | 13.4 | 18.0 |
| 2 | 9.3 | 10.6 |

Risk factors: Presence of visceral metastases, Karnofsky performance status <80%.

incorporation into platinum-based combination regimens.

## Paclitaxel

Paclitaxel emerged initially as one of the effective single-agent drugs (Table 65.3).[29–34] The paclitaxel/carboplatin combination rapidly found its way into routine clinical practice because of its modest toxicity profile.[29–34] However, a randomized phase III study comparing the doublet with MVAC, conducted by the Eastern Cooperative Oncology Group (ECOG), was closed prematurely due to poor accrual when the limited efficacy of the doublet paclitaxel/carboplatin seen in several phase II trials became apparent.[25] It is not possible to interpret the results of this study because it failed to reach its accrual goal.

## Gemcitabine

Gemcitabine also revealed activity in locally advanced and metastatic urothelial cell cancer. Complete responses were noted even in patients previously treated with cisplatin.[35–38] In view of the synergistic effects between cisplatin and gemcitabine and the mild toxicity profile of gemcitabine, the two-drug combination of gemcitabine and cisplatin was soon evaluated.[39] Initial studies produced results similar to those with MVAC (Table 65.4).[35–42] Based on these results, a large randomized trial in which the MVAC regimen was compared with the

combination of gemcitabine and cisplatin (GC), both delivered every 4 weeks, was conducted. The study was designed to demonstrate a 4-month improvement in survival benefit with GC. The two treatment arms turned out to be very similar in terms of median survival (13.8 months for GC and 14.8 months for MVAC ), time to progression (7.4 months in both arms), and overall response rate (46% and 49%, respectively). Fewer patients on GC than on MVAC had grade 3/4 neutropenia (71% versus 82%, respectively), neutropenic fever (2% versus 14%), grade 3/4 mucositis (1% versus 22%), and hospital admissions (9 admissions for a total of 33 days versus 49 admissions for a total of 272 days). The toxic death rate was 1% with GC and 3% with MVAC. More GC than MVAC patients had grade 3/4 anemia and thrombocytopenia. One limitation of this large randomized study was that the better safety and tolerability of GC was not reflected in the quality of life (QoL) results.[43] Although this trial was not designed to show the equivalence of the two regimens, many researchers have interpreted the results as showing therapeutic noninferiority and determined that any difference in survival was unlikely to be sufficiently large to offset the improvement in toxicity with GC.[26]

In an attempt to improve the thrombocytopenic toxicity profile of GC which occurred around day 15, small phase II trials have evaluated a 3-week program of GC in which cisplatin is given either concomitantly on

**Table 65.3** Paclitaxel in advanced urothelial cancer

| Lead author | Year | Other therapy | Taxol (mg/m²) | Response rate (%) | Prior therapy |
|---|---|---|---|---|---|
| Iu[29] | 1995 | Methotrexate, cisplatin | 200 + G-CSF | 40 | Yes |
| Roth[30] | 1994 | Ifosfamide | 250 + G-CSF | 42 | No |
| Sweeney[31] | 1999 | Ifosfamide | 135 + G-CSF | 23 | Yes |
| Vaughn[32] | 1997 | Carboplatin | 200 | 64 | No |
| Zielinski[33] | 1998 | Carboplatin | 175 | 65 | No |
| Redman[34] | 1998 | Carboplatin | 200 | 52 | No |

G-CSF, granulocyte colony-stimulating factor.

**Table 65.4** Gemcitabine in advanced urothelial cancer

| Lead author | Year | Prior therapy | Response rate (%) | Gemcitabine (mg/m²) weekly × 3 q 4 weeks | Cisplatin (mg/m²) |
|---|---|---|---|---|---|
| Pollera[35] | 1994 | Yes | 27 | Above 1000 | |
| Stadler[36] | 1997 | No | 28 | 1200 | |
| Moore[37] | 1997 | No | 24 | 1200 | |
| Lorusso[38] | 1998 | Yes | 23 | 1200 | |
| Von der Masse[40] | 1999 | No | 42 | 1000 | 35 |
| Moore[41] | 1999 | No | 57 | 1000 | 70 |
| Kaufman[42] | 2000 | No | 41 | 1000 | 100, 75 |

day 1, or fractionated, and gemcitabine on days 1 and 8, recycling on day 21. This alteration did not modify the response rate. The indications of a better toxicity profile and fewer treatment delays will have to be confirmed in larger trials.[44,45]

## Docetaxel

Docetaxel has demonstrated activity in chemotherapy naive patients (31% response rate) and previously treated patients (13.3% response rate).[46,47] Although phase II studies of two-drug combinations of docetaxel with cisplatin (DC) have shown activity in untreated patients with response rates that are similar to MVAC, a recent randomized study reported by the Hellenic Group has shown inferior activity of the cisplatin/docetaxel combination compared to classical MVAC. Although this study was designed to detect a survival advantage for DC, the investigators instead observed that survival was inferior for patients treated with DC. Because performance status was not used in this trial as a prospective stratification variable, the treatment arms were not appropriately balanced. After adjusting for prognostic factors, difference in time to progression (TTP) remained significant (hazard ratio [HR] 1.61, p=0.005), whereas the survival difference was nonsignificant at the 5% level (HR 1.31, p=0.089).[22]

## Gallium nitrate and Ifosfamide

Gallium nitrate has activity as a single agent in the treatment of advanced bladder cancer, including activity in heavily pretreated patients. Partial responses were observed in 4 of 23 patients (17.4%) that received 350 $mg/m^2$/d or more for 5 days by continuous intravenous infusion.[48] Likewise, ifosfamide was evaluated in previously treated patients in whom it produced a 20% objective response rate. However, administration of ifosfamide at 1500 $mg/m^2$ with MESNA 750 $mg/m^2$/d for 5 days every 3 weeks resulted in significant renal and central nervous system toxicity.[49] The clinical activity obtained by combining ifosfamide with etoposide (14% response rate), paclitaxel (15% response rate in previously treated patients, 30.7% response rate in chemotherapy-naive patients), CMV (62.5% response rate), or vinblastine/gallium (44% response rate) is not justified in view of the significant toxicity.[50-53] To date, doublet ifosfamide-based regimens have no role in the routine therapy of advanced urothelial tumors.

## Carboplatin

Carboplatin exerted limited clinical activity as a single agent.[54] Carboplatin-based combinations were reported in the 1990s. The combination of carboplatin with methotrexate and vinblastine (carbo-MV and M-CAVI) have shown response rates of 30% to 40% and a median survival of 8–10 months. These results are inferior to those obtained with MVAC. Two underpowered,

randomized studies also suggested that carboplatin-based chemotherapy had suboptimal efficacy.[55,56] Similarly, cisplatin also seems to be more effective than carboplatin when combined with gemcitabine. In another underpowered randomized phase II trial, a response rate of 66% was achieved in patients treated with cisplatin/gemcitabine as compared with a response rate of only 35% with carboplatin/gemcitabine.[57]

## Lobaplatin and oxaliplatin

Lobaplatin, a third-generation platinum complex, demonstrated a 10% response rate in previously treated patients.[58] Oxaliplatin monotherapy has shown minimal activity in previously treated patients, but it is feasible to combine this with gemcitabine, with encouraging preliminary data in patients unfit for cisplatin.[59-61]

## Antifolate compounds

With regard to antifolate compounds, de Wit et al reported a response rate of 17% for trimetrexate in patients who had received prior chemotherapy.[62] Piritrexim, an oral second-generation antimetabolite, was tested in two studies. As a single agent in chemotherapy-naive patients, it demonstrated a 38% response rate, whereas in previously treated patients, partial response (PR) was obtained only at a rate of 23%.[63] This compound is now being evaluated with gemcitabine.[64]

Pemetrexed, a novel multitargeted antifolate (MTA) that inhibits multiple folate-dependent enzymes, achieved a 33% response rate in 22 chemonaive patients; however, there were two drug-related deaths.[65] It was also active in previously treated patients. A recent phase II trial as second line therapy (including relapses after adjuvant or neoadjuvant therapy) achieved an overall response rate of 27.7% (13 out of 47), with three patients obtaining CR. Of the responders, six were enrolled with prior adjuvant therapy within 12 months. Overall survival was 9.8 months.[66] A confirmatory second line trial is now planned.

## Vinflunine

Vinflunine is a new synthetically designed vinca alkaloid that has been recently studied in second line bladder cancer after platinum failure. Due to the reported activity of 16% response rate and a median survival of 6 months, a phase III second line multinational trial is presently ongoing, comparing this drug with best supportive care followed by treatment upon progression.[67,68]

## Irinotecan

Witte et al reported a response rate of 10% with irinotecan in patients that had previously received chemotherapy.[69] This agent is now being studied with gemcitabine in a phase II trial and as a single agent in the regimens of patients previously treated with a platinum-containing agent (Southwest Oncology Group).[70]

## NONPLATINUM-BASED REGIMENS

Both gemcitabine and the taxanes have been extensively evaluated in single-drug studies. In view of their toxicity profile, particularly the lack of nephrotoxicity, it is not surprising that multiple studies have been performed with this combination (Table 65.5).[71-79] Response ranges from 0% to 60% have been reported. This variability reflects diversity in patient prognostic factors and the effect of prior chemotherapy—lower responses when the combination was given for active disease, and higher when the combination was given after an adjuvant/neoadjuvant approach.[71-73,76-78]

## UNFIT PATIENTS

Most of the phase II and large phase III trials include patients with normal renal function and good performance status. Unfortunately, since this disease may interfere with kidney function, and often involves the elderly, many patients do not 'fit' with these good criteria.

Various strategies have been considered to avoid this problem, including modulation of cisplatin's nephrotoxicity by using nephroprotective agents, modifying the scheduling of cisplatin, using less cisplatin-intense regimens, or substituting carboplatin for cisplatin.[80] The emergence of active nontoxic agents enabled the design of other approaches for these patients. The ECOG reported on a 20.6% response rate with the combination of paclitaxel/carboplatin.[81] With gemcitabine-based regimens the response rates were gemcitabine/epirubicin, 46%; gemcitabine/vinorelbine, 47.6%; and gemcitabine/carboplatin, 44%.[82-84] This later trial was a dose-finding study with the combination of gemcitabine and carboplatin, and it was evaluated in clearly predefined 'unfit' bladder cancer patients: performance status >2 and/or creatinine clearance less than 60 ml/min. Using this combination, investigators reported a median time survival of 14.4 months in the 16 patients that were ineligible for a cisplatin-based regimen ('unfit' patient population). The preliminary results found on this phase II trial using the carboplatin/gemcitabine doublet prompted an EORTC randomized phase II/III trial (EORTC protocol 30986) comparing carboplatin/gemcitabine with M-CAVI in patients ineligible for cisplatin-based chemotherapy. This trial is presently ongoing.

It is important to mention that chronologic age should not exclude patients from the potential benefit of conventional cisplatin-based therapy, because elderly patients with adequate renal function tolerate conventional platinum-based chemotherapy as well as younger patients and may benefit equally.[85,86]

**Table 65.5** Gemcitabine/taxanes combination therapy in urothelial cancer

| Lead author | Gemcitabine | Paclitaxe | Docetaxel | Pts with prior therapy | No. pts | Response rate (%) | Median survival (months) |
|---|---|---|---|---|---|---|---|
| Sternberg[71] | 2000–3000 D 1 q 14 days | 150 D 1 q 14 days | | 41 | 41 | 60 | 14.4 |
| Kaufman[72] | 3000 D 1 q 14 days | 150 D 1 q 14 days | | 6 | 37 | 19 | |
| Meluch[73] | 1000 D 1, 8, 15 q 21 days | 200 D 1 q 21 days | | 15 | 54 | 54 | 14.4 |
| Parameswaran[74] | 1000 D 1, 8, 15 q 28 days | 110 D 1 q 28 days | | | 23 | 61 | |
| Srinivas[75] | 1000 D 1, 15 q 28 days | 110 D 1, 15 q 28 days | | | 17 | 65 | 7.5 |
| Garcia Del Muro[76] | 2000 D 1 q 14 days | | 65 D 1 q 14 days | 10 | 39 | 56 | |
| Friedland[77] | 1000 D 1, 8 q 21 days | | 75 D 1 q 21 days | 7 | 41 | 32 | 68% 1 year survival |
| Dreicer[78] | 800 D 1, 8 q 21 days | | 40 D 1, 8 q 21 days | 25 | 25 | 20 | |
| Gitlitz[79] | 800 D 1, 8, 15 q 28 days | | 60–80 D 1 q 28 days | | 27 | 33 | 12 |

## FUTURE DIRECTIONS

Several approaches are being investigated to improve the dismal outcome of advanced transitional cell carcinoma patients.[9,11–15,87] These approaches include the search for molecular treatment-response predicting markers, management of minimal/microscopic residual disease, dose-dense sequential approaches, incorporation of triple combination regimens, and targeted therapies.

## MOLECULAR TREATMENT-RESPONSE PREDICTING MARKERS

Alterations in p53 and pRb occur in approximately 50% and 35%, respectively, of bladder cancers and have been reported to correlate with high grade and stage.[88–90] There are conflicting reports regarding the relationship between chemosensitivity and p53, and several authors suggest that altered expression of p53 may be associated with resistance to MVAC, although others suggest the contrary. Paclitaxel can induce apoptosis, using p53 independent pathways.[91,92] Some studies have shown that the metastatic potential of bladder cancer correlates with the expression of several genes that regulate proliferation (EGFR) and angiogenesis (bFGF, VEGF, MMP9, and interleukin 8). Inhibition of the epidermal growth factor receptor type I pathway, either by physical receptor blockade, as with the monoclonal antibody IMC225, or with the tyrosine kinase inhibitor ZD1839, leads to demonstrable antitumor effects in animal models. Adding paclitaxel to EGFR-directed therapy produced a synergistic biologic effect on xenographs.[93,94] At present, none of the molecular markers has entered into routine clinical practice. Prospective studies of chemotherapy selection based on molecular markers are needed.

## RESIDUAL DISEASE POSTCHEMOTHERAPY

It is important to distinguish between 'minimal residual disease' after chemotherapy in patients who achieved a complete response to therapy (= microscopic), and radiographically detected minimal residual disease (= macroscopic), representing a good clinical PR to the treatment.

Regarding minimal residual disease postchemotherapy, researchers at the University of Texas M.D. Anderson Cancer Center have designed a phase II trial in which patients that have responded to initial cytotoxic chemotherapy are randomized to treatment with either docetaxel alone, or a combination of docetaxel and ZD1839 (Iressa). The objectives of this trial are to compare the proportion of patients free from progression 9 months after the start of consolidation therapy, testing the hypothesis that the antiproliferative, and especially the antiangiogenic, effects of concomitant docetaxel and Iressa will inhibit progression of residual disease following maximal response (complete response) to front-line chemotherapy.[94]

The postchemotherapy surgical resection of macroscopic residual disease could be a reasonable approach for some selected patients with small volume residual disease after chemotherapy. Patients that benefited most from this approach were those with a major response to chemotherapy, initially tumor confined to pelvic, bladder, regional lymph nodes, or with a solitary metastatic site. Postchemotherapy surgical resection of residual cancer extends the median survival of these patients to 31–37 months, and may result in disease-free survival in some patients that would otherwise die of disease.[95–97]

## SALVAGE THERAPY

Patients whose disease recurs following their initial chemotherapy are destined to die. Objective remission rates up to 30% have been reported with treatment based on paclitaxel, ifosfamide, gemcitabine, trimetrexate, piritrexim, pemetrexed, and vinflunine after cisplatinum-based therapy.[29–31,35,38,49,62,63,65–73,76–78]

There are limited data regarding salvage therapy following MVAC and no data after gemcitabine/ cisplatin. Since patients that relapse after MVAC (particularly if there was a 3–6 months' progression-free survival following the previous platinum-based chemotherapy) have responded again to the earlier same regimen, it could be suggested that their exposure again to gemcitabine/cisplatin after long-term disease-free progression (more than 6–12 months) could be a reasonable option. However, no definitive data exist in the literature.[98]

Until now, second line bladder cancer therapy is an unmet medical need with no data favoring monotherapy, polychemotherapy, or alternating therapy.[99] An alternative approach to identify early treatment failures has been suggested, with an early switch of therapy if there is not an at least 40% tumor reduction (the so-called 'play-the-winner-and-drop-the-loser' strategy). This not-yet-proved methodology is used to select one best treatment, or a best pair of treatments, as a two-stage strategy out of four different treatments.[100]

## DOSE-DENSE APPROACH

Based on the results obtained with the ITP[101] combination of ifosfamide, paclitaxel, and cisplatin, and on concepts derived from kinetic models studied in breast cancer, investigators from MSKCC have developed the concept of dose-dense sequential chemotherapy in bladder cancer using the two-drug regimen of doxorubicin and gemcitabine (AG), followed by the three-drug ITP regimen. In a phase I study with 15 patients, AG was well tolerated at all dose levels, and no grade 3 or 4 myelosuppression was observed.[102] In a phase II trial in 21 patients, the overall response rate reported was 86%. However, toxicity was significant. ITP increased the response seen after AG in six patients. This suggests noncross resistance for the two regimens. The same approach is being evaluated in patients with impaired renal function using AG, but followed by paclitaxel and carboplatin.[103]

## TRIPLET COMBINATIONS

Several triple combinations have been studies in urothelial cancer patients. Bajorin et al have reported the activity of the ITP combination.[101] They demonstrated a response rate of 68% and a median survival in the range of 20 months, which was reported initially as a 50% increment in survival compared historically to the original MVAC series. Taking in consideration the significant activity of paclitaxel and gemcitabine, either alone or in combination with cisplatin, their different mechanism of action, and their nonoverlapping toxicities, the Spanish Group (SOGUG) studied the feasibility of adding paclitaxel to the doublet of gemcitabine/cisplatin in a phase I/II trial. In 58 patients, an overall response rate of 78% was observed with a median survival time of 24 months for the phase I segment of the trial and 15.6 months for the phase II part of the study.[104] A similar triplet was also evaluated using carboplatin. Investigators at Wayne State University, Detroit, incorporated gemcitabine in the carboplatin/paclitaxel combination in a phase II trial with 49 previously untreated patients with advanced urothelial malignancy and normal renal function. Of the 47 patients assessable for response, 15 obtained a CR and 15 obtained a PR, for an overall response rate of 68%. The median survival was 14.7 months.[105] Other triplets reported to date are presented in Table 65.6.[106-113] A large global international study comparing cisplatin/gemcitabine/paclitaxel with the conventional GC doublet has now been closed to patient accrual (with 610 patients). This trial will shed light on the role of the triplets in the management of advanced urothelial tumors. Whether or not we can improve survival with the newer triplet regimen will depend upon the results of this phase III trial.

## TARGETED THERAPY

The family of epidermal growth factor receptors is among the most studied growth factor receptors in

**Table 65.6** Triplet combination chemotherapy in urothelial cancer

| Agents | No. pts with prior therapy | No. pts | Response rate (%) | Median survival time (months) |
|---|---|---|---|---|
| Cisplatin[104] Paclitaxel Gemcitabine | None | 58 | 77.6 | 15.8 |
| Cisplatin[106] Paclitaxel Gemcitabine | None | 29 | 52 | 10.7 |
| Cisplatin[107] Paclitaxel Gemcitabine | None | 15 | 66.6 | 13.5 |
| Cisplatin[108] Paclitaxel Ifosfamide | None | 44 | 68 | 20 |
| Cisplatin[29] Paclitaxel Methotrexate | 21 | 25 | 40 | |
| Cisplatin[109] Docetaxel Epirubicin | None | 30 | 66.7 | 14.5 |
| Carboplatin[105] Paclitaxel Gemcitabine | None | 47 | 68 | 14.7 |
| Carboplatin[110] Paclitaxel Gemcitabine | None | 26 | 47.6 | 7.1 |
| Carboplatin[78] Paclitaxel Gemcitabine | None | 15 | 53 | |
| Carboplatin[112] Docetaxel Gemcitabine | 6 | 13 | 38 | |
| Carboplatin[92] Paclitaxel Methotrexate | None | 32 | 56 | 15.5 |
| Gemcitabine[113] Paclitaxel Methotrexate | None | 20 | 45 | 18 |

bladder cancer[114] and several anti-EGFR strategies have been tested in urothelial patients. The activity of gefitinib (Iressa) has been analyzed in a recent phase II trial conducted by the Southwest Oncology Group in chemorefractory TCC of the bladder, with very limited results. Twenty-nine patients whose disease progressed after one chemotherapy regimen were treated with gefitinib and, of these, only one had a partial response. The estimated median progression-free survival was only 1.7 months.[115] Combination with gemcitabine/cisplatin resulted in excessive toxicity, and two patients died because of neutropenic infections. The toxicity was attributed to the fixed dose rate infusion of gemcitabine used in this Cancer and Leukemia Group B (CALGB) trial. The study is ongoing using the standard gemcitabine mode of administration.[116] As mentioned above, a trial combining docetaxel and Iressa for minimal residual disease following chemotherapy is also being conducted.[94]

The Her2/neu oncogene is another member of the epidermal growth factor receptor family. Its overexpression results in increased cell proliferation and an increase in metastatic potential. The Her2/neu oncogene contribution to the malignant phenotype of the cell is consistent with the high rates of expression in poorly differentiated tumors and with a poorer prognosis in breast cancer. Her2/neu is also overexpressed in bladder cancer. Overexpression was detected by immunohistochemistry in 28% of the primary tumors and in 53% of metastatic lymph nodes. Overexpression in the primary tumors consistently predicts overexpression in distant or regional metastasis, although some Her2/neu-negative primary tumors may show overexpression in their corresponding metastasis.[115] No prognostic implication was demonstrated in these bladder cancer patients. Discordant results regarding overexpression have been published, related to the diversity of the techniques used for the assays.[117] There are also conflicting results regarding gene amplification in these overexpressed Her2/neu tumors, ranging between 7% and 95%. The low amplification suggests that mechanisms other than gene amplification may account for the observed high protein overexpression.[118–120]

Preclinical and clinical data have shown marked enhancement of the antitumor activity of chemotherapy when combined with the monoclonal antibody against Her2/neu trastuzumab.[121] Thus, Hussain et al recently combined trastuzumab with the carboplatin/paclitaxel/gemcitabine triplet for patients with overexpressed Her2/neu and reported a 61% objective response rate in patients with advanced urothelial cancer.[122] It is too soon to define the role of Her2/neu blockage with chemotherapy. The response rate appears to be similar to the results obtained with cisplatin-based triplets (see Table 65.6).[29,78,92,104–110,112–113,118]

GW572016 is an oral, reversible, dual inhibitor of ErbB1 and ErbB2 receptors that has also been tested in second line urothelial cancer. All patients that were included in this trial had confirmed expression of ErbB1 and/or ErbB2 (1+, 2+ or 3+ by immunohistochemistry). However, limited numbers of patients included were finally eligible for response evaluation, with only 10%

being partial responders. Only one response was confirmed at 8 weeks.[123]

Several other strategies have been designed to target other elements involved in the activation of the cascade of biochemical and physiologic responses of the mitogenic signal transduction pathways. Preliminary results of the oral SCH66336 (a farnesyl protein transferase inhibitor) have indicated limited activity in previously treated patients with advanced/metastatic urothelial tract tumors.[124] Although this compound will not be further developed due to the inactivity seen in other indications, a study by the Early Clinical Study Group (ECSG) of the EORTC with the combination of SCH663366 and gemcitabine as second line in patients with advanced urothelial tract tumors revealed a 38.2 % encouraging response rate.[125]

Some clinical activity has been reported with several other compounds such as the histone deacetylase inhibitors.[126] In addition, cyclooxygenase 2 (COX2) might also be a therapeutic target in urothelial tumors. Although its expression had conflicting correlation with tumor grade or stage, in a subgroup of 62 patients that received chemotherapy, strong COX2 expression significantly correlated with poor overall survival.[127] Targeted therapy is discussed in more detail in Chapter 67.

## CONCLUSION

A review of abstracts published over the last 5 years (Table 65.7) indicates that most of the clinical activity in this relatively small patient population focuses on small phase II trials in various phases of the disease, many of which will never mature for routine clinical use. At the present time, the cisplatin/gemcitabine (CG) combination in a phase III trial has been demonstrated to be a valuable alternative to the classical MVAC regimen with similar efficacy and survival probabilities, but with the benefit of less toxicity.

Other new double and triple combinations have yet to define their activity in phase III trials. To date, there are no randomized data to show that any of these new

**Table 65.7** Published abstracts on urothelial cancer in the *Proceedings of the American Society of Clinical Oncology* (ASCO)

| ASCO | Phase II No. | Phase II No. pts | Phase III No. | Phase III No. pts | Unfit No. pts | Elderly No. pts | Salvage No. pts | Total No. pts |
|---|---|---|---|---|---|---|---|---|
| 2000 | 10 | 293 | 1 | 263 | 42 | | 48 | 556 |
| 2001 | 8 | 193 | | | | 27 | 15 | 193 |
| 2002 | 7 | 186 | | | 27 | 23 | 11 | 186 |
| 2003 | 7 | 276 | 2 | 309 | | 25 | 49 | 585 |
| 2004 | 7 | 279 | | | 36 | | 103 | 279 |

regimens improve patient survival as compared with either MVAC or CG. Strategies have been developed to minimize toxicity in patients that are 'unfit', 'elderly', or have 'compromised renal function'. Clinical trials should be designed to clearly distinguish among these three groups of patients. Outside a clinical trial, M-CAVI, carboplatin/gemcitabine, CBDCA/paclitaxel, gemcitabine/taxane or monotherapy with gemcitabine, CBDCA or a taxane could be used in 'unfit' patients in an individual basis. The new era of targeted therapy is being incorporated in the management of urothelial cancer with the hope of improving patient management in the not too distant future.

## REFERENCES

1. http://www.cancer.org/downloads/STT/CAFF2003PWSecured.pdf
2. Yagoda A. Chemotherapy of urothelial tract tumors. Cancer 1987;60:574–585.
3. Raghavan D, Shipley WU, Garnick MB, et al. The biology and management of bladder cancer. N Engl J Med 1990;322:1129–1138.
4. Harker WG, Meyers FJ, Freiha FS, et al. Cisplatin, methotrexate, and vinblastine (CMV): an effective chemotherapy regimen for metastatic transitional cell carcinoma of the urinary tract. A Northern California Oncology Group study. J Clin Oncol 1985;3:1463–1470.
5. Logothetis CJ, Dexeus FH, Chong C, et al. Cisplatin, cyclophosphamide and doxorubicin chemotherapy for unresectable urothelial tumors: the M.D. Anderson experience. J Urol 1989;141:33–37.
6. Sternberg CN, Yagoda A, Scher HI, et al. Preliminary results of M-VAC (methotrexate, vinblastine, doxorubicin and cisplatin) for transitional cell carcinoma of the urothelium. J Urol 1985;133:403–407.
7. Yagoda A. The role of cisplatin-based chemotherapy in advanced urothelial tract cancer. Semin Oncol 1989;16(4 Suppl 6):98–104.
8. Mead GM, Russell M, Clark P, et al. A randomized trial comparing methotrexate and vinblastine (MV) with cisplatin, methotrexate and vinblastine (CMV) in advanced transitional cell carcinoma: results and a report on prognostic factors in a Medical Research Council study. MRC Advanced Bladder Cancer Working Party. Br J Cancer 1998;78:1067–1075.
9. Sternberg CN, Yagoda A, Scher HI, et al. Methotrexate, vinblastine, doxorubicin, and cisplatin for advanced transitional cell carcinoma of the urothelium. Efficacy and patterns of response and relapse. Cancer 1989;64:2448–2458.
10. Tannock I, Gospodarowicz M, Connolly J, Jewett M. M-VAC (methotrexate, vinblastine, doxorubicin and cisplatin) chemotherapy for transitional cell carcinoma: the Princess Margaret Hospital experience. J Urol 1989;142(2 Pt 1):289–292.
11. Logothetis CJ, Dexeus FH, Finn L, et al. A prospective randomized trial comparing MVAC and CISCA chemotherapy for patients with metastatic urothelial tumors. J Clin Oncol 1990;8:1050–1055.
12. Boutan-Laroze A, Mahjoubi M, Droz JP, et al. M-VAC (methotrexate, vinblastine, doxorubicin and cisplatin) for advanced carcinoma of the bladder. The French Federation of Cancer Centers experience. Eur J Cancer 1991;27:1690–1694.
13. Loehrer PJ Sr, Einhorn LH, Elson PJ, et al. A randomized comparison of cisplatin alone or in combination with methotrexate, vinblastine, and doxorubicin in patients with metastatic urothelial carcinoma: a cooperative group study. J Clin Oncol 1992;10:1066–1073.
14. Bellmunt J, Ribas A, Eres N, et al. Carboplatin-based versus cisplatin-based chemotherapy in the treatment of surgically incurable advanced bladder carcinoma. Cancer 1997;80:1966–1972.
15. Saxman SB, Propert KJ, Einhorn LH, et al. Long-term follow-up of a phase III intergroup study of cisplatin alone or in combination with methotrexate, vinblastine, and doxorubicin in patients with metastatic urothelial carcinoma: a cooperative group study. J Clin Oncol 1997;15:2564–2569.
16. Gabrilove JL, Jakubowski A, Scher H, et al. Effect of granulocyte colony-stimulating factor on neutropenia and associated morbidity due to chemotherapy for transitional-cell carcinoma of the urothelium. N Engl J Med 1988;318:1414–1422.
17. Moore MJ, Iscoe N, Tannock IF. A phase II study of methotrexate, vinblastine, doxorubicin and cisplatin plus recombinant human granulocyte-macrophage colony stimulating factors in patients with advanced transitional cell carcinoma. J Urol 1993;150:1131–1134.
18. Loehrer PJ Sr, Elson P, Dreicer R, et al. Escalated dosages of methotrexate, vinblastine, doxorubicin, and cisplatin plus recombinant human granulocyte colony-stimulating factor in advanced urothelial carcinoma: an Eastern Cooperative Oncology Group trial. J Clin Oncol 1994;12:483–488.
19. Seidman AD, Scher HI, Gabrilove JL, et al. Dose-intensification of MVAC with recombinant granulocyte colony-stimulating factor as initial therapy in advanced urothelial cancer. J Clin Oncol 1993;11:408–414.
20. Scher HI, Geller NL, Curley T, Tao Y. Effect of relative cumulative dose-intensity on survival of patients with urothelial cancer treated with M-VAC. J Clin Oncol 1993;11(3):400–407.
21. Logothetis CJ, Finn LD, Smith T, et al. Escalated MVAC with or without recombinant human granulocyte-macrophage colony-stimulating factor for the initial treatment of advanced malignant urothelial tumors: results of a randomized trial. J Clin Oncol 1995;13(9):2272–2277.
22. Bamias A, Aravantinos G, Deliveliotis C, et al. Docetaxel and cisplatin with granulocyte colony-stimulating factor (G-CSF) versus MVAC with G-CSF in advanced urothelial carcinoma: a multicenter, randomized, phase III study from the Hellenic Cooperative Oncology Group. J Clin Oncol 2004;22:220–228.
23. Sternberg CN, de Mulder PH, Schornagel JH, et al. European Organisation for Research and Treatment of Cancer Genitourinary Tract Cancer Cooperative Group. Randomized phase III trial of high-dose-intensity methotrexate, vinblastine, doxorubicin, and cisplatin (MVAC) chemotherapy and recombinant human granulocyte colony-stimulating factor versus classic MVAC in advanced urothelial tract tumors: European Organisation for Research and Treatment of Cancer Protocol no. 30924. J Clin Oncol 2001;19:2638–2646.
24. Siefker-Radtke AO, Millikan RE, Tu SM, et al. Phase III trial of fluorouracil, interferon alpha-2b, and cisplatin versus methotrexate, vinblastine, doxorubicin, and cisplatin in metastatic or unresectable urothelial cancer. J Clin Oncol 2002;20:1361–1367.
25. Dreicer R, Manola J, Roth BJ, et al. Phase III trial of methotrexate, vinblastine, doxorubicin, and cisplatin versus carboplatin and paclitaxel in patients with advanced carcinoma of the urothelium. Cancer 2004;100:1639–1645.
26. von der Maase H, Hansen SW, Roberts JT, et al. Gemcitabine and cisplatin versus methotrexate, vinblastine, doxorubicin, and cisplatin in advanced or metastatic bladder cancer: results of a large, randomized, multinational, multicenter, phase III study. J Clin Oncol 2000;18:3068–3077.
27. Bajorin DF, Dodd PM, Mazumdar M, et al. Long-term survival in metastatic transitional-cell carcinoma and prognostic factors predicting outcome of therapy. J Clin Oncol 1999;17:3173–3181.
28. Bellmunt J, Albanell J, Paz-Ares L, et al. Pretreatment prognostic factors for survival in patients with advanced urothelial tumors treated in a phase I/II trial with paclitaxel, cisplatin, and gemcitabine. Cancer 2002;95:751–757.
29. Tu SM, Hossan E, Amato R, Kilbourn R, Logothetis CJ. Paclitaxel, cisplatin and methotrexate combination chemotherapy is active in the treatment of refractory urothelial malignancies. J Urol 1995;154:1719–1722.
30. Roth BJ, Dreicer R, Einhorn LH, et al. Significant activity of paclitaxel in advanced transitional-cell carcinoma of the urothelium: a phase II trial of the Eastern Cooperative Oncology Group. J Clin Oncol 1994;12:2264–2270.
31. Sweeney CJ, Williams SD, Finch DE, et al. A phase II study of paclitaxel and ifosfamide for patients with advanced refractory carcinoma of the urothelium. Cancer 1999;86:514–518.
32. Vaughn DJ, Malkowicz SB, Zoltick B, et al. Phase I trial of paclitaxel/carboplatin in advanced carcinoma of the urothelium. Semin Oncol 1997;24(1 Suppl 2):S2–47, S2–50.

33. Zielinski CC, Schnack B, Grbovic M, et al. Paclitaxel and carboplatin in patients with metastatic urothelial cancer: results of a phase II trial. Br J Cancer 1998;78:370–374.

34. Redman BG, Smith DC, Flaherty L, Du W, Hussain M. Phase II trial of paclitaxel and carboplatin in the treatment of advanced urothelial carcinoma. J Clin Oncol 1998;16:1844–1848.

35. Pollera CF, Ceribelli A, Crecco M, Calabresi F. Weekly gemcitabine in advanced bladder cancer: a preliminary report from a phase I study. Ann Oncol 1994;5:182–184.

36. Stadler WM, Kuzel T, Roth B, Raghavan D, Dorr FA. Phase II study of single-agent gemcitabine in previously untreated patients with metastatic urothelial cancer. J Clin Oncol 1997;15:3394–3398.

37. Moore MJ, Tannock IF, Ernst DS, Huan S, Murray N. Gemcitabine: a promising new agent in the treatment of advanced urothelial cancer. J Clin Oncol 1997;15:3441–3445.

38. Lorusso V, Pollera CF, Antimi M, et al. A phase II study of gemcitabine in patients with transitional cell carcinoma of the urinary tract previously treated with platinum: Italian Cooperative Group on Bladder Cancer. Eur J Cancer 1998;34:1208–1212.

39. Van Moorsel CJ, Veerman G, Vermorken JB, et al. Mechanisms of synergism between gemcitabine and cisplatin. Source Adv Exp Med Biol 1998;431:581–585.

40. Von der Maase H, Andersen L, Crino L, Weinknecht S, Dogliotti L. Weekly gemcitabine and cisplatin combination therapy in patients with transitional cell carcinoma of the urothelium: a phase II clinical trial. Ann Oncol 1999;10:1461–1465.

41. Moore MJ, Winquist EW, Murray N, et al. Gemcitabine plus cisplatin, an active regimen in advanced urothelial cancer: a phase II trial of the National Cancer Institute of Canada Clinical Trials Group. J Clin Oncol 1999;17:286–2881.

42. Kaufman D, Raghavan D, Carducci M, et al. Phase II trial of gemcitabine plus cisplatin in patients with metastatic urothelial cancer. J Clin Oncol 2000;18:1921–1927.

43. Lehmann J, Retz M, Stockle M. Is there standard chemotherapy for metastatic bladder cancer? Quality of life and medical resources utilization based on largest to date randomized trial. Crit Rev Oncol Hematol 2003;47:171–179.

44. Hussain SA, Stocken DD, Riley P, et al. A phase I/II study of gemcitabine and fractionated cisplatin in an outpatient setting using a 21-day schedule in patients with advanced and metastatic bladder cancer. Br J Cancer 2004;91:844–849.

45. Wilson JJ, Winquist E, Dorreen M, et al. A phase II trial of gemcitabine plus day 1 cisplatin given on a 21 day schedule in patients with advanced unresectable or metastatic bladder cancer. Proc Am Soc Clin Oncol 2002;21:151b.

46. McCaffrey JA, Hilton S, Mazumdar M, et al. Phase II trial of docetaxel in patients with advanced or metastatic transitional-cell carcinoma. J Clin Oncol 1997;15:1853–1857.

47. de Wit R, Kruit WH, Stoter G, et al. Docetaxel (Taxotere): an active agent in metastatic urothelial cancer; results of a phase II study in non-chemotherapy-pretreated patients. Br J Cancer 1998;78:1342–1345.

48. Seidman AD, Scher HI, Heinemann MH, et al. Continuous infusion gallium nitrate for patients with advanced refractory urothelial tract tumors. Cancer 1991;68:2561–2565.

49. Witte RS, Elson P, Bono B, et al. Eastern Cooperative Oncology Group phase II trial of ifosfamide in the treatment of previously treated advanced urothelial carcinoma. J Clin Oncol 1997;15:589–589.

50. Sweeney CJ, Williams SD, Finch DE, et al. A phase II study of paclitaxel and ifosfamide for patients with advanced refractory carcinoma of the urothelium. Cancer 1999;86:514–518.

51. Muller M, Heicappell R, Steiner U, Goessl C, Miller K. Side effects of chemotherapy for advanced urothelial carcinoma with etoposide and ifosfamide. Urol Int 1997;59:248–251.

52. Kyriakakis Z, Dimopoulos MA, Kostakopoulos A, et al. Cisplatin, ifosfamide, methotrexate and vinblastine combination chemotherapy for metastatic urothelial cancer. J Urol 1997;158:408–411.

53. Dreicer R, Propert KJ, Roth BJ, Einhorn LH, Loehrer PJ. Vinblastine, ifosfamide, and gallium nitrate—an active new regimen in patients with advanced carcinoma of the urothelium. A phase II trial of the Eastern Cooperative Oncology Group (E5892). Cancer 1997;79:110–114.

54. Raabe NK, Fossa SD, Paro G. Phase II study of carboplatin in locally advanced and metastatic transitional cell carcinoma of the urinary bladder. Br J Urol 1989;646:604–607.

55. Petrioli R, Frediani B, Manganelli A, et al. Comparison between a cisplatin-containing regimen and a carboplatin-containing regimen for recurrent or metastatic bladder cancer patients. A randomized phase II study. Cancer 1996;77:344–351.

56. Bellmunt J, Ribas A, Eres N, et al. Carboplatin-based versus cisplatin-based chemotherapy in the treatment of surgically incurable advanced bladder carcinoma. Cancer 1997;80:1966–1972.

57. Carteni G, Dogliotti L, Crucitta E, et al. Phase II randomized trial of gemcitabine plus cisplatin (GP) and gemcitabine plus carboplatin (GC) in patients (pts) with advanced or metastatic transitional cell carcinoma of the urothelium (TCCU). Proc Am Soc Clin Oncol 2003;22:A1543.

58. De Mulder P, Sternberg CN, Fossa S, et al. Lobaplatin in advanced urothelial tract tumors (EORTC 30931). Proc Am Soc Clin Oncol 1997;16:A1158.

59. Moore MJ, Winquist E, Vokes EE, Hirte H, Hoving H, Stadler WM. Phase II study of oxaliplatin in patients with inoperable, locally advanced or metastatic transitional cell carcinoma of the urothelial tract (TCC) who have received prior chemotherapy. Proc Am Soc Clin Oncol 2003;22:408 (Abstract 1638).

60. Culine S, Rebillard X, Iborra F, et al. Gemcitabine and oxaliplatin in advanced transitional cell carcinoma of the urothelium: a pilot study. Anticancer Res 2003;23:1903–1906.

61. Font A, Esteban E, Carles J, et al. Gemcitabine and oxaliplatin combination: a multicenter phase II trial in unfit patients with locally advanced or metastatic urothelial cancer. Proc Am Soc Clin Oncol 2004;22:A4544.

62. de Wit R, Kaye SB, Roberts JT, et al. Oral piritrexim, an effective treatment for metastatic urothelial cancer. Br J Cancer 1993;67:388–390.

63. Khorsand M, Lange J, Feun L, et al. Phase II trial of oral piritrexim in advanced, previously treated transitional cell cancer of bladder. Invest New Drugs 1997;15:157–163.

64. Dreicer R, Roth B, Wilding G. Perspectives in bladder cancer, supplement to Cancer. Overview of advanced urothelial cancer trials of the Eastern Cooperative Oncology Group. Cancer 2003;97(Suppl 8):2109–2114.

65. Paz-Ares L, Tabernero J, Moyano A, et al. A phase II of the multi-targeted antifolate, MTA (LY231514), in patients with advanced transitional cell carcinoma of the bladder. Proc Am Soc Clin Oncol 1998;17:A1307.

66. Sweeney C, Roth BJ, Kaufman DS, Nicol SJ. Phase II study of pemetrexed (pem) for second-line treatment of transitional cell cancer (tcc) of the bladder. Proc Am Soc Clin Oncol 2003;22:A1653.

67. Bui B, Theodore C, Culine S, et al. Preliminary results of a phase II study testing intravenous (iv) vinflunine (VFL) as second line therapy in patients with advanced transitional cell cancer (TCC) of the bladder. Proc Am Soc Clin Oncol 2003;22:A1571.

68. www.cancerbacup.org.uk

69. Witte RS, Propert KJ, Burch B, et al. An ECOG phase II trial topotecan (T) in previously treated advanced urothelial carcinoma (UC). Proc Annu Meet Am Soc Clin Oncol 1997;16:A115.

70. www.ClinicalTrials.gov

71. Sternberg CN, Calabro F, Pizzocaro G, et al. Chemotherapy with an every-2-week regimen of gemcitabine and paclitaxel in patients with transitional cell carcinoma who have received prior cisplatin-based therapy. Cancer 2001;92(12):2993–2998.

72. Kaufman D, Stadler W, Carducci M, et al. Gemcitabine and paclitaxel every two weeks: a multicenter phase II trial in locally advanced or metastatic urothelial cancer. Proc Am Soc Clin Oncol 2000;19:A1341.

73. Meluch AA, Greco FA, Burris HA 3rd, et al. Paclitaxel and gemcitabine chemotherapy for advanced transitional-cell carcinoma of the urothelial tract: a phase II trial of the Minnie pearl cancer research network. J Clin Oncol 2001;19:3018–3024.

74. Parameswaran R, Fisch MJ, Rafat H, et al. A Hoosier Oncology Group phase II study of weekly paclitaxel and gemcitabine in advanced transitional cell carcinoma (TCC) of the bladder. Proc Am Soc Clin Oncol 2001;20:A798.

75. Srinivas S, Guardino AE. Gemcitabine and paclitaxel chemotherapy effective for good risk advanced urothelial malignancies. Proc Am Soc Clin Oncol 2004;23:A4675.

76. Garcia Del Muro X, Marcuello E, Mellado B, et al. Phase II multicenter study of docetaxel plus gemcitabine as first-line treatment in advanced urothelial cancer. Proc Am Soc Clin Oncol 2003;22:A1643.

77. Friedland D, Gregurich MA, Belt R, et al. Phase II evaluation of docetaxel plus gemcitabine in patients with advanced unresectable urothelial cancer. Proc Am Soc Clin Oncol 2002;21:A2427.

78. Dreicer R, Manola J, Schneider DJ, et al. Phase II trial of gemcitabine and docetaxel in patients with advanced carcinoma of the urothelium: a trial of the Eastern Cooperative Oncology Group. Cancer 2003;97:2743–2747.

79. Gitlitz BJ, Baker C, Chapman Y, et al. A phase II study of gemcitabine and docetaxel therapy in patients with advanced urothelial carcinoma. Cancer 2003;98:1863–1869.

80. Chestera JD, Halla GD, Forsterb M, Protheroeb AS. Systemic chemotherapy for patients with bladder cancer—current controversies and future directions. Cancer Treat Rev 2004;30:343–358.

81. Vaughn D, Dreicer R, Manola J, et al. E2896 paclitaxel/carboplatin in advanced urothelial carcinoma and renal insufficiency: a phase II trial of the Eastern Cooperative Group. Proc Am Soc Clin Oncol 2000;19:A343.

82. Neri B, Di Cello V, Biscione S, et al. Phase II evaluation of gemcitabine (GEM) and epirubicin (EPI) in advanced bladder cancer. Proc Am Soc Clin Oncol 2000;19:A1380.

83. Turkolmez K, Beduk Y, Baltaci S, Gogus CA, Gogus O. Gemcitabine plus vinorelbine chemotherapy in patients with advanced bladder carcinoma who are medically unsuitable for or who have failed cisplatin-based chemotherapy. Eur Urol 2003;44:682–686.

84. Bellmunt J, de Wit R, Albanell J, Baselga J. A feasibility study of carboplatin with fixed dose of gemcitabine in 'unfit' patients with advanced bladder cancer. Eur J Cancer 2001;37:2212–2215.

85. Sella A, Logothetis CJ, Dexeus FH, Amato R, Finn L, Fitz K. Cisplatin combination chemotherapy for elderly patients with urothelial tumours. Br J Urol 1991;67:603–607.

86. Bamias A, Efstathiou E, Hamilos G, et al. Outcome of elderly patients following platinum-based chemotherapy for advanced urothelial cancer. Proc Am Soc Clin Oncol 2004;22:A4542.

87. Stadler WM, Hayden A, von der Maase H, et al. Long-term survival in phase II trials of gemcitabine plus cisplatin for advanced transitional cell cancer. Urol Oncol 2002;7:153–157.

88. Esrig D, Elmajian D, Groshen S, et al. Accumulation of nuclear p53 and tumor progression in bladder cancer. N Engl J Med 1994;331:1259–1264.

89. Chatterjee SJ, Datar R, Youssefzadeh D, et al. Combined effects of p53, p21, and pRb expression in the progression of bladder transitional cell carcinoma. J Clin Oncol 2004;22:1007–1013.

90. Slaton JW, Benedict WF, Dinney CP. P53 in bladder cancer: mechanism of action, prognostic value, and target for therapy. Urology 2001;57:852–859.

91. Sarkis AS, Bajorin DF, Reuter VE, et al. Prognostic value of p53 nuclear overexpression in patients with invasive bladder cancer treated with neoadjuvant MVAC. J Clin Oncol 1995;13:1384–1390.

92. Edelman MJ, Meyers FJ, Miller TR, et al. Phase I/II study of paclitaxel, carboplatin, and methotrexate in advanced transitional cell carcinoma: a well-tolerated regimen with activity independent of p53 mutation. Urology 2000;55:521–525.

93. Highshaw RA, McConkey DJ, Dinney CP. Integrating basic science and clinical research in bladder cancer: update from the first bladder Specialized Program of Research Excellence (SPORE). Curr Opin Urol 2004;14:295–300.

94. Inoue K, Slaton JW, Perrotte P, et al. Paclitaxel enhances the effects of the anti-epidermal growth factor receptor monoclonal antibody ImClone C225 in mice with metastatic human bladder transitional cell carcinoma. Clin Cancer Res 2000;6:4874–4884.

95. Herr HW, Donat SM, Bajorin DF. Post-chemotherapy surgery in patients with unresectable or regionally metastatic bladder cancer. J Urol 2001;165:811–814.

96. Siefker-Radtke AO, Walsh GL, Pisters LL, et al. Is there a role for surgery in the management of metastatic urothelial cancer? The M.D. Anderson experience. J Urol 2004;171:145–148.

97. Miller RS, Freiha FS, Reese JH, et al. Cisplatin, methotrexate and vinblastine plus surgical restaging for patients with advanced transitional cell carcinoma of the urothelium. J Urol 1993;150:65–69.

98. Kattan J, Culine S, Theodore C, Droz JP. Second-line M-VAC therapy in patients previously treated with the M-VAC regimen for metastatic urothelial cancer. Ann Oncol 1993;4:793–794.

99. Tu SM, Millikan RE, Pagliaro LC, et al. Treatment of refractory urothelial carcinoma with alternating paclitaxel, methotrexate, cisplatin (TMP) and 5-fluorouracil, α-interferon, cisplatin (FAP) Urol Oncol 2003;21:342–348.

100. Siefker-Radtke AO, Thall PF, Tannir NM, et al. Implementation of a novel statistical design to evaluate successive treatment courses for metastatic transitional cell carcinoma. A phase II trial at the M.D. Anderson Cancer Center. Proc Am Soc Clin Oncol 2004;22:A4543.

101. Bajorin DF, McCaffrey JA, Dodd PM, et al. Ifosfamide, paclitaxel, and cisplatin for patients with advanced transitional cell carcinoma of the urothelial tract. Final report of a phase II trial evaluating two dosing schedules. Cancer 2000;88:1671–1678.

102. Dodd PM, McCaffrey JA, Hilton S, et al. Phase I evaluation of sequential doxorubicin gemcitabine then ifosfamide paclitaxel cisplatin for patients with unresectable or metastatic transitional-cell carcinoma of the urothelial tract. J Clin Oncol 2000;18:840–846.

103. Novick S, Higgins G, Hilton S, et al. Phase I/II sequential doxorubicin plus gemcitabine followed by paclitaxel plus carboplatin in patients with transitional cell carcinoma and impaired renal function. Proc Am Soc Clin Oncol 2000;19:A1423.

104. Bellmunt J, Guillem V, Paz-Ares L, et al. Phase I/II study of paclitaxel, cisplatin, and gemcitabine in advanced transitional-cell carcinoma of the urothelium. J Clin Oncol 2000;18:3247–3255.

105. Hussain M, Vaishampayan U, Du W, Redman B, Smith DC. Combination carboplatin, paclitaxel and gemcitabine is an active treatment for advanced urothelial carcinoma. J Clin Oncol 2001;19:2527–2533.

106. Clark PE, Stindt D, Hall MC, et al. Phase II trial of gemcitabine, paclitaxel, and cisplatin in advanced transitional cell carcinoma. Proc Am Soc Clin Oncol 2004;22:A4610.

107. Hogan F, Lamm D, Schunn G, Kandzari S. Cisplatin (C), gemcitabine (G), and paclitaxel (P) for 50 poor-risk patients (pts) with advanced intra-pelvic (M0) or metastatic (M1) urothelial cancer. Proc Am Soc Clin Oncol 2002;21:A1702.

108. Bajorin DF, McCaffrey JA, Dodd PM, et al. Ifosfamide, paclitaxel and cisplatin for patients with advanced transitional cell carcinoma of the urothelial tract: final report of a phase II trial evaluating two dosing schedules. Cancer 2000;88:1671–1678.

109. Pectasides D, Visvikis A, Aspropotamitis A, et al. Chemotherapy with cisplatin, epirubicin and docetaxel in transitional cell urothelial cancer. Phase II trial. Eur J Cancer 2000;36:74–79.

110. Chahine GY, Kattan G, Farhat FS, et al. The weekly triplet: gemcitabine, carboplatin and paclitaxel as first line therapy for advanced urothelial cancer. ASCO Annual Meeting Proceedings (Post-Meeting Edition). J Clin Oncol 2004;22(Suppl 14):4704.

111. DiPaola RS, Rubin E, Toppmeyer D, et al. Gemcitabine combined with sequential paclitaxel and carboplatin in patients with urothelial cancers and other advanced malignancies. Med Sci Monit 2003;9:15–11.

112. Elizabeth H, Owen C, Shelton G, et al. Phase I/II study of docetaxel, gemcitabine, carboplatin in poor prognosis and previously treated patients with urothelial carcinoma. Proc Am Soc Clin Oncol 2000;19:A1376.

113. Law LY, Primo NL, Meyers FJ, et al. Platinum free combination chemotherapy in locally advanced and metastatic transitional cell carcinoma: phase I/II trial of gemcitabine, paclitaxel, methotrexate. Proc Am Soc Clin Oncol 2001;20:A767.

114. Mchugh LA, Leyshon Griffiths TR, Kriajevska M, Symonds RP, Mellon JK. Tyrosine kinase inhibitors of the epidermal growth factor receptor as adjuncts to systemic chemotherapy for muscle-invasive bladder cancer. Urology 2004;63:619–624.

115. Petrylak D, Faulkner JR, Van Veldhuizen PJ, Mansukhani M, Crawford ED. Evaluation of ZD1839 for advanced transitional cell carcinoma

(TCC) of the urothelium: a Southwest Oncology Group Trial. Proc Am Soc Clin Oncol 2003;22:A1619.

116. Philips G, Halabi S, Sanford B, Bajorin D, Small E. Phase II trial of cisplatin (C), fixed-dose rate gemcitabine (G) and gefitinib for advanced transitional cell carcinoma (TCC) of the urothelial tract: preliminary results of CALGB 90102. Proc Am Soc Clin Oncol 2004;23:A4540.

117. Jimenez RE, Hussain M, Bianco FJ Jr, et al. Her-2/neu overexpression in muscle-invasive urothelial carcinoma of the bladder: prognostic significance and comparative analysis in primary and metastatic tumors. Clin Cancer Res 2001;7:2440–2447.

118. de Pinieux G, Colin D, Vincent-Salomon A, et al. Confrontation of immunohistochemistry and fluorescent in situ hybridization for the assessment of HER-2/neu(c-erbb-2) status in urothelial carcinoma. Virchows Arch 2004;444:415–419.

119. Latifa Z, Wattersa AD, Dunna I, et al. HER2/neu gene amplification and protein overexpression in G3 pT2 transitional cell carcinoma of the bladder: a role for anti-HER2 therapy? Eur J Cancer 2004;40:56–63.

120. Piccart M. Closing remarks and treatment guidelines. Eur J Cancer 2001;37:30–33.

121. Slamon DJ, Leyland-Jones B, Shak S, et al. Use of chemotherapy plus a monoclonal antibody against HER2 for metastatic breast cancer that overexpresses HER2. N Engl J Med 2001;344:783–792.

122. Hussain M, Smith DC, Vaishampayan U, et al. Trastuzumab (T), paclitaxel (P), carboplatin (C) and gemcitabine (G) in patients with advanced urothelial cancer and overexpression of HER-2 (NCI study #198). Proc Am Soc Clin Oncol 2003;22:A1568.

123. Machiels J-P, Wülfing C, Richel DJ, et al. A single arm, multicenter, open-label phase II study of orally administered GW572016 as single-agent, second-line treatment of patients with locally advanced or metastatic transitional cell carcinoma of the urothelial tract. Interim analysis. Proc Am Soc Clin Oncol 2004;23:A4615.

124. Winquist E, Moore MJ, Chi K, et al. NCIC CTG IND.126: a phase II study of a farnesyl transferase inhibitor (SCH 66336) in patients with unresectable or metastatic transitional cell carcinoma of the urothelial tract failing prior chemotherapy. Proc Am Soc Clin Oncol 2001;20:A785.

125. Theodore C, Geoffrois L, Vermorken JB, et al. A phase II multicentre study of SCH66336 in combination with gemcitabine as second line treatment in patients with advanced/metastatic urothelial tract tumor. Proc Am Soc Clin Oncol 2003;22:A1667.

126. Kelly WK, Richon VM, O'Connor O, et al. Phase I clinical trial of histone deacetylase inhibitor: suberoylanilide hydroxamic acid administered intravenously. Clin Cancer Res 2003;9:3578–3588.

127. Wulfinga C, Eltzeb E, von Struenseea D, et al. Cyclooxygenase-2 expression in bladder cancer: correlation with poor outcome after chemotherapy. Eur Urol 2004; 45:46–52.

# Novel and emerging therapy

# Special considerations in the elderly patient 66

Gary R MacVicar, Maha Hussain

## INTRODUCTION

Over the past 100 years, life expectancy has increased significantly.[1,2] By the year 2030, 20.1% of the population of the United States is expected to be 65 years old or older, with the number of elderly individuals doubling to 70 million. It is also anticipated that the number of individuals over 75 years will triple and that the population of those over 85 years will double during this time period.[3] Considering that cancer is one of the most common causes of death among elderly individuals over the age of 65 years, and that half of all cancers occur in this segment of the population,[4] an increase in the numbers of elderly individuals requiring management of malignant disease is expected.

The majority of patients with bladder cancer are elderly. The peak age at presentation is 60–70 years old.[5] Currently, the average life expectancy for a 75-year-old is 11.3 years and for an 85-year-old it is 6.3 years.[6] Fewer than 15% of patients with invasive bladder cancer survive 2 years if left untreated and, for patients with localized disease who are surgical candidates, most deaths from bladder cancer occur within 3 years after cystectomy.[7] Considering these statistics, age alone should not determine treatment decisions for older patients with bladder cancer. Rather, decisions should be made on an individual basis, with a global assessment of multiple parameters, including functional status and comorbidities.

## SPECIAL CONSIDERATIONS

### AGING AND FRAILTY

Chronologically speaking, to age is simply to become old. With age comes a myriad of changes, including alterations in physiology, functional status, and cognition. Chronologic age may not accurately reflect the rate of decline of these changes. Age has been described as a continuum of stages, with independence declining into frailty, and frailty eventually giving way to pre-death. As these changes occur, individuals may become vulnerable to stressors so that energy reserves are reduced and activity is limited; they may also experience physiologic, functional, or cognitive deficits that influence the management of their medical care.

Frailty in the elderly is characterized by severe limitations that are not reversible.[8] Standard criteria defining frailty have not been established, but many investigators would agree on a few common factors (Box 66.1). Frail individuals are dependent on others for help in one or more activities of daily living, display three or more comorbid conditions, and suffer from at least one geriatric syndrome. Some would consider age over 85 as an additional criterion, or at least a reason to look for signs of frailty.[9] Therefore, 'frail' is a term that describes an individual with limited functional reserves. Frailty must not be confused with comorbidity or disability.

**Box 66.1** Criteria for Frailty

1. Dependent in one or more activities of daily living
2. Displays three or more comorbid conditions
3. Suffers from at least one geriatric syndrome:
   - Dementia
   - Delerium
   - Depression
   - Falls
   - Spontaneous bone fractures
   - Fecal incontinence
   - Neglect or abuse
   - Failure to thrive

Comorbidity is a risk factor for frailty, and disability is an outcome of frailty.[10]

## ASSESSMENT

Effective management of elderly patients with cancer requires an individualized assessment of the overall fitness of a patient and an understanding of the risks and benefits of treatment. While treatment may improve survival or palliate symptoms, the possibility exists of significantly harming patients with questionable functional reserves. Thus, in addition to age and life expectancy of an elderly patient, an accurate assessment of their functional reserves must be made when considering treatment options in order to avoid harm. Chronologic age and laboratory testing are not accurate predictors of life expectancy, functional reserve, or the risk of developing treatment-related complications in patients with cancer.[11] To help standardize the evaluation of elderly patients, assessment tools have been developed. These may assist clinicians in making appropriate treatment recommendations to elderly patients with bladder cancer.

Investigators have advocated the use of a comprehensive geriatric assessment (CGA) to more accurately evaluate elderly cancer patients prior to treatment.[12] Although no consensus exists as to the exact components of the CGA, in general it contains items that evaluate medical, functional, psychological, social, and environmental aspects of elderly individuals (Table 66.1).[13] Its use has been associated with an increased identification of unrecognized problems, development of prognostic geriatric variables, and improved treatment outcomes.[14] Ideally, a global assessment using the CGA assists clinicians in identifying three groups of patients:

- those that are functionally independent and without serious comorbidity
- those that are dependent in one or more instrumental activities of daily living and/or may present with one or two comorbid conditions
- those that are frail.

An individualized assessment can provide an appropriate recommendation of life-prolonging or palliative therapy.[15]

## FUNCTIONAL CONSIDERATIONS

Traditionally, oncologists have used functional status, which has been shown to be a predictor of response to chemotherapy and a measure of treatment-related toxicity, to assist in determining the appropriate treatment.[16] In geriatrics, functional status is assessed through basic and instrumental activities of daily living (ADLs). Basic ADLs consist of dressing, eating, ambulating, toileting, and hygiene; instrumental ADLs include shopping, housekeeping, accounting, food

**Table 66.1** Comprehensive geriatric assessment (CGA)

| CGA component | Means of assessment | Implications |
|---|---|---|
| Functional status | Basic activities of daily living (dressing, eating, ambulating, toileting, hygiene) Independent activities of daily living (shopping, housekeeping, accounting, food preparation, transportation) | Correlates with life expectancy, functional dependence, and tolerance of stress |
| Comorbidity | Number of comorbid conditions and comorbidity indices | Correlates with life expectancy and tolerance of stress |
| Mental status | Folstein Minimental Status Examination | Correlates with life expectancy and dependence |
| Emotional state | Geriatric Depression Scale | Correlates with survival, and may indicate motivation to receive treatment |
| Nutritional status | Mininutritional assessment | Possibly correlates with survival |
| Polypharmacy | Number and types of medication | Measure of risk of drug interactions |
| Geriatric syndromes | Delirium, dementia, depression, falls, incontinence, spontaneous bone fractures, neglect or abuse, failure to thrive | Correlates with survival and functional dependence |

Reprinted from Critical Reviews in Oncology/Hematology, Vol. 46, Balducci L. Geriatric Oncology, pp 211–220. Copyright (2003), with permission from Elsevier.

preparation, and transportation. Oncologists alternatively have used the Karnofsky performance status (KPS) and the Eastern Cooperative Oncology Group (ECOG) performance status scales to assess patients' functional capabilities. A KPS less than 80% is prognostic of a worse outcome for patients treated with methotrexate, vinblastine, doxorubicin, and cisplatin (MVAC) chemotherapy.[17] However, these scales are not as effective in the elderly because comorbidities may interfere with the measurement of performance status.[18] The use of the CGA has been shown to enhance the accuracy of the ECOG performance scale in predicting the functional status of elderly cancer patients,[19] and investigators recently included the CGA as part of their analysis of gemcitabine use in elderly bladder cancer patients.[20]

Elderly patients with bladder cancer frequently have preexisting comorbidities in addition to their malignancy. Smoking is a significant risk factor for bladder cancer, and many bladder cancer patients experience a number of tobacco-related illnesses, including chronic obstructive pulmonary disease, coronary artery disease, and peripheral vascular occlusive disease. Diabetes mellitus and its complications are prevalent in the elderly and may affect the choice of treatment. Dementia and depression are also encountered frequently in the elderly and may affect a patient's ability to make medical decisions. Bladder cancer itself may also present comorbidities, including renal impairment secondary to an obstructive uropathy, and anemia due to hematuria.

Comorbidity is independent from functional status in elderly oncology patients.[21] The prevalence of age-related changes increases dramatically after age 70,[15]

and, on average, elderly patients have three different diseases.[22,23] Several indices have been developed to assess comorbidity in the elderly, but no consensus exists as to which conditions should be included or how they should be scored. Two scales that are commonly used are the Charlson scale[24] and the Cumulative Illness Rating Scale–Geriatrics.[25] Regardless of which one is used, these indices have shown that the presence of comorbidities impacts negatively on cancer patients' survival,[26] and comorbidities may compromise an elderly individual's ability to tolerate chemotherapy.[27] Therefore, oncologists should actively address reversible comorbidities, such as anemia, depression or uncontrolled diabetes, in the effort to improve the results of treatment and general welfare of their patients.

The American Society of Anesthesiology (ASA) developed a classification scheme to categorize the physical status of patients undergoing surgical procedures.[28,29] The ASA score takes into account the presence and severity of comorbidities, but age is not a consideration (Box 66.2). It has been predictive of morbidity and mortality following surgical

**Box 66.2** American Society of Anesthesiology score

| Class | Description |
|---|---|
| I | Healthy patient |
| II | Mild systemic disease—no functional limitation |
| III | Severe systemic disease–definite functional limitation |
| IV | Severe systemic disease that is a constant threat to life |
| V | Moribund patient unlikely to survive 24 hours with or without operation |

**Table 66.2** Changes in pharmacokinetics with aging[32]

| Pharmacokinetic parameter | Changes with aging | Implications |
|---|---|---|
| Oral absorption | Mucosal atrophy<br>Decreased gut motility<br>Reduced splanchnic blood flow<br>Diminished secretion of digestive enzymes | Reduced rate of absorption |
| Volume of distribution | Changes in body composition:<br>    increased fat content and decreased water content<br>Albumin levels decrease<br>Incidence of anemia increases | Altered volume of distribution, peak concentration, and terminal half-life<br>Increased free fraction of active agent<br>Change in the pharmacokinetics of agents which are bound to red blood cells: anthracyclines, taxanes, epipodophyllotoxins |
| Hepatic function | Decreased liver mass with age<br>Decline in the activity of the cytochrome P450 system<br>Polypharmacy may inhibit or induce enzymes involved in the metabolism of chemotherapeutic agents<br>Decreased splanchnic blood flow | Decreased amounts of hepatic enzymes available to metabolize drugs<br><br>Lower clearance of agents which rely on blood flow for elimination |
| Renal function | Decline in glomerular filtration rate of 1 ml/min each year after 40<br>Decline in muscle mass with age | Inaccurate estimate of renal function by Cockcroft–Gault equation<br>Dose adjustments may need to be considered to avoid renal toxicity |

procedures,[30,31] and, in terms of bladder cancer patients, the ASA score has been predictive of major complications following cystectomy.[30] Some have suggested that patients with ASA scores of III or greater should undergo more extensive preoperative evaluations that aim to optimize correctable parameters and reduce operative risk.[30,31]

## PHYSIOLOGIC CONSIDERATIONS

With aging, physiologic changes occur that have an impact on management of bladder cancer. Age-related decline in organ function and changes in pharmacokinetics are of particular concern for patients considering chemotherapy (Table 66.2).[32] Reduced liver function alters the clearance of drugs that rely on hepatic metabolism for activation or elimination, and a reduction in the cytochrome P450 system may be further affected by polypharmacy, which is common among the elderly. Similarly, renal function declines with age, and nephrotoxic agents must be appropriately dosed in order to avoid unnecessary toxicity secondary to reduced renal elimination. Age-related changes of the gastrointestinal tract may result in a reduced rate of enteral absorption, which may become significant with the development of oral agents. Changes in body composition, albumin levels, and red blood cell concentration affect the volume of distribution, free-fraction, peak concentration, and half-life of many agents.[32]

Pharmacokinetic data regarding the use of specific cytotoxic therapies in the elderly are limited (Box 66.3),[32] and most drug information originates from studies that included younger patient populations.[33] Direct application of the data from these studies to the elderly may not be appropriate since it is acknowledged that older patients are more complex than younger patients. In addition to more comorbidities, elderly patients have tremendous variability in their underlying chronic health, nutritional status and the number of medications. Therefore they are at greater risk for drug interactions, and may experience more adverse effects.[34]

## TOXICITY OF CHEMOTHERAPY AND SUPPORTIVE CARE

With age, and particularly after 70, the risk of mucositis, myelosuppression, and cardiomyopathy, as well as central and peripheral neuropathy secondary to chemotherapy, increases.[15] However, despite experiencing toxicity, evidence exists that patients over 70 generally tolerate systemic chemotherapy with limited effects on independence, comorbidity, and quality of life.[35] The need exists for predictive models of chemotherapy tolerance that incorporate clinical measures. In a recent pilot study to determine predictors

**Box 66.3** Special considerations regarding chemotherapeutic agents in the elderly

1. Gemcitabine
   - Prolonged half-life in the elderly, but no dosing modification based on age
   - Dosing adjustments in hepatic and renal insufficiency have been published
   - Well tolerated as a single agent and should be considered for palliative purposes
   - Neutropenia and thrombocytopenia are common, and elderly are prone to myelosuppression
2. Methotrexate
   - Cleared by kidneys, and used with caution in the setting of renal insufficiency or advanced age
   - Increased risk of nephrotoxicity, gastrointestinal toxicity, and myelotoxicity with advanced age
   - Minimize toxicity with dose adjustments or leucovorin rescue
3. Doxorubicin
   - Increased risk of cardiotoxicity reported in the elderly
   - Dose-limiting myelosuppression
   - Dose adjustments necessary in the setting of hyperbilirubinemia
4. Epirubicin
   - Thought to be better tolerated than other anthracyclines with less nausea, vomiting, myelosuppression, and cardiac toxicity
   - Elderly patients have been shown to tolerate weekly dosing
5. Paclitaxel
   - Decreased clearance with age, but likely not clinically significant
   - Neurotoxicity and neuropathy concern for elderly with comorbidities (e.g. diabetes or gait disturbances)
   - Neurotoxicity may be decreased with amifostine or glutamic acid
6. Docetaxel
   - Increased toxic deaths in patients with hepatic insufficiency
   - Fluid retention associated with cumulative doses over 400 mg/m$^2$ in patients that do not receive dexamethasone prophylaxis
   - Taxanes undergo cytochrome P450 metabolism; pharmacokinetics altered by liver dysfunction and drug interactions
7. Cisplatin
   - Up to 90% cleared by the kidneys
   - Minimize renal toxicity with hydration
   - Ototoxicity can be a concern in elderly with baseline hearing loss
   - Renal insufficiency, magnesium wasting, nausea, peripheral neuropathy, ototoxicity, myelosuppression are potential toxicities
   - Amifostine may reduce some potential toxicities
8. Carboplatin
   - Cleared by the kidneys, but dose calculated by the Calvert formula, which accounts for creatinine clearance
   - Manufacturer recommends:
     a. initial doses of 250 mg/m$^2$ for CrCl <60 ml/min
     b. initial doses of 200 mg/m$^2$ for CrCl 16–40 ml/min

Based on data from Lichtman et al.[32]

of toxicity, pretreatment diastolic blood pressure and marrow invasion correlated independently with toxicity. Previous treatment with chemotherapy, lower body mass index, anemia, and thrombocytopenia were predictors of lower chemotherapy dose intensity.[36]

Guidelines regarding supportive care of elderly individuals have been published.[37] Of particular concern are the management and prevention of neutropenia with its associated risk of infection. Neutropenic infection-related mortality in lymphoma patients over 70 years of age has been estimated to be between 5% and 30%.[15] Furthermore, the majority of deaths and significant infections in older patients receiving chemotherapy occur during the first cycle.[38] The routine use of prophylactic growth factors should be considered in individuals over 70 who are receiving moderately toxic regimens. Additionally, anemia may lead to increased toxicity of chemotherapy, fatigue, and complications from medications or infections. Some have recommended that hemoglobin levels should be maintained at least at 12 g/dl with utilization of recombinant erythropoietin. Elderly patients with significant mucositis with resultant diminished oral intake or frequent diarrhea are at risk for dehydration, and they should be treated aggressively with fluid hydration. As previously mentioned, consideration should be given to an elderly patient's renal function, with dose modifications as necessary, to avoid toxicity and further renal impairment.[37]

## LOCALIZED OR LOCALLY ADVANCED DISEASE IN THE ELDERLY

### RADICAL CYSTECTOMY

Radical cystectomy is considered the standard of care for muscle-invasive disease in the United States. Although the procedure initially was thought to be associated with significant morbidity and mortality, follow-up of a large number of patients suggests otherwise. Stein et al reported the outcomes in a series of cystectomy patients with a median age of 66 years. They observed perioperative deaths in 2.5%, early complications in 28%, and an overall survival at 5 years of 66%.[7] Another series suggests that the operative mortality and complication rates for patients over 70 do not differ from those of patients under 70 year old.[39] Furthermore, evidence suggests that in the elderly population alternatives to cystectomy may be associated with greater morbidity and mortality and a worse quality of life.[40]

Comorbidity appears to play a significant role in outcomes following cystectomy in elderly patients. In the series by Stein et al, deaths occurring within the first 3 years following cystectomy were attributed to bladder cancer, but deaths occurring later were largely related to other comorbidities present in an elderly population.[7] While perioperative outcomes were not found to change with increased age in the series comparing cystectomy patients older than 70 with those younger than 70, an

over 5-year survival probability of 53% was reported for those over 70 compared to 63% reported for those under 70 years. Given that recurrence rates between the two groups were similar, this difference in survival may be attributable to comorbidities in the population.[39] Another report on a series of octogenarians with comorbidities who underwent cystectomy estimated that 26% of postoperative complications were attributable to underlying medical illnesses.[41] The ASA score has been used to better assess the effect of comorbidity on outcomes in elderly patients that undergo cystectomy. Results indicate that high-risk patients, based on an age of 75 years or older, with an ASA score of III or greater, are able to undergo cystectomy safely.[42]

Chronologic age alone should not determine whether cystectomy is feasible and appropriate. The surgeon must also weigh the fact that surgery may offer these patients a better chance for cure, perhaps with less morbidity than alternative options. While elderly patients may be able to undergo cystectomy safely, their comorbidities must be assessed objectively, and reversible conditions must be addressed seriously because comorbidities may affect both the immediate postoperative course and long-term survival.

### NEOADJUVANT AND ADJUVANT CHEMOTHERAPY

The use of neoadjuvant and adjuvant chemotherapy for patients with localized or locally advanced disease remains somewhat controversial, and largely only cisplatin-containing regimens have been reported in the perioperative period. Nonetheless, evidence exists to suggest that perioperative chemotherapy is beneficial in terms of survival.[43,44] Grossman et al recently reported a significant difference in median survival of 46 months for patients treated with cystectomy alone versus 77 months for patients that received three cycles of MVAC preoperatively.[43] Age did not appear to affect survival when patients were stratified by age less than or greater than 65 years. The median age in both treatment arms was 63 years, and the eldest patient receiving combined treatment was 79 years. Patients were excluded if renal, hepatic, or hematologic impairment was present and if a Southwest Oncology Group (SWOG) performance status was 2 or greater. Although no treatment-related deaths were reported, approximately one-third of patients experienced severe hematologic or gastrointestinal effects. MVAC did not appear to affect the chances of undergoing radical cystectomy nor risks of morbidity or mortality related to the procedure.[43,44] While the stratified age analysis suggests that perioperative chemotherapy may be equally efficacious in elderly and in younger patients, the significant toxicity of MVAC limits the use of this approach to the fittest elderly patients.

## RADIOTHERAPY-BASED MULTIMODALITY APPROACHES

The curative potential of radiotherapy alone for invasive bladder cancer is suboptimal. Historically, patients with surgically unresectable disease, or who are not surgical candidates because of medical comorbidities, have been considered for definitive radiotherapy. However, the elderly experience significant toxicity with radiation, and a 50% hospitalization rate due to gastrointestinal and urogenital side effects has been reported in patients 75 or more years old.[45] Additionally, studies have shown that as many as 70% of radiotherapy patients may experience a local recurrence, and that their 5-year survival rate is less than 40%.[46] Several phase II and phase III trials have suggested improved outcomes, at least in terms of local control, with the addition of chemotherapy.[47,48] Hypofractionated radiotherapy may be palliative in elderly bladder cancer patients.[49]

Bladder preservation protocols have been developed that incorporate tumor resection with chemotherapy and radiotherapy. Such a multimodality approach may be appropriate for elderly patients who are not surgical candidates or refuse cystectomy. A recent trial investigated a multimodality bladder-sparing approach for elderly patients that incorporated an initial transurethral resection (TUR) followed by systemic chemotherapy consisting of fluorouracil, epirubicin, and cisplatin.[48] Upon completion of chemotherapy, a follow-up TUR was performed, and, if residual disease was identified, then radiotherapy was planned. This study included 22 patients with a median age of 74 years, performance status as low as 60%, and medical contraindications to radical cystectomy. The overall response rate was 54.5%, with an actuarial median survival of only 11.6 months. Remarkably, the median relative dose intensities of the drugs were fairly high, with a median relative dose intensity of 96% for cisplatin. Toxicity was mainly hematologic and gastrointestinal in nature, and no toxic deaths occurred. The approach appears feasible, but the investigators note that their chemotherapy regimen was not as active as other existent regimens used in younger patients.[48] Thus multimodality treatment in the elderly is limited not only by ability to tolerate therapy but also by the availability of effective chemotherapy.

## TREATMENT OF METASTATIC DISEASE IN THE ELDERLY

Chemotherapy is the treatment of choice for metastatic bladder cancer. MVAC is considered by many to be the gold standard regimen to which newer chemotherapy combinations are to be compared. Its use is associated with significant myelosuppression, neutropenic sepsis, mucositis, and renal toxicity. Importantly, toxic death rates of approximately 4% have been reported consistently. However, it should be noted that age was not associated with outcomes in a cooperative group study that demonstrated superiority of MVAC over single-agent cisplatin and included patients as old as 79 in the combination chemotherapy arm.[50] Sella et al reported results in elderly bladder cancer patients aged 76–84 years who received cisplatin, methotrexate, and vinblastine (CMV) or MVAC. In patients treated for metastatic disease, 39% experienced septic complications, and 17% withdrew from the study because of toxicity of the drug. No treatment-related deaths were seen, and the efficacy of chemotherapy was comparable to that seen in younger patients.[51]

More recently, Bamias et al retrospectively analyzed outcomes in patients over 70 years old with inoperable locally advanced, metastatic, or recurrent bladder cancer who received one of four cisplatin- or carboplatin-based chemotherapy regimens, and they compared their outcomes with those in a similar cohort of patients under 70 years old.[52] A trend towards increased grade 3 or 4 neutropenia was identified, which did not reach statistical significance, in the over 70 population. However, 4.5% of patients over 70 years old who received docetaxel and cisplatin experienced neutropenic infections, whereas none of their under-70 counterparts experienced this complication. This difference was statistically significant. Notably, growth factor support was provided to a number of patients, and its use may explain the improved toxicity profile relative to the earlier studies. Interestingly, grade 3 or 4 renal toxicity was rare. Complete and overall response rates as well as median survival data were similar regardless of age. Importantly, a number of patients with an ECOG performance status of 2 or 3 were included, and, in a multivariate analysis, an ECOG performance status of 2 or 3 or hemoglobin less than 10 were independent prognostic factors. Patients over 70 years of age with a performance status of 0 or 1 and a hemoglobin greater than 10 had a median survival of 13.9 months. Alternatively, a performance status of 2 or 3 or a hemoglobin less than 10 resulted in a median survival of only 5 months. This analysis suggests that elderly patients may tolerate combination platinum-based therapy, but baseline characteristics such as performance status and hemoglobin may identify patients for whom less toxic therapy or palliative supportive care is more appropriate.[52]

As discussed, many elderly patients have comorbidities, and reduced cardiac function, renal insufficiency, or uncontrolled diabetes mellitus which would preclude patients from receiving MVAC or cisplatin-based therapy, even if they had an excellent performance status. The combination of gemcitabine and cisplatin (GC) has recently been shown to have an efficacy similar to that of MVAC with less significant toxicity, namely neutropenia, mucositis, and improved quality of life measures.[53] Many would consider this doublet to be a reasonable alternative to MVAC for elderly patients. However, cases of nephrotic syndrome and interstitial pneumonitis have been noted in elderly patients treated with this regimen.[54]

Effective alternatives to cisplatin-containing regimens are needed for elderly patients who are not candidates for cisplatin. Noncisplatin regimens incorporating newer agents, such as paclitaxel and gemcitabine, have demonstrated activity in bladder cancer. The combination of gemcitabine and carboplatin has been assessed in older patients with impaired renal function and poor performance status with promising response rates of 44% to 59% (Table 66.3).[55-58] Complete response rates were reported as high as 18%, and overall survival appears to be in the order of 10 months. Similarly, paclitaxel in combination with carboplatin has also shown activity in patients with renal impairment (Table 66.4).[59-61] Response rates appear to

be more variable with this doublet, but overall survival appears to be roughly 9 months.[59] Generally, both of these combinations were well tolerated with primarily hematologic toxicity in both regimens and neurologic toxicity with the paclitaxel doublet. Nevertheless, a few treatment-related deaths were reported. The apparent lower median survival with the latter two combinations may be a reflection of patient selection or lower efficacy; however, their use is acceptable when the treatment goals are strictly palliative.

Another noncisplatin doublet, paclitaxel and gemcitabine, has also been reported to have activity in bladder cancer, and some of the patients included in these studies were elderly or had a poor performance status (Table 66.5).[62-64] Response rates of 54% to 60% were observed, and a median overall survival of 14.4 months, which appears comparable to that with MVAC and GC, has been reported in two series. This doublet has been reasonably well tolerated, and toxicity has been primarily hematologic.[63,64] Notably, one group reported grade IV pulmonary toxicity in a few patients.[62]

**Table 66.3** Gemcitabine/carboplatin in bladder cancer patients with advanced age, comorbidity, or impaired renal function

| Lead author | No. pts | Age, years (median) | Performance status | CrCl (ml/min) | Gemcitabine | Carboplatin | RR (%) | CR (%) | Median OS |
|---|---|---|---|---|---|---|---|---|---|
| Llado[55] | 16 | 47–75 (68) | 18.8% WHO 2 | 5 pts >55 7 pts 30–55 4 pts <30 | 1000 mg/m² d 1, 8 | AUC 4.5 or 5 d 1 | 44 | 6 | NR |
| Carles[56] | 17 | 54–78 (69) | Range: 50–100% Mean: 80% (Karnofsky) | Range: 21–55 Mean: 45.4 | 1000 mg/m² d 1, 8 | AUC 5 d 1 | 53 | 12 | 10 mos |
| Shannon[57] | 17 | 54–78 (69) | 30% ECOG 2 | Range: 34–90 Mean: 56 | 1000 mg/m² d 1, 8 | AUC 5 d 1 | 59 | 18 | 10.5 mos |
| Nogue-Aliguer[58] | 41 | 52–85 (66) | 60–79%: 36.6% Median: 80% (Karnofsky) | 54% <60 | 1000 mg/m² d 1, 8 | AUC 5 d 1 | 56 | 15 | 10.1 mos |

Chemotherapy was given in 21-day cycles.
AUC, area under the curve (Calvert formula); CR, complete response; CrCl, creatinine clearance; d, day; ECOG, Eastern Cooperative Oncology Group; mos, months; NR, not reported; OS, overall survival; RR, response rate; WHO, World Health Organization.

**Table 66.4** Paclitaxel/carboplatin in bladder cancer patients with advanced age, comorbidity, or impaired renal function

| Lead author | No. pts | Age, years (median) | Performance status | CrCl (ml/min) | Paclitaxel | Carboplatin | RR (%) | CR (%) | Median OS |
|---|---|---|---|---|---|---|---|---|---|
| Redman[60] | 35 | 38–82 (66) | 11% ECOG 2 | NR | 200 mg/m² d 1 | AUC 5 d1 | 52 | 20 | 9.5 mos |
| Small[59] | 29 | 37–78 (68) | 7% ECOG 2 | Range: 36–125.6 Median: 61 | 200 mg/m² d 1 | AUC 5 d1 | 21 | 0 | 9 mos |
| Vaughn[61] | 37 | 34–82 (70) | 11% ECOG 2 | Range: 21.5–58.6 Median: 35.2 | 225 mg/m² d 1 | AUC 6 d1 | 24 | 8 | 7.1 mos |

Chemotherapy was given in 21-day cycles.
AUC, area under the curve (Calvert formula); CR, complete response; CrCl, creatinine clearance; d, day; ECOG, Eastern Cooperative Oncology Group; mos, months; NR, not reported; OS, overall survival; RR, response rate.

**Table 66.5** Paclitaxel/gemcitabine in bladder cancer patients with advanced age and comorbidity

| Lead author | No. pts | Age, years (median) | Performance status | Paclitaxel | Gemcitabine | RR (%) | CR (%) | Median OS |
|---|---|---|---|---|---|---|---|---|
| Meluch[64] | 54 | 33–88 (67) | 11% ECOG 2 | 200 mg/m² d 1 of 21 day cycles | 1000 mg/m² d 1, 8, 15 | 54 | 7 | 14.4 mos |
| Parameswaran[62] | 24 | 35–77 (65) | Range: 80–100% Median: 90% (Karnofsky) | 110 mg/m² d 1, 8, 15 of 28 day cycles | 1000 mg/m² d 1, 8, 15 | 61 | 39 | NR |
| Sternberg[63] | 41 | 32–78 (62) | Range: 40–100% Median: 70% (Karnofsky) | 150 mg/m² d 1 of 14 day cycles | 2500–3000 mg/m² d 1 | 60 | 28 | 14.4 mos |

Chemotherapy was given in 14-day,[63] 21-day,[64] and 28-day[62] cycles.

AUC, area under the curve (Calvert formula); CR, complete response; d, day; ECOG, Eastern Cooperative Oncology Group; mos, months; NR, not reported; OS, overall survival; RR, response rate.

Currently, the SWOG is investigating the utility and feasibility of this regimen in patients over the age of 70 with bladder cancer. This is a phase II study (S0028) in which patients are given gemcitabine 1000 mg/m² and paclitaxel 175 mg/m² on days 1 and 8 in 21-day cycles. Correlations between response, pharmacokinetics, and genetic polymorphisms are planned, and assessments of quality of life and comorbidity will be made.[65]

Single-agent chemotherapy should be considered for elderly patients that are unable to tolerate multiagent regimens and for whom treatment goals are strictly palliative. Paclitaxel, docetaxel, and gemcitabine are considered to be the most active single agents with modest toxicity profiles. Use of single-agent gemcitabine in the elderly has been reported.[20] In a series of 25 patients with a median age of 76 years treated with gemcitabine 1200 mg/m², a 40% response rate was observed with a median survival of 8 months. The functional status of the patient population was limited, considering that 52% were assessed as an ECOG 2 and that 32% were dependent in either an activity of daily living (ADL) or an instrumental activity of daily living (IADL). Toxicity was reasonable, and results suggest that single-agent gemcitabine can be given safely to elderly patients, and even in patients with limited functional status.[20]

## CONCLUSION

Regardless of disease stage, elderly patients with bladder cancer require special consideration. A body of evidence suggests that age alone should not exclude patients from standard therapies with the goal of cure or prolonging survival. However, elderly individuals should be carefully screened, at least in terms of comorbidities and functional status, to begin to determine their overall fitness and ability to tolerate treatment. On the other hand, frail individuals should be identified and treated with the goals of preserving quality of life and palliation of symptoms. Newer chemotherapeutic agents are better tolerated by the elderly than older ones, and clinical trials are needed to focus on the efficacy and safety of novel drug combinations in this population as the number of elderly individuals with bladder cancer is expected to increase significantly.

## REFERENCES

1. Murray CJ, Lopez AD. Alternative projections of mortality and disability by cause 1990–2020: Global Burden of Disease Study. Lancet 1997;349(9064):1498–1504.
2. Franceschi S, La Vecchia C. Cancer epidemiology in the elderly. Crit Rev Oncol Hematol 2001;39(3):219–226.
3. Yancik R, Ries LA. Aging and cancer in America. Demographic and epidemiologic perspectives. Hematol Oncol Clin North Am 2000;14:17–23.
4. Balducci L, Extermann M. Cancer and aging. An evolving panorama. Hematol Oncol Clin North Am 2000;14(1):1–16.
5. Raghavan D, Shipley WU, Garnick MB, Russell PJ, Richie JP. Biology and management of bladder Cancer N Engl J Med 1990;322(16):1129–1138.
6. Arias E. United States life tables, 2000. Natl Vital Stat Rep 2002;51(3):1–38.
7. Stein JP, Lieskovsky G, Cote R, et al. Radical cystectomy in the treatment of invasive bladder cancer: long-term results in 1,054 patients. J Clin Oncol 2001;19(3):666–675.
8. Hamerman D. Toward an understanding of frailty. Ann Intern Med 1999;130(11):945–950.
9. Balducci L, Corcoran MB. Antineoplastic chemotherapy of the older cancer patient. Hematol Oncol Clin North Am 2000;14(1):193–212, x–xi.
10. Fried LP, Tangen CM, Walston J, et al. Frailty in older adults: evidence for a phenotype. J Gerontol A Biol Sci Med Sci 2001;56(3):M146–156.
11. Balducci L, Stanta G. Cancer in the frail patient: a coming epidemic. Hematol Oncol Clin North Am 2000;14:235–250.
12. Bernabei R, Venturiero V, Tarsitani P, Gambassi G. The comprehensive geriatric assessment: when, where, how. Crit Rev Oncol Hematol 2000;33(1):45–56.
13. Balducci L. Geriatric oncology. Crit Rev Oncol Hematol 2003;46(3):211–220.
14. Extermann M. Studies of comprehensive geriatric assessment in patients with Cancer Cancer Control 2003;10(6):463–468.

15. Balducci L, Extermann M. Management of cancer in the older person: a practical approach. Oncologist 2000;5(3):224–237.

16. Rao AV, Seo PH, Cohen HJ. Geriatric assessment and comorbidity. Semin Oncol 2004;31(2):149–159.

17. Bajorin DF, Dodd PM, Mazumdar M, et al. Long-term survival in metastatic transitional-cell carcinoma and prognostic factors predicting outcome of therapy. J Clin Oncol 1999;17(10):3173–3181.

18. Balducci L, Beghe C. The application of the principles of geriatrics to the management of the older person with Cancer Crit Rev Oncol Hematol 2000;35(3):147–154.

19. Repetto L, Pietropaolo M, Gianni W. Comprehensive geriatric assessment in oncology: pro. Tumori 2002;88(1 Suppl 1):S101–102.

20. Castagneto B, Zai S, Marenco D, et al. Single-agent gemcitabine in previously untreated elderly patients with advanced bladder carcinoma: response to treatment and correlation with the comprehensive geriatric assessment. Oncology 2004;67(1):27–32.

21. Extermann M, Overcash J, Lyman GH, Parr J, Balducci L. Comorbidity and functional status are independent in older cancer patients. J Clin Oncol 1998;16(4):1582–1587.

22. Fried LP, Bandeen-Roche K, Kasper JD, Guralnik JM. Association of comorbidity with disability in older women: The Women's Health and Aging Study. J Clin Epidemiol 1999;52(1):27–37.

23. Overcash J. Symptom management in the geriatric patient. Cancer Control 1998;5(3 Suppl 1):46–47.

24. Charlson M, Szatrowski TP, Peterson J, Gold J. Validation of a combined comorbidity index. J Clin Epidemiol 1994;47(11):1245–1251.

25. Conwell Y, Forbes NT, Cox C, Caine ED. Validation of a measure of physical illness burden at autopsy: the Cumulative Illness Rating Scale. J Am Geriatr Soc 1993;41(1):38–41.

26. Extermann M. Measuring comorbidity in older cancer patients. Eur J Cancer 2000;36(4):453–471.

27. Piccirillo JF, Feinstein AR. Clinical symptoms and comorbidity: significance for the prognostic classification of cancer. Cancer 1996;77(5):834–842.

28. Saklad M. Grading of patients for surgical procedures. Anesthiology 1941;2:281–284.

29. American Society of Anesthesiologists. New classification of physical status. Anesthiology 1963;24:111.

30. Malavaud B, Vaessen C, Mouzin M, Rischmann P, Sarramon J, Schulman C. Complications for radical cystectomy. Impact of the American Society of Anesthesiologists score. Eur Urol 2001;39(1):79–84.

31. Wolters U, Wolf T, Stutzer H, Schroder T. ASA classification and perioperative variables as predictors of postoperative outcome. Br J Anaesth 1996;77(2):217–222.

32. Lichtman SM, Skirvin JA, Vemulapalli S. Pharmacology of antineoplastic agents in older cancer patients. Crit Rev Oncol Hematol 2003;46(2):101–114.

33. Yuen GJ. Altered pharmacokinetics in the elderly. Clin Geriatr Med 1990;6(2):257–267.

34. Lichtman SM, Skirvin JA. Pharmacology of antineoplastic agents in older cancer patients. Oncology 2000;14(12):1743–1755.

35. Chen H, Cantor A, Meyer J, et al. Can older cancer patients tolerate chemotherapy? A prospective pilot study. Cancer 2003;97(4):1107–1114.

36. Extermann M, Chen H, Cantor AB, et al. Predictors of tolerance to chemotherapy in older cancer patients: a prospective pilot study. Eur J Cancer 2002;38(11):1466–1473.

37. Balducci L, Yates J. General guidelines for the management of older patients with cancer. Oncology 2000;14(11A):221–227.

38. Balducci L. New paradigms for treating elderly patients with cancer: the comprehensive geriatric assessment and guidelines for supportive care. J Supportive Oncol 2003;1(Suppl 2):30–37.

39. Figueroa AJ, Stein JP, Dickinson M, et al. Radical cystectomy for elderly patients with bladder carcinoma: an updated experience with 404 patients. Cancer 1998;83(1):141–147.

40. Leibovitch I, Avigad I, Ben-Chaim J, Nativ O, Goldwasser B. Is it justified to avoid radical cystoprostatectomy in elderly patients with invasive transitional cell carcinoma of the bladder? Cancer 1993;71(10):3098–3101.

41. Stroumbakis N, Herr HW, Cookson MS, Fair WR. Radical cystectomy in the octogenarian. J Urol 1997;158(6):2113–2117.

42. Chang SS, Alberts G, Cookson MS, Smith JA Jr. Radical cystectomy is safe in elderly patients at high risk. J Urol 2001;166(3):938–941.

43. Grossman HB, Natale RB, Tangen CM, et al. Neoadjuvant chemotherapy plus cystectomy compared with cystectomy alone for locally advanced bladder cancer. N Engl J Med 2003;349(9):859–866.

44. Skinner DG, Daniels JR, Russell CA, et al. The role of adjuvant chemotherapy following cystectomy for invasive bladder cancer: a prospective comparative trial. J Urol 1991;145(3):459–464; discussion 464–467.

45. Sengelov L, Klintorp S, Havsteen H, Kamby C, Hansen SL, von der Maase H. Treatment outcome following radiotherapy in elderly patients with bladder cancer. Radiother Oncol 1997;44(1):53–58.

46. Pollack A, Zagars GZ. Radiotherapy for stage T3b transitional cell carcinoma of the bladder. Semin Urol Oncol 1996;14(2):86–95.

47. Coppin CM, Gospodarowicz MK, James K, et al. Improved local control of invasive bladder cancer by concurrent cisplatin and preoperative or definitive radiation. The National Cancer Institute of Canada Clinical Trials Group. J Clin Oncol 1996;14(11):2901–2907.

48. Veronesi A, Lo Re G, Carbone A, et al. Multimodal treatment of locally advanced transitional cell bladder carcinoma in elderly patients. Eur J Cancer 1994;30A(7):918–920.

49. Duchesne GM, Bolger JJ, Griffiths GO, et al. A randomized trial of hypofractionated schedules of palliative radiotherapy in the management of bladder carcinoma: results of Medical Research Council Trial BA09. Int J Radiat Oncol Biol Phys 2000;47(2):379–388.

50. Loehrer PJ Sr, Einhorn LH, Elson PJ, et al. A randomized comparison of cisplatin alone or in combination with methotrexate, vinblastine, and doxorubicin in patients with metastatic urothelial carcinoma: a Cooperative Group Study. J Clin Oncol 1992;10(7):1066–1073.

51. Sella A, Logothetis CJ, Dexeus FH, Amato R, Finn L, Fitz K. Cisplatin combination chemotherapy for elderly patients with urothelial tumours. Br J Urol 1991;67(6):603–607.

52. Bamias A, Efstathiou E, Hamilos G, et al. Outcome of elderly patients following platinum-based chemotherapy for advanced urothelial cancer. Proc Am Soc Clin Oncol 2004;23:4542a.

53. von der Maase H, Hansen SW, Roberts JT, et al. Gemcitabine and cisplatin versus methotrexate, vinblastine, doxorubicin, and cisplatin in advanced or metastatic bladder cancer: results of a large, randomized, multinational, multicenter, phase III study. J Clin Oncol 2000;18(17):3068–3077.

54. Elsaid A, Khaled H, Gaafar R, Abdelazim H. Cytotoxicity profile of gemcitabine in elderly patients. Proc Am Soc Clin Oncol 2000;19:1422a.

55. Llado A, Bellmunt J, Kaiser G. A dose finding study of carboplatin with fixed doses of gemcitabine in 'unfit' patients with advanced bladder cancer. Proc Am Soc Clin Oncol 2000;19:1354a.

56. Carles J, Nogue M, Domenech M, et al. Carboplatin–gemcitabine treatment of patients with transitional cell carcinoma of the bladder and impaired renal function. Oncology 2000;59(1):24–27.

57. Shannon C, Crombie C, Brooks A, Lau H, Drummond M, Gurney H. Carboplatin and gemcitabine in metastatic transitional cell carcinoma of the urothelium: effective treatment of patients with poor prognostic features. Ann Oncol 2001;12(7):947–952.

58. Nogue-Aliguer M, Carles J, Arrivi A, et al. Gemcitabine and carboplatin in advanced transitional cell carcinoma of the urinary tract: an alternative therapy. Cancer 2003;97(9):2180–2186.

59. Small EJ, Lew D, Redman BG, et al. Southwest Oncology Group Study of paclitaxel and carboplatin for advanced transitional-cell carcinoma: the importance of survival as a clinical trial end point. J Clin Oncol 2000;18(13):2537–2544.

60. Redman BG, Smith DC, Flaherty L, Du W, Hussain M. Phase II trial of paclitaxel and carboplatin in the treatment of advanced urothelial carcinoma. J Clin Oncol 1998;16(5):1844–1848.

61. Vaughn DJ, Manola J, Dreicer R, See W, Levitt R, Wilding G. Phase II study of paclitaxel plus carboplatin in patients with advanced carcinoma of the urothelium and renal dysfunction (E2896): a trial of the Eastern Cooperative Oncology Group. Cancer 2002;95(5):1022–1027.

62. Parameswaran R, Fisch MJ, Ansari RH. A Hoosier Oncology Group phase II study of weekly paclitaxel and gemcitabine in advanced transitional cell carcinoma of the bladder. Proc Am Soc Clin Oncol 2001;20:798a.

63. Sternberg CN, Calabro F, Pizzocaro G, Marini L, Schnetzer S, Sella A. Chemotherapy with an every-2-week regimen of gemcitabine and paclitaxel in patients with transitional cell carcinoma who have received prior cisplatin-based therapy. Cancer 2001;92(12):2993–2998.

64. Meluch AA, Greco FA, Burris HA 3rd, et al. Paclitaxel and gemcitabine chemotherapy for advanced transitional-cell carcinoma of the urothelial tract: a phase II trial of the Minnie Pearl Cancer Research Network. J Clin Oncol 2001;19(12):3018–3024.

65. Crawford ED, Wood DP, Petrylak DP, Scott J, Coltman CA Jr, Raghavan D. Southwest Oncology Group studies in bladder cancer. Cancer 2003;97(Suppl 8):2099–2108.

# Targeted therapy for bladder cancer

*Wassim Kassouf, Bernard H Bochner, Colin P Dinney*

## INTRODUCTION

Transitional cell carcinoma (TCC) of the bladder is the fifth most common solid tumor malignancy in the United States. The American Cancer Society has estimated approximately 13,180 people will die from TCC of the bladder in the United States in 2005, and most of these deaths will occur as the result of metastatic disease.[1] The standard treatment for operable invasive bladder cancer is radical cystectomy. Patients with metastatic TCC are usually treated with systemic chemotherapy.[2–5] Since the mid-1980s, the standard treatment for metastatic urothelial cancer has been methotrexate, vinblastine, adriamycin, and cisplatin (MVAC). Although high response rates are induced with combination chemotherapy, responses are usually short lived. Virtually all patients with distant metastatic bladder cancer succumb to the disease after a median survival duration of 18 months, even with the most effective available regimens.[3,4] Despite considerable effort to dose-escalate or otherwise modulate the components of MVAC, no improvement in survival has been realized.[6] Recently, paclitaxel, gemcitabine, and ifosfamide have been recognized for their activity against TCC, and many novel combination regimens have been reported.[7–13] Whereas some of these newer regimens are less toxic than MVAC, there is as yet no compelling evidence of improved patient survival.

In general, the treatment of metastatic epithelial cancers by classic cytotoxic chemotherapy has reached a therapeutic plateau, with an overall impact that falls short of the goal. Only for patients with germ cell cancers has the cytotoxic paradigm produced expectation of cure, and, even then, only when properly integrated with surgery and delivered by clinicians with an extremely refined knowledge of the relevant clinical biology. Apart from germ cell cancers, we find that, despite high response rates, even the 'chemosensitive' epithelial cancers (such as small cell carcinoma of the lung and cancers of the bladder and ovary) are generally incurable. What has been achieved is clinically significant palliation for many, and improved outcome as well as cure by adjuvant application of cytotoxic therapy to microscopic metastatic disease. Thus, while it is clear that cytotoxic chemotherapy remains an important aspect of combined therapy, the need for more effective treatment options remains. Fortunately, an improved understanding of the biology of malignancy is at last providing novel therapeutic approaches.

## TARGETED TREATMENTS FOR UROLOGIC MALIGNANCIES

Deregulation of cell-cycle and apoptotic pathways via mutation or altered expression of p53, p21/WAF-1, pRB, p27, and INK4A (p16) are necessary for uroepithelial transformation. In addition, members of the erbB family, vascular epidermal growth factor (VEGF), NFκB, Akt, PTEN, and cyclooxygenase 2 (COX2), are also implicated in the progression of the disease.[14] All of these molecules are potential targets for novel therapies. The most interesting targets, which are the focus of this chapter, include angiogenesis and aberrant signal transduction of specific growth factor receptors, i.e. epidermal growth factor receptor (EGFR) and HER2.

# ANGIOGENESIS AND BLADDER CANCER

Angiogenesis is characterized by increased endothelial cell proliferation and migration with new blood vessel formation. Tumor growth and metastasis depend on the development of a neovasculature in and around the tumor.[15-18] In the 1970s, Judah Folkman demonstrated that tumor cells interact with their environment to stimulate new vessel growth and that invasion and metastasis occur rapidly once neovascularization has occurred.[17,19] Such angiogenic tumors have higher vascular densities and immature vessels, which has a bearing on tumor biology, as the vascular architecture within areas of active angiogenesis is disorganized and irregular with permeable endothelial cell membranes.[18,20]

As is the case with most solid malignancies, angiogenesis plays a central role in the growth and progression of urothelial carcinoma. Over the past 25 years, the angiogenic nature of TCC of the bladder has been established through experimental findings and clinical observations. The angiogenic phenotype appears to be acquired at an early stage in the development of high-risk bladder tumors. The induction of a neovascular response in the preinvasive phase of tumor development is not unique to bladder carcinogenesis and may represent a necessary early step in the development of advanced disease.[21]

## PROGNOSTIC STUDIES OF MICROVESSEL DENSITY

Quantitative evaluations relating the extent of angiogenesis within bladder tumors to outcome have been performed using immunohistochemical endothelial cell markers (factor VIII, CD31, CD34). Several studies have documented an adverse relationship with increasing angiogenesis, disease recurrence, and patient survival. Although not all studies have demonstrated consistent findings, it appears that, as the level of tumor neovascularity increases, so does the biologic aggressiveness of the tumor.[22-26]

## ANGIOGENESIS INDUCERS

Multiple studies have documented that bladder cancers contain increased levels of angiogenic inducers compared to normal bladder tissues. In one of the earliest laboratory reports on the angiogenic nature of bladder cancer, Chodak et al demonstrated that bladder cancer, as opposed to normal bladder tissues, could induce a neovascular response in in vivo assays.[27] Bladder cancer patients were subsequently found to have high levels of excreted proangiogenic substances in their urine, further supporting the presence of endothelial cell inducers within bladder tumors.[28] Since these initial investigations, a wide variety of proangiogenic substances have been described in bladder cancer (Box 67.1). The specific inducer overexpressed within a given tumor may be cancer-type specific, as suggested by the finding that different tumor systems produce unique patterns of overexpressed inducers. Further highlighting the complexity of inducer overexpression in cancer, Crew et al reported that the extent of angiogenesis inducers expressed by bladder tumors may be produced in a stage-specific manner. Invasive T1 lesions were found to contain a four-fold increase in VEGF when compared to muscle-invasive tumors. In contrast, thymidine phosphorylase (TP) was markedly overexpressed in muscle-invasive disease, with an eight-fold increase in TP protein compared to superficial tumors.[29]

VEGF is one of the best characterized angiogenesis inducers. As a prognostic marker in bladder cancer, higher levels of VEGF in tumor tissue predict for an increased risk of progression of T1 disease, and elevated urinary levels are a marker of an increased risk of recurrence for patients with superficial lesions.[30] Recent clinical studies suggest that VEGF overexpression in prechemotherapy samples from patients with locally advanced urothelial cancer undergoing cystectomy and chemotherapy is a strong predictor for recurrence and death from bladder cancer.[31] This observation puts forward the important hypothesis that VEGF expression is mechanistically relevant to clinically aggressive bladder cancer, and provides the rationale for clinical investigation of interventions capable of blocking VEGF signaling. On the other hand, TP (responsible for the

---

**Box 67.1** Angiogenic inducers and inhibitors associated with bladder cancer

1. Inducers
   - Acidic fibroblastic growth factor (aFGF)[48,49]
   - Basic fibroblast growth factor (bFGF)[50-53]
   - Vascular epidermal growth factor (VEGF)[30,31,51,54-56]
   - Thymidine phosphorylase[32,33,57-60]
   - Scatter factor/hepatocyte growth factor[61,62]
   - Midkine[63]
   - Transforming growth factor-β1 and 2[64]
   - Angiogenin[64]
   - Interleukin 8 (IL8)[65]
   - Matrix metalloproteinases[38,40,66-68]
   - Fragments of hyaluronic acid[69-72]
   - Urokinase plasminogen activator[44,73]
   - Hypoxia inducible factors 1 and 2[74]
   - Cyclooxygenase 2[75]
   - Eukaryotic initiation factor 4E (EIF4E)[76]
2. Inhibitors
   - Thrombospondin[34,35]
   - Interferon-α (IFNα)[77,78]
   - BCG-induced: IFNγ, IP10, IL12[36]
   - Angiostatin[37]

breakdown of thymidine) plays a role in the generation of oxygen-free radicals, and can induce the expression of proteins involved in the induction of angiogenesis, including interleukin (IL) 8, matrix metalloproteinase (MMP) 1, and VEGF. Progressively increasing levels of TP activity have been found with increasing levels of invasion (superficial to high-grade invasive disease).[32] Additionally, the level of tumor-associated TP correlates with a decreased time-to-recurrence in superficial disease and decreased survival with more aggressive tumors.[33]

The inducers identified in tumors are derived from several possible sources, including direct production by bladder cancer cells, secretion from recruited stromal or immune cells, or release from stores located within the extracellular matrix.

## ANGIOGENESIS INHIBITORS

Under normal homeostatic conditions, limited active angiogenesis occurs within the bladder. A recognized mechanism of the angiogenic switch involves loss of production of endothelial cell inhibitory substances, thus tipping the balance between endothelial activation/inhibition in favor of active angiogenesis. Investigations into the role of inhibitors in cancer have demonstrated that thrombospondin (TSP) 1, a potent endogenous inhibitor of endothelial cell function, may play a central role in the switch that occurs during bladder cancer progression. Levels of TSP1 expression in invasive bladder cancers have been observed to correlate with the microvessel density within the primary tumor.[34] Downregulation of TSP1 was associated with a higher vascular density within the tumor, increased risk of recurrence, and decreased survival after radical cystectomy. Significantly lower levels of TSP1 in the culture media of bladder cancer cells were found compared to normal cultured urothelium.[35] The conditioned media from these cultures, tested in a rat corneal angiogenesis assay, demonstrated that normal bladder cells could not induce new blood vessel formation; however, the TSP1-deficient bladder cancer cell media were potently angiogenic.

Current treatments for TCC of the bladder, such as intravesical bacillus Calmette–Guérin (BCG), may work partly through inhibition of angiogenesis. Poppas et al found that the urine of patients undergoing BCG treatment for bladder cancer becomes increasing angioinhibitory.[36] Levels of the inhibitory proteins IL12, interferon-inducible protein 10 (IP10), and interferon-γ were increased in the urine of BCG-treated patients, suggesting that additional inhibitors of angiogenesis may participate in the angiogenic balance within the bladder. The role of other inhibitors of angiogenesis in bladder cancer remains less clear and is under active investigation. Angiostatin, an internal cleavage fragment of plasminogen, is a powerful endogenous inhibitor of angiogenesis. It has been found to have antitumor activity in several animal models and is currently under investigation in various phase I–III human studies. Angiostatin is active against bladder cancer, and can inhibit tumor growth in both superficial and invasive cancer models.[37] Replacement of other endogenous inhibitors such as endostatin, a cleavage fragment of collagen XVIII, also appears to inhibit bladder cancer growth.[38]

## MATRIX INTERACTIONS, ANGIOGENESIS, AND BLADDER CANCER

Interactions between extracellular matrix elements, cellular adhesion proteins, proteases, and accessory cells of the immune system play a key role in modulating the angiogenic response. The extracellular matrix, which provides a scaffold for cell migration, transmits a series of regulatory signals to the endothelial cell based on its composition and state of remodeling. Enzymes that degrade the matrix facilitate endothelial cell invasion by exposing protein motifs that are used by endothelial cells for attachment and migration. An important example is the regulatory mechanism involved in controlling the release of basic fibroblast growth factor (bFGF), which is found in large extracellular stores bound to proteoglycans located within the matrix of tumor tissues. Release from these extracellular sites involves a signaling cascade initiated by the tumor that results in the activation of enzymes which degrade and restructure the matrix (urokinase, heparanases, metalloproteinases), allowing bFGF to be utilized for endothelial cell activation. Compounds that block the activity of matrix-degrading enzymes, such as the tissue inhibitors of matrix metalloproteinases (TIMPs) are currently under investigation in clinical trials for their potential antitumor effect.

Several degradative enzymes have been identified as having important roles in the matrix remodeling of bladder cancer, and include the family of matrix metalloproteinases (MMPs), urokinase-type plasminogen activator (UPA), and tissue plasminogen activator. Studies of MMP2 (72 kDa, gelatinase A) and MMP9 (92 kDa, gelatinase B) in bladder cancer have shown an association with MMP2 and MMP9 and bladder tumor stage and grade,[39] although not all studies agree about their clinical relevance.[40] Urinary levels of MMP9 are sufficiently elevated in patients with superficial bladder cancer compared to healthy controls such that it may be useful as a marker of disease status.[38] The relationship between matrix-degrading enzymes, angiogenesis inducers, and inhibitors is quite complex. Oncogene activation (jun, fos, myb) and tumor suppressor gene inactivation (p53) have been found to increase the level of metalloproteinases associated with increased basement membrane degradation by tumor.[41,42]

UPA is a serine protease that functions to activate plasminogen to plasmin, which degrades the basement membrane of tissues. UPA is important in tumor migration and disease progression. Bladder tumors have been found to contain high levels of UPA.[43] The extent of UPA present within a tumor increases with tumor grade and pathologic stage. UPA tumor levels are predictive of recurrence risk in superficial bladder cancer,[43] and provide independent prognostic information.[44]

## ANGIOGENIC REGULATION AND THE ANGIOGENIC SWITCH IN BLADDER CANCER

The regulatory mechanisms responsible for controlling inducer and inhibitor expression and matrix degradation are receiving increasing attention in cancer research. It is now well established that activation of oncogenes and inactivation of tumor suppressor genes, in addition to their effects on cellular proliferation and apoptosis, can influence the angiogenic properties of cancer cells by altering the relative amounts of angiogenesis inhibitors, inducers, and matrix-degrading enzymes. The tumor suppressor gene p53 normally suppresses angiogenesis by increasing TSP1 expression, inducing degradation of hypoxia-inducible factor 1a (HIF1a), suppressing transcription of VEGF, and decreasing the expression of bFGF-binding protein. Several tumor suppressor genes experience frequent inactivation in high-grade and invasive bladder tumors, particularly the p53 and retinoblastoma tumor suppressor genes. P53 inactivation can lead to decreased expression of TSP1 and increased levels of VEGF.[34] Crew noted that p53 mutations were associated with increased VEGF expression and tumor angiogenesis.[30] In contrast, Reiher et al performed viral-mediated p53 gene replacement experiments into bladder cancer cell lines and noted no effect on TSP1 levels. These same studies, however, did identify that VEGF levels were decreased 5- to 50-fold in the higher VEGF-secreting cell lines following p53 expression.[45] Other tumor suppressor genes, or oncogenes with known regulatory activity on angiogenic substances such as p16, retinoblastoma, PTEN, and ras, have been found to play a role in tumor angiogenesis in other tumor systems; however, their role in bladder cancer is less clear.

## HYPOXIA

During tumor growth, blood vessels are needed to provide oxygen and nutrients, and remove metabolic waste products. As tumors enlarge, oxygen demands can outgrow their blood supply and a hypoxic state develops. Tumors have developed adaptations to hypoxia that provide metabolic and growth support to avoid cell death. One of the best documented adaptations is the hypoxia-related induction of proteins responsible for angiogenesis. Transcription factors, such as HIF1a, are key regulators of the hypoxia response cascade. Cell culture data demonstrate that HIF1a protein is increased in bladder cancer cells during experimentally induced hypoxia. Jones et al observed that HIF1a induction in bladder cell lines was associated with a corresponding increase in VEGF levels.[46] In concordance with the known differences in clinical behavior and genetic make-up, cell lines derived from superficial bladder tumors demonstrated different responses to hypoxia compared to invasive lines.

## ANTIANGIOGENIC THERAPY

A growing number of drugs are being developed that target tumor angiogenesis. Broadly, these agents are classified as direct or indirect inhibitors of tumor-induced blood vessel formation depending on their mechanism of action. Direct inhibitors target the endothelial cell population itself. This approach has the advantage of attacking a genetically stable cell population, perhaps limiting the risk for the subsequent development of drug resistance. Additionally, recent markers of actively proliferating tumor-associated blood vessels have been identified and may allow for specific targeted therapy, limiting injury (and side effects) to other cell types.[47] Indirect agents target the inducers that stimulate endothelial cell function by decreasing the expression of inducers or blocking their function, such as interfering with receptor function or signal transduction. Endogenous inhibitors have been identified that block the receptors of inducers directly or by decreasing their level of expression to limit endothelial cell activation.

Animal studies using different antiangiogenesis strategies have demonstrated the ability to limit TCC growth. Strategies have included the use of antibodies targeting specific inducers, such as VEGF, intravesical inhibitor administration (TNP470), and systemic inhibitor therapy (TNP470, angiostatin). Whereas multiple agents are under investigation in phase I–III development, specific indications for bladder cancer await future trials. Chemopreventive therapy, and definitive treatment for local or metastatic disease (alone or in combination with conventional chemotherapy agents), remain future potential indications for antiangiogenic therapy for bladder cancer. The tumoristatic nature of antiangiogenic agents makes it likely that long-term administration of agents capable of suppressing endothelial cell function will be required for adequate treatment. Potential morbidities, such as suboptimal wound healing, inhibition of the development of collateral vascularity in organs (such as the heart), and female sterility will need to be considered with long-term treatment. Additionally, the development of oral agents will facilitate the study and acceptance of chronic antiangiogenic treatment. As long-term systemic therapy presents financial and logistic difficulties, development of a gene therapy strategy that provides for long-term in vivo production of endothelial cell inhibitors is particularly appealing. Preclinical studies using inactivating lentiviral vectors to produce endostatin-overproducing bladder cancer cells have proven effective in limiting orthotopic bladder tumor growth and tumor-associated angiogenesis.[38]

The complexity of angiogenesis and its regulation have generated a number of potential targets for antiangiogenic therapy. Randomly targeting one factor or one particular pathway may have only limited clinical success as different angiogenic pathways may predominate within different tumors and even within the same tumor at different stages of development. A 'one size fits all' approach to antiangiogenic therapy is unrealistic, and ongoing efforts to delineate the crucial pathways within particular tumors remains the challenge to allow accurate and therapeutic targeting of a tumor's blood supply.

# EPIDERMAL GROWTH FACTOR RECEPTORS AND BLADDER CANCER

Many human tumors express high levels of growth factors and their receptors, which can be used as potential therapeutic targets. Tyrosine kinase (TK) receptors, including many growth factor receptors— such as the receptors for epidermal growth factor (EGF), insulin growth factor (IGF), platelet-derived growth factor (PDGF), vascular endothelial growth factor (VEGF), fibroblast growth factor (FGF), and hepatocyte growth factor (HGF)—have been found to be overexpressed in different tumor types. For many of these growth factor receptors, the degree of expression has been associated with the progression of cancer and a poor prognosis.[79–81]

Among the best studied growth factor receptors are the two members of the EGF receptor family: EGFR (ErbB1) and HER2/neu (ErbB2).

## BIOLOGIC ROLE OF THE EGF RECEPTOR FAMILY IN MALIGNANCY

EGF receptor and HER2 are plasma membrane glycoproteins that belong to the EGF receptor family (also known as type I receptor tyrosine kinases (TKs) or ErbB TK receptors). This receptor family is comprised of four closely related receptors: the EGF receptor itself (ErbB1/EGFR/HER1), ErbB2 (HER2/neu), ErbB3 (HER3), and ErbB4 (HER4). These receptors are composed of an extracellular binding domain, a transmembrane lipophilic segment, and an intracellular

protein TK domain with a regulatory carboxyl terminal segment.

The receptors exist as inactive monomers that homo- or heterodimerize (between EGFR and another member of the EGF receptor family) after ligand activation.[82] Following receptor dimerization, activation of the intrinsic protein TK activity, with autophosphorylation of tyrosine residues, occurs. These events result in the recruitment and phosphorylation of several intracellular substrates that initiate a cascade of events leading to cell-cycle progression and mitogenic signaling, as well as a number of other processes that are crucial to cancer progression.[83–85] Activation of the EGF receptor family (EGFR or HER2) has been identified as a key initiating event to a cascade of intracellular signaling leading to proliferation, cell survival, angiogenesis, and metastasis.[86]

## EGFR/HER1

EGFR is expressed, overexpressed, or dysregulated in many human solid tumors, including breast, ovarian, non small-cell lung (NSCL), colorectal, and head and neck cancers.[87–90] EGFR activation seems to promote tumor growth by increasing cell proliferation, motility, adhesion, and invasive capacity, and by blocking apoptosis.[91–93] In support of its important role in tumor biology, EGFR overexpression and dysregulation have been reported to be associated with indices of poorer prognosis in patients, and are associated with metastasis, late-stage disease, and resistance to chemotherapy, hormone therapy, and radiotherapy.[87,89,94–97]

Given the importance of EGFR in epithelial tumor biology, EGFR-targeted cancer therapies are currently being developed. Several potential points of intervention at the level of the extracellular receptor itself, as well as along the receptor's signaling pathway, have been identified. In recent years, the two strategies of EGFR-targeting agents (receptor TK inhibitors and monoclonal antibodies against the extracellular domain of the receptor) have been developed, alone or in combination with chemotherapy in several tumors.[98,99] Recent clinical trials have shown that such EGFR-targeted therapies have antitumor activity against a range of tumor types tested.

## EGFR EXPRESSION AND BLADDER CANCER PROGRESSION

Although the mechanism by which EGFR regulates tumor biology in bladder cancer is not clearly defined, it has been demonstrated that EGFR signaling regulates cellular proliferation, differentiation, survival, and invasion, and is implicated in the induction of tumor-induced angiogenesis and metastasis in TCC of the bladder.[100] High concentrations of biologically active EGF are found in the urine and can stimulate the growth and angiogenesis of TCC.[101] A study using a rat bladder cancer model showed that EGF in the urine induces cellular proliferation deep within the bladder wall.[102] Immunohistochemical studies have demonstrated that EGFR is overexpressed in human TCC compared to the normal urothelium, and that normally the urothelial cells which overexpress EGFR are found primarily in the basal layer of the urothelium.[102] However, in malignant and dysplastic urothelium, EGFR is expressed in all cell layers, possibly allowing for greater contact between the tumor cell and EGF.[103] These alterations in EGFR expression precede histologic evidence of cancer.[103]

Clinical studies evaluating the significance of EGFR expression in human TCC have shown that more than 50% of human TCCs overexpress the EGFR and that the level of expression directly correlates with tumor grade, stage, and survival.[104] In patients with superficial bladder cancer, EGFR expression correlates with multiplicity, time to disease recurrence, and overall recurrence rates.[104] EGFR expression also predicted for disease progression to muscle-invasive or metastatic TCC, and was an independent prognostic factor for death in a multivariate analysis. Patients with muscle-invasive TCC which overexpresses EGFR have only a 20% probability of long-term cancer-specific survival which is significantly worse than the survival of those whose tumors did not express EGFR.[105] The majority of metastases from TCC overexpress EGFR, and this expression is not downregulated by chemotherapy or radiation.[105] These studies emphasize the importance of EGFR overexpression in the development and progression of human TCC, and establish the rationale for the development of EGFR-directed therapy for human TCC.

## EGFR SIGNALING AND REGULATION OF CELLULAR PROLIFERATION, DEATH AND ANGIOGENESIS IN BLADDER CANCER

Therapy of human cancer cells with tyrosine kinase inhibitors or antibodies specific to the EGFR results in an antiproliferative effect, ranging from a mere slowing of cell division to cell-cycle arrest in the G1–S phase of the cell cycle. This cytostatic effect is due to inhibition of CDK2 activity and a decline in cyclin D levels, and upregulation of the cell-cycle inhibitor p27[Kip1] bound to CDK.[106–109]

Growth inhibition has also been documented in established human bladder cancer xenografts following therapy with cetuximab (IMC-C225), an EGFR blocker. Immunohistologic staining of tumors demonstrated a decrease in proliferating cell nuclear antigen accompanied by a rise in p27[Kip1]. These changes were accompanied by a marked inhibition of tumor growth. Apoptosis has also been implicated in EGFR signaling because, in several human cancer cell lines, cell-cycle arrest is followed by enhanced apoptosis.[110–112] Alternatively, elevations in caspase-3, -8, and -9 were observed in A431 squamous cell carcinoma following anti-EGFR therapy. In vivo, increased apoptosis in human TCC xenografts was observed following therapy with cetuximab, and the effect was enhanced by co-administration of paclitaxel. Thus, it is evident that a variety of proapoptotic mechanisms are activated when the EGFR signaling pathway is inhibited.

EGFR signaling and angiogenesis have been independently evaluated as targets for therapy, but the link between them has only recently been identified.[113–116] Using an orthotopic bladder cancer model, Perrotte et al reported the regression of established TCC growing in the bladders of nude mice following therapy with IMC-C225 due to a reduction in tumor-induced neovascularization secondary to the downregulation of tumor cell expression of the angiogenic factors VEGF, IL8, and bFGF.[117–119] Similar results were reported following the therapy of human squamous cell and pancreatic carcinoma xenografts with IMC-C225.[113,120] The mechanisms by which EGFR signaling pathways regulate VEGF, IL8, and bFGF are unclear, but it has been established that upregulation of these factors follows activation of the EGFR signaling pathways by EGF or tumor growth factor-$\alpha$ (TGF$\alpha$) and proceeds through both MAPK and Akt pathways.[109,111,113,114,121,122] EGFR activation also upregulates the production of proteolytic enzymes and MMPs and results in enhanced cell motility and invasion through Matrigel membranes.[123–134] Inoue et al provided a strong rationale for testing EGFR-directed therapy and cytotoxic therapy in patients with bladder cancer since taxol enhanced the antitumor activity of IMC-C225 in preclinical models.[135,136]

## THERAPEUTIC STRATEGIES AGAINST EGFR

### MONOCLONAL ANTIBODIES AGAINST THE EXTRACELLULAR DOMAIN OF THE EGFR

One of the most studied monoclonal antibodies (mAbs) against EGFR is IMC-C225, a human/murine chimeric monoclonal antibody. The effects of IMC-C225 include cell-cycle arrest, inhibition of angiogenesis, immunologic activity through antibody-dependent cellular cytotoxicity, and inhibition of tumor cell invasion and metastasis, as well as augmentation of the antitumor effects of chemotherapy and radiation therapy.[100,119,137–150] The demonstration that EGFR-targeted therapy may be an effective approach in cancer cells expressing the EGFR led to a series of clinical trials with anti-EGFR mAbs in patients with EGFR-positive tumors.[137,151-153] Of a series of anti-EGFR mAbs under clinical development, IMC-C225 is the one in a more advanced phase in clinical development, and shows particularly promising results.[138]

A series of phase I/II studies of IMC-C225 given alone or in combination with either chemotherapy or radiation therapy have now been completed.[154,155] In phase II studies, IMC-C225 has been shown to be capable of reverting chemotherapy resistance to CPT11 in colorectal cancer and cisplatin-based therapy resistance in head and neck tumors. Following the clinical observation that the addition of IMC-C225 induced responses in CPT11 refractory patients with colorectal carcinoma,[156] a phase II study in patients with advanced colorectal carcinoma and documented progression on CPT11 has been performed. The response rate was 22.5%, with a median duration of response of 186 days.[157] In a recent update of that trial, the median survival was reported to be 232 days.[158] A similar study has been done in head and neck tumors stable or progressing under cisplatin therapy with a response rate of 23%.[159] IMC-C225 plus gemcitabine has been studied in pancreatic carcinoma with a median time to progressive disease of 3.5 months, median overall survival of 6.75 months (202.5 days), and a 1-year overall survival rate of 32.5%.[160] Promising results have also been observed by the addition of IMC-C225 to radiation therapy in head and neck tumors.[161]

Other anti-EGFR mAbs are also being investigated. ABX-EGF is a fully humanized antihuman EGFR monoclonal antibody that inhibits the growth of human tumor xenografts and is in phase I clinical development.[162,163] EMD-72000, a fully humanized anti-EGFR mAb, is also currently being evaluated in phase I studies.[164] Bispecific antibodies against the EGFR with dual specificity (second binding to an immunologic effector cell) are also being studied as potential therapeutic tools.[165-167]

## THERAPEUTIC STRATEGIES AGAINST THE INTRACELLULAR DOMAIN OF THE EGFR

Over the last decade, drug discovery efforts have produced a variety of chemical structures that inhibit the EGFR tyrosine kinase, and several of these agents are currently under clinical development.[168,169] Tyrosine kinase inhibitors (TKIs) share some of their mechanisms of action with anti-EGFR mAbs, suggesting that blocking ligand binding with antibodies, or preventing kinase activation with specific inhibitors, results in a similar shutdown of EGFR-dependent processes.[170-178]

There are a number of EGF receptor compounds that are under clinical development. These agents are classified by their degree of receptor reversibility or irreversibility of action. ZD1839 and OSI-774 are reversible EGFR-specific TKIs and are furthest ahead in clinical development. ZD1839 (gefitinib or Iressa) is an orally active, selective EGFR TKI that has demonstrated antitumor activity against a variety of human cancer cell lines expressing EGFR, including ovarian, bladder, breast, and colon, and it is active in a range of xenograft models, including colon, NSCL, bladder and prostate.[158,179-181] In human xenograft models, ZD1839, like other EGFR inhibitors in combination with standard cytotoxic agents, resulted in both delayed tumor growth and tumor regression, irrespective of the level of EGFR, leading to enhanced survival.[177]

Phase I clinical studies have demonstrated that daily oral administration of ZD1839 is safe, and that the most common side effects were an acneiform skin rash and diarrhea, both generally mild and reversible on cessation of treatment.[99,182-184] In phase I trials with this targeted compound, investigators at Vall d'Hebron Hospital (Spain) have shown that orally administered ZD1839 inhibits the activation of EGFR and receptor-dependent processes in human skin, a well-characterized EGFR-dependent tissue that was chosen as a surrogate marker of drug effects on the EGFR.[185] ZD1839 as a single agent has shown antitumor effects against NSCL cancer (NSCLC) and prostate cancer.[99,182-184]

Phase II studies with two dose levels of ZD1839 (250 and 500 mg) have been completed in patients with NSCLC that had progressed after first or second line chemotherapy for advanced disease. The results of the first study (IDEAL 1) have been reported.[186] The overall response rate was 18.7% (95% CI: 13.7–24.7), and the overall disease control rate was 52.9% (95% CI: 45.9–59.8). The median progression-free survival was 84 days, with 34% of patients progression-free after 4 months; 78% also showed symptom improvement by the Lung Cancer Symptom Scale, and 52% showed improved quality of life by the Functional Assessment of Cancer Therapy–Lung (FACT-L). A similar US study has supported a role of ZD1839 in second and third line treatment in NSCLC.[187]

ZD1839 has also proven to be clinically safe when combined with cisplatin/gemcitabine and carboplatin/paclitaxel in the treatment of lung cancer.[188] As a consequence, these combinations in patients with NSCLC have been conducted in two multicenter, multinational phase III trials as first line treatment in nonoperable stage III and stage IV NSCLC. Patients received ZD1839 (250 or 500 mg/day) in combination with standard regimens of gemcitabine/cisplatin (trial INTACT 1) or paclitaxel/carboplatin (trial INTACT 2). Surprisingly, these trials did not confirm the preclinical synergy of the combination.[189,190] Recent published data have demonstrated that tumors that were sensitive to ZD1839 had a mutation in the EGFR, which may explain why the majority of tumors did not respond to ZD1839.[191,192] Screening for this mutation in bladder cancer may identify appropriate patients for ZD1839 therapy.

OSI-774 (Tarceva) is an orally available quinazoline that is a selective inhibitor of the EGFR. Similar to ZD1839, OSI-774 inhibited EGFR-dependent processes in skin and tumor biopsies.[193] Clinical responses were also seen, and the clinical activity of this compound has now been demonstrated in phase II studies conducted in patients with NSCLC, head and neck tumors, and ovarian carcinoma.[194] Another specific TKI, PKI 166, has been tested in oral squamous cancer cell lines and is now being evaluated in a phase I study.[195]

EKB is a representative of the second group of TKIs, the irreversible EGFR-specific TKIs. EKB-569 binds covalently and irreversibly to the EGFR.[196] The efficacy of this drug is currently being assessed.

Coexpression of the EGF receptor and the HER2 receptor occurs in tumors, a situation that leads to receptor heterodimerization and activation of downstream signaling.[87] Under those circumstances, a dual EGFR and HER2 inhibitor may have potential advantages by simultaneously targeting the two receptors. This group of reversible Pan-HER (EGFR family) TKIs is best exemplified by GW572016.[197,198] A relevant question is whether a dual inhibitor will really lead to a greater efficacy due to the promiscuity of paracrine interactions among receptors. A phase II trial with GW572016 as second line therapy for bladder and renal cell carcinoma is now ongoing.

The last group of TKIs is represented by CI-1033, a 4-anilinoquinazoline that belongs to the group of irreversible Pan-HER (EGFR family) TKIs. These compounds irreversibly inhibit in vitro the three catalytically active members of the EGFR family: EGFR, HER2, and HER4.[170] CI-1033 is currently under phase I evaluation.[199]

## HER2 (H2N)

The H2N gene is localized on chromosome 17q, and it encodes a 185 kDa transmembrane TK growth factor receptor.[200,201] While its ligand has not yet been identified, activation of the intracellular kinase is thought to play a role in cell differentiation, motility, and adhesion.[202]

Overexpression and amplification of the oncogene was first identified in a human breast carcinoma cell line and subsequently in approximately 30% of breast adenocarcinomas.[203,204] It has been repeatedly shown to be a prognostic marker in breast cancer, particularly in patients with positive lymph nodes.[205–207] Gene amplification, protein overexpression, or both, have been associated with worse outcome in breast and ovarian carcinoma.[204,205] The prognostic significance in other epithelial neoplasms, however, is less clear. Similarly, the prognostic significance of H2N overexpression in bladder urothelial carcinoma is largely unknown, mainly because of conflicting data in published reports.[80,208–215] Most studies have included both superficial and muscle-invasive disease in their study cohorts, so data concerning exclusively muscle-invasive disease are largely lacking.

Recently, with the advent of a recombinant humanized mAb anti-H2N (anti-p185[HER2/neu]), known as trastuzumab (Herceptin), assessment of H2N status has assumed therapeutic significance.[216] It has been demonstrated that this drug has resulted in clinical responses in patients with H2N overexpressing metastatic breast cancer, and there has been reported synergy between trastuzumab and both paclitaxel and cisplatin, drugs commonly used in the treatment of metastatic urothelial carcinoma.[217–220] Therefore, aside from its prognostic significance, accurate determination of H2N status in patients with bladder cancer may have therapeutic implications.

Overexpression of H2N in urothelial carcinoma has been reported to range from 2% to 74%.[80,208–215,221] Although studies have correlated H2N overexpression with more aggressive clinical behavior, some have found no significant prognostic association, and others have linked it to a better clinical outcome.[80,106,112,209–215] Differences in both the incidence of expression and its prognostic significance are very likely explained by different methodologies, including assessment of H2N status, i.e. detection of amplification versus detection of overexpression, method employed, i.e. polymerase chain reaction (PCR), fluorescent in situ hybridization (FISH), and immunohistochemistry (IHC), and definition of H2N positivity.

Jimenez et al[222] recently evaluated H2N overexpression by IHC, a method most commonly employed for breast cancer H2N-status determination, and with a widely used antibody, which is the basis for the commercially available Hercept test. This analysis was conducted in a well-characterized set of cystectomy specimens harboring muscle-invasive urothelial carcinomas and correlated with clinical outcome, thus evaluating its prognostic significance. Eighty cases of muscle-invasive urothelial carcinoma of the bladder treated by radical cystectomy with available follow-up were tested for H2N using IHC. Twenty-eight percent of primary tumors were H2N positive (2+ or 3+). The median survival of H2N-negative patients was 50 months, and 33 months for H2N-positive patients (p=0.46). Of the 80 cases, 60 had simultaneous or subsequent metastasis. H2N overexpression was present in 37% of primaries, 63% of lymph node metastases, and 86% of distant metastases. Forty-five percent of H2N-negative primaries had H2N-positive lymph node metastases, whereas 92% of H2N-positive primaries were associated with positive metastasis. The median survival of patients with H2N-negative versus H2N-positive lymph nodes was 24 and 28 months, respectively (p=0.39). H2N overexpression, in this study, did not predict survival when analyzed by its presence either in the primary tumor or in the regional lymph node metastasis.[222]

An important observation was the fact that determination of H2N status in urothelial carcinoma may depend on whether the assessment is done in primary or metastatic tumor. The incidence of H2N overexpression was significantly higher in metastatic tumors compared to primaries, and a fairly reproducible pattern of overexpression was identified when metastatic tumors were compared to their corresponding primary. This would imply a significant relationship between H2N overexpression and metastasis development, which, however, did not translate into prognostically significant data in the survival analysis. Others have also found evidence of H2N overexpression heterogeneity in bladder cancer.[223]

## THERAPEUTIC STRATEGIES AGAINST THE HER2 RECEPTOR

In preclinical studies, muMab 4D5, the murine version of trastuzumab, produced significant antiproliferative effects in vitro against human breast cell lines that overexpressed the H2N receptor, whereas it had no effect on cell lines that did not overexpress it.[224] Trastuzumab binds the extracellular domain of the H2N receptor with three times greater affinity than does muMab 4D5, and it induces an antibody-dependent cellular cytotoxicity against tumor cell lines.[225] The clinical benefit of trastuzumab was demonstrated in a recent phase III trial, which showed a more prolonged time to disease progression in patients treated with trastuzumab plus chemotherapy, compared to those treated with chemotherapy alone, in women with metastatic breast cancer with H2N overexpression.[226] Similarly, single-agent trastuzumab has been associated with a 15% response rate in patients with metastatic H2N-positive breast cancer.[217] However, trastuzumab has also been associated with a syndrome of myocardial dysfunction similar to that observed with anthracyclines.[217] It is thus apparent that accurate determination of H2N status is of high clinical relevance, as patients that would benefit most from trastuzumab-based therapy can be accurately identified, minimizing unnecessary risks to those that will not benefit from the drug.

There are no data documenting the efficacy of trastuzumab in the treatment of metastatic bladder cancer. However, the reported synergy between paclitaxel and trastuzumab in breast cancer,[139,227] between trastuzumab and cisplatin,[218,219] and the fact that both paclitaxel and cisplatin are part of the armamentarium of the medical management of metastatic bladder cancer, have prompted the testing of trastuzumab in bladder cancer. The rationale is further strengthened by the rate of H2N overexpression, as discussed previously. Based on these data and the activity of the combination regimen of paclitaxel, carboplatin, and gemcitabine, a multicenter, National Cancer Institute-sponsored phase II clinical trial is being conducted using the combination of trastuzumab, paclitaxel, carboplatin, and gemcitabine in the treatment of patients with metastatic urothelial cancer that overexpresses H2N.[228] The primary objective of the trial is to assess the safety of the combination. The secondary objectives include evaluation of: 1) complete and partial response rates; 2) median and overall survival; and 3) the percentage of patients with metastatic or recurrent bladder cancer that overexpresses H2N histologically (IHC and FISH) and serologically (ELISA).

The preliminary results of this trial indicate that urothelial cancers have a high rate of H2N overexpression (46%). H2N overexpression is identified only in TCCs and is primarily detected by IHC, with 12 (63%) of 19 H2N-positive tumors demonstrating a score of 3+. Only 16% of the H2N-positive tumors demonstrated H2N gene amplification, and only 26% were positive by ELISA. The preliminary response data suggest that objective responses occur despite low rates of H2N gene amplification. Among treated patients, myelosuppression was the most common toxicity. Accrual to this study is ongoing.

## OTHER NOVEL TARGETS

Tumor cell longevity has emerged as a potential avenue for cancer therapy. Telomerase is an enzyme that is protective against progressive erosion of chromosomal telomeres. It is often aberrantly expressed in bladder cancer (90%), and its inhibition may be a potential target for therapy.[229] Preclinical studies of anti-telomerase treatment demonstrated significant activity against bladder cancer in both in vitro and in vivo animal models.[230]

Another target that has been developed is gene therapy for bladder cancer. One candidate is the p53 tumor suppressor gene. It has been selected as a target for new therapeutic strategies to treat various malignancies because the expression of the p53 gene is altered in more cancers than any other known gene.[231] Introduction of the DNA using adenoviral (as opposed to retroviral and liposomal) vectors has received the greatest attention because of several advantages that include: 1) the ability to transduce both proliferating and quiescent cells; 2) a wide tissue tropism; 3) lack of integration into the host genome; 4) high-level transgene expression; 5) existence of efficient protocols for producing clinical-grade material at high concentrations; and 6) the established safety of adenoviral vaccines.[232,233] In vitro, cell viability was decreased upon p53 gene transfer in human bladder cancer cell lines, and synergy was noted when combined with cisplatin.[234] A phase I clinical trial demonstrated that intravesical instillation of adenovirus-mediated p53 gene transfer is safe, feasible, and biologically active when administered in multiple doses to patients with bladder cancer.[235] Future work must address the need for more efficient gene delivery systems and stronger transgene expression in the target tissue. Frequent genetic alterations in neoplasias have provided biologic targets for novel therapies. A rapidly increasing body of knowledge also provides evidence for multiple epigenetic alterations in cancer, which can complement or even precede genetic alterations. Histone deacetylase inhibitors represent a class of epigenetic agents that act by promoting acetylation of histones, leading in turn to uncoiling of chromatin and activation of a variety of genes implicated in the regulation of cell survival, proliferation, differentiation, and apoptosis. These are future potential agents in the treatment of cancer.[236]

Increased prostaglandin production correlates positively with cancer risk, and COX2, the inducible rate-limited enzyme for prostaglandin synthesis, is upregulated in bladder cancers. COX2 appears to play an important role in angiogenesis. Therapeutic inhibitors of COX2 (nonsteroidal anti-inflammatory drugs) are under active preclinical investigation as chemopreventive agents, and a clinical trial in bladder cancer is currently being undertaken.[237]

Bortezomib, a 20S proteasome inhibitor, is another drug that has shown significant antiproliferative activity in aggressive bladder cancer cells, and a clinical trial of bortezomib for patients with bladder cancer is being formulated.[238] Deregulation of cell-cycle and apoptotic pathways via mutation or altered expression of p53, p21/WAF-1, pRB, p27, and INK4A (p16) are necessary for uroepithelial transformation. In addition, members of the erbB family—VEGF, NFκB, Akt, and PTEN—are also implicated in the progression of the disease. All of these molecules are potential targets for novel therapies. Other potential targets include regulators of protein trafficking, farnesyl transferase inhibitors that affect the ras signaling pathway, mTOR inhibitors, antisense oligodeoxynucleotides, cyclin-dependent kinase, and protein kinase C inhibitors. These are just a few of the many targets that need to be further studied for their potential impact on cancer therapy.[239]

## CONCLUSION

Novel targeted therapy holds promise in improving the current results of bladder cancer treatment. Based on the success seen with targeted therapy, such as anti-HER2 mAbs (trastuzumab), there is great interest in assessing these agents in patients with bladder cancer. With an expanding list of potential biologic targets and limited patient resources, definitive, prospective, and highly selective trials are needed to address the value of a specific targeted agent. Unfortunately, despite promising preclinical data, there are no human data suggesting improved outcome by the integration of newer, targeted therapies. A prerequisite for the success of these trials is a clearly defined patient population, clearly defined endpoints, and rigorous statistical methods.

## REFERENCES

1. Jemal A, Murray T, Ward E, et al. Cancer statistics, 2005. CA: Cancer J Clin 2005;55:10–30.

2. Geller NL, Sternberg CN, Penenberg D, Scher H, Yagoda A. Prognostic factors for survival of patients with advanced urothelial tumors treated with methotrexate, vinblastine, doxorubicin, and cisplatin chemotherapy. Cancer 1991;67:1525–1531.

3. Sternberg CN, Yagoda A, Scher HI, et al. M-VAC (methotrexate, vinblastine, doxorubicin and cisplatin) for advanced transitional cell carcinoma of the urothelium. J Urol 1988;139:461–469.

4. Sternberg CN, Yagoda A, Scher HI, et al. Methotrexate, vinblastine, doxorubicin, and cisplatin for advanced transitional cell carcinoma of the urothelium. Efficacy and patterns of response and relapse. Cancer 1989;64:2448–2458.

5. Pagano F, Bassi P, Galetti TP, Meneghini A, Milani C, Artibani W, Garbeglio A. Results of contemporary radical cystectomy for invasive bladder cancer: a clinicopathological study with an emphasis on the inadequacy of the tumor, nodes and metastases classification. J Urol 1991;145:45–50.

6. Logothetis CJ, Finn LD, Smith T, et al. Escalated MVAC with or without recombinant human granulocyte-macrophage colony-stimulating factor for initial treatment of advanced malignant urothelial tumors: results of a randomized trial. J Clin Oncol 1995;13:2272–2277.

7. Roth BJ, Dreicer R, Einhorn LH, et al. Significant activity of paclitaxel in advanced transitional cell carcinoma of the urothelium: a phase II trial of the Eastern Cooperative Oncology Group. J Clin Oncol 1994;12:2264–2270.

8. Vaughn DJ, Malkowicz SB, Zoltick B, et al. Paclitaxel plus carboplatin in advanced carcinoma of the urothelium: an active and tolerable outpatient regimen. J Clin Oncol 1998;16:255–260.

9. Redman BG, Smith DC, Flaherty L, Du W, Hussain M. Phase II trial of paclitaxel and carboplatin in the treatment of advanced urothelial carcinoma. J Clin Oncol 1998;16:1844–1848.

10. Bajorin DF, McCaffrey JA, Hilton S, et al. Treatment of patients with transitional-cell carcinoma of the urothelial tract with ifosfamide, paclitaxel, and cisplatin: a phase II trial. J Clin Oncol 1998;16:2722–2727.

11. Von der Maase H, Hansen SW, Roberts JT, et al. Gemcitabine and cisplatin versus methotrexate, vinblastine, doxorubicin, and cisplatin in advanced or metastatic bladder cancer: results of a large randomized, multinational, multicenter, phase III study. J Clin Oncol 2000;17:3068–3077.

12. Bellmunt J, Guillem V, Paz-Ares L, et al. Phase I–II study of paclitaxel, cisplatin, and gemcitabine in advanced transitional-cell carcinoma of the urothelium. J Clin Oncol 2000;18:3247–3255.

13. Hussain M, Vaishampayan U, Du W, et al. Combination carboplatin, paclitaxel and gemcitabine is an active treatment for advanced urothelial carcinoma. J Clin Oncol 2001;19:2527–2533.

14. Cote RJ, Datar RH. Therapeutic approaches to bladder cancer: identifying targets and mechanisms. Crit Rev Oncol Hematol 2003;46(Suppl):S67–83.

15. Hanahan D, Weinberg R. The hallmarks of cancer. Cell 2000;100:57–70.

16. McCarthy SA, Kuzu I, Gatter KC, et al. Heterogeneity of the endothelial cell and its role in organ preference of tumour metastasis. Trends Pharmacol Sci 1991;12:462–467.

17. Folkman J. Tumor angiogenesis: therapeutic implications. N Engl J Med 1971;285:1182–1186.

18. Carmeliet P, Jain RK. Angiogenesis in cancer and other diseases. Nature 2000;407:249–257.

19. Folkman J. What is the evidence that tumors are angiogenesis dependent? [editorial]. J Natl Cancer Inst 1990;82:4.

20. Dvorak HF, Nagy JA, Feng D, et al. Vascular permeability factor/vascular endothelial growth factor and the significance of microvascular hyperpermeability in angiogenesis. Curr Top Microbiol Immunol 1999;237:97–132.

21. Hanahan D, Christofori G, Naik P, et al. Transgenic mouse models of tumour angiogenesis: the angiogenic switch, its molecular controls, and prospects for preclinical therapeutic models. Eur J Cancer 1996;32A:2386–2393.

22. Dickinson A J, Fox SB, Persad RA, et al. Quantification of angiogenesis as an independent predictor of prognosis in invasive bladder carcinomas. Br J Urol 1994;74:762–766.

23. Bochner BH, Cote RJ, Weidner N, et al. Angiogenesis in bladder cancer: relationship between microvessel density and tumor prognosis. J Natl Cancer Inst 1994,87:1603–1612.

24. Jaeger TM, Weidner N, Chew K, et al. Tumor angiogenesis correlates with lymph node metastases in invasive bladder cancer. J Urol 1995;154:69–71.

25. Philp EA, Stephenson TJ, Reed MW. Prognostic significance of angiogenesis in transitional cell carcinoma of the human urinary bladder [see comments]. Br J Urol 1996;77:352–357.

26. Chaudhary R, Bromley M, Clarke NW, et al. Prognostic relevance of micro-vessel density in cancer of the urinary bladder. Anticancer Res 1999;19:3479–3484.

27. Chodak GW, Haudenschild C, Gittes RF, et al. Angiogenic activity as a marker of neoplastic and preneoplastic lesions of the human bladder. Ann Surg 1980;192:762–771.

28. Chodak GW, Scheiner CJ, Zetter BR. Urine from patients with transitional-cell carcinoma stimulates migration of capillary endothelial cells. N Engl J Med 1981;305:869–874.

29. Crew JP, O'Brien TS, Harris AL. Bladder cancer angiogenesis, its role in recurrence, stage progression and as a therapeutic target. Cancer Metastasis Rev 1986;15:221–230.

30. Crew JP. Vascular endothelial growth factor: an important angiogenic mediator in bladder cancer. Eur Urol 1999;35:2–8.

31. Slaton JW, Millikan R, Inoue K, et al. Correlation of metastasis related gene expression and relapse-free survival in patients with locally advanced bladder cancer treated with cystectomy and chemotherapy. J Urol 2004;171:570–574.

32. Mizutani Y, Okada Y, Yoshida O. Expression of platelet-derived endothelial cell growth factor in bladder carcinoma. Cancer 1987;79:1190–1194.

33. Arima J, Imazono Y, Takebayashi Y, et al. Expression of thymidine phosphorylase as an indicator of poor prognosis for patients with transitional cell carcinoma of the bladder. Cancer 2000;88:1131–1138.

34. Grossfeld GD, Ginsberg DA, Stein JP, et al. Thrombospondin-1 expression in bladder cancer: association with p53 alterations, tumor angiogenesis, and tumor progression. J Natl Cancer Inst 1997;89:219–227.

35. Campbell SC, Volpert OV, Ivanovich M, et al. Molecular mediators of angiogenesis in bladder cancer. Cancer Res 1998;58:1298–1304.

36. Poppas DP, Pavlovich CP, Folkman J, et al. Intravesical bacille Calmette–Guérin induces the antiangiogenic chemokine interferon-inducible protein 10. Urology 1998;52:268–275.

37. Beecken WD, Fernandez A, Joussen AM, et al. Effect of antiangiogenic therapy on slowly growing, poorly vascularized tumors in mice. J Natl Cancer Inst 2001;93:382–387.

38. Kikuchi E, Menendez S, Ohori M, Cordon-Cardo C, Kasahara N, Bochner BH. Inhibition of orthotopic human bladder tumor growth by lentiviral gene transfer of endostatin. Clin Cancer Res 2004;10:1835–1842.

39. Bianco FJ Jr, Gervasi DC, Tiguert R, et al. Matrix metalloproteinase-9 expression in bladder washes from bladder cancer patients predicts pathological stage and grade. Clin Cancer Res 1998;4:3011–3016.

40. Grignon DJ, Sakr W, Toth M, et al. High levels of tissue inhibitor of metalloproteinase-2 (TIMP-2) expression are associated with poor outcome in invasive bladder cancer. Cancer Res 1996;56:1654–1659.

41. Grant GM, Cobb JK, Castillo B, et al. Regulation of matrix metalloproteinases following cellular transformation. J Cell Physiol 1996;167:177–183.

42. Ozdemir E, Kakehi Y, Okuno H, et al. Strong correlation of basement membrane degradation with p53 inactivation and/or MDM2 overexpression in superficial urothelial carcinomas. J Urol 1997;158:206–211.

43. Hasui Y, Marutsuka K, Nishi S, et al. The content of urokinase-type plasminogen activator and tumor recurrence in superficial bladder cancer. J Urol 1994;151:16–19.

44. Hasui Y, Marutsuka K, Asada Y, et al. Prognostic value of urokinase-type plasminogen activator in patients with superficial bladder cancer. Urology 1996;47:34–37.

45. Reiher FK, Ivanovich M, Huang H, et al. The role of hypoxia and p53 in the regulation of angiogenesis in bladder cancer. J Urol 2001;165:2075–2081.

46. Jones A, Fujiyama C, Blanche C, et al. Relation of vascular endothelial growth factor production to expression and regulation of hypoxia-inducible factor-1 alpha and hypoxia-inducible factor-2 alpha in human bladder tumors and cell lines. Clin Cancer Res 2001;7:1263–1272.

47. Brooks PC, Clark RAF, Cheresh DA. Requirement of vascular integrin avb3 for angiogenesis. Science 1994;264:569–571.

48. Chopin DK, Caruelle JP, Colombel M, et al. Increased immunodetection of acidic fibroblast growth factor in bladder cancer, detectable in urine. J Urol 1993;150:1126–1130.

49. Ravery V, Jouanneau J, Gil-Diez S, et al. Immunohistochemical detection of acidic fibroblast growth factor in bladder transitional cell carcinoma. Urol Res 1992;20:211–214.

50. Chodak GW, Hospelhorn V, Judge SM, et al. Increased levels of fibroblast growth factor-like activity in urine from patients with bladder or kidney cancer. Cancer Res 1988;48:2083–2088.

51. O'Brien T, Cranston D, Fuggle S, et al. Different angiogenic pathways characterize superficial and invasive bladder cancer. Cancer Res 1995;55:510–513.

52. Nguyen M, Watanabe H, Budson AE, et al. Elevated levels of the angiogenic peptide basic fibroblast growth factor in urine of bladder cancer patients. J Natl Cancer Inst 1993;85:241–242.

53. Gazzaniga P, Gandini O, Gradilone A, et al. Detection of basic fibroblast growth factor mRNA in urinary bladder cancer: correlation with local relapses. Int J Oncol 1999;14:1123–1127.

54. Campbell SC. Advances in angiogenesis research: relevance to urological oncology [see comments]. J Urol 1997;158:1663–1674.

55. Brown LF, Berse B, Jackman RW, et al. Increased expression of vascular permeability factor (vascular endothelial growth factor) and its receptors in kidney and bladder carcinomas. Am J Pathol 1993;143:1255–1262.

56. Chow NH, Liu HS, Chan SH, et al. Expression of vascular endothelial growth factor in primary superficial bladder cancer. Anticancer Res 1999;19:4593–4597.

57. O'Brien TS, Smith K, Cranston D, et al. Urinary basic fibroblast growth factor in patients with bladder cancer and benign prostatic hypertrophy. Br J Urol 1995;76:311–314.

58. O'Brien T, Cranston D, Fuggle S, et al. The angiogenic factor midkine is expressed in bladder cancer, and overexpression correlates with a poor outcome in patients with invasive cancers. Cancer Res 1996;56:2515–2518.

59. Kubota Y, Miura T, Moriyama M, et al. Thymidine phosphorylase activity in human bladder cancer: difference between superficial and invasive cancer. Clin Cancer Res 1997;3:973–976.

60. Brown NS, Jones A, Fujiyama C, et al. Thymidine phosphorylase induces carcinoma cell oxidative stress and promotes secretion of angiogenic factors. Cancer Res 2000;60:6298–6302.

61. Joseph A, Weiss GH, Jin L, et al. Expression of scatter factor in human bladder carcinoma. J Natl Cancer Inst 1995;87:372–377.

62. Tamatani T, Hattori K, Iyer A, et al. Hepatocyte growth factor is an invasion/migration factor of rat urothelial carcinoma cells in vitro. Carcinogenesis 1999;20:957–962.

63. O'Brien TS, Fox SB, Dickinson AJ, et al. Expression of the angiogenic factor thymidine phosphorylase/platelet-derived endothelial cell

growth factor in primary bladder cancers. Cancer Res 1996;56:4799–4804.

64. Eder IE, Stenzl A, Hobisch A, et al. Expression of transforming growth factors beta-1, beta 2 and beta 3 in human bladder carcinomas. Br J Cancer 1997;75:1753–1760.

65. Inoue K, Perrotte P, Wood CG, et al. Gene therapy of human bladder cancer with adenovirus-mediated antisense basic fibroblast growth factor. Clin Cancer Res 2000;6:4422–4431.

66. Papathoma AS, Petraki C, Grigorakis A, et al. Prognostic significance of matrix metalloproteinases 2 and 9 in bladder cancer. Anticancer Res 2000;20:2009–2013.

67. Nutt JE, Mellon JK, Qureshi K, et al. Matrix metalloproteinase-1 is induced by epidermal growth factor in human bladder tumour cell lines and is detectable in urine of patients with bladder tumours. Br J Cancer 1998;78:215–220.

68. Durkan GC, Nutt JE, Rajjayabun PH, et al. Prognostic significance of matrix metalloproteinase-1 and tissue inhibitor of metalloproteinase-1 in voided urine samples from patients with transitional cell carcinoma of the bladder. Clin Cancer Res 2001;7:3450–3456.

69. Lokeshwar VB, Block NL. HA-HAase urine test. A sensitive and specific method for detecting bladder cancer and evaluating its grade. Urol Clin North Am 2000;27:53–61.

70. Pham HT, Block NL, Lokeshwar VB. Tumor-derived hyaluronidase: a diagnostic urine marker for high-grade bladder cancer [published erratum appears in Cancer Res 1997;57(8):1622]. Cancer Res 1997;57:778–783.

71. Lokeshwar VB, Obek C, Soloway MS, et al. Tumor-associated hyaluronic acid: a new sensitive and specific urine marker for bladder cancer [erratum appears in Cancer Res 1998;58(14):3191]. Cancer Research 1997;57:773–777.

72. Lokeshwar VB, Young MJ, Goudarzi G, et al. Identification of bladder tumor-derived hyaluronidase: its similarity to HYAL1. Cancer Res 1999;59:4464–4470.

73. Hasui Y, Osada Y. Urokinase-type plasminogen activator and its receptor in bladder cancer [comment]. J Natl Cancer Inst 1997;89:678–679.

74. Talks KL, Turley H, Gatter KC, et al. The expression and distribution of the hypoxia-inducible factors HIF-1alpha and HIF-2alpha in normal human tissues, cancers, and tumor-associated macrophages. Am J Pathol 2000;157:411–421.

75. Yoshimura R, Sano H, Mitsuhashi M, et al. Expression of cyclooxygenase-2 in patients with bladder carcinoma. J Urol 2001;165:1468–1472.

76. Crew JP, Fuggle S, Bicknell R, et al. Eukaryotic initiation factor-4E in superficial and muscle invasive bladder cancer and its correlation with vascular endothelial growth factor expression and tumour progression. Br J Cancer 2000;82:161–166.

77. Slaton JW, Perrotte P, Inoue K, et al. Interferon-alpha-mediated down-regulation of angiogenesis-related genes and therapy of bladder cancer are dependent on optimization of biological dose and schedule. Clin Cancer Res 1999;5:2726–2734.

78. Dinney CP, Babkowski RC, Antelo M, et al. Relationship among cystectomy, microvessel density and prognosis in stage T1 transitional cell carcinoma of the bladder. J Urol 1998;160:1285–1290.

79. Lipponen P, Eskelinen M. Expression of epidermal growth factor receptor in bladder cancer as related to established prognostic factors, oncoprotein (c-erbB-2, p53) expression and long-term prognosis. Br J Cancer 1994;69:1120–1125.

80. Korkolopoulou P, Christodoulou P, Kapralos P, et al. The role of p53, MDM2 and c-erb B-2 oncoproteins, epidermal growth factor receptor and proliferation markers in the prognosis of urinary bladder cancer. Pathol Res Pract 1997;193:767–775.

81. Chow NH, Chan SH, Tzai TS, et al. Expression profiles of ErbB family receptors and prognosis in primary transitional cell carcinoma of the urinary bladder. Clin Cancer Res 2001;7:1957–1962.

82. Lemmon MA, Schlessinger J. Regulation of signal transduction and signal diversity by receptor oligomerization. Trends Biochem Sci 1994;19:459–463.

83. Pawson T. Signal transduction. Look at a tyrosine kinase. Nature 1994;372:726–727.

84. Alroy I, Yarden, Y. The ErbB signaling network in embryogenesis and oncogenesis: signal diversification through combinatorial ligand-receptor interactions. FEBS Lett 1997;410:83–86.

85. Riese DJ, Stern DF. Specificity within the EGF family/erbB receptor family signaling network. Bioassays 1998;20:41–48.

86. Bellmunt J, de Witt R, Albiol S, et al. New drugs and new approaches in metastatic bladder cancer. Crit Rev Oncol Hematol 2003;47:195–206.

87. Salomon DS, Brandt R, Ciardiello F, et al. Epidermal growth factor-related peptides and their receptors in human malignancies. Crit Rev Oncol Hematol 1995;19:183–232.

88. Cornianu M, Tudose N. Immunohistochemical markers in the morphological diagnosis of lung carcinoma. Rom J Morphol Embryol 1997;43:181–191.

89. Fox SB, Harris AL. The epidermal growth factor receptor in breast cancer. J Mammary Gland Biol Neoplasia 1997;2:131–141.

90. Ke LD, Adler-Storthz K, Clayman GL, et al. Differential expression of epidermal growth factor receptor in human head and neck cancers. Head Neck 1998;20:320–327.

91. Wells A. The epidermal growth factor receptor (EGFR): a new target in cancer therapy. Signal 2000;1:4–11.

92. Tysnes BB, Haugland HK, Bjerkvig R. Epidermal growth factor and laminin receptors contribute to migratory and invasive properties of gliomas. Invasion Metastasis 1997;17:270–280.

93. Kulik G, Klippel A, Weber MJ. Antiapoptotic signalling by the insulin-like growth factor 1 receptor, phosphatidylinositol 3-kinase, and Akt. Mol Cell Biol 1997;17:1595–1606.

94. Chen Z, Ke LD, Yuan XH, et al. Correlation of cisplatin sensitivity with differential alteration of EGFR expression in head and neck cancer cells. Anticancer Res 2000;20:899–902.

95. Hutcheson IR, Gee JMW, Barrow D, et al. Endocrine resistance in breast cancer can involve a switch towards EGFR signaling pathways and a gain of sensitivity to an EGFR-selective tyrosine kinase inhibitor, ZD1839. Presented at the Signal Transduction Pathways and Regulation of Gene Expression as Therapeutic Targets Meeting, Luxembourg, January 26–29, 2000 (abstract).

96. Wosikowski K, Silverman JA, Bishop P, et al. Reduced growth rate accompanied by aberrant epidermal growth factor signalling in drug resistant human breast cancer cells. Biochim Biophys Acta 2000;1497:215–226.

97. Akimoto T, Hunter NR, Buchmiller L, et al. Inverse relationship between epidermal growth factor receptor expression and radiocurability of murine carcinomas. Clin Cancer Res 1999;5:2884–2890.

98. Rubin MS, Shin DM, Pasmatier M, et al. Monoclonal antibody IMC-C225, an anti-epidermal growth factor receptor for patients with EGFR-positive tumors refractory to or in relapse from previous therapeutic regimens. Proc Am Soc Clin Oncol 2000;19:A474.

99. Ferry D, Hammond L, Ranson M, et al. Intermittent oral ZD 1839 (Iressa), a novel epidermal growth factor receptor tyrosine kinase inhibitor shows evidence of good tolerability and activity: final results from a phase I study. Proc Am Soc Clin Oncol 2000;19:A3.

100. Mendelsohn J, Dinney CPN. The Wilet F Whitmore, Jr, Lectureship: blockade of epidermal growth factor receptors as anticancer therapy. J Urol 2001;165:1152–1157.

101. Neal DE, Mellon K. Epidermal growth factor receptor and bladder cancer: a review. Urol Int 1992;48:365–371.

102. Messing EM. Growth factors and bladder cancer: clinical implications of the interactions between growth factors and their urothelial receptors. Semin Surg Oncol 1992;8(5):285–292.

103. Andrawis RI, Contrino J, Lindquist RR, Albertson PC, Manyak MJ, Kreutzer DL. Interleukin-8 expression and human bladder cancer: in situ and in vitro expression of IL-8 by human bladder cancer cells. J Urol 1997;157:28.

104. Chow N-H, Liu HS, Lee EI et al. Significance of urinary epidermal growth factor and its receptor expression in human bladder cancer. Anticancer Res 1997;17:1293–1296.

105. Nguyen PL, Swanson PE, Jaszez W, et al. Expression of epidermal growth factor receptor in invasive transitional cell carcinoma of the urinary bladder. A multivariate survival analysis. Am J Clin Pathol 1994;101(2):166–176.

106. Wu X, Rubin M, Fan Z, DeBlasio T, Soos T, Koff A, Mendelsohn J. Involvement of p27KIP1 in G1 arrest mediated by an anti-epidermal growth factor receptor monoclonal antibody. Oncogene 1996;12:1397–1403.

107. Nicholson RI, Gee JMW, Harper ME. EGFR and cancer prognosis. Eur J Cancer 2001;37:S9–S15.

108. Benjamin LE, Keshet E. Conditional switching of vascular endothelial growth factor (VEGF) expression in tumors: induction of endothelial cell shedding and regression of hemangioblastoma-like vessels by VEGF withdrawal. Proc Natl Acad Sci 1997;94:8761–8766.

109. Grugel S, Finkenzeller G, Weindel K, Barleon B, Marme D. Both v-Ha-Ras and v-Raf stimulate expression of the vascular endothelial growth factor in NIH 3T3 cells. J Biol Chem 1995;270:25915–25919.

110. Rozakis-Adcock M, Fernley R, Wade J, Pawson T, Bowtell D. The SH2 and SH3 domains of mammalian Grb2 couple the EGF receptor to the Ras activator mSos1. Nature 1999;363:83–85.

111. Gutman M, Singh RK, Xie K, Bucana CD, Fidler IJ. Regulation of interleukin-8 expression in human melanoma cells by the organ environment. Cancer Res 1995;55:2470–2475.

112. Huang SM, Bock JM, Harari PM. Epidermal growth factor receptor blockade with C225 modulates proliferation, apoptosis, and radiosensitivity in squamous cell carcinomas of the head and neck. Cancer Res 1999;59:1935–1940.

113. Maher PA. Modulation of the epidermal growth factor receptor by basic fibroblast growth factor. J Cell Physiol 1993;154:350–358.

114. Mothe I, Ballotti R, Tartare R, Kowalski-Chauvel A, van Obberghen E. Cross talk among tyrosine kinase receptors in PC12 cells: desensitization of mitogenic epidermal growth factor receptors by the neurotrophic factors, nerve growth factor and basic fibroblast growth factor. Mol Biol Cell 1993;4:737–746.

115. Goldman CK, Kim J, Wong WL, King V, Brock T, Gillespie GY. Epidermal growth factor stimulates vascular endothelial growth factor production by human malignant glioma cells: a model of glioblastoma multiforme pathophysiology. Mol Biol Cell 1993;4:121–133.

116. Xie H, Turner T, Wang MH, Singh RK, Siegal GP, Wells A. In vitro invasiveness of DU-145 human prostate carcinoma cells is modulated by EGF receptor-mediated signals. Clin Exp Metastasis 1995;13:407–419.

117. Dinney CP, Fishbeck R, Singh R, et al. Isolation and characterization of metastatic variants from human transitional cell carcinoma passaged by orthotopic implantation in athymic nude mice. J Urol 1995;154:1532–1538.

118. Mendelsohn J. Blockade of receptors for growth factors: an anticancer therapy. The Fourth Annual Joseph H Burchenal American Association for Cancer Research Clinical Research Award letters. Clin Cancer Res 2000;6:747–753.

119. Perrotte P, Matsumoto T, Inoue K, et al. Anti-epidermal growth factor receptor antibody C225 inhibits angiogenesis in human transitional cell carcinoma growing orthotopically in nude mice. Clin Cancer Res 1999;5:257–264.

120. Bruns CJ, Solorzano CC, Harbison MT, et al. Blockade of the epidermal growth factor receptor signaling by a novel tyrosine kinase inhibitor leads to apoptosis of endothelial cells and therapy of human pancreatic carcinoma. Cancer Res 2000;60:2926–2935.

121. Rak J, Mitsuhashi Y, Bayko L, Filmus J, Shirasawa S, Sasazuki T, Kerbel RS. Mutant ras oncogene upregulates VEGF/VPF expression: implications for induction and inhibition of tumor angiogenesis. Cancer Res 1995;55:4575–4580.

122. Kizaka-Kondoh S, Sato K, Tamura K, Nojima H, Okayama H. Raf-1 protein kinase is an integral component of the oncogenic signal cascade shared by epidermal growth factor and platelet-derived growth factor. Mol Cell Biol 1992;12:5078–5086.

123. Radinsky R, Aukerman S, Fidler IJ. The pathogenesis of cancer metastasis: relevance to biotherapy. In Oldham RK (ed): Principles of Cancer Biotherapy, 4th ed. Dordrecht: Kluwer, 2003.

124. Sehgal G, Hua J, Bernhard EJ, Sehgal I, Thompson TC, Muschel RJ. Requirement for matrix metalloproteinase-9 (gelatinase B) expression in metastasis by murine prostate carcinoma. Am J Pathol 1998;152:591–596.

125. Brandt BH, Roetger A, Dittmar T, et al. c-erbB-2/EGFR as dominant heterodimerization partners determine a mitogenic phenotype in human breast cancer cells. FASEB J 1999;13(14):1939–1949.

126. Thorne HJ, Jose DG, Zhang H, et al. EGF stimulates the synthesis of cell-attachment proteins in human breast cancer cell line PMC42. Int J Cancer 1987;40:207–212.

127. Lichtner R, Wiedemuth M, Noeske-Jungblut, C, et al. Rapid effects of EGF on cytoskeletal structures and adhesive properties of highly metastatic rat mammary adenocarcinoma cells. Clin Expression Metastasis 1993;11:243–251.

128. Chen P, Gupta K, Wells A. Cell movement elicited by EGF-R requires kinase and autophosphorylation but is separable from mitogenesis. J Cell Biol 1994;124:547–555.

129. Inoue K, Slaton JW, Perrotte P, et al. Paclitaxel enhances the effects of the anti-epidermal growth factor receptor monoclonal antibody ImClone C225 in mice with metastatic human bladder transitional cell carcinoma. Clin Cancer Res 2000;6:4874–4884.

130. Gum R, Wang H, Lengyel E, Juarez J, Boyd D. Regulation of 92 kDa type IV collagenase expression by the amino-terminal kinase- and the extracellular signal-regulated kinase-dependent signaling cascades. Oncogene 1997;4:1481–1493.

131. Zeigler ME, Chi Y, Schmidt T, Varani J. Role of ERK and JNK pathways in regulating cell motility and matrix metalloproteinase 9 production in growth factor-stimulated human epidermal keratinocytes. J Cell Physiol 1999;180:271–284.

132. Gum R, Lengyel E, Juarez J, Chen H, Sato H, Seiki M, Boyd D. Stimulation of 92-kDa gelatinase B promoter activity by ras is mitogen-activated protein kinase 1-independent and requires multiple transcription factor binding sites including closely spaced PEA3/ets and AP-1 sequences. J Biol Chem 1996;271:10672–10680.

133. Bond M, Fabunmi RP, Baker AH, Newby AC. Synergistic upregulation of metalloproteinase-9 by growth factors and inflammatory cytokines: an absolute requirement for transcription factor NF-kappa B. FEBS Lett 1998;435:29–34.

134. Himelstein BP, Koch CJ. Studies of type IV collagenase regulation by hypoxia. Cancer Lett 1998;124:127–133.

135. Inoue K, Slaton JW, Perrotte P, et al. Paclitaxel enhances the effects of the anti-epidermal growth factor receptor monoclonal antibody ImClone C225 in mice with metastatic human bladder transitional cell carcinoma. Clin Cancer Res 2000;6:4874–4884.

136. Slaton JW, Karashima T, Perrotte P, et al. Treatment with low-dose interferon-α restores the balance between matrix metalloproteinase-9 and E cadherin expression in human transitional cell carcinoma of the bladder. Clin Cancer Res 2001;7:2840–2853.

137. Aboud-Pirak E, Hurwitz E, Pirak ME, Bellot F, Schlessinger J, Sela M. Efficacy of antibodies to epidermal growth factor receptor against KB carcinoma in vitro and in nude mice. J Natl Cancer Inst 1980;80:1605–1611.

138. Goldstein NI, Prewett M, Zuklys K, Rockwell P, Mendelsohn J. Biological efficacy of a chimeric antibody to the epidermal growth factor receptor in a human tumor xenograft model. Clin Cancer Res 1995;1:1311–1318.

139. Fan Z, Shang BY, Lu Y, Chou JL, Mendelsohn J. Reciprocal changes in p27(Kip1) and p21(Cip1) in growth inhibition mediated by blockade or overstimulation of epidermal growth factor receptors. Clin Cancer Res 1997;3:1943–1948.

140. Peng D, Fan Z, Lu YTD, Scher H, Mendelsohn J. Anti-epidermal growth factor receptor monoclonal antibody 225 up-regulates p27KIP1 and induces G1 arrest in prostatic cancer cell line DU145. Cancer Res 1996;56:3666–3669.

141. Wu X, Fan Z, Masui H, Rosen N, Mendelsohn J. Apoptosis induced by an anti-epidermal growth factor receptor monoclonal antibody in a human colorectal carcinoma cell line and its delay by insulin. J Clin Invest 1995;95(4):1897–1905.

142. Petit AM, Rak J, Hung MC, et al. Neutralizing antibodies against epidermal growth factor and ErbB-2/neu receptor tyrosine kinases down-regulate vascular endothelial growth factor production by tumor cells in vitro and in vivo: angiogenic implications for signal transduction therapy of solid tumors. Am J Pathol 1997;151:1523–1530.

143. O-charoenrat P, Modjtahedi H, Rhys-Evans P, Court W, Box G, Eccles S. Epidermal growth factor-like ligands differentially up-regulate

matrix metalloproteinase 9 in head and neck squamous carcinoma cells. Cancer Res 2000;60:1121–1128.

144. O-charoenrat P, Rhys-Evans P, Court W, Box G, Eccles S. Differential modulation of proliferation, matrix metalloproteinase expression and invasion of human head and neck squamous carcinoma cells by c-erbB ligands. Clin Expression Metastasis 1999;17:631–639.

145. Matsumoto T, Perrotte P, Bar-Eli M, et al. Blockade of EGF-R signaling with anti-EGFR monoclonal antibody (Mab) C225 inhibits matrix metalloproteinase-9 (MMP-9) expression and invasion of human transitional cell carcinoma (TCC) in vitro and in vivo [abstract]. Proc Am Assoc Cancer Res 1998;39:A83.

146. Baselga J, Norton L, Masui H, et al. Antitumor effects of doxorubicin in combination with anti-epidermal growth factor receptor monoclonal antibodies. J Natl Cancer Inst 1993;85:1327–1333.

147. Baselga J, Norton L, Coplan K, Shalaby R, Mendelsohn J. Antitumor activity of paclitaxel in combination with anti-growth factor receptor monoclonal antibodies in breast cancer xenografts [abstract]. Proc Am Assoc Cancer Res 1998;35:2262.

148. Fan Z, Baselga J, Masui H, Mendelsohn J. Antitumor effect of anti-EGF receptor monoclonal antibodies plus cis-diaminedichloroplatinum (cis-DDP) on well established A431 cell xenografts. Cancer Res 1993;53:4637–4642.

149. Ciardiello FRB, Damiano V, De Lorenzo S, et al. Antitumor activity of sequential treatment with topotecan and anti-epidermal growth factor receptor antibody. Clin Cancer Res 1999;5:909–916.

150. Milas L, Mason K, Hunter N, et al. In vivo enhancement of tumor radioresponse by C225 antiepidermal growth factor receptor antibody. Clin Cancer Res 2000;6:701–708.

151. Kawamoto T, Sato JD, Le A, Polikoff J, Sato GH, Mendelsohn J. Growth stimulation of A431 cells by EGF: identification of high affinity receptors for epidermal growth factor by an anti-receptor monoclonal antibody. Proc Natl Acad Sci USA 1983;80:1337–1341.

152. Sato JD, Kawamoto T, Le AD, Mendelsohn J, Polikoff J Sato GH. Biological effect in vitro of monoclonal antibodies to human EGF receptors. Mol Biol Med 1983;1:511–529.

153. Rodeck U, Herlyn M, Herlyn D, et al. Tumor growth modulation by a monoclonal antibody to the epidermal growth factor receptor: immunologically mediated and effector cell-independent effects. Cancer Res 1987;47:3692–3696.

154. Cohen R, Falcey JW, Paulter VJ, Fetzer KM, Waksal HW. Safety profile of the monoclonal antibody (MOAB) IMC-C225, an anti-epidermal growth factor receptor (EGFR) used in the treatment of EGFR-positive tumors [abstract]. Proc Am Soc Clin Oncol 2000;19:474.

155. Khazaeli MB, LoBuglio AF, Falcey JW, Paulter VJ, Fetzer MK, Waksal HW. Low immunogenicity of a chimeric monoclonal antibody (MOAB), IMC-C225, used to treat epidermal growth factor receptor-positive tumors [abstract]. Proc Am Soc Clin Oncol 2000;19:207.

156. Rubin M, Shin D, Pasmantier M, et al. Monoclonal antibody (MoAb) IMC-C225, an anti-epidermal growth factor receptor (EGFR), for patients with EGFR-positive tumors refractory to or in relapse from previous therapeutic regimens [abstract]. Proc Am Soc Clin Oncol 2000;19:474.

157. Saltz L, Rubin M, Hochster H, et al. Cetuximab (IMC-C225) plus irinotecan (CPT-11) is active in CPT-11-refractory colorectal cancer (CRC) that expresses epidermal growth factor receptor (EGFR) [abstract]. Proc Am Soc Clin Oncol 2001;20:3.

158. Saltz L, Rubin M. Acne-like rash predicts response in patients treated with cetuximab (IMC-225) plus irinotecan (CPT-11) in CPT-11 refractory colorectal cancer that expresses EGFR. AACR-NCI-EORTC International Conference on Molecular Targets and Cancer Therapeutics, Miami Beach, FL, 2001.

159. Hong WK, Arquette M, Nabell L, Needle M, Waksal HW, Herbst RS. Efficacy and safety of the anti-epidermal growth factor antibody IMC-C225 in combination with cisplatin in patients with recurrent squamous cell carcinoma of the head and neck refractory to cisplatin containing chemotherapy [abstract]. Proc Am Soc Clin Oncol 2001;20:224.

160. Abbruzzese JL, Rosenberg A, Xiong Q, et al. Phase II study of anti-epidermal growth factor receptor (EGFr) antibody cetuximab (IMC-C225) in combination with gemcitabine in patients with advanced pancreatic cancer [abstract]. Proc Am Soc Clin Oncol 2001;20:130.

161. Bonner J, Ezequiel MP, Robert F, et al. Continued response following treatment with IMC-C225, an EGFr MoAb, combined with RT in advanced head and neck carcinoma [abstract]. Proc Am Soc Clin Oncol 2000;19:4.

162. Yang X-D, Jia X-C, Corvalan JRF, Wang P, Davis CG, Jakobovits A. Eradication of established tumors by a fully human monoclonal antibody to the epidermal growth factor receptor without concomitant chemotherapy. Cancer Res 1999;59:1236–1243.

163. Figlin R. Clinical results of the fully humanized anti-EGFR antibody in patients with advanced cancer. AACR-NCI-EORTC International Conference on Molecular Targets and Cancer Therapeutics, Miami Beach, FL, 2001.

164. Bier H, Hoffmann T, Hauser U, et al. Clinical trial with escalating doses of the antiepidermal growth factor receptor humanized monoclonal antibody EMD 72 000 in patients with advanced squamous cell carcinoma of the larynx and hypopharynx. Cancer Chemother Pharmacol 2001;47:519–524.

165. Negri DR, Tosi E, Valota O, et al. In vitro and in vivo stability and anti-tumour efficacy of an anti-EGFR/anti-CD3 F(ab')2 bispecific monoclonal antibody. Br J Cancer 1995;72:928–933.

166. Curnow RT. Clinical experience with CD64-directed immunotherapy. An overview. Cancer Immunol Immunother 1997;45:210–215.

167. Pfister DG, Lipton A, Belt R, et al. A phase I trial of the epidermal growth factor receptor (EGFR)-directed bispecific antibody (BsAB) MDX-447 in patients with solid tumors [abstract]. Proc Am Soc Clin Oncol 1999;18:433.

168. Levitzki A, Gazit A. Tyrosine kinase inhibition: an approach to drug development. Science 1995;267:1782–1785.

169. Fry DW, Kraker AJ, McMichael A, et al. A specific inhibitor of the epidermal growth factor receptor tyrosine kinase. Science 1994;265:1093–1095.

170. Fry DW, Bridges AJ, Denny WA, et al. Specific, irreversible inactivation of the epidermal growth factor receptor and erbB2, by a new class of tyrosine kinase inhibitor. Proc Natl Acad Sci USA 1998;95:12022–12027.

171. Moyer JD, Barbacci ES, Iwata KT, et al. Induction of apoptosis and cell cycle arrest by CP-358,774, an inhibitor of epidermal growth factor receptor tyrosine kinase. Cancer Res 1997;57:4838–4848.

172. Busse D, Doughty R, Ramsey T, et al. Reversible G(1) arrest induced by inhibition of the epidermal growth factor receptor tyrosine kinase requires up-regulation of p27(KIP1) independent of MAPK activity. J Biol Chem 2000;275:6987–6995.

173. Budillon A, Di Gennaro E, Barbarino M, et al. ZD1839, an epidermal growth factor receptor tyrosine kinase inhibitor, upregulates p27Kip1 inducing G1 arrest and enhancing the antitumor effect of interferon-α [abstract]. Proc Am Assoc Cancer Res 2000;41:4910.

174. Burns CJ, Solorzano CC, Harbison MT, et al. Blockade of the epidermal growth factor receptor signaling by a novel tyrosine kinase inhibitor leads to apoptosis of endothelial cells and therapy of human pancreatic carcinoma. Cancer Res 2000;60:2926–2935.

175. Ciardiello F, Caputo R, Bianco R, et al. Inhibition of growth factor production and angiogenesis in human cancer cells by ZD1839 ('Iressa'), a selective epidermal growth factor receptor tyrosine kinase inhibitor. Clin Cancer Res 2001;7:1459–1465.

176. Ciardiello F, Caputo R, Bianco R, et al. Antitumor effect and potentiation of cytotoxic drugs activity in human cancer cells by ZD-1839 (Iressa), an epidermal growth factor receptor-selective tyrosine kinase inhibitor. Clin Cancer Res 2000;6:2053–2063.

177. Sirotnak FM, Zakowsky MF, Miller VA, et al. Efficacy of cytotoxic agents against human tumor xenographs is markedly enhanced by coadministration of ZD1839 ('Iressa'), an inhibitor of tyrosine kinase. Clin Cancer Res 2000;6:4885–4892.

178. Williams K, Telfer B, Stratford I, Wedge, S. Combination of ZD1839 ('Iressa'), an EGFR tyrosine kinase inhibitor, and radiotherapy increases antitumour efficacy in a human colon cancer xenograft model [abstract]. Proc Am Assoc Cancer Res 2001;42:3840.

179. Woodburn JR, Wakeling A, Kelly H, et al. Preclinical studies with the oral epidermal growth factor receptor tyrosine kinase inhibitor (EGFR-TKI) ZD1839 ('Iressa') demonstrate significant anti-tumor activity. Presented at the Signal Transduction Pathways and Regulation of Gene Expression as Therapeutic Targets Meeting, Luxembourg, January 26–29, 2000.

180. Sedlacek HH. Kinase inhibitors in cancer therapy: a look ahead. Drugs 2000;59:435–476.

181. Dominguez-Escrig JL, Kelly JD, Neal DE, King SM, Davies BR. Evaluation of the therapeutic potential of the epidermal growth factor receptor tyrosine kinase inhibitor gefitinib in preclinical models of bladder cancer. Clin Cancer Res 2004;10:4874–4884.

182. Nakagawa K, Yamamoto N, Kudoh S, et al. A phase I intermittent dose-escalation trial of ZD1839 (Iressa) in Japanese patients with solid malignant tumours [abstract]. Proc Am Soc Clin Oncol 2000;19:183.

183. Baselga J, Herbst R, LoRusso P, et al. Continuous administration of ZD1839 (Iressa), a novel oral epidermal growth factor receptor tyrosine kinase inhibitor (EGFR-TKI), in patients with five selected tumor types: evidence of activity and good tolerability [abstract]. Proc Am Soc Clin Oncol 2000;19:177.

184. Ranson M, Hammond LA, Ferry D, et al. ZD1839, a selective oral epidermal growth factor receptor-tyrosine kinase inhibitor, is well tolerated and active in patients with solid, malignant tumors: results of a phase I trial. J Clin Oncol 2002;20:2240–2250.

185. Albanell J, Rojo F, Averbuch S, et al. Pharmacodynamic studies of the EGF receptor inhibitor ZD1839 ('Iressa') in skin from cancer patients: histopathological and molecular consequences of receptor inhibition. J Clin Oncol 2002;20:110–124.

186. Baselga J, Yano S, Giaccone G, et al. Initial results from a phase II trial of ZD1839 ('Iressa') as second- and third-line monotherapy for patients with advanced non-small-cell lung cancer (IDEAL 1). AACR-NCI-EORTC International Conference on Molecular Targets and Cancer Therapeutics, Miami Beach, FL, 2001, p 630A.

187. Kris MG, Natale RB, Herbs RS, et al. A phase II trial of ZD1839 ('Iressa') in advanced non-small cell lung cancer (NSCLC) patients who failed platinum- and docetaxel-based regimens (IDEAL 2) [abstract]. Proc Am Soc Clin Oncol 2002;21:292.

188. Miller VA, Johnson D, Heelan RT, et al. A pilot trial demonstrates the safety of ZD1839 (Iressa), an oral epidermal growth factor receptor tyrosine kinase inhibitor (EGFR-TKI), in combination with carboplatin and paclitaxel in previously untreated advanced non-small cell lung cancer [abstract]. Proc Am Soc Clin Oncol 2001;20:326.

189. Giaccone G, Herbst RS, Manegold C, et al. Gefitinib in combination with gemcitabine and cisplatin in advanced non-small-cell lung cancer: a phase III trial—INTACT 1. J Clin Oncol 2004;22:777–784.

190. Herbst RS, Giaccone G, Schiller JH, et al. Gefitinib in combination with paclitaxel and carboplatin in advanced non-small-cell lung cancer: a phase III trial—INTACT 2. J Clin Oncol 2004;22:785–794.

191. Lynch TJ, Bell DW, Sordella R, et al. Activating mutations in the epidermal growth factor receptor underlying responsiveness of non-small-cell lung cancer to gefitinib. N Engl J Med 2004;350:2129–2139.

192. Paez JG, Janne PA, Lee JC, et al. EGFR mutations in lung cancer: correlation with clinical response to gefitinib therapy. Science 2004;304:1497–1500.

193. Hidalgo M, Siu LL, Nemunaitis J, et al. Phase I and pharmacologic study of OSI-774, an epidermal growth factor receptor tyrosine kinase inhibitor, in patients with advanced solid malignancies. J Clin Oncol 2001;19:3267–3279.

194. Perez-Soler R, Chachoua A, Huberman M, et al. A phase II trial of the epidermal growth factor receptor (EGFR) tyrosine kinase inhibitor OSI-774, following platinum-based chemotherapy, in patients (pts) with advanced, EGFR-expressing, non-small cell lung cancer (NSCLC) [abstract]. Proc Am Soc Clin Oncol 2001;20:310.

195. Hoeskstra R. A phase I and pharmacological study of intermittent dosing of PKI 166, a novel EGFR tyrosine kinase inhibitor administered orally to patients with advanced cancer. AACR-NCI-EORTC International Conference on Molecular Targets and Cancer Therapeutics, Miami Beach, FL, 2001.

196. Torrance CJ, Jackson PE, Montgomery E, et al. Combinatorial chemoprevention of intestinal neoplasia. Nat Med 2000;6:1024–1028.

197. Keith BR, Allen PP, Alligood, KJ, et al. Anti-tumor activity of GW2016 in the ErbB-2 positive human breast cancer xenograft, BT-474 [abstract]. Proc Am Assoc Cancer Res 2001;42:4308.

198. Rusnak DW, Affleck K, Gilmer TM, et al. The effects of the novel EGFR/ErbB-2 tyrosine kinase inhibitor, GW2016, on the growth of human normal and transformed cell lined [abstract]. Proc Am Assoc Cancer Res 2001;42:4309.

199. Zinner RG, Nemunaitis JJ, Donato NJ, et al. A phase I clinical and biomarker study of the novel pan-erbB tyrosine kinase inhibitor, CI-1033, in patients with solid tumors. AACR-NCI-EORTC International Conference on Molecular Targets and Cancer Therapeutics, Miami Beach, FL, 2001.

200. Coussens L, Yang-Feng TL, Liao YC, et al. Tyrosine kinase receptor with extensive homology to EGF receptor shares chromosomal location with neu oncogene. Science 1985;230:1132–1139.

201. Popescu NC, King CR, Kraus MH. Localization of the human erbB-2 gene on normal and rearranged chromosomes 17 to bands q12–21.32. Genomics 1989;4:362–366.

202. Verbeek BS, Adriaansen-Slot SS, Vroom TM, et al. Overexpression of EGFR and c-erbB2 causes enhanced cell migration in human breast cancer cells and NIH3T3 fibroblasts. FEBS Lett 1998;425:145–150.

203. King CR, Kraus MH, Aaronson SA. Amplification of a novel v-erbB-related gene in a human mammary carcinoma. Science 1985;229:974–976.

204. Slamon DJ, Clark GM, Wong SG, Levin WJ, Ulrich A, McGuire WL. Human breast cancer: correlation of relapse and survival with amplification of the HER-2/neu oncogene. Science 1987;235:177–182.

205. Slamon DJ, Godolphin W, Jones LA, et al. Studies of the HER-2/neu proto-oncogene in human breast and ovarian cancer. Science 1989;244:707–712.

206. Borg A, Tandon AK, Sigurdsson H, et al. HER-2/neu amplification predicts poor survival in node-positive breast cancer. Cancer Res 1990;50:4332–4337.

207. Toikkanen S, Helin H, Isola J, Joensuu H. Prognostic significance of HER-2 oncoprotein expression in breast cancer: a 30-year follow-up. J Clin Oncol 1992;10:1044–1048.

208. Tetu B, Fradet Y, Allard P, Veilleux C, Roberge N, Bernard P. Prevalence and clinical significance of HER2/neu, p53 and Rb expression in primary superficial bladder cancer. J Urol 1996;155:1784–1788.

209. Lee SE, Chow NH, Chi YC, Tzai TS, Yang WH, Lin SN. Expression of c-erbB-2 protein in normal and neoplastic urothelium: lack of adverse prognostic effect in human urinary bladder cancer. Anticancer Res 1994;14:1317–1324.

210. Mellon JK, Lunec J, Wright C, Home CH, Kelly P, Neal DE. C-erbB-2 in bladder cancer: molecular biology, correlation with epidermal growth factor receptors and prognostic value. J Urol 1996;155:321–326.

211. Nguyen PL, Swanson PE, Jaszcz W, et al. Expression of epidermal growth factor receptor in invasive transitional cell carcinoma of the urinary bladder. A multivariate survival analysis. Am J Clin Pathol 1994;101:166–176.

212. Lipponen P, Eskelinen M, Syrjanen S, Tervahauta A, Syrjanen K. Use of immunohistochemically demonstrated c-erb B-2 oncoprotein expression as a prognostic factor in transitional cell carcinoma of the urinary bladder. Eur Urol 1991;20:238–242.

213. Underwood M, Bartlett J, Reeves J, Gardiner DS, Scott R, Cooke T. C-erbB-2 gene amplification: a molecular marker in recurrent bladder tumors? Cancer Res 1995;55:2422–2430.

214. Lonn U, Lonn S, Friberg S, Nilsson B, Silfversward C, Stenkvist B. Prognostic value of amplification of c-erb-B2 in bladder carcinoma. Clin Cancer Res 1995;1:1189–1194.

215. Vollmer RT, Humphrey PA, Swanson PE, Wick MR, Hudson ML. Invasion of the bladder by transitional cell carcinoma: its relation to histologic grade and expression of p53, MIB-1, c-erb B-2, epidermal growth factor receptor, and bcl-2. Cancer 1998;82:715–723.

216. Lewis GD, Figari I, Fendly B, Wong WL, Carter P, Gorman C, Shepard HM. Differential responses of human tumor cell lines to anti-p185HER2 monoclonal antibodies. Cancer Immunol Immunother 1993;37:255–263.

217. Cobleigh MA, Vogel CL, Tripathy D, et al. Multinational study of the efficacy and safety of humanized anti-HER2 monoclonal antibody in women who have HER2-overexpressing metastatic breast cancer that has progressed after chemotherapy for metastatic disease. J Clin Oncol 1999;17:2639–2648.

218. Pegram MD, Slamon DJ. Combination therapy with trastuzumab (Herceptin) and cisplatin for chemoresistant metastatic breast cancer: evidence for receptor-enhanced chemosensitivity. Semin Oncol 1999;26:89–95.

219. Pegram MD, Lipton A, Hayes DF, et al. Phase II study of receptor-enhanced chemosensitivity using recombinant humanized anti-p185HER2/neu monoclonal antibody plus cisplatin in patients with HER2/neu-overexpressing metastatic breast cancer refractory to chemotherapy treatment. J Clin Oncol 1998;16:2659–2671.

220. Albanell J, Codony-Servat J, Rojo F, et al. Activated extracellular signal-regulated kinases: association with epidermal growth factor receptor/transforming growth factor alpha expression in head and neck squamous carcinoma and inhibition by anti-EGF receptor treatments. Cancer Res 2001;61:6500–6510.

221. McCann A, Dervan PA, Johnston PA, Gullick WJ, Carney DN. c-erbB-2 oncoprotein expression in primary human tumors. Cancer 1990;65:88–92.

222. Jimenez RE, Hussain M, Bianco FJ Jr, et al. Her-2/neu overexpression in muscle-invasive urothelial carcinoma of the bladder: prognostic significance and comparative analysis in primary and metastatic tumors. Clin Cancer Res 2001;7:2440–2447.

223. Sauter G, Moch H, Moore D, et al. Heterogeneity of erbB-2 gene amplification in bladder cancer. Cancer Res 1993;53:2199–2203.

224. Shepard HM, Lewis GD, Sarup JC, et al. Monoclonal antibody therapy of human cancer: taking the HER2 protooncogene to the clinic. J Clin Immunol 1991;11:117–127.

225. Carter P, Presta L, Gorman CM, et al. Humanization of an anti-p185 HER2 antibody for human cancer therapy. Proc Natl Acad Sci USA 1992;89:4285–4289.

226. Hussain M, Smith DC, Al-Sukhun S, Vaishampyan U, Petrylak D. Preliminary results of Her-2/neu screening and treatment with trastuzumab (T), paclitaxel (P), carboplatin (C) and gemcitabine (G) in patients with advanced urothelial cancer (NCI#198) [abstract]. Proc Am Soc Clin Oncol 2002;21:800.

227. Slamon DJ, Leyland-Jones B, Shak S, et al. Use of chemotherapy plus a monoclonal antibody against HER2 for metastatic breast cancer that overexpresses HER2. N Engl J Med 2001;344:783–792.

228. Pegram M, Hsu S, Lewis G, et al. Inhibitory effects of combinations of HER-2/neu antibody and chemotherapeutic agents used for treatment of human breast cancers. Oncogene 1999;18:2241–2251.

229. Orlando C, Gelmini S, Selli C, Pazzagli M. Telomerase in urologic malignancy. J Urol 2001;66(2):666–673.

230. Koga S, Kondo Y, Komata T, Kondo S. Treatment of bladder cancer cells in vitro and in vivo with 2-5A antisense telomerase RNA. Gene Ther 2001;8(8):654–658.

231. Hollstein M, Rice K, Greenblatt MS, et al. Database of p53 gene somatic mutations in human tumors and cell lines. Nucleic Acids Res 1994;22:3551–3555.

232. Crystal RG. Transfer of genes to human early lessons and obstacles to success. Science 1995;270:404–410.

233. Slaton JW, Bennedict W, Dinney CP. P53 in bladder cancer: mechanism of action, prognostic value, and target for therapy. Urology 2001;57:852–859.

234. Pagliaro LC, Keyhani A, Liu B, Perrotte P, Wilson D, Dinney CP. Adenoviral p53 gene transfer in human bladder cancer cell lines: cytotoxicity and synergy with cisplatin. Urol Oncol 2003;21:456–462.

235. Pagliaro LC, Keyhani A, Williams D, et al. Repeated intravesical instillations of an adenoviral vector in patients with locally advanced bladder cancer: a phase I study of p53 gene therapy. J Clin Oncol 2003;21:2247–2253.

236. Rosato RR, Grant S. Histone deacetylase inhibitors in cancer therapy. Cancer Biol Therapy 2003;2:30–37.

237. Keller JJ, Giardiello FM. Chemoprevention strategies using NSAIDs and COX-2 inhibitors. Cancer Biol Ther 2003;2(4 Suppl 1):S140–149.

238. Kamat AM, Karashima T, Davis DW, et al. The proteasome inhibitor bortezomib synergizes with gemcitabine to block the growth of human 253J B-V bladder tumor in vivo. Mol Cancer Ther 2004;3(3):279–290.

239. Adjei AA, Rowinsky EK. Novel anticancer agents in clinical development. Cancer Biol Ther 2003;2(Suppl):S5–15.

# Treatment of non-TCC

# Bladder cancer gene therapy 68

*Zhiping Wang, William Benedict, Seth P Lerner, Ronald Rodriguez*

## INTRODUCTION

The efficacy of current strategies for bladder cancer is often insufficient, especially for advanced disease, recurrent superficial cancer, and treatment-resistant carcinoma in situ. Existing approaches for the treatment of nonmuscle-invasive bladder cancer are endoscopic, relying generally on cystoscopy and transurethral resection (TUR). While the overall efficacy of TUR is excellent, recurrences are common. Intravesical chemo or immunotherapy can serve as adjunctive treatment, as therapy for residual microscopic disease, or as a means of disease prophylaxis in which there is an elevated risk of recurrence. Nearly 50% to 70% of patients treated for nonmuscle-invasive disease develop recurrence, and as many as 20% progress to a more aggressive, potentially life-threatening phenotype. Intravesical chemotherapy has proven efficacy both in reducing the frequency of recurrence and in prolonging the time to recurrence, particularly for papillary disease, although it has assumed a more subordinate position to bacillus Calmette–Guérin (BCG) intravesical immunotherapy for high-grade disease. Nevertheless, optimization of BCG intravesical therapy remains a challenge, as does defining effective and practical alternative treatments for patients that fail standard therapies.[1] Most patients experience dysuria, urinary urgency, and hematuria, and some may suffer from granulomatous prostatitis, fever, and even systemic 'BCGosis'.

Invasive and metastatic bladder cancer remains a persistent clinical and scientific challenge. While radical cystectomy is the mainstay of treatment, morbidity may result from the removal of the bladder and adjacent structures or from the use of intestinal segments for urinary tract reconstruction after radical cystectomy.

Recently, Shipley and others have advocated the concept of 'bladder-sparing' treatment, combining aggressive TUR with radiation and chemotherapy.[2] Early results from such protocols suggest that, for the properly selected patient, long-term cancer control can be achieved with functional bladder preservation.[3] However, such protocols require rigorous follow-up and a willingness to progress to cystectomy when recurrences are identified. Bladder-sparing protocols are still considered experimental, and do not represent the conventional standard of care in the United States. The fact that bladder-sparing protocols are being actively developed, however, points to the underlying need for improved novel treatment methods, with less morbidity than cystectomy. Recent advances in genetics and molecular biology have led to multiple potential new novel approaches for cancer treatment.

Optimal development of any potential new therapy requires attention to those areas where the current standard is inadequate. Hence, there are at least three potentially useful areas for gene therapy development: 1) for the prevention of recurrent nonmuscle-invasive disease; 2) as an adjuvant for bladder salvage protocols; and 3) as an adjuvant for the systemic therapy of advanced or metastatic disease.

In this chapter we will evaluate the current gene transfer technologies available for bladder cancer therapeutics, and explore the future potential applications of these technologies as they relate to our clinical need.

# GENE THERAPY IN BLADDER CANCER

## BIOLOGIC BASIS

The development of cancer is fundamentally a derangement of the normal regulation of gene expression. Both genetic and epigenetic changes occur in bladder cancer. For example, one of the first oncogenes ever identified (activated ras) was found in an invasive and highly anaplastic bladder cancer cell line.[4] Other important molecular mechanisms include the inactivation of tumor suppressor genes which code for proteins that regulate cell growth, DNA repair or apoptosis. Several suppressor gene loci have been closely associated with bladder cancer, including p53 and RB. Progression in the development of bladder cancer can occur when there is amplification or overexpression of normal genes that encode for growth factors or their receptors. For example, when angiogenesis activators such as fibroblast growth factor 2 (FGF2) or vascular epidermal growth factor (VEGF) are secreted by tumors, neovascularity results. There are a myriad of mechanisms by which a bladder cancer can either form or progress into an invasive malignancy. However, despite the profound heterogeneity of these cancers, there are multiple shared features, which are still amenable to the development of targeted gene therapeutics.

## GENERAL CONCEPT

'Gene therapy', in the most simplistic terms, refers to the use of genetic materials (DNA or RNA) to affect a therapeutic end. The translation of this concept requires the transfer of these genetic materials into a cell in such a way as to correct the underlying defect or result in cancer cell death. In principle, since cancer is a disease of aberrant gene regulation, 'correction' of even one of the genetic defects might be able to reverse the disease process.

In general, gene transfer technologies can be grouped into viral versus nonviral techniques: viral gene transfer vehicles include, but are not limited to, adenoviruses, adeno-associated viruses, retroviruses, pox viruses, herpes viruses, influenza viruses, Newcastle viruses and, more recently, lentiviruses (a form of retroviruses); nonviral techniques include the gene gun (colloidal gold particles coated with DNA and injected into cells under high pressure helium), liposomal gene transfer, electroporation, and a variety of ternary complexes. The advantages and disadvantages of each of these different modalities are well described in multiple recent reviews[5,6] and a detailed accounting of each method is beyond the scope of this chapter. Currently, the viral gene transfer methods enjoy wider acceptance than the nonviral methods because they permit more efficient gene transfer with less direct toxicity. Unfortunately, the viral vectors also elicit a more potent immune response, which may limit systemic administration due to this toxicity. In this chapter, we will concentrate predominantly on the currently developed viral vectors, including the double-stranded DNA vector, adenovirus. However, it should be noted that substantial efforts are being directed to develop nonviral vectors, in order to circumvent the myriad of limitations inherent in viral vectors.

## GENE THERAPY FOR NONMUSCLE-INVASIVE DISEASE

Current treatment for patients with nonmuscle-invasive bladder cancer involves TUR, followed in some high-risk patients by adjuvant intravesical chemotherapy or BCG administration. The basic biologic response to BCG treatment can be divided into three major phases: 1) binding and uptake of the bacteria to the bladder mucosa; 2) an early phase inflammatory response; and 3) a delayed inflammatory response. The binding and uptake of the attenuated mycobacterium appears to be mediated in part through attachment to fibronectin, since soluble fibronectin or antifibronectin antibodies have been shown to inhibit BCG binding and uptake.[7,8] An intense immune response is generated within 8–24 hours of BCG treatment following internalization of the mycobacterium. This early response is characterized by an increase in a number of different cytokines including tumor necrosis factor-α, interleukin (IL) 1, IL2, IL12, and interferon-γ (IFNγ).[9] Since the absolute number and profile of the cytokine response varies from patient to patient, such changes are difficult to characterize in terms of their mechanism of action. Thus, depending on the setting, these cytokines may exert different biologic effects on cellular immunity (Th1), humoral immunity (Th2), or direct tumor cytotoxicity.

The fact that immune stimulation is inherently an amplified process has resulted in multiple strategies to incorporate gene transfer and immunotherapy into a single treatment. One of the initial approaches to this strategy was to genetically engineer BCG with a secreted fusion of the alpha antigen and the murine IL2 cytokine.[10] In this way, the BCG was the actual gene transfer vehicle, thus augmenting the immunostimulatory effect of BCG, in vitro, in this murine model. While the soluble IL2 could be added exogenously in order to provide added stimulation, the secreted form appeared to be more potent, presumably because of its action in the microenvironment of the actual BCG organism. More recently, several of the immunodominant antigens from BCG have been identified, cloned, and incorporated into a nonviral combined DNA vaccine.[11] In this model, the gene transfer was performed with electric currents in tissue culture (i.e. electroporation) and then the inherent immunostimulation of the bladder cancer cells assessed in a murine model. The immune stimulation was particularly enhanced when these mycobacterium antigens were combined with murine IL12. As before, these experiments were conducted in a murine model and much work remains to be done before such efforts can be translated into actual clinical trials.

Another interesting approach has been to use an adenoviral vector to secrete an immunostimulatory molecule, taking advantage of the inherent immunogenicity of adenoviruses and augmenting this activity for a therapeutic benefit. In this example, IFNα is secreted by a replication-defective adenoviral vector, administered intravesically in combination with the incipient Syn3 to increase adenoviral gene transfer (see below for further details regarding Syn3).[12,13] High local concentrations of IFNα were obtained with Ad-IFNα/Syn3, and sustained for several days, both in normal mouse urothelium and in human bladder cancer cells growing as superficial bladder tumors in nude mice using an orthotopic bladder model.[14] Marked tumor regression was observed and little or no cytotoxicity was detected in normal cells. Ad- IFNα also produced death of bladder cancer cell lines that were resistant to high concentrations of IFNα protein as well as providing evidence of a 'bystander effect', discussed in more detail below.

These strategies support the contention that gene transfer technologies should be developed as a means of augmenting current immunotherapy strategies for superficial bladder cancer. Clinical translation of these methods is currently ongoing. A more detailed accounting of immunogene therapy in urologic malignancies can be found in the review by Kausch et al.[15]

## GENE THERAPY FOR INVASIVE BLADDER CANCER

One of the earliest concepts employed in the development of cancer gene therapy was the so-called bystander effect.[16] In this paradigm, a given gene therapy approach does not need to achieve gene transfer into all the cells of a tumor, provided that those cells which are transduced are capable of killing their neighbors as well. In essence, if the collateral damage of a gene therapy strategy is sufficiently high, then even an inefficient gene transfer vehicle can result in substantial tumor control. Prototypical of the bystander suicide gene therapies is the herpes simplex thymidine kinase gene, which is capable of phosphorylating the inactive prodrug ganciclovir (GCV). This phosphorylated GCV derivative, when incorporated into newly synthesized DNA, results in DNA damage sufficient to trigger apoptosis.

Importantly, the phosphorylated nucleoside poisons are capable of traversing cell membranes and hence result in substantial bystander death for those cells in intimate contact with the transduced cells.

Sutton and colleagues[17] demonstrated that established murine bladder cancer tumors could be effectively treated by the combination of RSV-TK (thymidine kinase gene, under the control of the powerful Rous sarcoma virus promoter) and GCV. Tumor growth was markedly inhibited by a single treatment, resulting in a significant survival advantage for the treated mice. More recently, Freund and associates evaluated the efficacy, toxicity, and potential synergism of adenoviral-mediated TK/GCV gene therapy in combination with various cytotoxic chemotherapeutic agents in human bladder cancer cell lines. Interestingly, they observed that most of the combined strategies did not result in improved efficacy, suggesting the treatments utilized overlapping pathways to cell death. However, low concentrations of methotrexate did enhance the antitumor effects of low- and medium-dose TK/GCV gene therapy.[18]

Mutations in p53 are common in muscle-invasive bladder cancer, occurring in nearly 50% of tumors as indicated by altered expression with immunohistochemistry; when present, these mutations portend a poorer prognosis.[19] P53 is a tumor suppressor gene involved in the regulation of DNA repair, cell cycle regulation, and apoptosis. Mutation or inactivation of p53, therefore, may result in a wide variety of genetic rearrangements, predisposing to the malignant phenotype. Reconstitution of wild-type p53 via an adenovirus vector would therefore have the advantage of 'resensitizing' transformed cells to the normal physiologic processes leading to apoptosis, and possibly also confer enhanced sensitivity to radiation or chemotherapy. For example, the introduction of the wild-type p53 gene into the human muscle-invasive bladder cancer cell line HT1376 markedly enhanced sensitivity to cisplatin in vitro. Direct injection of the p53 adenoviral vector into subcutaneous HT1376 tumors established in nude mice, followed by intraperitoneal administration of cisplatin, induced massive apoptotic destruction of the tumors.[20]

Currently, there are two independent adenoviral-mediated p53 gene transfer products under clinical testing: INGN201 and SCH58500. INGN201 is in clinical development for the treatment of lung, breast, ovarian, bladder, liver, and brain cancers[21]; SCH58500 is in phase II/III testing for stage III ovarian cancer, phase II trials for hepatocellular and metastatic colorectal cancers, and phase I trials for a variety of other cancers, including bladder cancer.[22]

Pagliaro et al performed repeated intravesical instillations of INGN201 in a phase I study of patients with locally advanced bladder cancer. Thirteen patients received a total of 22 courses without dose-limiting toxicity. Specific transgene expression was detected in bladder biopsy tissue from two of seven assessable patients. Outpatient administration of multiple courses was feasible and well tolerated. A patient with advanced nonmuscle-invasive bladder cancer showed evidence of tumor response.[23] However, poor gene transfer efficiency was noted in this trial, prompting the conclusion that additional methods will be necessary to overcome the natural barrier function of urothelium against adenoviral gene transfer.

In addition, several groups have observed that invasive bladder cancer cells often lack expression of the adenovirus receptor CAR (Coxsackie and adenovirus receptor), potentially limiting the efficacy of adenoviral-mediated gene transfer for bladder cancer[24-26] (Figure 68.1). Fortunately, a polyamide detergent called Syn3 has recently been identified which appears to both overcome the glycosaminoglycan (GAG) barrier of the bladder and facilitate gene transfer of adenoviruses, even in the absence of normal adenoviral receptors.[13] Alternative methodologies have also been developed to retarget adenoviruses to other bladder cancer cell-surface proteins, such as epidermal growth factor receptor (EGFR),[27] through the use of bispecific antibodies or by highly engineered adenoviruses with modifications, allowing retargeting to other receptors.

Direct intravesical clinical testing of SCH58500 has been performed in patients with bladder cancer, demonstrating excellent transgene expression into the urothelium when combined with an early precursor to Syn3, called Big-CHAP.[12] Specific transgene expression, RNA, and protein expression of the p53 target gene p21/WAF1 were detected in tissues from seven of eight patients treated with intravesical instillation of SCH58500 but in none of three assessable patients treated with intratumoral injection of SCH58500.[28] Distribution studies after intravesical instillation of SCH58500 revealed both high transduction efficacy and vector penetration throughout the whole urothelium and into submucosal tumor cells. No dose-limiting toxicity was observed, and side effects were local and of a transient nature. Further testing, however, will be required to better define the potential utility of this type of strategy.

## NOVEL STRATEGIES UNDER DEVELOPMENT

### ONCOLYTIC ADENOVIRUSES

The normal life cycle of adenoviruses is lytic. Hence, as virus is propagated in target cells, those cells are destroyed in the process. Early adenoviral vectors were deleted in the regions which controlled replication

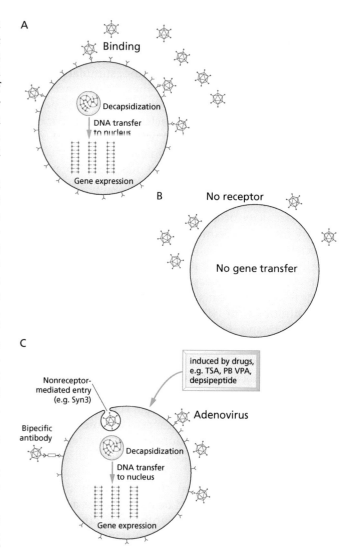

**Fig. 68.1**

Adenoviral gene transfer into bladder cancer cells. **A** Normal gene transfer: normal urothelium contains abundant receptors for adenovirus (CAR and αV integrins), allowing the viral particles to bind and internalize. After internalization, the virus protein coat is removed (decapsidization) and the protein–DNA complex transported to the nucleus, where gene expression occurs. **B** Poor gene transfer: high-grade, high-stage urothelial carcinomas often lack adenovirus receptors, hence gene transfer with normal adenoviral vectors is ineffective in these cell lines. **C** Methods of overcoming poor receptor expression: a number of techniques have been developed to counter poor CAR expression levels found in high-grade urothelial cancers, including the use of bispecific antibodies (which bridge the fiber knobs of the virus to some other membrane-bound epitope on the cell surface) or chemical disruption of the normal membrane barriers with polyamides (e.g. Syn3). Alternatively, certain differentiation-inducing drugs have been found to cause re-expression of CAR, including most histone deactylase inhibitors, such as suberoylanilide hydroxamic acid (SAHA), trichostatin A (TSA), pivanex (PB), valproic acid (VPA), and depsipeptide. (CAR, Coxsackie and adenovirus receptor.)

(E1A and E1B), so that the cells transduced would not be destroyed by lytic replication. However, more recently, it has been discovered that this lytic activity may be a useful strategy for cancer therapy. In the mid-1990s it was discovered that a naturally occurring mutant adenovirus, which lacked the E1B 55 kD gene, was capable of selectively replicating in cancer cells defective in the p53 axis, but not in normal cells.[29] This virus, termed ONYX-015, has been clinically tested in head and neck cancers. Similarly, it was found that tissue-specific replication could be achieved by replacing the regulatory sequences of the replication genes E1A and E1B with those of the prostate-specific antigen (PSA) regulatory sequences.[30] In this way, only cells which normally expressed PSA (e.g. prostatic epithelium) were capable of undergoing lytic adenoviral infection.

This strategy of conditionally replication competent adenovirus (CRAd) therapy for cancer has gained widespread popularity in the gene therapy community.[31] CRAd therapy derives part of its appeal from the fact that the therapeutic effect is amplified by local replication. Recently, D.C. Yu and colleagues demonstrated a bladder-specific CRAd with synergy when used in combination with certain taxanes.[32] Oncolytic replication was restricted to those cells which express the uroplakin II gene (UPII). Uroplakins (UPs) are a group of integral membrane proteins that are synthesized as the major differentiation products of mammalian urothelium. UPII gene expression is bladder specific and differentiation dependent.[33] Such combination strategies may prove particularly appealing for bladder salvage protocol development. In the long run, combination CRAd therapy and systemic chemotherapy will be developed, as there is strong biologic evidence that the two treatments provide synergy. However, such protocols will require new techniques to overcome specific and innate immunologic sequestration of the viruses when administered systemically.

## INHIBITION OF GENE EXPRESSION THERAPIES

Another novel strategy for selective tumor killing with gene transfer technologies involves the use of oligonucleotides, which are short sequence-specific DNA or RNA molecules designed to bind to the RNA of the target protein. Single-stranded antisense DNA oligonucleotides and, more recently, short double-stranded RNAs (RNAi) have been found to inhibit gene expression by binding to the target RNA and initiating degradation of the message before translation can occur. Hence, protein production is interrupted and target protein levels decrease. When double-stranded RNA is used, the total sequence size must be limited to less than

30 base pairs in order to prevent initiation of the interferon-mediated defense cellular response to potential viral pathogens. RNAi technology is still under early clinical development,[34] while antisense oligonucleotide (ASO) techniques have a well-established experimental and technical base that have already been tested in the clinical setting.[35]

Because these techniques can be tailored to eliminate or decrease expression of any particular gene product, ASOs can be used as a neoadjuvant before chemotherapy to help sensitize the tumor cells.[36] Most oncogenes—including EGFR, basic fibroblastic growth factor (bFGF), IL8, human telomerase (hTERT), and BCL2—can be targeted for antisense treatment in bladder cancer. For example, Hong et al observed that certain cisplatin-resistant bladder cancer T24 sublines (T24-R1 and T24-R2) had elevated levels of BCL2.[37] Even a short-term exposure of the T24 sublines to anti-BCL2 oligonucleotides restored chemosensitivity to cisplatin for these bladder cancer cells. Inoue et al reported on gene therapy of human bladder cancer with adenovirus-mediated antisense bFGF. Intralesional therapy with Ad-bFGF-AS decreased the in vivo expression of bFGF and matrix metalloproteinase type 9 (MMP9) mRNA and protein, reduced microvessel density, and enhanced endothelial cell apoptosis. Tumor growth was significantly inhibited by Ad-bFGF-AS, indicating that bFGF expression is a potential target for the therapy of bladder cancer.[38] Upregulation of BCL2 protein expression might be one of the mechanisms of cisplatin resistance in bladder cancer cells, and antisense BCL2 oligonucleotide may be helpful in chemotherapy for bladder cancer by reversing cisplatin resistance.[37]

## ANTIANGIOGENESIS STRATEGIES

Growth and metastasis of malignant tumors require angiogenesis. Inhibition of tumor-induced angiogenesis may represent an effective cytostatic strategy. Shichinohe et al utilized a vector based on the vesicular stomatitis virus (VSV-G, a lentivirus, similar in structure to the HIV virus) to efficiently transduce bladder cancer cells in vitro with both the angiostatin and endostatin genes.[39] Their vector demonstrated preferential gene transfer for the malignant bladder cells, while sparing normal endothelial cells, suggesting that they may ultimately have clinical utility in preferentially disrupting tumor vascularity. Alternatively, Inoue et al reported an antiangiogenesis strategy of gene therapy for human bladder cancer with adenovirus-mediated antisense bFGF. Intralesional therapy with Ad-bFGF-AS decreased the in vivo expression of bFGF and MMP9 mRNA and protein, reduced microvessel density, and enhanced endothelial cell apoptosis. Tumor growth was significantly inhibited by Ad-bFGF-AS, indicating that bFGF expression may be a reasonable target for bladder cancer gene therapy.[38]

## IMMUNOGENE THERAPY

Gene therapy using cytokines (cytokine immunogene therapy) may play an important role in immunotherapy. The co-stimulation of antitumor immune responses using cells modified with cytokine genes has been used in cancer immunotherapy. Several strategies have emerged, including:

- modification of tumor cells with cytokine genes ex vivo (whole tumor cell vaccines)
- ex vivo modification of other cell types for cytokine gene delivery
- delivery of cytokine genes into tumor microenvironments in vivo
- modification of dendritic cells with cytokine genes ex vivo.

Originally, single cytokine genes were used.[40] Introduction of genes encoding immunostimulatory cytokine(s) into cancer cells is known to enhance antitumor immunity. Similarly, injection of cells infected with adenovirus expressing IL12 or granulocyte-macrophage colony-stimulating factor (GM-CSF)—AdIL12 or AdGM-CSF—almost completely abolished tumorigenicity, and injection of AdGM-CSF into pre-established tumors significantly inhibited growth of the tumors injected. On the other hand, injection of AdIL12 into the pre-established tumors significantly inhibited growth of not only the tumors injected but also distant tumors, indicating induction of systemic antitumor immunity.[41] Similarly, mice with melanoma or breast carcinoma treated solely by intratumoral injections with allogeneic cells genetically modified to secrete IL2 were found to survive significantly longer than mice in various control groups.[42]

Studies from the Lattime laboratory have focused on using recombinant poxvirus encoding immune-enhancing cytokine genes given intravesically. Following preclinical validation, it has been shown in phase I clinical trials of vaccinia virus in melanoma (intralesionally)[43] and bladder (intravesically)[44] that efficient viral infection/transfection is achieved despite high levels of neutralizing antibody. Clinical testing of intravesical poxvirus recombinants with GM-CSF and the immune-stimulating TRICOM (LFA3, ICAM1, B7.1) in patients with advanced bladder cancer is currently ongoing (Cancer Therapy Evaluation Program No. 5585).

The density of tumor antigen in conjunction with major histocompatibility complex (MHC) class I molecules on the cell surface affects cytotoxic T cell (CTL) function in an active antitumor immune response. Thus, methods to enhance antigen expression/

presentation could augment the effect of cancer immune therapy. Increasing tumor immunogenicity may be key to inducing effective antitumor immunity. It has been shown that tumor immunogenicity can be enhanced through coupling cytokine expression with antigen presentation.[45] The MHC class II+/Ii– phenotype can be generated after adenoviral delivery of both an expressible gene for the MHC class II inducer and an antisense Ii-RNA construct in tumor cells. A single recombinant adenovirus with genes for IFNγ and an Ii-reverse gene construct (Ii-RGC)—rAV/IFNγ/Ii-RGC—efficiently induced the MHC class II+/Ii– phenotype. Injection of tumor nodules with rAV/Ii-RGC and rAV/CIITA/IFNγ, combined with a suboptimal dose of rAV/IL2, induced a potent antitumor immune response. The methods are adaptable for producing enhanced genetic vaccines, attenuated virus vaccines (e.g. vaccinia), and ex vivo cell-based vaccines (dendritic and tumor cells).[46]

Converting tumor cells to a MHC class II-positive, Ii protein-negative phenotype is another approach to increase tumor immunogenicity in tumor immunotherapy. MHC class II and Ii molecules were induced in tumor cells in situ following tumor injection of a plasmid containing the gene for the MHC class II transactivator (CIITA). Lipoprotein was suppressed by the antisense effect of an Ii-RGC.[47]

## POTENTIAL PROBLEMS TO BE OVERCOME

The major limitations of human gene therapy for cancer stem from two simple but profound observations:

- In order to cure a cancer by 'corrective' gene therapy, all cancer cells must be affected by the therapy. Currently, the efficiency of gene transfer in situ is poor, and 100% gene transduction of all cancer cells is not a realistic expectation.
- Urologic malignancies contain a wide variety of genetic derangements. Hence, no single gene pathway can be applied to 'correct' the underlying aberration in all bladder cancers. Because of the multiplicity of gene defects that occur in carcinogenesis, the selection of the most potent target for gene therapy will be difficult.

As sobering as these observations may be, however, there is still much room for optimism for the ultimate utility of gene therapy for cancer. While gene transfer efficiencies may be low, strategies which employ a bystander effect provide a means to amplify the efficacy of gene therapy strategies.[16] In addition, while no single genetic aberration can explain all urothelial malignancies, there are still multiple shared features which may render urothelial carcinomas susceptible to genetically based therapies.

One of the main concerns regarding the potential toxicity of many gene therapy strategies is the potential for toxic genes to be expressed in nontarget cells. While this is less of a concern for local intravesical instillation, it is a significant concern for the anticipated development of systemic gene therapy. In this sense, tissue- or tumor-specific gene expression is crucial for achieving successful results in suicide gene therapy.[48] Replication selective, tumor-specific viruses may present a novel approach for treating neoplastic disease. These vectors are designed to induce virus-mediated lysis of tumor cells after selective viral propagation within the tumor. Currently, the best-developed example of this type of strategy is a bladder-specific replication competent virus based on the uroplakin II promoter.[32]

L-plastin (LP) is constitutively expressed at high levels in malignant epithelial cells but is not expressed in normal tissues, except at low levels in mature hematopoietic cells. The LP promoter has been described as having tumor-specific gene expression in ovarian and bladder cancer cell lines and may prove to be another effective alternative for targeted gene therapy.[49] The transcription of therapeutic genes in cells infected by the AdLP vectors could be restricted to LP expression-positive ovarian carcinoma cells but would not be seen in the normal mesothelial cells of the peritoneal cavity.[49] Adenoviral vectors carrying therapeutic genes driven by the LP promoter would be of use in prodrug activating transcription unit gene therapy for cancer.

Telomerase activation is considered to be a critical step in carcinogenesis, and its activity is closely correlated with human telomerase reverse transcriptase (hTERT) expression. Hence the hTERT promoter has been characterized as a 'cancer-specific' promoter.[50] Zou et al reported that Ad-TERT displays cancer-specific E1A expression, virus replication, and cytolysis in in vitro experiments. In animal experiments, intratumoral administration of Ad-TERT demonstrates potent antitumoral efficacy in at least two xenograft models.[51] However, cancer cells are not alone in the expression of hTERT, as stem cells also require its expression, and other safeguards will need to be instituted.

Although the anatomic location of the bladder may appear to make it an ideal site for gene transfer, the inner layer of the urothelium is coated with a protective proteoglycan barrier. This GAG layer serves both to protect the bladder from unwanted entry of pathogens, and also to act as a significant impediment to gene transfer. Various strategies have been applied for improving the transduction efficacy of the therapeutic genes into the bladder cancer cells. These strategies include the modification of adenoviral fibers, cotransduction of incipient materials that enhance viral infectivity such as Syn3, and direct injection into the visible tumor.

Co-administration of 22% ethanol can enhance local adenoviral-mediated transgene expression in the normal and neoplastic bladder epithelium in rodents.[52] Similarly, Shimizu and colleagues have found that pretreatment of the bladder GAG layer with dilute hydrogen chloride results in markedly enhanced adenoviral gene transfer.[53] Prior to instillation of the adenoviral vector, normal bladders were pretreated with phosphate-buffered saline, which would destroy the mucosal GAG layer. Removing the GAG layer rendered the normal bladder highly susceptible to adenoviral gene transfer. Intravesical instillation of adenoviral vectors does not result in systemic infection.[53] However, even when the GAG layer has been disrupted, other factors, such as the relative deficiency of the adenoviral receptors (CAR) in transitional cell carcinoma may limit gene transfer. While this problem appears limiting, recent data from a variety of laboratories have demonstrated that certain drugs, such as histone deacetylase inhibitors (HDACI), are capable of causing re-expression of the adenovirus receptor in bladder cancer lines.[54] Interestingly, CAR upregulation appears to be tumor cell-specific, as other nonurothelial CAR-negative cell lines failed to demonstrate enhanced adenoviral gene transfer with the same treatments. These results provide a rational basis for combining HDACI therapy with gene therapy as a method of augmenting activity in bladder cancer.[55]

## THE FUTURE OF GENE THERAPY FOR BLADDER CANCER

Though much progress has been made in the translation of human gene therapy, this technology is still in its earliest stages of development. Currently, the most efficient vectors for gene transfer are viral based; however, such vectors invariably are highly immunogenic and are readily eliminated from the body when given systemically. In addition, many invasive bladder cancers lack expression of the receptors for adenovirus (CAR), although modifying the virus or combining viral-mediated gene therapy with an incipient can overcome this lack of expression.

The bladder is an easily accessible structure and systemic delivery may not always be required. Hence, early efforts for bladder cancer gene therapy are being focused on intravesical delivery. Direct intravesical treatment has low toxicity and thus can be readily combined with existing treatment. Many of the newer generation gene therapy treatments are synergistic with conventional therapies (e.g. radiation or chemotherapy). Furthermore, recombinant methodologies may also prove useful for augmenting conventional immunotherapies (e.g. BCG treatment). Future research directions will include development of more efficient vectors combined with conventional modalities for both prevention of recurrence and progression from nonmuscle-invasive disease, and also as an adjuvant to the development of bladder salvage protocols.

## REFERENCES

1. Witjes JA. Bladder carcinoma in situ in 2003: state of the art. Eur Urol 2004;45(2):142–146.
2. Shipley WU, Kaufman DS, Heney NM, Griffin PP, Althausen AF, Prout GR Jr. The integration of chemotherapy, radiotherapy and transurethral surgery in bladder-sparing approaches for patients with invasive tumors. Prog Clin Biol Res 1990;353:85–94.
3. Shipley WU, Kaufman DS, Zehr E, et al. Selective bladder preservation by combined modality protocol treatment: long-term outcomes of 190 patients with invasive bladder cancer. Urology 2002;60(1):62–67; discussion 67–68.
4. Taparowsky E, Suard Y, Fasano O, Shimizu K, Goldfarb M, Wigler M. Activation of the T24 bladder carcinoma transforming gene is linked to a single amino acid change. Nature 1982;300(5894):762–765.
5. Hughes RM. Strategies for cancer gene therapy. J Surg Oncol 2004;85(1):28–35.
6. Zhang WW. Development and application of adenoviral vectors for gene therapy of cancer. Cancer Gene Ther 1999;6(2):113–138.
7. Zhao W, Schorey JS, Bong-Mastek M, Ritchey J, Brown EJ, Ratliff TL. Role of a bacillus Calmette–Guérin fibronectin attachment protein in BCG-induced antitumor activity. Int J Cancer 2000;86(1):83–88.
8. Ratliff TL, Kavoussi LR, Catalona WJ. Role of fibronectin in intravesical BCG therapy for superficial bladder cancer. J Urol 1988;139(2):410–414.
9. Poppas DP, Pavlovich CP, Folkman J, et al. Intravesical bacille Calmette–Guérin induces the antiangiogenic chemokine interferon-inducible protein 10. Urology 1998;52(2):268–275; discussion 275–276.
10. Yamada H, Matsumoto S, Matsumoto T, Yamada T, Yamashita U. Murine IL-2 secreting recombinant Bacillus Calmette–Guérin augments macrophage-mediated cytotoxicity against murine bladder cancer MBT-2. J Urol 2000;164(2):526–531.
11. Lee CF, Chang SY, Hsieh DS, Yu DS. Treatment of bladder carcinomas using recombinant BCG DNA vaccines and electroporative gene immunotherapy. Cancer Gene Ther 2004;11(3):194–207.
12. Connor RJ, Engler H, Machemer T, et al. Identification of polyamides that enhance adenovirus-mediated gene expression in the urothelium. Gene Ther 2001;8(1):41–48.
13. Yamashita M, Rosser CJ, Zhou JH, et al. Syn3 provides high levels of intravesical adenoviral-mediated gene transfer for gene therapy of genetically altered urothelium and superficial bladder cancer. Cancer Gene Ther 2002;9(8):687–691.
14. Benedict W, Tao Z, Kim CS, et al. Intravesical Ad-IFN causes marked regression of human bladder cancer growing orthotopically in nude mice and overcomes resistance to IFN-alpha protein. Mol Ther 2004;10(3):525–532.
15. Kausch I, Ardelt P, Bohle A, Ratliff TL. Immune gene therapy in urology. Curr Urol Rep 2002;3(1):82–89.
16. van Dillen IJ, Mulder NH, Vaalburg W, de Vries EF, Hospers GA. Influence of the bystander effect on HSV-tk/GCV gene therapy. A review. Curr Gene Ther 2002;2(3):307–322.
17. Sutton MA, Berkman SA, Chen SH, et al. Adenovirus-mediated suicide gene therapy for experimental bladder cancer. Urology 1997;49(2):173–180.
18. Freund CT, Tong XW, Rowley D, et al. Combination of adenovirus-mediated thymidine kinase gene therapy with cytotoxic chemotherapy in bladder cancer in vitro. Urol Oncol 2003;21(3):197–205.
19. Smith ND, Rubenstein JN, Eggener SE, Kozlowski JM. The p53 tumor suppressor gene and nuclear protein: basic science review and relevance in the management of bladder cancer. J Urol 2003;169(4):1219–1228.
20. Miyake H, Hara I, Gohji K, Yamanaka K, Arakawa S, Kamidono S. Enhancement of chemosensitivity in human bladder cancer cells by adenoviral-mediated p53 gene transfer. Anticancer Res 1998;18(4C):3087–3092.
21. INGN 201. Ad-p53, Ad5CMV-p53, adenoviral p53, INGN 101, p53 gene therapy—Introgen, RPR/INGN 201. BioDrugs 2003;17(3):216–222.
22. Barnard DL. Technology evaluation: Sch-58500, Canji. Curr Opin Mol Ther 2000;2(5):586–592.
23. Pagliaro LC, Keyhani A, Williams D, et al. Repeated intravesical instillations of an adenoviral vector in patients with locally advanced bladder cancer: a phase I study of p53 gene therapy. J Clin Oncol 2003;21(12):2247–2253.
24. Li Y, Pong RC, Bergelson JM, et al. Loss of adenoviral receptor expression in human bladder cancer cells: a potential impact on the efficacy of gene therapy. Cancer Res 1999;59(2):325–330.
25. Sachs MD, Rauen KA, Ramamurthy M, et al. Integrin alpha(v) and coxsackie adenovirus receptor expression in clinical bladder cancer. Urology 2002;60(3):531–536.
26. Okegawa T, Pong RC, Li Y, Bergelson JM, Sagalowsky AI, Hsieh JT. The mechanism of the growth-inhibitory effect of coxsackie and adenovirus receptor (CAR) on human bladder cancer: a functional analysis of CAR protein structure. Cancer Res 2001;61(17):6592–6600.
27. van der Poel HG, Molenaar B, van Beusechem VW, et al. Epidermal growth factor receptor targeting of replication competent adenovirus enhances cytotoxicity in bladder cancer. J Urol 2002;168(1):266–272.
28. Kuball J, Wen SF, Leissner J, et al. Successful adenovirus-mediated wild-type p53 gene transfer in patients with bladder cancer by intravesical vector instillation. J Clin Oncol 2002;20(4):957–965.
29. McCormick F. Cancer-specific viruses and the development of ONYX-015. Cancer Biol Ther 2003;2(4 Suppl 1):S157–160.
30. Rodriguez R, Schuur ER, Lim HY, Henderson GA, Simons JW, Henderson DR. Prostate attenuated replication competent adenovirus (ARCA) CN706: a selective cytotoxic for prostate-specific antigen-positive prostate cancer cells. Cancer Res 1997;57(13):2559–2563.
31. Dobbelstein M. Replicating adenoviruses in cancer therapy. Curr Topics Microbiol Immunol 2004;273:291–334.
32. Zhang J, Ramesh N, Chen Y, et al. Identification of human uroplakin II promoter and its use in the construction of CG8840, a urothelium-specific adenovirus variant that eliminates established bladder tumors in combination with docetaxel. Cancer Res 2002;62(13):3743–3750.
33. Zhu HJ, Zhang ZQ, Zeng XF, Wei SS, Zhang ZW, Guo YL. Cloning and analysis of human uroplakin II promoter and its application for gene therapy in bladder cancer. Cancer Gene Ther 2004;11(4):263–272.
34. Mittal V. Improving the efficiency of RNA interference in mammals. Nat Rev Genet 2004;5(5):355–365.
35. Goodchild J. Oligonucleotide therapeutics: 25 years agrowing. Curr Opin Mol Ther 2004;6(2):120–128.
36. Duggan BJ, Gray S, Johnston SR, Williamson K, Miyaki H, Gleave M. The role of antisense oligonucleotides in the treatment of bladder cancer. Urol Res 2002;30(3):137–147.
37. Hong JH, Lee E, Hong J, Shin YJ, Ahn H. Antisense Bcl2 oligonucleotide in cisplatin-resistant bladder cancer cell lines. BJU Int 2002;90(1):113–117.
38. Inoue K, Perrotte P, Wood CG, Slaton JW, Sweeney P, Dinney CP. Gene therapy of human bladder cancer with adenovirus-mediated antisense basic fibroblast growth factor. Clin Cancer Res 2000;6(11):4422–4431.
39. Shichinohe T, Bochner BH, Mizutani K, et al. Development of lentiviral vectors for antiangiogenic gene delivery. Cancer Gene Ther 2001;8(11):879–889.
40. Kowalczyk DW, Wysocki PJ, Mackiewicz A. Cancer immunotherapy using cells modified with cytokine genes. Acta Biochim Pol 2003;50(3):613–624.
41. Tanaka K, Towata S, Nakao K, et al. Thyroid cancer immunotherapy with retroviral and adenoviral vectors expressing granulocyte macrophage colony stimulating factor and interleukin-12 in a rat model. Clin Endocrinol 2003;59(6):734–742.
42. Lichtor T, Glick RP. Cytokine immuno-gene therapy for treatment of brain tumors. J Neuro-oncol 2003;65(3):247–259.
43. Mastrangelo MJ, Maguire HC, McCue P, et al. A pilot study demonstrating the feasibility of using intratumoral vaccinia injections as a vector for gene transfer. Vaccine Res 1995;4:55–69.

44. Gomella LG, Mastrangelo MJ, McCue PA, Maguire HJ, Mulholland SG, Lattime EC. Phase I study of intravesical vaccinia virus as a vector for gene therapy of bladder cancer. J Urol 2001;166(4):1291–1295.

45. He X, Tsang TC, Luo P, Zhang T, Harris DT. Enhanced tumor immunogenicity through coupling cytokine expression with antigen presentation. Cancer Gene Ther 2003;10(9):669–677.

46. Hillman GG, Kallinteris NL, Li J, et al. Generating MHC Class II+/Ii– phenotype after adenoviral delivery of both an expressible gene for MHC Class II inducer and an antisense Ii-RNA construct in tumor cells. Gene Ther 2003;10(17):1512–1518.

47. Lu X, Kallinteris NL, Li J, et al. Tumor immunotherapy by converting tumor cells to MHC class II-positive, Ii protein-negative phenotype. Cancer Immunol Immunother 2003;52(10):592–598.

48. Yoshimura I, Ikegami S, Suzuki S, Tadakuma T, Hayakawa M. Adenovirus mediated prostate specific enzyme prodrug gene therapy using prostate specific antigen promoter enhanced by the Cre-loxP system. J Urol 2002;168(6):2659–2664.

49. Peng XY, Won JH, Rutherford T, et al. The use of the L-plastin promoter for adenoviral-mediated, tumor-specific gene expression in ovarian and bladder cancer cell lines. Cancer Res 2001;61(11):4405–4413.

50. Kawashima T, Kagawa S, Kobayashi N, et al. Telomerase-specific replication-selective virotherapy for human cancer. Clin Cancer Res 2004;10(1 Pt 1):285–292.

51. Zou W, Luo C, Zhang Z, et al. A novel oncolytic adenovirus targeting to telomerase activity in tumor cells with potent. Oncogene 2004;23(2):457–464.

52. Engler H, Anderson SC, Machemer TR, et al. Ethanol improves adenovirus-mediated gene transfer and expression to the bladder epithelium of rodents. Urology 1999;53(5):1049–1053.

53. Shimizu H, Akasaka S, Suzuki S, Akimoto M, Shimada T. Preferential gene transfer to BBN-induced rat bladder tumor by simple instillation of adenoviral vector. Urology 2001;57(3):579–584.

54. Hemminki A, Kanerva A, Liu B, et al. Modulation of coxsackie-adenovirus receptor expression for increased adenoviral transgene expression. Cancer Res 2003;63(4):847–853.

55. Sachs MD, Ramamurthy M, Poel Hvd, et al. Histone deacetylase inhibitors upregulate expression of the coxsackie adenovirus receptor (CAR) preferentially in bladder cancer cells. Cancer Gene Ther 2004;11(7):477–486.

# Treatment of non-TCC adenocarcinoma/sarcoma

# 69

*Sami Arap, Marco A Arap*

## INTRODUCTION

More than 90% of all bladder tumors are transitional cell carcinomas.[1] Nonurothelial bladder tumors are rare and account for less than 5% of all vesical tumors combined.[2] Despite the low incidence of nonurothelial bladder tumors, urologists should consider these tumors in the differential diagnosis of vesical neoplasms, especially in patients with unusual clinical presentations. Uncommon malignant bladder tumors are shown in Table 69.1. Other histologic types such as melanomas and lymphomas may also be found in the bladder but are extremely rare and account for less than 0.5% of all bladder malignancies.

## SQUAMOUS CELL CARCINOMAS

Squamous cell carcinomas (SCCs) are the second most prevalent epithelial neoplasms of the bladder and account for approximately 3% to 5% of bladder tumors in Western countries.[3] These tumors are usually aggressive and the most relevant common factor involved in the etiology of SCC is chronic bladder irritation, such as in patients with indwelling catheters

**Table 69.1** Uncommon malignant bladder tumors

| Tumor type | Percentage of bladder tumors |
|---|---|
| Squamous cell carcinomas | 3–5 |
| Adenocarcinomas | 0.5–2 |
| Small cell carcinomas | <0.5 |
| Sarcomas | <0.1 |

and those with neurogenic bladders that rely on clean intermittent catheterization.[4] A known pathogenesis of SCC is a chronic infection with *Schistosoma haematobium*. In countries with endemic schistosomiasis, SCC accounts for approximately 30% of cancers and is the second most common malignancy in women.[5] Schistosomiasis-related SCC is discussed elsewhere in this book.

Although partial squamous differentiation is common in cystectomy specimens, the diagnosis of SCC is only made in cases where no urothelial carcinoma is identified. Tumors may be well differentiated, expressing squamous features such as squamous pearls, keratohyaline granules and intercellular bridges, or poorly differentiated, with only focal squamous differentiation.

Patients with bladder SCC usually have a poor prognosis, mostly due to local invasion. The majority of patients have extravesical tumor extension at the time of diagnosis, and death is usually related to locally recurrent disease.[3] Treatment is therefore directed to local control of the disease with radical cystectomy and bilateral pelvic node dissection. Preoperative radiation for invasive (stages T2 and T3) SCC of the bladder can downstage the disease in 40% of patients.[6] Therefore, it may protect patients from pelvic recurrence, which is usually the main cause of death. In addition, chemotherapy with paclitaxel, carboplatin, and gemcitabine[7] proved to be effective as an adjuvant therapy for advanced SCC in other locations such as the head and neck, and may offer promise for patients with SCC of the bladder.

## ADENOCARCINOMAS

Pure adenocarcinoma of the bladder is the third most common type of epithelial tumor and represents 0.5%

to 2% of all bladder tumors. The definition of vesical adenocarcinomas is still controversial. However, the pathologic variations are tumors that form glandular structures resembling colonic adenocarcinomas (enteric type) and/or tumors that produce intra- (signet cell type) or extracellular mucin (mucinous type).[8]

Adenocarcinomas of the urinary bladder can be divided into three different subtypes depending on their origin. Adenocarcinomas may arise from a urachal remnant (urachal adenocarcinoma, UA), from metaplasia of the bladder urothelium (nonurachal adenocarcinoma, NUA), or from a metastatic site from another primary tumor such as from the rectum, prostate, stomach, breast, endometrium, or ovary.[1] NUAs arising from eutopic bladder urothelium account for between 0.4% and 3.9% of all bladder tumors, whereas primary UAs account for only 0.17% to 1.18% of those tumors.[9-12] Males are more frequently affected than females, with a ratio of approximately 7:3. Although there is no consensus regarding diagnostic criteria for UA, important clinicopathologic features include location to the bladder dome, a sharp demarcation between the tumor and surface epithelium, and exclusion of a primary adenocarcinoma that may have metastasized to the bladder.

The usefulness of separating adenocarcinomas of the bladder between UA and NUA types has yielded some discussion. Although it is believed that both tumors have the same pathogenesis (metaplasia changing the normal urothelium to a glandular type and ultimately to adenocarcinoma),[13-19] several differences are recognized between the two. In the series reported by Grignon et al,[8] patients with UA were significantly younger than those with NUA disease. Similarly, the mean ages in other studies were lower for patients with UA.[11,13] Several groups noted a striking difference in the clinical course between the two different subtypes. While patients with NUA tended to die rapidly within the first 2 years of diagnosis, those with UA died more regularly over a 10-year period.[8,14] Thomas et al, in a review of 52 cases, reported that 33% of patients with UA died of disease at 5 years compared with 71% of patients with NUA.[11]

Standard treatment for all vesical adenocarcinomas is radical cystectomy and bilateral pelvic node dissection, followed by urinary diversion.[20,21] In rare instances where patients have a well-differentiated, noninvasive UA localized to the bladder dome, partial cystectomy with removal of the urachus and umbilectomy may be considered.[8,11,13-15] The largest series for UA reported 5-year survival rates, ranging from 40% to 50% for patients with urachal adenocarcinomas.[22-24]

In the series from Siefker-Radtke et al, nodal status and surgical margins were significantly associated with survival.[25] In addition, although en bloc resection of the bladder dome, urachal ligament, posterior rectus abdominis fascia, and umbilicus was not statistically associated with survival, it is noteworthy that 13 of the 16 long-term survivors were treated with en bloc resections.[25] In this largest published series, no patient had disease confined to the epithelium or urachal ligament at presentation, with most patients showing locally advanced disease. In addition, more than 29% of all cases presented with positive nodal or systemic disease. Adjuvant treatment was, therefore, frequently employed and considered of importance in the management of UA.[25]

The most effective responses with chemotherapy were observed in patients receiving a combination of 5-fluorouracil and cisplatin, suggesting that a regimen for adenocarcinoma of the colon may be more beneficial for UA than the traditional urothelial cancer chemotherapy regimens.[25] Very few patients are included, however, to allow definitive conclusions to be made concerning the most appropriate regimen. Of the patients with metastases, almost half had bone involvement at diagnosis, which generally required radiation therapy and surgery.

For patients with NUA, radical cystectomy is usually the treatment of choice, as the tumor is often multifocal in origin.[11,20,21] Other treatment options such as radiotherapy, chemotherapy, and combinations thereof, have been described for these tumors, although bladder adenocarcinomas are usually considered to be radioresistant. There are a few published case reports describing different chemotherapy regimens for NUA with methotrexate, vinblastine, adriamycin, and cisplatin (MVAC),[26] or with the combination of cisplatin, mitomycin-C, etoposide, and tegafur-uracil.[27]

Prognosis is unfavorable for patients with NUA, with 5-year survival rates ranging between 30% and 60%.[8,14]

## SMALL CELL CARCINOMAS

Small cell carcinoma of the bladder is an extremely rare malignancy, accounting for less than 0.5% of all vesical tumors. It is also known as neuroendocrine carcinoma of the bladder and diagnosis is made with clinical and pathologic evaluation. However, special immuno-histochemical staining, such as neuron-specific enolase, chromogranin A, and synaptophysin, may also be valuable in the diagnosis of these tumors and in confirming their neuroendocrine origin.

Initial treatment for small cell carcinoma of the bladder is radical cystectomy and bilateral extended pelvic node dissection.[2] Despite aggressive treatment, prognosis is usually unfavorable with surgical therapy alone due to local invasion and distant metastasis. Trias and colleagues reported median patient survival of less than 1 year; extended survival of more than 5 years was very uncommon.[28] Another study of 22 patients with small cell carcinoma of the bladder showed a long-term

(6 years and beyond) recurrence-free survival rate of 23% for those with localized disease (pT2–4N0M0) treated by complete tumor resection.[29] Due to the poor prognosis of most patients treated by surgery alone, chemotherapy regimens should be evaluated for the treatment of small cell carcinoma of the bladder and strong consideration given to neoadjuvant chemotherapy.

## SARCOMAS

In adults, urinary bladder sarcomas are very rare, with an incidence of less than 0.1% of all bladder malignancies. They present most commonly in the sixth decade and are very aggressive tumors, with reported 5-years survival rates ranging from 40% to 60%.[30] The etiology of bladder sarcomas is unknown. However, association with schistosomiasis,[31] cyclophosphamide treatment,[32–34] and radiotherapy[35] has been previously documented. Bladder sarcomas are derived from connective cells and may be classified according to their origin (Table 69.2). This subclassification of bladder sarcomas employs special immunohistochemical techniques and is very important in the initial diagnosis, as it carries treatment and prognostic implications. Sarcomas are usually infiltrative and microscopic extension along anatomic tissue planes usually leads to early hematogenous dissemination, with metastasis found mainly in the lungs, liver, and bones.[36]

General treatment recommendations for bladder sarcomas have been based upon a relatively small number of cases that were managed with different protocols. No clear-cut conclusions can be drawn with tumors this rare. However, some treatment recommendations do exist. Initially, for tumors without signs of metastatic disease, surgical extirpation with margins is the treatment of choice in almost all cases.[34] Partial cystectomy can be considered for small tumors located in the bladder dome, but resection of the urachus, perivesical fat, and a 4–5 cm full-thickness

**Table 69.2** Subclassification of bladder sarcomas

| Sarcoma type | Percentage of sarcomas |
| --- | --- |
| Leiomyosarcomas | 50–60 |
| Rhabdomyosarcomas | 20–30 |
| Angiosarcomas | <2 |
| Carcinosarcoma | <1 |
| Fibrosarcomas | <1 |
| Malignant fibrous histiocytoma | <1 |
| Osteosarcomas | <1 |
| Chondrosarcomas | <0.5 |
| Liposarcomas | <0.5 |
| Plexoma | <0.5 |

bladder margin must be obtained due to the aggressive and infiltrative nature of sarcomas.[34,37] Tumors of any size involving the trigone and/or bladder neck are best treated by radical cystectomy. For tumors such as rhabdomyosarcomas, which have a high risk of pelvic lymph node spread, bilateral pelvic lymph node dissection is often recommended.

In an attempt to improve success rates for patients with bladder sarcomas, other treatment modalities such as radiotherapy, chemotherapy, and bone marrow transplantation have been undertaken.[34] These are usually part of a combined modality approach for patients with invasive or metastatic disease. Radiation has been recommended only for presumed or documented positive microscopic margins after resection of larger bulky tumors.[30,37] Cytoreductive preoperative chemotherapy with the combination of cisplatin and doxorubicin is encouraged by Ahlering and associates for patients with bulky or transmural disease. They also recommend two additional cycles of postoperative adjunctive chemotherapy in patients with pathologic stage P3A or positive nodal disease, as well as in patients whose tumors showed histologic evidence of sensitivity in the preoperative setting.[30] As for patients with adenocarcinomas, those with bladder sarcomas usually have a poor prognosis, unless diagnosis is made early in the course of the disease.

## LEIOMYOSARCOMA

Leiomyosarcoma is the most common type of bladder sarcoma in adults and is characterized histologically by interwoven bundles of spindle-shaped cells. Most patients are in their seventh decade and present with hematuria and obstructive voiding symptoms. Tumors may be related to a previous history of local radiation or chemotherapy for other malignancies.[38] Treatment of bladder leiomyosarcomas is usually challenging and depends on the clinical stage of the tumor. Patients with localized disease are treated ideally by wide local resection of the bladder. The most commonly used surgery is radical cystectomy with bilateral radical pelvic node dissection, followed by creation of a urinary diversion. In cases with locally advanced or metastatic disease, neoadjuvant chemotherapy may be employed. In a series from the University of Texas M.D. Anderson Cancer Center, 10 patients had locally advanced and 14 had metastatic bladder leiomyosarcomas and were treated with neoadjuvant chemotherapy. Among those with locally advanced disease, three patients had a complete response and one had a partial response. In addition, all patients presenting with locally advanced disease had resectable tumors after chemotherapy. The most common regimen used was doxorubicin and ifosfamide.[39]

Patients with metastatic disease are usually treated with similar chemotherapy regimens. In a multivariate analyses, only the Memorial Sloan-Kettering Cancer Center (MSKCC) stage was a significant predictor of disease-specific survival for adult bladder leiomyosarcomas.[39] Prognosis for bladder leiomyosarcomas is not as pessimistic as that for other sarcomas, as some patients are able to achieve long-term survival. The 5-year disease-specific survival rate may be higher than 60% in patients treated aggressively with a combination of radical surgery and chemotherapy.[36,39]

## RHABDOMYOSARCOMA

Rhabdomyosarcoma is a neoplasm that demonstrates evidence of skeletal muscle differentiation. About 5% of all rhabdomyosarcomas arise in the urinary bladder or prostate, and it is the most frequent tumor in children younger than 10 years old. Patients usually present with hematuria, incontinence and/or obstructive voiding symptoms. At cystoscopy, tumors may be infiltrative, nodular or polypoid (botryoid). Rhabdomyosarcomas are extremely rare in adults. The ideal treatment in children includes neoadjuvant polychemotherapy, followed by radical or partial resection of the bladder and prostate. Prognosis varies according to different variants of the tumor. Botryoid and spindle cell variants of embryonal rhabdomyosarcomas have the best prognosis. The conventional embryonal subtype has a less favorable prognosis, and alveolar and pleomorphic subtypes have a poor prognosis.[40]

## CARCINOSARCOMA

Carcinosarcomas of the urinary bladder are tumors characterized by the presence of both malignant epithelial and mesenchymal components.[41] Treatment is usually directed towards complete resection of the organ with circumferential margins. Prognosis is poor regardless of the treatment employed, and pathologic stage seems to be the best prognostic factor.[42]

## ANGIOSARCOMA

Angiosarcomas comprise approximately 2% of all soft tissue sarcomas and can arise in any location in the body.[43] Bladder angiosarcomas are exceedingly rare and one of the most aggressive cancers arising in the urinary bladder. Microscopically, angiosarcomas exhibit poorly differentiated packed endothelial cells with a primitive vascular organization,[44] and have the highest incidence of nodal metastasis among all sarcoma types.[45] Treatment recommendations for angiosarcomas in general involve radical surgery with wide margins and adjuvant radiotherapy for better local control of the disease, especially in patients with high-grade lesions.[43] However, angiosarcomas tend to be radioresistant,[43] and chemotherapy has been offered as palliation for patients with metastatic disease.[46]

## LIPOSARCOMA, OSTEOSARCOMA, ETC.

Other types of sarcoma, such as liposarcomas and osteosarcomas, are extremely rare and treatment must be decided on a patient-by-patient basis. The cornerstone of therapy is usually surgical removal of the tumor with wide margins, as for all the other types of sarcoma, in an attempt to prevent local recurrence.

## REFERENCES

1. Messing EM, Catalona W. Urothelial tumors of the urinary tract. In Walsh PC, Retik AB, Vaughan ED Jr, Wein AJ (eds): Campbell's Urology, 7th ed. Philadelphia: WB Saunders, 1998, pp 2327–2410.
2. Dahm P, Gschwend JE. Malignant non-urothelial neoplasms of the urinary bladder: a review. Eur Urol 2003;44:672–681.
3. Serreta V, Pomara G, Piazza F, Gange E. Pure squamous cell carcinoma of the bladder in western countries. Report on 19 consecutive cases. Eur Urol 2000;37:85–89.
4. Locke JR, Hill DE, Walzer Y. Incidence of squamous cell carcinoma in patients with long-term catheter drainage. J Urol 1985;133:1034–1035.
5. El-Sheikh SS, Madaan S, Alhasso A, Abel P, Stamp G, Lalani EN. Cyclooxygenase-2: a possible target in schistosoma-associated bladder cancer. BJU Int 2001;88:921–927.
6. Swanson DA, Liles A, Zagars GK, Preoperative irradiation and radical cystectomy for stages T2 and T3 squamous cell carcinoma of the bladder. J Urol 1990;143:37–40.
7. Hussain M, Vaishampayan U, Du W, Redman B, Smith DC. Combination paclitaxel, carboplatin, and gemcitabine is an active treatment for advanced urothelial cancer. J Clin Oncol 2001;19:2527–2533.
8. Grignon DJ, Ro JY, Ayala AG, Johnson DE, Ordoñes NG. Primary adenocarcinoma of the urinary bladder. A clinicopathologic analysis of 72 cases. Cancer 1991;67:2165–2172.
9. Ichikawa T. Remote results of bladder tumors. Jpn J Urol 1958;49:602–610.
10. Jacobo E, Loening S, Schmidt JD, et al. Primary adenocarcinoma of the bladder: a retrospective study of 20 cases. J Urol 1977;117:54–56.
11. Thomas DG, Ward AM, Williams JL. A study of 52 cases of adenocarcinoma of the bladder. Br J Urol 1971;43:4–15.
12. Jakse G, Schneider JM, Jacobi GH. Urachal signet-ring carcinoma, a rare variant of vesical adenocarcinoma: incidence and pathological criteria. J Urol 1978;120:764–766.
13. Mostofi FK, Thomson RV, Dean AL Jr. Mucous adenocarcinoma of the urinary bladder. Cancer 1955;9:741–758.
14. Anderström C, Johansson SL, von Schultz L. Primary adenocarcinoma of the urinary bladder. A clinicopathologic and prognostic study. Cancer 1983;52:1273–1280.
15. Abenoza P, Manivel C, Fraley EE. Primary adenocarcinoma of the urinary bladder: clinicopathologic study of 16 cases. Urology 1987;29:9–14.
16. Begg RC. The colloid adenocarcinomata of the bladder vault arising from the epithelium of the urachal canal: with a critical survey of the tumors of the urachus. Br J Surg 1931;18:422–466.
17. Patch FS, Rhea LJ. The genesis and development of Brunn's nests and their relation to cystitis cystica, cystitis glandularis, and primary adenocarcinoma of the bladder. Can Med Assoc J 1935;33:597–606.
18. Shaw JL, Gislason GJ, Imbriglia JE. Transition of cystitis glandularis to primary adenocarcinoma of the bladder. J Urol 1958;79:815–822.
19. Schubert GE, Pavkovic MB, Bethke-Bedurftig BA. Tubular urachal remnants in adult bladders. J Urol 1982;127:40–42.
20. Fuselier HA Jr, Brannan W, Ochsner MG, Matos LH. Adenocarcinoma of the bladder as seen at Ochsner medical institutions. South Med J 1978;71:804–806.
21. Kakizoe T, Matsumoto K, Andoh M, Nishio Y, Kishi K. Adenocarcinoma of urachus: report of 7 cases and review of literature. Urology 1983;21:360–366.

22. Ghoneim MA, el-Mekresh MM, el-Baz MA, el-Attar IA, Ashamallah A. Radical cystectomy for carcinoma of the bladder: critical evaluation of the results in 1,026 cases. J Urol 1997;158:393–399.

23. Fadl-Elmula I, Kytola S, Leithy ME, et al. Chromosomal aberration in benign and malignant bilharzias-associated bladder lesions analyzed by comparative genomic hybridization. BMC Cancer 2002;2:5–10.

24. Nakanishi K, Kawai T, Suzuki M, Torikata C. Prognostic factors in urachal adenocarcinoma. A study in 41 specimens of DNA status, proliferating cell-nuclear antigen immunostaining, and argyrophilic nucleolar-organizer region counts. Hum Pathol 1996;27:240–247.

25. Siefker-Radtke AO, Gee J, Shen Y, et al. Multimodality management of urachal carcinoma: the M.D. Anderson Cancer Center experience. J Urol 2003;169:1295–1298.

26. Queipo Zaragoza JA, Chicote Perez F, Borrell Palanca A, et al. Unusual bladder tumors: primary epidermoid carcinoma, adenocarcinoma, and sarcoma. Clinical behavior. Our experience. Actas Urol Esp 2003;27:123–131.

27. Kasahara K, Inoue K, Shuin T. Advanced adenocarcinoma of the urinary bladder successfully treated by the combination of cisplatinum, mitomycin-C, etoposide and tegafur-uracil chemotherapy. Int J Urol 2001;8:133–136.

28. Trias I, Agaba F, Condom E, et al. Small cell carcinoma of the urinary bladder. Presentation of 23 cases and review of 134 published cases. Eur Urol 2001;39:85–90.

29. Holmang S, Borghede G, Johansson SL. Primary small cell carcinoma of the bladder: a report of 25 cases. J Urol 1995;153:1820–1822.

30. Ahlering TE, Weintraub P, Skinner DG. Management of adult sarcomas of the bladder and prostate. J Urol 1988;140:1397–1399.

31. Alwan MH, Sayed M, Kamal MM. Schistosomiasis and sarcoma of the urinary bladder. Eur Urol 1988;15:139–140.

32. Carney CN, Stevens PS, Fried FA, et al. Fibroblastic tumor of the urinary bladder after cyclophosphamide therapy. Arch Surg 1982;106:247–249.

33. Rowland RG, Eble JN. Bladder leiomyosarcoma and pelvic fibroblastic tumor following cyclophosphamide therapy. J Urol 1983;130:344–346.

34. Parekh DJ, Jung C, O'Conner J, Dutta S, Smith ER Jr. Leiomyosarcoma in urinary bladder after cyclophosphamide therapy for retinoblastoma and review of bladder sarcomas. Urology 2002;60:164xii–164xiv.

35. Navon JD, Rahimzadeh M, Wong AK, et al. Angiosarcoma of the bladder after therapeutic irradiation for prostate cancer. J Urol 1997;157:1359–1360.

36. Russo P, Brady MS, Conlon K, et al. Adult urological sarcoma. J Urol 1992;147:1032–1036.

37. Swartz DA, Johnson DE, Ayala AG, Watkins DL. Bladder leiomyosarcoma: a review of 10 cases with 5-year followup. J Urol 1985;133:200–202.

38. Helpap B. Nonepithelial neoplasms of the urinary bladder. Virchows Arch 2001;439:497–503.

39. Rosser CJ, Slaton JW, Izawa JI, Levy LB, Dinney CPN. Clinical presentation and outcome of high-grade urinary bladder leiomyosarcomas in adults. Urology 2003;61:1151–1155.

40. Nigro KG, MacLennan GT. Rhabdomyosarcoma of the bladder and prostate. J Urol 2005;173:1365.

41. Wick MR, Swanson PE. Carcinosarcomas: current perspectives and a historical review of nosological concepts. Semin Diagn Pathol 1993;10:118–127.

42. Baschinsky DY, Chen JH, Vadmal MS, Lucas JG, Bahnson RR, Niemann TH. Carcinosarcoma of the urinary bladder—an aggressive tumor with diverse histogenesis. A clinicopathological study of 4 cases and review of the literature. Arch Pathol Lab Med 2000;124:1172–1178.

43. Mark R, Poen J, Tran L, et al. Angiosarcoma: a report of 67 patients and a review of the literature. Cancer 1996;77:2400–2406.

44. Engel JD, Kuzel TM, Moceanu MC, Oefelein MG, Schaeffer AJ. Angiosarcoma of the bladder: a review. Urology 1998;52:778–784.

45. Fong Y, Coit DG, Woodruff JM, et al. Lymph node metastasis from soft tissue sarcomas in adults. Analysis of data from a prospective database of 1772 sarcoma patients. Ann Surg 1993;217:72–77.

46. Budd G. Palliative chemotherapy of adult soft tissue sarcomas. Semin Oncol 1995;22:30–34.

# Treatment of squamous cell carcinoma 70

*Hassan Abol-Enein, Mohamed A Ghoneim*

## INTRODUCTION

Squamous cell carcinoma (SCC) of the bladder represents the second most common bladder malignancy in Western countries, comprising 2% to 5% of bladder tumors in most contemporary series. The male to female ratio is 1.4:1. Women tend to have more advanced disease when diagnosed. Spinal cord injuries, indwelling catheters, and chronic inflammation are among the most commonly noted risk factors. The relation between SCC and smoking has not been clearly established.[1]

Bilharziasis is the leading cause of SCC in areas where the disease is endemic. Egypt, Iraq, Zimbabwe, Yemen, Sudan, and middle Africa are the most affected areas.[2] The incidence of SCC in the last reported Egyptian series was 59% among patients with invasive bladder cancer. The male to female ratio was 4:1. The peak incidence of the disease occurs from the third to fifth decades.[3] The etiologic association between SCC and bilharziasis has been explained by DNA changes resulting from the presence of local chemical carcinogens, which are excreted in urine. Nitrosamines produced by chronic bacterial infections complicating urinary bilharziasis act as potent carcinogens. Furthermore, urinary stagnation, mechanical irritation, and metaplastic changes of the urothelium play an important role.[4]

## SQUAMOUS CELL CARCINOMA IN THE NONBILHARZIAL BLADDER

In the vast majority of patients the tumors are primary and there is no previous history of vesical malignancy.

By the time of diagnosis, the disease is often at a locally advanced stage. Superficial tumors are almost unknown. When Rundle et al reviewed the records of 114 patients with SCC of the bladder, they found that 97 (92%) had invasive tumors (T2–4) at the time of diagnosis, and that most of the tumors were high grade.[5]

The results reported after treatment with definitive external irradiation are uniformly poor.[5,6] Surgery appears to produce much better results. Richie and associates reported 5-year survival of 48% in 33 patients treated by radical cystectomy.[7] Tumor stage was identified as the most important predictor of outcome. Serretta et al reported on 19 patients with pure SCC of the bladder.[8] All had solitary, locally advanced tumors and were treated by radical cystectomy. Sixty-three percent of the treated patients died of locally recurrent bladder cancer at a mean follow-up of 52 months. Distant metastases were observed in only one patient.

Johnson and coworkers employed integrated preoperative radiation therapy followed by cystectomy and reported a 5-year survival rate of 34%.[9] A similar approach has been advocated by Swanson and colleagues.[10]

Patients with T2 disease have the highest survival rates. Furthermore, the results are better in patients whose tumors are downstaged by preoperative irradiation than in those in whom downstaging does not occur. However, no conclusions can be drawn about the efficacy of preoperative irradiation plus cystectomy for nonbilharzial SCC because too few patients treated in this way have been reported in the literature.[2] Because the tumor is uncommon, only a few cases are available for study, and it is extremely difficult to carry out well-controlled prospective studies to reach objective conclusions.

Squamous cell carcinoma of the bladder appears to be resistant to chemotherapy. A chemotherapy protocol effective against this disease has not yet been defined, and a role for adjuvant or neoadjuvant treatment has not been established.

Chemotherapy usually is not recommended because of the apparently low chemosensitivity of SCC of the bladder. Methotrexate, vinblastine, doxorubicin, and cisplatin (MVAC) chemotherapy has been evaluated in only a very few patients.[11]

Interestingly, SCC has a low incidence of distant metastasis, ranging from 8% to 10%.[12] The prognosis of SCC of the bladder is, however, dismal. Most patients die due to locoregional failure within 3 years. Distant metastases are more often the cause of death in patients with transitional cell carcinoma (TCC) than in those with SCC. Therefore, pelvic control for SCC is more important and is a major incentive to attempt local treatment, such as radical cystectomy, in order to reduce the incidence of pelvic recurrence.[4]

## PREVENTION AND EARLY DETECTION

Several screening protocols have been advocated in an attempt to diagnose tumors earlier and to improve outcome. Broecker et al[13] recommended annual cystoscopy and urine cytology in long-term paraplegics. Others have suggested routine random bladder biopsies every 1–2 years. Navon et al[14] do not routinely use urine cytology or random biopsies except in patients whose spinal cord injuries are more than 10 years old and in patients with recurrent or chronic urinary tract infections. Celis et al[15] showed that psoriasin (a calcium-binding protein expressed by squamous epithelia) is a potential marker of SCC. Other biomarkers, such as SCC antigen, BCL2 and p53 oncoproteins, may possibly have a role in the early diagnosis.[16] However, determination of the exact use of these new markers will require further studies to validate their role in early detection and follow-up of SCC of the bladder.

## SQUAMOUS CELL CARCINOMA IN THE BILHARZIAL BLADDER

## CLINICOPATHOLOGIC FEATURES

In most patients, disease is in an advanced stage at the time of initial diagnosis and, in 25% of cases, is inoperable.[4] This is partially explained by the overlapping of symptoms of bilharzial cystitis with early malignant cystitis.[17] When clinical staging was compared to pathologic findings, a clinical error of 37%

with a tendency for understaging was found. Recently, more than 86% of tumors have been found to be ≥P3 or P4. Most SCCs of the bladder are low-grade tumors. Lymph node involvement has been observed in 18.7% of cystectomy specimens.[3]

## TREATMENT

### CONSERVATIVE RESECTION

#### Endoscopic resection

In view of the tumor's bulk and its advanced stage, transurethral resection does not appear to be a feasible choice for definitive treatment, and there are no reports on results with this procedure in bilharzial bladder malignancy. Endoscopic resection is limited to obtaining biopsies for histopathologic diagnosis.

#### Segmental resection

Segmental resection is an attractive alternative that circumvents the physiologic and social inconveniences of urinary diversion and possible loss of sexual potency. However, local resection is feasible only under certain conditions: 1) when there is a solitary tumor that does not involve the trigone and is of a size allowing resection with an adequate margin of safety; and 2) when the remainder of the bladder mucosa is free of any associated precancerous lesions. These strict criteria are actually met in only a minority of cases. El-Hammady et al reported resectable bladder cancer in only 19 patients of 190 (10%).[18] Augmentation cystoplasty was required in five patients to increase residual bladder capacity. Five-year survival was 26.5%. Patients with low-grade tumors had roughly twice the survival rate of those with high-grade disease. On the other hand, Omar reported less favorable results in a series of 22 cases.[19] All patients with the exception of one experienced recurrence of tumor within 2 years. These differences in outcome may be related to a wide variability in selection criteria.

### RADICAL CYSTECTOMY

In view of the clinicopathologic characteristics and the natural history of this disease, radical cystectomy and urinary diversion provide the most logical treatment approach for patients with resectable tumors.[20,21] In men, the operation entails removal of the bladder, perivesical fat, peritoneal covering, prostate, seminal vesicles, and the endopelvic lymph nodes; in women, the bladder, urethra (if it is not used for orthotopic bladder substitution), uterus, and upper vagina, along with the pelvic cellular tissue and lymph nodes, are removed.

In a series of 138 cases, Ghoneim and associates reported a high postoperative mortality of 13.7%. This was due to peritonitis, adhesive intestinal obstruction, and hepatic failure. Cardiopulmonary complications were uncommon among this relatively young group of patients. In this series, reported in 1979, the overall 5-year survival was 32.6%. It was 43% and 30% in P1 and P2, and in P3 and P4, respectively. Patients with low-grade tumors had a 46% survival rate; those with high-grade disease had a 21% survival rate. Lymph node involvement reduced the 5-year survival rate to 20%.[21]

In a recent report of the results in 1026 cystectomy patients from an area where schistosomiasis is endemic, 59% of the tumors were SCC. Bilharzial ova were identifiable in 88% of the specimens. Extravesical extension was not significantly different between patients with SCC or TCC (13.5% and 14.9%, respectively). The overall 5-year survival rate of SCC patients was 50.3%. Only tumor stage, grade, and lymph node involvement had an independent and significant effect on survival. The latter reduced the survival rate by 50%.[3]

The poor results from these reports confirm that radical cystectomy alone is inadequate in dealing with the extent of local pathology. Adjuvant treatment directed to the pelvis might improve survival. Preoperative radiation therapy has been proposed as a possible treatment strategy in these patients.

## RADIATION THERAPY

The growth characteristics of carcinoma of the bilharzial bladder have been studied to evaluate their potential responsiveness to radiation.[22] Two growth features were demonstrated: 1) high cell mitotic rate with a potential doubling time of 6 days; and 2) an extensive cell loss factor. Tumors with such growth characteristics were expected to respond to radiation.[23] Nevertheless, early experiences with external beam therapy for definitive control of these tumors were disappointing.[24] Factors that have interfered with the efficacy of radiation treatment in these patients include coexisting bilharzial urologic lesions, which interfere with the local tissue tolerance and reduce local control as a result of considerable tumor bulk. Furthermore, the presence of radioresistant hypoxic tumor cells is suspected in light of the capillary vascular pattern of this cancer.[25]

## ADJUVANT PREOPERATIVE RADIATION

The aim of preoperative radiation is to sterilize microscopic tumor cells in the deeply infiltrating parts of the tumor as well as microextensions into the perivesical tissues and lymphatics. These small tumor foci theoretically may respond better to radiation

because they are oxygenated and composed of relatively small numbers of cells with a high mitotic index. These biologic factors and the pattern of treatment failures due to local pelvic recurrence have justified the use of preoperative radiotherapy.

Awaad and associates compared the results of cystectomy after preoperative administration of 40 cGy with those in a control group treated by cystectomy alone.[26] The reported 2-year survival rates showed significant improvement in the irradiated group. Ghoneim and colleagues compared the results of cystectomy after preoperative irradiation using 2000 cGy with those of cystectomy alone.[27] They treated 92 patients in two groups. Patients were followed for up to 60 months. Although patients that received preoperative radiation had better survival rates, this improvement did not approach statistical significance. In patients with low-stage tumors, regardless of grade, survival did not appear to be influenced by preoperative irradiation when compared with survival of patients with high-stage tumors.

The presence of a large proportion of hypoxic cells in bulky tumors could explain the modest improvement after radiation. To enhance the therapeutic value of irradiation treatment, misonidazole, a hypoxic cell sensitizer, was given before delivery of the radiation regimen. A three-arm randomized study was conducted to evaluate results with cystectomy alone, with 2000 cGy of radiation before cystectomy, and with the use of misonidazole as a radiosensitizer before radiation and cystectomy.[2] The 5-year survival rates in this trial are shown in Table 70.1. The addition of misonidazole did not provide any additional benefit to the patients receiving preoperative radiotherapy.[28]

## CHEMOTHERAPY

Several chemotherapeutic agents have been tried in the management of nonresectable SCC of the bilharzial bladder by Gad El-Mawla et al at the National Cancer Institute of Cairo University. All trials were phase II studies using single agents. The most promising results were obtained with epirubicin hydrochloride.[29] Neoadjuvant and adjuvant epirubicin chemotherapy was used in a prospective randomized study including 71 patients with invasive T2 and T3 bilharzial bladder cancers. Two-thirds of the treated patients had SCC. Patients were randomized to receive either two courses of epirubicin preoperatively plus four additional courses postoperatively (n=34) or radical surgery (n=37). At a median follow-up of 24 months, 25 patients from the chemotherapy group and 14 patients from the cystectomy group were alive and disease-free. The 2-year disease-free survival percentages were 73.5% and 37.9%, respectively (p=0.05).[30] Further long-term follow-up results were not published.

**Table 70.1** Comparison of 5-year survivals

| Patient characteristics | Cystectomy | 2000 cGy and cystectomy | Misonidazole, 2000 cGy, and cystectomy |
|---|---|---|---|
| Total number | 35 | 34 | 28 |
| Died postoperatively | – | – | – |
| Died from disease | 1 | 2 | 0 |
| Died from unknown causes | 11 | 4 | 7 |
| Living with disease | 9 | 8 | 4 |
| Free of disease ≥5 years | 14 | 20 | 17 |
| % survival | 40 | 58 | 60 |

In another multicenter study including 120 patients treated with neoadjuvant cisplatin and gemcitabine, patients with SCC did not have a better survival rate than patients treated with cystectomy alone.[31]

## PREVENTION AND EARLY DETECTION

Bilharzial bladder cancer is an example of a preventable malignant disease. Primary prevention entails control of bilharziasis through control of the snail (the intermediate host of the parasite) and mass treatment of the rural population with oral antibilharzial drugs.[32] Secondary prevention includes early detection using urinary cytology and selective screening of the population at risk. The yield of a screening study carried out in a rural area in Egypt was 2 per 1000 individuals.[33]

## CONCLUSION

Squamous cell carcinoma of the bladder is usually locally advanced by the time it is diagnosed. Radical cystectomy is the most reliable treatment modality. The majority of treatment failures are locoregional. Neither neoadjuvant/adjuvant chemotherapy nor radiotherapy has shown a survival benefit over cystectomy alone. Newer combination regimens such as paclitaxel, cisplatin, and gemcitabine may provide hope for the future, but thus far results have not been overly promising, and these newer agents should be further evaluated in randomized clinical trials.

## REFERENCES

1. Johansson SL, Cohen SM. Epidemiology and etiology of bladder cancer. Semin Surg Oncol 1997;13:291–298.

2. Ghoneim MA. Nontransitional cell bladder cancer. In Krane RJ, Siroky MB, Fitzpatrick JM (eds): Clinical Urology. Philadelphia: Lippincott, 1994, pp 679–687.

3. Ghoneim MA, El-Mekresh MH, El-Baz MA, et al. Radical cystectomy for carcinoma of the bladder: critical evaluation of the results in 1026 cases. J Urol 1997;158:393–399.

4. El-Bolkainy MN, Ghoneim MA, Mansour MA. Carcinoma of the bilharzial bladder in Egypt: Clinical and pathological features. Br J Urol 1972;44:561–570.

5. Rundle JSH, Hart AJL, McGeorge A, et al. Squamous cell carcinoma of the bladder: a review of 114 patients. Br J Urol 1982;54:522–526.

6. Bessett PL, Abell MR, Herwig KR. A clinicopathologic study of squamous cell carcinoma of the bladder. J Urol 1974;112:66–67.

7. Richie JP, Waisman J, Skinner DG, et al. Squamous carcinoma of the bladder: treatment by radical cystectomy. J Urol 1976;115:670–671.

8. Serretta V, Pomara G, Piazzo F, et al. Pure squamous cell carcinoma of the bladder in western countries. Eur Urol 2000;37:85–89.

9. Johnson DE, Schoenwald MB, Ayala AG, et al. Squamous cell carcinoma of the bladder. J Urol 1976;115:542–544.

10. Swanson DA, Liles A, Zagars GK. Pre-operative irradiation and radical cystectomy for stages T2 and T3 squamous cell carcinoma of the bladder. J Urol 1990;143:37–40.

11. Sternberg CN, Yagoda A, Scher HI, et al. Preliminary results of M-VAC (methotrexate, vinblastine, doxorubicin and cisplatin) for transitional cell carcinoma of the urothelium. J Urol 1985;133:403–407.

12. Wishnow KL, Dmochowski R. Pelvic recurrence after radical cystectomy without preoperative radiation. J Urol 1988;140:42–43.

13. Broecker BH, Klein FA, Hackler RH. Cancer of the bladder in spinal cord injury patients. J Urol 1981;125:196–197.

14. Navon JD, Soliman H, Khonsari F, et al. Screening cystoscopy and survival of spinal cord injured patients with squamous cell cancer of the bladder. J Urol 1997;157:2109–2111.

15. Celis JE, Rasmussen HH, Vorum H, et al. Bladder squamous cell carcinomas express psoriasin and externalize it to the urine. J Urol 1996;155:2105–2112.

16. Tsukamoto T, Kumamoto Y, Ohmura K, et al. Squamous cell carcinoma associated antigen in uro-epithelial carcinoma. Urology 1992;40:477–483.

17. Ghoneim MA, Mansour MA, El-Bolkainy MN. Staging of carcinoma of bilharzial bladder. Urology 1974;3:40–42.

18. El-Hammady SM, Ghoneim MA, Hussein ES, et al. Segmental resection for carcinoma of the bladder. Mansoura Med Bull 1975;3:191.

19. Omar SM. Segmental resection for carcinoma of the bladder. Egypt Med Assoc 1969;52:975.

20. Ghoneim MA, Awaad HK. Results of treatment in carcinoma of the bilharzial bladder. J Urol 1980;123:850–852.

21. Ghoneim MA, Ashamallah AG, Hammady S, et al. Cystectomy for carcinoma of the bilharzial bladder: 138 cases 5 years later. Br J Urol 1979;51:541–544.

22. Awaad HK, Hegazy M, Ezzat S, et al. Cell proliferation of carcinoma in bilharzial bladder: an autoradiology study. Cell Tissue Kinet 1979;12:513–520.

23. Denekamp J. The relationship between the cell loss factor and the immediate response to radiation in animal tumors. Eur J Cancer 1972;8:335–340.

24. Awaad HK. Radiation therapy in bladder cancer. Alex Med J Cancer 1958;4:118–131.

25. Omar AH, Shalaby MA, Ibrahim AH. On the capillary vascular bed in carcinoma of the urinary bladder. East Afr Med J 1975;51:34–41.

26. Awaad HK, Abdel Baki H, El-Bolkainy N, et al. Pre-operative irradiation of T3 carcinoma in bilharzial bladder. Int J Radiat Oncol Biol Phys 1979;5:787–794.

27. Ghoneim MA, Ashamallah AK, Awaad HK, et al. Randomized trial of cystectomy with or without pre-operative radiotherapy for carcinoma of the bilharzial bladder. J Urol 1985;134:266–268.

28. Denekamp J, McNally NJ, Fowler JF, et al. Misonidazole in fractionated radiotherapy: are many small fractions best? Br J Radiol 1980;53:981–990.

29. Gad El-Mawla N, Hamza MR, Zikri Z Kh, et al. Chemotherapy in invasive carcinoma of the bladder: a review of phase II trials in Egypt. Acta Oncol 1989;28:73–76.

30. Gad-El-Mawla N, Mansour MA, Eissa S, Ali NM, et al. A randomized pilot study of high-dose epirubicin as neoadjuvant chemotherapy in the treatment of cancer of bilharzial bladder. Ann Oncol 1991;2:137–140.

31. Khalid H, Zaghloul M, Ghoneim M, et al. Gemcitabin and cisplatin as a neoadjuvant chemotherapy for invasive bladder cancer. Proc Am Soc Clin Oncol 2003;22:411 (abstract 1652).

32. El-Bolkainy MN. Topographic pathology of cancer. Cairo University: The National Cancer Institute, 1998, pp 59–63.

33. El-Bolkainy MN, Ghoneim MA, El-Morsey BA, et al. Carcinoma of bilharzial bladder: diagnostic value of urine cytology. Urology 1974;3:319–323.

# Ancillary

# Pediatric bladder tumors 71

*Fernando A Ferrer, Michael Ritchey*

## INTRODUCTION

Bladder tumors in children are uncommon and their pathology differs from that of adults. Unlike adults, where transitional cell carcinoma is the most common cancer of the bladder, the most common malignant tumor in children is rhabdomyosarcoma. Environmental exposures, such as smoking, play a lesser role in causation and, although still poorly understood, genetic abnormalities are a more important causal factor. Treatment of children with rhabdomyosarcoma is determined through collaborative groups such as the Intergroup Rhabdomyosarcoma Study (IRS) or the International Society of Paediatric Oncology (SIOP). In this chapter we will review bladder/prostate rhabdomyosarcoma and also discuss the other rare bladder tumors seen in children.

## RHABDOMYOSARCOMA

### BACKGROUND

Rhabdomyosarcomas (RMS) may develop in any part of the body that contains embryonal mesenchyme, and can occur with or without the presence of concomitant skeletal muscle. It is estimated that rhabdomyosarcoma is the fifth most common solid tumor of childhood in the United States, representing 5% to 15% of all solid malignant tumors in children.[1] RMS accounts for 50% of all soft tissue sarcomas of childhood. The reported annual incidence in the US is 4.4/million Caucasian children and 1.3/million African–American children, with a slight male:female preponderance.[2]

The outcome of children with bladder/prostate RMS has improved significantly over the last few decades. This progress has largely been due to the collaborative trials conducted by the IRS. Presently, evaluation and treatment of children with bladder/prostate RMS is guided by the protocols set forth in IRS-V. Readers are referred to the Children's Oncology Group (COG) website (www.childrensoncologygroup.org) where the complete IRS treatment protocols are available. Access to this site is restricted to members, but nonmembers can access the site through the institutional COG primary investigator.

## ETIOLOGY AND GENETICS

The etiology of RMS is thought to be multifactorial. Both congenital and environmental factors have been identified. A genetic etiology can be inferred because of the association of RMS with neurofibromatosis, and Li–Fraumeni and basal cell nevus (Gorlin) syndromes.[3-5] Families with the Li–Fraumeni syndrome suffer from a variety of malignant diseases, including other sarcomas, breast carcinoma, brain tumors, adrenal carcinoma, and leukemia. This may be due to the association of Li–Fraumeni syndrome with loss of the tumor suppressor gene p53, on the short arm of chromosome 17.[6] Mutations of p53 have been identified in 10% of children with RMS.[7] Neurofibromatosis is a well-recognized disorder; however, basal cell nevus or Gorlin syndrome is less commonly discussed. This disorder is characterized by generalized overgrowth, developmental abnormalities of the skeleton, and a predisposition to both benign and malignant tumors. The syndrome results from germline mutations of the human homolog of the Drosophila segment polarity gene patched (ptc). Abnormal signaling via the ptc gene has also been associated with RMS.[8]

Recently, several important advances in our understanding of the molecular pathogenesis of RMS have been made. Specifically, Sorenson and coworkers reporting for the COG have documented the importance of PAX3-FKHR and PAX7-FKHR gene fusions in patients with alveolar RMS.[9] The authors evaluated the gene fusion status of 171 patients enrolled in IRS-IV, 78 of whom had alveolar histology. They found that these gene fusions are specific for alveolar RMS and that fusion status in these patients appears to be an important prognostic indicator. In patients with metastatic disease, PAX3-FKHR fusion resulted in a significantly higher rate of relapse and death. Patients with PAX3-FKHR fusion also seemed to have a greater predisposition for bone marrow metastasis. The authors speculate that the PAX3-FKHR oncoprotein may confer a survival advantage to tumor cells such as resistance to chemotherapy. Gene fusion evaluation will likely become standard in the evaluation and risk stratification of patients with Alveolar RMS.

Genetic analysis of RMS has identified some common alterations seen in this tumor, including the previously mentioned PAX3/7-FKHR fusion, expression of regulatory factors such as MYOD1 and myogenin, retinoblastoma pathway mutations, and p53 pathway mutations.[10] However, until recently, which individual or combined alterations could cause cell transformation was unknown. Sharp et al have reported that transgenic mice expressing inactivation of the cyclin-dependent kinase inhibitor/alternate reading frame (INK4a/ARF) associated with altered c-MET signaling undergo spontaneous development of rhabdomyosarcoma.[11] Deletions of INK4a/ARF have an effect on both retinoblastoma and p53 pathways which are known to be important in RMS. Hepatocyte growth factor/scatter factor (HGF/SF) is the ligand for the c-MET receptor tyrosine kinase oncogene. Mice with inactivated INK4a/ARF that overexpress HGF/SF were found to almost uniformly develop RMS with high penetrance and short latency. This important discovery begins to unravel the molecular basis for RMS, as well as providing a unique animal model for investigators.

Several environmental factors have been associated with RMS. These include herbicides, marijuana, cocaine, and maternal alcohol ingestion. A maternal history of radiation and prior stillbirth has also been associated with an increased risk.[12,13]

## PATHOLOGY

The most common sites for pelvic RMS are the bladder, prostate, and vagina. Grossly, RMS tends to be nodular,

firm, and well circumscribed, although microscopically it may infiltrate extensively into adjacent tissues. The tumors can present as a nodular mass emanating from the prostate or bladder, often in the area of the trigone. No other specific gross pathologic features are present except in the case of sarcoma botryoides. This subtype primarily arises in hollow organs, typically the vagina or bladder, with protrusion of tissue resembling a cluster of grapes into the viscous cavity. Patients with this type of tumor may present with prolapse of this tissue from the vaginal orifice or urethra.

The original histologic classification of Horne and Enterline included four different pathologic subtypes (Figure 71.1, Table 71.1): embryonal, alveolar, pleomorphic, and undifferentiated.[14] Although the basic system is still used today, pleomorphic tumors are now classified as undifferentiated. This change occurred when it was recognized that these lesions are anaplastic variants of the more common embryonal or alveolar subtypes.[15] Embryonal RMS is the most common subtype found in the bladder. Morphologically, the tumor resembles fetal striated muscle correlating to a gestational age of 7–10 weeks. The composition is mainly that of spindle-shaped cells with a central nucleus in an eosinophilic cytoplasm. Thirty percent of specimens exhibit cross-striation.[16] Sarcoma botryoides represents a subtype of embryonal tumor. As a group, the embryonal type comprises two-thirds of genitourinary RMS and 50% to 60% of all RMS in children.[2]

The alveolar subtype is the second most common, comprising 15% to 20% of RMS. It is most often seen in older children and histologically resembles 10–21 weeks' gestational age striated muscle. Specific histologic features include clusters of small round cells adhering to fibrosepta, giving the appearance of well-defined alveolar spaces. Unlike the embryonal subtype, cross-striations are uncommon. Alveolar RMS is more common in the extremities and trunk than the genitourinary tract.

The third most common histologic subtype of RMS is the undifferentiated subtype. These tumors are often very difficult to classify as they are made up of primitive small round cells and can be confused with Ewing's saroma. However, unlike in Ewing's sarcoma, these cells arise from soft tissue rather than from bone. They can be differentiated from Ewing's sarcoma by identifying expression of specific muscle proteins such as actin, myosin, desmin, and myoD.[17,18] Electron microscopy can identify Z bands associated with actin–myosin bundles and aid in the diagnosis.[19]

Histologic classification correlates strongly with outcome in RMS (Table 71.2). RMS can spread by local infiltration, and by lymphatic and hematogenous routes. Spread to local or regional lymph nodes is found in approximately 20% of patients at diagnosis.[20] Bladder/prostate tumors metastasize most commonly to

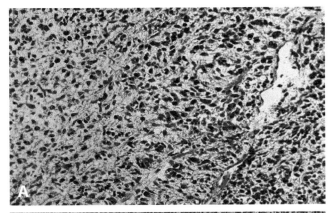

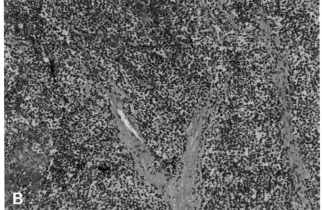

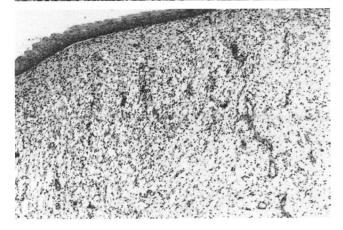

**Fig. 71.1**
Histologic images of common rhabdomyosarcoma variants.
**A** Embryonal. **B** Alveolar. **C** Botryoid. (Images courtesy of Dr
Steve Qualman, Children's Oncology Group, Biopathology
Center, Columbus, OH.)

the lung, marrow, and bone. Omentum is sometimes
involved, whereas metastases to other viscera (e.g. the
liver) are rare, as are metastases to the brain.[21-23]

## SIGNIFICANCE OF RHABDOMYOBLASTS

A current subject of controversy is the significance of
rhabdomyoblasts on post-treatment biopsy. Specifically,
do these represent active disease? Maturation of

**Table 71.1** Histologic classification of genitourinary rhabdomyosarcoma

| Histology | Prevalence (%) | Characteristics |
|---|---|---|
| Embryonal | 60–80 | Spindle ± round cells<br>Loose matrix<br>30% striations |
| Alveolar | 15–20 | Small round cells on fibrous septae<br>Rare striations |
| Pleomorphic | 1 | Varied cell shapes and sizes |
| Undifferentiated | 5–10 | Small round cells<br>Z bands on electron microscopy<br>Immunohistochemistry identification |

**Table 71.2** Outcomes based on histologic classification

| Histology | Prognosis | 5-year survival (%) |
|---|---|---|
| Sarcoma botryoides<br>Spindle cell | Favorable | 90 |
| Embryonal<br>Pleomorphic | Intermediate | 65–75 |
| Alveolar<br>Undifferentiated | Unfavorable | 40–55 |

rhabdomyoblasts after chemotherapy is a phenomenon
observed by various investigators; however, this
knowledge has not translated into a clear understanding
regarding this finding on post-treatment biopsy.[24] Atra
et al reported a group of patients with residual
'rhabdomyoblast' appearing cells that did not go on to
relapse during observation.[25] Subsequently, Heyn et al
reported on 2 of 14 patients that had maturing cells on
post-treatment biopsy that remained in remission.[26]
Analysis of postcystectomy specimens has also
demonstrated rhabdomyoblasts, along with a reduction
in cellularity in patients treated with chemotherapy,
suggesting that this pattern may be indicative of
response to therapy. More recently, Chertin and
coauthors reported the long-term follow-up of a child
with residual atypical cells after treatment with bladder
RMS that has not recurred after 5 years.[27]

Oretega et al followed six patients with post-
treatment biopsy showing mature rhabdomyoblasts.[28]
All six patients remained free of disease after a follow-up
period of 37–237 months. The authors emphasized the
importance of correctly identifying mature cells as those
with a large, smooth, solitary nucleus, no significant
pleomorphism, no mitotic activity, and the absence of
clusters of cells suggestive of growth from a common
precursor.[28]

Based on these reports it appears that a group of
patients will do well without further therapy despite
having rhabdomyoblasts on post-treatment biopsy.
Follow-up of these patients should include serial
imaging, cystoscopy, vaginoscopy, and biopsy if
indicated.

## EVALUATION AND STAGING

Patients with bladder/prostate RMS typically present with obstructive symptoms, including urinary retention, urgency, frequency, and incontinence. Gross or microscopic hematuria results when the tumor breaks through the mucosal layer of the genitourinary tract. Distant metastases occur in approximately 20% of patients at diagnosis, and occasionally patients present with systemic signs of malignancy.[22]

Abdominal ultrasound is usually obtained in children presenting with hematuria or obstructive voiding symptoms (Figure 71.2A). Definitive imaging of the bladder in bladder/prostate RMS requires magnetic resonance imaging (MRI) or computed tomography (CT) scan (Figure 71.2B). In up to 20% of cases, it is not possible to determine whether the site of origin is the bladder or the prostate. Diagnostic imaging needs to be performed in an accurate, reproducible way so that sequential imaging studies can be used to assess the efficacy of primary chemotherapy. Fine cut cross-sectional imaging is performed with and without contrast and accurate tumor measurements are taken along two axes. Regional lymph nodes should be assessed by retroperitoneal thin cut CT (Figure 71.3).

Chest imaging is necessary to exclude pulmonary metastases. Chest CT is indicated if lesions are seen on plain film or if skeletal or marrow evaluations are positive. Some authors argue that every child should undergo chest CT.[19] Imaging of the brain is not required for tumors limited to the genitourinary system. Box 71.1 summarizes the preoperative work-up of bladder/prostate RMS patients.

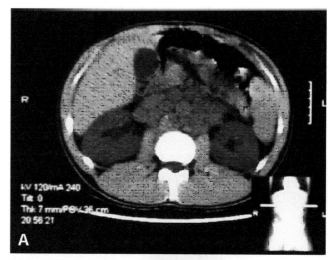

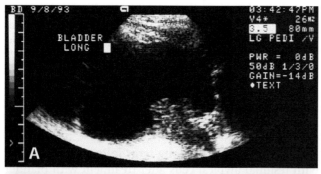

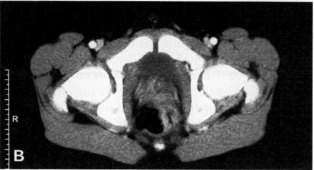

**Fig. 71.2**
**A** Ultrasound image demonstrating a bladder mass in a 12-year-old male confirmed to be rhabdomyosarcoma. **B** CT scan of the same patient confirming the presence of posterior/inferior bladder/prostate rhabdomyosarcoma.

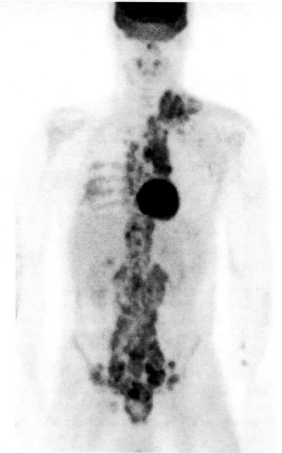

**Fig. 71.3**
**A** Retroperitoneal CT of a 16-year-old male with bladder/prostate rhabdomyosarcoma and bulky retroperitoneal adenopathy. **B** PET scan of the same patient demonstrating retroperitoneal adenopathy.

History and physical, size lesion

Complete blood count (CBC) with differential

Urinalysis

Electrolytes, creatinine (Cr), calcium (Ca), phosphate (PO₄)

Alkaline phosphatase, lactate dehydrogenase (LDH), bilirubin, serum glutamate pyruvate transaminase (SGPT)

MRI/CT of lesion

CT retroperitoneum

Chest x-ray/chest CT

Marrow aspirate ± bone scan

Endoscopic biopsy of the primary lesion may be attempted using a pediatric resectoscope or cold-cup biopsy forceps. Because the loop size of the pediatric resectoscope is small, multiple samples may be needed to make an accurate diagnosis. Cautery artifact can mimic spindle cell appearance to the inexperienced examiner or destroy the sample entirely. Low cutting current should be used when taking a loop biopsy.[29] Biopsy is best performed in conjunction with an onsite pathologist to evaluate frozen specimens and ensure adequate samples are obtained. If endoscopy reveals no mucosal abnormality appropriate for biopsy, or if frozen sections of the endoscopic biopsy are inconclusive, open biopsy should be undertaken if an intra-abdominal mass is present. Percutaneous tru-cut needle biopsy could result in needle tract seeding with tumor. If laparotomy is performed for biopsy, the surgeon should assess the pelvic and retroperitoneal nodes at or below the level of the renal arteries (see Table 71.3 for a complete listing of nodal basins). Follow-up studies to monitor progress of therapy are usually done by CT or MRI.[26]

In the past, two different staging systems have been used for patients with RMS. The IRS group has traditionally used a postsurgical staging system and SIOP has used a pretreatment TNM system. One of the objectives of IRS-V is the evaluation of the pretreatment TNM staging system. These systems are presented in Box 71.2 and Table 71.4. Table 71.5 summarizes the risk groups for treatment assignment.

## PRIOR IRS TRIALS AND UPDATE ON IRS-IV DATA

RMS was first described in 1850 by Wiener.[30] However, little was published on the treatment of RMS until the 1950s. At this time Horne and Enterline published a histologic classification system that is the basis for the system that is in use today.[14,31] As with most solid tumors, surgery was the only available therapy in the early 1900s. Subsequently, it was shown that outcomes were improved by multimodal therapy.[30,32,33] The effectiveness of combination therapy catalyzed the formation of large multicenter trials conducted by the IRS group. The focus of the IRS has been to refine treatment, improve outcomes, and limit morbidity.

### IRS-I

During the first IRS study (IRS-I) (1972–1978), primary anterior exenteration was the most common surgical procedure performed for patients with bladder/prostate tumors.[34,35] Patients that received up-front surgery followed by chemotherapy, with or without radiotherapy, had relatively favorable outcomes (78% overall survival). During the final years of this study, children began receiving a trial of primary chemotherapy directed towards the goal of bladder preservation. In IRS-I the bladder preservation rate at 3

**Table 71.3** Nodal basins for genitourinary rhabdomyosarcoma

| Site of primary | Regional nodal basin |
|---|---|
| Bladder/prostate | Pelvic + retroperitoneal nodes at or below level of renal arteries |
| Uterus/cervix | Pelvic + retroperitoneal nodes at or below level of renal arteries |
| Paratesticular | Pelvic + retroperitoneal lymph nodes at or below level of renal arteries |
| Vagina | Inguinal, retroperitoneal + pelvic nodes at or below common iliacs |
| Vulva | Inguinal nodes |
| Retroperitoneum/pelvis | Pelvic and retroperitoneal nodes |
| Perianal/perineal | Inguinal and pelvic nodes, may cross midline |

**Box 71.2** IRS grouping classification system for rhabdomyosarcoma

1. Group I
   - Localized disease, complete resection:
     a. confined to muscle/organ of origin
     b. beyond muscle/organ of origin
2. Group II
   - Regional disease, grossly resected:
     a. node negative but microscopic residual
     b. node positive, no residual
     c. node positive with microscopic residual ± node most distal to primary found with disease
3. Group III
   - Gross residual disease:
     a. after biopsy
     b. after attempted resection
4. Group IV
   - Distant disease

**Table 71.4** Revised pretreatment TNM classification

| Stage | Site | T | Size | N | M |
|-------|------|---|------|---|---|
| I | Orbit, head/neck, genitourinary (other than bladder/prostate) | T1 or T2 | A or B | N0 or NX | M0 |
| II | Bladder, prostate<br>Extremity<br>Intracranial<br>Trunk<br>Intrathoracic<br>Retroperitoneal<br>Biliary<br>Perineal | T1 or T2 | A | N0 or NX | M0 |
| III | Same as Stage II | T1 or T2 | A or B | N1 Any N | M0M0 |
| IV | Any | T1 or T2 | A or B | Any N | M1 |

**Table 71.5** IRS-V risk stratified treatment system

| Risk protocol | Stage | Group | Site | Size | Age (years) | Histology | Metastasis | Nodes | Treatment |
|---------------|-------|-------|------|------|-------------|-----------|------------|-------|-----------|
| Low, subgroup A (D9602) | 1 | I | Favorable | A or B | <21 | EMB | M0 | N0 | VA |
| | 1 | II | Favorable | A or B | <21 | EMB | M0 | N0 | VA + XRT |
| | 1 | III | Orbit only | A or B | <21 | EMB | M0 | N0 | VA + XRT |
| | 2 | I | Unfavorable | A | <21 | EMB | M0 | N0 or NX | VA |
| Low, subgroup B (D9602) | 1 | II | Favorable | A or B | <21 | EMB | M0 | N1 | VAC + XRT |
| | 1 | III | Orbit only | A or B | <21 | EMB | M0 | N1 | VAC + XRT |
| | 1 | III | Favorable (excluding orbit) | A or B | <21 | EMB | M0 | N0 or N1 or NX | VAC + XRT |
| | 2 | II | Unfavorable | A | <21 | EMB | M0 | N0 or NX | VAC + XRT |
| | 3 | I or II | Unfavorable | A | <21 | EMB | M0 | N1 | VAC (+ XRT, Gp II) |
| | 3 | I or II | Unfavorable | B | <21 | EMB | M0 | N0 or N1 or NX | VAC (+ XRT, Gp II) |
| Intermediate (D9803) | 2 | III | Unfavorable | A | <21 | EMB | M0 | N0 or NX | VAC ± Topo + XRT |
| | 3 | III | Unfavorable | A | <21 | EMB | M0 | N1 | VAC ± Topo + XRT |
| | 3 | III | Unfavorable | A | <21 | EMB | M0 | N0 or N1 or NX | VAC ± Topo + XRT |
| | 1, 2, or 3 | I, II or III | Favorable or unfavorable | A or B | <21 | ALV/UDS | M0 | N0 or N1 or NX | VAC ± Topo + XRT |
| | 4 | I, II, III, or IV | Favorable or unfavorable | A or B | <10 | EMB | M1 | N0 or N1 | VAC ± Topo + XRT |
| High (D9802) | 4 | IV | Favorable or unfavorable | A or B | ≥10 | EMB | M1 | N0 or N1 | CPT11, VAC + XRT |
| | 4 | IV | Favorable or unfavorable | A or B | <21 | ALV/UDS | M1 | N0 or N1 | CPT11, VAC + XRT |

ALV/UDS, alveolar/undifferentiated sarcoma; CPT11, irinotecan; EMB, embryonal; Topo, topotecan; VA, vincristine/actinomycin; VAC, vincristine/actinomycin/cyclophosphamide; XRT, radiation therapy.

years was about 23%.[36] Hence, survival was often attained at the cost of radical exenterative procedures that were associated with substantial complications.[37,38]

IRS-I also demonstrated that lymph node dissection and adjuvant therapy benefited patients with bladder/prostate RMS and positive lymph nodes.[39,40]

## IRS-II

IRS-II (1979–1984) established the routine use of chemotherapy and/or radiotherapy prior to surgery. It was hoped that primary chemotherapy would lessen the number of patients requiring exenterative surgery.[41]

About 10% of patients achieved relapse-free survival with chemotherapy alone. Overall survival was reported at approximately 80%, not significantly improved over IRS-I. Disappointingly, the rate of survival with an intact 'functional' bladder was 25%.[41,42] Similarly, a contemporaneous study by SIOP resulted in 30% survival with an intact bladder.

## IRS-III

IRS-III (1985–1992) achieved significant improvements in bladder/prostate RMS patient outcomes. Chemotherapy was standardized to include doxorubicin, cisplatin, and etoposide. Additionally, the timing of radiotherapy was fixed at 6 weeks after induction therapy. The use of primary or delayed partial cystectomy with the goal of bladder preservation was emphasized. Overall survival was approximately 83%.[42] The proportion of patients that retained bladder function at 4 years rose to 60%. However, detailed or formal assessment of bladder functionality was not performed (see below).[43,44] Data from IRS-III suggested that bladder complications occurred more frequently in radiated patients.[44]

In summary, IRS-III showed that conservative surgery after primary chemotherapy, with or without radiation therapy (XRT), could produce excellent disease-free survival and reduce morbidity.

## IRS-IV

The bladder function outcomes of 88 bladder/prostate RMS patients treated during IRS-IV (1993–1997) have recently been reported by Arndt et al.[45] Seventy percent of these tumors were identified as arising from the bladder. Event-free survival at a mean of 6.1 years' follow-up was 77%, with an overall 6-year survival of 82%. Seventy-four patients had XRT for local tumor control, and 55 patients retained bladders without relapse. Of the entire group only 36 (40%) have 'normal' bladder function. It is important to note that 'normal' was defined by responses to a nonvalidated questionnaire, raising the possibility that the true extent of bladder dysfunction is underestimated.

Survival for patients with bladder/prostate RMS enrolled in IRS-IV was 81%.[46] IRS-IV was the first study to evaluate the use of a TNM pretreatment staging system. Additionally, IRS-IV data concluded that hyperfractionated radiation did not provide an outcome advantage over standard conformal XRT.[47]

# CURRENT TREATMENT, IRS-V

The current protocol, IRS-V, is designed to treat patients based on stratification into low-, intermediate-, and high-risk protocols. The low-risk protocols are similar to those of previous IRS studies but new protocols are in place for intermediate- and high-risk patients.

## SURGICAL MANAGEMENT

Initial treatment of patients with bladder/prostate RMS may involve management of urethral or ureteral obstruction. Bladder outlet obstruction is initially managed by urethral catheterization. Suprapubic drainage is contraindicated because of the potential for tract seeding. If ureteral obstruction is present, internal stent placement avoids the discomfort of percutaneous

nephrostomy (PCN); however, tumor mass or distortion of the trigone may necessitate PCN. It is important to relieve obstruction promptly to optimize renal function during chemotherapy.

Bladder preservation is a principal goal of therapy. The initial operation is usually an endoscopic or open biopsy for diagnosis. If a bladder tumor can be completely resected with partial cystectomy, and preservation of bladder and urethral function assured, it may be removed at the initial operation. Performance of ureteral reimplantation or bladder augmentation may be required in conjunction with a partial resection of the bladder. The latter procedures are typically performed when partial cystectomy is performed after cytoreductive chemotherapy. Radical exenteration should not be carried out as a primary operation for bladder/prostate tumors. Response of prostatic tumors to chemotherapy may allow prostatectomy to be performed with complete gross and/or microscopic tumor removal and preservation of the urethra and bladder.

## RISK BASED TREATMENT

Molecular information is used to stratify treatment by risk groups for many pediatric cancers. The risk categorization schema for RMS, however, is based on clinical staging information. A brief overview of risk-based adjuvant therapy follows. Readers are referred to the IRS-V protocols for a detailed description of chemotherapy and radiation therapy regimens for low-, intermediate- and high-risk groups.

## LOW-RISK GROUP (D9602)

Patients with embryonal or botryoid tumors are assigned to the low-risk category if the tumor is:

- ≤5 cm in diameter and completely resected
- ≤5 cm and completely resected and there is microscopic residual disease and negative lymph nodes; or ≤5 cm or >5 cm, completely resected or microscopic disease, regardless of nodal status.

Chemotherapy for patients in low-risk group A (tumor ≤5 cm, complete resection, clinically nodes negative) includes dactinomycin (AMD) and vincristine (VCR) for 3 weeks. Patients with nonalveolar, nonundifferentiated sarcoma histology will continue on AMD and VCR for a total of 45 weeks. Patients in low-risk group B (tumor ≤5 cm, microscopic residual disease; or tumor ≤5 cm, positive nodes or tumor >5 cm regardless of nodal status if complete resection/ microscopic disease) will receive VCR, AMD and cyclophosphamide (VAC). Patients with no residual tumor (clinical group I) will not receive XRT. Patients with microscopic residual tumor (clinical group II, N0) will receive 36 Gy of XRT.

## INTERMEDIATE-RISK GROUP (D9803)

The intermediate-risk group comprises patients with nonmetastatic alveolar RMS or undifferentiated sarcoma in clinical groups I–III and those with embryonal tumors in clinical group III. Patients less than 10 years of age who are clinical group IV/embryonal histology are also included in this group.

In the intermediate-risk group, the likelihood of bladder preservation decreases to 25% to 45% of cases based on IRS-II and IRS-III data. Complete resection at the initial procedure is often impossible. As with low-risk group patients, radical resection procedures (e.g. pelvic exenteration) should be delayed if response to therapy is observed. The number of second look and exenterative procedures is greater in this group. Chemotherapy in this group is stratified between those receiving VAC versus VAC alternating with topotecan. Topotecan is a topoisomerase inhibitor which has displayed substantial activity against RMS in xenograft models and human studies.[48,49] XRT is typically started at week 12, usually 2 weeks after second-look surgery.

### Second-look surgery or delayed primary resections

Patients undergoing chemotherapy should be assessed for feasibility of complete resection of the primary tumor at week 12. Patients that achieve complete clinical response (CR) or partial response (PR) status, and selected nonresponders (NR)/stable disease (SD) patients, are candidates for second-look surgery. Second-look surgery is performed to confirm clinical response, evaluate pathologic response to therapy, and to remove residual tumor, if possible. For patients with a CR, biopsy at the site of the original mass to confirm the radiologic findings is performed. Patients with proven residual tumor after completion of all therapy, or in those with early progression of disease after therapy has been initiated, should be considered for complete cystoprostatectomy.

## HIGH-RISK GROUP (D9802)

The high-risk group includes children with metastatic disease who are more than 10 years of age with embryonal RMS and all children with metastatic alveolar or undifferentiated histology. In this grouping, the initial procedure is biopsy only. Complete resection of the primary tumor is rarely indicated and should be deferred for 3–6 months when metastatic disease is controlled. Bladder-sparing surgery may be feasible if chemotherapy and/or XRT have caused shrinkage of larger, previously unresectable tumors. Radical exenteration is reserved for children with persistent local tumor and no metastatic disease after treatment.

Patients with disseminated disease in IRS-V will receive a relatively new agent, irinotecan (CPT11), in combination with VAC. Irinotecan has shown significant activity in in vitro studies and in animal xenografts of RMS.[50-52] As irinotecan is believed to work synergistically with VCR, these agents have been combined in an upfront window in IRS-V.[53]

## OUTCOMES

Overall, survival for patients treated for bladder/prostate RMS has increased steadily from 30% to approximately 80% over the course of the IRS studies.[42] Most recently, Arndt and coworkers looked at the IRS-IV data and found a 77% event-free survival at 6 years.[45] This has largely been due to improvement of therapeutic agents. At this point in time, many of the goals of current therapy involve reduction of comorbidity. However, many questions remain regarding the efficacy of therapy.

### HAVE BLADDER PRESERVATION STRATEGIES BEEN PROVEN TO BE EFFECTIVE?

Prior studies have shown that bladder salvage is possible in approximately 60% of patients after primary chemotherapy.[38,44,54] However, the recent report by Arndt and coworkers calls into question the function of these preserved bladders. Retaining the bladder should not be the only goal. Another major objective of pediatric cancer trials should be documenting the function of preserved bladders in children treated for RMS.[25]

To date only one study has used the 'gold standard'—urodynamic evaluation—to investigate bladder function in children treated for pelvic RMS. Yeung et al evaluated 11 children with pelvic RMS, of whom 7 had involvement of the bladder or prostate.[55] After mean follow-up of 6.6 years, only 4 of the 11 children had a normal voiding pattern. These four children had not received pelvic XRT. All 7 of the children that were irradiated had nocturnal enuresis, continuous dribbling, an abnormal bladder capacity, and/or an abnormal voiding pattern. In addition, four of the children displayed evidence of hydronephrosis, two of whom required reconstructive surgery.

In four children, urodynamic studies were completed. All four cases displayed a reduced functional bladder capacity. None of the children displayed detrusor instability and peak uroflow rates were normal (14–27 ml/second). Only one child had decreased bladder compliance. The observation that the most significant bladder impairment was a reduced functional capacity is surprising, as one would expect that reduced compliance would be found if radiation-induced fibrosis alone was the culprit.

The remainder of the published literature regarding bladder outcomes in children treated for RMS consists of anecdotal reports. No objective studies, upper tract imaging, or even standardized questionnaires have been regularly used. In a report from the IRS, Hays and coworkers reviewed the outcomes of 40 patients treated for primary bladder RMS. Partial cystectomy was performed in 33 of the 40 patients.[44] The extent of partial cystectomy ranged from 15% to 80% of the bladder mucosal surface. All 40 patients received chemotherapy and many received cyclophosphamide in conjunction with XRT. Information regarding bladder function was obtained by patient survey. Only 1 of 11 survivors treated without radiation therapy had urinary symptoms. Nine of the 19 irradiated patients had symptoms suggesting a small or contracted bladder. Several patients reported urinary incontinence and some were documented to have vesicoureteral reflux. Further analysis of this group suggested that patients receiving greater than 40 Gy radiation had a higher incidence of bladder symptoms. All three patients receiving greater than 50 Gy had bladder complications.

El-Sherbiny and coworkers reported on the outcome of 30 children treated for pelvic RMS with the intent of bladder preservation. They noted that bladder function had been preserved in 11 of the 12 patients that underwent partial cystectomy. The authors explain that bladder function was assessed on the basis of an interview with the children's parents, urographic studies, and post-void residuals. No specific details as to the nature of the questionnaire or the radiographic findings were documented, and urodynamics were not used.[56]

Silvan and coworkers reported on bladder function in a group of 10 children treated for RMS.[54] All but one child received 40 Gy of radiation. Of the 10 children, 8 are alive with functioning bladders after a period of observation ranging from 5.7 to 18.4 years. Hemorrhagic cystitis was the most significant complication but children treated early on did not receive Mesna. No specific analysis of bladder function or continence was documented in this study.[57] Heij et al published their results of treating children with pelvic RMS. These authors emphasize treatment with chemotherapy and conservative surgery, reserving radiotherapy only for tumor recurrence.[58] In their review of 25 patients, radiotherapy was given to only eight patients. All nonirradiated patients are reported to have done well. The authors concluded that primary chemotherapy, followed by limited surgical resection (with the use of radiotherapy in patients that relapse) can provide long-term successful bladder preservation.

While the IRS-IV data suggest that significant impairment of bladder function may exist after treatment of bladder RMS, only one study has reported urodynamic data on bladder function in a limited number of children. An association of dysfunction with total radiation dose has been suggested, but this remains unproven. Future studies should focus on careful evaluation of bladder function in patients with pelvic disease. Other complications that can ensue in patients treated for RMS include nephrotoxicity,[44] cardiotoxicity, sexual dysfunction, and infertility.

## TIMING AND NECESSITY OF RADIATION THERAPY?

Radiation therapy is a standard component of current IRS protocols for all patients with bladder/prostate RMS except those with stage I disease (low-risk group A). Some authors have questioned the need for radiotherapy prior to surgery.[58,59] They have suggested that chemotherapy followed by complete surgical resection with negative margins will achieve satisfactory local tumor control, obviating the need for XRT. In addition, many surgeons believe that XRT makes extirpative surgery and reconstruction more difficult and increases complications. This is in addition to its known general morbidity such as growth retardation, organ malformation, secondary malignancy, etc.

Merguerian et al advocated for delayed radiotherapy based on their experience in a group of children with lower urinary tract sarcoma.[59] The authors presented 13 patients with bladder/prostate RMS. IRS risk groups were III in 10 and IV in 3. The authors used a protocol that included chemotherapy, followed by surgery. Radiotherapy was reserved only for patients with residual or metastatic disease. Using this schema they reported a survival rate of 80% among their group III patients; 6 of 10 did not receive radiation, one of whom had positive margins. The majority of these patients had prostate lesions, and many underwent prostatectomy, urethrectomy and partial cystectomy. Despite favorable outcomes, the limited number of patients in this single center experience mandate cautious interpretation of these conclusions.

In contrast to the above report is the recently reported combined experience of SIOP and the Italian Cooperative Group (ICG). They presented preliminary data comparing patients that did and did not receive XRT. In total, 54 of 105 patients did not receive XRT as part of their initial therapy. It was observed that patients that did not receive XRT had a poorer 5-year event-free survival (64%) when compared to those that had XRT (79%), p=0.02. No difference was noted in the overall 5-year survival statistics.[60] This finding is also supported by limited data from IRS-IV data. In IRS-IV, 14 of 62 (22%) patients that received XRT went on to have tumor recurrence as compared to 3 of 9 (33%) patients that did not receive XRT.[61] Finally, the German cooperative studies (CWS81) found that hyperfractionated radiotherapy begun earlier resulted in a lower relapse rate than chemotherapy alone.[62]

In summary, available data support the recommendation for XRT in patients with bladder/prostate RMS.

## EARLY VERSUS DELAYED SURGICAL RECONSTRUCTION?

Despite advances in therapy, select patients will require total or near total cystectomy as a component of their treatment. The question for these patients is: When and how should they be reconstructed?

Duel et al reported their experience with initial urinary diversion followed by delayed continent reconstruction for patients achieving long-term cure.[63] The authors favored formation of nonrefluxing transverse or sigmoid colon conduits in order to avoid irradiated bowel segments. Later, these segments can be incorporated in continent catheterizable reconstructions. Others have advocated for combining continent reconstruction at the time of extirpative surgery. Lander et al described the use of Le Bag continent reconstructions in three children, one of whom was 26 months of age. Despite initially negative frozen section analysis, permanent sections revealed residual viable tumor requiring local radiation and chemotherapy.[64] Similarly, Merguerian et al performed reconstruction at the time of cystectomy. They noted that a frozen section is an unreliable predictor of residual disease. Several of their patients had residual disease requiring adjuvant therapy or reoperation.[59] In light of the latter observation, the wisdom of proceeding with a continent reconstruction before confirming adequacy of local control should be questioned. Hensle and Chang reported on success with early reconstruction but suggested that timing of reconstruction should be considered on an individual basis, and that early reconstruction should only be performed if it is certain that no further local therapy will be required.[65]

While early reconstruction is feasible, it needs to be judiciously applied. In addition to the aforementioned issues, the extent of bowel damage from irradiation may not be apparent at the initial surgery. Finally, delayed reconstruction allows assurance that a durable cure has been attained and that the patient is mature enough to implement self-catheterization.[65]

## FUTURE DIRECTIONS

Evaluation for gene fusion resulting in production of PAX3-FKHR oncoprotein will likely become standard in risk stratification of patients with RMS. This will allow molecular staging to factor into the risk-based stratification of treatment.

Other broadly applied anticancer strategies are being evaluated in RMS. For example, anti-vascular endothelial growth factor (VEGF) antibodies have been shown to have a dramatic effect on RMS growth in animal models.[66] The role of VEGF and other proangiogenic molecules, such as basic fibroblast growth factor (bFGF) and interleukin 8 (IL8), are currently being explored.[67]

Currently, under the auspices of COG, antisense therapy directed at the antiapoptotic, proto-oncogene BCL2, in conjunction with chemotherapy, is being tried for children with relapsed solid tumors. As our understanding of the molecular events involved in RMS progresses, we will hopefully see progress in this poorly understood malignancy.

## TRANSITIONAL CELL CARCINOMA IN CHILDREN

Transitional cell carcinoma (TCC) of the bladder is an extremely uncommon lesion in children. It is particularly rare in the first decade of life. In a review of TCC, Javadpor and Mostofi found 40 lesions amongst 10,000 patients under the age of 20.[68] Only one of these occurred before 10 years of age. In a more recent review of the literature, Serrano-Durba et al noted five cases occurring in children under the age of 10 years out of a total of 13 cases.[69] Prior series have shown that the tumor occurs predominantly in males with a ratio of 9:1 or higher. Occasionally, these tumors may be associated with cyclophosphamide treatment.[70]

The most common presenting symptom is painless gross hematuria. Irritative voiding symptoms, recurrent urinary tract infections, and microscopic hematuria have also been reported.[71] Diagnosis of this lesion has most commonly been made using ultrasonography. In some series, ultrasound has been purported to be 100% sensitive for this diagnosis.[69,71] Intravenous pyelography has no role in the diagnosis of this tumor nowadays, and the resolution of CT scanning may not be adequate. Definitive diagnosis is made by cystoscopy and biopsy which simultaneously will allow for treatment. Approximately 90% of cases are isolated lesions but rare multifocal lesions have been reported.[69,71-73] Pathologic analysis typically reveals grade 1 lesions in 80% of cases. A much smaller percentage of cases are classified as grade 1-2; lesions invading through the lamina propria are rare.[71,74,75] Due to the low grade, intravesical therapy is not indicated, and transurethral resection or fulguration is the treatment of choice. Recurrence is uncommon, with published rates of approximately 2% to 5%. Despite the low recurrence rate, periodic surveillance of these children is recommended throughout childhood.

Surveillance after the occurrence of TCC in a child is not standardized. Because of the low grade of lesions, cytology has a limited role. Therefore, microscopic urinalysis looking for hematuria and periodic bladder sonography are the mainstays. Serrano-Durba and coworkers have proposed urinalysis every 3 months, followed by sonography and cytology every 6 months.

Unlike adults, cystoscopy in children requires anesthesia so surveillance cystoscopy has been considered necessary only in cases where the previous studies are positive. However, the rare child with a high-grade tumor clearly should have regular endoscopic evaluation.

## OTHER RARE LESIONS

### MALIGNANT LESIONS

Urachal adenocarcinoma is a lesion usually seen in adults but has been reported in children.[76,77] Patients typically present with hematuria. The tumor arises from the urachus and invades into the bladder. Its location in the dome of a hollow viscus results in advanced disease at presentation. Treatment consists of primary surgery, and prognosis is generally poor in advanced cases. No standardized adjuvant therapy protocols currently exist.[76,77]

Adenocarcinoma has been reported in patients with a history of bladder exstrophy. These lesions occur mostly in patients that have not had modern reconstruction of their bladder or those undergoing ureterosigmoidostomy. In patients with ureterosigmoidostomy, the incidence of cancer is high and related to the duration of follow-up.[78] No standard surveillance is currently recommended for patients undergoing modern-staged or one-stage reconstruction of exstrophy. Patients with ureterosigmoidostomy should undergo routine surveillance endoscopy.[79–81]

Leiomyosarcoma is a rare malignant lesion of the bladder in children.[82] Tumor size and pathologic appearance impact on prognosis. Treatment consists primarily of local excision.[83,84]

### NONMALIGNANT LESIONS

Inflammatory myofibroblastic tumor (pseudotumor of the bladder) is a benign lesion that can mimic rhabdomyosarcoma. Presenting symptoms are similar for both and, radiologically, the lesions may be indistinguishable (Figure 71.4). The tumors consist of a spindle cell proliferation with myofibroblastic differentiation in a collagen stroma with inflammatory infiltrates (Figure 71.5). The lesion is differentiated from malignant spindle cell lesions such as leiomyosarcoma by the absence of atypical mitosis, cytologic atypia, tumor necrosis, and lack of necrosis at the tumor margin.[85] Chromosome 2p23 rearrangements involving the ALK gene have been recently detected in these tumors.[86]

Although nonmetastatic, these lesions have the potential to be locally aggressive and can recur despite

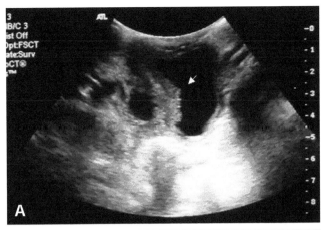

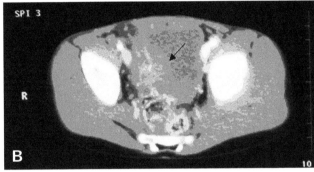

**Fig. 71.4**
**A** Ultrasound image of an inflammatory myofibroblastic tumor (IMT) projecting into the lumen of the bladder. **B** CT scan of the same patient depicting IMT and associated mucosal abnormality in the bladder. Radiographic diagnosis was rhabdomyosarcoma.

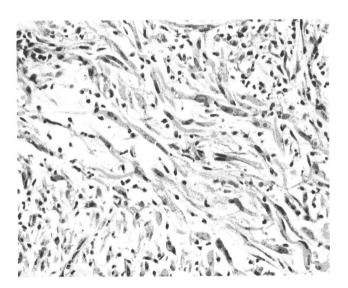

**Fig. 71.5**
Hematoxylin and eosin section of inflammatory myofibroblastic tumor of the bladder in a 4-year-old male.

perceived adequate resection.[87] While extirpative surgery remains the mainstay of treatment, recently there has been substantial interest and apparent success with the use of cyclooxygenase 2 inhibitors to reduce tumor burden prior to surgery.[88] The risk of recurrence mandates that periodic long-term surveillance be performed.

Hemangiomas of the bladder can also be confused for malignant lesions. These lesions are extremely rare and can present with hematuria or obstructive symptoms. Radiographically, they can easily be confused with RMS of the bladder (Figure 71.6). Treatment consists of local resection only, which can often be accomplished by partial cystectomy.[89] In some cases, once the diagnosis is confirmed, laser ablation can be successfully performed (Fig. 71.7).

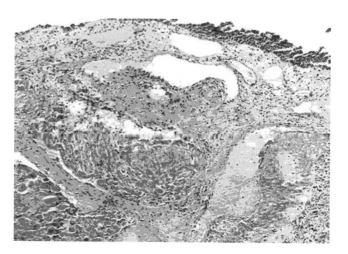

**Fig. 71.7**
Unremarkable urothelium with underlying prominent and dilated blood vessels containing organizing and organized thrombi, consistent with arteriovenous malformation (hematoxylin and eosin stain, 20×). (Image courtesy of Dr Fabiola S Balarezo.)

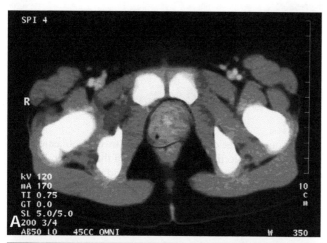

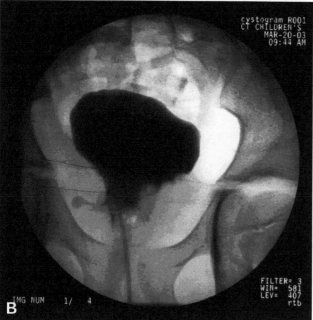

**Fig. 71.6**
A CT scan of a young female with a large hemangioma of the bladder neck. B Voiding cystourethrogram of the same patient.

Nephrogenic adenomas of the bladder are an uncommon cause of irritative symptoms, hematuria and an associated bladder mass.[90] Typically, these tumors resemble papillary lesions and are associated with prior surgery or inflammation.[91] Once the pathologic diagnosis is confirmed by the presence of tubular structures within the lamina propria, treatment is possible by endoscopic fulguration and antimicrobials.[91]

## REFERENCES

1. Young JL Jr, Miller RW. Incidence of malignant tumors in U.S. children. J Pediatr 1975;86(2):254–258.
2. Maurer HM, Moon T, Donaldson M, et al. The intergroup rhabdomyosarcoma study: a preliminary report. Cancer 1977;40(5):2015–2026.
3. Li FP, Fraumeni JF Jr, Mulvihill JJ, et al. A cancer family syndrome in twenty-four kindreds. Cancer Res 1988;48(18):5358–5362.
4. Pappo AS, Shapiro DN, Crist WM. Rhabdomyosarcoma. Biology and treatment. Pediatr Clin North Am 1997;44(4):953–972.
5. Hartley AL, Birch JM, Blair V, et al. Patterns of cancer in the families of children with soft tissue sarcoma. Cancer 1993;72(3):923–930.
6. Malkin D, Li FP, Strong LC, et al. Germ line p53 mutations in a familial syndrome of breast cancer, sarcomas, and other neoplasms. Science 1990;250(4985):1233–1238.
7. Diller L, Sexsmith E, Gottlieb A, Li FP, Malkin D. Germline p53 mutations are frequently detected in young children with rhabdomyosarcoma. J Clin Invest 1995;95(4):1606–1611.
8. Hahn HW, Wojnowski L, Zimmer AM, Hall J, Miller G, Zimmer A. Rhabdomyosarcomas and radiation hypersensitivity in a mouse model of Gorlin syndrome. Nat Med 1998;4:619–622.
9. Sorensen PH, Lynch JC, Qualman SJ, et al. PAX3-FKHR and PAX7-FKHR gene fusions are prognostic indicators in alveolar rhabdomyosarcoma: a report from the children's oncology group. J Clin Oncol 2002;20(11):2672–2679.
10. Cavenee WK. Muscling in on rhabdomyosarcoma. Nat Med 2002;8(11):1200–1201.
11. Sharp R, Recio JA, Jhappan C, et al. Synergism between INK4a/ARF inactivation and aberrant HGF/SF signaling in rhabdomyosarcomagenesis. Nat Med 2002;8(11):1276–1280.

12. Grufferman S, Schwartz AG, Ruymann FB, Maurer HM. Parents' use of cocaine and marijuana and increased risk of rhabdomyosarcoma in their children. Cancer Causes Control 1993;4(3):217–224.

13. Hartley AL, Birch JM, Blair V, et al. Foetal loss and infant deaths in families of children with soft-tissue sarcoma. Int J Cancer 1994;56(5):646–649.

14. Horne R, Enterline W. Rhabdomyosarcoma: a clinical–pathological study and classification of 39 cases. Cancer 1958;11:181.

15. Kodet R, Newton WA Jr, Hamoudi AB, et al. Childhood rhabdomyosarcoma with anaplastic (pleomorphic) features. A report of the Intergroup Rhabdomyosarcoma Study. Am J Surg Pathol 1993;17(5):443–453.

16. Tsokos M, Webber BL, Parham DM, et al. Rhabdomyosarcoma. A new classification scheme related to prognosis. Arch Pathol Lab Med 1992;116(8):847–855.

17. Dodd S, Malone M, McCulloch W. Rhabdomyosarcoma in children: a histological and immunohistochemical study of 59 cases. J Pathol 1989;158(1):13–18.

18. Parham DM, Webber B, Holt H, et al. Immunohistochemical study of childhood rhabdomyosarcomas and related neoplasms. Results of an Intergroup Rhabdomyosarcoma study project. Cancer 1991;67(12):3072–3080.

19. Wilcox DT. Rhabdomyosarcoma. In Gearhart JP, Rink RC, Mouriquand PDE (eds): Pediatric Urology. Philadelphia: WB Saunders, 2001, pp 885–895.

20. Lawrence W Jr, Hays DM, Heyn R, et al. Lymphatic metastases with childhood rhabdomyosarcoma. A report from the Intergroup Rhabdomyosarcoma Study. Cancer 1987;60(4):910–915.

21. Wexler L, Helman L. Rhabdomyosarcoma and the undifferentiated sarcomas. In Pizzo P, Poplack D (eds): Principles and Practice of Pediatric Oncology. Philadelphia: Lippincott-Raven, 1997, pp 799–829.

22. Raney RB Jr, Tefft M, Maurer HM, et al. Disease patterns and survival rate in children with metastatic soft-tissue sarcoma. A report from the Intergroup Rhabdomyosarcoma Study (IRS)-I. Cancer 1988;62(7):1257–1266.

23. Ruymann FB, Newton WA, Ragab AH, et al. Bone marrow metastases at diagnosis in children and adolescents with rhabdomyosarcoma. A report from the Intergroup Rhabdomyosarcoma Study. Cancer 1984;53(2):368–373.

24. Molenaar WM, Oosterhuis JW, Kamps WA. Cytologic 'differentiation' in childhood rhabdomyosarcomas following polychemotherapy. Hum Pathol 1984;15(10):973–979.

25. Atra A, Ward HC, Aitken K, et al. Conservative surgery in multimodal therapy for pelvic rhabdomyosarcoma in children. Br J Cancer 1994;70(5):1004–1008.

26. Heyn R, Newton WA, Raney B, et al. Preservation of the bladder in patients with rhabdomyosarcoma. J Clin Oncol 1997;15(1):69–75.

27. Chertin B, Reinus C, Koulikov D, Rosenmann E, Farkas A, Chertin B. Post-chemotherapy microscopic residual prostate rhabdomyosarcoma: long-term conservative follow-up. Pediatr Surg Int 2002;18(1):68–69.

28. Ortega JA, Rowland J, Monforte H, et al. Presence of well-differentiated rhabdomyoblasts at the end of therapy for pelvic rhabdomyosarcoma: implications for the outcome. J Pediatr Hematol Oncol 2000;22(2):106–111.

29. Snyder HM, D'Angio GL, Evans AE, Raney RB. Pediatric oncology. In Walsh PC, Retik AB, Vaughan EAJW (eds): Campbell's Urology, 7th ed. Philadelphia: WB Saunders, 1998, pp 2210–2256.

30. Wiener E. Rhabdomyosarcoma. In O'Neil JA et al (eds): Pediatric Surgery, 5th ed. St Louis: Mosby, 1998, pp 431–445.

31. Pack G, Eberhart W. Rhabdomyosarcoma of the skeletal muscle: report of a 100 cases. Surgery 1952;32:1032.

32. Stobbe GDH. Embryonal rhabdomyosarcoma of the head and neck in children and adolescents. Cancer 1950;3:826.

33. Pinkel D, Pickren J. Rhabdomyosarcoma in children. JAMA 1961;175:293–298.

34. Raney B Jr, Heyn R, Hays DM, et al. Sequelae of treatment in 109 patients followed for 5 to 15 years after diagnosis of sarcoma of the bladder and prostate. A report from the Intergroup Rhabdomyosarcoma Study Committee. Cancer 1993;71(7):2387–2394.

35. Johnson DG. Trends in surgery for childhood rhabdomyosarcoma. Cancer 1975;35(Suppl 3):916–920.

36. Raney RB Jr, Gehan EA, Hays DM, et al. Primary chemotherapy with or without radiation therapy and/or surgery for children with localized sarcoma of the bladder, prostate, vagina, uterus, and cervix. A comparison of the results in Intergroup Rhabdomyosarcoma Studies I and II. Cancer 1990;66(10):2072–2081.

37. Michalkiewicz EL, Rao BN, Gross E, et al. Complications of pelvic exenteration in children who have genitourinary rhabdomyosarcoma. J Pediatr Surg 1997;32(9):1277–1282.

38. Hays DM. Bladder/prostate rhabdomyosarcoma: results of the multi-institutional trials of the Intergroup Rhabdomyosarcoma Study. Semin Surg Oncol 1993;9(6):520–523.

39. Lawrence W Jr, Hays DM, Moon TE. Lymphatic metastasis with childhood rhabdomyosarcoma. Cancer 1977;39(2):556–559.

40. Tefft M, Hays D, Raney RB Jr, et al. Radiation to regional nodes for rhabdomyosarcoma of the genitourinary tract in children: is it necessary? A report from the Intergroup Rhabdomyosarcoma Study No. I (IRS-I). Cancer 1980;45(12):3065–3068.

41. Maurer HM, Gehan EA, Beltangady M, et al. The Intergroup Rhabdomyosarcoma Study-II. Cancer 1993;71(5):1904–1922.

42. Crist W, Gehan EA, Ragab AH, et al. The Third Intergroup Rhabdomyosarcoma Study. J Clin Oncol 1995;13(3):610–630.

43. Lobe TE, Wiener E, Andrassy RJ, et al. The argument for conservative, delayed surgery in the management of prostatic rhabdomyosarcoma. J Pediatr Surg 1996;31(8):1084–1087.

44. Hays DM, Raney RB, Wharam MD, et al. Children with vesical rhabdomyosarcoma (RMS) treated by partial cystectomy with neoadjuvant or adjuvant chemotherapy, with or without radiotherapy. A report from the Intergroup Rhabdomyosarcoma Study (IRS) Committee. J Pediatr Hematol Oncol 1995;17(1):46–52.

45. Arndt C, Rodeberg D, Breitfeld PP, Raney RB, Ullrich F, Donaldson S. Does bladder preservation (as a surgical principle) lead to retaining bladder function in bladder/prostate rhabdomyosarcoma? Results from Intergroup Rhabdomyosarcoma Study IV. J Urol 2004;171(6 Pt 1):2396–2403.

46. Crist WM, Anderson JR, Meza JL, et al. Intergroup Rhabdomyosarcoma Study-IV: results for patients with nonmetastatic disease. J Clin Oncol 2001;19(12):3091–3102.

47. Donaldson SS, Meza J, Breneman JC, et al. Results from the IRS-IV randomized trial of hyperfractionated radiotherapy in children with rhabdomyosarcoma—a report from the IRSG. Int J Radiat Oncol Biol Phys 2001;51(3):718–728.

48. Houghton PJ, Houghton JA, Myers L, Cheshire P, Howbert JJ, Grindey GB. Evaluation of N-(5-indanylsulfonyl)-N'-(4-chlorophenyl)-urea against xenografts of pediatric rhabdomyosarcoma. Cancer Chemother Pharm 1989;25:84–88.

49. Vietti T, Crist W, Ruby E, et al. Topotecan window in patients with rhabdomyosarcoma (RMS): an IRSG study [abstract]. Proc Am Soc Clin Oncol 1997;16:510a.

50. Houghton P, Chesire PJ, Hallman J, et al. Efficacy of topoisomerase I inhibitors, topotecan and irinotecan, administered at low doses in protracted schedules to mice bearing xenografts of human tumors. Cancer Chemother Pharmacol 1995;36:393–403.

51. Dancey J, Eisenhauer E. Current perspectives on camptothecins in cancer treatment. Br J Cancer 1996;74:327–338.

52. Stewart C, Zamboni W, Crom W, et al. Topoisomerase I interactive drugs in children with cancer. Inv New Drugs 1996;14:37–47.

53. Thompson J, George EO, Poquette CA, et al. Synergy of topotecan in combination with vincristine for treatment of pediatric solid tumor xenografts. Clin Cancer Res 1991;5:3617–3631.

54. Andrassy RJ, Hays DM, Raney RB, et al. Conservative surgical management of vaginal and vulvar pediatric rhabdomyosarcoma: a report from the Intergroup Rhabdomyosarcoma Study III. J Pediatr Surg 1995;30(7):1034–1036; discussion 1036–1037.

55. Yeung CK, Ward HC, Ransley PG, et al. Bladder and kidney function after cure of pelvic rhabdomyosarcoma in childhood. Br J Cancer 1994;70(5):1000–1003.

56. El-Sherbiny MT, El-Mekresh MH, El-Baz MA, Ghoneim MA. Paediatric lower urinary tract rhabdomyosarcoma: a single-centre experience of 30 patients. BJU Int 2000;86(3):260–267.

57. Silvan AM, Gordillo MJ, Lopez AM, et al. Organ-preserving management of rhabdomyosarcoma of the prostate and bladder in children. Med Pediatr Oncol 1997;29(6):573–575.

58. Heij HA, Vos A, de Kraker J, Voute PA. Bladder preservation in pelvic rhabdomyosarcoma. Lancet 1995;345(8952):141–142.

59. Merguerian PA, Agarwal S, Greenberg M, Bagli DJ, Khoury AE, McLorie GA. Outcome analysis of rhabdomyosarcoma of the lower urinary tract. J Urol 1998;160(3 Pt 2):1191–1194; discussion 1216.

60. Audry OO, Capelli C, Martelli H, et al. The role of conservative surgery in bladder/prostate rhabdomyosarcoma: an update of experience of the SIOP [abstract]. European Society of Pediatric Urology (ESPU), 2000.

61. Ardnt C. Personal communication, 2003.

62. Koscielniak E, Harms D, Henze G, et al. Results of treatment for soft tissue sarcoma in childhood and adolescence: a final report of the German Cooperative Soft Tissue Sarcoma Study CWS-86. J Clin Oncol 1999;17(12):3706–3719.

63. Duel BP, Hendren WH, Bauer SB, et al. Reconstructive options in genitourinary rhabdomyosarcoma. J Urol 1996;156(5):1798–1804.

64. Lander EB, Shanberg AM, Tansey LA, et al. The use of continent diversion in the management of rhabdomyosarcoma of the prostate in childhood. J Urol 1992;147(6):1602–1605.

65. Hensle TW, Chang DT. Reconstructive surgery for children with pelvic rhabdomyosarcoma. Urol Clin North Am 2000;27(3):489–502, ix.

66. Ferrara N. VEGF and the quest for tumour angiogenesis factors. Nat Rev Cancer 2002;2(10):795–803.

67. Pavlakovic H, Havers W, Schweigerer L. Multiple angiogenesis stimulators in a single malignancy: implications for anti-angiogenic tumour therapy. Angiogenesis 2001;4(4):259–262.

68. Javadpour N, Mostofi FK. Primary epithelial tumors of the bladder in the first two decades of life. J Urol 1969;101(5):706–710.

69. Serrano-Durba A, Dominguez-Hinarejos C, Reig-Ruiz C, Fernandez-Cordoba M, Garcia-Ibarra F. Transitional cell carcinoma of the bladder in children. Scand J Urol Nephrol 1999;33(1):73–76.

70. Samra Y, Hertz M, Lindner A. Urinary bladder tumors following cyclophosphamide therapy: a report of two cases with a review of the literature. Med Pediatr Oncol 1985;13(2):86–91.

71. Hoenig DM, McRae S, Chen SC, et al. Transitional cell carcinoma of the bladder in the pediatric patient. J Urol 1996;156(1):203–205.

72. Khasidy LR, Khashu B, Mallett EC, et al. Transitional cell carcinoma of bladder in children. Urology 1990;35(2):142–144.

73. Quillin SP, McAlister WH. Transitional cell carcinoma of the bladder in children: radiologic appearance and differential diagnosis. Urol Radiol 1991;13(2):107–109.

74. Paduano L, Chiella E. Primary epithelial tumors of the bladder in children. J Urol 1988;139(4):794–795.

75. Scott AA, Stanley W, Worshaw GF, et al. Aggressive bladder carcinoma in an adolescent. Report of a case with immunohistochemical, cytogenetic, and flow cytometric characterization. Am J Surg Pathol 1989;13(12):1057–1063.

76. Rankin LF, Allen GD, Yuppa FR, Pirozzi MJ, Hajjar JR. Carcinoma of the urachus in an adolescent: a case report. Bladder tumours in children: the late presentation of adenocarcinoma in bladder exstrophy. J Urol 1993;150(3 Pt 1):1472–1473.

77. Sheldon CA, Clayman RV, Gonzalez R, et al. Malignant urachal lesions. J Urol 1984;131(1):1–8.

78. Khan MN, Naqvi AH, Lee RE. Carcinoma of sigmoid colon following urinary diversion: a case report and review of literature. World J Surg Oncol 2004;2(1):20.

79. Krishnamsetty RM, Rao MK, Hines CR, et al. Adenocarcinoma in exstrophy and defunctional ureterosigmoidostomy. J Ky Med Assoc 1988;86(8):409–414.

80. Jakobsen BE, Olesen S. Bladder exstrophy complicated by adenocarcinoma. Dan Med Bull 1968;15(8):253–256.

81. Eraklis AJ, Folkman MJ. Adenocarcinoma at the site of ureterosigmoidostomies for exstrophy of the bladder. J Pediatr Surg 1978;13(6D):730–734.

82. Weitzner S. Leiomyosarcoma of urinary bladder in children. Urology 1978;12(4):450–452.

83. Goldschneider KR, Forouhar FA, Altman AJ, Yamase HT, Walzak MP Jr. Diagnostic pitfalls in the diagnosis of soft tissue bladder tumors in pediatric patients. Ann Clin Lab Sci 1990;20(1):22–27.

84. Lack EE. Leiomyosarcomas in childhood: a clinical and pathologic study of 10 cases. Pediatr Pathol 1986;6(2–3):181–197.

85. Horn LRS, Biesold M. Inflammatory pseudotumor of the ureter and urinary bladder. Pathol Res Pract 1997;193:607–612.

86. Debiec-Rychter MMP, Hagemeijer A, Pauwels P. ALK-ATIC fusion in urinary bladder inflammatory myofibroblastic tumor. Genes Chromosomes Cancer 2003;38:187–190.

87. Janik JS, Janik JP, Lovell M, et al. Recurrent inflammatory pseudotumors in children. J Pediatr Surg 2003;38:1491–1495.

88. Appelbaum H. Personal communication, 2004.

89. Legraverend JM, Canarelli JP, Boudailliez B, et al. [Cavernous hemangioma of the bladder in children. Apropos of a case]. Ann Urol (Paris) 1986;20(4):265–266.

90. Ritchey ML. Nephrogenic adenoma of the bladder: a report of 8 cases. J Urol 1984;131:537–539.

91. Kay R, Lattanzi C. Nephrogenic adenoma in children. J Urol 1985;133(1):99–101.

# Bladder cancer: internet resources 72

A Karim Kader, Laurence Klotz

## INTRODUCTION

*Nam et ipsa scientia potestast est.* (For knowledge itself is power.)

In the history of mankind, information has never been as abundant and accessible as it is today. Patients have traditionally sought medical information through their friends and family, primary care physicians, specialists, lay press, and scientific media. Today, they also access the internet.

The internet has revolutionized the quantity of information and access to it. A search engine such as Google used to look up "bladder cancer" will identify over 792,000 sites within 0.17 seconds. There is a vast range in the quality of this information. Patients and their families have embraced this new technology. However, many urologists, trained in a predigital era, have reacted slowly.

This chapter will briefly review the history of the internet and provide suggestions for counseling patients about the optimal use of the internet. It also includes a review of resources currently available to physicians treating patients with bladder cancer. This is not an exhaustive review of the bladder cancer web sites, although some key sites are highlighted.

## HISTORY OF THE INTERNET

The internet is approximately 20 years old. It was first conceived of by Leonard Kleinrock in 1961. At that time he was a PhD candidate at Massachusetts Institute of Technology (MIT) whose thesis proposal involved the flow of information packets between nodes. In the late 1960s he joined the staff at University of California Los Angeles (UCLA) where Vinton Cerf was a PhD candidate. Vinton began working on packet-switching networks sponsored by the Defense Advanced Research Projects Agency (DARPA). The project became known as the Advanced Research Project Agency Network (ARPANET).[1]

The first network involved nodes (servers) at UCLA, University of Utah, Stanford Research Institute, and the University of California Santa Barbara. Shortly after the initiation of this first network, Vinton met Robert Kahn from the computer technology company BBN (Bolt, Beranek, and Newman). In 1971 Ray Tomlinson, also of BBN, invented the first e-mail program for sending messages over this network, which now included 15 nodes and 23 hosts (terminals accessing the network).[2]

In 1974, Cerf, together with Kahn, invented the transmission control protocol (TCP) that later, together with the internet protocol (IP), became the basis for the protocol used by today's internet. These visionaries are the fathers of the internet.

In 1984, the domain name system was introduced and the number of hosts topped 1000. In 1991, the World Wide Web system was introduced and the internet was accessed by some 617,000 hosts. Today, there are more than 200 million hosts,[3] accessing over 3 billion web pages.[4]

MD Consult, a physician-focused medical resource site, was started in 1997. The first archived articles on the internet from the *Journal of Urology* date back to 1998.

With increasing file transfer speeds and newer technologies, delivery of picture, sound, and video information has become possible. The growth and complexity of the internet has vastly outstripped the expectations of the founders. In the early 1980s Bill Gates is reported to have said, '640K ought to be enough for anybody.'[5] The development and success of the internet is a remarkable testament to the ingenuity and creative potential of human beings. It is one of the great inventions of all time. It affords an opportunity to further human communication and understanding in all fields of human endeavor, not the least of which includes the diagnosis and treatment of bladder cancer.

## PATIENT RESOURCES

A diagnosis of cancer is perceived by patients to be a catastrophe and results in a flood of emotions in patients and their loved ones. Patients experience a loss of control over their lives and seek to regain that control. One way of seizing this control is to arm themselves with information. More than 20% of urology patients seek information on the internet.[6] The internet explosion has resulted in an expansion of sites, of varying quality. In the worst case, these offer dangerous advice. There is no peer-review process established for medical-based web pages.

There are, however, resources available to evaluate the quality of web-based information. This is a new field of research. One such site is provided by the University of California at Berkeley (www.lib.berkeley.edu/TeachingLib/Guides/internet/Evaluate.html). The site suggests that quality can be assessed by determining the credentials of the author, identify potential sources of bias, and determining accuracy. The site poses the following questions:

1. Author
   - Are the authors' names provided?
   - What are their titles? Are they specialists, physicians, allied health professionals or lay people?
   - What is their level of training?
   - Have you seen their names on any other resources?
2. Affiliation
   - Who is the sponsor of the web site? Is it a university department, a company or an individual?
   - Check the link: extensions such as .edu are normally associated with educational institutions, .gov with governments, and .org with nonprofit organizations.
3. Audience
   - Who is the intended audience?
4. Currency
   - How current is the web site?
   - Is it dated?

5. Accuracy: There is not as yet a universally accepted way of assessing the accuracy of information on bladder cancer sites. Lee et al have recently published an excellent review of the medical accuracy of various bladder cancer web sites identified using a variety of search engines.[7] They developed a checklist of items (based on practice guidelines from the National Comprehensive Cancer Network) that should be included in a web site to be considered complete. This list includes general information and information about risk factors, prevention, screening, diagnosis, staging, treatment, urinary diversion, prognosis, surveillance, recurrence, and research and support groups.

A little knowledge can be a dangerous thing. Bladder cancer is a complex disease. A concern associated with patient-directed research is the possibility that misconceptions will grow from patients' inability to fully understand the information presented. The barrage of technical information at such an emotionally charged time may contribute to an inability to incorporate the facts into a decision regarding treatment options. Another risk is that the patient may become dogmatic about specific treatments. This may result in patients demanding (or rejecting) a certain course of action.

An additional problem is the well-known difficulty of moving from the general to the specific. Each patient comes with a unique set of circumstances that in many cases require tailored therapy. Even the best web site cannot address these issues.

Conversely, when used with an appreciation for its inherent limitations, the internet can be a powerful tool for patients. It may provide patients with access to valuable information regarding natural history, risk factors, means of staging, and treatment options. As a result, patients may be able to calm themselves, avoid risky behavior, ask more educated questions, and be better able to make informed decisions regarding their care. Questions regarding management of complications may be efficiently dealt with by a well-organized internet site. Furthermore, these sites may prompt the patient to turn to patient and family support networks that can help them deal with the emotional vulnerability associated with a diagnosis of cancer. They may also facilitate a patient's ability to recruit family support in dealing with adverse quality of life effects related to stomas, incontinence, erectile dysfunction, and chemotherapy. Information on ancillary supports (e.g. stoma therapists, financial support for appliances, etc.) and clinical trials is also available.

Urologists treating bladder cancer should familiarize themselves with a list of appropriate and worthwhile sites. Endorsing these sites initiates the peer-review process. Patients should be cognizant that bladder cancer is an evolving field, and a site that is not updated regularly may be offering inappropriate advice. An attractive alternative, especially for urologists in a group practice, is to design a web page that identifies the most valuable information. Links to sites that the urologist feels are trustworthy can be included.

A collection of excellent web sites dealing with bladder cancer can be found in Table 72.1. This table includes some of the web sites judged to be the most accurate by Lee et al as well as some of the favorites named in an informal poll of our patients.

Some urologists have been slow to adopt the internet as a means of enhancing communication with patients. While this may be due to the multiple demands on available time due to practice, research, and teaching, it more likely reflects the truism, 'It's hard to teach an old dog new tricks.' Incorporating internet resources into practice is not something that is often taught in residency or emphasized during training. Clearly, however, in this 21st century, the resources and pervasiveness of the internet mandate that urologists embrace this technology so that its potential is exploited.

## PHYSICIAN RESOURCES

Clinicians do use the internet for accessing scientific literature. Most of the major urology journals are available on line, and several links are presented in Box 72.1. MD Consult (www.mdconsult.com), a paid service provided by the publishing house Elsevier, gives access to *Campbell's Urology* as well as the *Urology Clinics of North America* online.

The United States National Library of Medicine (NLM) has developed a bibliographic database of more than 4600 journals dating back to 1966. Medline (Medical Literature, Analysis and Retrieval System Online) has more than 11 million entries, with over 500,000 new entries annually. It may be accessed in a variety of different ways. The most common ways currently being used include the NLM's Pubmed web site (www.ncbi.nlm.nih.gov/pubmed), which is a free service; the paid Ovid system, which is available directly through the company (www.ovid.com) or through most university medical libraries; and MD Consult. In addition to its access to scientific literature, MD Consult has patient handouts. These have not been peer reviewed and require careful assessment prior to distribution to patients.

To access a variety of sites, or to refine a search to a very specific topic, an efficient and comprehensive search engine is invaluable. Several search engines are available (Box 72.2). The most commonly used is Google (www.google.com), which performs more than 250 million searches per day.[8] This search engine has

---

**Box 72.1** Internet links to urology journals

*BJU International*: www.bjui.org

*European Urology*: www.journals.elsevierhealth.com/periodicals/eururo

*Journal of Urology*: www.jurology.com

*Urology*: www.goldjournal.net

*UroOncology*: www.ingentaconnect.com/content/tandf/guro

*World Journal of Urology*: www.springeronline.com/sgw/cda/frontpage/0,11855,5-10085/70-1049544-0,00.html

---

**Box 72.2** Internet search engines

Google: www.google.com

Yahoo: www.yahoo.com

Ask Jeeves: www.askjeeves.com

AllTheWeb: www.alltheweb.com

HotBot: www.hotbot.com

---

**Table 72.1** Web sites dealing with bladder cancer

| Site | Link | Comments |
|---|---|---|
| NIH (National Institutes of Health) | www.nci.nih.gov/cancerinfo/types/bladder | Comprehensive, accurate, resources for patients and clinicians<br>Gives patients important questions to ask<br>Has access to complementary medicine<br>Fantastic access to trial information<br>Somewhat complicated |
| AUA (American Urologic Association) | www.urologyhealth.org/adult/index.cfm?cat=03&topic=37 | Good information on what to expect including side effects<br>Good drawings<br>Links are not as comprehensive<br>Site not that attractive |
| ACS (American Cancer Society) | www.cancer.org/docroot/cri/content/cri_2_4_1x_what_is_bladder_cancer_44.asp | Accurate information, well organized<br>Somewhat difficult to find from home page |
| Bladder Cancer WebCafé | www.blcwebcafe.org | Great comprehensive site, particularly from a patient's perspective<br>Good access to support |
| MedlinePlus | www.medlineplus.gov | Good links<br>Information easily found |

more than 3 billion indexed sites and features a full service calculator, a dictionary, a phone directory, and many other helpful online tools.

Access to some sites is fee based and may be cumbersome to use, requiring multiple key strokes, 'log-ins', and passwords. Alternatively, university medical libraries are a valuable resource, and may be accessed by students, faculty, and alumni effortlessly and cost effectively. With a single 'log-in', it is possible to gain access to Ovid for a Medline search and access full-text online versions of most, if not all, of the relevant publications.

At times it may be necessary to look up information about unfamiliar medications that patients are taking concurrently with their bladder cancer treatment. There are numerous sites that give access to such information. Examples of free sites include RxList.com (www.rxlist.com) and the drug information site of Medlineplus (www.nlm.nih.gov/medlineplus/druginformation.html). Access to this information may be placed in a Palm Pilot format using the free or paid services of Epocrates (www.epocrates.com) or the paid service of Tarascon (www.tarascon.com).

Apart from providing access to information, the internet has facilitated other valuable advances in medicine, including:

- wireless transmission of patient information, including films and pathology; this has allowed remote consultation and has ushered in the era of telemedicine[9]
- research surveys are now easily conducted over the internet[10]
- access to genetic and protein database information is now available[11]
- the advent of laparoscopy and robotics, telementoring, and telesurgery, permitting surgical educators and surgeons to work from a remote location[12]
- multi-institutional clinical trials may be coordinated over the internet.[13]

With the vast amount of information on the internet, one of the biggest challenges facing the urologist is the time-consuming endeavor of selecting high-quality sites. A collaborative team effort by colleagues circulating valuable sites among themselves will result in a database of useful sites. Once the database is established, monitoring of quality and currency would be required. We hope that this chapter has provided a basis for such initiatives.

## CONCLUSION

Bladder cancer is a disease that poses numerous diagnostic and treatment challenges. The internet has the potential to help both patients and physicians navigate these complexities by providing information to patients and by facilitating access to information for clinicians. It is also used as a research tool and most recently has been exploited to teach and perform surgeries. These advances come with potential pitfalls, including poor-quality information, loss of patient confidentiality, and risks to patient safety.

In contrast to many purported improvements in healthcare, which require major resource commitments, the internet is (mostly) free. A small investment of time will afford rational and peer-review-based exploitation of the extensive information resource on the internet. The internet has the potential to contribute to significant improvements in the management of patients with bladder cancer.

## REFERENCES

1. Hobbes R. 2004 Hobbes' Internet Timeline Version 8.0. 2004. Available: www.zakon.org/robert/internet/timeline.
2. Cerf V, Aboba B. How the internet came to be. Vinton Cert as told to Bernard Aboba. 1993. Available: www.netvalley.com/archives/mirrors/cerf-how-inet.txt.
3. Internet Systems Consortium. Internet domain survey, January 2004. Available: www.isc.org/index.pl?/ops/ds/reports/2004-01.
4. Tyler N, Krane D. Google press release: Google offers immediate access to greater than 3 billion web documents. 2001. Available: www.google.com/press/pressrel/3billion.html.
5. Bill Gates Quotes: Jokes-Jokes.net. 2003. Available: www.jokes-jokes.net/Bill-Gates-Quotes.html.
6. Hellawel GO, Turner KJ, Le Monnier KJ, Brewster S F. Urology and the internet an evaluation of internet use by urology patients and of information available on urological topics. BJU Int 2000;86:191–194.
7. Lee CT, Smith CA, Hall JM, Waters WB, Biermann JS. Bladder cancer facts: accuracy of information on the internet. J Urol 2003;170:1756–1760.
8. Sullivan D. SearchEngineWatch: Searches Per Day. 2003. Available: http://searchenginewatch.com/reports/article.php/2156461.
9. Kuo RL, Aslan P, Dinlenc CZ, et al. Secure transmission of urologic images and records over the internet. J Endourol 1999;13:141–146.
10. Kim HL, Hollowell CMP, Patel RJ, Bales GT, Clayman RV, Gerber GS. Use of new technology in endourology and laparoscopy by American urologists: internet and postal survey. Urology 2000;56:760–765.
11. Wolfe KH, Li WH. Molecular evolution meets the genomics revolution. Nat Genet 2003;33(Suppl 2):255–265.
12. Rodrigues Netto N, Mitre AI, Lima SV, et al. Telementoring between Brazil and the United States: initial experience. J Endourol 2003;17:217–220.
13. Lallas CD, Preminger GM, Pearle MS, et al. Internet based multi-institutional clinical research: a convenient and secure option. J Urol 2004;171:1880–1885.

*Mary Ellen Haisfield-Wolfe*

## INTRODUCTION

Providing patients and their significant others with adequate information and support from the time of diagnosis facilitates better adjustment and improves coping and quality of life for cancer patients.[1-4] A support group is one avenue of support. More than 25 million Americans are estimated to have participated in a support group at some time in their lives, with approximately 10 million presently participating.[5] Support groups specifically for cancer patients were not seen until the 1970s. One of the earliest reported cancer support groups was the 'I Can Cope' Program, which has demonstrated a significant impact on participants' anxiety levels, disease-related knowledge, and sense of life meaning.[6]

## ABOUT SUPPORT GROUPS

The purpose of a support group is to give support and information to persons with common problems. These groups are focused on patients' needs and form around specific cancer types. Support group programs provide inherent mutual support in a safe environment, foster relationships among members, provide a sense of belonging, communicate experiential knowledge, and teach coping skills.[7-11]

The characteristics of a support group can vary widely. Support groups can be professionally or patient-led, with either an open- or closed-ended format. Groups are generally small, consisting of 5–10 members, with these gatherings providing more in the way of support and comfort than promotion of change for their members.[4,7]

Support groups may include therapy, counseling, self-help, education, and psycho-education. The most common focus is support and education. More recently, support groups have expanded from solely face-to-face groups to internet support groups. It is widely recognized that females and individuals with a higher average income are more likely to be in a support group.[12-16] Predictors for the use of support groups are more formal education and physician referral.[17] Factors influencing attendance are geographic distance, a tendency to join voluntary associations, experience with professional mental health counseling, age, and marital status.[18]

Support group participation is beneficial and has been significantly associated with fewer mood disturbances, fewer maladaptive coping responses, and reduced psychological distress.[4,19] Ferlic et al reported improved adjustment and self-concept at the end of 2 weeks in a support group, which returned to baseline within 6 months.[20] Common reasons cited for support group participation were mental distress and a desire to obtain help in coping with an illness. Participants have reported liking support groups in that they provide an opportunity to ventilate feelings and the 'all in the same boat phenomenon'.[19,21]

Reasons for not participating in a support group are sufficient support from family members, friends or doctors, and not knowing about the existence of support groups.[17] Individuals participating in social interactions may experience negative effects such as pressures to conform, stresses to reciprocate obligations, feeling overwhelmed, and finding open communication a threatening experience.[22] Consequently, potential negative outcomes of support groups include member distress and decline in functioning. Participants have reported aspects of group membership they disliked as the short-term nature of the group, group monopolizers, and membership compositions with others different from themselves in age, diagnosis, or stage of illness.[19] A problem with irregular group attendance has also been reported.[22]

The efficacy of support groups has not been adequately studied, and one reason may be that cancer patients experience a variety of clinical courses, illnesses, and trajectory. One qualitative study reported the outcomes of support group experiences as valuable for reconceptualization of the person's personal identity and life story, and enhancement of self-expression and decision-making.[23]

## CYBERSUPPORT

Within the past several years support groups have emerged on the internet, presenting new opportunities for patients to communicate with healthcare professionals and other patients. The internet creates connections between persons through the use of online support groups and listservs. No longer is the size of a group or geographic distance a barrier to participation. A large portion of online self-help activity takes place between 7:00 pm and 1:00 am.[24] Advantages of online groups are that participants have more control over when and how much support they receive, and group members can choose to remain anonymous.

## SEX TALK

Communication of sexuality was examined in a prostate cancer support group.[25] Men in the structured meetings rarely discussed sex unless it was addressed. This research concluded that the omission of sexuality was related to the structure of the meeting rather than men not being interested. Topics that men reported as being important were sex as a priority, sex as spontaneous, and men renegotiating sexuality in a wide variety of ways with their partners. These are important findings for men recovering sexually after cancer treatment.

## SUPPORT GROUPS FOR PATIENTS WITH BLADDER CANCER

The *United Ostomy Association* (UOA) helps ostomy patients through mutual aid and emotional support. They provide information to patients and the public, they will put people in touch with local support groups and ostomy nurses, and will send volunteers to visit new ostomy patients. They have several national networks including Continent Diversions Network, Gay and Lesbian Ostomated, and Young Adults (see United

Ostomy Association Inc, Suite 200, 19772 MacArthur Boulevard, Irvine CA 92612-2405 at 1-800-826-0826; www.uoa.org). For worldwide information contact the International Ostomy Association at www.ostomy.org, and for continent diversions (including support group information) contact www.ostomyalternative.org. There are support groups in every state and most cities.

The *American Urological Association Foundation* (formerly the American Foundation for Urologic Disease) supports research, provides education to patients, the general public, and health professionals, and offers patient support services for those who have or may be at risk for a urologic disease or disorder. They provide information on urologic disease and dysfunction, including bladder health, prostate cancer, treatment options, and sexual function (see American Urological Association Foundation, 1000 Corporate Boulevard, Linthicum, MD 21090 at Toll Free (US only) 1-866-RING AUA; at 1-866-746-4282; admin@afud.org or http://www.afud.org).

The *Bladder Cancer WebCafé* is an online community created by and for patients with bladder cancer to help users navigate through bladder cancer information and 'find the best path on a difficult journey'. The site contains e-mail discussion groups, an online nurse, and an interactive storyboard. The site provides advice for newly diagnosed patients on treatment, chemoprevention, and survival guides (see http://blcwebcafe.org).

## CANCER SUPPORT GROUPS

Many organizations offer support groups for people diagnosed with cancer and their family members or friends. The National Cancer Institute fact sheet *National Organizations That Offer Services to People With Cancer and Their Families* lists many cancer-concerned organizations that can provide information about support groups. The fact sheet is available on the internet at http://cis.nci.nih.gov/fact/8_1.htm, or can be ordered from the Cancer Information Service at 1-800-4-CANCER (1-800-422-6237).

The following groups are supported by the American Cancer Society (ACS):

- The *Cancer Hope Network* provides individual support to cancer patients and their families by matching them with trained volunteers who have undergone and recovered from a similar cancer experience. Such matches are based on the type and stage of cancer, treatments used, side effects experienced and other facts (see Cancer Hope Network, Two North Road, Chester, NJ 07930 at 1-877-467-3638; www.cancerhopenetwork.org).
- The *National Coalition for Cancer Survivorship* (NCCS) is a network of groups and individuals that offer

support to cancer survivors and their loved ones. It provides information and resources on cancer support, advocacy, and quality of life issues (see The National Coalition for Cancer Survivorship, Suite 770, 1010 Wayne Avenue, Silver Spring, MD 20910-5600 at 1-877-622-7937; www.canceradvocacy.org).

- *Vital Options® International TeleSupport® Cancer Network* is a southern California-based not-for-profit cancer communication, support, and advocacy organization dedicated to using technology to help people cope with cancer. Its mission is to facilitate a global cancer dialogue. The organization holds a weekly syndicated call-in radio talk show called The Group Room® which provides a forum for patients, long-term survivors, family members, physicians, and therapists to discuss cancer issues. A live simulcast of 'The Group Room' can be heard by logging onto the Vital Options web site (see Vital Options® International TeleSupport® Cancer Network, Suite 645, 15821 Ventura Boulevard, Encino, CA 91436 at 1-800-477-7666; www.vitaloptions.org).

- The *Wellness Community* provides free psychological and emotional support to cancer patients and their families. They offer support groups facilitated by licensed therapists, stress reduction and cancer education workshops, nutrition guidance, exercise sessions, and social events (see The Wellness Community, Suite 412, 35 East Seventh Street, Cincinnati, OH 45202 at 1-888-793-9355; www.wellnesscommunity.org).

## REFERENCES

1. Manfredi C, Czaja R, Price J, Buis M, Janiszcewski R. Cancer patients search for information. Monogr J Natl Cancer Inst 1993;14:93–104.
2. Harris KA. The informational needs of patients with cancer and their families. Cancer Pract 1998;6:39–46.
3. Cunningham AJ, Edmonds G. Which cancer patients benefit from a brief-group, coping skills program? Int J Psychiat Med 1993;23(4):383–398.
4. Krupnick JL, Rowland J, Goldberg R, Ursula D. Professionally-led support groups for cancer patients: an intervention in search of a model. Int J Psychiat Med 1993;23(3):275–294.
5. Kessler RC, Mickelson KD, Zhao S. Patterns and correlates of self-help group membership in the United States. Social Policy 1997;27:27–44.
6. Johnson J. The effects of a patient education course on persons with a chronic illness. Cancer Nurs 1982;5:117–123.
7. Kurtz LF. Self-Help and Support Groups: A Handbook for Practitioners. London: Sage, 1997.
8. Schopler J, Galinsky M. Support groups as open systems: model for practice and research. Health Social Work 1993;18(3):195–207.
9. Stearns NM, Lauria MM, Hermann JF, Fogelberg PR. Oncology Social Work: A Clinician's Guide. Atlanta, GA: The American Cancer Society, 1993.
10. Posluszny DM, Hyman KB, Baum A. Group interventions in cancer. The benefits of social support and education on patients' adjustment. In Tindale RS (ed): Theory and Research on Small Groups. New York: Plenum Press, 1998, pp 87–105.
11. Fawzy FI, Fawzy NW, Canada AL. Psychoeducational intervention programs for patients with cancer. In Baum A, Anderson BL (eds): Psychosocial Interactions for Cancer. Washington, DC: The American Psychological Association, 2001.
12. Bond CR, Daiter S. Participation in medical self-help groups. In Lieberman MA, Borman LD (eds): Self-Help Groups for Coping with Crisis. San Francisco: Jossey-Bass, 1979, pp 164–180.
13. Borman L. Self-help skills: leadership in self-help mutual aid groups. Citizen Participation 1982;3:30–31.
14. Edwards G, Hensman C, Hawker F, Williamson V. Who goes to Alcoholics Anonymous? Lancet 1966;2(459):382–384.
15. Fried B. Alcoholics Anonymous as a self-help group: institutionalized but not professionalized. Unpublished manuscript, University of Chicago, 1976.
16. Durman EC. Role of self-help in service provisions. J Appl Behav Sci 1976;12:433–444.
17. Eakin E, Strycker L. Awareness and barriers to use of cancer support and information resources by HMO patients with breast, prostate or colon cancer: patients and provider perspectives. J Psycho-Oncol 2001;10:103–113.
18. Galinsky M, Schopler J. Negative experiences in support groups. Social Work in Health Care 1994;20(1):77–95.
19. Glajchen MM, Magen R. Evaluating process, outcome and satisfaction in community-based cancer support groups. Social Work in Groups 1995;18(1):27–40.
20. Ferlic M, Goldman A, Kennedy BJ. Group counseling in adult patients with advanced cancer. Cancer 1979;43:760–766.
21. Plass A, Koch U. Participation of oncological outpatients in psychosocial support. J Psycho-Oncol 2001;10:511–520.
22. Bauman G, Siegel R. Factors associated with cancer patients' participation in support groups. J Psycho-Oncol 1992;10(3):1–20.
23. Gray RE, Davis M, Phillips C. Breast cancer and prostate cancer self-help groups: reflections on differences. J Psycho-Oncol 1996;5(2):137–142.
24. Ferguson T. Health Online: How to Find Health Information Support Groups and Self-help Communities in Cyberspace. Reading, MA: Perseus, 1996.
25. Arrington M. Thinking inside the box: on identity, sexuality, prostate cancer, and social support. J Aging Identity 2000;5(3):151–158.

# Education and counseling of the cystectomy patient

74

*Joanne Walker*

## INTRODUCTION

Shock and disbelief are common initial reactions to the diagnosis of muscle-invasive bladder cancer. Many people regard this diagnosis as a death sentence. Their reactions are shaped by actual statistics,[1] but more so by their personal past experiences with cancer. Rare is the person that does not have a friend or family member who died 'a horrible death' from cancer.

As the now 'patient' moves through the healthcare system and the maze of testing and polysyllabic medical terms, options are offered and decisions must be made. There is little time to focus on the inner process of grieving that must also be accomplished. The stages of this process mirror Kubler-Ross's stages of death and dying.[2] The person with bladder cancer must work through the anger and disbelief to eventually accept that life, if it is to continue, will be forever altered.

This chapter will focus on those people that will have cystectomy with urinary tract reconstruction as their treatment option. Most commonly, this reconstruction will involve a stoma with an external appliance, although the numbers that choose orthotopic neobladders or catheterizable neobladders are increasing. Wherever possible, people providing support to the patient should be included in discussions, teaching, and counseling.

## HISTORICAL PERSPECTIVE

The person with a urinary tract reconstruction presents the caregiver with a constellation of needs in the cognitive, affective, and psychomotor arenas. Such a degree of adjustment is required that an entire nursing specialty has developed to meet the needs of this group.

In 1958, Rupert B. Turnbull of the Cleveland Clinic Foundation trained a former patient with an ileostomy to care for ostomy patients. This 'trainee', Norma Gill, is credited, along with Dr. Turnbull, of founding the first school of enterostomal therapy in 1961 in response to a demand for caregivers with this specialized training.[3] Ms. Gill is also credited with being a founder of the World Council of Enterostomal Therapy, which first met in Milan, Italy, in 1978. She was instrumental in helping to organize the many patient-led support groups into what is currently the United Ostomy Association (UOA).[4]

In 1977, at the UOA annual conference, the International Association for Enterostomal Therapy (IAET) presented an 'Ostomate Bill of Rights' to the House of Delegates' meeting (Box 74.1). It was adopted by the UOA at that meeting.

---

**Box 74.1** Ostomate Bill of Rights

The ostomate shall:
1. be given preoperative counseling
2. have an appropriately positioned stoma site
3. have a well-constructed stoma
4. have skilled postoperative nursing care
5. have emotional support
6. have individual instruction
7. be informed on the availability of supplies
8. be provided with information on community resources
9. have posthospital follow-up and life-long supervision
10. benefit from team efforts of health care professionals
11. be provided with information and counsel from the ostomy association and its members.

As is evident, ostomy care as we know it derived from an informed public—a public which demonstrated that, along with a life saved, the quality of that life must be ensured.

## ROLE OF THE SPECIALTY NURSE

### PREOPERATIVE

Consistent with the Ostomate Bill of Rights, ideally the relationship between the wound ostomy and continence nursing (WOCN) nurse (formerly the enterostomal therapy nurse) and the patient begins well before the proposed operative procedure.

The WOCN nurse may clarify points about surgical options, assess cognitive ability, and determine the patient's unique style of learning and coping with stressors. Information about past positive or negative experiences with stress is discussed at this time. Points of particular interest are preconceived ideas the person might have about an 'ostomy', history of depression or mental illness, and support systems in place (family, religion, etc.), as well as where the person is in terms of grieving the loss and exactly what that loss is perceived to be.

Those people who find strength through communion with others may be questioned as to whether they would find a support group or 'ostomy visitor' helpful (see Chapter 73), whereas those who prefer to cope individually may be most helped by internet resources (see Chapter 72) and printed materials. Information about all of the resources should be offered preoperatively, postoperatively, and again during follow-up. The need for formal counseling may be determined at this time.

Although it is sometimes helpful to know the person's level of formal education, simply asking questions about how the person learns or prefers to gain knowledge may be far more useful.[5]

Manual dexterity will be important with any reconstruction requiring application of an appliance or catheterization. If adaptations or occupational therapy referrals will be needed, these issues may be addressed at this time.

Questioning the patient regarding activities that they plan to pursue post-recovery is helpful in determining the type of appliance needed, but more so to discover how the patient perceives that their life will be altered.

Physical assessment of the patient to determine an appropriate stoma site is critical. Factors to consider in choosing a stoma site include the following.[6]

1. Location within the rectus muscle: It is commonly believed that the incidence of hernia is decreased if the stoma is placed here; however, placing the stoma mid-rectus as opposed to laterally (within centimeters of the edge) decreases the likelihood of shifting abdominal planes under the pouch seal with resultant instability and pouch leakage.
2. Avoidance of scars, skin folds, natural waistline, umbilicus, and bony prominences, which would interfere with pouch adhesion.
3. Surface area adequate to affix an appliance.
4. Need for braces or special positioning which might require upper quadrant placement.
5. Site not affected by movement.

The above factors are ones that cannot be altered. However, other factors—for example, clothing considerations such as belt line, and visibility to the patient—can be adapted if necessary.

In general, upper quadrant sites should be avoided where possible: although all the criteria above may be met by choosing a high site, the ability of the patient to disguise the pouch with clothing is greatly diminished. The patient should always be included in the process of site selection for assessment of life style, clothing and visual considerations.

After discussion and examination of the abdomen, the WOCN nurse may mark the suggested site in such a way as to not be obliterated by activities of daily living prior to surgery. Methods vary with institution and range from indelible pen with film dressing cover to scratching the skin with a 25 G needle. The surgeon has ultimate responsibility for site determination, and the patient should be made aware preoperatively that the suggested site may be affected by intraoperative considerations.

Frequently patients have additional questions after the initial meeting with the WOCN nurse, and it is therefore appropriate to give reading material, videotapes, and contact information at this time. Occasionally patients request an appliance to try with various articles of clothing and activity.

The PLISSIT model is a helpful one to follow in guiding counseling in the domain of sexual functioning (Box 74.2). If the patient is given permission to do so, questioning about sexual functioning occurs during the initial meeting and is elaborated subsequently. The cancer patient facing potentially destructive surgery expects a forthright discussion from the physician regarding percentages of postoperative sexual dysfunction as well as what forms of therapy are available should dysfunction occur. Questions addressed to the nurse tend to focus on intimacy and

| **Box 74.2** The PLISSIT model | |
|---|---|
| **P**: | permission |
| **LI**: | limited information |
| **SS**: | specific suggestion |
| **IT**: | intensive therapy |

acceptance issues, such as how to discuss these matters with a partner. Patients frequently have concerns about hurting themselves, about preferable positions, how to prevent appliance leakage, and how to disguise the appliance. Their partners generally have the same concerns, including fear of harming the cancer patient. Many people perceive the stoma as very delicate and easily injured. Appliance covers and camouflaging undergarments help allay fears about these issues with both partners.

Fear and worry about sexual activity occasionally stem from a lack of understanding of basic sexual functioning and anatomy. Although patients may have heard which parts will be removed, they are frequently unaware of the implications (e.g. men equating sterility with impotence). Decreased libido and lack of energy are common sequelae of cancer and surgery and are not specific to this group.

Regardless of the type of reconstruction, male patients frequently have decreased or absent erections. Sexual functioning may improve up to 24 months after surgery. Male patients should be counseled that they will have the sensation of orgasm, but ejaculation will be 'dry' or without fluid. Oral medications, penile injections, suction devices, and implants are available to enhance erections. Male patients with orthotopic neobladders may have the additional concern of urinary incontinence during sexual activity. This may be addressed by using a condom or waterproof underpadding, depending on the extent of leakage and comfort level with the partner.

Female patients may have sexual dysfunction related to a postoperative shortened or narrowed vagina and/or vaginal dryness. Simple water-soluble lubricating jelly may be all that is needed, although vaginal forms and topical or oral hormone therapy may be required.

There are brochures available through local cancer societies, which may be helpful in answering patient questions and offering suggestions.

## POSTOPERATIVE

If appropriate assessment and counseling have occurred preoperatively, the patient will expect that the teaching/learning and process of adjustment will begin soon after surgery.

The patient may need to retreat emotionally at this time and, with a precipitous drop in preoperative adrenaline, a low mood may be evident. Signs of anger and depression may be exhibited. The reality of the cancer diagnosis and bodily changes necessitated by it become clear. The thought of learning a new way of elimination while awaiting a pathology report, and enduring operative and gas pains as well as sleep deprivation, commonly overwhelm the patient. Ongoing emotional support remains critical. The body

of information and technical skills necessary for independent care must be separated into small manageable steps. Merely visualizing the stoma and realizing it is now a part of the body may be all that a patient can absorb during the first lesson. All lessons should be supplemented with written information and audiovisuals where possible. Many fine self-care tapes are available through ostomy product manufacturers.

In addition to resolution of the issues identified preoperatively, and the involvement of appropriate interdisciplinary team members, the basics of ostomy care are taught during the hospitalization. These basics include:

1. choosing a comfortable, hypoallergenic and dependable appliance
2. locations and means of obtaining supplies
3. skin care
4. pouch application
5. system management during sleep
6. adaptation for activity, travel, and seasons.

Urostomy care is focused on a system which causes the least need for life style change and reduces extrinsic factors, which may lead to urinary tract infection.[7] Such care consists of:

1. thorough cleansing of the peristomal skin with a nongreasy, nonperfumed soap, thorough rinsing, and gentle drying
2. pouch change at least every 4 days
3. ensuring the pouch opening is no more than 1/16″ larger than the stoma
4. the use of additional adhesives, caulking products, belts, flexible or convex pouches as needed for flush stomas or uneven peristomal areas
5. the use of skin protective products such as barrier films for sensitive individuals
6. drainage system use or routine for wakening to manage urinary output during sleep hours
7. adequate fluid intake of noncaffeine beverages (fluid intake should be such that the urine is light yellow in color).

The patient is also instructed to contact the urologist and/or WOCN nurse if the urine becomes bloody, foul, or diminished in volume after leaving the hospital.

Peristomal skin problems in the early postoperative period are common—a yeast rash after antibiotics is often seen and generally easily treated with antifungal powders; however, the use of cream or ointment under an appliance should be avoided as it will affect its adhesion.

Acanthosis or pseudoverrucous lesions may develop later in the course of recovery, are precipitated by alkaline urine, and are managed with both oral and topical acidifying agents.

Mucocutaneous separation is seen more frequently in debilitated or previously radiated patients and may interfere with the pouching system. The deficit, if shallow, may be managed with karaya powder; if it is deep, it may require an absorbent packing such as calcium alginate with a moisture-proof covering.

## CONCLUSION

The person with a urinary diversion because of invasive bladder cancer will best negotiate the torturous route from denial and anger, through bargaining and depression, with the benefit of a multidisciplinary team of caregivers who communicate well with the patient and with each other, who respect the unique contribution of each member, and who freely share information.

REFERENCES

1. Schoenberg MP. The Guide to Living with Bladder Cancer. Baltimore: Johns Hopkins Press, 2000.
2. Kubler-Ross E. On Death and Dying. New York: Macmillan, 1969.
3. Colwell J, Goldberg M, Carmel J. Roles of the Ostomy Nurse Specialist. Historical Perspectives, Role Potential. Fecal and Urinary Diversions, Management Principles. St Louis: Mosby, 2004.
4. UOA web site. www.uoa.org/ostomy_rights.htm.
5. Knowles MB. The Modern Practice of Adult Education. New York: Association Press, 1970.
6. Hampton BG, Bryant RA. Ostomies and Continent Diversions: Nursing Management. St Louis: Mosby Year Book, 1992.
7. Annon JS. The PLISSIT model: a proposed conceptual scheme for the behavioral treatment of sexual problems. Sex Educ Ther 1972;2:1–15.
8. Walker JM, Haldeman K. Report of a study: factors affecting urinary tract infection in patients with urinary diversions. AUAA Annual Meeting, San Antonio, 1992.

# Index

**Notes:** Please note that as the subject of this book is bladder cancer, all entries refer to this disease unless otherwise stated. Also entries followed by 'f' and 't' refer to figures and tables/boxed material respectively.
**Abbreviations:** To save space in the index, the following abbreviations have been used: BCG - bacillus Calmette–Guérin; VEGF - vascular endothelial growth factor; MVAC - methotrexate/vinblastine/adriamycin/cisplatin combined chemotherapy; TURBT - transurethral resection of bladder tumor

For Product Safety Concerns and Information please contact
our EU representative GPSR@taylorandfrancis.com Taylor & Francis
Verlag GmbH, Kaufingerstraße 24, 80331 München, Germany

T - #0298 - 160425 - C808 - 279/216/37 - PB - 9780367391225 - Gloss Lamination